D1175309

PHYSICAL REHABILITATION
of the
INJURED ATHLETE

PHYSICAL REHABILITATION
of the
INJURED ATHLETE

THIRD EDITION

James R. Andrews, M.D.

Clinical Professor of Surgery
University of Alabama at Birmingham School of Medicine
Division of Orthopaedic Surgery
Medical Director, American Sports Medicine & Orthopaedic Center
Orthopaedic Surgeon, Alabama
Sports Medicine & Orthopaedic Center
Birmingham, Alabama

Gary L. Harrelson, Ed.D., A.T.,C.

Adjunct Assistant Professor
Athletic Training Education Program
The University of Alabama
Manager, Educational Services and Technology
DCH Health System
Tuscaloosa, Alabama

Kevin E. Wilk, P.T.

Adjunct Assistant Professor
Programs in Physical Therapy
Marquette University
Milwaukee, Wisconsin
National Director, Research and Clinical Education
HealthSouth Rehabilitation Corporation
Associate Clinical Director
HealthSouth Sports Medicine and Rehabilitation Center
Director of Rehabilitative Research
American Sports Medicine Institute
Birmingham, Alabama

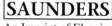
SAUNDERS
An Imprint of Elsevier

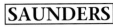

An Imprint of Elsevier

170 S. Independence Mall
300 E
Philadelphia, PA 19106-3399

PHYSICAL REHABILITATION OF THE INJURED ATHLETE   ISBN 0-7216-0014-X

© 2004, 1998, 1991 Elsevier Inc. All rights reserved.

No part of this publication may be reproduced or transmitted in any form or by any means, electronic or mechanical, including photocopy, recording, or any information storage and retrieval system, without permission in writing from the publisher.

Permissions may be sought directly from Elsevier Inc. Rights Department in Philadelphia, USA: phone: (+1)215 238 7869, fax: (+1) 215238 2239, email: healthpermissions@elsevier.com. You may also complete your request on-line via the Elsevier Science homepage (http://www.elsevier.com, by selecting "Customer Support" and then "Obtaining Permissions.")

Notice

Medicine is an ever-changing field. Standard safety precautions must be followed but as new research and clinical experience broaden our knowledge, changes in treatment and drug therapy may become necessary or appropriate. Readers are advised to check the most current product information provided by the manufacturer of each drug to be administered to verify the recommended dose, the method and duration of administration, and contraindications. It is the responsibility of the treating physician, relying on experience and knowledge of the patient, to determine dosages and the best treatment for each individual patient. Neither the Publisher nor the author assumes any liability for any injury and/or damage to persons or property arising from this publication.

The Publisher

Library of Congress Cataloging in Publication Data

Physical rehabilitation of the injured athlete /
  [edited by] James R. Andrews, Gary L. Harrelson, Kevin E. Wilk – 3rd ed.
    p.   cm.
   Includes bibliographical references and index.
   ISBN 0-7216-0014-X
    1. Sports injuries–Treatment. 2. Sports physical therapy. I. Andrews, James R. (James Rheuben), 1942-II. Harrelson, Gary L. III. Wilk, Kevin E.
  [DNLM: 1. Athletic Injuries–rehabilitation. 2. Physical Therapy Techniques. QT 261 P578 2004]
RD97-P49 2004.
617.1′027–dc21

                                                          2003053884

Acquisitions Editor: Daniel Pepper
Publishing Services Manager: Joan Sinclair
Project Manager: Mary Stermel

Printed in USA
Last digit is the print number: 9   8   7   6   5   4   3   2

To Noah, who at age 4 never had the writing/editing of this book on his "radar" screen, but hopefully the time I chose to carve out to be present with you was. Thanks for allowing me to once again view a complex world in a simplistic manner through your presence in my life.

Love, Dad (GLH)

CONTRIBUTORS

Christopher Arrigo, M.S., P.T., ATC
National Director of Clinical Services
HealthSouth Corporation
Birmingham, AL
Shoulder Rehabilitation; Elbow Rehabilitation

Turner A. "Tab" Blackburn, M.Ed., P.T., ATC
Adjunct Assistant Professor
Department of Orthopedics
Executive Director
Tulane Institute of Sports Medicine
Tulane University School of Medicine
New Orleans, Louisiana
Functional Training and Advanced Rehabilitation

Jake Bleacher, M.S.P.T., C.S.C.S.
Physiotherapy Associates—Scottsdale Sports Clinic
Scottsdale, Arizona
Proprioception and Neuromusclar Control

Terese L. Chmielewski, Ph.D., P.T., S.C.S.
Assistant Professor
Department of Physical Therapy
University of Florida
Gainesville, Florida
Rehabilitation Considerations for the Female Athlete

Gray Cook, M.S. P. T., O.C.S., C.S.C.S.
Director of Orthopedic and Sports Physical Therapy
Dunn, Cook, and Associates
Danville, Virgina
Functional Training and Advanced Rehabilitation

Anthony Cuoco, D.P.T., M.S., C.S.C.S.
Staff Physical Therapist and Research Associate
PRO Sports Physical Therapy
Scarsdale, New York
Plyometric Training and Drills

R. Barry Dale, Ph.D., P.T., ATC, C.S.C.S.
Assistant Professor
Department of Physical Therapy
University of South Alabama
Mobile, Alabama
Principles of Rehabilitation

George J. Davies, D.P.T., M.Ed., P.T., S.C.S., ATC, L.A.T., C.S.C.S.
Professor
Armstrong Atlantic State University
Savannah, Georgia
Professor Emeritus
University of Wisconsin–LaCrosse
LaCrosse, Wisconsin
Consultant, Clinician, and Co-Director
Sports Physical Therapy Residency Program
Gundersen Lutheran Sports Medicine
LaCrosse, Wisconsin
Application of Isokinetics in Testing and Rehabilitation

Todd S. Ellenbecker, M.S., P.T., O.C.S., S.C.S., C.S.C.S.
Clinic Director
Physiotherapy Associates—Scottsdale Sports Clinic
Scottsdale, Arizona
*Proprioception and Neuromusclar Control; Application
    of Isokinetics in Testing and Rehabilitation*

Reed Ferber, Ph.D., ATC, C.A.T.(C)
Post-Doctoral Fellow
Human Performance Laboratory
Faculty of Kinesiology
University of Calgary
Calgary, Alberta, Canada
Rehabilitation Considerations for the Female Athlete

Julie M. Fritz, Ph.D., P.T., ATC
Assistant Professor
Department of Physical Therapy
University of Pittsburgh
Pittsburgh, Pennsylvania
Low Back Rehabilitation

James B. Gallaspy, BS, M.Ed., ATC
Associate Professor Emeritus
The University of Southern Mississippi
Hattiesburg, Mississippi
Hamstring, Quadriceps and Groin Rehabilitation

Greg Gardner, Ed.D., ATC
Clinical Associate Professor of Athletic Training
Associate Director, School of Nursing
The University of Tulsa
Tulsa, Oklahoma
Hamstring, Quadriceps and Groin Rehabilitation

Gary L. Harrelson, Ed.D, ATC
Adjunct Professor
The University of Alabama
Tuscaloosa, Alabama
Manager
Educational Services and Technology
DCH Health System
Tuscaloosa, Alabama
Physiologic Factors of Rehabilitation
Measurement in Rehabilitation
Range of Motion and Flexibility
Principles of Rehabilitation
Shoulder Rehabilitation

Todd Hooks PT, MTC
Physical Therapist
Integrity Rehab Group
Birmingham, Alabama
Cervical Spine Rehabilitation

Barbara J. Hoogenboom, M.H.S., P.T., S.C.S., ATC
Assistant Professor of Physical Therapy
Grand Valley State University
Grand Rapids, Michigan
Functional Training and Advanced Rehabilitation

Jeff G. Konin, M.Ed., ATC, M.P.T.
Assistant Athletic Director for Sports Medicine
Assistant Professor of Health Sciences
James Madison University
Harrison, Virginia
Adjunct Professor
Nova Southeastern University
Fort Lauderdale, Florida
Range of Motion and Flexibility

Deidre Leaver-Dunn, Ph.D., ATC
Associate Professor
Director
Athletic Training Education Program
The University of Alabama
Tuscaloosa, Alabama
Principles of Rehabilitation
Range of Motion and Flexibility

Bob Mangine, P.T., ATC
NovaCare
Florence, Kentucky
Physiological Factors of Rehabilitation

Mark A. Merrick, Ph.D., ATC
Director
Athletic Training Division
The Ohio State University
Columbus, Ohio
The Efficacy of Modalities in Rehabilitation

Edward P. Mulligan, M.S., P.T., S.C.S., ATC
Clinical Instructor
Department of Physical Therapy
The University of Texas Southwestern Medical Center
Dallas, Texas
Assistant Vice President
National Director of Clinical Education
HealthSouth Rehabilitation Corporation
Grapevine, Texas
Foot, Ankle, and Leg Rehabilitation

Dale G. Pease, B.S., M.S., Ph.D.
Associate Professor
Department of Health and Human Performance
University of Houston
Houston, Texas
Psychological Factors of Rehabilitation

Greg Pitts, M.S., O.T.R./L C.H.T.
Clinical Director
Kentucky Hand and Physical Therapy, PLLC
Lexington, Kentucky
Wrist and Hand Rehabilitation

Michael M. Reinold, P.T., ATC
Coordinator of Rehabilitative Research and Clinical
    Education
HealthSouth Rehabilitation
American Sports Medicine Institute
Birmingham, Alabama
Biomechanical Consideration in Rehabilitation

Elizabeth Swann, Ph.D., ATC
Program Director
Athletic Training
Nova Southeastern University
Fort Lauderdale, Florida
Measurement in Rehabilitation

Jill M. Thein-Nissenbaum, M.P.T.
Faculty Associate
Instructor
Musculoskeletal Track
University of Wisconsin–Madison
Madison, Wisconsin
Aquatic Rehabilitation

Timothy F. Tyler, M.S., P.T., ATC
Clinical Research Associate
The Nicholas Institute of Sports Medicine and Athletic
    Trauma
Lenox Hill Hospital
New York, New York
Plyometric Training and Drills

Tim L. Uhl, Ph.D., ATC P.T.
Assistant Professor
Division of Athletic Training
University of Kentucky
Lexington, Kentucky
Wrist and Hand Rehabilitation

Michael L. Voight, D.H.Sc., P.T., O.C.S., S.C.S., ATC
Professor
School of Physical Therapy
Belmont University
Nashville, Tennessee
Functional Training and Advanced Rehabilitation

Mark Weber, Ph.D., ATC, P.T., S.C.S.
Professor
Department of Physical Therapy
School of Health Related Professions
University of Mississippi Medical Center
Jackson, Mississippi
Knee Rehabilitation

Kevin Wilk, P.T.
HealthSouth Sports Medicine and Rehabilitation
Birmingham, Alabama
Rehabilitation Consultant
Tampa Bay Devil Rays Baseball Club
Tampa Bay, Florida
Shoulder Rehabilitation; Elbow Rehabilitation

Jason Willoughby, O.T.R./L.
Kentucky Hand and Physical Therapy, PLLC
Lexington, Kentucky
Wrist and Hand Rehabilitation

William Woodall, Ed.D., P.T., ATC, S.C.S.
Associate Professor
Department of Physical Therapy
School of Health Related Professions
University of Mississippi Medical Center
Jackson, Mississippi
Knee Rehabilitation

PREFACE

Therapeutic rehabilitation use to be a product of philosophies based on tradition handed down through the years from clinician to clinician. These concepts were usually based on the premise, "Well, it has always worked for me," with the subsequent blending of these philosophies and/or exercises into therapeutic rehabilitation programs without an underlying scientific rationale for their implementation. Many early rehabilitation concepts and exercises were extrapolated from scientific models using biomechanical principles without empirical research data to support the theories. Today, 5 years since the second edition of this book and 10 years since its initial publication the plethora of research to support the scientific underpinnings for rehabilitation principles and concepts for the physically active is astounding. As orthopaedic surgical techniques have advanced to aid the injured athlete to return to their former level of competition, so has the scientific bases for implementing and sequencing therapeutic exercises along a continuum of care. This 3rd edition of *Physical Rehabilitation of the Injured Athlete* incorporates this ever expanding scientific bases for rehabilitation of the physically active.

So, Why a 3rd edition? What has changed? What is new? What is cutting edge? As in the previous editions we have attempted to bring together contributors who are experts in the field of athletic rehabilitation and many have the monumental task of both practicing clinically and the desire or responsibility to share their research, knowledge and experience with others through their writing. We have also used many new contributors to give you a different perspective on the content. Furthermore, as with the previous editions, the primary audience for this text is the practicing clinician. Yet we realize that this book is used as a textbook in many educational settings, thus we have also attempted to address the content and format from that perspective as well.

Specifically, outside the new text dimensions and format, what content changes and additions will you find in this third edition?

- The rehabilitation protocols have been updated to reflect the current research and state of practice. We have found that the rehabilitation protocols are a huge feature for this book. Our purpose for inclusion of the protocols is to provide a set of parameters for rehabilitation and are by no means "the only way to do it." Rather, advancement through a rehabilitation program should be based on clinical findings such as the athlete's pain tolerance level, joint effusion, and achievement of specific criteria before the rehabilitation program is advanced. Additionally, surgeons vary their surgical techniques for specific lesions and this must be considered when developing a rehabilitation regimen. Rehabilitation can by no means be "cookbooked," with a program developed for every injury for every athlete. Each athlete brings a unique set of personal qualities that must be addressed by the clinician to facilitate the athlete's rehabilitation.

- New chapters have been added on Cervical Spine Rehabilitation, Biomechanics of Shoulder and Knee Rehabilitation, Female Considerations in Rehabilitation, Proprioception and Neuromuscular Control, Plyometrics, and Functional Training and Advanced Rehabilitation. The later three have been expanded to their own chapters to adequately reflect the exponential growth in these areas.

- The rehabilitation guidelines for those surgical techniques that have come to the forefront over the past 5 years such as reconstruction of the anterior cruciate ligament reconstruction using the semitendonious tendon and the laser capsular shrinkage technique for unstable shoulders. Those surgical techniques that are no longer as prevalent as they once were have been deleted.

- The chapter on modalities has changed from a "How to Use", "How to Apply", "Indications/Contraindications" to more of a clinical efficacy model based on current research findings.

- We have strived for a new look and feel with this 3rd edition with the hope that it is more user friendly than its two predecessors.

It is our hope that this third edition of *Physical Rehabilitation of the Injured Athlete* will serve as a reference for clinicians as well as a text for students interested in the area of athletic rehabilitation. We further hope that this book will serve as a clinician's reference source to improve their clinical practice as well as providing students with the basic knowledge for the development and implementation of rehabilitation programs for the injured athlete.

JAMES R. ANDREWS, M.D.
GARY L. HARRELSON, Ed.D., ATC
KEVIN WILK, P.T.

CONTENTS

CHAPTER 1

PSYCHOLOGIC FACTORS OF REHABILITATION

Dale G. Pease, Ph.D.

CHAPTER OBJECTIVES

At the end of this chapter the reader will be able to:

- Explain the relationship of psychologic traits to potential for injury in sport participation.
- Explain the importance of life stress factors in relation to athletic injury.
- Recognize potential postinjury psychologic responses.
- Identify psychologic coping and adherence strategies for use in the postinjury period.
- Explain the role of slumps and the potential for burnout in relation to athletic injuries.

Although coaches, athletes, and spectators have recognized that physical injury is an inherent risk factor of sport and exercise participation, the psychologic aspects of participation and injury have often been overlooked. Until recently, many individuals in sports treated the body and mind as a dichotomous unit, resulting in the development of training programs that focused on the body and, in some cases, that treated the mind with scorn. Following the lead taken by those in other fields of medicine, practitioners of sports medicine have moved toward a more holistic approach. It has been recognized that the psychologic state of the athlete is as important, and sometimes more important, than the athlete's physical state (Fig. 1-1).

Research involving psychologic factors related to injury susceptibility and rehabilitation is still in its early stages. Numerous interacting variables such as types of sports, level of participation, time of season, team role, types of injuries, and psychologic states pre- and postinjury have made understanding of the psychologic role in injury difficult. Also important to recognize is the fact that most of this research has focused on acute injuries and not on injuries resulting from overuse. What has been learned is that there is great variability among athletes for the reasons summarized in Box 1-1. Although many of the studies cited in this chapter investigated intact teams or specific groups of athletes, we know it is important to view each athlete as unique to fully understand his or her psychologic responses to the threat of injury and to actual injury, especially during the recovery period.

PSYCHOLOGIC RISK FACTORS
Personality Factors

"The athlete is just injury prone!"

This statement, heard from coaches and spectators, often implies that the athlete in question has personal factors that increase susceptibility to injury. Are there psychologic factors that could help sports medicine personnel identify athletes who are more prone to injury than others? Early research on this question focused on personality dispositions, sometimes referred to as traits, measured by paper/pencil instruments such as the Cattell 16 PF.[8] These personality studies investigated traits such as introversion–extroversion,* locus of control,† self-concept, anxiety, aggressiveness, and dominance. For example, it was believed that an athlete with a strong anxiety trait would have greater body tension and be less able to focus effectively on critical information involving performance, thus becoming more susceptible to injury or that athletes with an external locus of control, who would perceive themselves as having less control over the events around them, would thus have a greater potential for injury. By identifying certain psychologic traits as contributors to potential injury, an athlete with such traits might be advised to select sports with a low-injury risk factor or to take special precautions if participating in a sport with a high-injury risk factor.

---

*Introverts tend to withdraw into themselves (introversion), whereas extroverts extend or seek out external stimulation (extroversion).

†Locus of control is the responsibility people feel for their behavior by referring to internal causes (e.g., attributed to their own actions) or to external causes, in which they have little control over the events in their lives.

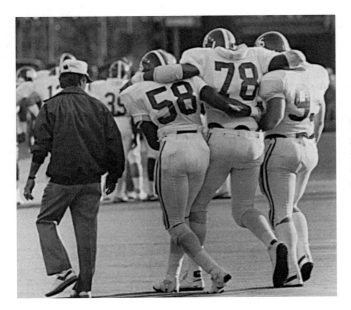

Figure 1-1. Risk factors have been recognized as inherent with sport participation. Until recently, the athlete's body and mind were treated as a single unit, with the latter receiving little or no attention. (From Philpot, D. [1986]: Evaluation of the injured ankle. Sports Med. Update, 1:5.)

Results of research using the trait approach have shown limited significant findings involving the relationship of psychologic traits and the occurrence of athletic injuries. It was found that football players who were more "tender-minded" and reserved were more susceptible to injury.[16,17] Contrary to this finding, a study of women volleyball players found that players with higher levels of tough-mindedness (e.g., assertiveness or independence) were found to experience a higher rate of severe injuries than athletes who were more tender-minded.[34] This study supported a previous study reporting that female basketball players with a higher incidence of injury scored more positively on self-concept and identity and on physical and personal self-factors than noninjured female players.[35] It was suggested that these injured volleyball and basketball players were more likely to take risks because of greater self-confidence and consequently their potential for injury was increased. Other studies have reported a significant relationship between internal locus of control and injury in elite gymnasts but not in nonelite gymnasts.[20] Petrie[25] reported trait anxiety to be positively related to injury rate in starting football players but not in nonstarting players. These are a few examples of the studies investigating the

relation of personality factors to injury. For a more comprehensive review, see Williams.[30]

Although some studies have given support to the notion that there is a relationship between identified personality traits and the occurrence of injury, other studies have produced mixed or contrary results. Most researchers at the present time believe that the evidence is inconclusive for prediction and intervention purposes and that other factors need investigation. However, the role one's personality plays in relation to injury should not be ignored as will be observed in the stress model discussed in the next section.

Life Stress Model

As a result of a lack of consistent and significant findings from trait studies, the research focus shifted to exploring the relationship of stress to injury. The concept that stressful life events may be related to the occurrence of athletic injuries was initially based on reports in the general medical literature. Studies have shown a positive relationship between stressful life events, especially those with high negative stress, and the occurrence of injury and disease. In general, high life stress is believed to wear down an individual's ability to adapt or cope. Using this research, Anderson and Williams[2] developed a theoretic stress model that recently has been somewhat revised to show the interaction effect among personality, an individual's history, and coping resources[32] (Fig. 1-2).

This model includes the personality traits previously discussed and presents these traits as factors that interact with an individual's history of stress events and coping resources or as a factor that may have a direct impact on the stress response. More recently, Williams[30] has suggested that personality factors such as sensation seeking,

---

Box 1-1

What Makes Each Athlete Different?

- Past experiences
- Value systems
- Expectations
- Coping skills
- Support systems
- Physical attributes
- Psychologic attributes

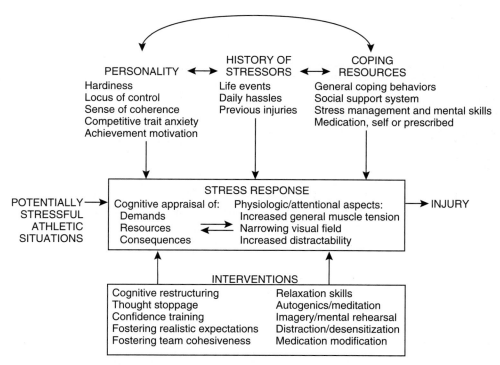

Figure 1-2. A model of stress and athletic injury. (Modified from Anderson, M.B., and Williams, J.M. [1988]: A model of stress and athletic injury: Prediction and prevention. J. Sport Exerc. Psychol., 10:297. Copyright 1988 by Human Kinetics Publishers, Inc. Reprinted by permission.)

mood states, aggression, anger, and self-concept should be included in this model. The model should be reviewed to understand the proposed factors contributing to and interacting with the stress response. It is also referred to later in this chapter.

In general, the relationship between life stress and athletic injury appears to be substantial. Williams[30] reported that 30 of 35 studies assessing life events, which involved different sports and competitive levels, found some significant relation between life stress and injury. She further reported that approximately two thirds of the studies found some relationship between life stress and injury severity. These studies involved an array of sports including football, figure skating, baseball, gymnastics, wrestling, soccer, and track and field. Although we often think of life stress resulting from major events (e.g., a death in the family or a divorce), a recent study[11] investigated the role of minor events, which were referred to as "hassles" (daily hassles), in sport injury. Injured athletes were found to have had a significant increase in hassles for the week before injury whereas noninjured athletes had no significant increase in hassles.

Additional examples of studies that have investigated the life stress relationship to sport injuries are as follows. Bramwell and associates[5] studied the life changes of 79 varsity college football players for 1- and 2-year periods before their playing season and found that a greater percentage of injuries occurred in those in the high life

change group. In their study of two college football teams, Passer and Seese[23] found a significant relationship between negative life stress and injury on one team but not on the other. Studies of elite female gymnasts revealed that stressful life events are related significantly to both the number and severity of injuries.[18] In this study, factors such as anxiety, loss of control, and self-concept were not significant predictors of injury. Although several studies have noted a relationship between high life stress (especially negative stress) and injuries, a study involving male and female intercollegiate volleyball players showed no relationship between life stress and injury.[33] The type of sport and the predominant types of injuries, especially the severity of the injury and lost participation time, found in a sport may be important variables in the stress–injury relationship, but there is very limited research addressing this hypothesis.

In the studies mentioned in the preceding paragraph the primary focus was on negative life events. However, positive life events can also create stress that has been related to athletic injury.[3,14] Events such as being named a team leader, which increases the team responsibility role, being named to a preseason all-star team, or receiving a performance award may increase the performance expectations of the athlete, resulting in increased levels of stress and making the athlete more prone to injury. Williams and Anderson[32] stated that the stress response is not determined just by the life stress demands, but by how the

---

Box 1-2

Sources of Life Stress*

Examples of negative life stress:	Examples of positive life stress:
• Death of a significant other • Illness of significant other • Breakup of a relationship • Loss of job/team position • Potential illness or injury to self • Previous injury • Academic failure or threat of failure • Daily hassles	• Made captain of the team or a starter • Moved up a competitive level (e.g., junior varsity to varsity) • Received media recognition for previous performance • Experienced changes in what others expect because of success of a sibling • Made all-star team • Had a new significant other (boyfriend/ girlfriend)

*Remember it may not be the event itself, such as those listed, but how the athlete perceives the demands of the event and his or her ability to cope with it.

---

athlete perceives these demands and his or her ability to cope with them. See Box 1-2 for a listing of some positive and negative stress factors.

To explore this stress–injury relationship further, the physiologic and psychologic changes in response to stress must be understood, as shown in a model by Nideffer[22] (Fig. 1-3). In regard to physiologic changes, there is increasing concern about the muscle tension produced as a result of the stress response. Increased tension in the antagonistic and agonistic muscle groups results in a reduction of flexibility and loss of motor coordination. Another significant factor related to increased muscular tension is a slowed reaction time, which reduces the

athlete's ability to respond to environmental events. Therefore, the maintenance of appropriate muscle tension to achieve a desired result appears to be essential in the prevention of injuries.

By studying the Nideffer model (Fig. 1-3), one can see that an important psychologic variable is the ability of the athlete to select and process information, because stress has been shown to narrow or switch the attentional focus. For example, a player under heavy stress in football might not process information in the peripheral areas of the visual field, resulting in a lack of response to oncoming physical contact (e.g., greater potential for a blind-side hit). Another important aspect of attentional focus involves

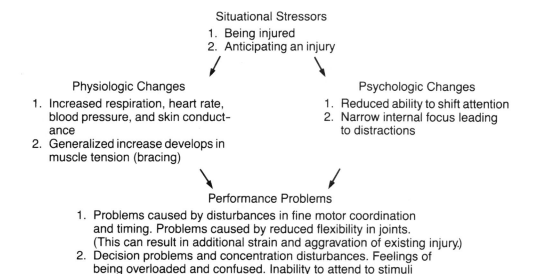

Situational Stressors
1. Being injured
2. Anticipating an injury

Physiologic Changes
1. Increased respiration, heart rate, blood pressure, and skin conductance
2. Generalized increase develops in muscle tension (bracing)

Psychologic Changes
1. Reduced ability to shift attention
2. Narrow internal focus leading to distractions

Performance Problems
1. Problems caused by disturbances in fine motor coordination and timing. Problems caused by reduced flexibility in joints. (This can result in additional strain and aggravation of existing injury.)
2. Decision problems and concentration disturbances. Feelings of being overloaded and confused. Inability to attend to stimuli relevant to the task because of physiologic distractions. Inability to shift attention from one focus to another.

Figure 1-3. Physical and psychologic changes accompany increases in pressure as a result of injury or the fear of injury. Problems in performance resulting from stress and reduced physiologic and psychologic flexibility can become chronic. Disturbances in physical flexibility affect concentration and, as the athlete becomes upset at his or her own failure (frustration or anxiety increases), the attentional and physiologic disturbances become stronger and more intractable. (Modified from Nideffer, R.M. [1983]: The injured athlete: Psychological factors in treatment. Orthop. Clin. North Am., 14:373-385.)

what the athlete was thinking at the time of injury. The Nideffer model proposes that an athlete under stress, especially negative stress, might be thinking about the events causing the emotional stress and not thinking about what is currently happening in the environment. Therefore, the athlete does not process relevant information that could result in a protective response. For example, a linebacker in football who has just learned of the divorce plans of his parents might be thinking of what his future holds (internal focus) and not attending well to information involving what is happening on the field (external focus). Hence, there would be a greater potential for injury for this athlete.

In support of the Nideffer model, Williams and Anderson[31] found significant deterioration with all perceptual variables in high stress conditions compared with low stress conditions. Athletes with high negative life stress experienced slower central visual reaction time and greater peripheral narrowing than athletes with low life event stress. Further, this study supported the interactive nature of the previously presented Anderson and Williams model. The lowest perceptual sensitivity was found in males who were low in social support, low in coping skills, and high in negative life stress. A similar interaction was found for females in their ability to detect central visual cues. This distractibility in the central and peripheral visual fields certainly increases the injury risk factor.

The importance of attentional focus in athletic injuries must include interest in recent studies involving the psychologic phenomenon of mood congruence. It has been shown that we attend, encode, and retrieve information that is congruent with our mood state.[4] For example, if the mood state of the athlete described above is depression, resulting from knowledge of his parents' divorce, the information he is attending to probably contains affect-congruent information. In this case, it is negative information from the environment (external focus) and negative thoughts (internal focus) that are affecting his thought process and not the game happenings.

If the mood state is anger as a result of the divorce plans, high levels of activation would be expected, which also disrupt the attentional ability and the processing of relevant information. With the occurrence of either emotion, depression or anger, the ability to control attention and process correct information is inhibited, thus increasing his potential for injury. The ability to control attention and block out irrelevant information depends greatly on the individual, with wide variation among athletes.

From the Anderson and Williams model, a history of stressors is an important consideration. For the athlete returning to competition after recovery from injury, the role of attentional focus and muscular tension can be a major problem. Fear or worry about a second injury can place an athlete's thought processing in an internal mode, causing increased muscular tension. There has been interest in the role of psychologic hardiness as it relates to return from injury. Hardiness can be defined as a combination of commitment, control, and challenge on the part of an individual and seems to be a moderating factor in the stress–illness relationship.[19] It is believed that athletes who exhibit greater qualities of this trait are better able to control the attentional processing of information and in turn reduce the potential for occurrence of a second injury. At present, however, not enough studies have been done on hardiness and its relationship to injury to be able to reach definite conclusions.

Fatigue, the final factor to be discussed here, has been recognized as a contributor to injury from the physical aspect. Usually, however, fatigue has been regarded as only a physical factor, and mental fatigue may be more important. The ability to maintain a high level of concentration (attention) requires a large amount of energy and, combined with a demanding training program, attention is reduced as both physical and mental fatigue sets in. Reduced attention results in slowed response times and, combined with the loss of neuromuscular coordination, increases the potential for injury.

In moving beyond the general physical effects of stress, as discussed above, recent research has shown the importance of the social support systems available in the ability of the athlete to cope with the stress response that has been shown to be related to the incidence of injury. Petrie[24] reported that female collegiate gymnastics in low social support conditions were most vulnerable to the effects of life stress, which was positively related to the incidents of injury. In a second study with collegiate football players, Petrie[25,26] reported a significant relationship for starting players on the teams involved. The number of severe injuries, the days missed due to injury, and the games missed were related to negative life stress with social support serving as a moderating variable. In other words, if the athlete had a strong social support system around him or her, the life stressors encountered would not result in as high an injury potential. This relationship of social support to stress and injury did not exist for nonstarting players. It is also important to note that Petrie reported that players with high social support and low life stress were more likely to experience injury than those reporting low levels of support with low life stress. One explanation is that under low stress/high support conditions, athletes may have a greater sense of confidence and security and therefore exhibit greater risk-taking behaviors, which would increase the potential for injury to occur. From the current research it appears that social support is an important moderating variable in either high or low life stress situations to the potential for injury in sport situations.

Thus, current studies involving psychologic risk factors and injury support the importance of the stress response (as presented in the Anderson and Williams model, Fig. 1-2).

CLINICAL PEARL #1

It appears that a positive relationship exists between stressful life events, especially those with high negative stress, and the occurrence of injury and disease.

CLINICAL PEARL #2

Although life stress is most often thought to result from negative happenings, positive happenings can also produce stress that can influence life experiences.

OCCURRENCE OF INJURY

"Whistle blows—an athlete is down—coaches, players, and spectators are standing/looking; medical personal are rushing to the player." This can be the beginning of psychologic turmoil for the athlete and the significant others around him or her.

When an athlete is injured, the primary focus of athletic trainers, coaches, teammates, physicians, parents, and even the spectator is generally on tangible evidence of the injury: "How severe is the injury?" "Will surgery be required?" These questions are followed by others: "How long will the athlete be out of competition?" "Who will replace this athlete in the lineup?" And, if the athlete is in a critical position (e.g., quarterback or pitcher), many of the significant people working with this athlete might think of the season "going down the drain."

Immediate treatments, such as cryotherapy and immobilization, are usually provided quickly, followed by a rehabilitation program that includes a regimen for regaining strength and flexibility. Although the physical needs of an injured athlete are being taken care of, other major needs that may create more pain than the physical aspect of the injury are often overlooked. If an athlete is injured, his or her thoughts and feelings are often disregarded or given a low priority. These thoughts and feelings, reflecting on past experiences involving injury to self or others and how this injury may change the future, can produce psychologic pain that is greater and lasts longer than the physical pain. Well-intended comments to an injured athlete (e.g., "you will be okay" or "just hang in there") are often heard, but these do not really address the psychologic problems the athlete is experiencing.

Emotional Responses

As the initial physical pain of the injury subsides, the athlete encounters an array of psychologic reactions. Emotional responses, such as "why me?," "why now?," and "this can't be happening," take over the thoughts of the athlete. Other emotions, such as anger, depression, anxiety, and panic, are common responses. Sometimes these emotions cannot be

expressed overtly by the athlete, because this type of behavior is unacceptable in the "macho" world of athletics. When an athletic career is interrupted or perhaps terminated as a result of an injury, the years of expectations and hard work seem wasted and a strong emotional response, overt or hidden, must be expected and dealt with.

Although an injury can be psychologically devastating to many athletes, some athletes view the injury with relief. For these athletes, the injury provides them with attention and support from others that they may not have been receiving before the injury. For others, the injury relieves the pressure to perform, and the respite from training and competition may be welcomed. This gives the athlete a chance to enjoy other aspects of life and provides time for reevaluating his or her commitment to the sport. The idea that an athlete may obtain satisfaction from an injury, however, is often difficult for the athletic trainer and especially a coach to understand. With the emphasis on sports in today's society, resulting in enormous pressure on the athlete to perform and be successful, there is increasing evidence that more athletes are using this method of coping with some of these pressures.[6,7]

As stated previously, various psychologic responses can be observed immediately after injury and can continue long after recovery. The nature and intensity of these responses depend on several factors, such as the type of injury, its importance to performing the skills essential to the sport, the time of injury in regard to the season and major competitive events, and the importance of participation to the athlete. The major variable related to these factors seems to be the athlete's perception of the injury and its effect on the future. Although the injury might seem minor to the athletic trainer or physician, the athlete might believe that it is more severe and therefore could exhibit emotional responses that seems unwarranted to others. Of significance here is acceptance by the athlete of the athletic trainer's or physician's appraisal of the injury. If the athlete lacks confidence in the ability of medical personnel to appraise and treat the injury properly, he or she can reject and ignore the medical advice, resulting in a stronger negative emotional response.

Lynch[21] reported that severely injured athletes go through emotional stages of denial, anger, bargaining, depression, and acceptance. This suggested orderly process for emotional behavior after injury, often referred to as a stage model, has not been supported in a recent review of athletic injury research.[6] It was found that the emotional reactions to injury vary among individual athletes, depending on the stress resulting from the athlete's appraisal of the injury. Personal (e.g., motivation, coping skills, self-esteem, and personality) and situational (e.g., injury severity, timing, impact on daily lives, and social pressures) factors cause athletes to alternate among emotional states and reflect feelings of fear, panic, and even learned helplessness. There are often behavioral indications suggesting that the

---

Box 1-3

Signs of Adjustment Problems

- Emotional displays of anger, depression, confusion, or apathy
- Obsession with the question, "When will I be able to play again?"
- Denial—athlete leads you to believe the injury is no big deal
- History of coming back too fast from injury
- Exaggerated storytelling or bragging about accomplishments

- Dwelling on minor somatic complaints
- Remarks about letting the team down or feeling guilty
- Dependence on therapist—hanging around athletic training room
- Withdrawal from teammates, coaches, or friends
- Rapid mood swings or changes in behavior
- Statements indicating feeling of helplessness to impact recovery

Adopted from Petitpas, A., and Danish, S. (1995): Caring for injured athlete. *In* S. Murphy, S. (ed.), Sport Psychology Interventions. Champaign, IL, Human Kinetics, pp. 255-281.

---

athlete is experiencing psychologic stress in dealing with his or her injury (Box 1-3).

What about gender differences? Do male and female athletes respond differently to injury? Most athletic injury studies have not included a gender comparison in the study of the emotional responses of injured athletes. In one of the very few reports comparing gender behaviors, Quackenbush and Crossman,[27] studied recovering athletes at three sports medicine clinics and found significant emotional differences between male and female athletes. Female athletes were found to express more emotional responses, both positive and negative, than male athletes. Immediately after injury both male and female athletes were equally frustrated, angry, and discouraged; male athletes were more irritable whereas female athletes were more cooperative, optimistic, and hopeful. During the recovery period female athletes showed more positive signs toward returning to practice. These researchers concluded that socialization differences have an impact on the expression of psychologic feelings and thoughts, suggesting that gender of the injured athlete must be a consideration in the psychologic component of the rehabilitation process.

CLINICAL PEARL #3

The acceptance by the athlete of the athletic trainer's and physician's appraisal of the injury is important. If the athlete lacks confidence in the ability of medical personnel to appraise and treat the injury properly, he or she can reject and ignore the medical advice, resulting in a stronger negative emotional response.

Social Support Systems: Recovery Phase

The psychologic responses mentioned above, coupled with the physical pain resulting from the injury, result in a threat to self-esteem and induce feelings of incompetence that may have a major influence on the recovery period.

This seems to be especially true if the athlete has no strong social support system available. During recovery the stress resulting from the injury can be a major problem—remember it is the perceived stress experienced by the athlete that is important. For example, the coach may plan for the injured athlete to return to his or her starting position after recovery and may discuss these plans with the athlete. If the athlete perceives the starting role to be in jeopardy, however, there can be additional stress on the athlete that others may not observe or understand. This stress, from whatever source, causes increased muscle tension and can reduce the circulatory system's ability to supply blood to the injured area. This stress can also reduce the ability of the athlete to perform the simple physical movement patterns necessary for rehabilitation

Of prime importance in providing medical services to an athlete during recovery is identifying and developing a strong social support system. Extensive medical research has shown the value of support systems as buffers or moderators of the negative stress resulting from disease or injury. Results of studies involving sports settings have also suggested a positive relationship between desired athlete behaviors during the recovery period and the support provided by significant others.[10,12] Weiss and Troxell[29] presented a strong case for the role of the athletic trainer in the support system. The presence and positive support of others who understand the needs of the athlete and why certain behaviors are occurring are valuable in helping the athlete cope with various problems during the recovery period. This understanding is especially necessary because the injured athlete might be depressed and, as a result, could reject the efforts of people close to him or her. Within a short period, however, this same athlete may be seeking assurance and reinforcement from these same individuals. Those in the support system, which must include the athletic trainer, physical therapist, and physician, therefore play an extremely important role in understanding and guiding the athlete through the emotional times during recovery.

CLINICAL PEARL #4

Of prime importance in providing medical services to an athlete during recovery is identifying and developing a strong social support system.

ADHERENCE AND RECOVERY PROBLEMS

During the recovery period a disturbing behavior of the athlete sometimes emerges. The athlete misses assigned therapy sessions or, when attending the session, does not put forth the necessary effort for effective rehabilitation. Brewer[7] reported estimates of athlete adherence to sport injury rehabilitation programs ranging from 40% to 91%. The lack of commitment becomes extremely disturbing to coaches, athletic trainers, physical therapists, teammates, and others who are influenced by this behavior. As stated before, some of this behavior by athletes may be due to their seeing the occurrence of an injury as a positive event, in that it may relieve them of the pressures of competition, gain them attention, or allow them time to reevaluate the importance of sports participation.

Research by Duda and colleagues[10] represents one of the few studies investigating why athletes do not adhere to rehabilitation programs. Their study involved 40 intercollegiate athletes who had sustained a sport injury of at least second-degree severity that resulted in scheduled rehabilitation sessions for 3 weeks or more. They measured the attendance, completion of the exercise protocol, and observed exercise intensity of the injured athletes. The study showed that perceived value of the treatment, social support, degree of self-motivation, and task involvement in sports are significant predictors of adherence behaviors. Brewer[7] identified additional personal variables associated with adherence problems such as pain tolerance, tough-mindedness, and internal health locus of control. He also listed situational factors associated with adherence such as clinical environment, scheduling of treatments, and expectations of health care personal as important adherence factors.

CLINICAL PEARL #5

In some instances rehabilitation adherence problems with athletes may be due to their seeing the occurrence of an injury as a positive event, in that it may relieve them of the pressures of competition, gain them attention, or allow them time to reevaluate the importance of sports participation.

Educating the Athlete

How do these factors relate to the participation of a sports medicine team in treatment of an injury? Educating the athlete about the nature and value of the treatment is a responsibility of the athletic trainer, physical therapist, and physician, with the aid of the coach and parents. Often, treatments and drug therapy are prescribed without providing the person receiving the treatment with information about how it influences the rehabilitation process.

This problem arises because it is often assumed that the athlete already knows why a treatment is prescribed or because, when large numbers of players are involved, such as a football team, there is not enough time to provide individual attention. The importance of providing the athlete with information about the rehabilitation program was found by Udry[28] with athletes after knee surgery. Athletes seeking information about the injury or rehabilitation program adhered to a greater extent than athletes who did not seek such information. The educational process is part of the responsibility of those who provide social support in the recovery period.

Motivational Factors in Adherence

Two factors—self-motivation and task involvement—are sometimes the most misunderstood variables when one is working with athletes, because most people assume that highly successful athletes have high levels of self-motivation and a high degree of involvement and commitment to their sport. This assumption is not true, however; some athletes with great natural abilities have low-need achievement levels and a limited commitment to the sport for which they are recognized. Such athletes usually lack self-directed goals that can help provide the intrinsic drive necessary to gain maximum value from their natural abilities. Therefore, when this type of athlete is injured, the lack of internal drive and goals results in problems with adherence to a prescribed rehabilitation program, which takes time and effort to complete. Also, the lack of adherence could be the result of the athlete's not viewing the reward system (extrinsic motivation) as providing the necessary returns for overcoming the lack of internal motivation to complete the rehabilitation program successfully.

The adherence variables described earlier are consistent with those found in the medical literature.[9] However, studies on adherence in sports are limited, and there are still many questions to be answered to understand this problem. These include type of sport, gender of athlete, time during the season when the injury occurs, and perceived cause of the injury. Injury is an inherent variable in sports participation, so factors that influence the adherence to rehabilitation programs are important for the effective functioning of a sports medicine team.

A behavioral observation reported by coaches and athletic trainers after an athlete is injured and returns to competition is that the athlete does not have the same intensity and dedication to the sport as observed before the injury. This loss of focus and intensity can contribute to adherence problems but becomes more serious on return to practice and competition.

It is generally believed that the athlete has a fear of being reinjured, and to some extent this is true. It may also be the case, however, that the athlete has had time to reflect on the role of sports in his or her life, has questioned its importance and rewards, and, as a result, has established new priorities. One athlete, currently in her middle teens, after having to take time off from swimming because of a car accident injury, reported that "I never thought there were so many other fun things to do." This swimmer had been attending twice-a-day workouts for the past 10 years of her life, and everything she did was related to swimming. The "time out" gave her a chance to participate in other activities and changed her thinking about the importance of sports in her life.

Athletic trainers, coaches, and significant others play important roles in the recovery period. Their understanding of the problems that an athlete can encounter during this period is critical to satisfactory recovery. They can provide the motivation to help the athlete adhere to rehabilitation programs and to return to practice and competition with a positive mental attitude (Fig. 1-4). Successful sports medicine personnel understand and provide the athlete needed education and psychologic support in the areas listed in Box 1-4.

ADHERENCE COPING STRATEGIES

In reviewing the Anderson and Williams model (Fig. 1-2) you will find that there are two aspects showing the importance of coping strategies. The first is listed under coping resources, where the importance of social support systems, stress management and mental skills, and general coping behaviors is shown to mediate life stress factors and to interact directly with the stress response. The second aspect of the model deals with the interventions that can be used in response to stress. Although this model was designed to explain the psychologic phenomena involved as antecedents of an injury, the model is also useful for

understanding the psychologic interventions for dealing with postinjury responses. Although the model presents several general interventions, three basic interventions will be discussed.

Goal Setting

Goal setting has consistently been found to be one of the most powerful motivational tools when one works with athletes. With the injured athlete, the long-term goal is returning the athlete to preinjury performance levels. However, the short-term goals are more important. In the next 3 to 4 weeks, what does the athlete need to achieve in terms of increased strength, flexibility, range of movement, and even improved psychologic state? In establishing short-term goals one must measure the current performance level and establish a level of performance that can with effort reasonably be achieved in the 3- to 4-week period. A specific plan must be established with athlete input such as the amount of weight, types of lifts, and number of repetitions that must be performed. Short-term goals such as "do your best" and "work as hard as you can" are not good goals and do not provide the necessary motivation to perform. At the end of the predetermined time period an assessment must be done, and if the goals have been achieved, celebrate and establish new goals. If the goals have not been achieved, assess why, and establish new goals that the athlete has a better chance of achieving. Although goal setting is important from a motivational perspective, it also can be an important tool in controlling the behavior so that an athlete does not overdo in an attempt to return to competition too soon.

Visualization/Imagery

The use of mental skills referred to a visualization (seeing with the mind's eye) or, even better, imagery (using all senses, i.e., visual, kinesthetic, auditory, tactile, olfactory,

Figure 1-4. The return of an athlete to his or her sport involves not only the physical rehabilitation program, but also the athlete's mental health. Of the support personnel available, the athletic trainer can be the best qualified to address these concerns. (Photo by John Rawlston, News-Free Press.)

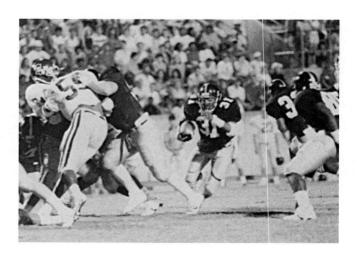

Box 1-4

Reminders for the Sports Medicine Team in Working with the Injured Athlete

Important rehabilitation concerns:	To be successful in achieving these rehabilitation concerns, you must
• Athlete must feel understood • Athlete must accept the reality of the injury • Athlete must understand the rehabilitation plan • Athlete must adhere to the rehabilitation plan	• Build rapport with the injured athlete • Educate the athlete about the rehabilitation process • Teach athlete coping skills • Identify and help develop the athlete's social support system

and gustatory, to re-create or create an experience in the mind) can be an important tool in the rehabilitation process. Visualization/imagery can be used for stress management through inducing relaxation and thereby reducing muscle tension and increasing blood flow. For example, Green[13] has shown how athletes trained in the use of imagery can potentially reduce stress, which may lead to injury, and more important here how imagery can be used during the rehabilitation process. Direct benefits have been shown by Ievleva and Orlick,[15] who found the use of healing imagery related to faster healing of knee injuries in patients. Visualization/imagery can be used to reduce the fear of reinjury when the athlete returns to competition. In addition, use of visualization/imagery can help the athlete stay in contact with his or her sport by mentally practicing game skills and strategies. However, athletes must be trained to use this skill.

Self-Talk

Often the injured athlete is consumed with negative thoughts about what happened and about his or her future. These negative thoughts must be countered by using positive statements. If allowed to predominate, negative thoughts can produce negative mood states such as depression and anxiety and slow the healing process. It is important to work with the athlete to develop positive statements related to improvement or the effort being put forth to be used when negative feelings and thoughts enter the mind. For more in-depth information on interventions the reader is referred to a new book *Doing Sport Psychology* edited by Anderson.[1]

SLUMPS AND INJURIES

Most athletes experience declines in performance at some time, commonly referred to as "slumps." These can result from physical, technical, or psychologic problems or from some combination of these. The prescription for a slump can range from "work harder and work your way through it" to a "time out," during which the athlete has a period of total rest from the sport. How do athletic injuries and psychologic variables further relate to slumps?

Probably the most common cause of a slump is a physical factor. Fatigue caused by overtraining and injury, especially nagging minor injuries that receive little attention, creates problems in the execution of a skill and results in a lower performance level. As the athlete senses the declining physical performance, psychologic factors resulting in anxiety, loss of concentration, and confidence become a major source of future problems.

The increased anxiety results in greater muscle tension, which interferes with coordination in the muscular system and results in a lower performance level, and in increased risk of further injury. Because a slump can be extremely draining, it can further add to the general fatigue factor, and the athlete's ability to concentrate on important information can be hindered still more.

Sometimes slumps are the result of problems that are not directly related to sport participation. Marital or financial problems or family illness could be the cause of a slump. Again, the problem of lack or loss of concentration increases the potential for injury to occur. In some cases the athlete may use the injury as a means of explaining the slump and to escape the pressure of performance and the need to explain the real problem to others.

It is therefore important that the members of the sports medicine team do not write off a slump as only a psychologic problem related to athletic performance. Often the antecedents to the observed psychologic responses, such as injury, fatigue, or outside influences, are the true sources of the slump.

SUMMARY

■ Personality factors have been found to be associated with frequency and severity of injury, but should not be used for predication or intervention purposes.

■ Life-stress has been shown to have a strong association with injury, and certain personality factors, coping skills, and injury history can serve as stress moderators.

■ Emotional responses ranging from depression, anger, anxiety, and even panic must be considered normal responses to an injury that threatens the future career of an athlete.

■ Social support systems are important in both the prevention of injury and during the rehabilitation phase after injury.

■ Adherence by the athlete to the rehabilitation program will vary greatly, depending on factors such as the athlete's goals, task involvement, and perceived value of treatment.

■ Adherence to the rehabilitation program can be increased by educating the athlete about the injury and the treatment and through strong social support systems.

■ Educating the athlete in the use of effective coping strategies (e.g., goal setting, imagery, self-talk, and relaxation) can address both physical and psychologic problems.

■ Most important is the role of the clinician in providing not only the physical treatment component but also the knowledge and skill to assess and remediate the psychologic responses associated with injury.

REFERENCES

1. Anderson, M.B. (2000): Doing Sport Psychology. Champaign, IL, Human Kinetics.
2. Anderson, M.B., and Williams, J.M. (1988): A model of stress and athletic injury: Prediction and prevention. J. Sport Exerc. Psychol., 10:294-306.
3. Blackwell, B., and McCullagh, P. (1990): The relationship of athletic injury to life stress, competitive anxiety and coping resources. Athl. Train., 25, 23-27.
4. Blaney, P.H. (1986): Affect and memory: A review. Psychol. Bull., 99:229-246.
5. Bramwell, S.T., Masuda, M., Wagner, N.N., and Holmes, T.H. (1975): Psychosocial factors in athletic injuries: Development and application of the social and athletic readjustment rating scale. J. Human Stress, 1:6-20.
6. Brewer, B.W. (1994): Review and critique of models of psychological adjustment to athletic injury. J. Appl. Sport Psychol., 6:87-100.
7. Brewer, B.W. (2001): Psychology of sport injury rehabilitation. In: Singer, R., Hausenblas, H., and Janelle, C. (eds.): Handbook of Sport Psychology, 2nd ed. New York, John Wiley and Sons, pp.787-809.
8. Cattell, R.B. (1965): The Scientific Analysis of Personality. Baltimore: Penguin Books.
9. Dishman, R.K. (1986): Exercise compliance. A new view for public health. Physician Sportsmed., 14:127-145.
10. Duda, J.L., Smart, A.E., and Tappe, M.K. (1989): Predictors of adherence in the rehabilitation of athletic injuries: An application of personal investment theory. J. Sport Exerc. Psychol., 11:367-381.
11. Fawkner, H.J., McMurray, N.E., and Summers, J.J. (1999): Athletic injury and minor life events: A prospective study. J. Sci. Med. Sport, 2:117-124.
12. Fisher, A.C., Domm, M.A., and Wuest, D.A. (1988): Adherence to sports-injury rehabilitation programs. Physician Sportsmed., 16:47-52.
13. Green, L.B. (1992): The use of imagery in the rehabilitation of injured athletes. Sport Psychologist, 6:416-428.
14. Hanson, S.J., McCullagh, P., and Tonymon, P. (1992): The relationship of personality characteristics, life stress, and coping resources to athletic injury. J. Sport Exerc. Psychol., 14:262-272.
15. Ievleva, L., and Orlick, T. (1991): Mental links to enhanced healing: An exploratory study. Sport Psychologist, 5:25-40.
16. Irwin, R.F. (1975): Relationship between personality and the incidence of injuries to high school football participants. Dissertation Abstr. Int., 36:4328A.
17. Jackson, D.W., Jarrett, H., Bailey, D., et al. (1978): Injury prediction in the young athlete: A preliminary report. Am. J. Sports Med., 6:6-14.
18. Kerr, G., and Minden, H. (1988): Psychological factors related to the occurrence of athletic injuries. J. Sport Exerc. Psychol., 109:167-173.
19. Kobasa, S.C., Maddi, S.R., and Puccetti, M.C. (1982): Personality and exercise as buffers in the stress–illness relationship. J. Behav. Med., 5:391-404.
20. Kolt, G., and Kirkby, R. (1996): Injury in Australian female competitive gymnasts: A psychological perspective. Aust. J. Physiother., 42, 121-126.
21. Lynch, C.P. (1988): Athletic injuries and the practicing sport psychologists: Practical guidelines for assisting athletes. Sport Psychologist, 2:161-167.
22. Nideffer, R.M. (1983): The injured athlete: Psychological factors in treatment. Orthop. Clin. North Am., 14:373-385.
23. Passer, M.W., and Seese, M.D. (1983): Life stress and athletic injury: Examination of positive versus negative events and three moderator variables. J. Human Stress, 9:11-16.
24. Petrie, T.A. (1992): Psychosocial antecedents of athletic injury: The effects of life stress and social support on women collegiate gymnasts. Behav. Med., 18:127-138.
25. Petrie, T.A. (1993): The moderating effects of social support and playing status on the life stress-injury relationship. J. Appl. Sport Psychol., 5:1-16.
26. Petrie, T.A. (1993): Coping skills, competitive trait anxiety, and playing status: Moderating effects on the life stress-injury relationship. J. Sport Exerc. Psychol., 15:261-274.
27. Quackenbush, N., and Crossman, J. (1994): A study of emotional responses. J. Sport Behav., 17:178-187.
28. Udry, E. (1997): Coping and social support among injured athletes following surgery. J. Sport Exerc. Psychol., 19:71-90.
29. Weiss, M.R., and Troxell, R.K. (1986): Psychology of the injured athlete. Athletic Training, 21:104-110.
30. Williams, J.M. (2001): Psychology of injury risk and prevention. In: Singer, R., Hausenblas, H., and Janelle, C. (eds.): Handbook of Sport Psychology, 2nd ed. New York, John Wiley and Sons, pp. 766-786.
31. Williams, J.M., and Anderson, M.B. (1997): Psychosocial influences on central and peripheral vision and reaction time during demanding tasks. Behav. Med., 26:160-167.
32. Williams, J.M., and Anderson, M.B. (1998): Psychosocial antecedents of sport injury: Review and critique of the stress and injury model. J. Appl. Sport Psych., 10:5-25.

33. Williams, J.M., Tonymon, P., and Wadsworth, W.A. (1986): Relationship of stress to injury in intercollegiate volleyball. J. Human Stress, 12:38-43.

34. Wittig, A.F., and Schurr, K.T. (1994): Psychological characteristics of women volleyball players: Relationships with injuries, rehabilitation, and team success. Pers. Soc. Psychol. Bull., 20:322-330.

35. Young, M.L., and Cohen, D.A. (1981): Self-concept and injuries among high school basketball players. J. Sports Med., 21:55-61.

CHAPTER 2

PHYSIOLOGIC FACTORS OF REHABILITATION

Bob Mangine, M.Ed.P.T., ATC
Gentian Nuzzo, P.T.
Gary L. Harrelson, Ed.D., ATC

CHAPTER OBJECTIVES

At the end of this chapter the reader will be able to:

- Explain the body's chemical, metabolic, permeability and vascular changes that occur as a result of trauma.
- Explain how different joint structures respond to the inflammatory process.
- Summarize the effect that immobilization has on muscle, periarticular connective tissue, articular cartilage, ligaments and bone.
- Describe the sequela of events that result in synovitis.
- Describe the process that can result in arthrofibrosis.
- Summarize how muscle, periarticular connective tissue, articular cartilage, ligaments and bone respond to exercise following a period of immobilization.
- Explain the therapeutic benefits of the use of CPM.
- List several ways to help deter the deleterious effects of immobilization to specific body structures.

The effects of immobilization on bone and connective tissue have been widely reported in the literature. The evolution from immobilization to implementation of early motion programs has become accepted practice in the orthopedic community. The proper use of specific exercises can accelerate the healing process, whereas the lack of exercise during the early stages of rehabilitation can result in long-term functional impairment. Caution must be observed, however, because exercise that is too vigorous can also result in undesired effects of healing tissues. Immobilization initially results in loss of tissue substrate, with a subsequent loss of basic tissue components. The reversibility of these changes appears to depend on the length of immobilization.

To understand the body's response to immobilization and remobilization, its normal reaction to injury must be addressed. The sequence of events that transpire after trauma occurs to a joint can cause cartilage degradation, chronic joint synovitis, and stretching of the joint capsule as a result of increased effusion.

REACTION TO INJURY

Inflammation is the body's response to injury, and, optimally, it results in healing of tissues by replacement of damaged and destroyed tissue, with an associated restoration of function.[52] Repeated injury or microtrauma to a specific region can cause a cumulative effect, resulting in adverse effects to the joint and its surrounding structures. The inflammatory response is the same, regardless of the location and nature of the injurious agent, and consists of chemical, metabolic, permeability, and vascular changes, followed by some form of repair.[85]

Figure 2-1 illustrates the primary and secondary injuries affiliated with trauma and the associated inflammation and repair processes. Primary injury is the result of trauma that directly injures the cells themselves. Secondary injury (sometimes referred to as secondary hypoxia) is precipitated by the body's response to trauma. This response includes decreased blood flow to the traumatized region as a result of vasoconstriction, which decreases the amount of oxygen to the injured area. Thus, additional cells die because of secondary hypoxia; these dead cells organize and ultimately form a hematoma.

Cell degeneration or cell death perpetuates the release of potent substances that can induce vascular changes. The most common of these substances is histamine, which increases capillary permeability and allows the escape of fluid and blood cells into the interstitial spaces. In the

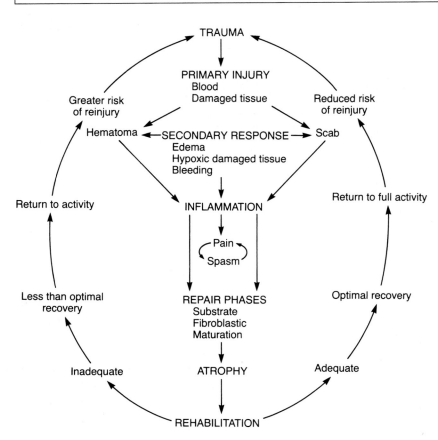

Figure 2-1. Cycle of athletic injury. (From Booher, J.M., and Thibodeau, G.A. [1989]) Athletic Injury Assessment. St. Louis, Times Mirror/Mosby College Publishing.)

noninjured state, plasma and blood proteins escape from capillaries by osmosis and diffusion into the interstitial spaces but are reabsorbed. This homeostasis is maintained by colloids present within the blood system. However, trauma leads to increased capillary permeability as a result of the release of cell enzymes, allowing blood plasma and proteins to escape into surrounding tissues. Concurrently, the concentration of colloids greatly increases in the surrounding tissues, thus reversing the colloidal effect. Rather than the colloids' pulling fluid back into the capillaries, the presence of the colloids outside the vessels causes additional fluid to be pulled into the interstitial tissues, resulting in swelling and edema.

The body's reaction after injury is to mobilize and transport the defense components of the blood to the injured area. Initially, blood flow is reduced, allowing white blood cells to migrate to the margins of the blood vessels. These cells adhere to the vessel walls and eventually travel into the interstitial tissues. Once in the surrounding tissues, the white cells remove irritating material by the process of phagocytosis. Neutrophils are the first white blood cells to arrive, and they normally destroy bacteria. However, because bacteria are not usually associated with athletic injuries, these neutrophils die.[85] Then, macrophages appear and phagocytize the dead neutrophils, cellular debris, fibrin, red cells, and other debris that may impede the repair process.[85] Unfortunately, the destruction of the neutrophils results in the release of

active proteolytic enzymes (i.e., enzymes that hasten the hydrolysis of proteins into simpler substances), which can attack joint tissues, into the surrounding inflammatory fluid.[61] Although this is the natural response of ridding the body of toxic or foreign materials, prolongation of this process can damage surrounding joint structures.

After the inflammatory debris has been removed, repair can begin. Cleanup by the macrophages and repair often occur simultaneously. However, for repair to occur, enough of the hematoma must be removed to permit ingrowth of new tissue. Thus, the size of the hematoma or the amount of the exudate is directly related to the total healing time. If the size of the hematoma can be minimized, healing can begin earlier and total healing time is reduced.[85]

CLINICAL PEARL #1

The primary role of the rehabilitation specialist during the acute phase of injury is to decrease inflammation and prevent damaging secondary effects such as decreased range of motion, decreased muscle strength, and prolonged edema. The presence of inflammation must be regarded with caution, because too much activity can prolong the inflammation and increase pain. Inflammation is controlled with ice, rest, and electrical stimulation such as electrical galvanic stimulation or transcutaneous electrical stimulation. Secondary effects are prevented with gentle range-of-motion exercises, isometrics, and prevention of maladaptive postures or gait patterns.

Response of Joint Structures to Injury

As a result of the inflammatory process, each joint structure responds differently to injury (Fig. 2-2). The reaction of the synovial membrane to injury involves the proliferation of surface cells, an increase in vascularity, and a gradual fibrosis of the subsynovial tissue. Post-traumatic synovitis is not uncommon after most injuries. Continued mechanical irritation can produce chronic synovitis, which results in the reversal of normal synovial cell ratios.[61,129] Changes in synovial fluid occur as a result of alterations in the synovial membrane. Cells are destroyed as a consequence of the synovitis; the white blood cells ingest lysosomes and proteolytic enzymes. This ingestion and the subsequent death of white blood cells in the transudate result in the further release of proteolytic enzymes. The overall consequence is the spawning of a vicious inflammatory cycle, which can keep reactive synovitis active for some time, even without further trauma (Fig. 2-3).[18] As chronic posttraumatic effusions occur, changes of the synovial membrane can continue, with progressing sclerotic alterations as a sequel.[143] If conservative treatment consisting of anti-inflammatory medications, rest, aspiration, and cold applications does not relieve the symptoms, a synovectomy may be necessary.

Articular cartilage lesions within a synovial joint or meniscus lesions within the knee, whether acute or chronic, are invariably accompanied by increased synovial effusion. Surgical correction is often required to prevent secondary damage to other joint structures from prolonged inflammation. After the problem has been corrected, the synovial irritation usually subsides. If, however, the problem is left uncorrected, tissues not injured by the original trauma can be damaged from the prolonged inflammation, resulting in progressive degradation of the synovial membrane.

Fortunately, once the inflammation begins to abate, synovial tissue can regenerate remarkably well, an ability that possibly stems from its excellent blood supply and origin. Synovium regenerates completely within several months into tissue that is indistinguishable from the normal tissue.[61] Acute and chronic synovitis directly affects the amount and content of synovial fluid produced. Synovitis can result in an increased protein level within the synovial fluid. In addition, chronic synovitis can cause a decrease in synovial fluid viscosity and a decrease in the concentration of hyaluronic acid.[25] The concentration of hyaluronic acid is directly related to synovial fluid viscosity. Minor joint trauma results in no change in either the concentration or the molecular weight of the hyaluronic acid.[25] As trauma severity increases, however, the hyaluronic acid concentration decreases to levels below normal, and when the inflammatory process becomes sufficiently disruptive, joint-lining cells fail not only to

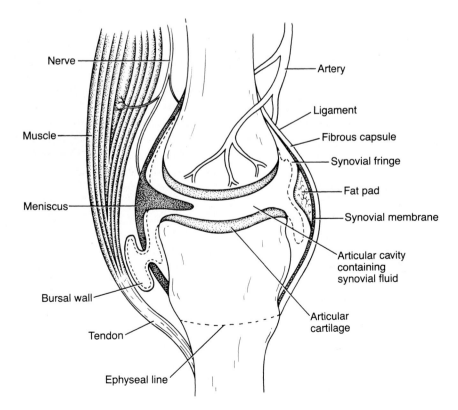

Figure 2-2. Synovial joint structures. (From Wright, V., Dowson, D., and Kerry, J. [1973]: The structure of joints. Int. Rev. Connect. Tissue Res., 6:105-125.)

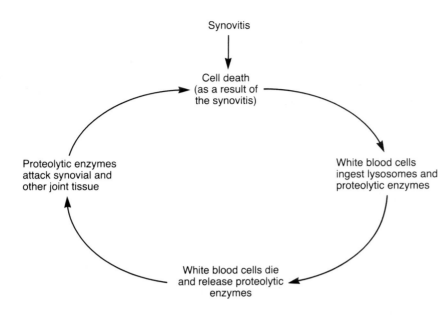

Figure 2-3. Continued mechanical irritation of a joint can result in chronic synovitis that is perpetuated by a vicious inflammatory cycle. This keeps the reactive synovitis alive even without further trauma.

maintain hyaluronic acid concentration but also to maintain normal polymer weight.[25]

A hemarthrosis, or bleeding into a joint, can have an effect on the joint structures. When a vascular joint structure is damaged, the synovial fluid has a lower sugar concentration, blood clots can be detected in the synovial fluid, and fibrinogen, can be detected as a result of bleeding into the joint. Although the average time for natural evacuation of a hemarthrosis is about 4 days,[124] it depends on individual factors such as the magnitude of injury, the nature of the structures injured, and the individual's activity level after injury. The presence of blood in a joint has a damaging effect on articular cartilage, with a potentially irreversible decrease in proteoglycan synthesis.[125] In addition, younger individuals with a hemarthrosis have been shown to have a greater decrease in proteoglycan synthesis and a slower return to normal rates of synthesis.[123]

The absorption rate of solutions from the joint space is inversely proportional to the size of the solutes; the larger the molecules, the slower the clearance. Clinically, absorption from a joint is increased by active or passive range of motion, massage, intra-articular hydrocortisone, or acute inflammation, whereas the effect of external compression is variable.[150]

The reaction of the joint capsule to injury is similar to that of the synovial membrane. If the inflammatory process continues, the joint capsule eventually becomes a more fibrous tissue, and effusion into the joint cavity can lead to stretching of the capsule and its associated ligaments. The higher the hydrostatic pressure and volume of effusion, the faster the fluid reaccumulates after aspiration.[61,62] Conversely, a significant rise in intra-articular hydrostatic pressure contributes to joint damage by stretching the capsule and associated ligaments.

The load-carrying surfaces of the synovial joint are covered with a thin layer of specialized connective tissue,

referred to as articular cartilage. The response of the articular cartilage to trauma is not unlike that of the other structures within the joint. The mechanical properties of articular cartilage are readily affected by enzymatic degradation of cartilage components. This can occur after acute inflammation, synovectomy, immobilization, or other seemingly minor insults.[140] When articular cartilage loses its content of proteoglycan (a protein aggregate that helps establish the resiliency and resistance to deformation of articular cartilage), the physical properties of the cartilage are changed; this renders the collagen fibers susceptible to mechanical damage.[140] The opposite is also true: if a joint loses the collagen of the outer layer of articular surface, the proteoglycans beneath are subject to damage. As a result of either of these two types of degradation, articular cartilage can erode and leave denuded bone, resulting in early, irreversible osteoarthritis or degenerative joint disease (Fig. 2-4).

The reduction of post-traumatic joint effusion is paramount in the early rehabilitation process and is important in the restoration of joint kinematics. Prolonged effusion, if left unchecked, can result in reactive synovitis, damage of the joint capsule, and degradation of articular cartilage. The early use of mobilization techniques such as continuous passive motion and modalities such as cryotherapy and vasopneumatic compression can aid in reducing joint effusion.

EFFECTS OF IMMOBILIZATION
Muscle

One of the first and most obvious changes that occur as a result of immobilization is loss of muscle strength. This correlates with a reduction in muscle size and a decrease in tension per unit of muscle cross-sectional area.[15,98,99] MacDougall and colleagues[99] reported that 6 weeks of elbow cast immobilization results in a greater than 40%

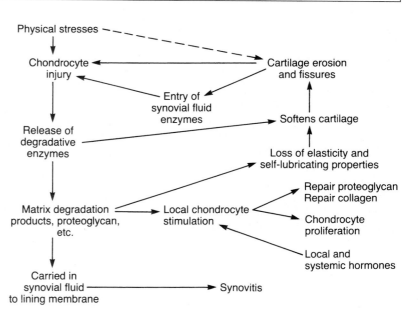

Figure 2-4. Postulated final pathway of cartilage degeneration. (From Howell, D.S. [1976]: Osteoarthritis—Etiology and pathogenesis. *In:* American Academy of Orthopaedic Surgeons: Symposium on Osteoarthritis [1976]. St. Louis, C.V. Mosby.)

decrease in muscle strength. This strength deficit is correlated with a loss of fiber cross-sectional area and with an associated decrease in muscle mass. The quadriceps muscle cross-sectional area may decrease from 21% to 26% with 4 to 6 weeks of immobilization in an individual without a pathologic condition.[160] It is important to note that immobilization atrophy is due to a loss of fiber cross-sectional area not to a loss of fibers, as is seen in elderly persons.[148]

The rate of loss appears to be most rapid during the initial days of immobilization. Structural and metabolic changes in muscle cells have been documented with as little as 2 hours of immobilization.[91,95] Lindboe and Platou[95] reported that in humans, muscle fiber size is reduced by 14% to 17% after 72 hours of immobilization. After 5 to 7 days of immobilization, the absolute loss in muscle mass appears to slow considerably.[7,12] The amount of training before immobilization may dramatically decrease the amount of atrophy during immobilization.[7]

Both slow-twitch (type I) and fast-twitch (type II) muscle fibers atrophy. It is generally accepted that there is a selective decrease in type I (slow-twitch) fibers.[54,55] However, conflicting evidence is found in the literature.[87] After immobilization, the contractile ability of type I fibers is more adversely affected than that of type II fibers.[55,59,170,180] The decreased contractile ability of type I fibers, rather than decreased fiber proportion, may be more clinically relevant. This implies that exercises with decreased intensity and increased frequency should be used after immobilization. This is particularly relevant in an athlete who is specifically conditioned to aerobic activity, because there is a more dramatic decrease in the percent area of type I fibers. These studies only evaluated the effect of immobilization of muscle fiber composition; not the combined effect of injury and immobilization. Muscle fiber atrophy after injury or surgery may be different from that which occurs when a healthy muscle is immobilized.

There are changes in the mechanical properties of the myotendinous junction as a result of immobilization. The contact area between the muscle cells and the collagen fibers of the tendon is decreased by 50%.[77] There is also a decrease in the glycosaminoglycan content of the myotendinous junction.[77] These changes can predispose the myotendinous junction to injury after immobilization. A dramatic increase in activity after immobilization may lead to a secondary tendinopathy.

In addition to causing changes in muscle size and volume, immobilization also results in histochemical changes. These include a reduction in the levels of adenosine triphosphate (ATP), adenosine diphosphate, creatine, creatine phosphate, and glycogen and a greater increase in lactate concentration with work. Furthermore, the rate of protein synthesis decreases within 6 hours of immobilization.[14,16,99,100,157]

Immobilization also causes an increase in muscle fatigability as a result of decreased oxidative capacity. Reductions occur in maximum oxygen consumption, glycogen levels, and high-energy phosphate levels.[14,15,26,99,103] Rifenberick and Max[121] reported fewer mitochondria in atrophic muscle and a significant decrease in mitochondrial activity by day 7 postimmobilization, causing a reduction in cell respiration and contributing to decreased muscle endurance (Box 2-1).

It appears that there is selective muscle atrophy with immobilization. For example, immobilization of the thigh is often associated with selective atrophy of the quadriceps femoris muscle.[66] Although the knee is the area traditionally noted for selective atrophy, this phenomenon can also be observed in the triceps brachii of an immobilized elbow. Clinically, one can observe that quadriceps atrophy is

Box 2-1

Summary of the Effects of Immobilization on Muscle

- Decrease in muscle fiber size
- Change in muscle resting length
- Decrease in size and number of mitochondria
- Decrease in total muscle weight
- Increase in muscle contraction time
- Decrease in muscle tension produced
- Decrease in resting levels of glycogen and adenosine triphosphate (ATP)
- More rapid decrease in ATP level with exercise
- Increase in lactate concentration with exercise
- Decrease in protein synthesis

greater than that of the hamstrings. This is supported by evidence on computed tomographic scanning that despite a significant loss of quadriceps cross-sectional area, there is no significant difference in hamstring or adductor muscle cross-sectional area after 5 weeks of immobilization.[66]

The selective atrophy seen in the quadriceps femoris and the triceps brachii with immobilization of the knee and elbow, respectively, may be due to their roles as primarily one-joint muscles. Three of the four heads of the quadriceps only cross the knee joint, and two of the three triceps heads only cross the elbow joint. In contrast, all heads of the biceps and the hamstrings cross two joints. The biceps and hamstrings are therefore "less" immobilized by having all portions contract across one of the two joints they cross (the hip or the shoulder), which may be the reason muscle cross-sectional area is preserved in these muscles.[180]

CLINICAL PEARL #2

The muscle volume of the thigh decreases after immobilization, but the subcutaneous adipose tissue volume does not change. This can mask the amount of quadriceps atrophy and invalidates girth measures as a tool for measuring atrophy.[65] Girth measurements also do not distinguish between muscle groups and therefore can underestimate the amount of quadriceps atrophy. Girth measurements do not correlate with strength deficits.

Reflexive inhibition, or arthrogenous muscle wasting, can contribute to selective muscle atrophy, particularly of the quadriceps, after trauma or surgery to a joint. Pain has traditionally been regarded as the general cause of reflex inhibition. The perception and fear of pain can greatly affect muscular strength. Athletes who fear that muscle contraction will result in pain may be very apprehensive about contracting those particular muscles, but severe inhibition of muscle strength is seen even after pain subsides.[136] At 1 to 2 hours after arthrotomy and meniscectomy, there is a 62% decrease in quadriceps electromyographic (EMG) activity.[137] This is due to reflexive inhibition. A significant amount of anesthetic injected into the knee may decrease (but not eliminate) inhibition temporarily, but the effects are lost after 4 to 5 hours.[137] Ten to 15 days after surgery, there is a decrease in quadriceps EMG action of 35%.[137] Whether this is due to reflexive inhibition or disuse atrophy is unclear. Pain has been shown to inhibit strength in patients with preoperative shoulder pathologic changes, but postoperative reflex inhibition has not been investigated.[11,67,81]

In studies investigating arthrogenous muscle wasting, the level of quadriceps activation is typically determined through EMG testing. The degree of unilateral quadriceps inhibition is then judged by the difference in maximum voluntary activation between the two limbs. There is no method to directly measure inhibition, so it is therefore indirectly quantified by EMG testing. This may not be a valid measure of true reflex inhibition during the first few hours after injury or surgery. After injury, reflex inhibition leads to muscle atrophy. Once the inhibition had left, muscle weakness due to disuse or immobilization atrophy will continue. Caution must be used when one generalizes the findings of studies pertaining to arthrogenous muscle weakness.

The nature of the surgical procedure performed may have an effect on the amount of arthrogenous muscle wasting after surgery. Advances in technology have led to the use of a less invasive arthroscope for many procedures that previously required an arthrotomy. A significant decrease in quadriceps muscle electromyographic action is seen after an arthrotomy of the knee. Although this decrease in EMG action is still present after arthroscopy of the knee, the magnitude of the change is much decreased.[60] A two-portal arthroscopy, rather than a three-portal arthroscopy, produces a lesser decrease in quadriceps strength after surgery.[147] Clinically, patients undergoing an arthroscopic procedure would be expected to recover at a more rapid rate, but consideration must be given to the specific surgical procedure. In general, patients who have undergone less invasive procedures (arthroscopy) will initially recover faster than those who have had more invasive procedures (arthrotomy), but the long-term outcome is usually the same. This has been demonstrated at the knee[118] and shoulder.[156]

Tourniquet ischemia has also been thought to contribute to quadriceps shutdown. When a tourniquet is used to provide a relatively bloodless field during surgery, the pressure required to staunch blood flow is also enough to damage the tissues being compressing. The use of a tourniquet, although necessary, leads to postoperative EMG changes[8,134] and increased quadriceps atrophy.[8] Nonroutine complications from tourniquet use include compression neuropraxia, wound hematoma, tissue necrosis, vascular injury, and compartment syndrome.[165]

Research has shown that distension of a knee with plasma can lead to quadriceps shutdown and subsequent quadriceps weakening in normal individuals, even in the absence of pain.[27,70,80,144,181] Young and associates[180] and others[80] have reported that injection of small volumes of fluid (20 to 30 ml) into normal knees results in 60% quadriceps inhibition, with the inhibition increasing as infusion increases. Spencer and associates[144] found the threshold amount of effusion for reflexive shutdown to be between 20 and 30 ml for the vastus medialis and between 50 and 60 ml for the vastus lateralis and rectus femoris. The decreased threshold for the vastus medialis can contribute to patellar tracking problems when the knee is even slightly effused. Inhibition is directly related to the degree of effusion and increases as the amount of effusion increases.[49] With a chronically effused joint, aspiration of the effusion does not demonstrate any difference in quadriceps inhibition.[72] This may be attributed to concomitant disuse atrophy.

Joint angle has also been shown to have an effect on quadriceps inhibition. In normal knees, the highest quadriceps EMG action is obtained with the knee in the shortened position, or full extension.[86] Stratford[149] reported that effusion inhibits quadriceps contraction less when the knee is in 30's of flexion than when it is fully extended. Similar results have been found even after arthrotomy with meniscectomy, in that isometric quadriceps contraction is inhibited less in flexion than in extension.[86,136,148] This has been postulated to occur because intra-articular pressure is less when the knee is in 30's of flexion versus full extension.[42,70,92,93,136] Despite higher EMG action being obtained with the knee in flexion, it is not desirable to perform all exercises in the clinic in a flexed knee position. On the contrary, this information emphasizes to the clinician the importance of training the quadriceps in a fully extended position to overcome the biomechanical disadvantage.

The length at which the muscle is immobilized also affects selective atrophy. Tardieu and colleagues[153] suggested that muscle fibers under stretch lengthen by adding sarcomeres in series, whereas those immobilized in a shortened position lose sarcomeres. Thus, when a muscle is immobilized in a lengthened position, the length of the muscle fibers increases to accommodate the muscle's new length, along with other connective tissue changes. A similar adjustment in sarcomere number occurs with muscle that is immobilized in a shortened position; the length of the fibers decreases, and the number of sarcomeres is reduced to achieve the physiologic change.[169] Immobilization of a muscle in a shortened position leads to increased connective tissue and reduced muscle extensibility.[153] Muscle immobilization in a lengthened position maintains muscle weight and fiber cross-sectional area better than does immobilization in a shortened position.[69,71] This theoretically explains selective atrophy of the quadriceps when the knee is immobilized in full extension. Because the knee is usually immobilized in an extended or slightly flexed position, the hamstrings are placed in a lengthened position and the quadriceps are in a shortened position. These positions help to preserve muscle cross-sectional area and strength, but the sarcomeres will no longer be able to shorten enough to achieve maximal extension. Clinically, the position of the joint cannot be the only factor that influences muscle atrophy; for example, in the shoulder that is immobilized in internal rotation, the external rotators (the rotator cuff muscles) still demonstrate marked atrophy.

CLINICAL PEARL #3

One of the factors that may also influence reflex inhibition is the muscle spindle. When a muscle is immobilized in a shortened or lengthened position, the spindle will assume a new resting length.[33] The muscle in the shortened position will then have a greater resistance to stretch, and the muscle immobilized in the lengthened position will have a decreased contractile ability. This is especially true at the shoulder, which is typically immobilized in internal rotation, and at the elbow, which is typically immobilized in flexion. The shortened position facilitates the shortened muscles (elbow flexors and shoulder internal rotators) and may account for the decreased strength in the shoulder external rotators and elbow extensors. Treatment for these joints should include facilitatory techniques for the lengthened muscles and inhibitory techniques for the shortened muscles. The shortened muscles should be stretched often but gently, because quick or aggressive stretching can cause a facilitatory response. Isometric contractions can also preserve the tension in the muscle spindle while allowing healing of damaged tissues.

Despite the fact that the knee is typically immobilized in extension, patients tend to hold the knee in a slightly flexed position, either sitting with the hips flexed or supine with the pelvis posteriorly tilted, which shortens the hamstrings. Hamstring stretches to increase the resting length of the spindle are an important part of a knee rehabilitation program after immobilization. Increasing the length of the hamstrings will decrease the amount of resistance the quadriceps must contract against to achieve full knee extension. Stretching of the posterior capsule may also be required if the knee is held in a flexed position.

CLINICAL PEARL #4

Despite the increased preservation of quadriceps muscle cross-sectional area and increased EMG action in flexion, this is not the preferential position for immobilization of the knee after injury or surgery. If the knee is immobilized in flexion, full passive extension must be maintained by passively extending the knee to 0°s several times per day (barring medical or surgical precautions.) This ensures that the quadriceps will maintain proper length to allow shortening of the muscle to full knee extension.

Active quadriceps exercises should be done in full extension for several reasons. Full active knee extension is needed for a proper gait pattern during initial contact (heel strike). A quadriceps contraction in full extension allows maximal superior glide of the patella in the trochlear groove, preventing patella infera. If a patient does not have full active extension, he or she must be taught to self-superiorly glide the patella to preserve length of the patellar tendon. If a patient does not have full passive knee extension after immobilization, a motion complication program should be initiated.

Periarticular Connective Tissue

Periarticular connective tissue consists of ligaments, tendons, synovial membrane, fascia, and joint capsule. As a result of immobilization, injury, or surgery, biochemical and histologic changes occur in periarticular tissue around synovial joints, which may result in arthrofibrosis. Arthrofibrosis has been referred to as ankylosis, joint stiffness, or joint contracture.[63] It is a term that describes the excessive formation of scar tissue around a joint after a surgical procedure or traumatic injury.[116,145] The characteristic feature is the formation of scar tissue within the joint capsule, the synovium, or the intra-articular spaces.[68]

The two main components of fibrous connective tissue are the cells and an extracellular matrix. The matrix consists primarily of collagen and elastin fibers and a nonfibrous ground substance. Fibrocytes, located between the collagen fibers in fibrous connective tissue, are the main collagen-producing cells. As collagen fibers mature, intra- and intermolecular bonds or cross-links are formed, and these increase in number, thereby providing tensile strength to the fibers.[45] On the basis of the arrangement of its collagen fibers, connective tissue is commonly classified into two types: irregular and regular.[57] The irregular type of connective tissue is characterized by fibers running in different directions in the same plane.[31] This arrangement is of functional value for capsules, aponeuroses, and sheaths, which are physiologically stressed in many directions.[31,57] Conversely, in regularly arranged tissues, collagen fibers run more or less in the same plane and in the same linear direction.[31] This arrangement affords great tensile strength to ligaments and tendons, which physiologically receive primarily unidirectional stress.[31]

The extracellular matrix is often referred to as ground substance and is composed of glycosaminoglycans (GAGs) and water. To understand the changes that occur with immobilization it is important to be familiar with GAGs and their effect on connective tissue extensibility. Four major GAGs are found in connective tissue: hyaluronic acid, chondroitin-4-sulfate, chondroitin-6-sulfate, and dermatan sulfate. Generally, GAGs are bound to a protein and are collectively referred to as proteoglycans. In connective tissue, proteoglycans combine with water to form a proteoglycan aggregate.[22]

Water constitutes 60% to 70% of the total connective tissue content. GAGs have enormous water-binding capacity and are responsible for this large water content. Together, GAGs and water form a semifluid viscous gel in which collagen and fibrocytes are embedded. Hyaluronic acid with water is thought to serve as a lubricant between the collagen fibers.[3,57,151] This lubricant maintains a distance between the fibers, thereby permitting free gliding of the fibers past each other and perhaps preventing excessive cross-linking. Such free gliding is essential for normal connective tissue mobility.[3]

The sliding of collagen fibers across each other, the collagen weave pattern, and the cross-links all can be illustrated by the Chinese finger-trap analogy.[31] When tension is applied to the Chinese finger trap, the trap lengthens to a certain point, as the straw-weave patterns of the trap move across one another (Fig. 2-5). If tension continues to increase when the end point of the trap is reached, the straw fibers will begin to fail. This illustration is not unlike how body connective tissue functions.

Arthrofibrosis is induced primarily by immobilization after trauma to the joint, which results in a significant reduction in GAG content with subsequent water loss, contributing to abnormal cross-link formation and joint restriction. In addition, within the joint space and recesses, there is excessive connective tissue deposition in the form of fatty fibers, which later mature to form scar tissue that adheres to intra-articular surfaces and restricts motion further.[31]

The most significant reduction of GAG content occurs within the matrix. Akeson and associates[1-3,5] reported a 40% decrease in hyaluronic acid and 30% decreases in chondroitin-4-sulfate and chondroitin-6-sulfate; collagen mass decreases by about 10%, and collagen turnover increases, with accelerated degradation and synthesis (Box 2-2).

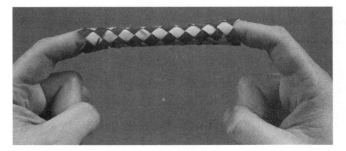

Figure 2-5. Chinese finger trap. The trap can be used to illustrate the sliding of collagen fibers over each other in normal connective tissue.

Box 2-2

Summary of the Effects of Immobilization on Connective Tissue

- Reduction in water and GAG content, which decreases the extracellular matrix
- Reduction in extracellular matrix, which is associated with a decrease in lubrication between fiber cross-links
- Reduction in collagen mass
- Increase in rate of collagen turnover, degradation, and synthesis
- Increase in abnormal collagen fiber cross-links

The pathophysiology of arthrofibrosis appears to be the reduction in the semifluid gel as a result of loss of GAG and water, causing a decrease in the critical fiber distance between collagen fibers.[31] Friction is created between fibers, thus reducing collagen extensibility. It has recently been suggested that arthrofibrosis may be a result of an increase in the expression of collagen IV, which forms a fibrous network between collagen I and III fibrils. Collagen IV forms irregular cross-links between the collagen fibrils, which decreases the ability of the fibrils to slide (Fig. 2-6).[182] Recent evidence suggests that arthrofibrosis may be a result of an autoimmune reaction.[17]

Currently, arthrofibrosis most commonly affects the knee joint, particularly as a complication after anterior cruciate ligament (ACL) reconstructive surgery, in which

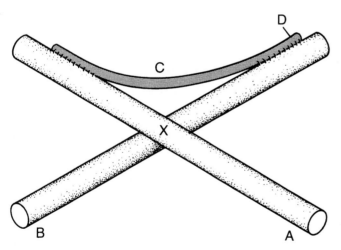

Figure 2-6. Idealized model of the interaction of collagen cross-links at the molecular level. A and B, pre-existing fibers; C, newly synthesized fibril; D, cross-links created as the fibril becomes incorporated into the fiber; X, point at which adjacent fibers are normally freely movable past each other. (From Akeson, W.H., Armiel, D., and Woo, S. [1980]: Immobility effects of synovial joints: The pathomechanics of joint contracture. Biorheology, 17:95, with permission from Elsevier Science Ltd, The Boulevard, Langford Lane, Kidlington 0X5 1GB, UK.)

the operative knee develops a thicker joint capsule and a secondary flexion contracture. Arthrofibrosis of the knee joint is characterized by a lack of flexion as well as extension (the most commonly involved motion is extension). Prolonged joint immobilization is the most recognized risk factor for the development of arthrofibrosis. Microscopic examination of a knee with arthrofibrosis shows a proliferation of fibroblasts and an associated accumulation of extracellular matrix. The principal component of the matrix is type I collagen that is specifically found as an unorganized network of fibers.[4] Although these findings are well recognized, the etiology underlying the formation of the exuberant scar tissue is less clear.

With a lack of experimental studies and suitable animal models, the pathophysiology of arthrofibrosis remains poorly understood. However, several theories have been proposed to explain and prevent this condition. Several authors[64,138] have recommended delaying reconstructive surgery on acutely injured ACLs until the knee joint recovers from the initial trauma. It is theorized that the synovitis that occurs after the initial injury, which is then compounded with the synovitis after surgical reconstruction, may predispose the joint to arthrofibrosis. The authors suggest that surgery be delayed until the hemarthrosis and synovitis have decreased, range of motion is restored, and the patient has active control of the quadriceps. ACL reconstruction is not an emergency surgical procedure, and better outcomes are seen with preoperative rehabilitation to decrease the initial response to injury.

Fibrosis results from increased numbers of collagen-synthesizing cells (from proliferation and from recruitment), increased synthesis by existing cells, or deficient collagen degradation with continued collagen synthesis.[164] Injury-induced inflammation precedes the repair process, therefore, precise regulation and control of the inflammatory response will have a direct impact on the timing and amount of fibrosis during healing. Recently, it has been suggested that an immune response is the cause of the capsulitis that leads to excessive connective tissue proliferation.[26] This supports the theory that the excessive intra-articular deposition of connective tissue is a result of consecutive inflammatory phases after trauma to the joint. This has clinical implications; if the rehabilitation is overly aggressive, it can cause increased inflammation and potentially worsen this process. Long-duration, low-load techniques should be used to increase range of motion and decrease the potential for an inflammatory response.[101] The location of the fibrous lesions has a relationship with the amount of motion loss in terms of knee flexion. Fibrous connective tissue bands in the suprapatellar pouch is the primary area for limitation of flexion.[101] Flexion can also be limited by a patella infera or by a shortening of the patellar tendon. This can be prevented by superior mobilization of the patella on a daily basis.[152] Extension of the knee is limited by a shortening of the posterior capsule.

It has been shown that arthrofibrotic tissue matures over time, and maturation is complete by about 6 months after onset. However, although the tissue matures over time, a progressive loss of range of motion has not been seen.[101] Attempts to lengthen the tissues will be less successful as time passes due to the maturation and decreased remodeling capability of the tissues.[9] Efforts to treat arthrofibrosis conservatively are likely to fail after 6 months have passed.[101] Figure 2-7 illustrates the sequelae leading to arthrofibrosis or return to activities.

CLINICAL PEARL #5

Early recognition of arthrofibrosis is important, and its prevention is paramount. Arthrofibrosis has been associated with Dupuytren's disease and diabetes. Patients with these conditions, as well as patients who appear to have an excess amount of fibrous tissue at other joints, should be viewed as having a risk for developing arthrofibrosis. It is a useful clinical test to examine the joint play at another synovial joint, such as a metacarpophalangeal joint, to determine whether the patient is systemically hyper- or hypomobile. Clinically, hypermobile individuals rarely develop arthrofibrosis.

Joint motion is essential in the prevention of contractures and the formation of adhesions within joints. Physical forces and motion modulate the synthesis of proteoglycans and collagen in normal joints. Stress and motion also influence the deposition of newly synthesized collagen fibers, allowing proper orientation of collagen to resist tensile stress. Motion appears to inhibit periarticular tissue contractures by the following mechanisms[174]:

1. Stimulating proteoglycan synthesis, thereby lubricating and maintaining a critical distance between existing fibers
2. Ordering (rather than randomizing) the disposition of new collagen fibers to resist tensile stress
3. Preventing formation of anomalous cross-links in the matrix by preventing a stationary fiber-fiber attitude at intercept points

The matrix changes associated with immobilization (noted above) are relatively uniform in ligaments, capsules, tendons, and fasciae. These changes involve extracellular water loss and GAG depletion, along with collagen cross-link changes.

Articular Cartilage

Articular cartilage is a thin covering on the ends of bones that creates the moving surfaces of synovial joints.[168] It varies from 1 to 7 mm in thickness, with the cartilage covering larger, weight-bearing joints (e.g., hip and knee joints) being thicker than that covering smaller, non–weight-bearing joints.[168,175] Articular cartilage consists of fibers, ground substance, and cells. The fibers are composed primarily of type II collagen and make up 57% to 75% of the dry weight of the cartilage.[161] Collagen provides the tensile strength of articular cartilage and aids the gliding of opposing articular surfaces. The ground substance is similar to that of periarticular tissue and consists of water (70% to 80%) and proteoglycans (15% to 30%).[35,61,167] Proteoglycans have a unique bond with water and allow articular cartilage to resist and distribute compressive forces. The quantity of proteoglycans in articular cartilage depends on joint

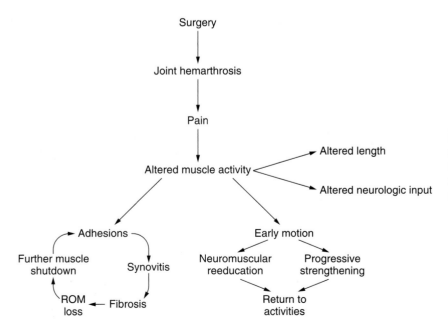

Figure 2-7. Arthrofibrotic loop. A key to avoiding arthrofibrosis is early motions and muscle "turn-on" through neuromuscular reeducation and progressive muscle strengthening. ROM = range of motion.

location, with weight-bearing joints having a higher proteo-glycan content than non–weight-bearing joints.[158] Both collagen and proteoglycans are produced by chondrocytes, the cells that are in articular cartilage.

As a result of immobilization, articular cartilage undergoes structural, biochemical, and physiologic changes at the cellular and ultrastructural levels.[168] Consistently reported changes include the following: fibrillation, fraying, cyst formation, varying degrees of chondrocyte degeneration, atrophy in weight-bearing areas, sclerosis, and cartilage resorption. There are also decreases in the proteoglycan GAG content, which decreases the ability of cartilage to resist compressive forces. These changes are generally permanent, but the length of immobilization is important in determining whether the articular changes are irreversible.

Articular cartilage is avascular, and its nutritional requirements are met through diffusion and osmosis. Diffusion occurs through a hydraulic pressure gradient. This pressure is increased by weight bearing or joint movement. Low hydraulic pressure has no effect, whereas constant pressure interferes with nutrition.[168] High intermittent pressure loading does not contribute much to the diffusion rate. Joint motion, however, increases the diffusion rate to three to four times the static level.[102] This implies that in the absence of weight bearing, motion must be present to preserve articular cartilage integrity. The opposite (weight bearing without range of motion) is not desirable, however, compressive forces on only the weight-bearing aspects of the immobilized joint can cause severe articular damage.[73]

The effects of immobilization depend on the position in which the joint is immobilized. A flexed knee position produces greater chondrocyte necrosis and degeneration of the articular cartilage than an extended position.[59] This result may be due to the increased compression and intra-articular pressure in the fully flexed position. The position of immobilization is not as critical in the upper extremities, because they contain primarily non–weight-bearing joints.

The effects of immobilization on articular cartilage can be separated into contact and noncontact effects. In contact areas, the seriousness of the changes depends mainly on the degree of compression. In noncontact areas, it depends on the ingrowth of connective tissue on the articular surface.[75] Constant compression of articular cartilage decreases the synovial fluid diffusion rate and leads to pressure necrosis and chondrocyte death.[119,162] Whether the lesions are reversible depends directly on the duration of continuous compression.[131] Also, loss of contact between opposed articular surfaces in weight-bearing and non–weight-bearing joints appears to lead to degenerative changes, suggesting a functional relationship between joint motion and normal articular cartilage surface contact[56,162] (Box 2-3).

Intermittent joint loading appears to have a critical role in maintaining healthy articular cartilage. The formation

---

Box 2-3

Summary of the Effects of Immobilization on Articular Cartilage

- Decrease in chondrocyte size
- Decrease in capability of chondrocytes to synthesize proteoglycan
- Softening of articular cartilage
- Decrease in articular cartilage thickness
- Adherence of fibrofatty connective tissue to cartilage surfaces
- Pressure necrosis at points of cartilage-cartilage contact

---

and circulation of synovial and interstitial fluids are stimulated with intermittent joint loading and retarded in its absence. Because synovial fluid is important in cartilage nourishment and lubrication, intermittent pressure can facilitate chondrocyte nourishment and is important for cell function.[20,34,37] Conversely, joint immobilization in which the joint is constantly loaded or unloaded can compromise the metabolic exchange necessary for proper structure and function, eventually leading to cartilage degradation and eburnation.[40,89,139,157] Immobilization of knees in extension leads to irreversible and progressive osteoarthritis. The compression between articular surfaces increases in the immobilized knee and, after 4 weeks of immobilization, reaches a level that is three times greater than the initial level.[162]

CLINICAL PEARL #6

Roth and associates[127] found that prolonged knee immobilization after an ACL reconstruction leads to significant patellofemoral chondromalacia and that immediate mobilization prevented patellofemoral degeneration. It may be assumed that immobilization after other forms of surgery leads to articular changes as well. Although it is important to begin motion and gentle strengthening exercises after surgery, it is important that the clinician remember that there is the potential for the articular surfaces to be compromised. Moderate activity after immobilization has been shown to stimulate articular surface regeneration, but strenuous activity can reduce the proteoglycan content of articular cartilage.[82] Do not "over-rehabilitate" the articular surfaces with too much activity too soon.

Ligaments

Ligaments undergo the same changes in structure as do other elements in periarticular tissue. However, because of the function of ligaments and because of the bone-ligament interface, additional factors must be considered to understand the response of ligaments to immobilization.

Like bone, a ligament appears to remodel in response to the mechanical demands placed on it. Stress results in a stiffer, stronger ligament, whereas inactivity yields a weaker, more compliant structure.[24] These changes in properties appear to be caused more by an alteration in the mechanical properties of ligaments[6] and by subperiosteal resorption at the bone-ligament junction than by actual ligament atrophy.[110] With immobilization, the bone-ligament junction is at increased risk for injury, rather than the mid-substance of the ligament. The alterations in ligament collagen lead to a decrease in the tensile strength of the ligament and thus reduce the ability of ligaments to provide joint stability (Box 2-4).

Immobilization of the ligaments of the knee has been widely studied. It is well established in the literature that the amount of time the ligament is immobilized is much shorter than the amount of remobilization time necessary for the ligament to reach its pre-immobilization strength.[174,177] The reconditioning process must provide progressive stresses that overload the ligament enough to stimulate regeneration, but the stresses must be controlled to prevent cumulative microtrauma. The effects of immobilization on ligament structure and function may be specific to each particular ligament.

With immobilization, the medial collateral ligament (MCL) decreases in cross-sectional area and ultimate stress load.[177] These effects are assumed to depend on the exact position of the knee joint. The MCL is taut in full extension, so the assumption is that if the knee is immobilized with the MCL in a shortened position, a tighter ligament would be provided. Research has shown[13,154,166] that a reconstructed MCL has increased creep, or lengthening per unit stress, with immobilization rather than with full motion. This has implications for rehabilitation after MCL injury or reconstruction. After MCL injury or reconstruc-

tion, the knee should be placed in a position of slight flexion, so that extension is preserved, but the ligament is not under stress. Progressive motion should be allowed several times per day, however, to prevent creep and loss of cross-sectional area. Although this research only involves the MCL, it is likely that the same biomechanical principles may be applied to the lateral collateral ligament.

The effects of immobilization on the ACL have been widely studied. The specific effects are difficult to measure consistently due to the complex fiber orientation of the ligament. For the rehabilitation specialist, it is enough to note that there is increased risk for damage to the ACL after immobilization and that the amount of reconditioning necessary to restore the ligament is much greater than the time of immobilization. A discussion of the effects of immobilization after reconstruction is not warranted due to the widespread use of early aggressive range of motion exercises and rehabilitation after reconstruction.

The menisci also undergo degenerative changes with immobilization, and this degeneration is directly related to the amount of time the joint was immobilized.[112] In an animal model, the blood flow to the menisci after injury was increased fivefold. However, there was no increase in blood flow when the joint was immobilized.[19] Currently, healing is thought to depend on an adequate blood supply, and immobilization may therefore delay healing of the meniscus. Knee joint immobilization decreases the proteoglycan and water contents of the meniscus,[30] which changes its ability to distribute compressive forces. In the absence of weight bearing, active joint motion has been shown to decrease the loss of ligament and meniscal mass.[84]

Box 2-4

Summary of Response of Ligaments to Immobilization

- Significant decrease in linear stress, maximum stress, and stiffness
- Decrease in cross-sectional area of the ligament fibril, resulting in reduction of fibril size and density
- Increased synthesis and degradation of collagen resulting in increased turnover rate
- Disruption of the parallel arrangement of collagen
- Reduction in load and in energy-absorbing capabilities of the bone-ligament complex
- Decrease in GAG level
- Increase in osteoclastic activity at the bone-ligament junction, causing an increase in bone resorption in that area

Data from Refs. 1, 12, 46, 108, 109, 172, and 177.

CLINICAL PEARL #7

When a ligament reconstruction (not a primary repair) is performed, the graft undergoes neovascularization and ligamentization. This process begins at about 3 to 7 weeks postoperatively for a patellar tendon autograft.[23,43,128] This is the time when the graft is weakest, and the rehabilitation specialist must take care not to overstress the graft during this period. Bone to bone healing occurs faster than bone to tendon healing, which implies that rehabilitation should be less aggressive for an ACL reconstruction with a hamstring autograft than that with a patellar tendon autograft.[114] At 6 months postoperatively the patellar tendon autograft is indistinguishable from a normal ACL,[135] and the mechanical properties are not different, These findings imply that return to full activity may occur at this time, but other factors such as strength, dynamic control, balance, and psychologic readiness must be considered.

Bone

The effects of immobilization on bone are similar to those on other connective tissues. A consistent finding in response to diminished weight bearing and muscle contraction is bone loss. Bone changes can be detected as early as 2 weeks after immobilization.[58,101,158] Although the pathogenesis of immobilization osteoporosis is unclear, animal studies have shown decreased bone formation and increased bone resorption.[21,44,50,88]

Bone hardness decreases steadily with the duration of immobilization, dropping to 55% to 60% of normal by 12 weeks.[146] There is also a decline in elastic resistance—the bone becomes more brittle and thus more susceptible to fracture.

It appears that mechanical strain influences osteoblastic and osteoclastic activity on the bone surface.[38] Bone loss from disuse atrophy occurs at a rate 5 to 20 times greater than that resulting from metabolic disorders affecting bone.[104] The primary cause of this immobilization osteoporosis appears to be the mechanical unloading, which may be responsible for the inhibition of bone formation during immobilization.[176] Therefore, non–weight-bearing immobilization of an extremity should be limited to as short a period as possible.

CONTINUOUS PASSIVE MOTION

Salter,[130] in 1970, originated the biologic concept of continuous passive motion (CPM) of synovial joints to stimulate healing, regenerate articular tissue, and avoid the harmful effects of immobilization.[96] In 1978, Salter and Saringer (who was an engineer) collaborated to develop the first CPM device for humans.[130] A CPM machine is an electrical, motor-driven device that helps support the injured limb. It is used to move a joint at variable rates through progressively increasing ranges of motion; no muscular exertion is required of the patient.

Salter and colleagues[130,131] provided the first histologic evidence in support of CPM. They reported[130,133] that CPM significantly stimulates healing of articular tissues, including cartilage, tendons, and ligaments; it prevents adhesions and joint stiffness; it does not interfere with healing of incisions over the moving joint; and it influences the regeneration of articular cartilage through neochondrogenesis.

Compared with immobilization of tendons, CPM has proved to be effective in increasing linear and maximum stress, linear load, and ultimate strength for tendons.[96] Salter and Minster[132] have also reported preliminary results for semitendinous tenodesis for MCL reconstruction in experimental animals, in which increased strength was reported after use of CPM. The application of early tensile forces appears to facilitate the proper alignment of collagen fibers during the initial healing process. Also, decreases in medication requests and in wound edema and effusion in operative knees were reported in patients undergoing CPM.[105] The greatest benefit of CPM appears to be the prevention of articular cartilage degradation. Salter[130] reported that there appears to be more rapid and

complete healing in cartilage defects in rabbits when CPM is used.

CPM has received widespread attention for use in pathologic conditions of the knee. However, CPM machines have been developed for the shoulder as well. Raab and colleagues[117] found increased range of motion and decreased pain with the use of CPM after rotator cuff repair, although there was no difference in combined outcome measures at 3 months postoperatively. Lastayo and co-workers[90] found no difference in outcomes between subjects who used a CPM machine or those who had a friend or relative perform manual range-of-motion exercises, indicating that the presence of passive motion is more important than the mode of delivery.

It is well established in the literature that the use of CPM is not associated with a significant difference in outcome measures at approximately 4 weeks postoperatively.[36,47,126] However, when the short-term effects of CPM are examined, subjects undergoing CPM regain their motion faster and with less pain than those who are not undergoing CPM.[106] While there may be no long-term difference, CPM appears to be beneficial to the patient in the short term (Box 2-5).

Use of CPM units is considered an acceptable practice after most orthopedic procedures. Although initially designed for the lower extremities, CPM units are available for the upper extremities as well. CPM has helped to counteract the deleterious effects of immobilization by allowing early motion because it can be used in a protected range of motion. Some indications for the use of CPM include ligament reconstruction or repair, total joint replacement, joint contracture release, tendon repair, open reduction of fractures, and articular cartilage defects.

EFFECTS OF REMOBILIZATION

Physical forces provide important stimuli to tissues for the development and maintenance of homeostasis.[171] The lack of or denial of mobilization results in deleterious effects on bone, muscle, connective tissue, and articular cartilage. The advent of CPM in the late 1970s and early 1980s

---

Box 2-5

Benefits of the Early Use of Passive Motion

- No deleterious effects on the stability of the ligament
- Decrease in joint swelling and effusion
- Decrease in pain medication taken
- Faster regaining of knee range of motion
- Reduced muscle atrophy

Data from Refs. 28, 48, 106, 111, and 179.

provided an impetus for the initiation of early motion to repair tissues and for using early electrical stimulation of muscle to decrease atrophy and promote early muscle reeducation. In addition, the emergence of hinged braces, which allow early protected motion, has helped foster early mobilization.

Early motion and loading and unloading of joints through partial weight bearing promote the diffusion of synovial fluid to nourish articular cartilage, meniscus, and ligaments. Moreover, research has shown that motion enhances this trans-synovial nutrient flow.[93,102,120] Regardless of the cell-stimulating mechanism, it is clear that the fibroblasts and chondrocytes respond to physical forces by increasing their rate of synthesis, and extracellular degradation of matrix components is similarly controlled.[1]

Immobilization is still used, however, in the treatment of many ligamentous reconstructions and fractures. It is not known whether the deleterious effects of prolonged immobilization can be reversed with remobilization techniques. These structural changes generally appear to depend on the duration and angle of immobilization and on the weight-bearing status.

CLINICAL PEARL #8

Rehabilitation protocols for specific injuries and surgical procedures are popular and commonly used. These protocols must be seen as guidelines and not as rules. Each patient's condition must be taken into account when one determines appropriate progression of activities. Objective and subjective findings are used to determine the patient's tolerance of a new activity. Signs of intolerance include increased effusion, pain, erythema, or an inability to perform a task correctly. These are signs that the activity should be modified or delayed.

Muscle

Many researchers have investigated the process of remobilization after immobilization. Application of the results of these studies to an injured or postoperative patient population must be done with caution, however, because injury may compound the effects of immobilization. It is critical to consider how the specific injury or surgical procedure and the length of immobilization will affect the return rate of muscle strength.

To achieve gains in muscle strength, the principle of overload must be used.[76] Overload involves application of a stimulus that is greater than the stimulus the muscle is accustomed to. This principle must be used with caution in an injured population, however, because excessive overload can be detrimental to healing tissues.

The return of quadriceps strength after knee surgery has been widely investigated. With ACL reconstruction, there appears to be a greater loss of quadriceps strength with bone-patellar tendon-bone autografts than with semitendinosus-gracilis autografts.[78,141] Despite quadriceps weakness being associated with patellar tendon-bone autografts, only a slight amount of hamstring weakness is associated with semitendinosus-gracilis autografts.[79] This may be due to the previously discussed reasons for quadriceps predisposition to atrophy. After ACL reconstruction with patellar tendon-bone autografts, quadriceps strength has been found to be less than 50% of that of the contralateral side 3 months postoperatively[178] and 72% to 78% of that of the contralateral side from 6 to 12 months postoperatively.[78,178] Six months after ACL reconstruction with a semitendinosus-gracilis autograft, quadriceps strength has been found to be 88% of that of the contralateral side, and hamstring strength has been found to be 90% of that of the contralateral side.[79] In both a human[113] and an animal model,[182] this type of reconstruction in a female patient,[10,178] and older age are factors for increase risk of prolonged muscle weakness after surgery.

Shoulder strength after rotator cuff injury has been studied. In shoulders with a rotator cuff tear, strength is decreased by one third to two thirds for abduction, flexion, and external rotation.[67,81] Strength is decreased by one third 6 months after repair and becomes comparable to that of the contralateral side at 1 year after repair.[122] Shoulder strength is positively correlated with the size of the rotator cuff tear.[122]

It has been theorized that electrical muscle stimulation (EMS) can provide enough muscle activity to deter atrophy and the deleterious effects of immobilization on muscle. EMS has been investigated primarily as a tool to preserve muscle strength and cross-sectional area after knee surgery, particularly with ACL reconstruction. EMS has been shown to preserve quadriceps cross-sectional area and protein synthesis for an immobilized injured knee[51,107] when combined with traditional rehabilitation exercises.[29,39,141] EMS has also been shown to be associated with a more normalized gait pattern postoperatively.[142] This may be particularly effective in women.[10]

Some literature reports do not support the effectiveness of EMS in preserving muscle strength after injury or surgery.[115] This lack of support may be due to the type and individual parameters of electrical stimulation used. EMS is comparable to voluntary exercise only when the exercises are required to be performed at the same intensity as the EMS.[94] In addition, EMS is only effective when it is used at a level strong enough to produce a contraction that is greater than that which the patient has voluntarily. Biofeedback training has been shown to be as effective as EMS for recovery of quadriceps strength.[32]

CLINICAL PEARL #9

EMS can have a clinical benefit when a patient does not have active full knee extension. This can be especially helpful if the patient is immobilized in a flexed position. The patient must apply the EMS on a regular basis (three to five times a day at home) with the knee in full extension during each use and full range of motion is preserved.

EMS will only benefit the patient when it is strong enough to produce a contraction in a shortened position than that which the patient has voluntarily.

Many clinicians use EMS for the quadriceps after knee surgery or injury. However, EMS can help preserve motion and allow early neuromuscular reeducation at other joints. Functional electrical stimulation is used on the rotator cuff of patients who have a subluxated shoulder after a cerebral injury.

Articular Cartilage

The effects of remobilization on articular cartilage seem to be time dependent. Many studies have examined the effects of remobilization on articular cartilage after a period of immobilization. The period of remobilization required to restore articular cartilage structure and function is significantly longer than the immobilization period required to cause those changes.[83,159] Kiviranta and associates[82,83] found that 50 weeks of remobilization after 11 weeks of immobilization is not sufficient to restore GAG content. Haapala and colleagues[53] used a similar protocol to demonstrate the inability of 50 weeks of remobilization to reverse cartilage softening in the cartilage of immature beagles. This indicates that younger individuals may have long-term damage in their articular surfaces from immobilization. Evans and co-workers[41] reported alterations in cartilage such as matrix fibrillation, cleft formation, and ulceration that are not reversible in rats after immobilization for up to 90 days. They noted, however, that soft tissue changes are reversible if the period of immobilization does not exceed 30 days. Clinically, it is rare that an extremity would be immobilized for longer than the 30 days that is required to cause irreversible damage.

The remobilization process after immobilization must consist of controlled stresses. Although moderate activity after a period of immobilization causes increases in cartilage thickness and proteoglycan content, strenuous activity can cause damage to the articular structures.[82] It is important to watch for signs of intolerance to a new activity. Signs of intolerance include increased effusion or edema, erythema, pain, or inability to complete a task correctly.

Bone

Immobilization results in disuse osteoporosis, which may not be reversible on remobilization of the limb. The reversibility is related to the severity of changes and to the length of immobilization. Permanent osseous changes appear to occur with an immobilization period exceeding

12 weeks.[181] Even though bone lost in the first 12 weeks is regained, the period of recovery is at least as long as and may be many times longer than the immobilization period.[22] The most effective means of modifying osteoporosis caused by reduced skeletal loads appears to be through exercise. Isotonic and isometric exercises decreased bone loss in subjects who were exposed to prolonged periods of weightlessness and bed rest.[97,163] Activity increases bone formation in these situations and can hasten recovery after return to a normal loading environment. If an appropriate environment can be maintained during immobilization of a limb, the deleterious effects of disuse on bone can be partially prevented, and rehabilitation can be accelerated.[22]

Ligaments

Remobilization after immobilization of ligaments occurs in an asynchronous fashion. It appears that the bone-ligament junction recovers at a much slower rate than do the mechanical or midsubstance properties of the ligament.[172,173] Cabaud and colleagues[24] have reported that ligament strength and stiffness in rat ACLs can increase with endurance-type exercises. Others have noted similar results.[74,75] Moreover, not only does the ligament injury result in weaker mechanical properties at midsubstance and at the bone-ligament complex, but nontraumatized ligaments become weaker as a result of immobilization. These weakened ligament mechanical properties must be considered when a rehabilitation program is being planned.

Recovery from immobilization depends on the duration of immobilization. Woo and associates[172] noted that 1 year of remobilization is required before the architectural components of the MCL-tibia junction return to normal after 12 weeks of immobilization. Noyes[109] reported in primates that after 5 months of remobilization following total body immobilization, ligament strength only partially recovers, although ligament stiffness and compliance parameters return to control values. It was reported that 12 months are required for complete recovery of ligament strength parameters.[109] Tipton and co-workers[155] observed a recovery of 50% of normal strength in a healing ligament by 6 months, of 80% after 1 year, and of 100% after 1 to 3 years, depending on the type of stresses placed on the ligament and on the prevention of repeated injury.

It appears that properties of ligaments return to normal with remobilization, but this depends on the duration of the immobilization, with the bone-ligament junction taking longer to return to normal after immobilization.

Connective Tissue

Few studies have documented the effects of remobilization after immobilization on formation of cross-links.[31] Movement maintains lubrication and critical fiber distance within the matrix and ensures an orderly deposition of collagen fibrils, thereby preventing abnormal cross-link formation.[31] Often, for range of motion to be restored, forceful manipulation that breaks the intracapsular fibrofatty adhesions may have to be performed.[31] Although range of motion is restored, it has been speculated that there is peeling of the fibrofatty tissue from the bone ends, with ragged edges of adhesions remaining in the joint.[37, 41] There is also increased joint inflammation from the manipulation, enhancing the potential for chronic synovitis.

SUMMARY

Motion problems should be detected early, joint endfeel should be assessed by palpation, and the reason for the motion problem should be determined. If manipulation is the treatment of choice, it should be performed early in the recovery process to decrease the amount of joint damage resulting from a manipulation and to prevent connective tissue changes from becoming morphologic changes.

The deleterious effects of immobilization on bone and connective tissue have been widely reported. The efficacy of early, controlled mobilization to allow orderly organization of collagen along lines of stress and to promote healthy joint arthrokinematics is supported by many studies. Acute injury that is not treated adequately by early concentration on decreasing joint effusion and pain and restoration of normal joint arthrokinematics can result in a vicious inflammatory cycle; this perpetuates the degradation of articular cartilage by the enzymes released after cell death. This articular cartilage damage is a secondary injury induced by inadequate attention to decreasing the severity of the early inflammatory process.

The harmful effects of immobilization on muscle are the most obvious changes. Muscle atrophy can be detected as early as 24 hours after immobilization. Muscle responds to immobilization by decreases in muscle fiber size, total muscle weight, mitochondria size and number, muscle tension produced, resting levels of glycogen and ATP, and protein synthesis. With exercise, there is an increase in the muscle contraction time and in the lactate level.

Muscle shutdown is a phenomenon generally seen after immobilization, but it can also be readily detected after most surgical procedures. It is observed in the quadriceps muscle after knee surgery. Although many reasons for muscle shutdown have been postulated, it appears to be affected by one or more of the following factors: joint effusion, angle of joint immobilization, periarticular tissue damage from surgery or trauma, and the H reflex.

Immobilization leads to biochemical and histochemical changes in the periarticular tissue, ultimately contributing to arthrofibrosis. Immobilization-induced arthrofibrosis has been widely documented, although the exact mechanism is still speculative. Connective tissue usually responds to immobilization by a reduction in water and glycosamino-glycan content; a decrease in the extracellular matrix, which leads to a reduction in the lubrication between fiber cross-links; a decrease in collagen mass; an increase in collagen turnover, degradation, and synthesis rates; and an increase in abnormal collagen fiber cross-links.

Ligaments are similarly affected by immobilization. It appears that the bone-ligament junction undergoes an increase in osteoclastic activity, resulting in a weaker junction. There is also ligament atrophy, with a corresponding decrease in linear stress, maximum stress, and stiffness.

The greatest effect from immobilization appears to be on the articular cartilage. The intermittent loading and unloading of synovial joints promotes the metabolic exchange necessary for the proper structure and function of articular cartilage. Joint immobilization, in which articular cartilage is in constant contact with opposing bone ends, can cause pressure necrosis. Conversely, noncontact between joint surfaces can promote ingrowth of connective tissue into the joint. Diminished weight bearing and loading and unloading of an extremity also cause an increase in bone resorption in that area.

CPM devices allow early joint motion, with no detrimental side effects. CPM has a significantly stimulating effect on healing articular tissues, including cartilage, tendons, and ligaments, and also prevents joint adhesions and stiffness. Patients using CPM devices have shown decreases in joint hemarthrosis and in requests for pain medication.

Tissues appear to recover at different rates with remobilization after immobilization, with muscle recovering the fastest. Although few studies on the effects of remobilization on immobilized connective tissue have been performed, it has been proved that early mobilization maintains lubrication and a critical fiber distance among collagen fibrils in the matrix, thus preventing abnormal cross-link formation. After immobilization, articular cartilage and bone respond the least favorably to remobilization. Changes in articular cartilage depend on the length and angle of immobilization. Prolonged immobilization can result in irreversible changes in articular cartilage.

Early protected motion and weight bearing, as healing restraints allow, are therefore advocated to avoid the deleterious effects of immobilization and to deter the secondary problems perpetuated by immobilization.

REFERENCES

1. Akeson, W.H., Amiel, D., and Abel, M.F. (1987): Effects of immobilization on joints. Clin. Orthop., 219:28-37.
2. Akeson, W.H., Amiel, D., and LaViolette, D. (1967): The connective tissue response to immobility: A study of the chondrotin-4- and 6-sulfate and dermatan sulfate changes in periarticular connective tissue of control and immobilized knee of dogs. Clin. Orthop., 51:183-197.
3. Akeson, W.H., Amiel, D., and Woo, S. (1980): Immobility effects of synovial joints: The pathomechanics of joint contracture. Biorheology, 17:95-110.

4. Akeson, W.H., Woo, S.L.Y., and Amiel, D. (1973): The connective tissue response to immobility: Biochemical changes in periarticular connective tissue of the immobilized rabbit knee. Clin. Orthop., 93:356-362.

5. Akeson, W.H., Woo, S.L.Y., and Amiel, D. (1984): The chemical basis of tissue repair. In: Hunter, L.Y., and Funk, F.J. (eds.), Rehabilitation of the Injured Knee. St. Louis, C.V. Mosby, pp. 93-148.

6. Amiel, D., Woo, S.L.Y., Harwood, F.L., and Akeson, W.H. (1982): The effect of immobilization on collagen turnover in connective tissue: A biochemical-biochemical correlation. Acta Orthop. Scand., 53:325-332.

7. Appell, H.J. (1986): Morphology of immobilized skeletal muscle and the effects of a pre- and postimmobilization training program. Int. J. Sports Med., 7:6-12.

8. Arciero, R.A., Scoville, C.R., Hayda, R.A., and Snyder, R.J. (1996): The effect of tourniquet use in anterior cruciate ligament reconstruction. A prospective, randomized study. Am. J. Sports Med., 24:758-764.

9. Arem, A.J., and Madden, J.W. (1976): Effects of stress on healing wounds: Intermittent noncyclical tension. J. Surg. Res., 20:93-102.

10. Arvidsson, I., Arvidsson, H., Eriksson, E., and Jansson, E. (1986): Prevention of quadriceps wasting after immobilization: An evaluation of the effect of electrical muscle stimulation. Orthopedics, 9:1519-1528.

11. Ben-Yishay, A., Zuckerman, J.D., Gallagher, M., and Cuomo, F. (1994): Pain inhibition of shoulder strength in patients with impingement syndrome. Orthopedics, 17:685-688.

12. Binkley, J.M., and Peat, M. (1986): The effects of immobilization on the ultrastructure and mechanical properties of the medial collateral ligament of rats. Clin. Orthop. Rel. Res., 203:301-308.

13. Boorman, R.S., Shrive, N.G., and Frank, C.B. (1998): Immobilization increases the vulnerability of rabbit medial collateral ligament autografts to creep. J. Orthop. Res., 16:682-689.

14. Booth, F.W. (1987): Physiological and biochemical effects of immobilization on muscle. Clin. Orthop. Rel. Res., 219:15-20.

15. Booth, F.W., and Kelso, J.R. (1973): Effect of hindlimb immobilization on contractile and histochemical properties of skeletal muscle. Pflugers Arch., 342:231-238.

16. Booth, F.W., and Seider, M.J. (1979): Recovery of skeletal muscle after 3 months of hindlimb immobilization in rats. J. Appl. Physiol., 47:435-439.

17. Bosch, U., Ziechen, J., and Skutek, M. (2001): Arthrofibrosis in the result of a T-cell mediated immune response. Knee Surg. Sports Trauma Arthrosc., 9:282-289.

18. Bozdech, Z. (1976): Posttraumatic synovitis. Acta Chir. Orthop. Traumatol. Cech., 43:244-247.

19. Bray, R.C., Smith, J.A., and Eng, M.K. (2001): Vascular response of the meniscus to injury: Effects of immobilization. J. Orthop. Res., 19:384-390.

20. Broom, N.D., and Myers, D.B. (1980): A study of the structural response of wet hyaline cartilage to various loading situations. Connect. Tissue Res., 7:227-237.

21. Burdeaux, B.D., and Hutchinson, W.J. (1953): Etiology of traumatic osteoporosis. J. Bone Joint Surg. [Am.], 35:479-488.

22. Burr, D.B., Frederickson, R.G., and Pavlinch, C. (1984): Intracast muscle stimulation prevents bone and cartilage deterioration in cast-immobilized rabbits. Clin. Orthop. Rel. Res., 189:264-278.

23. Butler, D.L., Grood, E.S., and Noyes, F.R. (1989): Mechanical properties of primate vascualrized versus nonvascularized patellar tendon grafts, changes over time. J. Orthop. Res., 7:68-79.

24. Cabaud, H.E., Chatty, A., and Gildengorin, V. (1980): Exercise effects on the strength of the rat anterior cruciate ligament. Am. J. Sports Med., 8:79-86.

25. Castor, C.W., Prince, R.K., and Hazelton, M.J. (1966): Hyaluronic acid in human synovial effusions: A sensitive indicator of altered connective tissue cell function during inflammation. Arthritis Rheum., 9:783-794.

26. Cooper, R.R. (1972): Alternatives during immobilization and regeneration of skeletal muscle in cats. J. Bone Joint Surg. [Am.], 54:919-953.

27. DeAndrade, J.R., Grant, C., and Dixon, A. (1965): Joint distension and reflex inhibition in the knee. J. Bone Joint Sug. [Am.], 47:313-322.

28. Dehert, W.J., O'Driscoll, S.W., van Royen, B.J., and Salter, R.B. (1988): Effects of immobilization and continuous passive motion on postoperative muscle atrophy in mature rabbits. Can. J. Surg., 31:185-188.

29. Delitto, A., Rose, S.J., and McKowen, J.M. (1988): Electrical stimulation versus voluntary exercise in strengthening thigh musculature after anterior cruciate ligament surgery. Phys. Ther., 68:660-663.

30. Djurasovic, M., Aldridge, J.W., and Grumbles, R. (1998): Knee joint immobilization decreases aggrecan gene expression in the meniscus. Am. J. Sports Med., 26:460-466.

31. Donatelli, R., and Owens-Burkhart, A. (1981): Effects of immobilization on the extensibility of periarticular connective tissue. J. Orthop. Sports Phys. Ther., 3:67-72.

32. Draper, V., and Ballard, L. (1991): Electrical stimulation versus electromyographic biofeedback in the recovery of quadriceps femoris muscle function following anterior cruciate ligament surgery. Phys. Ther., 71:455-461.

33. Edin, B.B., and Vallbo, A.B. (1988): Stretch sensitization of human muscle spindles. J. Physiol., 400:101-111.

34. Ekholm, R. (1955): Nutrition of articular cartilage: A radioautographic study. Acta Anat., 24:329-338.

35. Elliot, R.J., and Gardner, D.L. (1979): Changes with age of the glycosaminoglycans of human cartilage. Ann. Rheum. Dis., 38:371-377.

36. Engstrom, B., Sperber, A., and Wredmark, T. (1995): Continuous passive motion in rehabilitation after anterior cruciate ligament reconstruction. Knee Surg. Sports Trauma Arthrosc., 3:18-20.

37. Enneking, W.F., and Horowitz, M. (1972): The intra-articular effects of immobilization on the human knee. J. Bone Joint Surg. [Am.], 54:973-985.

38. Epker, B.N., and Frost, H.M. (1965): Correlation of bone resorption and formation behavior of loaded bone. J. Dent. Res., 44:33-41.

39. Eriksson, E., and Haggmark, T. (1979): Comparison of isometric muscle training and electrical stimulation supplementing isometric muscle training in the recovery after major knee ligament surgery. Am. J. Sports Med., 7:169-171.

40. Eronin, I., Videman, T., Friman, C., and Michelesson, J.E. (1978): Glycosaminoglycan metabolism in experimental osteoarthritis caused by immobilization. Acta Orthop. Scand., 49:329-334.

41. Evans, E.B., Egger, G.W.N., Butler, M., and Blumel, J. (1960): Experimental immobilization and remobilization of rat knee joints. J. Bone Joint Surg. [Am.], 42:737-758.

42. Eyring, E.J., and Murray, W.R. (1964): The effect of joint position on the pressure of intra-articular effusion. J. Bone Joint Surg. [Am.], 46:1235-1241.

43. Falconiero, R.P., DiStefano, V.J., and Cook, T.M. (1998): Revacularization and ligamentization of autogenous anterior cruciate ligament grafts in humans. Arthroscopy, 14:197-205.

44. Fleisch, H., Russell, R.G., Simpson, B., and Muhlbauer, R.C. (1969): Prevention by a diphosphonate of immobilization osteoporosis in rats. Nature, 223:211-212.

45. Fujimoto, D., Moriquichi, T., Ishida, T., and Hayashi, H. (1978): The structure of pyridinoline, a collegan cross link. Biochem. Biophys. Res. Commun., 84:52-57.

46. Gamble, J.G., Edwards, C.C., and Max, S.R. (1984): Enzymatic adaptation in ligaments during immobilization. Am. J. Sports Med., 12:221-228.

47. Gasper, L., Farkas, C., Szepesi, K., and Csernatony, Z. (1997): Therapeutic value of continuous passive motion after anterior cruciate replacement. Acta Chir. Hung., 36:104-105.

48. Gebhard, J.S., Kabo, J.M., and Meals, R.A. (1993): Passive motion: The dose effects on joint stiffness, muscle mass, bone density, and regional swelling. A study in an experimental model following intra-articular injury. J. Bone Joint Surg. [Am.], 75:1636-1647.

49. Geborek, P., Moritz, U., and Wollheim, F.A. (1989): Joint capsular stiffness in knee arthritis. Relationship to intraarticular volume, hydrostatic pressures, and extensor muscle function. J. Rheumatol., 16:1351-1358.

50. Geiser, M., and Trueta, J. (1985): Muscle action, bone rarefaction, and bone formation. J. Bone Joint Surg. [Br.], 40:282-311.

51. Gibson, J.N., Smith, K., and Rennie, M.J. (1988): Prevention of disuse muscle atrophy by means of electrical muscle stimulation: Maintenance of protein synthesis. Lancet, 7:767-770.

52. Golden, A. (1980): Reaction to injury in the musculoskeletal system. In: Rosse, C., and Clawson, D.K. (eds.), The Musculoskeletal System in Health and Disease. New York, Harper & Row, pp. 89-93.

53. Haapala, J., Arokoski, J., and Pirttimaki, J. (2000): Incomplete restoration of immobilization induced softening of young beagle knee articular cartilage after 50-week remobilization. Int. J. Sports Med., 21:76-81.

54. Haggmark, T., Eriksson, E., and Jansson, E. (1986): Muscle fiber type changes in human skeletal muscle after injuries and immobilization. Orthopedics, 9:181-185.

55. Haggmark, T., Jansson, E., and Eriksson, E. (1981): Fiber type area and metabolic potential of the thigh muscle in man after knee surgery and immobilization. Int. J. Sports Med., 2:12-17.

56. Hall, M.C. (1963): Cartilage changes after experimental relief of contact in the knee of the mature rat. J. Bone Joint Surg. [Am.], 45:36-44.

57. Ham, A.C., and Cormack, D. (1979): Histology, Vol. 8. Philadelphia, J.B. Lippincott.

58. Hardt, A.B. (1972): Early metabolic responses of bone to immobilization. J. Bone Joint Surg. [Am.], 54:119-124.

59. Hayashi, K. (1996): Biomechanical studies of the remodeling of knee joint tendons and ligaments. J. Biomech., 29:707-716.

60. Hess, T., Gleitz, M., and Hopf, T. (1995): Changes in muscular activity after knee arthrotomy and arthroscopy. Int. Orthop., 19:94-97.

61. Hettinga, D.L. (1979): I. Normal joint structures and their reaction to injury. J. Orthop. Sports Phys. Ther., 1:16-22.

62. Hettinga, D.L. (1979): II. Normal joint structures and their reaction to injury. J. Orthop. Sports Phys. Ther., 1:83-88.

63. Hugheston, J.C. (1985): Complications of anterior cruciate ligament surgery. Orthop. Clin. North Am., 16:237-240.

64. Hunter, R.E., Mastrangelo, J., and Freeman, J.R. (1996): The impact of surgical timing on postoperative motion and stability following anterior cruciate ligament reconstruction. Arthroscopy, 12:667-674.

65. Ingemann-Hansen, T., and Halkjaer-Kristensen, J. (1977): Lean and fat composition of the human thigh. The effects of immobilization in plaster and subsequent physical training. J. Rehabil. Med., 9:67-72.

66. Ingemann-Hansen, T., and Halkjaer-Kristensen, J. (1980): Computerized tomographic determination of human thigh components. The effects of immobilization in plaster and subsequent physical training. Scand. J. Rehab. Med., 12:27-31.

67. Itoi, E., Minagawa, H., and Solo, T. (1997): Isokinetic strength after tears of the supraspinatus tendon. J. Bone Joint Surg. [Br.], 79:77-82.

68. Jackson, D.W., and Shafer, R.K. (1987): Cyclops syndrome: Loss of extension following intra-articular anterior cruciate ligament reconstruction. Arthroscopy, 6:171-178.

69. Jarvinen, M.J., Einola, S.A., and Virtanen, E.O. (1992): Effect of the position of immobilization upon tensile properties of rat gastrocnemius muscle. Arch. Phys. Med. Rehab., 73:253-257.

70. Jayson, M.I.V., and Dixon, A. (1970): Intra-articular pressure in rheumatoid arthritis of the knee. III. Pressure changes during joint use. Ann. Rheum. Dis., 29:401-408.

71. Jokl, P., and Konstadt, S. (1983): The effect of limb immobilization on muscle function and protein composition. Clin. Orthop., 174:222-229.

72. Jones, D.W., Jones, D.A., and Newham, D.J. (1987): Chronic knee effusion and aspiration: The effect on quadriceps inhibition. Br. J. Rheumatol., 26:370-374.

73. Jozsa, L., Jarvinen, M., Kannus, P., and Reffy, A. (1987): Fine structural changes in the articular cartilage of the rat's knee following short-term immobilization in various positions: A scanning electron microscopical study. Int. Orthop., 11:129-133.

74. Jurvelin, J., Helminen, H.J., and Laurisalo, S. (1985): Influences of joint immobilization and running exercise on articular cartilage surfaces of young rabbits. Acta Anat., 122:62-68.

75. Jurvelin, J., Kiviranta, I., Tammi, M., and Helminen, J.H. (1986): Softening of canine articular cartilage after immobilization of the knee joint. Clin. Orthop. Rel. Res., 207:246-252.

76. Kannus, P., Jozsa, L., and Jarvinen, T.L. (1998): Free mobilization and low- to high-intensity exercise in immobilization-induced muscle atrophy. J. Appl. Physiol., 84:1418-1424.

77. Kannus, P., Jozsa, L., and Kvist, M. (1992): The effect of immobilization on myotendinous junction: An ultrastructural, histochemical and immunohistochemical study. Acta Physiol. Scand., 144:387-394.

78. Keays, S.L., Bullock-Saxton, J., and Keays, A.C. (2000): Strength and function before and after anterior cruciate reconstruction. Clin. Orthop. Rel. Res., 373:174-183.

79. Keays, S.L., Bullock-Saxton, J., Keays, A.C., and Newcombe, P. (2001): Muscle strength and function before and after anterior cruciate ligament reconstruction using semitendinosis and gracilis. Knee, 8:229-234.

80. Kennedy, J.C., Alexander, I.J., and Hayes, K.C. (1982): Nerve supply of the human knee and its functional importance. Am. J. Sports Med., 10:329-335.

81. Kirschenbaum, D., Coyle, M.P., and Leddy, L.P. (1993): Shoulder strength with rotator cuff tears: Pre- and postoperative analysis. Clin. Orthop. Rel. Res., 288:174-178.

82. Kiviranta, I., Tammi, M., and Jurvelin, J. (1992): Articular cartilage thickness and glycosaminoglycan distribution in the canine knee joint after strenuous running exercise. Clin. Orthop. Rel. Res., 283:302-308.

83. Kiviranta, I., Tammi, M., and Jurvelin, J. (1994): Articular cartilage thickness and glycosaminoglycan distribution in the young canine knee joint after remobilization of the immobilized limb. J. Orthop. Res., 12:161-167.

84. Klein, L., Heiple, K.G., and Torzilli, P.A. (1989): Prevention of ligament and meniscus atrophy by active joint motion in a non-weight-bearing model. J. Orthop. Res., 7:80-85.

85. Knight, K. (1976): The effects of hypothermia on inflammation and swelling. Athl. Train., 11:7-10.

86. Krebs, D.E., Staples, W.H., Cuttita, D., and Zickel, R.E. (1983): Knee joint angle: Its relationship to quadriceps femoris activity in normal and post-arthrotomy limbs. Arch. Phys. Med. Rehab., 64:441-447.

87. Labarque, V.L., Op't Eijnde, B., and Van Leemputte, M. (2002): Effect of immobilization and retraining on torque-velocity relationship of human knee flexor and extensor muscles. Eur. J. Appl. Physiol., 86:251-257.

88. Landry, M., and Fleisch, H. (1964): The influence of immobilization on bone formation as evaluated by osseous incorporation of tetracyclines. J. Bone Joint Surg. [Br.], 46:764-771.

89. Langenskiold, A., Michelsson, J.E., and Videman, T. (1979): Osteoarthritis of the knee in the rabbit produced by immobilization: Attempts to achieve a reproducible model for studies on pathogenesis and therapy. Acta Orthop. Scand., 50:1-14.

90. Lastayo, P.C., Wright, T., Jaffe, R., and Hartzel, J. (1998): Continuous passive motion after repair of the rotator cuff: A prospective outcome study. J. Bone Joint Surg., 80:1002-1111.

91. Leivo, I., Kauhanen, S., and Michelsson, J.E. (1998): Abnormal mitochondria and sarcoplasmic changes in rabbit skeletal muscle induced by immobilization. APMIS, 106:1113-1123.

92. Levick, R.J. (1983): Joint pressure-volume studies: Their importance, design and interpretation. J. Rheumatol., 10:353-357.

93. Levick, R.J. (1983): Synovial fluid dynamics: The regulation of volume and pressure. In: Holborrow, E.J., and Maroudas, V. (eds.), Studies in Joint Disease, London, Pitman Medical, pp. 153-240.

94. Lieber, R.L., Silva, P.D., and Daniel, D.M. (1996): Equal effectiveness of electrical and volitional strength training for the quadriceps femoris muscles after anterior cruciate ligament surgery. J. Orthop. Res., 14:131-138.

95. Lindboe, C.F., and Platou, C.S. (1984): Effects of immobilization of short duration on muscle fiber size. Clin. Physiol., 4:183-188.

96. Loitz, B.J., Zernicke, R.F., and Vailas, A.C. (1989): Effects of short-term immobilization versus continuous passive motion on the biomechanical and biochemical properties of the rabbit tendon. Clin. Orthop., 244:265-271.

97. Lynch, T.N., Jensen, R.L., and Stevens, D.M. (1967): Metabolic effects of prolonged bed rest: Their modification by simulated altitude. Aerosp. Med., 38:10-20.

98. MacDougall, J.D., Elder, G.C.B., and Sale, D.G. (1980): Effects of strength training and immobilization on human muscle fibers. Eur. J. Appl. Physiol., 43:25-34.

99. MacDougall, J.D., Ward, G.R., Sale, D.G., and Sutton, J.R. (1977): Biochemical adaptation of human skeletal muscle to heavy resistance training and immobilization. J. Appl. Physiol., 43:700-703.

100. Maier, A., Crockett, J.L., and Simpson, D.R. (1976): Properties of immobilized guinea pig hindlimb muscles. Am. J. Physiol., 231:1520-1526.

101. Mariani, P.P., Santori, N., and Rovere, P. (1997): Histological and structural study of the adhesive tissue in knee fibroarthrosis: A clinical-pathological correlation. Arthroscopy, 13:13-18.

102. Maroudes, A., Bullough, P., Swanson, S., and Freemna, M. (1968): The permeability of articular cartilage. J. Bone Joint Surg. [Br.], 50:166-177.

103. Max, S.R. (1972): Disuse atrophy of skeletal muscle: Loss of functional activity of mitochondria. Biochem. Biophys. Res. Commun., 46:1394-1398.

104. Mazess, R.B., and Whedon, G.D. (1983): Immobilization and bone. Calcif. Tissue Int., 35:265-267.

105. McCarthy, M.R., Buxton, B.P., and Yates, C.K. (1993): Effects of continuous passive motion on anterior laxity following ACL reconstruction with autogenous patellar tendon grafts. J. Sports Rehab., 2:171-178.

106. McCarthy, M.R., Yates, C.K., Anderson, M.A., and Yates-McCarthy, J.L. (1993): The effects of immediate continuous passive motion on pain during the inflammatory phase of soft tissue healing following anterior cruciate reconstruction. J. Orthop. Sports Phys. Ther., 17:96-101.

107. Morrissey, M.C., Brewster, C.E., Shields, C.L., and Brown, M. (1985): The effects of electrical stimulation on the quadriceps during postoperative knee immobilization. Am. J. Sports Med., 13:40-45.

108. Newton, P.O., Woo, S.L., and Kitabayashi, L.R. (1990): Ultrastructural changes in knee ligaments following immobilization. Matrix, 10:314-319.

109. Noyes, F.R. (1977): Functional properties of knee ligaments and alterations induced by immobilization. Clin. Orthop. Rel. Res., 123:210-242.

110. Noyes, F.R., Mangine, R.E., and Barber, S. (1974): Biomechanics of ligament failure. II. An analysis of immobilization, exercise, and reconditioning effects in primates. J. Bone Joint Surg. [Am.], 56:1406-1418.

111. Noyes, F.R., Mangine, R.E., and Barber, S. (1987): Early knee motion after open and arthroscopic anterior cruciate ligament reconstruction. Am. J. Sports Med., 15:149-160.

112. Ochi, M., Kanda, T., Sumen, Y., and Ikuta, Y. (1997): Changes in the permeability and histologic findings of rabbit menisci after immobilization. Clin. Orthop. Rel. Res., 334:305-315.

113. Osteras, H., Augestad, L.B., and Tondel, S. (1998): Isokinetic muscle strength after anterior cruciate ligament reconstruction. Scand. J. Med. Sci. Sports, 8:279-282.

114. Papageorgiou, C.D., Benjamin, C., and Abramowitch, S.D. (2001): Multidisciplinary study of the healing of an intraarticular anterior cruciate ligament in a goat model. Am. J. Sports Med., 29:620-626.

115. Paternostro-Sluga, T., Fialka, C., and Alacamliogliu, Y. (1999): Neuromuscular electrical stimulation after anterior cruciate ligament surgery. Clin. Orthop., 368:166-175.

116. Paulos, L., Rosenberg, T., and Drawbert, J. (1987): Infrapatellar contracture syndrome: An unrecognized cause of knee stiffness with patella entrapment and patella infera. Am. J. Sports Med., 15:331-342.

117. Raab, M.G., Rzeszutko, D., O'Conner, W., and Greatting, M.D. (1996): Early results of continuous passive motion after rotator cuff repair: A prospective, randomized, blinded, controlled study. Am. J. Orthop., 25:214-220.

118. Rabb, D.J., Fischer, D.A., and Smith, J.P. (1993): Comparison of arthroscopic and open reconstruction of the anterior cruciate ligament. Early results. Am. J. Sports Med., 21:680-683.

119. Radin, E.L., Paul, I.L., and Pollock, D. (1970): Animal joint behavior under excessive loading. Nature, 266:554-555.

120. Renzoni, S.A., Amiel, D., Harwood, F.L., and Akeson, W.H. (1984): Synovial nutrition of knee ligaments. Trans. Orthop. Res. Soc., 9:277-283.

121. Rifenberick, D.H., and Max, S.R. (1974): Substrate utilization by disused rat skeletal muscles. Am. J. Physiol., 226:295-297.

122. Rokito, A.S., Zuckerman, J.D., Gallagher, M.A., and Cuomo, F. (1996): Strength after surgical repair of the rotator cuff. J. Shoulder Elbow Surg., 5:12-17.

123. Roosendaal, G., Tekoppele, J.M., and Vianen, M.E. (2000): Articular cartilage is more susceptible to blood induced damage at young than at old age. J. Rheumatol., 27:1740-1744.

124. Roosendaal, G., Vianen, M.E., and Marx, J.J. (1999): Blood-induced joint damage: A human in vitro study. Arthritis Rheum., 42:1025-1032.

125. Roosendall, G., Vianen, M.E., and van der Berg, H.M. (1997): Cartilage damage as a result of hemarthrosis in a human in vitro model. J. Rheumatol., 24:1350-1354.

126. Rosen, M.A., Jackson, D.W., and Artwell, E.A. (1992): The efficacy of continuous passive motion in the rehabilitation of anterior cruciate ligament reconstruction. Am. J. Sports Med., 20:122-127.

127. Roth, J.H., Mendenhall, H.V., and McPherson, G.K. (1988): The effect of immobilization on goat knees following reconstruction of the anterior cruciate ligament. Clin. Orthop. Rel. Res., 229:278-282.

128. Rougraff, B.T., and Shelbourne, K.D. (1999): Early histologic appearance of human patellar tendon autografts used for anterior cruciate ligament reconstruction. Knee Surg. Sports Trauma Arthrosc., 7:9-14.

129. Roy, S., Ghadially, F.N., and Crane, W.A.J. (1966): Synovial membrane and traumatic effusion: Ultrastructure and autoradiography with tritiated leucine. Ann. Rheumatol. Dis., 25:259-271.

130. Salter, R.B. (1989): The biologic concept of continuous passive motion of synovial joints. Clin. Orthop., 242:12-25.

131. Salter, R.B., and Field, P. (1960): The effects of continuous compression on living articular cartilage. J. Bone Joint Surg. [Am.], 42:31-49.

132. Salter, R.B., and Minster, R.R. (1982): The effect of continuous passive motion on a semitendinous tenodesis in the rabbit knee (Abstract). Orthop. Trans., 6:292.

133. Salter, R.B., Simmonds, D.F., and Malcolm, B.W. (1975): The effect of continuous passive motion on the healing of articular cartilage defects: An experimental investigation in rabbits (Abstract). J. Bone Joint Surg. [Am.], 57:570.

134. Saunders, K.C., Louis, D.L., Weingarden, S.I., and Waylonis, G.W. (1979): Effect of tourniquet time on postoperative quadriceps function. Clin. Orthop. Rel. Res., 143:194-199.

135. Scranton, P.E., Lanzer, W.L., and Ferguson, M.S. (1998): Mechanism of anterior cruciate neovascularization and ligamentization. Arthroscopy, 14:702-716.

136. Shakespeare, D.T., Stokes, M., Sherman, K.P., and Young, A. (1983): The effect of knee flexion on quadriceps inhibition after meniscectomy. Clin. Sci., 65:64P-65P.

137. Shakespeare, D.T., Stokes, M., Sherman, K.P., and Young, A. (1985): Reflex inhibition of the quadriceps after menisectomy: Lack of association with pain. Clin. Physiol., 5:137-144.

138. Shelborne, K.D., Wilchkens, J.H., Mollabashy, A., and DeCarlo, M. (1991): Arthrofibrosis in acute anterior cruciate ligament reconstruction: The effect of timing on reconstruction and rehabilitation. Am. J. Sports Med., 19:332-336.

139. Sherman, K.P., Young, A., Stokes, M., and Shakespeare, D.T. (1984): Joint injury and muscle weakness. Lancet, 2:646-651.

140. Sldege, C.B. (1975): Structure, development, and function of joints. Clin. Orthop. Clin. North Am., 6:619-628.

141. Snyder-Mackler, L., Delitto, A., Bailey, S.L., and Stralka, S.W. (1995): Strength of the quadriceps femoris muscles and functional recovery after reconstruction of the anterior cruciate ligament: A prospective, randomized clinical trial of electrical stimulation. J. Bone Joint Surg. [Am.], 77:1166-1173.

142. Snyder-Mackler, L., Ladin, Z., Schepsis, A.A., and Young, J.C. (1991): Electrical stimulation of the thigh muscles after reconstruction of the anterior cruciate ligament: Effects of electrically elicited contraction of the quadriceps femoris and hamstring muscles on gait and on strength of the thigh muscles. J. Bone Joint Surg. [Am.], 73:1025-1036.

143. Soren, A., Rosenbauer, K.A., Klein, W., and Hugh, F. (1973): Morphological examinations of so-called postraumatic synovitis. Beitr. Pathol., 1950:11-30.

144. Spencer, J.D., Hayes, K.C., and Alexander, I.J. (1984): Knee joint effusion and quadriceps inhibition in man. Arch. Phys. Med. Rehab., 65:171-177.

145. Sprangue, N.F., O'Conner, R.L., and Fox, J.M. (1982): Arthroscopic treatment of postoperative knee fibroarthrosis. Clin. Orthop., 166:165-172.

146. Steinberg, F.U. (1980): The Immobilized Patient: Functional Pathology and Management. New York, Plenum Press.

147. Stetson, W.B., and Templin, K. (2002): Two versus three portal technique for routine knee arthroscopy. Am. J. Sports Med., 30:108-111.

148. Stokes, M., and Young, A. (1984): The contribution of reflex inhibition to arthrogenous muscle weakness. Clin. Sci., 67:7-14.

149. Stratford, P. (1981): Electromyography of the quadriceps femoris muscles in subjects with normal knees and acutely effused knees. Phys. Ther., 62:279-289.

150. Stravino, V.D. (1972): The synovial system. Am. J. Phys. Med., 51:312-320.

151. Swann, D., Radin, E., and Nazimiec, M. (1976): Role of hyaluronic acid on joint lubrication. Ann. Rheum. Dis., 33:318-326.

152. Tamberello, M., Mangine, R.E., and Personius, W. (1982): Patella hypomobility as a cause of extensor lag. Presented at Total Care of the Knee: Before and After Injury (Cybex Conference), Overland Park, KS, May 17-19, 1985.

153. Tardieu, C., Tabary, J.C., Tabary, C., and Tardieu, G. (1982): Adaptation of connective tissue length in immobilization in the lengthened and shortened positions in cat soleus muscle. J. Physiol., 78:214-217.

154. Thornton, G.M., Boorman, R.S., Shrive, N.G., and Frank, C.B. (2002): Medial collateral ligament autografts have increased creep response for at least two years and early immobilization makes this worse. J. Orthop. Res., 20:346-352.

155. Tipton, C.M., James, S.L., and Mergner, W. (1970): Influence of exercise on strength of medial collateral knee ligament of dogs. Am. J. Physiol., 218:894-902.

156. T'Jonck, L., Lysens, R., and De Smet, L. (1997): Open versus arthroscopic subacromial decompression: Analysis of one-year results. Physiother. Res. Int., 2:46-61.

157. Trias, A. (1961): Effects of persistent pressure on articular cartilage. J. Bone Joint Surg. [Am.], 43:376-386.

158. Uhthoff, H.K., and Jaworski, Z.F.G. (1978): Bone loss in response to long-term immobilization. J. Bone Joint Surg. [Br.], 60:420-429.

159. Van, H., Lillich, J.D., and Kawcak, C.E. (2002): Clinical evaluation of the effects of immobilization followed by remobilization and exercise on the metacarpophalangeal joint in horses. Am. J. Vet. Res., 63:282-288.

160. Veldhuizen, J.W., Verstappen, F.T., and Vroemen, J.P. (1993): Functional and morphological adaptations following four weeks of knee immobilization. Int. J. Sports Med., 14:283-287.

161. Venn, M.F. (1979): Chemical composition of human femoral and head cartilage: Influence of topographical position and fibrillation. Ann. Rheum. Dis., 38:57-62.

162. Videman, T. (1981): Changes of compression and distances between tibial and femoral condyles during immobilization of rabbit knee. Arch. Orthop. Trauma Surg., 98:289-294.

163. Vogt, F.B., Mack, P.B., and Beasley, W.G. (1965): The effect of bed rest on various parameters of physiological function. Part XII. The effect of bed rest on bone mass and calcium balance. Washington, DC, National Aeronautics and Space Administration.

164. Wahl, S., and Renstrom, R. (1991): Fibrosis in soft-tissue injuries. In: Leadbetter, W., Buckwalter, J., and Gordon, S. (eds.), Sports-Induced Inflammation: Clinical and Basic Science Concepts. Park Ridge, IL, American Academy of Orthopaedic Surgeons, pp. 63-82.

165. Wakai, A., Winter, D.C., Street, J.T., and Redmond, P.H. (2001): Pneumatic tourniquets in extremity surgery. J. Am. Acad. Orthop. Surg., 9:345-351.

166. Walsh, S., Frank, C., Shrive, N., and Hart, D. (1993): Knee immobilization inhibits biomechanical maturation of the rabbit medial collateral ligament. Clin. Orthop. Rel. Res., 297:253-261.

167. Weiss, C. (1979): Normal and osteoarthritic articular cartilage. Orthop. Clin. North Am., 10:175-189.

168. Westers, B.M. (1982): Review of the repair of defects in articular cartilage: Part I. J. Orthop. Sports Phys. Ther., 3:186-192.

169. Williams, P.E., and Goldspink, G. (1978): Changes in sarcomere length and physiological properties in immobilized muscle. J. Anat., 127:459-468.

170. Witzmann, F.A., Kim, D.H., and Fitts, R.H. (1982): Hindlimb immobilization: Length-tension and contractile properties of skeletal muscle. J. Appl. Physiol., 53:335-345.

171. Wolf, J. (1982): Das Gesetz der Transformation der Knochen. Berlin, A. Hirschwald.

172. Woo, S., Gomez, M.A., and Sites, T.J. (1987): The biomechanical and morphological changes in the medial collateral ligament of the rabbit after immobilization and remobilization. J. Bone Joint Surg. [Am.], 69:1200-1211.

173. Woo, S., Inoue, D.M., McGurk-Burleson, E., and Gomez, M.A. (1987): Treatment of the medial collateral ligament injury. II: Structure and function of canine knees in response to differing treatment regimes. Am. J. Sports Med., 15:22-29.

174. Woo, S., Matthew, J.V., and Akeson, W.H. (1975): Connective tissue response to immobility. Arthritis Rheum., 18:257-264.

175. Wright, V., Dowson, D., and Kerr, J. (1973): The structure of joints. Int. Rev. Connect. Tissue Res., 6:105-125.

176. Wronski, T., and Morey, E.R. (1982): Skeletal abnormalities in rats induced by simulated weightlessness. Metab. Bone Dis., 4:69-74.

177. Yasuda, K., and Hayashi, K. (1999): Changes in the biomechanical properties of tendons and ligaments from joint disuse. Osteoarthritis Cartilage, 7:122-129.

178. Yasuda, K., Ohkoshi, Y., Tanabe, Y., and Kaneda, K. (1992): Quantitative evaluation of knee instability and muscle strength after anterior cruciate ligament reconstruction using patellar tendon and quadriceps tendon. Am. J. Sports Med., 20:471-475.

179. Yates, C.K., McCarthy, M.R., Hirsch, H.S., and Pascale, M.S. (1992): Effects of continuous passive motion following ACL reconstruction with autogenous patellar tendon grafts. J. Sports Rehab., 1:121-131.

180. Young, A., Stokes, M., and Iles, J.F. (1987): Effects of joint pathology on muscle. Clin. Orthop., 219:21-27.

181. Young, D.R., Niklowitz, W.J., and Steele, C.R. (1983): Tibial changes in experimental disuse osteoporosis in the monkey. Calcif. Tissue Int., 35:304-308.

182. Ziechen, J., van Griensven, M., and Albers, I. (1999): Immunohistochemical localization of collagen VI in arthrofibrosis. Arch. Orthop. Trauma Surg., 119:315-318.

CHAPTER 3

BIOMECHANICAL IMPLICATIONS IN SHOULDER AND KNEE REHABILITATION

Michael M. Reinold, P.T., ATC

CHAPTER OBJECTIVES

At the end of this chapter the reader will be able to:

- Summarize the importance of a thorough knowledge of the biomechanical factors associated with rehabilitation.
- Describe the best rehabilitation exercises to elicit recruitment of the glenohumeral and scapulothoracic musculature.
- Explain the normal function of the supraspinatus and deltoid musculature during various ranges of motion.
- Identify which shoulder exercises produce the most amount of supraspinatus activity with the least amount of deltoid activity.
- Explain the effect of pathologic changes on shoulder biomechanics.
- Identify which exercises produce co-contraction of the quadriceps and hamstrings musculature.
- Explain the tibiofemoral shear forces observed during open kinetic chain and closed kinetic chain exercises.
- Describe the in vivo forces on the anterior cruciate ligament during open kinetic chain, closed kinetic chain, bicycle, and stair-climbing exercises.
- Explain the normal arthrokinematics of the patellofemoral joint.
- Summarize the stress on the patellofemoral joint during open kinetic chain and closed kinetic chain exercises.
- Select safe and appropriate exercises for the glenohumeral musculature, scapulothoracic musculature, anterior cruciate ligament, posterior cruciate ligament, and patellofemoral joint.

The biomechanical analysis of rehabilitation exercises has gained recent attention in sports medicine and orthopedic practice. Several investigators have sought to quantify the kinematics, kinetics, and electromyographic (EMG) activity during common rehabilitation exercises in an attempt to fully understand the implications of each exercise on the arthrokinematics and soft tissues of the shoulder and knee. Advances in understanding of the biomechanical factors of rehabilitation have led to enhancement of rehabilitation programs that place minimal strain on specific healing structures while returning the injured athlete to competition as quickly and safely as possible. The purpose of this chapter is to provide an overview of the biomechanical implications associated with rehabilitation of the athlete's shoulder and knee.

BIOMECHANICAL IMPLICATIONS OF SHOULDER REHABILITATION

The glenohumeral joint exhibits the greatest amount of motion of any articulation in the human body, although little inherent stability is provided by its osseous configuration. Functional stability is accomplished through the integrated functions of the joint capsule, ligaments, and glenoid labrum, as well as the neuromuscular control and dynamic stabilization of the surrounding musculature, particularly the rotator cuff muscles.[2,8,20,48] The rotator cuff musculature maintains stability by compressing the humeral head into the concave glenoid fossa during upper extremity motion.[59] Thus, the glenohumeral muscles play a vital role in normal arthrokinematics and asymptomatic shoulder function.

Rehabilitation programs for the shoulder joint often focus on restoring maximum strength and muscular balance, particularly of the rotator cuff and scapulothoracic joint. The majority of research on shoulder biomechanics has focused on quantifying the EMG activity of particular muscles during common rehabilitation exercises, the goal of which is to determine the most optimal exercise to recruit specific muscle activity.

ELECTROMYOGRAPHIC ANALYSIS OF SHOULDER EXERCISES

Townsend and associates[53] conducted one of the first comprehensive studies analyzing the EMG activity of the shoulder musculature during rehabilitation exercises. Dynamic fine-wire EMG activities of the four rotator cuff muscles, pectoralis major, latissimus dorsi, and three portions of the deltoid were studied in 15 healthy male subjects during 17 common shoulder exercises. The authors quantified the exercises that produced the most activity for each specific muscle (Table 3-1).

For the anterior deltoid, exercises involving elevation of the shoulder, such as scaption with internal rotation (empty can), scaption with external rotation (full can), and forward flexion produced the greatest amount of activity at approximately 70% manual muscle test (MMT). This was also consistent with results for the middle deltoid, although exercises in the prone position involving horizontal abduction produced approximately 80% MMT. The posterior deltoid showed the greatest amount of activity in the prone position during exercises such as horizontal abduction and rowing at approximately 90% MMT.

Similar to the anterior deltoid, the supraspinatus muscle was most active during shoulder elevation movements, although the military press (from 0 to 30°) produced the greatest amount of supraspinatus activity with 80% MMT. Comparing the empty can and full can exercises, the authors found 74% MMT during the empty can and 64% MMT during the full can.

The exercises with the most activity of the subscapularis muscle also included those involving shoulder elevation, although at moderate intensity of approximately 55% MMT. Interestingly, the side-lying internal rotation exercise was not found to produce significant activity in the subscapularis, although the similar exercise of internal rotation at 0° abduction with exercise tubing was shown to have 52% maximal voluntary contraction by Hintermeister and colleagues.[21] Others have recommended motions involving lifting the hand off the lower back and motions that replicate a tennis forehand with internal rotation and horizontal adduction.

The infraspinatus and teres minor muscles showed similar results with high activity during the side-lying external rotation exercise (85% for infraspinatus and 80% for teres minor). Exercises in the prone position involving horizontal abduction also produced high activity of the external rotators with up to 88% MMT (range 68% to 88% MMT) activity of the infraspinatus during prone horizontal abduction with external rotation.

The press-up exercise was found to elicit the most activity of the latissimus dorsi (55% MMT) and the pectoralis major (84%). This is consistent with the prime function of shoulder depression for each of these muscles. In comparison, the push-up produced 64% MMT for the pectoralis major.

Townsend and associates[53] studied 17 exercises and recommended inclusion of the empty can exercise, shoulder flexion, prone horizontal abduction with external rotation, and the press-up in shoulder rehabilitation programs based on the high activity for each muscle examined during these exercises.

Several research studies have since expanded on the work of Townsend and associates.[53] In particular, researchers have sought to compare the effectiveness of several exercises for the external rotators, supraspinatus, deltoid, and scapulothoracic musculature. The following sections will discuss each one in detail.

External Rotators

The overhead throwing athlete requires the rotator cuff to maintain an adequate amount of glenohumeral joint congruency for asymptomatic function.[58] Strength of the infraspinatus and teres minor is integral during the overhead throwing motion to develop a compressive force equal to body weight at the shoulder joint to prevent distraction.[13] Andrews and Angelo[1] found that overhead throwers most often present with rotator cuff tears located from the mid-supraspinatus posterior to the midinfraspinatus area, which they believed to be a result of the compressive force produced to resist distraction, horizontal adduction, and internal rotation at the shoulder during arm deceleration. Thus, the external rotators are muscles that often appear weak and are affected by different shoulder pathologic conditions such as internal impingement,[25,54] joint laxity, labral lesions, and rotator cuff lesions,[42,47] particularly in overhead throwing athletes.[56,61] Consequently, many authors have advocated emphasis on external rotation strengthening during rehabilitation or athletic conditioning programs to enhance muscular strength, endurance, and dynamic stability in overhead throwing athletes.

Several studies have been published to document the EMG activity of the glenohumeral musculature during specific shoulder exercises.[3,5,7,18,30,32,35,41,53,65] Variations in experimental methodology have resulted in conflicting outcomes and controversy in exercise selection. As previously discussed, Townsend and associates[53] evaluated infraspinatus and teres minor activity during 17 shoulder exercises. The authors determined that the exercise eliciting the most EMG activity for the infraspinatus muscle was prone horizontal abduction with external rotation (88% MMT), and the most effective exercise for the teres minor muscle was side-lying external rotation (80% MMT).

Table 3-1

Electromyographic Analysis of Glenohumeral Musculature

Muscle	Exercise	Peak (% MMT ± SD)	Duration (% Exercise)	Peak Arc Range (°)
Anterior deltoid	Scaption IR	72 ± 23	50	90-150
	Scaption ER	71 ± 39	30	90-120
	Flexion	69 ± 24	31	90-120
	Military press	62 ± 26	50	60-90
	Abduction	62 ± 28	31	90-120
Middle deltoid	Scaption IR	83 ± 13	70	90-120
	Horiz. abd. IR	80 ± 23	38	90-120
	Horiz. abd. ER	79 ± 20	57	90-120
	Flexion	73 ± 16	31	90-120
	Scaption ER	72 ± 13	58	90-120
	Rowing	72 ± 20	43	90-120
	Military press	72 ± 24	38	90-120
	Abduction	64 ± 13	31	90-120
	Deceleration	58 ± 20	27	90-60
Posterior deltoid	Horiz. abd. IR	93 ± 45	63	90-120
	Horiz. abd. ER	92 ± 49	57	90-120
	Rowing	88 ± 40	57	90-120
	Extension	71 ± 30	44	90-120
	External Rot.	64 ± 62	43	60-90
	Deceleration	63 ± 28	27	60-90
Supraspinatus	Military press	80 ± 48	50	0-30
	Scaption IR	74 ± 33	40	90-120
	Flexion	67 ± 14	31	90-120
	Scaption ER	64 ± 28	25	90-120
Subscapularis	Scaption IR	62 ± 33	22	120-150
	Military press	56 ± 48	50	60-90
	Flexion	52 ± 42	23	120-150
	Abduction	50 ± 44	23	120-150
Infraspinatus	Horiz. abd. ER	88 ± 25	71	90-120
	External rot.	85 ± 26	43	60-90
	Horiz. abd. IR	74 ± 32	38	90-120
	Abduction	74 ± 23	31	90-120
	Flexion	66 ± 15	23	90-120
	Scaption ER	60 ± 21	38	90-120
	Deceleration	57 ± 17	27	90-60
	Push-up (hands together)	54 ± 31	38	90-60
Teres minor	External rot.	80 ± 14	57	60-90
	Horiz. abd. ER	74 ± 28	57	60-90
	Horiz. abd. IR	68 ± 36	43	90-120
Pectoralis major	Press-up	84 ± 42	75	½ pk-pk
	Push-up (hands apart)	64 ± 63	50	60-30
Latissimus dorsi	Press-up	55 ± 27	50	pk-1 sec

From Townsend, H., Jobe, F.W., Pink, M., and Perry, J. (1991): Electromyographic analysis of the glenohumeral muscles during a baseball rehabilitation program. Am. J. Sports Med., 19:264-272.
*Ranked by intensity of peak arc.
MMT, manual muscle test; SD, standard deviation; Horiz. abd., horizontal abduction; IR, internal rotation; ER, external rotation; pk, peak.

Similarly, Blackburn and associates[5] performed EMG analysis of rotator cuff muscles in 28 healthy subjects during a series of 23 common posterior rotator cuff strengthening exercises. The authors reported high levels of EMG activity of the infraspinatus (80% EMG activity) and teres minor (70% EMG activity) when the prone horizontal abduction movement at 90 and 100° of abduction with full external rotation was performed by 28 healthy subjects.

Conversely, Greenfield and colleagues[18] compared shoulder rotational strength in the scapular and frontal planes during isokinetic testing in 20 healthy subjects. The authors reported that there were no significant differences in internal rotation strength between positions; however, external rotation strength was significantly higher in the scapular plane, suggesting that the plane of the scapula may be a more effective position to exercise the external rotators.

Ballantyne and colleagues[3] compared the EMG activity of the external rotators during side-lying external rotation with external rotation in the prone position at 90° of abduction in 40 subjects. The authors reported similar EMG findings of the infraspinatus and teres minor during both exercises with approximately 50% normalized activity for each muscle. Conversely, in the previously cited study by Blackburn and associates,[5] the authors compared side-lying external rotation and prone external rotation exercises and noted greater EMG activity during prone external rotation for the infraspinatus (prone 80%, side-lying 30%) and teres minor (prone 88%, side-lying 45%).

We have recently analyzed several different exercises commonly used to strengthen the external rotators to determine the most effect exercise and position to recruit muscle activity of the posterior rotator cuff (Reinold et al., American Sports Medicine Institute unpublished data, 2002). Integrated EMG activities of the infraspinatus, teres minor, supraspinatus, posterior deltoid, and middle deltoid of 10 asymptomatic subjects (5 male and 5 female; mean age 28.1 years; range 22 to 38 years) were analyzed during seven exercises: prone horizontal abduction at 100° of abduction, full external rotation and prone external rotation at 90° of abduction, standing external rotation at 90° abduction, standing external rotation at 45° in the scapular plane, standing external rotation at 0° of abduction, standing external rotation at 0°

of abduction with a towel roll, and side-lying external rotation at 0° of abduction.

Based on the results of this study, the exercise that elicited the most combined EMG activity for the infraspinatus and teres minor was side-lying external rotation (infraspinatus 62% maximum voluntary isometric contraction [MVIC], teres minor 62%), followed closely by external rotation in the scapular plane (infraspinatus 53%, teres minor 64%), and finally prone external rotation in the 90-degree abducted position (infraspinatus 56%, teres minor 41%) (Table 3-2).

Exercises in the 90-degree abducted position are often incorporated to simulate the position and strain on the shoulder during similar overhead activities such as throwing. This position produced moderate activity of the external rotators but also increased activity of the deltoid and supraspinatus to stabilize the shoulder. It appears that the amount of infraspinatus and teres minor activity progressively decreases as the shoulder moves into an abducted position, whereas activity of the supraspinatus and deltoid increases. This may imply that as the arm moves into a position of less shoulder stability, the supraspinatus and deltoid are active to assist in the external rotation movement while providing some degree of glenohumeral stability through muscular contraction.

In the standing position external rotation at 90° of abduction may have a functional advantage over 0° of abduction, and in the scapular plane because of the close replication of this position in sporting activities, the combination of abduction and external rotation places strain on the shoulder's capsule, particularly the anterior band of the inferior glenohumeral ligament.[43,49] When the arm is not in an abducted position, external rotation places less strain on this portion of the joint capsule. Therefore, although muscle activity was low to moderate during external

Table 3-2

Peak Muscle Activity during External Rotation exercises (% MVIC, mean ± SD)

	Prone Horizontal Abduction (100°, full ER)	Prone ER (90° Abduction)	Standing ER 90° (90° Abduction)	Standing ER Scapular Plane	Standing ER 0°	Standing ER 0° with Towel	Side-Lying ER	Significance*
Supraspinatus	82 ± 37	68 ± 33	57 ± 32	32 ± 24	41 ± 39	41 ± 37	51 ± 47	a,c,d,e
Middle deltoid	82 ± 32	49 ± 15	55 ± 23	38 ± 19	11 ± 7	11 ± 6	36 ± 23	a,b,c,f
Posterior deltoid	88 ± 33	79 ± 31	59 ± 33	43 ± 30	27 ± 27	31 ± 27	52 ± 42	a,c,d,f,g
Infraspinatus	39 ± 17	56 ± 30	59 ± 38	53 ± 24	40 ± 15	51 ± 14	62 ± 13	h
Teres minor	41 ± 24	41 ± 22	33 ± 18	64 ± 51	34 ± 14	46 ± 22	62 ± 31	

*Significant finding exercise ($p < 0.050$): a = prone horizontal abduction > ER 90°, ER scapular plane, ER 0°, ER 0° with towel, sidelying ER; b = prone horizontal abduction > prone ER; c = prone ER > ER 0° and ER 0° with towel; d = prone ER > ER scapular plane; e = prone ER > side-lying ER; f = 90° ER > ER 0° and ER 0° with towel; g = side-lying ER > ER 0° and ER 0° with towel; h = side-lying ER > prone horizontal abduction.
MVIC, maximum voluntary isometric contraction; ER, external rotation.

rotation at 0° of abduction, this rehabilitation exercise may be worthwhile when strain of the inferior glenohumeral ligament is a concern. Side-lying external rotation may be the most optimal exercise to strengthen the external rotators based on the highest amount of EMG activity observed during this study.

Theoretically, external rotation at 0° of abduction with a towel roll provides both the low capsular strain and also a good balance between the muscles that externally rotate the arm and the muscles that adduct the arm to hold the towel. Our clinical experience has shown that adding a towel roll to the external rotation exercise provides assistance to the patient by ensuring that proper technique is observed without muscle substitution (Fig. 3-1). With the addition of a towel roll to the exercise a tendency toward higher activity of the posterior rotator cuff was seen consistently as well. An approximately 20% to 25% increase in infraspinatus and teres minor EMG activity was noted with the use of a towel roll.

Furthermore, external rotation in the scapular plane may be an effective exercise during rehabilitation because of the moderate amount of muscular activity of each of the muscles tested, with a moderate amount of capsular strain in

the 45° abducted position (Fig. 3-2). This exercise may offer a compromise between strengthening and stabilization.

CLINICAL PEARL #1

The exercises that produced the greatest amount of activity of the external rotators were side-lying external rotation, external rotation in the scapular plane, and external rotation at 90° abduction (both standing and in the prone position).

CLINICAL PEARL #2

As the angle of arm elevation increases during shoulder external rotation exercises, the amount of supraspinatus and deltoid activity increases while the amount of infraspinatus and teres minor activity decrease.

CLINICAL PEARL #3

Adding a towel roll to ER at 0° of abduction results in higher activity of EMG activity of the infraspinatus and teres minor.

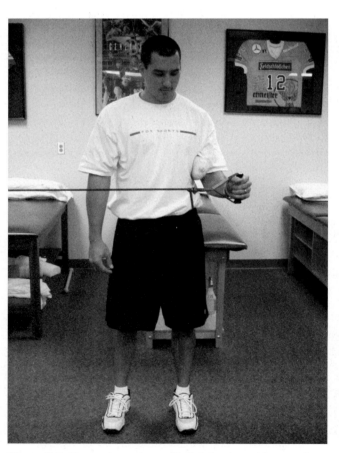

Figure 3-1. External rotation at 0° of abduction with a towel roll placed between the arm and the body.

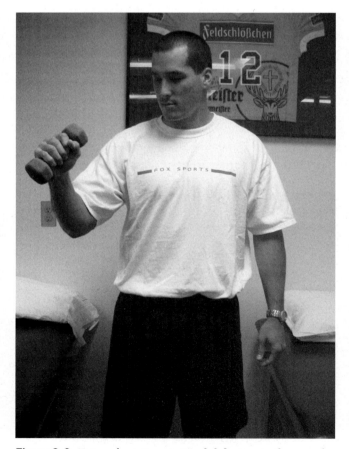

Figure 3-2. External rotation at 45° of abduction in the scapular plane.

Supraspinatus and Deltoid

Numerous investigators have studied the EMG activity of the supraspinatus during rehabilitation exercises. Controversy exists regarding the optimal exercise to elicit muscle activity. Jobe and Moynes[26] were the first to recommend elevation in the scapular plane with internal rotation, or the empty can exercise. The authors recommended this exercise for supraspinatus strengthening because of the high EMG activity observed during this movement. The recommendation of the empty can exercise was further strengthened by the work of Townsend and associates[53] who reported greater amounts of EMG activity of the supraspinatus and deltoid muscles during the empty can exercise compared with those seen with elevation in the scapular plane with external rotation or the full can exercise, although statistical analysis was not performed to compare exercises (see Table 3-1).

In clinical studies, numerous authors have suggested that the empty can exercise may provoke pain in many patients by encroaching the soft tissue within the subacromial space during this impingement type maneuver. Numerous authors have since compared the empty can exercise with several other common supraspinatus exercises to determine whether exercises that place the shoulder in less of a disadvantageous position elicit similar amounts of supraspinatus activity.

Blackburn and associates[5] compared the EMG activity of the rotator cuff during several exercises and reported no significant differences in supraspinatus activity during the empty can and full can exercises. However, the authors did report a statistically significant increase in supraspinatus activity during the prone horizontal abduction at 100° with full external rotation exercise (Fig. 3-3).

Worrell and associates[65] compared the amount of supraspinatus activity during the empty can exercise

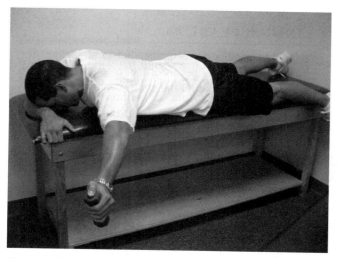

Figure 3-3. Prone horizontal abduction at 100° abduction and full external rotation.

recommended by Jobe and Moynes[26] and the prone horizontal abduction exercise recommended by Blackburn and associates.[5] The authors used fine-wire EMG and hand-held dynamometer measurements in 22 healthy subjects. The authors reported greater supraspinatus activity during the prone exercise although less total force production than the empty can exercise. The authors hypothesized that although supraspinatus activity was greater in the prone position, a greater amount of surrounding muscular activity was noted during the empty can exercise.

The effect of increased deltoid activity during arm elevation is a concern for the rehabilitation specialist, especially when a patient with subacromial impingement or rotator cuff pathologic conditions is being rehabilitated. Morrey and colleagues[37] examined the resultant force vectors of the deltoid and supraspinatus during arm elevation at various degrees of motion. Deltoid activity alone exhibited a superiorly orientated force vector from 0 to 90° and a compressive force on the glenohumeral joint at 120 to 150°. Conversely, the supraspinatus muscle produced a consistent compressive force throughout the range of elevation (Fig. 3-4). In patients with subacromial impingement, weak posterior rotator cuff muscles, inefficient dynamic stabilization, or rotator cuff pathologic changes, exercises that produce high levels of deltoid activity, may be detrimental because of the amount of superior humeral head migration observed when the rotator cuff does not efficiently compress the humeral head within the glenoid fossa. Therefore, exercises are often chosen to minimize the opportunity for the deltoid to overpower the rotator cuff musculature during arm elevation.

Based on the hypothesis of Worrell and associates,[65] Malanga and colleagues[32] examined the EMG activity of the supraspinatus and deltoid muscles during the empty can and prone exercises in 17 healthy subjects. The authors reported no significant differences in supraspinatus EMG activity during the two exercises (107% empty can, 94% prone). However, a statistically significant increase in posterior deltoid EMG activity was observed during the prone exercise (76% empty can, 96% prone) and significantly greater anterior deltoid EMG activity during the empty can exercise (96% empty can, 65% prone). Middle deltoid EMG activity was high during both exercises (104% empty can, 111% prone).

In a similar study, Kelley and colleagues[29] compared the isometric EMG activity of supraspinatus and deltoid muscles during the full can and empty can exercises in 11 healthy subjects. The authors again reported no significant difference in supraspinatus activity; however, they did note that the least amount of surrounding muscle activity was observed during the full can position and therefore recommended this position for manual muscle testing of the supraspinatus.

Takeda and associates[52] examined the most effective exercise for strengthening of the supraspinatus using

The authors developed a rank order of exercises that elicited the greatest amount of serratus activity. The three exercises that were suggested were the push-up with a plus

supraspinatus may allow superior migration of the numeral head, rather than glenohumeral joint compression, causing impingement within the subacromial space.

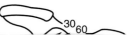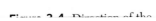

Table 3-4

Electromyographic Analysis of Scapulothoracic Musculature

Muscle	Exercise	Duration Qualified (% of Exercise)	Peak Arc (% MMT ± SD)	Peak Arc Range	Function
Upper trapezius	Rowing	75	112 ± 84	Isometric*	Retraction
	Military press	27	64 ± 26	150-peak	Upward rotation
	Horiz abd. w/ER	33	75 ± 27	Isometric*	Retraction
	Horiz. abd. (neutral)	33	62 ± 53	90-peak	Retraction
	Scaption	23	54 ± 16	120-150	Upward rotation
	Abduction	31	52 ± 30	90-120	Upward rotation
Middle trapezius	Horiz. abd. (neutral)	78	108 ± 63	90-peak	Retraction
	Horiz. abd. w/ER	67	96 ± 73	Peak-90	Retraction
	Extension (prone)	27	77 ± 49	Neutral-30	Retraction
	Rowing	33	59 ± 51	90-120	Retraction
Lower trapezius	Abduction	50	68 ± 53	90-150	Upward rotation
	Rowing	50	67 ± 50	120-150	Retraction
	Horiz. abd. w/ER	33	63 ± 41	90-peak	Retraction
	Flexion	23	60 ± 18	120-150	Upward rotation
	Horiz. abd. (neutral)	33	56 ± 24	90-peak	Retraction
	Scaption	23	60 ± 22	120-150	Upward rotation
Levator scapulae	Rowing	78	114 ± 69	Isometric*	Retraction
	Horiz. abd. (neutral)	67	96 ± 57	Isometric*	Retraction
	Shrug	63	88 ± 32	Isometric*	Elevation
	Horiz. abd. w/ER	33	87 ± 66	Isometric*	Retraction
	Extension (prone)	36	81 ± 76	Isometric*	Elevation
	Scaption	46	69 ± 46	120-150	Retraction
Rhomboids	Horiz. abd. (neutral)	33	66 ± 38	90-peak	Retraction
	Scaption	25	65 ± 79	120-150	Retraction
	Abduction	31	64 ± 53	90-150	Retraction
	Rowing	30	56 ± 46	Isometric*	Retraction
Middle serratus anterior	Flexion	69	96 ± 45	120-150	Up. rot./protract.
	Abduction	54	96 ± 53	120-150	Up. rot./protract.
	Scaption	58	91 ± 52	120-150	Up. rot./protract.
	Military press	64	82 ± 36	150-peak	Up. rot./protract.
	Push up w/a plus	28	80 ± 38	Plus man.	Up. rot./protract.
	Push up hands apart	21	57 ± 36	Last arc of push up	Up. rot./protract.
Lower serratus anterior	Scaption	50	84 ± 20	120-150	Up. rot./protract.
	Abduction	54	74 ± 65	120-150	Up. rot./protract.
	Flexion	31	72 ± 46	120-150	Up. rot./protract.
	Push up with a plus	67	72 ± 3	Chest moving away from floor	Up. rot./protract.
	Push up hands apart	21	69 ± 31	Isometric as the chest was near the floor	Up. rot./protract.
	Military press	36	60 ± 42	120-150	Up. rot./protract.
Pectoralis minor	Press up	75	89 ± 62	Isometric*	Depression
	Push up with a plus	34	58 ± 45	Plus man.	Protraction
	Push up with hands apart	50	55 ± 34	2nd to last arc	Protraction

*Isometric contractions were at the extreme of the range of motion.
MMT, manual muscle test; SD, standard deviation; Horiz. abd., horizontal abduction; IR, internal rotation; ER, external rotation; Up. rot./protract., upward rotation and protraction.
From Moseley, J.B., Jr, Jobe, F.W., Pink, M., et al. (1992): EMG analysis of the scapular muscles during a shoulder rehabilitation program. Am. J. Sports Med., 20:128-134.

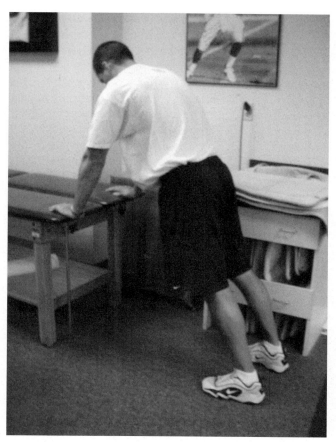

Figure 3-6. Push-up on a table top with a plus. The patient is instructed to fully protract their shoulder blade at the top of the push-up.

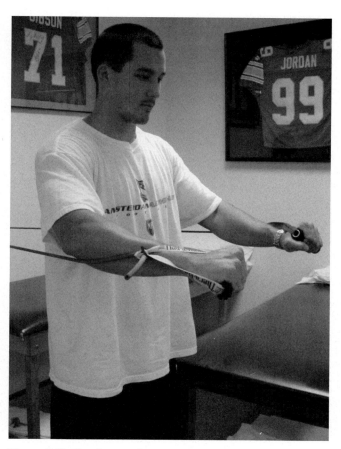

Figure 3-7. The dynamic hug exercise. Using resistance, the patient horizontally adducts the shoulder at 60° of elevation while protracting the scapula.

McMahon and associates[36] compared the EMG activity of the rotator cuff and scapulothoracic muscles in 15 normal shoulders and 23 shoulders with anterior instability. Subjects performed EMG testing of abduction, scaption, and forward flexion before surgical intervention for unidirectional anterior stabilization. The authors reported a statistically significant decrease in supraspinatus activity during abduction and scaption from 30 to 60° in subjects with instability. During all three movements, a statistically significant decrease in serratus anterior activity was also observed in subjects with instability. This occurred in the range of 30 to 120° of abduction and at 0 to 120° of scaption.

The authors suggested that the decreased amount of supraspinatus activity may result in disadvantageous superior humeral head migration and affect the amount of abnormal glenohumeral translation. Blasier and colleagues[6] reported that the supraspinatus muscle is highly active in shoulder joint stabilization, with an 18% reduction of force needed for subluxation of the glenohumeral joint when the supraspinatus muscle was not active.

Furthermore, the finding of decreased serratus anterior activity is also important in patients with shoulder instability. Decreased serratus anterior activity has also been observed in baseball pitchers with anterior instability[17] and swimmers with shoulder pain.[49] The authors suggested that the decreased amount of serratus anterior activity may result in an inability to position the scapula in an upward position during shoulder elevation and thus alter the position and length-tension relationship of the static and dynamic stabilizers of the shoulder.

CLINICAL PEARL #5

EMG activity of the rotator cuff is decreased in shoulders with subacromial impingement and anterior shoulder instability.

CLINICAL PEARL #6

Based on the EMG results of these studies, the Thrower's Ten Exercise Program (see Appendix A) is recommended for athletes to strengthen the glenohumeral and scapulothoracic muscles need to perform competitively.

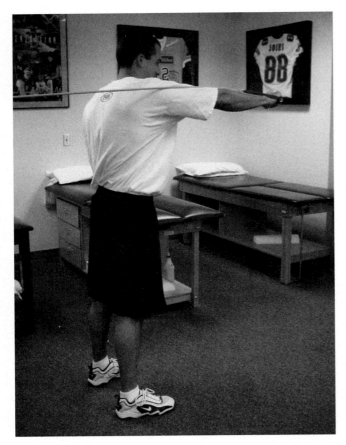

Figure 3-8. The standing serratus anterior punch exercise. The patient protracts the shoulder blade against resistance.

BIOMECHANICAL IMPLICATIONS OF KNEE REHABILITATION

Several methods of biomechanical analysis have been used to study rehabilitation of the knee, including cadaveric, electromyographic, kinematic, kinetic, mathematical modeling, and in vivo strain gauge measurements. To best evaluate these studies, it is helpful to delineate the findings based on the tissue or structure being examined, such as the anterior cruciate ligament (ACL), posterior cruciate ligament (PCL), and patellofemoral joint.

Anterior Cruciate Ligament

The majority of biomechanical research during rehabilitation of the knee has focused on the ACL. The efficacy of open kinetic chain (OKC) and closed kinetic chain (CKC) exercises have been heavily scrutinized after years of theoretical and anecdotal assumptions. Markolf and colleagues[33] examined the effect of compressive loads on cadaveric knees to simulate body weight. The authors reported that compressive forces reduce strain on the ACL compared with OKC exercises, thus providing a protective mechanism. Fleming and associates[16] investigated this

theory with in vivo strain gauge measurements within the ACL. The use of in vivo strain gauge measurements within the ACL have allowed a method of direct measurement of ACL strain during activity. The authors noted that strain on the ACL increased from −2.0% during non–weight bearing to 2.1% in a weight-bearing position. Although an increase in ACL strain was observed in a weight-bearing position, it is still unclear whether a 2% strain is detrimental to the healing ACL graft, although clinical experience has shown that early weight bearing has not resulted in poor functional outcomes in ACL reconstructions postoperatively.

CKC exercises have also been theorized to reduce ACL strain by providing co-contraction of the hamstrings and quadriceps. Wilk and co-workers[60] examined the EMG activity of the quadriceps and hamstrings during the CKC squat, leg press, and OKC knee extension. The authors noted that co-contraction occurred from 30 to 0° during the ascent phase of the squat, when the body is positioned directly over the knees and feet, but did not occur at other ranges of motion or during the CKC leg press or OKC knee extension. Thus, not all CKC exercises produce a co-contraction of the quadriceps and hamstrings. Rather, it appears that several factors affect the muscle activation during CKC exercises including knee flexion angle, body position relative to the knee, and the direction of movement (ascending or descending). Clinically, exercises performed in an upright and weight-bearing position with the knee flexed to approximately 30°, such as squats and lateral lunges, may be used during knee rehabilitation to promote co-contraction of the quadriceps and hamstrings.

Wilk and co-workers[60] also used mathematical modeling to estimate the shear forces at the tibiofemoral joint during the squat, leg press, and knee extension exercise (Fig. 3-9). The authors report that a posterior tibiofemoral shear force was observed during the entire range of motion during both CKC squatting and leg press (peak 1500 N), and during deep angles of OKC knee extension from 100 to 40° (peak 900 N). Anterior tibiofemoral shear force (peak 250 N) and theoretically ACL strain were observed during the OKC knee extension exercise from 40 to 10°.

Similar to the results of Wilk and co-workers,[60] Beynnon and associates[4] reported that the greatest amount of ACL strain (2.8%) occurred during 40 to 0° during OKC knee extension using in vivo strain-gauge measurements. This strain was found to significantly increase in a linear fashion with the application of an external 45-N boot (3.8%). However, the authors also reported ACL strain during the CKC squat exercise of 3.6%. In contrast, the application of external loading did not significantly increase the amount of strain on the ACL (4.0%). Based on the results of these studies,[4,16,60] both OKC and CKC exercises are performed, although the patient is often limited to 90 to 40° during the OKC knee extension when heavy resistance is applied.

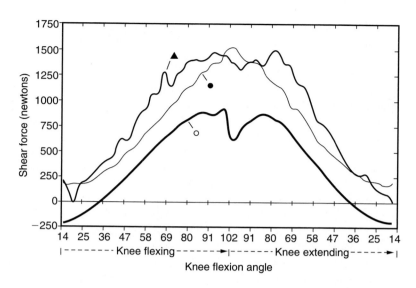

Figure 3-9. Shear forces at the tibiofemoral joint during the squat (filled triangles), leg press (small points), and knee extension exercise (open circles). (From Wilk, K.E., Escamilla, R.F., Fleisig, G.S., et al. [1996]: A comparison of the tibiofemoral joint forces and electromyographic activity during open and closed kinetic chain exercises. Am. J. Sports Med., 24:518-527.)

Also commonly used during ACL rehabilitation are the bicycle and stair-climbing machines. Fleming and colleagues[14] analyzed six different bicycle-riding conditions, manipulating speed and power. The authors found no significant differences between conditions with a minimal mean ACL strain of 1.7%. The greatest amount of strain was observed when the knee reached the greatest amount of extension. Similarly, Fleming and colleagues[15] analyzed two cadences of stair climbing (80 and 112 steps per minute) and noted a similar 2.7% strain on the ACL. Again, the most amount of strain was observed during terminal knee extension. Thus, both bicycling and stair climbing are safe exercises with low strain on the ACL compared with other rehabilitation exercises (Table 3-5). Furthermore, the greatest amount of strain was observed as the knee moved into terminal knee extension similar to the results of Wilk and co-workers[60] and Beynnon and associates[4] during OKC and CKC exercises.

CLINICAL PEARL #7

Open kinetic chain knee extension may be performed from 90° to 40° with progressive resistance to minimize strain on the ACL.

CLINICAL PEARL #8

Weight bearing and closed kinetic chain exercises may be performed immediately without placing excessive strain on the ACL.

CLINICAL PEARL #9

Closed kinetic chain exercise in the upright position with the knee flexed to 30° (such as squatting and lateral lunges) may be used to promote co-contraction of the quadriceps and hamstrings.

CLINICAL PEARL #10

Bicycling and stair climbing may be performed with minimal strain on the ACL.

Posterior Cruciate Ligament

Historically, the results of rehabilitation after injury of the PCL have been mixed. Poor functional outcomes have

Table 3-5

In Vivo Strain on the Anterior Cruciate Ligament*

Exercise	Strain (%)
Isometric quadriceps contraction at 15°	4.4
Squatting with resistance	4.0
Active knee flexion with resistance	3.8
Lachman test (150 N of anterior shear at 30°)	3.7
Squatting without resistance	3.6
Active knee flexion without resistance	2.8
Quadriceps and hamstring co-contraction at 15°	2.7
Isometric quadriceps contraction at 30°	2.7
Stair climbing	2.7
Anterior drawer test (150 N anterior shear at 90°)	1.8
Stationary bicycle	1.7
Quadriceps and hamstrings co-contraction at 30°	0.4
Passive knee range of motion	0.1
Isometric quadriceps contraction at 60° and 90°	0.0
Quadriceps and hamstrings co-contraction at 60° and 90°	0.0
Isometric hamstring contraction at 30°, 60°, and 90°	0.0

*Modified from Fleming, B.C., Beynnon, B.D., Renstrom, P.A., et al. (1999): The strain behavior of the anterior cruciate ligament during stair climbing: an in vivo study. Arthroscopy, 15:185-191.

often been attributed to residual laxity present after surgical reconstruction. The biomechanics of the tibiofemoral joint during exercise must be understood so that the rehabilitative process will not create deleterious effects on the PCL. Posterior tibiofemoral shear forces that occur during specific activities such as level walking,[39] ascending and descending stairs,[38] and resisted knee flexion exercises[28,50] have been previously documented.[55,57] Level walking and descending stairs have a relatively low posterior tibiofemoral shear force of 0.4 × body weight (BW) and 0.6 × BW, respectively (Table 3-6). However, high posterior shear force has been noted during several commonly performed activities of daily living such as climbing stairs (1.7 × BW at 45° of knee flexion)[9,38] and squatting (3.6 × BW at 140° of knee flexion) that may have an effect on residual laxity postoperatively. Further studies show that isometric knee flexion at 45° places a posterior shear force of 1.1 × BW on the tibiofemoral joint.[50]

Tremendous shear forces on both the PCL and the tibiofemoral joint occur during OKC resisted knee flexion. Posterior tibial displacement is attributed to the high EMG activity of the hamstring muscle while resistive knee flexion is performed. Lutz and colleagues reported a maximum shear force of 1780 N at 90° of flexion, 1526 N at 60°, and 939 N at 30° during isometric knee flexion (Fig. 3-10). Kaufman and associates[28] also noted a PCL load of 1.7 × BW at 75° of flexion during the isokinetic knee flexion exercise. Because PCL stress increases with knee flexion angle, isolated OKC knee flexion exercises should be avoided for at least 8 weeks postoperatively and until symptoms subside nonoperatively.

Excessive stress on the PCL has also been observed during deeper angles of OKC knee extension. Several studies have proved that resisted knee extension at 90° of flexion causes a posterior tibiofemoral shear force and potential stress on the PCL.[10,27,28,31,60] Wilk and co-workers[60] documented a posterior shear force from 100 to 40° with resisted OKC knee extension (see Fig. 3-9). The highest amount of stress on the PCL existed at angles of 85 to 95° during knee flexion. Conversely, the lowest amount of posterior shear force occurred from 60 to 0° of resisted knee extension.[60] Kaufman and associates[28] also reported

that posterior shear forces take place until 50 to 55° of knee flexion. Furthermore, Jurist and Otis[27] also documented stress on the PCL at 60° of flexion during an isometric knee extension exercise when resistance was applied at the proximal tibia. To reduce the excessive posterior shear force placed on the PCL, OKC resisted knee extension should be performed from 60 to 0°.[55,57]

The stress applied to the PCL while CKC exercises are performed is relative to the knee flexion angle produced during the exercise. Wilk and co-workers[60,63] reported an increase in posterior shear force as the knee flexion angle increases during CKC exercise (see Fig. 3-9). Meglan and associates[34] also documented a linear increase in posterior shear force from 40 to 100° of knee flexion during the front squat maneuver. Therefore, to reduce PCL stress during CKC exercises, leg presses and squats are performed from 0 to 60° of the knee flexion.[55,57]

CLINICAL PEARL #11

Open kinetic chain knee flexion produces high posterior tibiofemoral shear forces and should initially be limited to minimize strain on the PCL.

CLINICAL PEARL #12

Open kinetic chain knee extension may be performed from 60° to 0° to minimize strain on the PCL.

CLINICAL PEARL #13

Closed kinetic chain exercise may be performed from 0° to 30°, progressing to 0° to 45°, and 0° to 60° as the patient's condition improves, to minimize strain on the PCL.

Patellofemoral Joint

When one is rehabilitating a patient with a known lesion of the patellofemoral joint, it is important to first understand the normal patellofemoral joint arthrokinematics. Articulation between the inferior margin of the patella and the femur begins at approximately 10 to 20° of knee flexion.[23]

Table 3-6

Posterior Tibiofemoral Shear Forces

Source	Activity	Knee Angle (°)	Force (× Body Weight)
Kaufman et al.[28]	60°/s flexion isokinetic	75	1.7
	180°/s flexion isokinetic	75	1.4
Morrison[39]	Level walking	5	0.4
Morrison[38]	Descending stairs	5	0.6
	Ascending stairs	45	1.7
Smidt[50]	Isometric flexion	45	1.1

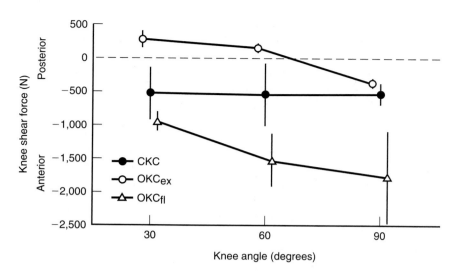

Figure 3-10. Shear force at the tibiofemoral joint during squatting, knee extension and knee flexion. (From Lutz, G.E., Palmitier, R.A., An, K.N., and Chao, E.Y. [1993]: Comparison of tibiofemoral joint forces during open and closed kinetic chain exercises. J. Bone Joint Surg., 75A:732-735.)

As the knee proceeds into greater degrees of knee flexion, the contact area of the patellofemoral joint moves proximally along the patella. At 30°, the area of patellofemoral contact is approximately 2.0 cm.[2,23] The area of contact gradually increases as the knee is flexed. At 90° of knee flexion the contact area increases up to 6.0 cm.[2,23]

Alterations in the Q angle are often associated with patellofemoral disorders and may alter the contact areas and thus the amount of joint reaction forces of the patellofemoral joint. Huberti and Hayes[22] examined in vitro patellofemoral contact pressures at various degrees of knee flexion from 20 to 120°. The maximum contact area occurred at 90° of knee flexion with a force estimated to be 6.5 × BW. An increase or decrease in the Q angle of 10° resulted in increased maximum contact pressure and a smaller total area of contact throughout the range of motion. This information may be applied when one prescribes rehabilitation interventions so that exercises are performed in ranges of motion that place minimal strain on damaged structures.

The effectiveness and safety of OKC and CKC exercises during patellofemoral rehabilitation have been heavily scrutinized in recent years. Whereas CKC exercises replicate functional activities such as ascending and descending stairs, OKC exercises are often desired for isolated muscle strengthening when specific muscle weakness is present.[62]

Steinkamp and associates[51] analyzed patellofemoral joint biomechanics during leg press and extension exercises in 20 normal subjects. Patellofemoral joint reaction force, stress, and moments were calculated during both exercises (Fig. 3-11). From 0 to 46° of knee flexion, patellofemoral joint reaction force was less during the CKC leg press. Conversely, from 50 to 90° of knee flexion, joint reaction forces were lower during the OKC knee extension exercise. Joint reaction forces were minimal at 90° of knee flexion during the knee extension exercise.

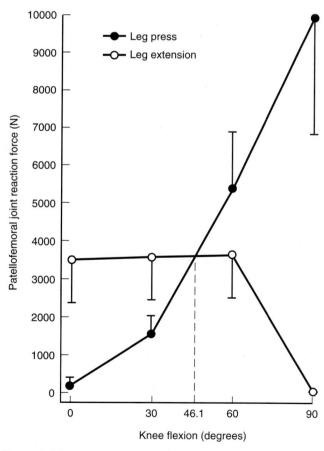

Figure 3-11. Patellofemoral joint reaction forces during the leg press and leg extension exercises. (From Steinkamp, L.A., Dillingham, M.F., Markel, M.D., et al. [1993]: Biomechanical considerations in patellofemoral joint rehabilitation. Am. J. Sports Med., 21:438-444.)

Escamilla and co-workers[12] observed the patellofemoral compressive forces during OKC knee extension and CKC leg press and vertical squat. Results were similar to the findings of Steinkamp and associates[51]; OKC knee extension produced significantly greater forces at angles less than 57° of knee flexion whereas both CKC activities produced significantly greater forces at knee angles greater than 85°.

When analyzing the biomechanics of the OKC knee extension, Grood and colleagues[19] reported that quadriceps force was greatest near full knee extension and increased with the addition of external loading. The small patellofemoral contact area observed near full extension, as previously discussed, and the increased amount of quadriceps force generated at these angles may make the patellofemoral joint more susceptible to injury. As the knee approaches terminal extension, the large magnitude of the quadriceps is focused onto a more condensed location on the patella. When one applies the results of Steinkamp and associates,[51] Escamilla and co-workers,[12] and Grood and colleagues,[19] it appears that during OKC knee extension, as the contact area of the patellofemoral joint decreases, the force of quadriceps pull subsequently increased, resulting in a large magnitude of patellofemoral contact stress being applied to a focal point on the patella. In contrast, during CKC exercises, the quadriceps force increases as the knee continues into flexion. However, the area of patellofemoral contact also increases as the knee flexes, leading to a wider dissipation of contact stress over a larger surface area.

Recently, Witvrouw and associates[64] prospectively studied the efficacy of OKC and CKC exercises during nonoperative patellofemoral rehabilitation. Sixty patients participated in a 5-week exercise program consisting of either OKC or CKC exercises. Subjective pain scores, functional ability, quadriceps and hamstring peak torque, and hamstring, quadriceps, and gastrocnemius flexibility were all recorded before and after rehabilitation as well as at 3 months after intervention. Both treatment groups reported a significant decrease in pain, an increase in muscle strength, and an increase in functional performance at 3 months after intervention.

Thus, it appears that both OKC and CKC exercises may be used to maximize the outcomes for patients with patellofemoral joint problems if performed within a safe range of motion. Exercises are based on the clinical assessment. If CKC exercises are less painful than OKC exercises, then that form of muscular training is encouraged. Additionally, in postoperative patients, regions of articular cartilage wear is carefully considered before an exercise program is designed. Mostly we allow OKC exercises such as knee extension from 90 to 40° of knee flexion. This range of motion provides the lowest amount of patellofemoral joint reaction forces while exhibiting the greatest amount of patellofemoral contact area. CKC

exercises such as the leg press, vertical squats, lateral step-ups, and wall squats (slides) are performed initially from 0 to 30° and then progressed to 0 to 60° where patellofemoral joint reaction forces are lowered. As patient symptoms subside, the ranges of motion that are performed are progressed to allow greater muscle strengthening in larger ranges. Exercises are progressed based on the patient's subjective reports of symptoms and the clinical assessment of swelling, ROM, and painful crepitus.

CLINICAL PEARL #14

Open kinetic chain knee extension may be performed from 90° to 40° to produce the lowest amount of patellofemoral joint reaction forces with the greatest amount of patella surface contact.

CLINICAL PEARL #15

Closed kinetic chain exercise may be performed initially at 0° to 45°, progressing to 0° to 60° as the patient's condition improves, to produce the lowest amount of patellofemoral joint reaction forces.

CLINICAL PEARL #16

Exercise prescription should be based on location of the symptoms and symptom reproduction during exercises.

A thorough understanding of the biomechanical factors associated with rehabilitation is necessary to return the injured athlete to competition as quickly and safely as possible. Various factors are associated with specific pathologic conditions that will alter the rehabilitation program to minimize stress on healing structures. Knowledge of the biomechanical implications discussed in this chapter may be used when rehabilitation programs are designed for patients with rotator cuff, ACL, PCL, and patellofemoral joint pathologic conditions.

SUMMARY

Overview

- Knowledge of the biomechanical implications to rehabilitation is a vital component to successful treatment prescription.
- Exercises vary based on the specific pathologic conditions.

Shoulder Rehabilitation

- Several exercises may be effective in the strengthening of the rotator cuff, glenohumeral, and scapulothoracic musculature.

■ Shoulder rehabilitation exercises may be adjusted or performed in different positions to minimize activity of and strain on specific healing structures.

■ The diagnosis of specific shoulder pathologic conditions may have an effect on the biomechanics of the shoulder.

Knee Rehabilitation

■ Not all closed kinetic chain exercises produce co-contraction of the quadriceps and hamstring muscles.

■ The amount of co-contraction varies depending on several factors including body position and direction of movement (ascent and descent phases).

■ The use of both open and closed kinetic chain exercises may be advantageous in the rehabilitation of anterior cruciate ligament, posterior cruciate ligament, and patellofemoral joint pathologic conditions if performed in safe ranges of motion that apply minimal stress on the injured structures.

REFERENCES

1. Andrews, J.R., and Angelo, R.L. (1988): Shoulder arthroscopy for the throwing athlete. Tech. Orthop., 3:75.
2. Apreleva, M., Hasselman, C.T., Debski, R.E., et al. (1998): A dynamic analysis of glenohumeral motion after simulated capsulolabral injury. J. Bone Joint Surg. [Am.], 80:474-480.
3. Ballantyne, B.T., O'Hare, S.J., Paschall, J.L., et al. (1993): Electromyographic activity of selected shoulder muscles in commonly used therapeutic exercises. Phys. Ther., 73:668-677.
4. Beynnon, B.D., Johnson, R.J., Flemming, B.C., et al. (1997): The strain behavior of the anterior cruciate ligament during squatting and active flexio-extension: A comparison of an open and closed kinetic chain exercise. Am. J. Sports Med., 25:823-829.
5. Blackburn, T.A., McLeod, W.D., and White, B. (1990): EMG analysis of posterior rotator cuff exercises. Athl. Train., 25:40-45.
6. Blasier, R.B., Guldberg, R.E., and Rothman, E.D. (1992): Anterior shoulder stability: Contributions of rotator cuff forces and the capsular ligaments in a cadaveric model. J. Shoulder Elbow Surg., 1:140.
7. Bradley, J.P., and Tibone, J.E. (1991): Electromyographic analysis of muscle action about the shoulder. Clin. Sports Med., 10:805.
8. Cain, P.R., Mutsehler, T.A., and Fu, F.H. (1987): Anterior stability of the glenohumeral joint. A dynamic model. Am. J. Sports Med., 15:144-148.
9. Clancy, W.G. (1988): Repair and reconstruction of the posterior cruciate ligament. In: Chapman, M.W. (ed.): Operative Orthopaedics. Philadelphia, J.B. Lippincott, pp. 2093-2107.
10. Daniel, D.M., Stone, M.L., Barnett, P., et al. (1988): Use of quadriceps active test to diagnose posterior cruciate ligament disruptions and measure posterior laxity of the knee. J. Bone Joint Surg., 70:386-390.
11. Decker, M.J., Hintermiester, R.A., Faber, K.J., and Hawkins, R.J. (1999): Serratus anterior muscle activity during selected rehabilitation exercises. Am. J. Sports Med., 27:784-791.
12. Escamilla, R.F., Fleisig, G.S., Zheng, N., et al. (1998): Biomechanics of the knee during closed kinetic chain and open kinetic chain exercises. Med. Sci. Sports Exerc., 30556-30569.
13. Fleisig, G.S., Barrentine, S.W., Escamilla, R.F., and Andrews, J.R. (1996): Biomechanics of overhand throwing with implications for injuries. Sports Med., 21:421-437.
14. Fleming, B.C., Beynnon, B.D., Renstrom, P.A., et al. (1998): The strain behavior of the anterior cruciate ligament during bicycling: an in vivo study. Am. J. Sports Med., 26:109-118.
15. Fleming, B.C., Beynnon, B.D., Renstrom, P.A., et al. (1999): The strain behavior of the anterior cruciate ligament during stair climbing: an in vivo study. Arthroscopy, 15:185-191.
16. Fleming, B.C., Renstrom, P.A., Beynnon, B.D., et al. (2001): The effect of weightbearing and external loading on anterior cruciate ligament strain. J. Biomech., 34:163-170.
17. Glousman, R., Jobe, F., Tibone, J., et al. (1988): Dynamic electromyographic analysis of the throwing shoulder with glenohumeral instability. J. Bone Joint Surg. [Am.], 70:220-226.
18. Greenfield, B.H., Donatelli, R., Wooden, M.J., and Wilkes, J. (1990): Isokinetic evaluation of shoulder rotational strength between the plane of the scapula and the frontal plane. Am. J. Sports Med., 18:124-128.
19. Grood, E.S., Suntay, W.J., Noyes, F.R., and Butler, D.L. (1984): Biomechanics of the knee-extension exercise. Effect of cutting the anterior cruciate ligament. J. Bone Joint Surg., 66A:725-734.
20. Harryman, D.T., II, Sidles, J.A., Clark, J.A., et al. (1990): Translation of the humeral head on the glenoid with passive glenohumeral motion. J. Bone Joint Surg., 72A:1334-1343.
21. Hintermeister, R.A., Lange, G.W., and Schultheis, et al. (1998): Electromyographic activity and applied load during shoulder rehabilitation exercises using elastic resistance. Am. J. Sports Med., 26:210-220.
22. Huberti, H.H., and Hayes, W.C. (1984): Patellofemoral contact pressures. J. Bone Joint Surg., 66A:715-724.
23. Hungerford, D.S., and Barry, M. (1979): Biomechanics of the patellofemoral joint. Clin. Orthop., 144:9-15.
24. Itoi, E., Kido, T., Sano, A., et al. (1999): Which is more useful, the "full can test" or the "empty can test," in detecting the torn supraspinatus tendon. Am. J. Sports Med., 27:65-68.
25. Jobe, F.W., Kvitne, R.S., and Giangarra, C.E. (1989): Shoulder pain in the overhand or throwing athlete. The relationship of anterior instability and rotator cuff impingement. Orthop. Rev., 18:963-975.
26. Jobe, F.W., and Moynes, D.R. (1982): Delineation of diagnostic criteria and a rehabilitation program for rotator cuff injuries. Am. J. Sports Med., 10:336-339.
27. Jurist, K.A., and Otis, J.C. (1985): Anteroposterior tibiofemoral displacements during isometric extension efforts. Am. J. Sports Med., 13:254-258.
28. Kaufman, K.R., An, K.N., Litchy, W.J., et al. (1991): Dynamic joint forces during knee isokinetic exercise. Am. J. Sports Med., 19:305-316.
29. Kelly, B.T., Kadrmas, W.R., and Speer, K.P. (1996): The manual muscle examination for rotator cuff strength: An electromyographic investigation. Am. J. Sports Med., 24:581-588.
30. Kronberg, M., Nemeth, G., and Brostrom, L.A. (1990): Muscle activity and coordination in the normal shoulder—An electromyographic study. Clin. Orthop., 257:76-85.
31. Lutz, G.E., Palmitier, R.A., An, K.N., and Chao, E.Y. (1993): Comparison of tibiofemoral joint forces during open and closed kinetic chain exercises. J. Bone Joint Surg., 75A:732-735.

32. Malanga, G.A., Jenp, Y.N., Growney, E.S., and An, K.A. (1996): EMG analysis of shoulder positioning in testing and strengthening the supraspinatus. Med. Sci. Sport Exerc., 28:661-664.

33. Markolf, K.L., Gorek, J.F., Kabo, J.M., and Shapiro, M.S. (1990): Direct measurement of resultant forces in the anterior cruciate ligament. An in vitro study performed with a new experimental technique. J. Bone Joint Surg. [Am.], 72:557-567.

34. Meglan, D., Lutz, G., and Stuart, M. (1993): Effects of closed kinetic chain exercises for ACL rehabilitation upon the load in the capsular and ligamentous structures of the knee. Presented at the Orthopedic Research Society Meeting, San Francisco, February 15-18.

35. McCann, P.D., Wootten, M.E., Kadaba, M.P., and Bigliani, L.U. (1993): A kinematic and electromyographic study of shoulder rehabilitation exercises. Clin. Orthop., 288:179-188.

36. McMahon, P.J., Jobe, F.W., Pink, M.M., et al. (1996): Comparative electromyographic analysis of shoulder muscles during planar motions: Anterior glenohumeral instability versus normal. J. Shoulder Elbow Surg., 5:118-123.

37. Morrey, B.F., Itoi, E., and An, K.N. (1998): Biomechanics of the shoulder. In: Rockwood, C.A., and Matsen, F.A. (eds): The Shoulder, 2nd ed. W.B. Saunders, Philadelphia, pp. 233-276.

38. Morrison, J.B. (1969): The biomechanics of the knee joint in various knee activities. Biomech. Eng., 4:573-578.

39. Morrison, J.B. (1970): The biomechanics of the knee joint in relation to normal walking. J. Biomech., 3:51.

40. Moseley, J.B., Jr., Jobe, F.W., Pink, M., et al. (1992): EMG analysis of the scapular muscles during a shoulder rehabilitation program. Am. J. Sports Med., 20:128-134.

41. Moynes, D.R., Perry, J., Antonelli, D.J., et al. (1986): Electromyographic motion analysis of the upper extremity in sports. Phys. Ther., 66:1905-1911.

42. Neer, C.S., II, Craig, E.V., and Fukuda, H. (1983): Cuff tear arthropathy. J. Bone Joint Surg. [Am.], 65A:1232.

43. O'Brien, S.J., Neves, M.C., Arnoczky, S.P., et al. (1990): The anatomy and histology of the inferior glenohumeral ligament complex of the shoulder. Am. J. Sports Med., 18:449-456.

44. Poppen, N.K., and Walker, P.S. (1978): Forces at the glenohumeral joint in abduction. Clin. Orthop., 135:165-170.

45. Reddy, A.S., Mohr, K.J., Pink, M.M., et al. (2002): Electromyographic analysis of the deltoid and rotator cuff muscles in person with subacromial impingement. J. Shoulder Elbow Surg., 9:519-523.

46. Reinold, M.M., Ellerbusch, M.T., Barrentine, S.W., et al. (2002): Electromyographic analysis of the supraspinatus and deltoid muscles during rehabilitation exercises. J. Orthop. Sports Phys. Ther., 32:A-43.

47. Rockwood, C.A., Matsen, F.A., eds. (1990): The Shoulder. Philadelphia, W.B. Saunders, pp. 755-795.

48. Saha, A.K. (1971): Dynamic stability of the glenohumeral joint. Acta Orthop. Scand., 42:491-505.

49. Scovazzo, M.L., Browne, A., Pink, M., et al. (1991): The painful shoulder during freestyle swimming. An electromyographic cinematographic analysis of twelve muscles. Am. J. Sports Med., 19:577-582.

50. Smidt, G.L. (1973): Biomechanical analysis of knee extension and flexion. J. Biomech., 6:79-83.

51. Steinkamp, L.A., Dillingham, M.F., Markel, M.D., et al. (1993): Biomechanical considerations in patellofemoral joint rehabilitation. Am. J. Sports Med., 21:438-444.

52. Takeda, Y., Kashiwaguchi, S., and Endo, K. (2002): The most effective exercise for strengthening the supraspinatus muscle: Evaluation by magnetic resonance imaging. Am. J. Sports Med., 30:374-381.

53. Townsend, H., Jobe, F.W., Pink, M., and Perry, J. (1991): Electromyographic analysis of the glenohumeral muscles during a baseball rehabilitation program. Am. J. Sports Med., 19:264-272.

54. Walch, G., Boileau, P., Noel, E., and Donell, T. (1992): Impingement of the deep surface of the infraspinatus tendon on the posterior glenoid rim. J. Shoulder Elbow Surg., 1:239-245.

55. Wilk, K.E. (1994): Rehabilitation of isolated and combined posterior cruciate ligament injuries. Clin. Sports Med., 13:649-677.

56. Wilk, K.E., Andrews, J.R., Arrigo, C.A., et al. (1993): The internal and external rotator strength characteristics of professional baseball pitchers. Am. J. Sports Med., 21:61-66.

57. Wilk, K.E., Andrews, J.R., Clancy, W.G., et al. (1999): Rehabilitation programs for the PCL-injured and reconstructed knee. J. Sport Rehab., 8:333-361.

58. Wilk, K.E., and Arrigo, C. (1993): Current concepts in the rehabilitation of the athletic shoulder. J. Orthop. Sports Phys. Ther., 18:365-378.

59. Wilk, K.E., Arrigo, C.A., and Andrews, J.R. (1997): Current concepts: The stabilizing structures of the glenohumeral joint. J. Orthop. Sports Phys. Ther., 25:364-379.

60. Wilk, K.E., Escamilla, R.F., Fleisig, G.S., et al. (1996): A comparison of the tibiofemoral joint forces and electromyographic activity during open and closed kinetic chain exercises. Am. J. Sports Med., 24:518-527.

61. Wilk, K.E., Meister, K., and Andrews, J.R. (2002): Current concepts in the rehabilitation of the overhead throwing athlete. Am. J. Sports Med., 30:136-151.

62. Wilk, K.E., and Reinold, M.M. (2001): Closed kinetic chain exercises and plyometric activities. In: Bandy, W.D. and Sanders, B. (eds.): Therapeutic Exercise: Techniques for Intervention. Baltimore, Lippincott Williams & Wilkins, pp. 179-211.

63. Wilk, K.E., Zheng, N., Fleisg, G.S., et al. (1997): Kinetic chain exercise: Implication for the ACL patient. J. Sport Rehab., 6:125-143.

64. Witvrouw, E., Lysens, R., Bellemans, J., et al. (2000): Open versus closed kinetic chain exercises for patellofemoral pain. A prospective, randomized study. Am. J. Sports Med., 28:687-694.

65. Worrell, T.W., Corey, B.J., York, S.L., and Santiestaban J. (1992): An analysis of supraspinatus EMG activity and shoulder isometric force development. Med. Sci. Sports Exerc., 24:744-748.

CHAPTER 4

THERAPEUTIC MODALITIES AS AN ADJUNCT TO REHABILITATION

Mark A. Merrick, Ph.D., ATC

CHAPTER OBJECTIVES

At the end of this chapter the reader will be able to:

- Identify which modalities are effective and clinically useful for particular pathologic conditions.
- Identify incorrect modality application techniques that can compromise their clinical effectiveness.
- Choose the appropriate clinical use(s) for a specific modality.
- Explain the effect that cryotherapy application has on certain biologic functions in the acute care of an injury.
- Explain the effect that compression and elevation have on certain biologic functions in an acute injury.
- Choose appropriate modalities based on their clinical efficacy for use during the rehabilitation process.
- Explain when to initiate, modify, and discontinue modality protocols based on patient needs and rehabilitative goals.

One of biggest conceptual errors made by students and novice clinicians is thinking that rehabilitation is a post–acute injury process. Inexperienced students tend to self-organize the care of athletic injuries into an evaluation phase, a management phase, and a rehabilitative phase and they see these phases as being distinctly different from each other. Although this organizational scheme is not entirely incorrect, advanced practitioners tend to think of all of these components of postinjury care as part of a rehabilitative continuum. Advanced practitioners are able to recognize that a quick and accurate evaluation leads to a more rapid initiation of acute management, which, in turn, leads to an easier and more rapid return to function. This view of rehabilitation as a continuum, beginning with injury and ending with a return to full function (when possible), is essential when the goal is to safely return an athlete to competition in the briefest time possible after an injury.

When clinicians recognize the interrelated nature of evaluation, management, and rehabilitation, they can dramatically alter the injury's prognosis. Appropriate therapeutic techniques applied at the appropriate times can radically reduce complicating factors, such as edema and neuromuscular inhibition, that confound the patient's return to normal function. To this end, therapeutic modalities are a critically important set of tools whose use can play a central role throughout the rehabilitative continuum. Like all tools however, modalities have specific uses in specific situations and are of little benefit when used for the wrong reason, with the wrong technique, or at the wrong time. At their best, therapeutic modalities are an exceptionally useful complement to the rehabilitative process but are not a replacement for it. At their worst, therapeutic modalities can be blindly applied and ineffective tools, wasting the time of both the patient and clinician. In this chapter, we will explore the general use, rehabilitative timing, and specific application of therapeutic modalities. More importantly, we will examine the literature regarding the clinical efficacy of common therapeutic modalities to identify which appear to be effective and which do not.

GENERAL PRINCIPLES WITH THEAPEUTIC MODALITIES

What Are Modalities and Why Use Them?

Although most clinicians would readily identify therapeutic ultrasound as a modality, far fewer would identify surgery as one; but they should. In fact, a great many treatments can and should be considered to be therapeutic modalities. The when, why, and how of therapeutic modalities require that we first understand what modalities are.

Simply stated, modalities are therapeutic techniques. These include dissimilar things such as surgery, medications, and psychologic counseling, none of which is appropriate for independent use by allied health practitioners such as athletic trainers or physical therapists. The modalities with which we are more familiar and that are more appropriate for our use are generally referred to as *therapeutic modalities* and mostly include physical agents such as heat, cold, sound, electromagnetic energy, massage, and compression. These physical agents are appropriate for application by clinicians in any of several different professions, although their actual use is generally governed by the practice acts of individual states. Many therapeutic modalities including ultrasound, diathermy, lymphedema pumps, LASERs, and others are classified as medical devices and are therefore regulated in the United States by the Center for Devices and Radiological Health, part of the Food and Drug Administration (FDA) (http://www.fda.gov/cdrh/consumer/mda/index.html).

Modalities as Part of a Comprehensive Rehabilitative Program

The single most important point to remember about therapeutic modalities is that they are tools and should never be used as replacements for a comprehensive rehabilitative program. Modalities are an adjunct to rehabilitation. That is, they can *help* a clinician and patient to accomplish a goal, but therapeutic modalities generally do not accomplish goals in isolation. Instead, they should be combined with other rehabilitative techniques (especially therapeutic exercise) and should not be viewed as a replacement for these techniques.

A common fault is to mistake modality use for rehabilitation. Modality use can be a part of rehabilitation, but it is not equivalent to rehabilitation. For example, using only ice massage before practice for someone with patellar tendonitis is not the same as using a comprehensive rehabilitative program that involves counteracting chronic inflammation, minimizing sclerosis, correcting biomechanics, improving strength, endurance, and power, and limiting overuse.

When to Use Modalities

Like any tool, a therapeutic modality should be used for a specific purpose. You would use a screwdriver to tighten a screw but not to drive-in a nail. Likewise, you would use cryotherapy to counteract acute inflammation but not to counteract the range of motion loss associated with prolonged immobilization. Although it seems obvious, the key to using modalities appropriately is to match the specific physiologic effects of the modality with the specific rehabilitative goal for the patient. The obvious corollary to this is that if the physiologic effects of the modality do not match the rehabilitative goals then the modality should not be used, or if the goals have been met then the modality should be discontinued. Although these principles are almost self-evident, it is not uncommon for novice clinicians to make the mistake of using a modality without

having a specific goal in mind or failing to discontinue use of a modality after the goal for which it was chosen has been achieved.

Comprehensive rehabilitative programs are always patient specific and should never be blindly generalized protocols. For example, a "cookbook" protocol for the rehabilitation of an ankle sprain makes far less sense than a protocol that is based on the specific problems and limitations of your specific patient for his or her specific injury. Patients who present with similar injuries do not necessarily have the same set of problems. For example, one might have more effusion than the other or one might have better range of motion than the other. Therefore, because the problems are usually somewhat different, the goals would also be somewhat different, and therefore the use of modalities would also be somewhat different. Once identified, the rehabilitative goals are prioritized and sequenced. For example, we generally work to restore range of motion before we work to restore muscular endurance or power. Because goals are prioritized and sequenced with different goals being emphasized at different points in the rehabilitative program, modality usage should also change at different points in the rehabilitative program.

Generally, practitioners do a fine job of identifying patient problems, creating specific goals related to these problems, and choosing modalities to help achieve these goals. A difference between novice and advanced practitioners, however, is that advanced practitioners are also skilled at determining when a modality should be discontinued. In the current era in which health insurance providers are attempting to limit billed charges, it is important for rehabilitative programs to be cost-effective, and the efficient and effective use of therapeutic modalities is an important piece of a cost-effective program. Inexperienced practitioners often continue to use a modality even after the goal has been achieved because they lack a goal-oriented focus in modality use. To avoid this error, practitioners should ask themselves four questions before each modality treatment (Box 4-1).

How to Use Modalities

This chapter is not intended to be a substitute for a formal course in therapeutic modality application. That topic is somewhat more comprehensive, and there are a few very good texts on modalities[23,37,130,151,162] that provide a greater level of instruction in modality application. In this chapter we will instead review the general elements common to all modality applications and will discuss some specific aspects of application and efficacy for each modality presented.

Legal and Appropriate Use of Modalities

First and foremost, a majority of states have specific practice acts for rehabilitation professionals such as physicians,

Box 4-1

Questions to Ask before Every Modality Treatment

1. What is the specific goal I am trying to achieve today by using this modality?
2. Am I using the best available modality (and correct application technique) to achieve this goal?
3. What specific criteria am I looking for to indicate that I should stop today's treatment with this modality?
4. What specific criteria am I looking for to indicate that I have finished using this modality as part of this patient's treatment plan? (This final question is often overlooked.)

athletic trainers, and physical therapists. These practice acts typically govern therapeutic modality usage. Therefore, practitioners should familiarize themselves with the specific details of their state practice acts before using any therapeutic modalities. A general provision in most practice acts is that practitioners are required to have specific training in both therapeutic modality theory and the application techniques for these modalities. A good principle to follow is that you should never use a therapeutic modality that you have not been specifically trained to use. Although this seems obvious, it is particularly relevant for students. Students should not apply therapeutic modalities until they have completed the relevant coursework to support their use of modalities.

Another important aspect of the legal and appropriate use of modalities involves prescriptions for treatment. In most states, prescriptions for outpatient rehabilitation are required and, in some, prescriptions are required for athletic trainers practicing in the settings of high school, collegiate, or professional sports. Again, there is no substitute for thoroughly reviewing the requirements of your specific state practice act. Although specific prescriptions for each modality are sometimes required, often they are not and the use of therapeutic modalities is left to the professional judgment of the clinician. However, there are some modalities, particularly those involving pharmaceutical delivery (iontophoresis or phonophoresis), that almost always require a specific prescription.

As is true with any rehabilitative procedure, practitioners assume some degree of liability with the use of therapeutic modalities. To maximize patient safety and to minimize the liability associated with the use of therapeutic modalities, a number of policies and procedures should be adopted (Box 4-2).

Application Procedures

Although the specific application procedures for each therapeutic modality differ, there are some commonalities to all modality treatments. One of the most important of these, actively involving the patient in his or her own care, is often overlooked. Before you apply any modality, you should explain its use thoroughly to the patient. Such explanations allow the patient to make informed decisions about consent to treatment. Similarly, they also help the patient to understand the specific goals and effects of the treatment. This also helps patients to understand any potentially harmful complications, such as excessive heating and lets patients know that they should tell you if they have discomfort with a treatment so that you can modify it before a problem arises. You should also ask patients if they have any questions about the use of the modality in their treatment. An additional bonus of involving the patient in his or her own care is that patients who feel like partners in their own care often comply with their rehabilitative programs. Box 4-3 lists some common things you should explain to the patient before modality application.

In addition to making the patient a partner in his or her own care, another commonality with all modality treatments is in the actual setup for the treatment. The physical preparations for modality usage involve two items. The

Box 4-2

Suggested Policies and Procedures for Modality Application

- Good professional judgment must be used. The exercise of good professional judgment and the application of a modality that you have not been trained to use are mutually exclusive. Therefore, modalities should only be used by those formally trained (and legally permitted) to use them.
- Every piece of equipment for a modality must be in good working order and be recently calibrated to ensure its safe use.
- Every planned modality treatment for every patient should be evaluated to ensure that it is appropriate with regard to the indications and contraindications for the modality.
- Every modality treatment should be monitored for both safety and efficacy throughout the course of treatment. Treatments causing adverse effects should be immediately discontinued, as should treatments that are not effective.
- Unattended modality treatments are obviously to be avoided as are patient self-applications of most modalities.

Box 4-3

Patient Education before Modality Treatments

- Which modality is to be used: For example, "We're going to use some ice on your knee for about 20 minutes after your exercise today."
- The specific goal for the modality/what the modality does: For example, "The ice helps to reduce any inflammation we may have caused today, and it also helps to reduce your soreness."
- Rule-out contraindications: For example, "Do you have any circulatory or neurologic problems such as Raynaud's disease?"
- Explain what the patient should expect: For example, "It will feed really cold, and it will probably be a little bit uncomfortable until you get used to it."
- Explain the precautions and the reasons to discontinue the treatment this time: For example, "You shouldn't feel any pain, numbness, or tingling down in your leg or foot, but if you do let me know right away and I'll take the ice off."
- Explain the criteria for discontinuing the use of this modality overall: For example, "We'll quit using the ice if it's not giving the result we want or when you quit having inflammation or soreness after your exercises."

first of these is the preparation of the patient. Before any other aspect of patient preparation, you should determine whether a prescription for the modality treatment is required and present and if the prescription has expired or the number of permissible treatments has been exceeded. Once this step is completed, the remainder of patient preparation generally involves reviewing the specific goal for the treatment with the indications for the modality, ensuring that there are no contraindications present and reviewing the patient's previous response to the treatment (ask them), and the patient's consent to the treatment. The outcome of any previous treatments should also be reviewed. Physical preparation of the patient generally involves removing or adjusting clothing as necessary for the specific modality and positioning the patient as comfortably as possible. This last aspect is critically important when modality treatments are given for more than just a few minutes.

The second aspect of physical preparation is the physical setup of the modality equipment and treatment area. First and foremost, the patient's safety must be ensured through a quick but complete safety checkout of the equipment and area before every modality use (Box 4-4). After the equipment safety checkout is completed, you should make sure you have all of the necessary accessories for the treatment present before you actually begin the treatment.

Postapplication Procedures

Just as there are commonalities in the setup for all modality treatments, there are also commonalities in the post-treatment procedures. Most of these are obvious and include removing the patient from any equipment, returning the equipment to its appropriate storage area, and assisting the patient with wiping off any treatment-related water, gel, or other materials as necessary. The most important aspects of the postapplication period are less obvious and are often overlooked, particularly in competitive athletic settings. The first of these is record keeping. It is absolutely critical that practitioners record the treatment parameters used with the modality application. Recording the parameters allows a different practitioner to continue the course of treatment if you are unavailable. Without such a record, other practitioners are either forced to guess your protocol or ask the patient what has been done. At no time should a practitioner ever have to ask the patient which treatment parameters have been used because even the most involved of patients cannot be expected to understand the parameters or explain them correctly. It is also important to make specific notes of any complications that occurred with the treatment as well as noting the patient's response to the treatment.

Another postapplication procedure often overlooked is reviewing the response to the modality treatment to determine whether the goal of use of the modality has been

Box 4-4

Equipment Checklist before Modality Application

- Check the condition of any patient cables or electrodes and ensure they meet required standards.
- Confirm that the equipment is operational.
- Confirm that patient safety switches are operational.
- For electrical modalities, ensure that the equipment is properly grounded and that the equipment is only used with outlets equipped with ground-fault circuit interrupters.
- Evaluate the treatment area to make sure that there are no hazards present such as standing water or unstable treatment tables.

met, whether the treatment has been effective, or whether the treatment should be continued. A plan for discontinuing the modality treatment should be in place to help with this last question.

SEPARATING FACTS FROM FICTION

Now that we have reviewed the basics of therapeutic modalities, their use, and their general application procedures, we can begin the more important aspect of this chapter: determining whether or not specific modalities are effective and clinically useful. We will see that a number of modalities commonly used in clinical settings may not be as effective as once thought and that the clinical efficacy of modalities that are known to be useful can be easily compromised by incorrect application techniques. Unfortunately, practitioners apply many ineffective or unnecessary modality treatments. The unnecessary, incorrect, or inappropriate use of modalities has been a recent topic of discussion for clinicians and researchers as well as for health insurance providers who are carefully scrutinizing outcomes of research to determine whether or not they should reimburse for certain treatments with certain modalities. There are also several very effective therapeutic modalities, such as shortwave diathermy and low-power LASERs, that are not in common use in our clinics because we are either not sufficiently aware of them, not trained to use them, or not able to afford to purchase equipment to use them. To adequately examine the efficacy of therapeutic modalities, we need to first review a few basic principles about modality research.

Modality Research

In examining the history of modality use, one obvious trend is that clinical practice has almost always preceded scientific research. That is, clinicians pass along anecdotes about how they have used modalities and the results they have observed. This has led to a great deal of modality folklore that has very little basis in fact. We really did not see a meaningful body of scientific research related to therapeutic modalities until the last few decades. This modality research has been conducted by scientists and clinicians from a number of different professional fields including early work by physicians such as Lewis[105] who examined cold and Lehmann[99,100,102] who examined heat. Most of the more recent research has been conducted by researchers from allied health fields such as athletic training and physical therapy. In fact, the overwhelming majority of recent research in the clinical use of therapeutic modalities has been completed by athletic trainers, yet there are still states in which athletic trainers are prohibited from using these modalities.

The commonly observed trend of clinical practice preceding scientific inquiry with therapeutic modalities has

greatly influenced modality research. Many, if not most, modality researchers began their careers as clinicians. This clinician background has resulted in the use of many clinically relevant and relatively unsophisticated dependent variables in research on modalities. These clinical variables typically include factors such as range of motion, strength (usually isometric or isokinetic), swelling, pain/soreness, and various functional measures. There is also a body of research that has gone beyond clinical variables and examined slightly more basic variables such as temperature, electromyographic activity, blood flow, and tissue stiffness. In recent years, there are also a small number of laboratories examining very basic variables such as cell metabolism, protein expression, gene expression, and cell proliferation.

The simpler and more clinical variables have obvious value to clinicians and are very useful in establishing outcomes, a type of research that is very useful for supporting reimbursement activities. Unfortunately, these variables are generally less useful for helping to establishing modality theory. Most clinical variables are, at best, secondary manifestations of the effects of modalities. That is, modalities generally do not directly produce the effects seen in clinical variables, but rather they produce these clinical effects indirectly. For example, continuous ultrasound treatments do not improve range of motion directly. Instead, continuous ultrasound causes vibration between molecules in the tissue. The vibrations increase the tissue temperature.[25,43,99,102] The increased tissue temperature may allow tissues to become more elastic.[57,100] Increased elasticity may in turn allow stretching techniques to be more effective. More effective stretching may finally improve range of motion.

The indirect relationship between most modalities and clinical variables presents problems in establishing theories because identification of clinical variables is easily confounded. That is, there are many factors that might influence the clinical variables and that can potentially mask or intensify the effects of the modality. The more steps that occur between the believed direct effect and the clinical variable of the modality, the greater is the chance that something can become confounded along the way. If this happens, we may not be able to observe a strong effect that we can use to support or refute the underlying theory regarding the modality. Likewise, the more steps that occur between the clinical variable and the direct effect, the greater are the number of opportunities for a methodologic mistake to prevent the desired outcome. When we are examining only a relatively limited number of modality protocols and we do not see an effect, it is difficult and probably inappropriate to make broad generalizations about the modality. A recent and important example of this was a review on ultrasound by Robertson and Baker[155] (Table 4-1). The conclusion drawn in this review was that therapeutic ultrasound was not an effective adjunct for improving range of motion or decreasing pain. The effect

Table 4-1

Robertson and Baker's "A Review of Therapeutic Ultrasound: Effectiveness Studies"

Robertson and Baker[155] reviewed 35 ultrasound studies from peer-reviewed journals between 1975 and 1999. Because of small sample size or other problems, they were forced to discard 25 of the studies and therefore reported findings based on 10 articles reporting clinical outcomes. Of these 10 articles, only two reported that ultrasound was better than placebo. Robertson and Baker concluded that the literature shows that ultrasound is no more effective than placebo.

At first glance, this study appears to be a damning condemnation of the clinical use of ultrasound. Upon closer examination however, this study actually becomes a good case in drawing poor conclusions because of poor data. In a letter to the editor in the February 2002 issue of *Physical Therapy*, Draper[40] pointed out that 8 of the 10 studies used in this review had serious methodologic flaws that rendered them virtually useless in describing the clinical efficacy of ultrasound (see below). Just as an automobile appears to be useless as a means of transportation if you are stepping on the wrong pedal, ultrasound appears to be useless as a modality if you use the wrong parameters.

Problem Area	Problematic Protocol Used	Problem with the Protocol
Effective radiating area (ERA)	Thermal ultrasound to an area 5 times the size of the faceplate	The ERA is always smaller than the ultrasound faceplate and the treatment area should be no larger than twice the ERA to cause an effective increase in temperature.
	Thermal ultrasound to an area 10-25 times the size of the faceplate	
	Thermal ultrasound to an area 10 times the size of the faceplate	
	Nonthermal ultrasound to an area 10 times the size of the faceplate	There is no published evidence that nonthermal ultrasound to such a large area produces an increase in healing.
Ultrasound frequency	1 MHz ultrasound used to treat superficial tissues (epicondylagia)	1 MHz ultrasound is effective at depths of 2.5 to 5 cm. The epicondyles are considerably more superficial and should have been treated with 3 MHz ultrasound.
Treatment time	1 MHz ultrasound applied for a 3-minute treatment to test joint mobility with a treatment size at least 12 times as large as the ERA	This would not have produced any meaningful temperature change because of the huge treatment area. Even with an appropriate treatment area, it would only be estimated to produce a 1.2°C temperature increase. A temperature increase of at least 3-4°C would be required to produce elasticity changes.
	7 of the 10 studies used a 25% pulsed duty cycle; treatment times varied from 2 to 15 minutes	The two studies that did show an effect of ultrasound both used 14-minute treatment times. The shorter treatment times probably explain the lack of effect.

From Robertson, V., and Baker, K. (2001): A review of therapeutic ultrasound: Effectiveness studies. Phys. Ther., 81:1339-1350.

of this review has been a reluctance of outpatient practitioners to use therapeutic ultrasound because they fear that insurance providers, in the wake of this article, might not reimburse for such treatments. Unfortunately, in the research studies reviewed in this article clinical variables and rather ineffective ultrasound application protocols were used, and most did not produce a positive effect.[40] The use of substandard ultrasound protocols meant that there would have been a smaller than expected direct effect of ultrasound. A smaller than expected effect would have been further diluted because there were a number of physiologic steps between the presumed effect of the ultrasound and the clinical variables studied. In fact, in examining the methods used in the studies from this review, it is clear that most were wholly inappropriate and were very unlikely to cause a useful effect and, not surprisingly, no useful effects were seen.[40]

Although much of the existing modality research has focused on clinical variables, there are a surprisingly large number of modality effects that are commonly accepted by clinicians but that have little scientific support. In some cases there is even scientific evidence to the contrary, yet these widely held clinical beliefs still persist. One common example of this is cold-induced vasodilation with cryotherapy. There are similarly incorrect beliefs still circulating regarding contrast baths for edema reduction[64,134-136] and transcutaneously applied microcurrent for muscle injuries.[21,123,175] These will be discussed later in the chapter.

CLINICAL PEARL #1

Cold-induced vasodilation, the notion that cryotherapy treatments can cause blood flow to increase above base-line levels, is still touted as an effect of cryotherapy by some clinicians.[105] In fact, you still may occasionally hear someone incorrectly suggest that you should not use cold for more than about 30 minutes to avoid this phenomenon. In fact, cryotherapy does not increase blood flow above baseline levels at all.[91] This has been repeatedly demonstrated[5,33,65,66,80,91] for more than 60 years!

Where to Go from Here

In the future, modality research needs to accomplish two important tasks. First, we need to establish a body of suitable outcomes research to document the efficacy of our modality treatments. Although we are continuing to learn about the physiologic effects of modalities, there is a wholly inadequate body of outcomes research related to the use of these modalities. Research is sorely needed to confirm whether our physiologically based treatments actually improve the outcomes of the patients we treat. This outcomes research must examine multiple protocols for each modality to refine our clinical techniques and maximize the benefits that our patients receive. Second, we need research that focuses more on the direct effects that we think are caused by the modalities. Generally, this means more research on the basic science variables that we think are the root of the clinical effects. Once we establish and understand the very basic effects caused by our modalities, we will be better able to refine our treatments to maximize the clinical benefits of modalities treatments. For example, we are very confident that cryotherapy is useful in minimizing the unwanted consequences of acute injury. However, we are not completely certain of the precise mechanisms by which this modality is effective. Although there are a number of articles that have proposed theories, these theories have yet to be confirmed. In fact, we do not yet know the answers to basic questions about cryotherapy such as how cold we need to make the injured tissues or how long we should apply the cold to be most effective. Answering the basic questions of how a modality works physiologically will allow us to better examine the clinically relevant questions of how to maximize the benefit of the modality.

MODALITIES FOR ACUTE CARE
Modality Goals for Acute Care

The use of therapeutic modalities with acute injuries is governed by a specific set of clinical goals (Table 4-2). The

Table 4-2

Goals and Modalities for Acute Injury Care

Acute Care Goal	Modality Choices
Reduce pain	Cryotherapy, TENS
Minimize edema formation	Cryotherapy, compression, elevation, microcurrent(?)
Minimize bleeding	Cryotherapy, compression, elevation
Minimize secondary injury	Cryotherapy
Minimize acute inflammation	Cryotherapy, microcurrent(?)
Prevent further injury	Immobilization/protection

TENS, transcutaneous electrical nerve stimulation.

most important of these goals is thought to be limiting the total quantity of tissue damage associated with the injury.[90,125] Because we know that the time required for tissue healing partially depends on the quantity of tissue damaged, a smaller amount of damaged tissue should translate into a quicker repair and faster return to activity.

When an injury occurs, the immediate tissue damage associated with that injury is referred to as *primary injury*.[86,88-90,125] This damage includes disruption of a variety of structures including ligamentous, tendinous, muscular, vascular, nervous, and bony tissues. Because primary injury occurs immediately with the trauma, it has already occurred before we even evaluate the injury. There is nothing that we can do to limit the magnitude of this primary tissue damage apart from immobilizing the injured area to prevent further tearing of partially torn tissues. However, primary damage is not the end of the story. The pathophysiologic response to primary injury can lead to additional tissue damage, known as *secondary injury*, in tissues that were otherwise not initially injured.[86,88-90,125] For example, a disruption of blood flow resulting from an injury to vascular tissues can lead to ischemic injury of the otherwise uninjured tissues they supply. Although ischemia is probably one of the leading causes of secondary injury, there are actually a number of other suggested causes as well. Unlike primary injury, secondary injury may be inhibited by our acute interventions. For example, there is some evidence that immediate cryotherapy inhibits secondary injury after acute trauma.[129] By limiting secondary injury, we limit the total quantity of injured tissue and should thereby reduce the time necessary to repair the damage and return to activity.

A second but equally important goal of acute modality usage is to limit the sequelae of the acute inflammatory response. Because acute inflammation occurs with every injury to perfused tissues, we can expect to see all five signs of inflammation to some extent.[108] These signs, redness, heat, pain, edema, and loss of function, can lead to an unnecessarily prolonged time for healing. By limiting these signs, particularly the pain and edema, we can restore function sooner and thereby return our patients to activity sooner. Likewise, the biochemical consequences of acute inflammation include the release of a number of damaging enzymes and radicals[108] that are capable of producing additional tissue damage (see Chapter 2). Obviously, limiting the quantity or activity of these damaging molecules could help to reduce the total quantity of damaged tissue and therefore lead to quicker repair.

Cryotherapy

The traditional management of acute injuries is described by the acronym R.I.C.E., which stands for *rest*, *ice*, *compression*, and *elevation*.[23,37,63,130,151,162] Cryotherapy, the therapeutic use of cold, is by far the most commonly used and probably the most effective modality for managing acute musculoskeletal injuries.[33,86,88,89,92,93,104,111,129] There is almost certainly no more familiar modality to practitioners than the ice bag; however, in clinical practice, cryotherapy takes many forms and can be used to help accomplish a variety of goals, in both acute and post–acute injuries. From a scientific standpoint, there is perhaps no modality that we know more about; even so, our understanding of cryotherapy is somewhat more limited than you probably imagine. In this section, we will discuss only the acute use of cryotherapy. Its post–acute injury use in facilitating early exercise will be discussed in conjunction with the other post–acute injury modalities later in the chapter.

Description

Cryotherapy is one of the most broadly defined of the therapeutic modalities. Quite simply, it involves the therapeutic application of cold. There are many different forms of cold therapy commonly found in clinical practice and there are new forms being developed and marketed continually. Although one of the most common forms of cryotherapy is the ice bag, cold modalities also include ice massage, ice slush immersions, cold-water immersion, frozen gel packs, vapocoolant sprays, cold-compression devices, and even "instant" cold packs. Note that virtually all of these involve the *local* use of cold application rather than the *global* (whole body) application of cold. The physiology of local cooling is somewhat different from that of global cooling, and this local cooling is of most interest in rehabilitation.

The wide array of cryotherapy options reflects both the obvious efficacy of this modality and our inadequate understanding of what constitutes an ideal treatment. All of these various forms of cryotherapy are capable of cooling tissues to differing extents; however, there are only limited data to suggest which of these forms of cryotherapy is the most effective.[7,127,128,138,168,177]

How We Think It Works

Like all modalities, cold treatments produce a variety of physiologic effects (Table 4-3). These physiologic effects

Table 4-3

Physiologic Effects and Clinical Uses

Physiological Effect	Clinical Use
Reduced temperature	↓ secondary injury, ↓ edema formation, ↓ bleeding, ↓ pain
Reduced metabolic rate	↓ secondary injury
Reduced perfusion	↓ bleeding, ↓ edema formation
Reduced inflammation	↓ secondary injury, ↓ edema formation, ↓ pain

↓ = decrease.

can be easily translated in goals for cryotherapy treatments.[89] Although we generally discuss each of these effects separately, we need to remember that they all occur simultaneously. Therefore, we need to consider all of the effects of a modality when we use it and we need to balance the desired effects with the unwanted effects to determine whether the use of the modality is judicious or if it is inadvisable.

Temperature Reduction

The most easily recognizable effect of cryotherapy is a reduction in tissue temperature. In fact, virtually all of the effects that we observe with cryotherapy are a direct result of this tissue temperature change. In the past 10 years alone, a great deal of cryotherapy research has used temperature reduction as the variable of interest.[7,27,30,64,69,78,97,109,111,127,128,134,136-139,142,145,146,153,168,177] Most of these studies have examined skin temperature (Fig. 4-1), but there is also a growing body of literature

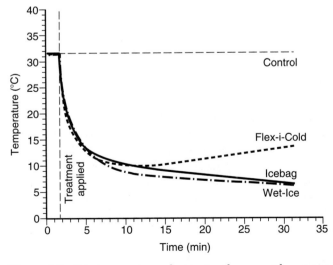

Figure 4-1. Skin temperatures during cryotherapy with various cold modalities. (From Merrick, M., Jutte, L., and Smith, M. [2003]: Cold modalities with different thermodynamic properties produce different surface and intramuscular temperatures. J. Athl. Train., 38:28-33.)

describing deep tissue temperatures during cryotherapy (Fig. 4-2). From this literature, we know that during many forms of cryotherapy the skin can easily reach single digit temperatures (°C) and that intramuscular temperature change is quite variable, depending on the depth at which temperature is measured and the duration of the treatment. Typical intramuscular temperatures during most forms of cryotherapy are in the range of 25° to 31°C.

The most important factor that determines the tissue temperature change during cryotherapy is heat transfer.[89,127] An important concept to remember when we speak of tissue cooling is that cold cannot be transferred because cold is merely the absence of heat. Heat is transferred from one body to another with the net transfer always in the direction of high heat moving toward lower heat. Therefore, bodily tissues (high heat) are cooled because they lose heat that is absorbed by the cold modality (low heat); the greater the ability of a cold modality to absorb heat, the greater is its potential for reducing tissue temperatures.

The heat-absorbing capacity of cold modalities is determined by a number of factors (Box 4-5). Cold modalities with more mass can absorb more heat than those with a small mass. Similarly, the greater the contact area is, the greater the heat transfer that occurs. Greater temperature differences also lead to more rapid heat transfer. Conversely, the greater the tissue thickness is, particularly for adipose layer thickness, the slower the heat transfer.

One of the most important factors controlling heat transfer is the specific heat of the tissue and modality. The specific heat is the amount of heat necessary to raise

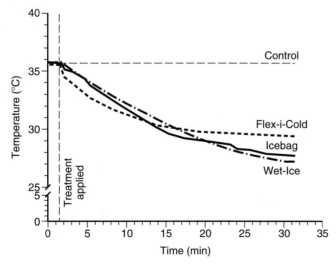

Figure 4-2. Temperatures 1 cm deep to the adipose layer during cryotherapy with various cold modalities. (From Merrick, M., Jutte, L., and Smith, M. [2003]: Cold modalities with different thermodynamic properties produce different surface and intramuscular temperatures. J. Athl. Train., 38:28-33.)

Box 4-5

Factors That Determine the Heat-Absorbing Capacity of a Cold Modality

- Mass of the modality
- Size of the contact area
- Temperature difference between the modality and the tissue
- Distance across which heat must be transferred (tissue thickness)[89,127]

---

the temperature of 1 kg of the material by 1°K (or 1°C because the units are the same size).[62,89,107,127] The greater the specific heat is, the more energy that is required to raise the temperature of the material. Therefore, materials with a greater specific heat can absorb more heat energy per degree of temperature change than materials with a lower specific heat. Perhaps even more important is whether or not the cold modality goes through a change of state (solid to liquid) when it absorbs heat. Changes of physical state occur at specific temperatures. For example, ice at 0°C becomes water as it melts. The amount of heat required to cause this change of state during melting is known as the *heat of fusion* and is much higher than the specific heat of the material.[62,89,107,127] For example, at 0°C the specific heat of ice is 2090 J $\bullet$ kg^{-1} $\bullet$ °C^{-1}, and the specific heat of water at the same temperature is 4190 J $\bullet$ kg^{-1} $\bullet$ °C^{-1}, whereas the heat of fusion for ice melting to water is 333,000 J $\bullet$ kg^{-1}. In other words, a cold modality changing from ice at 0°C into water at 0°C absorbs roughly 80 times as much heat as raising the temperature of cold water from 0°C to 1°C!

CLINICAL PEARL #2

From a thermodynamics standpoint, it is clear that modalities that undergo a phase change (e.g., ice) are capable of absorbing more heat than those that do not (e.g., frozen gel). This notion recently received some clinical support when it was demonstrated that lower skin and intramuscular temperatures are observed when ice-based modalities are used than when flexible gel cold packs are used.[127] Another important factor in tissue temperature reduction is the use of compression. Cryotherapy used in combination with compression has been shown to produce greater temperature reductions than cryotherapy used alone.[7,28]

In addition to the thermodynamic properties of the modality itself, the tissue temperatures observed during cryotherapy also largely depend on factors related to the tissues being treated. Of these factors, the thickness of the adipose layer at the treatment site appears to be the most important.[78,139,145] In a recent noteworthy study, Otte and colleagues[145] compared the treatment duration required to produce a uniform temperature change in patients with differing adipose layer thicknesses (Fig. 4-3). Remarkably, to produce an identical temperature drop of 7°C in the quadriceps muscle with an ice bag application, subjects with anterior thigh skin folds of 11 to 20mm required 23 minutes whereas subjects with skin folds of 31 to 40 mm required an almost unthinkable 59 minutes! Clearly, the days of "one duration fits all" for cryotherapy treatments are long gone.

Metabolic Rate Reduction

Perhaps the most important goal of acute cryotherapy is a reduction in the metabolic rate of the cooled tissue. Such a reduction in metabolic rate would be quite beneficial in improving the ability of a tissue to survive the proposed secondary injury events that follow primary trauma.[86,88-90,108,125,129] Although the exact mechanics of secondary injury are still being defined, it is clear that several of its suggested mechanisms would be altered by a change in temperature. For example, one of the two most common theories is that secondary injury results from the activity of damaging enzymes and/or free-radicals that are released during the inflammatory process.[89,90,125] We know that the rate of chemical reactions is reduced at lower temperatures,[61] so lowering the temperature of a tissue with cryotherapy would reduce the rate of activity of the detrimental enzymes or radicals and thereby reduce the quantity of damage that they cause. Likewise, the other suggested principal mechanism of secondary injury is that

it is the result of postinjury ischemia.[89,90,125] We know that without oxygen, tissues fail metabolically in a relatively short period of time.[61,108] A reduction in temperature and its related drop in metabolic rate have been clearly shown to reduce the demand of a tissue for oxygen and thereby improve tissue survival under such conditions.[61,108,124]

The temperature-dependent alteration in metabolic rate is generally described using a physical chemistry concept referred to as Q_{10}.[61,108] The Q_{10} is simply the change in the rate of chemical reactions observed with a 10°C change in temperature as calculated using the Arrhenius equation. In physiology, Q_{10} is generally used to describe metabolic rate and is most commonly determined by examining either O_2 consumption or NH_3 excretion. A common misconception among biologists is that $Q_{10} = 2$; that is, the rate of reaction doubles with each 10°C temperature increase. In fact, Q_{10} is somewhat variable and depends on the organism, specific temperature range and metabolic pathway of interest. It generally falls between 1.2 and 2.5. That is, increasing temperature by 10°C will lead to an increase in the reaction rate of 1.2 to 2.5 times (i.e., a 20% to 150% increase). Although normally defined for an increase in temperature, we can also use Q_{10} to understand the physiologic effect of cryotherapy, where we decrease temperature and therefore metabolic rate. For example, let us arbitrarily say that the Q_{10} is 1.5 for increasing temperature from 27 to 37°C. This would mean that metabolic rate increases by 1.5 times for this temperature increase (i.e., a 50% increase). If we were to apply cryotherapy to a tissue whose temperature is 37°C to decrease it to 27°C, the metabolic rate would then be reduced by 1.5 times, or 50%.

Although a decline in metabolic rate is clearly an important aspect of the acute use of cryotherapy, there is still much we do not know in this area. For example, although the arguments for the role of damaging enzymes and free-radicals are getting stronger, most of this research has been performed in organs and neurologic tissues, and we still know very little about the progression of secondary injury in musculoskeletal tissues.[125] Likewise, postinjury ischemia theories have not yet been well examined.

CLINICAL PEARL #3

Gaps in the area of research on ischemia lead to several significant shortcomings in our current understanding of cryotherapy. We do not yet have a definitive answer about the most effective tissue temperature, cryotherapy duration, or on/off ratio for using cryotherapy for acute injury treatments.

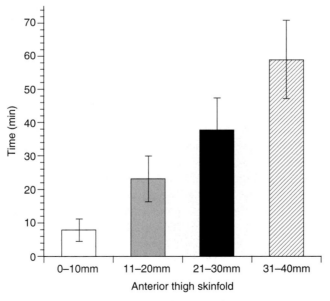

Figure 4-3. Cryotherapy duration required to reduce thigh intramuscular temperature by 7°C in subjects with differing adipose thicknesses. (From Otte, J., Merrick, M., Ingersoll, C., and Cordova, M. [2002]: Subcutaneous adipose tissue thickness alters cooling time during cryotherapy. Arch. Phys. Med. Rehab., 83:1501-1505.)

Perfusion/Blood Flow

As was true with metabolic rate, perfusion is also reduced with a decline in tissue temperature.[5,65,66,80,91,117] The decrease in blood flow is an effect of constriction of the vessel walls in response to cold. There are still some practitioners and even educators who suggest that cold can also cause a dilation of blood vessels. This concept, known as cold-induced vasodilation[89,91,105] does not occur and is discussed in Box 4-6.

As vessels become colder, their muscular walls begin to contract, causing the vessel to constrict in diameter. The constriction is generally thought to be more pronounced in arteries and veins with smaller diameters and in the arterioles and venules. The constriction does not occur in capillaries because their walls are single-cell thick endothelium and do not contain muscular tissue that can contract. Vasoconstriction causes a decrease in blood flow that has been well documented over the past few decades.[5,33,65,66,80,91,117] A decrease in blood flow is a mixed blessing and causes a dilemma for injury management theory. On the beneficial side, less blood flow would translate to less hemorrhaging from damaged vessels, less edema formation, and decreased accumulation of inflammatory cells that might cause secondary injury. These would all contribute to improved outcomes of the injury. On the detrimental side, less blood flow would also mean less delivery of O_2 and nutrients and less removal of metabolic waste products. These could all worsen the secondary damage after injury. In fact, the topical application of cold only reduces blood flow and does not completely prevent it. Therefore, because cold application probably does not impose too great an ischemic stress, the pros are thought to outweigh the cons.

Inflammation

It is well accepted that cryotherapy inhibits inflammation,[26,33,51,86,88,89,92-94,104,129,142] but the specific effects of cold on inflammation are somewhat complex because inflammation itself is extremely complex. Most introductory texts[12,23,37,63,89,130,151,162] describe inflammation in terms of its vascular events, chemical events, and cellular events, and all three of these are altered by acute cryotherapy. The vascular events of inflammation, most notably vasodilation, are counteracted by the vasoconstriction that results from cold treatments as already described. The chemical events—the release of more than 100 chemicals that mediate the inflammatory process—are also affected by cold.[108] Although the effects of cold have not been explored for the majority of these inflammatory chemicals, we do know that the release or activity of several of the key inflammatory chemicals is inhibited during cryotherapy. The cellular events of inflammation are marked by the early activity of neutrophils, which gradually gives way over a period of hours into the activity of macrophages.[61,108] Through a cold-induced reduction in metabolism, the activities of all of these cells are reduced. This is thought to be quite beneficial in the early stages of inflammation in which neutrophils dominate, but less useful later on when the macrophages are active in removing inflammatory debris in preparation for tissue repair. Neutrophils account for roughly 60% to 70% of all circulating white blood cells.[61,108] Their primary function is to fight an expanding bacterial infection by phagocytizing the bacteria and releasing a variety of damaging chemicals and

---

Box 4-6

Facts about Cold-Induced Vasodilation

As is the case with virtually every modality, there are a number of anecdotal beliefs about cryotherapy that do not stand up to scrutiny in the laboratory. Unfortunately, modality myths have great tenacity and refuse to die quietly, and the myth about cold-induced vasodilation (CIVD) is no exception, even though the idea was discredited by Knight more than 20 years ago.[91] Some clinicians and even a few modality instructors still cite CIVD, sometimes called rebound vasodilation, as an important physiologic effect of cryotherapy. CIVD is generally described as an increase in blood flow, above baseline levels, that accompanies cryotherapy treatments. This phenomenon is often used as a rationale for limiting cryotherapy treatments to less than 20 to 30 minutes in duration. Originally, the notion of CIVD grew from a study by Lewis in 1930,[105] in which he described cyclical fluctuations in finger temperature during immersion in ice water. He did not examine blood flow or vessel diameter and his subjects were probably hypothermic as a result of being underdressed in a very cold room. He observed that finger temperature fluctuated, becoming warmer after a period of immersion in cold water. This was incorrectly translated to mean increased blood flow and was a popular rationale for cryotherapy in rehabilitation for a number of years.

In fact, CIVD does not occur. Limb blood flow during cryotherapy is clearly depressed and never increases above baseline as long as the temperature is below normal.[5,33,65,66,80,91] However, as is often the case with misunderstood ideas, there is a hint of truth buried in the legend of CIVD. That hint is known as the *Hunting response*.[16,34,55] During local hypothermic conditions, we see a clear and profound vasoconstriction in vessels with muscular walls such as arterioles. However, during prolonged local hypothermia, the degree of vasoconstriction in these vessels fluctuates and the resulting blood flow show cyclical increases and decreases. The important thing to note is that this blood flow cycling occurs at flow levels that are considerably less than their normal baseline.[16,34,55,89,91] Said another way, the cyclical increase in blood flow during prolonged hypothermia does not approach the pre-cryotherapy baseline blood flow and certainly does not go above baseline levels. Therefore, practitioners can use cryotherapy for longer than 15 to 30 minutes without fear of hyperperfusing acutely inflamed tissues.

free-radicals, the immune system equivalent of hand grenades, to destroy additional bacteria. They are also very active in amplifying the overall immune response by releasing an assortment of chemical messengers. Because most musculoskeletal athletic injuries do not involve open wounds and infection, the activity of neutrophils with these injuries is generally greater than is necessary and can lead to unwanted secondary damage to otherwise uninjured tissues[112,125] (see Chapter 2). The use of cryotherapy to retard neutrophil activity and thereby limit this damage is a promising area of future cryotherapy research.

Edema

One of the most important physiologic effects of acute cryotherapy is its ability to retard the formation of edema/effusion.[5,65,66,80,91,117] The primary mechanism by which cryotherapy retards edema formation is thought to be its effect on Starling forces.[88,89] These are the forces that cause fluid movement across the capillary wall, with two forces causing fluid to escape from the vessel and two forces attempting to retain fluid in the vessel. Under normal circumstances, the balance of these forces is such that a small amount of fluid is constantly escaping and being collected by the lymphatic system. When an injury occurs the tissue osmotic pressure, one of the escape forces, is thought to dramatically increase because of the release of free protein and other molecules from the damaged tissue. This would shift the balance of forces even further in the direction of fluid loss and edema formation. Cryotherapy is thought to minimize the total tissue damage, hindering the release of free protein and thereby the increase in tissue osmotic pressure. Coupled with the lowered blood flow resulting from vasoconstriction and cryotherapy this results in a decrease in the other escape force, capillary hydrostatic pressure. With both escape forces reduced, but not completely eliminated, the formation of edema or effusion is lessened, but not entirely prevented. Obviously, compression is a critical adjunct to cold in limiting the formation of edema and is discussed separately in this chapter.

CLINICAL PEARL #4

The popular phrase "ice reduces swelling" is not used here and with good reason. *Swelling* is a troublesome word because it is sometimes used as a noun in place of edema or effusion or it can be used as an action verb meaning that fluid is accumulating. Cold reduces the formation of edema, but does not remove edema that is already present.

The problem with the phrase "ice reduces swelling" is that it is misleading and is often misunderstood. It is well accepted that cryotherapy retards the accumulation of fluid both intra- and extra-articularly.[5,65,66,80,91,117] However, cryotherapy by itself does not remove fluid that has accumulated. Cryotherapy and compression in combination are somewhat effective in removing accumulated fluid, but this is probably a function of the compression and not the cold.[95,96,160,174]

Pain

Aside from selected pharmaceuticals, no modality is more effective than cryotherapy in managing both the acute and chronic pain associated with athletic injuries.[89] There are three primary theories that attempt to explain the pain-relieving efficacy of cold, and, in fact, all three probably occur simultaneously (Box 4-7).[23,37,89,130,151,162]

Ironically, although cold is an outstanding pain control modality, its application actually can be quite painful. This is particularly true of cryotherapy treatments that involve immersion in ice water for patients who are not accustomed to the treatment. The pain with cold application can be initially intense but often subsides after several minutes. Repeated applications over a period of days or weeks generally leads to better tolerance by patients as they grow accustomed to the treatment.[89,132,164]

Neuromuscular Effects

The neuromuscular effects of cryotherapy are generally not used as a goal for cryotherapy treatments for acute injuries but can be quite useful in managing muscle spasms and in rehabilitation. They are discussed with the rehabilitative use of cryotherapy.

Box 4-7

Three Theories That May Explain Cold's Pain-Relieving Efficacy

Gate control theory: The first and best known of these is gate control theory, in which the cold causes stimulation of A-β afferent nerve fibers which, in turn, inhibit pain transmission on second-order neurons through gating at the substantia gelatinosa in the dorsal root ganglion of the spinal cord.

Reduction in nerve conduction velocity: Nerve conduction velocity has been shown to be reduced by as much as 30% after typical cryotherapy treatments.[87,89,162] Slower conduction would translate into a diminished sensation of pain.

Reduction in sensitivity to pain receptors: A lesser known theory is that local cold application reduces the sensitivity of pain receptors much in the same way that it reduces sensitivity of touch and pressure receptors.[61,89]

Techniques and Dosage

At the present time, we use cryotherapy under the assumption that colder tissue temperatures are better, provided that we do not cause tissue freezing and frostbite. Therefore, the aim of cryotherapy treatments for acute injuries is to reduce tissue temperature as greatly and quickly as possible.

Topical Application and Insulating Barriers

The most common application technique for cryotherapy is the direct application of a cold modality, usually an ice bag or frozen gel pack, to the injured area with some sort of a compressive wrap, generally an elastic bandage or plastic wrap (Table 4-4). As a general rule, cold packs made from ice are superior to frozen gel packs for the thermodynamic reasons discussed earlier.[127] Ice-based cold packs are also generally safer than frozen gel packs. It is possible to cause further injury with cryotherapy, and there are three primary ways that patients are injured (Box 4-8).

Typically, ice bags are made from either cubed or crushed ice produced by an ice machine and stored in an unrefrigerated hopper below the ice machine. Because this ice is not stored in a refrigerated container, it is continually melting. Melting ice, by definition, has a temperature of 0°C, and because heat is being added to the ice from the tissues being treated, it is physically impossible for such ice to freeze the skin and cause frostbite.[89,168] For this reason, ice bags made from ice stored in unrefrigerated hoppers should be directly applied to the skin without the addition of an insulating layer. The same cannot be said for ice stored in a freezer or frozen gel packs, however. Because their temperatures will probably be less than 0°C, they pose a risk of causing frostbite and therefore require

some type of barrier, such as a wet elastic wrap, between the pack and the skin.[89] Unfortunately, such barriers have been shown to severely limit the ability of the modality to cool the tissues and therefore are assumed to meaningfully impair the efficacy of the modality.[168]

CLINICAL PEARL #5

As a general rule, use a barrier only when applying a cold modality that has been stored at a temperature of less than 0°C. Cubed or crushed ice stored in an unrefrigerated hopper does not meet this criterion because it is continually melting as heat is being added to the ice from the tissues being treated and, thus, no barrier should be used.

Cold Combined with Compression

One of the most overlooked aspects of applying ice packs for acute injury is the use of compression. Practitioners are taught to treat injury with ice, compression, and elevation (ICE), and the compression and elevation are used to retard edema formation. However, we often overlook the fact that the compression also plays a valuable role in the cooling. When we use compression in combination with cryotherapy, we observe that deep tissue temperatures cool more rapidly and that lower temperatures can be achieved (Fig. 4-4).[7,128] Merrick and colleagues[128] were the first to describe this combined effect on cooling and they speculated that the improved cooling resulted from the combination of better contact between the tissue and the modality and from a compression induced reduction in blood flow.

Gaining in popularity are devices that automatically combine cryotherapy and compression (Fig. 4-5). These devices, considered to be lymphedema pumps for regulatory

Table 4-4

Common Application Techniques for Acute Cryotherapy

Cold Modality	Application Technique	Comments
Ice bag	Apply directly to skin, use compression wrap and elevation (ICE), duration depends on adipose and should be 20 to 40 minutes for most athletes.	Crushed ice conforms better than cubed ice. Ice from an unrefrigerated bin on an ice machine will not cause frostbite, but ice directly from a freezer may. Use appropriate caution.
Ice immersion	Submersion in water with ice. Consider using a thin layer of elastic tape for compression (less insulating than elastic bandages).	Durations not scientifically described, but most mimic ice bag durations.
Frozen gel pack	Do NOT apply directly to skin. Use compression wrap and elevation. Duration should be 20 to 40 minutes for most athletes.	Because these are stored in a freezer at temperatures less than 0°C, they can cause frostbite. They also rewarm much more quickly than ice bags.
Vapocoolant sprays	Use for spray and stretch technique for muscle spasms and trigger points.	Not used for most injuries (sprains, strains, fractures, contusions, etc.). These can quickly cause frostbite so care must be used.

Box 4-8

Three Ways to Cause Further Injury with Cryotherapy

- It is possible to cause injury by using too much compression over too small an area, creating a tourniquet-like effect. For this reason, compression wraps should not be applied with more than moderate force, generally defined as 45 to 50 mm Hg.
- Extended use of cryotherapy over superficial portions of peripheral nerves can cause injury. In several cases, nerve palsy has been caused by cryotherapy treatments, typically over the common peroneal nerve on the lateral aspect of the knee or the ulnar nerve at the medial aspect of the elbow. When using cryotherapy over these areas, we must diligently monitor the treatment, control the compression, and limit the treatment duration.
- Cold-induced injury is frostbite. Frostbite occurs when tissue has been destroyed by freezing. For frostbite to occur, the tissues must be cooled to the point where ice crystals begin to form. This occurs when the tissue temperature drops to less than 0°C and is accelerated by greater than required compression. Therefore, care must be used with cold modalities that are colder than 0°C and compression should be carefully applied.

purposes by the FDA, typically use a fluid-filled (hydraulic) sleeve that is filled with cold water to provide both cooling and compression. Many of these devices use partitioned sleeves that either fill sequentially in an effort to move edematous fluids proximally or use different pressure in each partition (gradient pressure) for the same purpose. Most devices allow the clinician to control the compression pressure and some also allow for control of the temperature of the water used for the compression. Although these devices make sense intuitively, as with nearly all therapeutic modalities, there are few data available describing their clinical outcomes.

Cold Immersion

Cold immersion treatments can be performed with either cold water, typically in the form of a cold whirlpool, or with an ice and water bath. There are two important advantages of ice immersion over ice packs.[89] First, immersion treatments can be used to treat larger areas and do so more uniformly. Second, immersions allow for heat transfer through water, which has much greater thermal conductivity than ice packs. This greater thermal conductivity may allow for more rapid cooling. There are disadvantages to cold immersion treatments as well. The first of these is that it is nearly impossible to use elevation when immersion treatments are used. The second disadvantage of immersion treatments is that the water develops thermal gradients. Thermal gradients are regions where the water has been heated by the somewhat warmer tissues that are being immersed. The water around these tissues becomes warmer than the rest of the water in the immersion container. As these regions of water are warmed, they are less able to absorb heat and a reduction in cooling occurs. To avoid this gradient effect, the water should periodically be mixed throughout the treatment. Patients typically do not enjoy the mixing, however, because it brings colder water

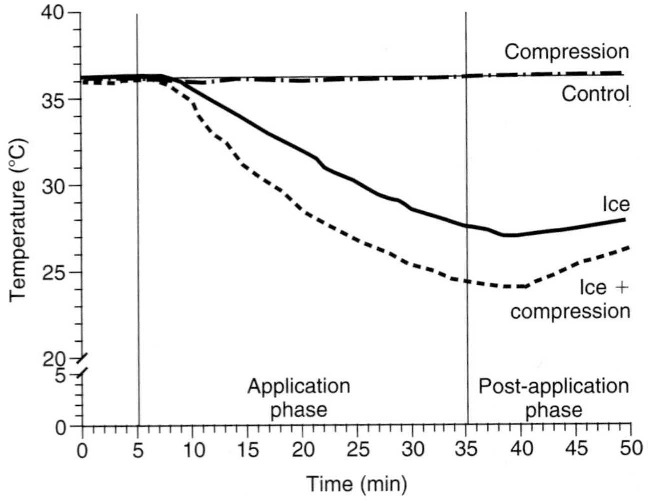

Figure 4-4. Compression improves the cooling ability of cryotherapy treatments. (From Merrick, M., Knight, K., Ingersoll, C., and Potteiger, J. [1993]: The effects of ice and compression wraps on intramuscular temperatures at various depths. J. Athl. Train., 28:236-245.)

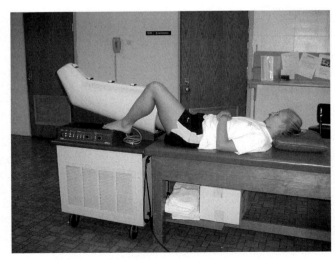

Figure 4-5. Lymphedema pumps that combine cold and compression are a valuable tool in managing acute injury.

back into contact with their limb and is somewhat uncomfortable.

Ice and water baths, often referred to as ice slushes, are considerably more uncomfortable to patients than cold water baths, but their lower temperatures make them a more effective choice. Patient tolerance of ice slush treatments for the foot and ankle can be improved by the use of toe covers, which prevent the cold water from coming in direct contact with the toes.[132]

CLINICAL PEARL #6

When making an ice slush, put the ice in first, then add water to the ice analogous to the way you would add milk to breakfast cereal. The ice should just begin to float so that, when the limb is added, the ice surrounds the area to be treated.

Ice Massage

Ice massage, the rubbing of a block of ice against the tissue, is an effective and common, but somewhat messy, practice (Fig. 4-6). Towels must be used beneath the treated tissues because the ice is constantly melting, but the water is not collected in the ice bag. Ice massage treatments are generally of briefer duration than ice pack or cold immersion treatments and are capable of producing similar intramuscular temperatures. Care must be taken to avoid using excessive pressure over peripheral nerves.

Spray and Stretch

A somewhat different type of cryotherapy treatment is known as "spray and stretch" and is used to cause brief, intense cooling to relieve myofascial pain and spasm. The technique has also been used to treat muscle cramps, but this use has not been examined in the literature. The spray and stretch technique involves the application of a vapocoolant spray, typically Ethyl Chloride (Gebauer Company, Cleveland, OH) or Fluori-Methane (Gebauer Company), which rapidly cools the skin during evaporation. Ethyl Chloride is very flammable and therefore use of the nonflammable Fluori-Methane is becoming more popular. Fluori-Methane contains chlorofluorocarbons, which can deplete the ozone layer; however, the United States Environmental Protection Agency has granted it a nonessential class I product exemption for clinical use.

The technique involves spraying of the vapocoolant liquid in parallel strokes over the skin overlying a muscle with myofascial trigger points and then immediately stretching the muscle (Fig. 4-7). The brief, intense cooling is thought to act as a distracting neurologic stimulus that may cause reflexive motor inhibition allowing for more effective stretching.

Future Questions

For all that we have learned about cryotherapy, answers to the most important questions still elude us. The vast majority of cryotherapy research has used clinically convenient or easy to measure variables such as temperature. We now know a great deal about the skin and intramuscular temperature responses with cryotherapy. For example, we know that skin temperature drops almost immediately and that muscle temperature does not begin to fall until 3 to 5 minutes into the treatment. We also know that once the cold modality is removed, the skin temperature begins to immediately climb but deep tissue temperature actually continues to fall for nearly 5 minutes. We know that after cryotherapy treatments, temperature does not return to normal for more than 1 hour in resting subjects. But we do not yet know the temperature we need a tissue to reach to have a positive outcome with cryotherapy, and we certainly do not yet know the optimum intramuscular temperature to retard secondary injury or inflammation. To answer these

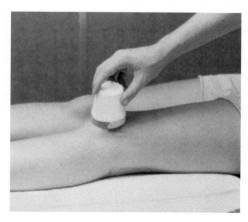

Figure 4-6. Ice massage effectively produces local cooling in discrete areas, making it an excellent treatment choice for overuse syndromes.

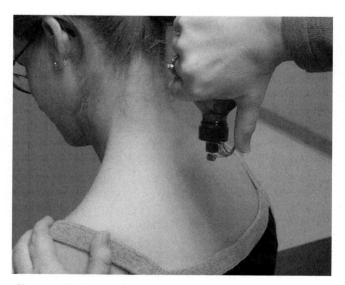

Figure 4-7. Spray and stretch technique with Fluori-Methane.

critically important questions, we will need to examine variables related to secondary injury or inflammation itself.

Because we do not yet know the optimum temperature we need to reach during cryotherapy, we also do not know how long our cryotherapy treatments should be applied to produce this temperature. We know that there is a point of diminishing return with cryotherapy duration. In examining the time required for rewarming of the skin after cryotherapy, researchers have shown that longer cold applications lead to longer rewarming periods only up to a point.[109,133] Applications that exceeded 30 minutes had rewarming times that were nearly identical to those with 30-minute applications. We also know that adipose layer thickness is an important factor that we need to consider in choosing application duration. In fact, to produce a typical cryotherapy effect for many of our athletes, we need to double or even triple the treatment durations that are commonly in use now[145] (see Fig. 4-3). A third important question about cryotherapy is related to these first two. We do not yet know how often we need to reapply cold modalities. A typical recommendation is 20 minutes per hour for the first 5 or 6 hours after injury; however, there are few data to support any specific on-off cycling for cryotherapy.[146]

Compression

Compression, the application of external pressure, is a commonly used adjunct to acute cryotherapy, but also has usefulness in isolation. Compression, the "C" in R.I.C.E., is one of the cornerstones of traditional acute injury management, although it has not been well studied. The effectiveness of compression is thought to be largely related to its effect on Starling forces, the forces governing transcapillary fluid movement,[2,13,58,96,117] although compression has other useful effects not related to these forces.[7,38,96,128,174] In this section, we will discuss only the acute use of compression. Its post–acute injury use in resolving existing edema will be discussed in conjunction with the other post–acute injury modalities later in the chapter.

Description

Compression involves the application of external pressure to a tissue or tissues in either a circumferential or focal manner. Although the most common forms of compression involve circumferential application with either an elasticized bandage or elastic tape, there are actually quite a few other compression modalities available.[176] Among the best of these are the pneumatic or hydraulic lymphedema pumps that provide circumferential compression in either a constant or intermittent manner. Pneumatic lymphedema pumps use air to fill a compression garment, providing nearly uniform circumferential compression. Hydraulic lymphedema pumps, on the other hand, use water or some other liquid to fill the compression garment. Although many of the early lymphedema pumps used

single-chamber compression garments, most contemporary units use multichambered garments, allowing for sequential filling (distal to proximal), gradient compression (more pressure in distal chambers than in proximal chambers), or both. For acute injury management, an important advantage is found with hydraulic pumps because they allow for the use of precooled water, which provides concurrent cryotherapy. Both pneumatic and hydraulic lymphedema pumps are considered to be medical devices and are therefore regulated by the FDA through the Center for Devices and Radiological Health.

How We Think It Works

Compression produces several physiologic effects that can be used to explain its effectiveness. As was the case with cryotherapy, these effects probably do not work in isolation but instead work in concert to produce our desired outcome. There are three primary means by which we think compression is effective in managing acute injuries.[89] One of these is that compression increases the cooling efficacy of cryotherapy as discussed earlier in the section on cryotherapy.[7,128] The other two mechanisms involve resisting the formation of edema. The first of these anti-edema mechanisms is a manipulation of Starling forces.[2,13,117] The second involves lessening the bleeding from vessels damaged during the injury.[113]

Starling Forces

The most common explanation for the obvious effects of compression on retarding the formation of edema is through its effect on Starling forces (Table 4-5).[36,61,89,108] These forces, sometimes called capillary filtration forces, govern the movement of plasma from the vascular system into the extravascular space through the intact walls of the capillaries.[61,108] Under normal homeostatic conditions, there are three forces, capillary hydrostatic, tissue hydrostatic, and tissue osmotic, that cause fluid to migrate from the capillary into the extravascular space and there is one force, capillary osmotic, that resists the extravascular migration of fluid. Normally a net loss of fluid from the vascular system occurs because there is a slight imbalance in the Starling forces in which the "out" forces causing fluid loss from the capillary are slightly larger than the "in" forces. As discussed in the section on cryotherapy, acute injury causes a dramatic increase in the out forces through both a decrease in plasma osmotic pressure and an increase in interstitial osmotic pressure. These pressure changes result from the loss of plasma proteins into the surrounding tissues and from the release of free-proteins from cells damaged by the injury.

External compression is thought to work primarily by increasing the tissue hydrostatic pressure, reducing the magnitude of the pro-edema pressure gradient. Reduction of this gradient would lessen the fluid loss from the vascular system and therefore retard the

Table 4-5

Starling Equilibrium for Capillary Fluid Exchange*

Force	Description	Direction	Mean Value	Effect of Injury
Capillary hydrostatic	Fluid pressure from inside the capillary	Vascular fluid loss	−17.3 mm Hg	−17.3 mm Hg (no change)
Interstitial osmotic	Osmotic pressure exerted by extravascular solutes	Vascular fluid loss	−8 mm Hg	−28 mm Hg
Interstitial hydrostatic	Extravascular fluid pressure in the tissue	Vascular fluid loss†	−3 mm Hg	+4 mm Hg
Capillary osmotic	Osmotic pressure exerted by intravascular solutes	Vascular fluid retention	+28 mm Hg	+14 mm Hg
	Net force under normal conditions	Vascular fluid loss	−0.3 mm Hg	−27.3 mm Hg

Adapted from Guyton, A.C. (1991): Textbook of Medical Physiology, 8th ed. Philadelphia, W.B. Saunders, pp. 149-203, Knight, K.L. (1985): Cryotherapy in Sport Injury Management. Champaign, IL, Human Kinetics, pp. x, 301; and Majno, G., and Joris, I. (1996): Cells, Tissues, and Disease: Principles of General Pathology. Cambridge, MA, Blackwell Scientific.
*Negative values = outward force; positive values = inward force.
†Normally there is a negative (outward) interstitial hydrostatic force (a partial vacuum) that helps hold tissue layers together, but as edema accumulates, this vacuum disappears, allowing tissues to separate and retain even more fluid. The fluid eventually develops positive pressure and can even occlude vessels if the pressure is great enough.

formation of edema. Note, however, that external pressure is unlikely to completely compensate for the increase in tissue osmotic pressure and therefore some edema can be expected to form even with the use of external compression.

Perfusion/Blood Flow

The edema or effusion associated with injury does not form solely from plasma fluid and protein that leaks through intact capillary walls. A significant portion of the fluid accumulation associated with injury is from blood that spills out of blood vessels damaged in the injury. This blood causes most of the ecchymosis seen in the injured area over the days after the injury. Compression is effective in the management of this blood loss in several ways. First, it reduces the quantity of blood flow to the damaged vessels and therefore limits the volume of blood available to be spilled from these vessels. Second, compression slows the rate of flow, allowing for more rapid development of the fibrin scaffolding that eventually forms a clot and stops the blood loss.[61,108]

Technique and Dosage

There is very little in the literature to describe the appropriate compression technique or dosage in managing acute injuries. Most often, compression is used in combination with cryotherapy, and the duration is determined based on the cryotherapy and not the compression. There is a small body of research examining typical compression pressures with elastic wraps and surface pressures of 40 to 50 mm Hg have been reported.[171] These pressures correspond to applying an elastic bandage with a medium stretch for which roughly one half of the stretch capacity of the wrap is used during application. There is evidence that compression in this pressure range improves the cooling

observed with cryotherapy by producing both lower tissue temperatures and slightly faster cooling.[7,128] There is also evidence that varying application pressures have little effect on tissue temperatures.[159]

Compression can be increased by the use of focal compression, such as that achieved with a felt or foam "horseshoe" pad. This can be very useful in limiting the accumulation of fluid at specific sites, such as around the malleoli with ankle injuries or in the peripatellar region with knee injuries.

In addition to compression wraps, the other common form of compression used with acute injuries is lymphedema pumps, typically combined with cryotherapy. The application of these devices for acute injury management have not been well described and ideal parameters have not yet been identified, but typical guidelines are 20 to 40 minutes of intermittent compression with a 30- to 40-second inflation time and a 20- to 30-second deflation or rest time. Appropriate application pressure for these devices is not yet clear, but manufacturers have recommended pressures between 50 and 90 mm Hg. However, these recommendations are generally intended for the post–acute injury removal of edema rather than for retarding the formation of edema. On the other hand, there is a good argument for using pressures that are just below the patient's diastolic blood pressure in an effort to use as much pressure as possible without occluding the vasculature.

Future Questions

Obviously, the use of compression in acute injuries is a very common clinical practice. However, very few researchers have attempted to describe the physiologic effects of compression and even fewer have examined its use in the management of acute injuries. This leaves many questions still unexamined. Among the most important of these would be appropriate pressure, appropriate duration, the effectiveness of intermittent versus continuous compression, use of intermittent cycling parameters, and the importance of compression or elevation in retarding edema formation.

Elevation

Description

Elevation, the "E" in R.I.C.E., is the least studied of the trio of ice, compression, and elevation, but its use is widespread in acute injury management. Elevation of an injured body part can be accomplished in a variety of ways, ranging from specially designed treatment tables to simple, on-the-field techniques such as resting an injured ankle on a football helmet or equipment bag.

How We Think It Works

The underlying premise with elevation is that gravity will limit the amount of blood delivered to the acutely injured area. Limiting blood flow to the injured area immediately after the injury is perceived to have three benefits. First, it would help to control bleeding from damaged vessels, and this would be a benefit in terms of limiting edema and hematoma formation as described earlier in this chapter. Second, it would alter the transcapillary Starling forces in the injured area by reducing capillary hydrostatic pressure, one of the major forces causing fluid to move from the vessel out into the extravascular space. This has obvious implications for retarding edema formation. The third and most often overlooked benefit is that reduced blood flow and reduced capillary hydrostatic pressure would also limit the transport of neutrophils to the injury site. Neutrophils are the most numerous cells in the leukocyte population, and they play a vital role in the early intensification of the inflammatory process. They are also thought to be among the most likely villains in secondary injury. Limiting the delivery of neutrophils and other pro-inflammatory agents at the injury site would be of potential benefit in limiting the total amount of tissue damage and inflammation that would have to be resolved before repair could take place.

Future Questions

Unfortunately, the magnitude of actual benefits from elevation has not been described. Although the arguments for elevation are intuitive and make good physiologic sense, it is unclear whether elevation plays an important role, a minor role, or no role in improving outcomes from injury. Therefore, there are several important questions to be examined including the effects of elevation on edema formation, the magnitude and duration of elevation necessary, and a relative comparison of the importance of elevation and compression. For example, a number of clinicians treat acute ankle sprains by applying elastic tape

compression wraps and then immersing the ankle in an ice bath. The more rapid cooling with the ice bath compared with an ice bag may be of some benefit; however, use of the gravity-dependent position goes against the commonly accepted importance of elevation. The actual importance of the elevation needs to be established to resolve this clinical dilemma.

Other Modalities?

There are other modalities for which claims of efficacy in the management of acute injuries are being made, and some of these appear to have some degree of promise. High-voltage electrical current has been proposed as an acute treatment, which has been suggested to limit the retraction of endothelial cells, thus minimizing the increases in vascular permeability that accompany acute inflammation.[9,39,79,118,165,167] However, the efficacy of this approach in the actual management of acute musculoskeletal injuries in humans has not been well examined, and therefore claims about outcome must be made sparingly. Another valuable adjunct to acute injury management is transcutaneous electrical nerve stimulation.

MODALITIES FOR REHABILITATION
Modality Goals for Rehabilitation

Whereas the goals for acute injury management are centered on the immediate sequelae of the injury including minimizing additional tissue damage, retarding the acute inflammatory process, retarding the formation of edema, and minimizing pain, the goals for the rehabilitative use of modalities are somewhat different (Table 4-6). In post–acute injury rehabilitation, the goals are mostly focused on removing the unwanted remnants of inflammation, repairing the tissue, and restoring more normal physiologic function of the repaired tissue. This is an important distinction that the inexperienced practitioner does not recognize. To make appropriate modality choices, you must first understand the stage of the patient's injury in the progression of injury and what the next logical stage would be. It is vital to understand that all injuries progress through a predefined set of stages and that these stages are sequential and progressive. That is, you cannot truly begin to restore normal function in an acutely inflamed tissue until you first control the inflammation, second remove the inflammatory debris and fluid, and third repair the damage.

Generally, your goal should be to move to the next stage of the injury. When signs of acute inflammation are present, your modality choices should focus on minimizing the inflammation. When examination reveals that the acute phase of inflammation has been controlled, your modalities choices should focus on removing the unwanted debris left over from inflammation and promoting tissue repair. When

Table 4-6

Goals and Modalities for Rehabilitative Care

Rehabilitative Phase	Goals for Modality Use	Modality Choices
Post–acute	Remove edema and inflammatory debris	Intermittent compression, thermotherapy, ultrasound(?), massage, electrotherapy, exercise
	Retard atrophy	Exercise, electrotherapy
Repair/regeneration	Increase perfusion/oxygen delivery	Thermotherapy, ultrasound, shortwave diathermy, exercise, hyperbaric oxygen
	Increase healing stimulus	Exercise, ultrasound, low-power laser, microcurrent(?)
	Retard atrophy	Exercise, electrotherapy
Restore function (early)	Limit pain	Pre-activity cryotherapy, cryokinetics, TENS, electrotherapy, microcurrent(?)
	Counteract neuromuscular inhibition	Pre-activity cryotherapy, cryokinetics, electrotherapy
	Restore ROM	Thermotherapy, ultrasound, shortwave diathermy, joint mobilization, ROM exercise
	Restore adequate muscular strength, power, and endurance for activities of daily living	Exercise, electrotherapy
	Minimize recurrence of inflammation after activity	Post activity cryotherapy & compression
Restore function (middle)	Reduce preactivity stiffness as needed	Pre-activity thermotherapy
	Increase muscular strength, power, and endurance to functional/competitive levels	Exercise Only
	Restore muscular speed	Exercise only
	Restore cardiopulmonary endurance	Exercise only
	Minimize recurrence of inflammation after activity as needed	Postactivity cryotherapy and compression
Restore function (late)	Reduce preactivity stiffness as needed	Preactivity thermotherapy
	Restore agility	Exercise only
	Restore sport specific skills	Exercise only
	Controlled sport activity	Exercise only
	Uncontrolled sport activity	Exercise only
	Minimize recurrence of inflammation after activity as needed	Postactivity cryotherapy and compression

TENS, transcutaneous electrical nerve stimulation; ROM, range of motion.

you have been successful in removing the debris and promoting tissue repair, you should focus on remodeling the new tissue and restoring adequate function for mobility and activities of daily living. When these are established, then you can address goals related to a return to competition. Fortunately, most athletic injuries are able to be progressed through the early phases quickly, and athletes are often able to begin addressing competitive function early in the postinjury timeline. Keep in mind the fact that modality choices and rehabilitative goals for each of these phases are not mutually exclusive. There is almost never a clear dividing point between these phases on examination of the patient, and likewise there is no clear dividing point between the rehabilitative goals and the modalities that can help us to achieve them. However, there should often be a degree of overlap between goals and therefore an overlap

in modalities. This is particularly true in the repair and remodeling phases. For example, we know that appropriate rehabilitation can influence both the quantity and orientation of scar tissue made by the body. To use modalities and controlled exercise to minimize the quantity of scar tissue produced and at the same time to improve the strength of that scar tissue has a great benefit.

The role of traditional therapeutic modalities is almost exclusively limited to the earlier phases of rehabilitation, and the later phases concerned with restoring athletic performance almost exclusively depend on exercise as the modality of choice (Table 4-6). Modality usage in the later phases of rehabilitation is seldom more than preactivity thermotherapy with an aim of increasing perfusion and decreasing stiffness or postactivity cryotherapy with a goal of minimizing any activity-related inflammation. This notion is tied very closely to the beginning of this chapter where the importance of having criteria for the discontinuation of a modality was discussed. When a modality is used to accomplish a specific goal, the modality can and should be discontinued when that goal has been accomplished or when the modality is no longer effective for the patient. For example, if you are using electrotherapy for muscle re-education and to overcome postinjury inhibition, you can discontinue its use when neuromuscular function appears normal and you are ready to begin resistance training.

CLINICAL PEARL #7

The hallmark of an experienced practitioner is using modalities for a specific purpose and replacing them with more appropriate measures when the goal has been met and they are no longer needed.

Cryotherapy

Description

We have already addressed cryotherapy for acute injury management in great detail earlier in the chapter. The rehabilitative use of cryotherapy is somewhat different, however. Cryotherapy is used with two main purposes and at two different times in a rehabilitation session. First and most commonly, it is used to minimize any inflammation that develops as a result of the rehabilitation session and is applied after the session. For this purpose, cryotherapy use is virtually identical to that already described for the management of acute injuries. The second use of cryotherapy rehabilitatively is to control pain and neuromuscular inhibition.[70,71,89,97] When used for this purpose, cryotherapy is typically used before activity or is alternated with activity, a highly effective technique known as *cryokinetics*.[89,150]

How We Think It Works
Pain

Cryokinetics is perhaps the single most effective rehabilitative technique for the early restoration of function after joint injuries, particularly ankle sprains.[89] In this technique, several bouts of cryotherapy and exercise are alternated within a single rehabilitative session, usually very early after injury as discussed later. The preliminary rationale for the dramatic effectiveness of cryokinetics was that the cold reduced pain. Pain is thought to cause neuromuscular inhibition, and this inhibition is thought to be the primary limiting factor in a patient's ability to perform rehabilitative exercise in the early postinjury period. We know that early exercise is the most important modality in our arsenal and the sooner that controlled rehabilitative exercise can be initiated, the faster the progression of the injured tissue toward normal function and presumably the better the outcome. We know that cold is effective in reducing pain and most other sensations as well. Therefore, if cold reduces pain and pain causes inhibition, then cold should help to overcome inhibition and therefore allow the patient to begin controlled rehabilitative exercise at an earlier point in the rehabilitative process.

Cold actually plays a contradictory role with pain. Anyone who has placed their bare feet into an ice slush can tell you with great detail that cold can absolutely cause pain. On the other hand, if you have ever burned your finger and then held it under running cold water you can also testify to the fact that cold reduces pain. So how do we explain the contradiction? First, cold-induced pain seems to be much more common with ice slush immersions than with any other form of cryotherapy, although no explanation for this other than frequent observation has been offered. The magnitude of the pain also appears to be inversely related to the temperature of the ice bath. Also, those with injury-related pain are often observed to tolerate cold applications better than do normal, uninjured subjects. It appears that when pain is already present, cold acts to inhibit that pain whereas when cold is applied to patients without pain, the cold itself becomes uncomfortable.

The primary suggestions of how cryotherapy may inhibit pain lie in the effects of cold on neurologic function. Cryotherapy has been shown to decrease nerve transmission in pain fibers and decrease the excitability of free nerve endings, some of the most important pain receptors.[87] Cold also has been shown to cause asynchronous transmission in pain fibers, cause the release of endorphins, and inhibit spinal nerve conduction. All of these are capable of altering the perception of pain.[89]

Neuromuscular Effects

Because cold reduces nerve conduction velocity on both afferent and efferent nerves, its effect is not limited to altering sensory function. Motor function is altered as well. The changes in motor function have often been overlooked, but have some important implications for clinicians.

Among the more controversial neuromuscular effects of local cryotherapy is whether or not cold decreases maximal force production. The literature on the subject is mixed.[8,17,30,75,81,82,87] Force production has been reduced, both isometrically and with both concentric and eccentric force. In a few studies on isometric force, an increase in force production was noted roughly 60 to 80 minutes after cold treatment, but concentric or eccentric force was not adequately examined. The authors speculated that the increase was the result of either increased temperature or increased blood flow to the limbs after the removal of the cold. These explanations seem unlikely because intramuscular temperatures remain depressed from some time after cryotherapy.

The initial decrease in strength after cryotherapy has created concern in some clinicians about the appropriateness of preactivity cryotherapy. They have questioned whether we are placing athletes at risk for injury by having them practice or compete under circumstances in which nerve conduction velocity and maximal strength are diminished. In an effort to address this issue, there is a growing body of research reporting the effects of cryotherapy on proprioception.[8,81,82,87,154,166,169] As is often the case, the literature is divided with some studies showing no alterations in proprioception or functional performance and some showing a decline in functional performance. Unfortunately, the body of research in this area is still small, so a definitive answer has yet to be determined. However, because maximal strength is seldom used and because a clear detriment to performance has not been shown, many believe that it is safe to use cryotherapy before activity.

Some of the most exciting new cryotherapy research relates to motor neuron pool availability.[70,71,97] After injury, we see a period of neuromuscular inhibition that results in motor weakness, impaired coordination of motor activities, and impaired proprioception. Clearly, these impairments present a significant hurdle in the early rehabilitation of injuries. One of the more common research strategies for examining inhibition is to look at the availability of the motor neuron pool. Under normal circumstances, we voluntarily can recruit only a portion of our total motor neuron pool. The body does not allow total recruitment of the pool because the forces that would be generated would cause us to pull muscles off their bony attachments and cause fractures and other injuries. During an injury and the subsequent postinjury rehabilitative period, the percentage of the motor neuron pool that can be recruited is less than normal and can be quantified by measurement of the Hoffman reflex (H-reflex).[70,71,97]

In several recent studies, neuromuscular inhibition, indicated by a diminished H-reflex, has been artificially created by causing a joint effusion through injection of sterile saline into the synovial space.[70] The results of this research strongly suggest that neuromuscular inhibition after injury is not only related to pain (as suggested in cryokinetics theory) but is also related to joint effusion. Interestingly, the use of cryotherapy has been shown not only to counteract this effusion-induced reduction in motor neuron pool availability, but also to actually lead to motor neuron pool facilitation.[71,97] That is, cold application actually increased the amount of the motor neuron pool that was available for recruitment. This suggests that cryotherapy can be used not only to counter the pain that limits early rehabilitation after injury, but it can also be used to overcome the neuromuscular inhibition after injury as well. Perhaps even more interesting, Krause and colleagues[98] demonstrated that cryotherapy-induced facilitation also occurs when the cold modality is placed on a different body part, away from the injury (different dermatome). They showed that knee effusion-induced reduction in motor neuron pool availability was counteracted by

applying cryotherapy to the armpit! This suggests that the facilitation is mediated by the central nervous system rather than by action on local nerves. On the other hand, members of this same research group[147] have also shown that artificial effusion–induced inhibition is not present in the contralateral limb, so there is still much to learn in this area.

Techniques and Dosage

Many cryotherapy techniques were discussed in the section on acute management. Those presented here are more appropriate for rehabilitative use than for acute use.

Cold Whirlpool

An old favorite among therapeutic modalities is the whirlpool and virtually no athletic health care facility is without one. Cold whirlpools use water that is typically as cold as is available from the tap, typically around 50 to 60°F.[23,37,89,101,130,151,162] Some clinicians add ice to the whirlpool to reduce its temperature, but to date no ideal temperature has been stated in the literature. Whirlpools function by using a turbine to circulate the water around the body part, but they would probably be just as effective without the turbine. The key feature of the whirlpool is the water temperature itself and not the fact that the water is moving.[89] Cold whirlpools were not discussed in the acute management section of this chapter because most are probably too warm to work well for acute injuries and other cold modalities are likely to be more effective.[114-116] Cold whirlpools are very well suited to the rehabilitative use of cryotherapy, however, because the emphasis is not placed on cooling a tissue as quickly as possible or to the greatest degree possible. Typical cold whirlpool treatments last from 15 to 30 minutes, mimicking the durations of other cold treatments such as ice bags, but again, there is little evidence to suggest that this duration is most appropriate.

An important safety consideration with whirlpools is that they should be appropriately grounded and only connected to ground fault circuit interrupted (GFCI) circuits. Whenever possible, it is recommended that an electrician be employed to disconnect the turbine on/off switch on the whirlpool and instead connect the whirlpool to a GFCI circuit with a timer switch that is out of the reach of the patient in the whirlpool. This prevents the patient from operating the switch while standing in the water and also provides an effective means for controlling the duration of the treatment. This second benefit is probably more important with warm whirlpool treatments because athletes tend to not want to get out of the whirlpool.

Cryokinetics

Cryokinetics is a rehabilitative technique that includes alternating bouts of cryotherapy and exercise (Box 4-9). The technique is used primarily in the early phases of a rehabilitative program in an attempt to allow exercise to

Box 4-9

A Typical Cryokinetics Protocol for an Ankle Sprain

Note that each exercise bout becomes progressively more difficult. When used correctly, by the 4th or 5th bout you should encounter exercises your patient is unable to complete. At that point, back off to the most difficult task they can complete and have them complete the bouts. Activities should mirror the actual requirements of the athlete's sport participation.[89]

Activity	Duration	Description
Ice slush immersion	15-20 minutes	Ice immersion until numb, 20 minutes maximum
Exercise bout 1	2-5 minutes	Non–weight-bearing exercise: PROM, AROM, RROM as tolerated
Ice slush immersion	5 minutes	Ice immersion until numb, 5 minutes maximum
Exercise bout 2	2-5 minutes	Weight-bearing exercise: proprioceptive exercises including weight-shifting, wobble boards (two feet then one foot, in-line walking (without a limp)
Ice slush immersion	5 minutes	Ice immersion until numb, 5 minutes maximum
Exercise bout 3	2-5 minutes	More difficult weight-bearing exercise including walking in curves or zig-zags (without a limp), toe raises (two feet, then one foot), in-place hopping
Ice slush immersion	5 minutes	Ice immersion until numb, 5 minutes maximum
Exercise bout 4	2-5 minutes	More difficult weight-bearing activities including in-line jogging and curve or zig-zag jogging (without a limp), hopping over a line or in a square pattern
Ice slush immersion	5 minutes	Ice immersion until numb, 5 minutes maximum
Exercise bout 5	2-5 minutes	More difficult weight-bearing activities including in-line running, curve running, running and cutting, sprint starts and stops, jump stops, backwards running
Ice slush immersion	5 minutes	Ice immersion until numb

PROM, passive range of motion; AROM, assisted range of motion; RROM, resistive range of motion.

be initiated sooner than might otherwise be possible because of pain and neuromuscular inhibition.[89,150] It is often started as soon as the day after the injury or even the day of the injury for relatively minor injuries. It is particularly useful for joint sprains, particularly ankle sprains, but is not as effective with muscle injuries. The cold helps to lessen the pain and reverse the inhibition, allowing for exercise to occur. It has been suggested that early cryokinetics can cut days or even weeks from the rehabilitation of an ankle sprain. The real benefits from cryokinetics are found in the exercise because exercise is the single most important modality available to cause positive changes after injury.

A typical cryokinetics regimen involves five bouts of exercise with cryotherapy treatments to produce numbing in between. The patient begins with a cryotherapy treatment, ideally an ice slush immersion, until the injured body part is numb. The duration is typically 12 to 20 minutes for this initial bout of cryotherapy. After the initial cryotherapy, the patient completes an exercise bout until the numbness begins to wear off, typically 2 to 5 minutes. Then the patient goes back in the ice slush until the injured body part is again numb, which typically is 5 minutes for these re-numbing treatments. When the part is numb again, the patient completes a second bout of

exercise until the numbness begins to wear off in 2 to 5 minutes. Patients continue this pattern of cold and exercise until they have completed five bouts of exercise with each bout becoming progressively more difficult. When they complete the exercise, they conclude with a final 5-minute ice immersion (Box 4-9).

Knight[89] suggested that the key to cryokinetics is not the time spent performing the activity nor the number of repetitions, but rather it is the performance of progressively more difficult exercises without pain. Cryokinetics appears to work primarily by allowing the patient to overcome some of the neuromuscular inhibition produced by the injury. By completing progressively more difficult exercises, the neuromuscular system is forced to function at a higher and higher level and thereby reestablishing the motor control pathways that are critical for a return to normal function.

Superficial Thermotherapy

Description

Heating modalities are generally classified by their depth of effective heating and are considered to be superficial or deep.[12,23,37,101,130,151,156,162] Superficial thermotherapy, the use of superficially applied heat, is an extremely common modality in the rehabilitative setting. In fact, it is so common that it may be our most overused rehabilitative modality. Like all modalities, superficial thermotherapy should be used to accomplish a specific goal and should not be used as a "cure-all" modality. The goals for which superficial thermotherapy are most appropriately used include improving range of motion, increasing circulation, and reducing pain or the sense of tightness that is often associated with injured tissues.

CLINICAL PEARL #8

Thermotherapy should only be used when the examination of the patient suggests that acute inflammation has passed and that the patient's injury is in the waste removal and repair phases or beyond.

How We Think It Works
Range of Motion

First and foremost, the range of motion effects for all thermal modalities are not a direct function of the modality itself. Instead, the thermal modality should be seen as an adjunct that allows other techniques, such as stretching or joint mobilization, to be more effective. In isolation, thermal modalities are not effective in altering range of motion limitations. However, the combination of thermal modalities with specific techniques to improve range of motion can be effective when used correctly.

The correct use of thermal modalities for range of motion effects involves elevating the temperature of the tissue that limits the range of motion into a range where it becomes more elastic and its length can be effectively altered. This means that, first, the choice of modality must be made based upon the depth of the limiting tissue and, second, the modality needs to be capable of producing adequate tissue temperatures. Superficial thermal modalities are generally capable of elevating tissue temperatures down to a depth of roughly 1 to 2 cm, making them appropriate for only the most superficial of tissues.[101,130,162] The tissue temperature required depends on the type of tissue. For collagenous tissues such as tendon, ligament, and scar, tissue temperatures between 39° to 45°C (102° to 113°F) are required.[57,100] Muscle tissue, on the other hand, because it is able to change length easily, causes range of motion limitations as a function of resting muscle tone rather than structural elements such as collagen fibers. To date, the appropriate temperatures to best facilitate residual changes in muscle length has not been described, but they are probably less than those required for collagenous tissues.

Achieving an elevated temperature is only a piece of the equation. The key to effective therapy is to apply the stretching or joint mobilization while the tissue is in the target temperature range, typically just 2 to 3 minutes.[42,47,157]

Increasing Circulation

Circulatory changes are observed with all thermal modalities, both hot or cold. The degree of circulatory change depends upon the tissue temperature achieved and the quantity of tissue being heated. Superficial thermotherapy increases tissue temperature and produces a vasodilation effect in the small arteries, arterioles, venules, and veins. These vascular effects are only seen in superficial vessels.[61] There is some debate about the actual mechanism which causes the vessels to dilate, but the most commonly cited rationales involve local metabolites, nitric oxide signaling, and spinal reflexes.[10,32,61] A strong argument for spinal reflexes as an explanation is that some degree of dilation occurs in the contralateral limb during these treatments even though there are no changes in the metabolic demand on these contralateral tissues.[61]

The dilation of the vessels allows for increased perfusion of the capillary beds fed by the arterioles. Note however that the vasodilation does not occur in the capillary beds themselves. Capillaries have a vessel wall that is a single cell thick, and these cells are endothelium and not smooth muscle. Because capillaries have no muscular layer, they cannot actively dilate or constrict.

Reducing Pain

Pain reduction with superficial thermotherapy is perhaps the primary reason why this modality is so popular with patients. Hot packs simply feel good, and most patients enjoy them. This can lead to problems when all your athletes think they need a hot pack before every practice. As is the case with any modality, you should use superficial thermotherapy only when you have a specific therapeutic goal rather than finding a goal to apply so your athlete can use thermotherapy.

Thermotherapy treatments have many of the same effects on nerve function as cryotherapy treatments. They decrease peripheral nerve conduction velocity, inhibit most nerve receptors, and alter spinal nerve conduction.[37,130] Even with these changes, the most likely explanation for the pain-reducing effects of thermotherapy is their stimulation of cutaneous temperature receptors, which may help to reduce pain through a gait control mechanism.[37,130]

Techniques and Dosage
Hot Packs

The most common form of superficial thermotherapy is the application of moist heat packs, typically hot Hydrocollator packs. These are canvas packs that are partitioned into cells that are filled with silica gel or a similar substance that is capable of absorbing a large quantity of water. These packs are immersed in hot water

(160° to 170°F). By absorbing the hot water, the packs are able to retain heat for an extended period of time. When these packs are applied, some type of barrier must be used between them and the skin because they will cause burns if applied directly. Generally, a terrycloth pack is used; however, towels also work nicely. Even with a Hydrocollator pack, towels are often used initially and are removed as the pack cools. Application duration has not been well studied, but typical applications range from 20 to 30 minutes and produce skin temperatures in excess of 40° to 41°C and muscle temperatures of approximately 38°C.

CLINICAL PEARL #9

It is unlikely that Hydrocollator packs will produce adequate temperature to improve collagen elasticity in any tissues except the most superficial connective tissues with little overlying adipose.

Paraffin Bath

Paraffin baths—melted paraffin with a small amount of mineral oil (7 parts paraffin and 1 part mineral oil)—are another common form of superficial thermotherapy. Paraffin, because of its low specific heat, allows considerably greater thermal conduction than water of the same temperature. The mineral oil is used to lower the melting temperature of the paraffin to a point where it can be used safely with patients. Paraffin baths are typically used to treat the hands or feet and are best for areas that can be dipped into the paraffin. Although some have suggested that paraffin can be applied with a brush to larger areas, these areas are better treated with hot packs. Paraffin bath temperatures are typically in the range of 118° to 126°F and the most common application technique involves dipping the hand or foot into the paraffin 7 to 12 times to form a wax "glove," then covering the glove with a plastic bag and wrapping it with towels to help retain the heat. The duration for this method is generally 15 to 20 minutes. A less used but more effective alternative involves immersing the hand or foot directly in the bath for 5 to 15 minutes. This method is used less often because the risk of burns is increased.

Whirlpools

Warm whirlpools, like their cold counterparts, are extremely common in athletic health care settings. They are most beneficial in reducing the perception of soreness that occurs a few days after strenuous exertion or the stiffness in a recently immobilized body part but can be used for any superficial thermal modality purpose. The temperature of a warm whirlpool generally depends on the body part to be treated. Temperatures of extremity whirlpools are generally hotter (102° to 106°F) than are those of whole body immersion whirlpools (98° to 102°F). They are

sometimes used in the cleaning of skin wounds and an anti-infective agent such as povidone-iodine solution is generally added for this purpose. When they are used in wound care, great diligence must be used in cleaning the whirlpool between patients.

Fluidotherapy

Although less common than moist heat techniques such as hot packs or paraffin, fluidotherapy is another effective superficial thermal modality. Fluidotherapy involves the circulation of heated air and dry cellulose particles through a cabinet into which the body part is inserted into a nylon sleeve. The air and cellulose act as a fluid, floating the body part as though it were in water and transferring heat to it through convection. The temperature used in fluidotherapy is typically in the range of 100° to 118°F, and treatment durations are usually 20 minutes. Fluidotherapy devices come in a variety of sizes and configurations to accommodate different body parts, and many also have sleeves through which the practitioner can insert his or her hands to perform manual therapy during the treatment.

Future Questions

Although the use of superficial thermal modalities is very common, there is actually very little good research about their specific physiologic effects and even less about their efficacy in improving patient outcomes. The common 15- to 30-minute applications are more a matter of tradition than a data-driven guideline. The appropriate temperatures to use and tissue target temperature sought are also an area for which little definitive data exist. These modalities are prime targets for future research that examines their duration, frequency of use, and appropriate tissue temperatures.

Ultrasound

Description

Aside from cryotherapy, there is probably no modality about which more current research has been completed than for therapeutic ultrasound. The unfortunate reality about this research, however, is that there is still a great deal we do not know and a good amount of controversy about clinical outcomes.[40,41,120-122,155] Ultrasound, simply defined, is the use of acoustic energy at a frequency beyond the audible range (>30,000 Hz). Ultrasonic energy is used for many different purposes, some of which, like ultrasonic cleaning, have little to do with healing. Medical ultrasound is the application of ultrasonic energy for medical purposes, and it has two general categories. The first is imaging ultrasound, in which ultrasonic energy at frequencies between 1,000,000 Hz (1 MHz) and 10 MHz, is used to capture images of deep structures such as the heart or major blood vessels. A MEDLINE search using the term *ultrasound* will produce predominantly imaging ultrasound literature. Therapeutic ultrasound, on the other hand, is the use of ultrasonic energy to cause specific changes in tissues in an effort to improve healing or alter their function.

Although therapeutic ultrasound can theoretically use any of thousands of frequencies between 800 kHz and 3 MHz, two predominant frequencies, 1 and 3 MHz, are most commonly used. The acoustic energy is created when an alternating electrical current is applied to a neutral crystal, usually lead zirconate-titanate, causing the crystal to vibrate through an electropiezo effect. The vibrating crystal is tightly adhered to a metal plate on the transducer of the ultrasound device and sound waves are transmitted from the crystal through the metal plate and into the tissue. Generally a coupling medium is used to facilitate acoustic energy transmission.

We tend to conceptualize therapeutic ultrasound as either being thermal or nonthermal based on the intensity and duty cycle parameters that we select. In fact, the combination of intensity and duty cycle produces a continuum in which thermal ultrasound is at one end and nonthermal is at the other. Most of the time, our treatments are somewhere in between. We collectively characterize thermal ultrasound as a deep heating modality, although this characterization may be misplaced for 3 MHz ultrasound because it is commonly thought to heat to depths between 0.8 and 1.6 cm.[43,101,126,163]

How We Think It Works

The answer to this question about how we think therapeutic ultrasound works is somewhat complex because we use ultrasound for several different goals. We use thermal ultrasound with goals related to circulation, range of motion/tissue extensibility, calcium deposit reabsorption, and driving medications through the skin. Nonthermal ultrasound is gaining popularity for goals related to edema resolution, tissue regeneration, and fracture healing.

Thermal Ultrasound

Because it is more commonly used, we will begin with thermal ultrasound, that is, using ultrasound to cause a temperature increase in tissues. For ultrasound to cause a rise in tissue temperature, the acoustic energy must be absorbed. This absorption of acoustic energy is greater in tissues with higher protein content and at the interface between different types of tissue, particularly between bone and muscle.[99,100,102] For the temperature to increase, the rise in temperature produced by the ultrasound must be greater than the removal of that heat by conduction to other tissues and by the influx of unheated blood and carrying away of heated blood. Typically, thermal ultrasound is produced by a combination of higher ultrasound intensity and greater duty cycle (the percentage of time that acoustic energy is being produced by the transducer).

The most common use of thermal ultrasound is to augment techniques to improve range of motion. As was the case with superficial thermal modalities, ultrasound by itself is not adequate to effect a change in range of motion. Instead, ultrasound is used in an attempt to alter the elasticity of restricting tissues so that efforts to stretch them will be more effective.[42,47,122,157]

CLINICAL PEARL #10

Ultrasound does not effectively produce range of motion changes by itself; it is only effective as an adjunct to techniques such as stretching or joint mobilization and even then only if they are performed while the tissue temperature is still elevated in the therapeutic range.

There have been many studies in which this therapeutic range has been studied and clinical parameters to produce therapeutic temperatures have been described. Most of the early work was completed by Lehmann and colleagues in the 1960s through the early 1980s.[99-102] In several papers, they and others[57,100,101] attempted to identify the temperature range for elasticity changes in collagenous tissues and reported that the therapeutic range was somewhere between 39° or 40°C and 45°C. Temperatures less than 39° or 40°C did not produce significant elasticity changes and temperatures greater than 45°C often caused tissue damage. Later, Lehmann paraphrased this range in relative terms; that is, he described it in terms of the temperature change rather than the absolute temperatures.[101] A very important and often overlooked aspect of this early temperature-defining work was that the temperature range was not studied in vivo, it was not studied in humans, and the initial paper examining elasticity and temperature changes did not use ultrasound![57] In fact, the therapeutic temperature range was determined using excised sections of rat tail tendon in a heated bath at various temperatures. Although we commonly apply the data from this study to therapeutic ultrasound, we are actually making a relatively significant leap of faith that most clinicians do not realize they are making.

The relative description of temperature change first suggested by Lehmann[101] has gained a great deal of popularity recently with the extensive work of Draper and colleagues[41-45,47,48,157] whose papers often state that a "vigorous heating" temperature increase of 3° to 4°C is required for elasticity changes. As a general rule, thinking of relative temperature change as a clinical goal may be problematic, however. Many tissues commonly treated with ultrasound have baseline temperatures of approximately 35.5°C, and some baseline temperatures have been recorded that are less than 35°C.[122] For these tissues, a 4°C temperature change barely reaches the lower bound of the therapeutic range or may not reach it at all. In a recent article, Merrick and colleagues[126] observed that neurologically normal subjects reported that a distinct heating sensation was experienced with thermal ultrasound and that this sensation became uncomfortable to the point of discontinuing the treatments when temperatures exceeded 41°C. They speculated that this observation, although unconfirmed, may eventually form the basis of a clinical guideline for thermal ultrasound treatments in which the beginning of patient discomfort might serve as an indicator that the temperature has reached the therapeutic range.

The period of time when the temperature is in the therapeutic range has been described as the *stretching window*.[47,157] The stretching window with ultrasound has been reported to last only 2 to 3 minutes and researchers suggested that stretching should begin even before the conclusion of the ultrasound treatment. It has been clearly demonstrated that stretching at a lower magnitude for a longer period of time is more effective than shorter stretches of greater magnitude.[57,100,148] It has also been reported that the stretching window was briefer for superficial structures (3 MHz)[47] than it was with deeper structures (1 MHz).[157]

The literature directly examining ultrasound and stretching is very sparse and in the small amount of research on the topic very little promise is seen. Ultrasound applied to the calf of subjects with nonpathologic conditions produced little benefit during stretching compared with stretching alone (only a 3° difference in dorsiflexion).[42] Also, the benefits of the ultrasound were not residual; that is, there was no difference at the beginning of the session on the next day. The lack of good findings here may be a function of how ultrasound was used in the study rather than a failure of the modality.[120,122] The treatment area for ultrasound is normally limited to twice the effective radiating area of the crystal and this generally represents a volume of tissue roughly the same as two rolls of 35-mm photographic film for 1 MHz ultrasound. This is a relatively small volume of tissue compared with the total volume of the ankle plantar flexors. By heating only a portion of the total muscle group and by using subjects without an existing range of motion limitation, it is quite possible that the lack of effect in this study was related to the methodology. Similarly, the heating was mostly in muscle tissue rather than in collagenous tissues such as the Achilles tendon, and there are presently no data to suggest how heating of muscle affects range of motion, particularly in normal subjects. For these reasons and because we know that temperature does indeed affect the elasticity of collagenous connective tissues, ultrasound should be further examined in range of motion studies in which the volume of tissue and type of tissue are best suited to ultrasound treatments.

Thermal ultrasound through its increase in temperature can also lead to circulatory changes through vasodilation, and this increased blood flow may last as long as 45 to 60 minutes.[18] These circulatory changes, coupled with the case study–based notion that continuous ultrasound tended to cause reabsorption of calcium from bony deposits has made ultrasound popular for the treatment of bone spurs and other bony deposits. In particular, ultrasound has been used for bursitis and a variety of tendinopathies as well as for myositis ossificans. In fact, the actual efficacy of ultrasound for this purpose is still in question and has not been examined aside from case study literature in which no specific cause for resolution could be identified.[23]

Nonthermal Ultrasound

Nonthermal ultrasound is somewhat less familiar to most practitioners than its thermal counterpart, but is gaining in popularity. By convention, most nonthermal ultrasound treatments are accomplished by using a pulsed duty cycle. That is, the acoustic energy emitted by the transducer is "pulsed" so that it has an "on" period during which acoustic energy is emitted and an "off" period during which no energy is emitted. A 20% duty cycle with relatively normal intensity is probably the most common protocol, but some machines allow a number of pulsed options. The idea is that the heat produced by the ultrasound is allowed to dissipate before it produces a meaningful rise in tissue temperature. An alternative and increasingly more popular means of producing nonthermal ultrasound is to use a continuous (100% on time) duty cycle with a very low ultrasound intensity. There are inadequate data to compare the two approaches to date.

Nonthermal ultrasound is used primarily when the goal is to augment the repair or regeneration of damaged tissue. Although the work is preliminary, there are a number of strong studies that appear to support this use. Nonthermal ultrasound has been suggested to increase the regeneration of muscle tissue and bony tissue and aid in the healing of slow-to-heal skin ulcers.[20,22,60,73,85] This work is still very preliminary and much of it was conducted in animal models or in patients who are very different than the athletic patients we typically see. Therefore, caution should be used in applying these findings to the sports medicine area. Likewise, we do not yet know if nonthermal ultrasound is most effective when used as a pulsed protocol or a low-intensity continuous protocol although investigations of this topic are underway.

Phonophoresis

Another common use for therapeutic ultrasound is the transcutaneous delivery of medications, a technique known as phonophoresis. Since its introduction in 1954, phonophoresis has become a very popular clinical technique in the management of musculoskeletal injuries in athletes.[121] Unlike its cousin iontophoresis, phonophoresis is thought to drive whole molecules through the skin and into the underlying tissue and bloodstream.[18] If effective, phonophoresis would have the benefit of providing local medication delivery without the problems associated with injection or with the side effects often associated with oral medications. Transport of a drug across the skin barrier is limited by its ability to cross the outermost layer of the skin, the stratum corneum. Because this layer is composed of dead stratified squamous epithelial tissue, its permeability depends greatly on its level of hydration. Removal of a portion of the stratum corneum by abrasion greatly increases drug absorption until the layer is reestablished in 2 to 3 days. The easiest path for drug passage through the skin is through hair follicles, sebaceous glands, and sweat ducts with the follicles serving as the primary route of transmission. Heating the skin before phonophoresis increases the rate of drug transmission, enhancing local delivery.[121] On the other hand, heating immediately after phonophoresis increases the rate of drug absorption by the vascular system, decreasing local delivery but enhancing systemic delivery.

Phonophoresis is somewhat controversial, however.[6,19,28,35,84,121] In several studies, phonophoresis has been shown to increase the diffusion of hydrocortisone across the skin and into skeletal muscle and nervous tissue, and there are several studies showing positive clinical effects. On the other hand, most hydrocortisone preparations for phonophoresis have been suggested to be poor transmitters of ultrasound (Table 4-7). In one abstract ultrasound with hydrocortisone preparations produced intramuscular temperatures similar to those of standard ultrasound, however.[54] This leads to ongoing confusion about the efficacy of phonophoresis, and clearly it is an area in dire need of additional investigation.

Techniques and Dosage

To understand this section, a few ultrasound parameters will be discussed in relation to their effect on the treatment. First, the frequency of the acoustic energy (usually 1 or 3 MHz) determines the effective depth of the treatment. Lower-frequency ultrasound (i.e., 1 MHz) has a more collimated acoustic energy beam that results in a greater depth of heating than higher frequency ultrasound (i.e., 3 MHz). We generally describe the effective depth of heating in terms of half-value depths. A half-value depth is the depth at which 50% of the ultrasound energy has been absorbed by the tissue. The half-value depth of 1 MHz ultrasound is greater (2.3 cm) than that of 3 MHz ultrasound (0.8 cm).[163] Ultrasound devices have been shown to produce effective heating at depths of at least up to twice the half-value depth (i.e., around 5 cm for 1 MHz and around 2 cm for 3 MHz).[43,163]

Other important parameters for ultrasound include the spatial averaged intensity, often referred to simply as intensity. The spatial averaged intensity is the total amount of acoustic energy emitted by the transducer averaged over the effective radiating area (ERA) of the transducer. The ERA is simply the area of the transducer

Table 4-7

Ultrasound Transmission by Phonophoresis Media

Product	Transmission Relative to Water (%)
Media that transmit ultrasound (US) well	
Lidex gel, fluocinonide 0.05%[a]	97
Thera-Gesic cream, methyl salicylate 15%[b]	97
Mineral oil[c]	97
US gel[d]	96
US lotion[e]	90
Betamethasone 0.05%[f] in US gel[d]	88
Media that transmit US poorly	
Diprolene ointment, betamethasone 0.05%[g]	36
Hydrocortisone (HC) powder 1%[h] in US gel[d]	29
HC powder 10%[h] in US gel[d]	7
Cortril ointment, HC 1%[i]	0
Eucerin cream[j]	0
HC cream 1%[k]	0
HC cream 10%[k]	0
HC cream 10%[k] mixed with equal weight US gel[d]	0
Myoflex cream, trolamine salicylate 10%[l]	0
Triamcinolone acetonide cream 0.1%[k]	0
Velva HC cream 10%[h]	0
Velva HC cream 10%[h] with equal weight US gel[d]	0
White petrolatum[m]	0
Other	
Chempad-L[n]	68
Polyethylene wrap[o]	98

Reprinted from Cameron, M.H., and Monroe, L.G. (1992): Relative transmission of ultrasound by media customarily used for phonophoresis. Phys. Ther., 72:147. With the permission of the APTA.
[a]Syntex Laboratories Inc, 3401 Hillview Ave, PO Box 10850, Palo Alto, CA 94303.
[b]Mission Pharmacal Co, 1325 E Durango, San Antonio, TX 78210.
[c]Pennex Corp, Eastern Ave at Pennex Dr, Verona, PA 15147.
[d]Ultraphonic, Pharmaceutical Innovations Inc, 897 Frelinghuysen Dr, Newark, NJ 07114.
[e]Polysonic, Parker Laboratories Inc, 307 Washington St, Orange, NJ 07050.
[f]Pharmfair Inc, 100 Kennedy Dr, Hauppauge, NY 11788.
[g]Schering Corp, Galloping Hill Rd, Kenilworth, NJ 07033.
[h]Purepac Pharmaceutical Co, 200 Elmora Ave, Elizabeth, NJ 07207.
[i]Pfizer Labs Division, Pfizer Inc, 253 E 42nd St, New York, NY 10017.
[j]Beiersdorf Inc, PO Box 5529, Norwalk, CT 06856-5529.
[k]E Fougera & Co, 60 Baylis Rd, Melville, NY 11747.
[l]Rorer Consumer Pharmaceuticals, Div of Rhône-Poulenc Rorer Pharmaceuticals Inc, 500 Virginia Dr, Fort Washington, PA 19034.
[m]Universal Cooperatives Inc, 7801 Metro Pkwy, Minneapolis, MN 55420.
[n]Henley International, 104 Industrial Blvd, Sugar Land, TX 77478.
[o]Saran Wrap, Dow Brands Inc, 9550 Zionsville Rd, Indianapolis, IN 46268.

that is actually emitting the acoustic energy. The ERA is related to the size of the crystal and not the area of the sound head that contacts the patient. In fact, the ERA is always smaller than the patient contact area of the sound head. The intensity of the ultrasound is one of two major factors that determine the temperature rise. Higher intensities translate into higher temperatures. The other major determinant of temperature rise is the duty cycle already discussed.

A final important parameter for ultrasound is the beam nonuniformity ratio (BNR). The BNR of an ultrasound transducer is simply the ratio of the peak intensity at any point on the sound head to the average intensity. Because ultrasound crystals do not have perfect structures, "hot spots" are produced on the crystal where more energy is emitted than in other spots. The lower the BNR, the more uniform the crystal and the more comfortable the treatment to the patient. BNRs of more than 5:1 are generally considered to be unacceptable in modern equipment and BNRs of less than 4:1 should be sought. The BNR and ERA of the ultrasound transducer are generally found on a label on the transducer head or lead wire. Most ultrasound manufacturers report only the average BNR for a sample of their devices rather than reporting the BNR for each device.

Although not really considered a treatment parameter, another important consideration in ultrasound application is the coupling medium selected. Coupling media are used between the tissue being treated and the patient contact surface of the ultrasound transducer in an effort to facilitate the transfer of acoustic energy. Ultrasound is not well propagated through the air and without a coupling medium, a large amount of the energy is actually reflected at the transducer surface and may actually cause damage to the ultrasound transducer. Although there are many choices of coupling media, not all are equally effective. To allow comparison, the transmission capacity for media are usually expressed in terms relative to the transmission with distilled water (Table 4-7). Some commonly used media, such as hydrocortisone powder in ultrasound gel, have actually been shown to have poor transmission of ultrasound. Interestingly, although 10% hydrocortisone cream in ultrasound gel has been shown to only transmit 7% as much ultrasound as distilled water, ultrasound treatments coupled with

this medium appear to produce tissue temperature similar to those with ultrasound gel alone.[54] This apparent contradiction is puzzling and requires further study. Similarly, indirect ultrasound, for which the transducer and the body part are both immersed in water, has been shown to produce smaller temperature effects than directly coupled ultrasound. This may be a function of the temperature of the water and needs further exploration.

Perhaps more than any other research group, Draper and colleagues reported a great deal of information related to establishment of guidelines for the use of thermal ultrasound.[39,41,43,45-47,50,157] Their findings and those of other laboratories are summarized in Box 4-10. In an often cited paper Draper and co-workers[43] described temperature changes with continuous ultrasound at both 1 and 3 MHz at different depths and at different intensities. The observations from this study were that for 1 MHz ultrasound, an intensity of 2.0 W/cm^2 for 10 minutes was required to reach the therapeutic range and for 3 MHz an intensity of 2.0 W/cm^2 required only 3 minutes to reach the therapeutic range. An interesting set of observations was reported separately by Holcomb and Joyce[68] and by Merrick and colleagues[126] who each compared different brands of ultrasound devices using identical parameters. They each reported that not all devices produced the same results and that one brand of device in particular (Omnisound 3000) produced substantially greater temperature increases than the others. Merrick and colleagues[126] went on to suggest that because the commonly accepted parameters described by Draper and colleagues to produce therapeutic temperature changes were determined using an Omnisound device, these parameters may not be adequate for other brands of devices and either greater intensities or greater durations are probably required with other devices. Recommendations for effective ultrasound treatments are found in Box 4-11.

Future Questions

Although there are several major questions about ultrasound still to be answered, none is more important right now than the question of clinical outcome data. To date, there are virtually no quality outcome data for therapeutic ultrasound as was highlighted in a review by Robertson and Baker[155] earlier in the chapter (Table 4-1). Although

Box 4-10

Pertinent Research Findings on the Clinical Use of Ultrasound for Thermal Purposes

- Subcutaneous fat plays little or no role in determining ultrasound dosage.[49]
- Many (if not most) clinicians do not use an adequate ultrasound intensity.[41,43]
- Indirect (underwater) ultrasound does not produce the same temperature effect as direct ultrasound with coupling gel.[50]
- Precooling of tissues negates the thermal effects of ultrasound.[48]

Box 4-11

Recommendations for Effective Thermal Ultrasound Treatments

Parameter	Why It Is Important	Recommended Value
Sound frequency	It controls the depth of heating.	Use 1 MHz for tissues between 2.5 and 5 cm deep and 3 MHz for tissues up to 2.5 cm deep.
Duty cycle	It helps to determine whether the heat can accumulate.	Continuous (100% duty cycle) should be used.
Treatment area	Diluting the treatment over too large an area negates the heating effect. It is like using a candle to heat a bathtub full of water.	The treatment area should be no larger than twice the effective radiating area of the crystal (ERA). Note: the ERA is smaller than the patient contact area of the sound transducer.
Spatial averaged intensity	It determines the degree of heating. Higher intensities produce greater heating.	For 1 MHz ultrasound, the intensity should be at least 1.5 W/cm^2 and 2.0 W/cm^2 is recommended. For 3 MHz ultrasound, 1.5 W/cm^2 is recommended.
Treatment duration	It determines whether a thermal effect can be expected.	For 1 MHz treatments at 2.0 W/cm^2, the duration should be roughly 10 minutes. For 3 MHz treatments at 1.5 W/cm^2, the duration should be roughly 4 to 6 minutes. It may be possible to use patient sensation as a guide to duration. The patient should feel a heating sensation that approaches discomfort when the therapeutic range is reached.
BNR	It determines the patient's comfort and may contribute to heating rate.	Devices with lower BNRs are more comfortable and appear to heat tissue more quickly. Look for a BNR of 4:1 or less; lower is better.

BNR, beam nonuniformity ratio; ERA, effective radiating area.

they are to be commended for their attempts to describe the outcomes literature for ultrasound, Robertson and Baker created a problem in that their review suggested that the data do not support the clinical efficacy of therapeutic ultrasound. Although they reviewed the available literature, the only studies available for their use had serious methodologic flaws that included dramatic problems with the size of the treatment area, the intensity used, and the duration used.[40] These flaws were of such magnitude that positive clinical outcomes could not have been expected to occur. Thus, when data from these problematic studies are strictly used, the only logical conclusion would be that ultrasound is not effective. Since the publication of this review, a number of articles, editorials, and policy statements have called for the end of ultrasound as a clinical treatment. However, these calls for the death of ultrasound are probably a bit premature. There is growing evidence that when used appropriately, ultrasound does indeed produce some significant physiologic changes. However, quality clinical trials with good methodologies are desperately needed to document whether these effects seen in the laboratory translate into positive outcomes for the patient.

Shortwave Diathermy

Description

Shortwave diathermy is another deep heating thermal modality, and it is probably the best thermal modality available to the practitioner.[119] It is also a modality about which many practitioners have significant reservations, some of which are well founded and others of which are not. Shortwave diathermy uses shortwave (10 to 100 MHz) electromagnetic energy to cause an increase in tissue temperature. To avoid radiofrequency interference with communications frequencies, the Federal Communications Commission regulates the available frequencies of shortwave diathermy available and has allocated three frequencies for medical use (13.56, 27.12, and 40.68 MHz).

Shortwave diathermy devices are not commonly found in athletic health care facilities, and we rarely spend much time on this modality in our education programs. In fact, many of those teaching modality courses have never used diathermy on a patient. In many cases, diathermy education consists of a brief discussion of indications and effects and a more pointed discussion of the risks, contraindications, and precautions. The net result is that many practitioners are unfamiliar with diathermy and are apprehensive about using it on their patients. Likewise, we have been taught (incorrectly) that ultrasound can produce similar effects and is safer.

CLINICAL PEARL #11

Shortwave diathermy is probably safer than most practitioners suspect and appears to be considerably more effective than the other deep thermal modalities at our disposal.

How We Think It Works

All diathermies produce temperature changes through resistance to the passage of electromagnetic energy through the tissue being treated.[11,14,45,56,83,119] For shortwave diathermy, this passage of energy can lead to therapeutic temperature changes to depths of 6 to 8 cm. As with ultrasound, continuous shortwave diathermy (CSWD) produces greater temperature increases than does pulsed shortwave diathermy (PSWD).[83] However, unlike ultrasound, PSWD can indeed cause therapeutic temperature changes and is actually the most commonly used form.

The effects of diathermy are essentially the same as those for the other deep thermal modalities we have addressed and include temperature changes and their resulting effects on nerve function, circulation, tissue repair, and tissue elasticity. The real benefit of shortwave diathermy is that it accomplishes all of these effects to a much greater degree than the other deep thermal modalities that we use.[56] For example, a typical 1 MHz therapeutic ultrasound treatment can cover a treatment area with roughly the volume of two rolls of 35-mm photographic film. This is fine if you are treating a small injury, but it becomes a significant limitation if you are trying to treat the entire low back or the hamstring muscle of a running back. With shortwave diathermy, on the other hand, you are able to treat a volume of tissue roughly equivalent to a full bowl of breakfast cereal. The dramatic difference in the volume of tissue treated allows the effective use of shortwave diathermy in places where ultrasound cannot be effective.[42,46,56]

Techniques and Dosage

Although there are several application systems for PSWD, the most common of them is the induction method. In this setup, an electromagnetic field is generated by passing an electrical current through a coiled cable electrode, and the patient is placed into this field. Unlike the conductance method of diathermy, the patient is not actually a part of the electrical circuit. The resistance of a tissue to the passage of this electromagnetic field causes the temperature increase. There are two main configurations for the inductance method. In one a cable electrode that is coiled on top of or around the body part is used. In the other the cable is precoiled into a "drum" that is usually on a

swing-arm attached to the unit. The drum setup is very popular because it is the easiest and safest to use.

The most common frequency for PSWD is 27.12 MHz, and there are quite a few devices available on the market, although most are expensive and typically cost up to 10 times as much as a top-of-the-line ultrasound device. The parameters for most units are consistent and include a 20-minute treatment duration and pulsed delivery at 800 bursts/sec with a 400-fsec burst width. Average outputs of less than 38 W are considered to be nonthermal whereas higher outputs are thermal.

Shortwave diathermy has risks and drawbacks. Aside from the hefty price for the device, many practitioners have safety concerns related to both the patient and the clinician. Many safety concerns involved inadvertent burning of the patient. Patient burns typically result from clinician errors such as not checking precautions and contraindications (e.g., metal jewelry or implants or a lack of sensation in the treatment area) or allowing perspiration to accumulate (water heats preferentially). Burns are also more common with CSWD than with PSWD, particularly when one is using capacitance-type electrodes with which the patient becomes part of an electrical circuit. Microwave diathermy units, which are less common and not discussed in this chapter, can cause burns because the energy is reflected at tissue interfaces and forms standing waves that result in hot spots. Fortunately, most of the newer diathermy units are PSWD units operating at 27.12 MHz with induction electrodes that are no more likely to cause burns than are hot Hydrocollator packs.

A more pertinent safety-related concern with diathermy treatments involves stray electromagnetic energy from the units.[103,110,119] In diathermy treatments electromagnetic fields are used to produce thermal changes in the treated tissues. Unfortunately, these fields can extend beyond the area being treated. Martin and colleagues[110] examined stray electromagnetic energy from both shortwave and microwave diathermy units. They reported that continuous shortwave units and microwave units have stray electromagnetic fields above recommended levels for a distance of about 1 m surrounding cables and electrodes. Pulsed shortwave units, which are more common, had stray fields above recommended levels for a distance of about 0.5 m surrounding the electrodes. It has been suggested that repeated exposure to these stray fields may cause adverse health effects in clinicians, and appropriate care should be taken.

Electrical Stimulation

Description

People have been passing electrical currents through their bodies for healing purposes for thousands of years. In the last century researchers made a systematic attempt to describe the effects of such therapeutic uses of electricity and to organize them to make them useful. Much as was the case with cryotherapy, we have collectively learned that there are a number of different forms and therapeutic uses of electricity, and their popularity in athletic health care facilities is growing. The recent growth in the use of electrotherapy is probably related to manufacturing improvements in electrotherapy devices that make them easier to use and provide more treatment options than were available before. Although this growth has certainly bolstered the clinical use of electrotherapy, it has also created a strong tendency to use "cookbook" electrotherapy protocols rather than protocols based on specific goals for the patient. In fact, many clinicians now learn to use only preset protocols that are factory programmed onto the machine, and they have great difficulty in creating a custom protocol to accomplish their goals. Worse yet, many of the factory preset protocols for electrotherapy devices have little or no basis in basic research or outcomes data and may not be effective at all. Similarly, there is a great deal of inconsistency across manufacturers' terminology such that practitioners must first translate the instruction manuals into a common set of terms before they can understand them. For these reasons, it is important that practitioners have a good understanding of the basic principles of electrotherapy and the ability to apply these to produce desired outcomes. This section provides a basic framework and description of electrotherapy, but it cannot be a substitute for a comprehensive course in therapeutic modalities.

How We Think It Works
Electricity Fundamentals and Terminology

A basic familiarity with electricity is assumed for this discussion, but a brief review of a few essential concepts that influence the clinical use of electrotherapy is provided here.[62] First, *electricity* is the flow of electrons from an area of high concentration to an area of lower concentration. Because electrons carry a negative charge, the area of high electron concentration has a negative charge or negative polarity and the area of low concentration has a positive charge or positive polarity. Therefore, electricity flows from a negatively charged area, called the *negative pole* or *cathode*, to a positively charged area, called the *positive pole* or *anode*. An electrically conductive pathway connecting the negative pole to the positive pole is called a *circuit*. Electrotherapy treatments work by making the targeted tissues a part of this circuit. The flow of electricity along a circuit is known as *current*. Electrical currents can either be continuous, like water constantly running through a garden hose, or interrupted, like turning the spigot for our garden hose on and off quickly and repeatedly so that you get separate spurts of water through the hose. The amount of electricity flowing along the circuit is measured in amperes and is analogous to the volume of water in the garden hose. The force that moves the electrons along the circuit is referred to as voltage and is

analogous to water pressure in our garden hose. The relationship between force and flow (voltage and current) is described by Ohm's law (Box 4-12).

For most of our uses of clinical electrotherapy, the direction of the current flow (i.e., which end of the circuit is positive or negative) is seldom as important as ensuring that current actually flows through the target tissue in sufficient amounts to cause the physiologic response we are seeking. The flow of current is always unidirectional, from the negative pole to the positive pole. If the two poles at the ends of the circuit never change polarity while the current is on, then the direction of current flow is constant, and we call this *direct current* (DC). If the two poles at the ends of the circuit switch polarity, the direction of the current flow also switches, and this is called *alternating current* (AC). AC is the type of current available from electrical wall outlets, and it switches direction at a constant rate of 60 cycles/sec (60 Hz) in North America. DC is the type of current that is available from a battery.

By connecting the electrical circuit to an oscilloscope, we can visualize the shape, or waveform, of the current (Fig. 4-8). The waveform for DC would be entirely on one side of the horizontal baseline and would continue along indefinitely until the current is turned off (Fig. 4-8A). Because the current is always moving in one direction, the charge would always have the same polarity and would remain on one side of the baseline. DC can therefore be said to have a single phase and is often called *monophasic current*. With AC, the waveform would initially be on one side of the baseline, and then switch to the other side when the direction of the current and therefore the polarity alternated (Fig. 4-8B). The graph would repeat this switching as long as the current is flowing. Thus, AC can be said to have two phases (one positive and one negative) and is therefore often called *biphasic current*. A third type of current, *polyphasic current*, actually has three or more phases and is typically produced by simultaneously overlaying an interrupted current over a continuous biphasic current called a carrier frequency. Common examples of polyphasic waveform devices are interferential stimulators and Russian stimulators.[173]

If we turn the current on and off repeatedly, we would have individual phases with periods of no current flow (no charge) between them (Fig. 4-8C) and this is often called

Box 4-12

Ohm's Law

$$I = \frac{V}{R}$$

I = current flow (in amps)
V = driving force (in volts)
R = resistance to current flow (in Ohms)

The greater the driving force, the greater the flow of current

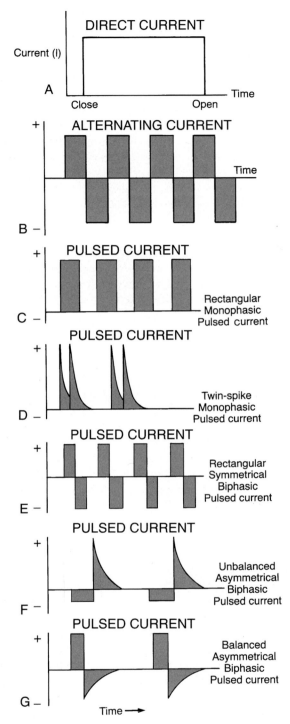

Figure 4-8. Graphic representation of the three types of electrical current. *A,* Direct current. *B,* Alternating current. *C* through *G,* Pulsed currents. (Modified from Robinson, A.J. [1989]: Basic concepts and terminology in electricity. *In:* Snyder-Mackler, L., and Robinson, A.J. [eds.]: Clinical Electrophysiology. Baltimore, Williams and Wilkins, pp. 9, 11, 13.)

pulsed or *interrupted current.* The majority of electrotherapy devices use interrupted current, although there are a few exceptions that are discussed later in the chapter. Electrotherapy devices allow the practitioner to control the number of these individual pulses per second (pps; pulse rate). With low pulse rates (<30), pulsing muscle contractions can be caused. By increasing the pulse rate to between 30 and 50 pps the muscle contraction appears smooth and sustained. A muscle that is contracting in a smooth and sustained fashion is said to be in tetany. Even higher pulse rates are often used and also cause tetanic contractions. You will note (Fig. 4-8*D-G*) that by using different combinations of polarity, voltage, and phase duration, we can control the shape of each phase. Common phase shapes are rectangular or square (Fig. 4-8*E*), spiked or twin spiked (Fig. 4-8*D*), asymmetrical (Fig. 4-8*F* and *G*), in which the positive phase and negative phase have different shapes, and sinusoidal (Fig. 4-9). If the positive phase and negative phases have the same voltage (height), the waveform is said to be balanced (Fig. 4-8*G*).

In examining a waveform, we use a specific set of terms to describe the phases and pulses (Fig. 4-9). A *phase* is a single positively or negatively charged bolus of current, whereas a *pulse* is several consecutive phases that are continuous. All currents have at least one phase, but pulses are seen only with interrupted current and are separated from each other by brief intervals where no phase is present. The height, or amplitude, of each phase represents the voltage (the driving force for the current). The width of each phase represents the phase duration or phase width, usually in milliseconds. A related concept is pulse width, the combined duration of all of the phases within a single pulse of interrupted current. Related to phase and pulse widths are phase and pulse intervals, the duration between phases where there is no current (phase interval) or between pulses where there is no current (pulse interval). *Phase interval* and *pulse interval* are terms that are sometimes used interchangeably.

The lack of consistency in terminology across manufacturers and textbooks is an ongoing problem in electrotherapy and this leads us to a fourth, and sometimes confusing, waveform concept called *frequency.* The frequency of a waveform can mean two very different things. Technically it represents the number of cycles per second for the current. A cycle, also called a period, is one complete waveform including all of its phases. In clinical usage, the term frequency more commonly means the number of pulses per second and is also called the pulse rate. Remember that a pulse is several consecutive cycles of a current in an interrupted current. For example, if you use the electricity coming from your wall outlet, it is a continuous sinusoidal biphasic current with a frequency of 60 Hz. Now, say that you are using an outlet connected to a switch and you manually turn the current on and off 10 times per second. The resulting current would be an

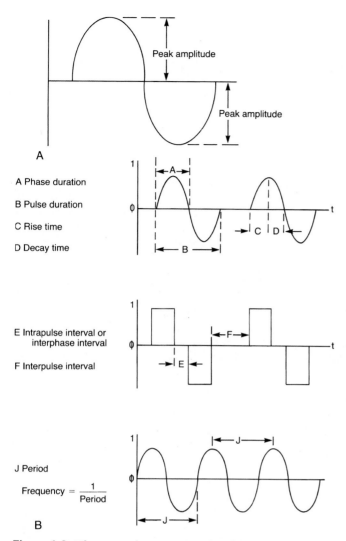

Figure 4-9. Electricity characteristics. (Modified from Robinson, A.J. [1989]: Basic concepts and terminology in electricity. *In:* Snyder-Mackler, L., and Robinson, A.J. [eds.]: Clinical Electrophysiology. Baltimore, Williams and Wilkins, p. 15.)

interrupted sinusoidal biphasic current with a frequency of 60 Hz and a pulse rate of 10 Hz. Obviously this terminology can be somewhat confusing, and most clinicians and manufacturers generally use *frequency* to mean *pulse rate* and the actual frequency of the current being interrupted is ignored.

Although the scientific study of electrotherapy is progressing, we do not know as much about the physiology of this modality as we do for cryotherapy, superficial thermotherapy, or ultrasound, and the precise mechanisms by which electrotherapy is effective have not yet been described. As was the case for these better-studied modalities, there is a conspicuous lack of outcomes research for electrotherapy as well. Even though the literature is still sparse, there are a number of rehabilitative goals for which electrotherapy has been suggested to be effective (Box 4-13),

most of which are related to the ability of electricity to depolarize nerves. There are also some proposed effects that are related to the electrical charge fields around the electrodes and that do not rely on nerve depolarization.

Muscle Reeducation

Neuromuscular function is altered through inhibition after injury as previously discussed with rehabilitative cryotherapy. In fact, the great majority of early muscular strength and power loss after an injury is thought to result from neurologic inhibition rather than from more morphologic causes such as loss of muscle mass. Muscular strength and power losses are seen immediately after injury before a loss of muscle mass has even occurred. In fact, the loss of muscle mass as an explanation for the loss of strength only becomes valid after several weeks have passed. The goal of muscle reeducation is to counteract postinjury inhibition in an attempt to allow for more normal use of the surrounding musculature. By reducing the degree of inhibition seen in these muscles in the early period after injury, earlier and more functional exercise can begin, and this exercise is the most important tool in returning the athlete to competition. Muscle reeducation is sometimes thought of as helping a muscle to "remember" how to contract. Similarly, reeducation can be used to help reestablish neuromuscular pathways after periods of immobilization or even to help correct pathologic neuromuscular patterns such as those that are seen when a patient compensates for gait or postural abnormalities. An additional means by which electrotherapy can help with reeducation is by overcoming the inhibition associated with the injury.[70]

The primary means by which electrotherapy is thought to be an effective tool for muscle reeducation is through the recruitment of motor units that are not otherwise being recruited. The muscle tissue is not directly caused to contract, however. Instead, the electrical current stimulates motor neurons to depolarize and thereby causes contraction of their respective muscle fibers. By artificially recruiting these motor units through stimulation of the motor nerves, it is thought that we may somehow overcome the inhibitory stimuli that are interfering with their voluntary recruitment at some location up the neurologic tree.[70] Although there is common anecdotal agreement about the efficacy of muscle reeducation, very little research has been done to directly examine its effects.

Retard Atrophy

As was the case with muscle reeducation, electrotherapy used to retard atrophy is based on the ability of electrical current to cause muscle contraction.[4,143] During disuse, immobilization, or paralysis, the relative inactivity of the muscles leads them to atrophy. Likewise, a lack of muscle contraction–induced stress on the bones can also cause them to atrophy, eventually to the point at which they can become fragile if the disuse is of sufficient

Box 4-13

Common Therapeutic Goals for Electrotherapy

Goal	Rationale
Muscle reeducation	Retrain firing patterns or overcome neuromuscular inhibition in intact muscles after injury or pathologic change. The mechanism is thought to be related to increasing the quantity of motor units recruited or decreasing the inhibition of the motor nerves that is preventing normal function.
Retard atrophy	Cause the muscle to contract in an effort to reduce the atrophy effects of immobilization or paralysis.
Retard edema formation	Limit the formation of edema during acute inflammation by inhibiting the increase in vascular permeability with sensory level stimulation.
Remove edema	Remove edema that is already present through a muscle-pump mechanism with motor-level stimulation.
Reduce pain	Interfere with the transmission or perception of pain through a variety of different electrotherapy approaches.
Reduce spasm	Reduce acute spasms by either reducing the contraction frequency of the muscle or by fatiguing the muscle until it fails (very uncomfortable). Electrotherapy can also be used in managing the spasticity associated with neuromuscular diseases or spinal cord trauma.
Increase strength	Increase muscle force output in nonpathologic tissue by causing hypertrophy of the muscle. Although muscular strength can be improved with motor level stimulation, the protocols required are very uncomfortable and are not nearly as effective as resistance exercise. This is not generally an appropriate goal for electrotherapy.
Increase range of motion	A commonly cited but misleading goal. Electrotherapy can be effective in reducing muscle spasticity or edema and thereby countering ROM loss associated with them, but electrotherapy is not an effective means of improving ROM by itself.
Transport medications	Iontophoresis: Deliver medications by driving electrically charged ions through the skin.
Tissue healing	Microcurrent: There is some evidence that microcurrent may augment tissue repair with fractures or slow-healing skin ulcerations. The mechanism has yet to be described.

duration. Electrotherapy is often used if prolonged immobilization is anticipated, such as with casting for fractures or with paralysis. The premise is that electrotherapy can be used to cause low-intensity isometric contractions of the muscle that can retard the progression of atrophy without compromising the immobilization. Note that the word *retard* was used rather than *prevent*. Prevention implies that we can completely counteract the atrophy that is occurring (Box 4-14). Instead, we are more likely to slow its progression.

Edema Management

The management of edema with electrotherapy can take two different forms. The first of these is retarding the formation of the edema. The second is removing edema that is already present. The technique is different for each strategy, and each technique should only be used in the correct situation. For example, the use of electrotherapy to retard the formation of edema should only be used in the period during which edema is forming immediately after the injury. Use of this approach once a large area of edema is already present may actually inhibit the removal of that edema.

Sensory level, high-voltage pulsed electrical stimulation applied directly to the area of the injury has been shown to limit the volume of edema after uniform injuries in an animal model.[9,79,118,165,167] There have been two proposed mechanisms for this retarding of edema through the application of electrotherapy. The first is that the current combats the increasing permeability of the capillaries during the initial acute inflammatory response and thereby reduces the efflux of fluid from the circulatory system into the injured tissues. As explained in Chapter 2, one of the major events of the acute inflammatory response is a marked increase in capillary permeability that results from the release of numerous chemical mediators. The permeability increase occurs when adjacent endothelial cells in capillaries do not adhere to each other as tightly as they normally do. This makes the capillaries "leaky" and allows the transcapillary Starling forces to exert an even greater influence. The second and less accepted of the proposed mechanisms is that pulsed monophasic current causes vascular spasm that limits the delivery of fluid to the injured area. Regardless of the suggested physiologic explanation for the effectiveness of the technique, the protocol used is very specific and requires a specific waveform. This protocol is outlined in the section on technique and dosage later in this chapter. One of the key elements of the protocol is the timing in relation to injury. This approach is only effective when it is begun

Box 4-14

Three Reasons Why Electrotherapy Cannot Completely Prevent Atrophy

- The scenario in which electrotherapy is typically used to retard atrophy involves prolonged and purposeful immobilization. In such situations, strong muscle contractions are generally to be avoided so that displacement of the immobilized structures does not take place. Therefore, we tend to use mild isometric contractions that will retard atrophy, but not prevent it.
- Second, and probably more importantly, the pattern of motor unit recruitment with electrical stimulation appears to be quite different from that seen with voluntary contraction. In volitional contractions, smaller diameter motor neurons supplying small muscle fibers of small motor units are recruited first and larger neurons with larger and stronger motor units are recruited later as needed for greater muscle force. With electrical stimulation, this order appears to be reversed so that larger diameter motor neurons are recruited first and smaller diameter fibers are recruited less and only when sufficient voltage is used.[23,37,151,162] This different pattern of muscle recruitment leads to a variable rate of atrophy for which the smaller motor neuron motor units, which are responsible for fine motor tasks, atrophy at a faster rate than the larger motor neuron motor units that are responsible for gross motor tasks.
- A third reason why we appear to be unable to completely prevent atrophy is related to the athletic ability and training level of athletes. Even if we were not concerned about the consequences of displacing our immobilized tissue with strong contractions, it is unlikely that we could produce strong enough contractions to prevent all muscle loss in injured athletes. By the nature of their extensive training and conditioning programs, athletes have considerably larger muscle masses and force-producing capacities than the patient in general. The differential recruitment of motor units with electrical stimulation implies that we are not likely to be able to generate sufficient muscle force with electrical stimulation to provide an adequate stimulus to retain the muscle mass that has been produced by extensive resistance training.

before significant edema has formed. Therefore, the time window for initiating this modality is quite literally the first few minutes after the injury.

In addition to retarding the formation of edema during acute inflammation, electrotherapy can also be a valuable adjunct in the removal of edema that is already present. The proposed mechanism by which existing edema is removed is somewhat different from that for retarding the formation of edema, however. Whereas retarding the formation of edema was based on limiting the permeability of the vasculature, such a strategy may actually hinder our ability to remove edema. Once, present, edema is removed by the lymphatic system rather than the circulatory system. The removal requires that the edematous fluid be absorbed into lymph capillaries where it flows to larger collecting vessels and eventually to one of the lymphatic ducts where the fluid is returned to the circulatory system. If we limit the permeability of the lymphatic capillaries, a potential outcome of the edema retardation electrotherapy protocol, we may actually hinder the movement of fluid into the lymphatic system and therefore reduce our effectiveness of edema removal.

Instead of using protocols focused on altering permeability, edema removal protocols focus on moving fluid into the lymphatic system and then moving it along the lymphatic vessels and away from the injury site.[29,53,59,67,140,141] This is accomplished by motor level electrical stimulation with which muscles are caused to contract in a pulsing fashion using interrupted current. Each muscle contraction exerts external pressure on the lymphatic vessels. The squeezing of the lymphatic vessels causes the fluid in them to move. This strategy for edema removal is sometime

called the *muscle pump strategy*. When fluid reaches the collecting vessels of the lymphatic system, its flow essentially becomes unidirectional because of the presence of one-way valves within the vessels. Much like the valves located in the veins, pressure exerted on the lymphatic vessel from muscular contractions causes the upstream valve to close and the downstream valve to open, allowing the fluid to only flow back toward the circulatory system. Because fluid moves with each muscular contraction, electrotherapy pulse rates that are less than the level needed for tetany are used. Tetanic contractions would only produce a single pressure pulse and would not be expected to move as much fluid as repetitive contractions.

CLINICAL PEARL #12

Although electrotherapy can be a useful adjunct to edema removal, the role of exercise in removing edema should not be overlooked. Exercise also causes muscle pumping, typically in more muscles than are used with electrotherapy alone.

Pain Management

The management of pain with electrotherapy is among the most common, best documented, and most successful uses of this modality.[3,15,24,52,72,74,76,77,131,144,152] Much of the pain reduction literature deals with a subform of electrotherapy called *transcutaneous electrical nerve stimulation* (TENS). TENS typically involves the use of pulsed, sensory level stimulation to interfere with the transmission of pain signals in the spinal cord through a mechanism known as gait control. Gait control uses sensory information on A-β afferent nerves to interfere with the transmission of pain on A-δ and C afferent fibers. To be effective, adequate stimulation of the A-β fibers must occur. The literature suggests that this is most likely to occur with pulse rates between 60 and 150 pps, and pulse rates of 100 to 150 pps are most common.[23,37,162] Because of the high pulse rates this protocol is called *high-frequency TENS*. High-frequency TENS units generally use a short pulse duration (20 to 60 μsec) combined with a 50- to 100-Hz frequency of stimulation. Additionally, the combination of sensory level TENS and cryotherapy has been shown to provide greater pain relief than either of these modalities used individually.

Although the gait control strategy is certainly the most common, it is not the only strategy for controlling pain with electrotherapy. Motor level stimulation with a high-voltage (>150 V) stimulator can be used to stimulate the release of endogenous opiate-like substances from nerve fibers. Sometimes this protocol is referred to as *low TENS* because of its low pulse rate (2 to 4 pps). The patient is often uncomfortable during application but experiences pain relief after the treatment. This is somewhat different from conventional high-frequency TENS with which pain relief is usually experienced during the treatment and for a short time after. The release of opiates strategy is not as common as the gate control strategy; however, it may provide longer-lasting pain relief.

Another pain relief technique with electrotherapy involves the use of a sensory level polyphasic current known as *interferential current*.[72,76,77] Interferential current is actually the combination of two different biphasic currents that are out of phase with each other. The two currents each have different frequencies and are carried on two different circuits (or channels) that are applied more or less perpendicular to each other. The differing frequencies of the currents and the fact that they are out of phase with each other produce a constantly changing waveform in the region where the currents cross. The key feature of interferential electrotherapy is this constantly changing waveform. Because the waveform is constantly changing, the body has a very difficult time accommodating to it. Accommodation is the process by which the sensory system learns to ignore sensory stimuli that are unchanging. For example, persons married for more than a few months no longer sense their wedding ring against their finger. The body has a reasonably good ability to accommodate to electrotherapy, particularly sensory level electrotherapy. This accommodation reduces the efficacy of the treatments. With interferential electrotherapy, the constantly changing waveform reduces the accommodation and allows the treatment to be more effective than fixed waveform treatments. The mechanism for pain relief is thought to be the same as that for high-frequency TENS. In fact, many TENS units now use modulated waveforms that change throughout the treatment in an attempt to overcome accommodation.

Spasticity Management

The management of spasticity is among the more commonly cited uses of electrotherapy, although it is generally less applicable with athletic injuries than with other conditions such as neurologic lesions. The management of spasticity associated with neurologic lesions often involves stimulating the antagonist muscles and relying on reciprocal relaxation. In fact, in the vast majority of the literature on electrotherapy for spasticity the focus is on this type of spasticity, which results from spinal cord trauma, cerebral vascular accidents, brain trauma, and disease.[158] Because these lesions are not common with athletic injuries, they will not be discussed further in this chapter. On the other hand, the management of muscle spasm associated with athletic injuries is a common use of electrotherapy and needs to be addressed, although the literature describing it is very sparse.

There are two predominant strategies for managing athletic injury–related acute muscle spasm with electrotherapy, although only one of them is very tolerable to the patient. The more tolerable of the two strategies involves using motor level stimulation to the spastic muscles in an attempt to alter their contraction frequency. Recall that the rate of firing of the motor units determines whether the contraction of a muscle will be pulsing or smooth (tetanic). Smooth contractions occur with firing rates greater than 30 to 50 pps. When a muscle is in spasm, it is generally contracting smoothly and continuously. By using a muscle stimulator with relatively high intensity and a less than tetanic pulse rate, it may be possible to slow the firing rate and cause the spasm to stop. The other and probably more effective strategy involves using the stimulator to fatigue the muscle to the point where the spasm ceases. This strategy has been shown to be effective, but it is not very comfortable and most patients may not tolerate it well. Generally the technique involves the use of high pulse rate stimulation at a maximally tolerable intensity from a high-voltage stimulator to recruit as many motor units as is possible. This will eventually lead to muscular fatigue, and the spasm will lessen or stop altogether. Although this technique is uncomfortable, it can be made more comfortable and more effective if it is combined with a static stretch of the affected muscles. Cryotherapy is also a common adjunct in this technique.

Increasing Strength

Although electrotherapy can indeed be used to improve strength, this is among the most often misapplied uses of this modality. To understand this application of electrotherapy, we must first make a distinction between the use of electrotherapy for muscle reeducation versus the use of electrotherapy for increasing strength. As discussed earlier, muscle reeducation involves using electrotherapy to overcome neuromuscular inhibition that is interfering with normal muscle function. Said another way, muscle reeducation involves using an electrical stimulator to try to improve pathologic muscle function by reestablishing the normal and appropriate neurologic pathways for muscle contraction. This is different from using a stimulator to improve muscle strength.

When we use a stimulator to improve strength, we are not trying to overcome inhibition or other neuromuscular pathologic changes. Instead, we are using electrotherapy to strengthen tissue that has normal neuromuscular function but that is not as strong as we would like it to be. Said another way, muscle strengthening with electrotherapy is about causing an overload to the contractile elements within muscle in an attempt to cause them to adapt by becoming stronger. This is precisely the same goal that we have with resistance training to improve muscle strength, but the catch is that resistance training is considerably more effective for this goal than is electrotherapy.

To strengthen muscle tissue, regardless of the method, the muscle must exert more force than it is accustomed to exerting. This principle is known as *overload*. Overload of a muscle can be accomplished in two ways: increasing the rate of firing of motor units and recruiting a larger number of motor units.[61] During resistance training, the body's strategy is to do both, but to predominantly favor recruiting more motor units. In fact, during exercise, the body varies its motor unit recruitment pattern. At the beginning of an exercise, the smaller diameter motor neurons of the fine control motor units are recruited. If more force is required, then the larger diameter motor neurons controlling the stronger but less finely controlled motor units are recruited. As the muscle begins to fatigue, the fine control motor units fail first and additional large motor units are recruited until they eventually fail. This is why we start to see some shaking and less coordination as muscles get fatigued during resistance training. When a muscle stimulator is used, however, we see a different pattern of recruitment.[23,37,162]

A muscle stimulator also improves strength by depending on overload and uses both a high rate of motor unit firing and measures aimed to recruit more motor units. In strengthening with electrotherapy, a pulse rate at or near the maximum available for the stimulator is used in an effort to produce as high a rate of motor unit firing as possible. Also, as high an intensity (voltage) as is tolerable is used because higher intensities lead to better penetration of the nerve by the electrical current and therefore recruitment of an increased number of motor units. The unfortunate catch in this strategy, however, is that motor unit recruitment with electrotherapy appears to operate backwards from normal voluntary recruitment. With electrotherapy, the motor units that are of larger diameter and that are closer to the surface of the nerve are preferentially

recruited. These same motor units appear to be stimulated over and over, rather than different motor units being recruited as some of them fatigue, as is the case with normal exercise. This repeated firing of the same motor units is the reason that muscular fatigue is experienced so quickly with electrical stimulation and not so quickly with exercise. The repeated recruitment of a limited set of motor units also limits the effectiveness of electrotherapy-based strengthening programs. Strengthening adaptations are essentially limited to the motor units that are being recruited, and with electrotherapy fewer motor units are recruited than with active exercise. Although some degree of strengthening of normal tissue can occur with electrotherapy, the strengthening is not as effective as active exercise in a resistance training program. Therefore, the use of electrotherapy for muscle reeducation is recommended in athletic therapy, but the use of electrotherapy as a tool to strengthen muscles that have normal function is not.

Increasing Range of Motion

Many texts on modalities suggest that electrotherapy can be used to improve range of motion, and it certainly can do so, but not in the way we are usually seeking with athletic injuries. The use of electrotherapy to improve range of motion is appropriate and effective in only a few limited situations. The most common of these is for a patient with neurologic trauma or disease that results in spasticity. For example, it is not uncommon to see spasticity in the gastrocnemius and soleus muscles of a patient with a spinal cord injury. Such spasticity leads to a lack of ankle dorsiflexion range of motion. Electrotherapy to the dorsiflexors can be used to both stimulate them and to inhibit the gastrocnemius and soleus. This would allow greater dorsiflexion range of motion because of the reduction in spasticity of the plantarflexors. Although useful in some patients with neurologic conditions, this type of range of motion improvement is of little value in the rehabilitation of common athletic injuries. A situation that is of more use with athletic injuries is improving range of motion that is limited by pain, edema, or both. As discussed earlier, electrotherapy can be used in the management of these conditions and may result in an indirect improvement in range of motion as well.

Iontophoresis of Pharmaceuticals

Iontophoresis, the use of an electrical current to deliver medications through the skin is another common form of electrotherapy. This technique has some real advantages in that it can be used to deliver medications locally without having to inject them. This can be particularly useful for patients with fear of needles or for pediatric patients. In fact, iontophoresis with local anesthetics is gaining popularity as a preinjection technique to lessen the discomfort of pediatric immunizations. Although potentially advantageous, there is also some controversy over iontophoresis in the literature.[1,18,31,106,149,161,170,172] There are conflicting reports as to whether iontophoresis delivers enough medication to a deep enough tissue depth to be effective for many conditions. Also, outcomes data for iontophoresis are limited, and the technique has not been adequately demonstratied to have much benefit in patients with musculoskeletal injuries.

Iontophoresis requires a very specific type of electrical current and is not possible with typical muscle stimulators. To use electrical current to move medications, the medications must dissociate into electrically charged ions in solution. When an electrical current is applied to the medication solution, the charge at each electrical pole repels the medication ions with like charges and attracts the ions with opposite charges. Therefore, it is critical that the medication be applied to the electrode that has the same polarity as the ion of interest in the medication. Likewise, only a direct (monophasic) current can be used because alternating (biphasic) currents would both repel and retract the medication, producing no net transport through the skin. The current used also needs to be continuous. Interrupted currents do not repel the drug long enough for it to travel through the skin. For these reasons, iontophoresis stimulators are different from other electrotherapy devices and are designed expressly for use in iontophoresis. These devices are equipped with single-use electrodes and deliver low-intensity direct current in a monopolar setup as described later. The dosage is typically the product of the treatment duration and the amount of current used and is expressed in milliampere minutes. The specific dosage depends on the medication being used and treatments last typically between 10 and 20 minutes although they can be longer if lower amounts of current must be used because the patient does not tolerate the direct current well. A new iontophoresis device, the IontoPatch, was introduced in April 2001 and is somewhat different. Instead of the typical 10- to 20-minute treatment with low to moderate amounts of current, the treatment duration with the IontoPatch is much longer (usually 24 hours) and at an extremely low level of current delivered from a self-contained battery in the patch. The lower level of current means fewer complications in terms of skin burns, and anecdotal reports have been very favorable although research results are lacking because the device is so new.

A relatively small number of medications, usually corticosteroids, are commonly used with iontophoresis in athletic medicine settings. However, from a technical standpoint, any medication that dissociates into ions in solution to produce the desired effects could be used. The most commonly used medications are found in Table 4-8.

Clinical Considerations

The specific waveform chosen for electrotherapy can be critical in some cases and can make very little difference in others. One of the hallmarks of a skilled practitioner is an understanding of the difference, which requires familiarity with the fundamentals of electricity and the terminology defined earlier as well as an understanding of the following concepts. First, we have already discussed the fact that waveforms can be monophasic (DC), biphasic (AC), or polyphasic (a mixed waveform such as interferential current). We have also discussed the fact that waveforms can be either continuous or interrupted. These points can be combined to produce some general classes of waveforms that have impacts on clinical treatments.

Continuous versus Interrupted Current

Continuous currents are found in very few devices and are used in very specific situations. The first of these is for iontophoresis for which a continuous monophasic current is used. Continuous currents must be used in this situation because interrupted currents do not have a sufficient duration of current flow to move ions across the skin. A second situation for which continuous current is used is for stimulation of denervated muscle to prevent disuse atrophy. In this situation, continuous current is used because the longer current duration makes it easier to cause depolarization of what little remains of the motor nerves or perhaps even the muscle itself. Aside from these two situations, continuous currents are normally only found as biphasic carrier frequencies in polyphasic currents. In these currents, they are normally used to create a perpetually changing waveform to help overcome accommodation as is the case with both interferential current and a waveform used for strengthening known as MFBurstAC or Russian current.[173]

Polarity

Electrotherapy devices that offer monophasic waveforms can be readily distinguished from biphasic or polyphasic waveforms because of their ability to select a polarity for the treatment electrodes. Because biphasic and polyphasic waveforms have both positively and negatively charged phases that alternate, no specific polarity can be assigned to the electrodes. In fact, there are very few situations in which the specific polarity of the electrodes makes a clinical difference; however it does make a very big difference in a few. For example, iontophoresis can only be accomplished with a continuous monophasic current and even then only when the drug is applied to the correct electrode. Another situation in which polarity clearly matters is in the stimulation of denervated muscle for preventing disuse atrophy; however, this is a topic that is less important in rehabilitation of athletic injuries. A third situation in which polarity has been suggested to make a difference is in electrotherapy to retard the formation of edema. In this situation, cathodal (negative polarity) stimulation has been shown to be effective as discussed later. There is little evidence to suggest that

Table 4-8

Ions and Radicals from Nonsteroidal Drugs

Ion or Radical (Charge)	Features*
Magnesium (+)	From magnesium sulfate (Epsom salts), 2% aqueous solution; excellent muscle relaxant, good vasodilator, mild analgesic
Mecholyl (+)	Familiar derivative of acetylcholine, 0.25% ointment; powerful vasodilator, good muscle relaxant and analgesic; used with discogenic low back radiculopathies and sympathetic reflex dystrophy
Iodine (−)	From Iodex ointment, 4.7%; bactericidal, fair vasodilator, excellent sclerolytic agent; used successfully with adhesive capsulitis ("frozen shoulder"), scars
Salicylate (−)	From Iodex ointment with methyl salicylate, 4.8% ointment (if desired without the iodine, can be obtained from Myoflex ointment, [trolamine salicylate, 10%] or from a 2% aqueous solution of sodium salicylate powder); a general decongestant, sclerolytic, and anti-inflammatory agent; used successfully with frozen shoulders, scar tissue, warts, and other adhesive or edematous conditions
Calcium (+)	From calcium chloride, 2% aqueous solution; believed to stabilize the irritability threshold in either direction, as dictated by the physiologic needs of the tissues; effective with spasmodic conditions, tics, "snapping joints"
Chlorine (−)	From sodium chloride, 2% aqueous solution; good sclerolytic agent; useful with scar tissue, keloids, burns
Zinc (+)	From zinc oxide ointment, 20% trace element necessary for healing; especially effective with open lesions and ulcerations
Copper (+)	From 2% aqueous solution of copper sulfate crystals; fungicide, astringent, useful with intranasal conditions (e.g., allergic rhinitis—hay fever), sinusitis, and dermatophytosis (athlete's foot)
Lidocaine (+)	From Xylocaine, 5% ointment; anesthetic and analgesic, especially with acute inflammatory conditions (e.g., bursitis, tendinitis, tic douloureux, and temporomandibular joint pain)
Lithium (−)	From lithium chloride or carbonate, 2% aqueous solution; effective as an exchange ion with gouty tophi and hyperuricemia†
Acetate (−)	From acetic acid, 2% aqueous solution; dramatically effective as a sclerolytic exchange ion with calcific deposits‡
Hyaluronidase (+)	From Wydase crystals in aqueous solution, as directed; for localized edema
Tap water (+/−)	Usually administered with alternating polarity, sometimes with glycopyrronium bromide in hyperhidrosis
Ringer's solution (+/−)	With alternating polarity; used for open decubitus lesions
Citrate (+)	From potassium citrate, 2% aqueous solution; reported effective in rheumatoid arthritis
Priscoline (+)	From benzazoline hydrochloride, 2% aqueous solution; reported effective with indolent ulcers
Antibiotics: gentamicin sulfate (+)	8 mg/ml; for suppurative ear chondritis

From Kahn, J. (1987): Non-steroid iontophoresis. Clin. Manage., 7:15. Reprinted from CLINICAL MANAGEMENT with the permission of the American Physical Therapy Association.

*All solutions are 2%; ointments are also low-percentage compounds. The literature and clinical reports confirm that the lower the percentage, the more effective the ionic exchange and transfer. Whether this is purely a physical chemistry phenomenon or an example of the Arndt-Schultz law, which states that "the smaller the stimulant, the greater the physiological response," remains to be proven.
†The lithium ion replaces the weaker sodium ion in the insoluble sodium urate tophus, converting it to soluble lithium urate.
‡The acetate radical replaces the carbonate radical in the insoluble calcium carbonate calcific deposit, converting it to soluble calcium acetate.

polarity is an important consideration in the management of pain or in the ability to produce contractions in innervated muscle tissue.

Unipolar versus Bipolar

One of the easiest to understand yet most misunderstood application techniques related to electrotherapy is unipolar versus bipolar electrode configuration. A unipolar electrode configuration means that the active effects of the stimulator are seen in only the electrodes attached to one of the two electrical poles. Bipolar configuration means that the active effects of the stimulator are seen in the electrodes attached to both poles. Recall that to have an electrical circuit, you must have a pathway for electricity to flow from one pole (negative) to another pole (positive). In DC these poles maintain a constant polarity and in AC they switch polarity. For the purpose of electrode configuration, the actual polarity of the electrode does not matter except in the cases discussed earlier. Whether or not an electrode displays "active effects" of the current depends on the current density under the electrode, and this is determined by the combination of current intensity and size of the electrode. For a given amount of current, a bigger electrode will have that current more spread out over a larger area and a smaller electrode will have that current spread out over a smaller area. The amount of current per unit of area is the current density. To have an active effect, such as causing sensory or motor stimulation, the current density must be adequate. The smaller the electrode is, the greater the current density, and therefore greater stimulation effects will be seen. Conversely, the larger the electrode is, the smaller the current density, and therefore little or no stimulation effect will be seen.

In a unipolar configuration, current density is manipulated using electrode size. One pole has a relatively small electrode (or several small electrodes) and the other pole has a relatively large electrode usually called a dispersive electrode. Because the dispersive electrode has a large area, it has a small current density that does not produce active effects. Unipolar configurations are standard on monophasic high-voltage stimulators and are very useful for situations in which you want to move the active electrode, such as with trigger point stimulation. Bipolar configurations use similarly sized electrodes at both poles, so similar effects are seen at both electrodes. Bipolar configurations are more common on newer devices and biphasic stimulators. Bipolar configurations are useful for situations in which you do not plan to move the electrodes or if exposing enough skin to use a dispersive electrode may compromise a patient's modesty.

The names *unipolar* and *bipolar* can sometimes be confusing because they sound similar to polarity. However, unipolar and bipolar configurations have absolutely nothing to do with the polarity of the electrical current under the electrode. Although we do typically see unipolar arrangements as the standard electrode setup on monophasic high-voltage stimulators, this is actually a matter of convention rather than necessity. In fact, any stimulator can be used with either a unipolar or bipolar configuration. The choice of which one to use is really a matter of clinical convenience rather than association with a specific stimulator. To convert a unipolar configuration to a bipolar configuration, one would simply replace the large dispersive electrode with an electrode similar in size to the other active electrode. Similarly, a greater effect can be produced with a stimulator by merely using smaller electrodes. To convert a bipolar configuration to a unipolar configuration, one would simply replace one of the active electrodes with a larger dispersive electrode. One unique unipolar setup involves using electrotherapy during immersion in water, such as a whirlpool or ice slush. In this case, a relatively small electrode is attached to a motor point of a body part that is immersed in water (e.g., the gastrocnemius muscle). This small (active) electrode must be attached to a motor point that is out of the water. The other electrode lead wire is immersed in the water along with the body part. The water acts as a very large dispersive electrode and the small electrode acts as an active electrode. This technique is usually used with edema retarding or removing protocols.

Current Modulation

In addition to the manipulations of electrical currents already discussed, there are a number of other current modulations that are common. Current modulation is simply an alteration to the waveform of the current. It includes items already discussed such as use of interrupted current as well as a few other alterations we will discuss here. It is used for a variety of reasons such as counteracting accommodation, increasing patient comfort, minimizing fatigue, or making contraction easier.

Among the most common modulations is varying the pulse rate of an interrupted current to minimize accommodation. Most contemporary stimulators have built-in preset protocol to modulate pulse rate. Typically, these vary the pulse rate up and down within a specific band of frequencies that corresponds to a desired effect. For example, among the more common preset protocols is one that varies the pulse rate up and down between 1 and 10 pps, obviously in the subtetanic range if used with muscle contraction. With sufficient intensity, this setting would cause the muscle to visibly twitch at a varying rate that would not become a tetanic contraction. Similar preset protocols can be found in the pulse rate range just above the threshold for tetany and also at much higher frequencies that are commonly used for pain management or muscle strengthening.

Another common modulation is ramping the intensity with an interrupted current. When a ramp setting is used, the current is not at its maximum intensity when it first comes on. Instead, each successive pulse of current increases slightly in intensity until the desired maximum is reached. The ramp setting allows the user to specify the length of time it takes for the maximum to be reached. Some devices also allow a ramp setting for when the current is ending. Ramp settings are used to increase patient comfort because it is generally more tolerable for the patient to ramp up to the maximum current rather than receiving the total current all at once.

Another modulation related to patient comfort is controlling the pulse width. There is an indirect relationship between the pulse duration (width) and the pulse amplitude (the intensity) when causing a muscle contraction. For patients who have a hard time tolerating high amplitudes, the amplitude can be reduced to tolerable levels and the pulse width increased to still cause muscle contraction. Increasing pulse width can also improve the ability to cause a contraction in other situations as well.

The use of on-time and off-time is another common modulation with electrotherapy. Recall that muscle stimulators cause the recruitment of the same set of motor units over and over again. Because this does not match the normal physiologic recruitment pattern for motor units, it often leads to rapid fatigue in the muscle. Although there are some protocols in which fatigue is desirable, such as when one is trying to overcome spasticity, muscle fatigue is to be avoided with most electrotherapy protocols. For this reason, many stimulators provide the practitioner with the ability to have either *continuous* current flow or current flowing for a period of time followed by a rest period with no flow of current. This type of modulation is often called *interrupted,* but it should not be confused with interrupted current as discussed previously. Normally when we speak of current interruption we mean that there are discreet pulses of current with brief (microseconds to milliseconds) intervals of no current. When we use on and off modulation, we get current during the on-time, and this current is pulsed at whatever pulse rate setting we have chosen. Likewise, the continuous setting on most stimulators produces a constant flow of interrupted (pulsed) current, rather than a noninterrupted current. Obviously, the terminology is confusing and the confusion becomes worse when different manufacturers use their own terminology. There is little consensus on the correct durations for on-time or off-time or even the correct on/off ratio. Although research is required to better explore this parameter, many clinicians anecdotally report using a 1:1 ratio or less on-time than off-time.

Intensity

The intensity setting controls the amplitude (voltage) of the waveform and therefore controls the quantity of current flowing through the circuit. Recall that the relationship between force and flow (voltage and current) is describe by Ohm's law (Box 4-12). The greater the intensity, or driving force, the greater the flow of current will be. Although most contemporary stimulators provide the user with a read-out of intensity or current levels, using a numerical value can be misleading. Because of variability in electrode placement, electrode size, skin conductivity, moisture, and other factors, the voltage used for one treatment to cause muscle contraction would not necessarily cause the same degree of contraction for a different treatment in the same patient. For this reason, it is more useful to think of intensity levels

in terms of their effects rather than their numerical value. Perhaps the easiest scheme involves classifying intensity progressively as subsensory, sensory, motor, and noxious (Table 4-9).

Techniques and Dosage

In this chapter only a general framework for electrotherapy techniques is presented. For more complete and detailed information, a full text on modalities should be consulted. To simplify this section, general strategies and parameters are summarized in Table 4-10. There are very few data on appropriate treatment durations for most protocols. By convention, most are 15 to 30 minutes in duration unless otherwise noted.

Future Questions

There are many remaining questions about electrotherapy because there actually is very little research that has been conducted to examine specific combinations of parameters to determine their efficacy. Similarly, there are also very few quality outcome studies available. There is currently some very promising work in the areas of retarding edema formation and in the management of pain. Similarly, iontophoresis has also been examined sporadically, and conflicting results have been reported. As a general statement, electrotherapy as a whole remains a vast and little explored modality with many areas for further study.

SUMMARY
Introduction

■ Modalities have specific uses in specific situations and are of little benefit when used for the wrong reason, with the wrong technique, or at the wrong time. At their best, therapeutic modalities are an exceptionally useful complement to the rehabilitative process, but are not a replacement for it.

■ The key to using modalities appropriately is to match the specific physiologic effects of the modality with the specific rehabilitative goal for the patient.

■ Practitioners should familiarize themselves with the specific details of their state practice acts before using any therapeutic modalities.

Table 4-9		
Classification of Intensity Level by Its Effects		
Subsensory level	The current is not perceived by the patient. This level is rarely used outside of microcurrent electrotherapy.	
Sensory level	The patient can feel the current, but the current does not cause muscle contraction.	
Motor level	Motor levels of intensity cause muscle contractions. As the name implies, noxious levels of intensity are rather uncomfortable and are rarely if ever used, but they provide the maximum tolerable level of muscle contraction.	

Table 4-10

General Electrotherapy Parameters Common for Athletic Injury Rehabilitation

Goal	Waveform	Pulse Rate°	Intensity†	On-Time/Off-Time
Muscle reeducation	Interrupted, shape matters little	Subtetanic	Motor	Yes
Retard atrophy in innervated tissue	Interrupted, shape matters little	Tetanic	Motor	Yes
Retard edema formation	Interrupted monophasic	Supertetanic (120 pps reported)	Sensory (10% below motor threshold)	Use recurrent 30-minute bouts with 60 minutes between
Remove edema	Interrupted, shape matters little	Subtetanic (usually <10 pps)	Motor	Yes
Reduce pain	High TENS	Tetanic to supertetanic (50 to 100 pps)	Sensory	No
	Low TENS (45 minutes +)	Subtetanic (2 to 4 pps)	Motor/noxious	No
	Interferential	Variable, see device instructions	Sensory	No
Reduce spasm	Interrupted, shape matters little	Subtetanic	Motor	No
	Interrupted, shape matters little	Supertetanic	Motor/noxious	No
Improve strength	Interrupted or MF-BurstAC (Russian)	Supertetanic	Noxious	Yes
Iontophoresis	Continuous monophasic	N/A	As tolerated	N/A

*Pulse rates are as follows: subtetanic = <30 pps; tetanic = 30 to 50 pps (produces smooth contraction); supertetanic = >100 pps and higher.
†Intensity levels are as follows: sensory = perceived by patient; motor = causes strong but tolerable contraction; noxious = maximum tolerable intensity.
TENS, transcutaneous electrical nerve stimulation.

Modality Research

■ There are a number of modalities commonly used in clinical settings that may not be as effective as once thought, and the clinical efficacy of modalities that are known to be useful can be easily compromised by incorrect application techniques.

■ The general trend is that clinical practice almost always precedes scientific research in regard to modality usage.

■ Most research on the therapeutic value of modalities has concentrated on clinically relevant types of data, which are indirect measures of the effectiveness of a modality and are important in establishing outcomes data versus the direct effect, which is important in establishing modality theory.

■ There are a number of modality effects that are commonly accepted by clinicians but that have little scientific support. In some cases there is scientific evidence to the contrary, yet these widely held clinical beliefs still persist.

Modalities for Acute Care

■ The two primary goals of modality usage with acute injures are limiting the total quantity of tissue damage associated with an injury and limiting the sequelae of the acute inflammatory response.

Cryotherapy

■ Data support the fact that the application of cold reduces local skin and intramuscular temperature, the metabolic rate of the cooled tissue, and blood flow, inhibits inflammation, retards the formation of edema/effusion, and helps manage pain.

■ We do not yet have a definitive answer about the most effective tissue temperature, cryotherapy duration, or on/off ratio for using cryotherapy for acute injury treatments.

■ Cold-induced vasodilation is a misnomer; in fact, cryotherapy does not increase blood flow above baseline levels at all.

■ Cryotherapy used in combination with compression has been shown to produce greater temperature reductions than cryotherapy used alone.

■ Ice bags made from ice stored in unrefrigerated hoppers should be directly applied to the skin without the addition of an insulating layer. Frozen gel packs or ice stored in a freezer, however, should have some type of appropriate barrier between the patient and the skin.

Compression

- It is believed that compression is effective in managing acute injuries by increasing the cooling efficacy of cryotherapy, manipulating the Starling forces, and reducing bleeding from vessels damaged during the injury.
- There is little scientific evidence to support specific recommendations on pressure and duration, use of intermittent versus continuous compression, or use of intermittent cycling parameters and the importance of compression or elevation in retarding edema formation.

Elevation

- The premise for elevation is based on gravity limiting the amount of blood delivered to an acutely injured area, which would result in the occurrence of several positive physiologic events. Unfortunately, the magnitude of the actual benefits from elevation has not been described in the literature.

Modalities for Rehabilitation

- In post–acute injury rehabilitation, the goals are mostly focused on removing the unwanted remnants of inflammation, repairing the tissue, and restoring more normal physiologic function of the repaired tissue.
- When a modality is used to accomplish a specific goal, the modality can and should be discontinued when that goal has been accomplished or when the modality is no longer effective for the patient.

Cryotherapy

- Cold reduces pain, and pain is one cause of inhibition; therefore, cold should help to overcome inhibition, allowing the patient to begin controlled rehabilitative exercise at an earlier point in the rehabilitative process. This is also the primary basis for the efficacy of cryokinetics.
- There is some early evidence that cryotherapy facilitates the motor neuron pool, which helps overcome neuromuscular inhibition after injury.

Superficial Thermotherapy

- Superficial thermotherapy techniques should be used as an adjunct, along with stretching or joint mobilization techniques, to improve range of motion.
- These types of modalities do increase superficial circulation and reduce pain.
- Further research still needs to address their duration, frequency of use, and appropriate tissue temperatures.

Ultrasound

- Thermal ultrasound is used primarily to augment techniques to improve range of motion although the literature directly examining the efficacy of ultrasound and stretching is very sparse.
- Nonthermal ultrasound is primarily used when the goal is to augment the repair or regeneration of damaged tissue. There is scientific evidence to support this use.
- Not all coupling mediums for ultrasound are equally effective.

Phonophoresis

- The research regarding the efficacy of phonophoresis is mixed at this point.

Shortwave Diathermy

- This is probably the best thermal modality available to the practitioner today and can be used to treat, therapeutically, a much larger area than ultrasound.

Electrical Stimulation

- The most promising uses of electrical stimulation are for pain management, muscle reeducation, and aiding in retarding the formation of and removal of edema.
- Some degree of strengthening of normal tissue can occur with electrotherapy, but the strengthening is not as effective as active exercise in a resistance program.

Iontophoresis

- There are conflicting reports on whether iontophoresis delivers enough medication to a deep enough tissue depth to be effective for many conditions. Also, outcomes data for iontophoresis are limited and have not yet adequately demonstrated that the technique is of much benefit to patients with musculoskeletal injuries.

REFERENCES

1. Anderson, C., Morris, R., Boeh, S., Panus, P., et al. (2003): Effects of iontophoresis current magnitude and duration on dexamethasone deposition and localized drug retention. Phys. Ther., 83:161-170.
2. Angus, J.C., Prentice, W.E., and Hooker, D. (1994): A comparison of two intermittent external compression devices and their effect on post acute ankle edema. J. Athl. Training, 29:179.
3. Ardic, F., Sarhus, M., and Topuz, O. (2002): Comparison of two different techniques of electrotherapy on myofascial pain. J. Back Musculoskeletal Rehab., 16:11-16.
4. Baldi, J., Jackson, R., Moraille, R., and Mysiw, W. (1998): Muscle atrophy is prevented in patients with acute spinal cord injury using functional electrical stimulation. Spinal Cord, 36:463-469.
5. Barcroft, H., and Edholm, O.G. (1943): The effect of temperature on blood flow and deep temperature in the human forearm. J. Physiol., 102:5-20.

6. Bare, A., McAnaw, M., Pritchard, A., et al. (1996): Phonophoretic delivery of 10% hydrocortisone through the epidermis of humans as determined by serum cortisol concentrations. (Including commentary by Robinson, A.J., and Echternach, J.L., with author response.) Phys. Ther., 76:738-749.

7. Barlas, D., Homan, C., and Thode, H.J. (1996): In vivo tissue temperature comparison of cryotherapy with and without external compression. Ann. Emerg. Med., 28:436-439.

8. Benoit, T., Martin, D., and Perrin, D. (1996): Hot and cold whirlpool treatments and knee joint laxity. J. Athl. Train., 31:242-244.

9. Bettany, J.A., Fish, D.R., and Mendel, F.C. (1990): High-voltage pulsed direct current: Effect on edema formation after hyperflexion injury. Arch. Phys. Med. Rehab., 71:677-681.

10. Bickford, R., and Duff, R. (1953): Influence of ultrasonic irradiation on temperature and blood flow in human skeletal muscle. Circ. Res., 1:534-538.

11. Birkett, J. (1999): Soft tissue healing and the physiotherapy management of lower limb soft tissue injuries. Phys. Ther. Rev., 4:251-263.

12. Bracciano, A.G. (2000): Physical Agent Modalities: Theory and Application for the Occupational Therapist. Thorofare, NJ, Slack, pp. viii, 160.

13. Brewer, K.D. (1990): The effects of intermittent compression and cold on edema in postacute ankle sprains. Unpublished masters thesis, University of North Carolina, Chapel Hill, NC.

14. Bricknell, R. and Watson, T. (1995): The thermal effects of pulsed shortwave therapy. BJTR pull-out physiotherapy supplement on electrotherapy. Br. J. Ther. Rehab., 2:430-434.

15. Brosseau, L., Milne, S., Robinson, V., et al. (2002): Efficacy of the transcutaneous electrical nerve stimulation for the treatment of chronic low back pain: A meta-analysis. Spine, 27:596-603.

16. Brown, R.T., and Baust, J.G. (1980): Time course of peripheral heterothermy in a homeotherm. Am. J. Physiol., 239:R126-R129.

17. Burke, D., MacNeil, S., Holt, L., et al. (2000): The effect of hot or cold water immersion on isometric strength training. J. Strength Cond. Res., 14:21-25.

18. Byl, N. (1995): The use of ultrasound as an enhancer for transcutaneous drug delivery: Phonophoresis. Phys. Ther., 75:539-553.

19. Byl, N.N., McKenzie, A., Halliday, B., et al. (1993): The effects of phonophoresis with corticosteroids: A controlled pilot study. J. Orthop. Sports Phys. Ther., 18:590-600.

21. Byl, N.N., McKenzie, A.L., West, J.M., et al. (1994): Pulsed microamperage stimulation: A controlled study of healing of surgically induced wounds in Yucatan pigs. Phys. Ther., 74:201-213; discussion 213-218.

22. Byl, N.N., McKenzie, A.L., West, J.M., et al. (1992): Low-dose ultrasound effects on wound healing: A controlled study with Yucatan pigs. Arch. Phys. Med. Rehab., 73:656-664.

23. Cameron, M. (1999): Physical Agents in Rehabilitation: From Research to Practice. Philadelphia, W.B. Saunders.

24. Carroll, D., Moore, R., McQuay, H., et al. (2003): Transcutaneous electrical nerve stimulation (TENS) for chronic pain. The Cochrane Library, Oxford, Update Software.

25. Chan, A., Myrer, J., Measom, G., and Draper, D. (1998): Temperature changes in human patellar tendon in response to therapeutic ultrasound. J. Athl. Train., 33:130-135.

26. Chapman-Jones, D., and Hill, D. (2002): Novel microcurrent treatment is more effective than conventional therapy for chronic Achilles tendinopathy: Randomised comparative trial. Physiotherapy, 88:471-480.

27. Chesterton, L., Foster, N., and Ross, L. (2002): Skin temperature response to cryotherapy. Arch. Phys. Med. Rehab., 83:543-549.

28. Conner-Kerr, T., Franklin, M., Kerr, J., et al. (1998): Phonophoretic delivery of dexamethasone to human transdermal tissues: A controlled pilot study. Eur. J. Phys. Med. Rehab., 8:19-23.

29. Cook, H., Morales, M., La, R.E., et al. (1994): Effects of electrical stimulation on lymphatic flow and limb volume in the rat. Phys. Ther., 74:1040-1046.

30. Cornwall, M. (1994): Effect of temperature on muscle force and rate of muscle force production in men and women. J. Orthop. Sports Phys. Ther., 20:74-80.

31. Costello, C., and Jeske, A. (1995): Iontophoresis: Applications in transdermal medication delivery. Phys. Ther., 75:554-563.

32. Crockford, G., Hellon, R., and Parkhouse, J. (1962): Thermal vasomotor response in human skin mediated by local mechanisms. J Physiol., 161:10-15.

33. Curl, W.W., Smith, B.P., Marr, A., et al. (1997): The effect of contusion and cryotherapy on skeletal muscle microcirculation. J. Sports Med. Phys. Fitness, 37:279-286.

34. Daanen, H.A., d.L. Van, F.-J, Romet, T.T., and Ducharme, M.B. (1997): The effect of body temperature on the hunting response of the middle finger skin temperature. Eur. J. Appl. Physiol. Occup. Physiol., 76:538-543.

35. Darrow, H., Schulthies, S., Draper, D., et al. (1999): Serum dexamethasone levels after Decadron phonophoresis. J. Athl. Train., 34:338-341.

36. Dawson, D. (1997): Pathophysiology of focal ischemic injury: An overview. Top. Emerg. Med., 19:63-78.

37. Denegar, C. (2000): Therapeutic Modalities for Athletic Injuries. Champaign, IL, Human Kinetics.

38. Dervin, G., Taylor, D., and Keene, G. (1998): Effects of cold and compression dressings on early postoperative outcomes for the arthroscopic anterior cruciate ligament reconstruction patient. J. Orthop. Sports Phys. Ther., 27:403-406.

39. Dolan, M., Thornton, R., Fish, D., and Mendel, F. (1997): Effects of cold water immersion on edema formation after blunt injury to the hind limbs of rats. J. Athl. Train., 32:233-237.

40. Draper, D. (2002): Don't disregard ultrasound yet—The jury is still out. Phys. Ther., 82:190-191.

41. Draper, D. (1998): Guidelines to enhance therapeutic ultrasound treatment outcomes. Athl. Ther. Today. 3:7-11, 28-19, 55.

42. Draper, D., Anderson, C., Schulthies, S., and Ricard, M. (1998): Immediate and residual changes in dorsiflexion range of motion using an ultrasound heat and stretch routine. J. Athl. Train., 33:141-144.

43. Draper, D., Castel, J., and Castel, D. (1995): Rate of temperature increase in human muscle during 1 MHz and 3 MHz continuous ultrasound. J. Orthop. Sports Phys. Ther., 22:142-150.

44. Draper, D., Harris, S., Schulthies, S., et al. (1998): Hot-pack and 1-MHz ultrasound treatments have an additive effect on muscle temperature increase. J. Athl. Train., 33:21-24.

45. Draper, D., Knight, K., Fujiwara, T., and Castel, J. (1999): Temperature change in human muscle during and after pulsed short-wave diathermy. (Including commentary by Byl, N., with author response.) J. Orthop. Sports Phys. Ther., 29:13-22.

46. Draper, D., Miner, L., Knight, K., and Ricard, M. (2002): The carry-over effects of diathermy and stretching in developing hamstring flexibility. J. Athl. Train., 37:37-42.

47. Draper, D., and Ricard, M. (1995): Rate of temperature decay in human muscle following 3 MHz ultrasound: The stretching window revealed. J. Athl. Train., 30:304-307.

48. Draper, D., Schulties, S., Sorvisto, P., and Hautala, A. (1995): Temperature changes in deep muscles of humans during ice and ultrasound therapies: An in vivo study. J. Orthop. Sports Phys. Ther., 21:153-157.

49. Draper, D., and Sunderland, S. (1993): Examination of the law of Grotthus-Draper: Does ultrasound penetrate subcutaneous fat in humans? J. Athl. Train., 28:246, 248-250, 278-249.

50. Draper, D., Sunderland, S., Kirkendall, D., and Ricard, M. (1993): A comparison of temperature rise in human calf muscles following applications of underwater and topical gel ultrasound. J. Orthop. Sports Phys. Ther., 17:247-251.

51. Edwards, D., Rimmer, M., and Keene, G. (1996): The use of cold therapy in the postoperative management of patients undergoing arthroscopic anterior cruciate ligament reconstruction. Am. J. Sports Med., 24:193-195.

52. Ellis, B. (1996): A retrospective study of long-term users of transcutaneous electrical nerve stimulators. Br. J. Ther. Rehab., 3:88-93.

53. Faghri, P., Hovorka, C., and Trumbower, R. (2002): From the field. Reducing edema in the lower extremity of hemiplegic stroke patients: A comparison of non-pharmacological approaches. Clin. Kinesiol. J. Am. Kinesiother. Assoc., 56:51-60.

54. Fahey, S., Smith, M., Merrick, M., Ingersoll, C., and Sandrey, M. (2000): A comparison of hydrocortisone cream to powder in increasing intramuscular tissue temperature during phonophoresis treatments. J. Athl. Train., 35:S-47.

55. Gardner, C.A., and Webb, R.C. (1986): Cold-induced vasodilatation in isolated, perfused rat tail artery. Am. J. Physiol., 251:H176-H181.

56. Garrett, C., Draper, D., and Knight, K. (2000): Heat distribution in the lower leg from pulsed short-wave diathermy and ultrasound treatments. J. Athl. Train., 35:50-55.

57. Gersten, J. (1955): Effect of ultrasound on tendon extensibility. Am. J. Phys. Med., 34:662.

58. Gilbart, M., Oglivie-Harris, D.J., Broadhurst, C., and Clarfield, M. (1995): Anterior tibial compartment pressures during intermittent sequential pneumatic compression therapy. Am. J. Sports Med., 23:769-772.

59. Giudice, M. (1990): Effects of continuous passive motion and elevation on hand edema. Am. J. Occup. Ther., 44:914-921.

60. Gum, S., Reddy, G., Stehno-Bittel, L., Enwemeka, C. (1997): Combined ultrasound, electrical stimulation, and laser promote collagen synthesis with moderate changes in tendon biomechanics. Am. J. Phys. Med. Rehab., 76:288-296.

61. Guyton, A.C. (1991): Textbook of Medical Physiology, 8th ed. Philadelphia, W.B. Saunders, pp. 149-203.

62. Halliday, D., and Resnick, R. (1988): Fundamentals of Physics, 3rd ed. New York, John Wiley & Sons, pp. 464-475.

63. Hecox, B., Andemicael Mehreteab, T. and Weisberg, J. (1994): Physical agents: A comprehensive text for physical therapists. Norwalk, CT, Appleton & Lange, pp. xv, 473.

64. Higgins, D., and Kaminski, T. (1998): Contrast therapy does not cause fluctuations in human gastrocnemius intramuscular temperature. J. Athl. Train., 33:336-340.

65. Ho, S., Coel, M., Kagawa, R., and Richardson, A. (1994): The effects of ice on blood flow and bone metabolism in knees. (Including commentary by Johnson, R.J. with author response.) Am. J. Sports Med., 22:537-540.

66. Ho, S., Illgen, R., Meyer, R., et al. (1995): Comparison of various icing times in decreasing bone metabolism and blood flow in the knee. Am. J. Sports Med., 23:74-76.

67. Holcomb, W. (1997): A practical guide to electrical therapy. J. Sport Rehab., 6:272-282.

68. Holcomb, W., and Joyce, C. (2003): A comparison of temperature increases produced by 2 commonly used ultrasound units. J. Athl. Train., 38:24-27.

69. Holcomb, W., Mangus, B., and Tandy, R. (1996): The effect of icing with the Pro-Stim Edema Management System on cutaneous cooling. J. Athl. Train., 31:126-129.

70. Hopkins, J., Ingersoll, C., Edwards, J., and Klootwyk, T. (2002): Cryotherapy and transcutaneous electric neuromuscular stimulation decrease arthrogenic muscle inhibition of the vastus medialis after knee joint effusion. J. Athl. Train., 37:25-31.

71. Hopkins, J., and Stencil, R. (2002): Ankle cryotherapy facilitates soleus function. J. Orthop. Sports Phys. Ther., 32:622-627.

72. Hou, C., Tsai, L., Cheng, K., et al. (2002): Immediate effects of various physical therapeutic modalities on cervical myofascial pain and trigger-point sensitivity. Arch. Phys. Med. Rehab., 83:1406-1414.

73. Houghton, P. (1999): Effects of therapeutic modalities on wound healing: A conservative approach to the management of chronic wounds. Phys. Ther. Rev., 4:167-182.

74. Hsueh, T., Cheng, P., Kuan, T., and Hong, C. (1997): The immediate effectiveness of electrical nerve stimulation and electrical muscle stimulation on myofascial trigger points. Am. J. Phys. Med. Rehab., 76:471-476.

75. Jameson, A., Kinzey, S., and Hallam, J. (2001): Lower-extremity-joint cryotherapy does not affect vertical ground-reaction forces during landing. J. Sport Rehab., 10:132-142.

76. Johnson, M., and Tabasam, G. (1999): A double-blind placebo controlled investigation into the analgesic effects of inferential currents (IFC) and transcutaneous electrical nerve stimulation (TENS) on cold-induced pain in healthy subjects. Physiother. Theory Pract., 15:217-233.

77. Johnson, M., and Tabasam, G. (2003): An investigation into the analgesic effects of interferential currents and transcutaneous electrical nerve stimulation on experimentally induced ischemic pain in otherwise pain-free volunteers. Phys. Ther., 83:208-223.

78. Jutte, L., Merrick, M., Ingersoll, C., and Edwards, J. (2001): The relationship between intramuscular temperature, skin temperature, and adipose thickness during cryotherapy and rewarming. Arch. Phys. Med. Rehab., 82:845-850.

79. Karnes, J., Mendel, F., Fish, D., and Burton, H. (1995): High-voltage pulsed current: Its influence on diameters of histamine-dilated arterioles in hamster cheek pouches. Arch. Phys. Med. Rehab., 76:381-386.

80. Karunakara, R., Lephart, S., and Pincivero, D. (1999): Changes in forearm blood flow during single and intermittent cold application. J. Orthop. Sports Phys. Ther., 29:177-180.

81. Kimura, I., Gulick, D., and Thompson, G. (1997): The effect of cryotherapy on eccentric plantar flexion peak torque and endurance. J. Athl. Train., 32:124-126.

82. Kinzey, S., Cordova, M., Gallen, K., et al. (2000): The effects of cryotherapy on ground-reaction forces produced during a functional task. J. Sport Rehab., 9:3-14.

83. Kitchen, S., and Partridge, C. (1992): Review of shortwave diathermy continuous and pulsed patterns. Physiotherapy, 78:243-252.

84. Klaiman, M., Shrader, J., Danoff, J., et al. (1998): Phonophoresis versus ultrasound in the treatment of common musculoskeletal conditions. Med. Sci. Sports Exerc., 30:1349-1355.

85. Kloth, L., and McCulloch, J. (1996): Promotion of wound healing and electrical stimulation. Adv. Wound Care J. Prev. Healing, 9:42-45.

86. Knight, K., Brucker, J., Stoneman, P., and Rubley, M. (2000): Muscle injury management with cryotherapy. Athl. Ther. Today, 5:26-30, 32-23, 64.

87. Knight, K., Okuda, I., Ingersoll, C., and Edwards, J. (1997): The effects of cold applications on nerve conduction velocity and muscle force (Abstract). J. Athl. Train., 32:S-5.

88. Knight, K.L. (1985): Cryotherapy: Theory, Technique, and Physiology, 1st ed. Chattanooga, TN, Chattanooga Corp. Education Division, pp. ix, 188.

89. Knight, K.L. (1985): Cryotherapy in Sport Injury Management. Champaign, IL, Human Kinetics, pp. x, 301.

90. Knight, K.L. (1976): Effects of hypothermia on inflammation and swelling. Athl. Train. JNATA, 11:7-10.

91. Knight, K.L., Aquino, J., Johannes, S.M., and Urban, C.D. (1980): A re-examination of Lewis' cold-induced vasodilatation in the finger and the ankle. Athl. Train. JNATA, 15:238-250.

92. Knight, K.L., Thoma, D.B., Fink, D., et al. (1996): Cryotherapy for First Aid. Champaign, IL: Human Kinetics.

93. Knight, K.L., Thoma, D.B., Fink, D., et al. (1996): Cryotherapy for Rehabilitation. Champaign, IL, Human Kinetics.

94. Konrath, G., Lock, T., Goitz, H., and Scheidler, J. (1996): The use of cold therapy after anterior cruciate ligament reconstruction: A prospective, randomized study and literature review. Am. J. Sports Med., 24:629-633.

95. Kraemer, W., Bush, J., Wickham, R., et al. (2001): Continuous compression as an effective therapeutic intervention in treating eccentric-exercise-induced muscle soreness. J. Sport Rehab., 10:11-23.

96. Kraemer, W., Bush, J., Wickham, R., et al. (2001): Influence of compression therapy on symptoms following soft tissue injury from maximal eccentric exercise. J. Orthop. Sports Phys. Ther., 31:282-290.

97. Krause, B., Hopkins, J., Ingersoll, C., et al. (2000): The relationship of ankle temperature during cooling and rewarming to the human soleus H reflex. J. Sport Rehab., 9:253-262.

98. Krause, B., Hopkins, J., Ingersoll, C., et al. (2000): The effects of ankle and axillary cooling on the human soleus Hoffman reflex (Abstract). J Athl. Train., 35:S-58.

99. Lehmann, J., deLateur, B, Stonebridge, J., and Warren, C. (1967): Therapeutic temperature distribution produced by ultrasound as modified by dosage and volume of tissue exposed. Arch. Phys. Med. Rehab., 47:662-666.

100. Lehmann, J., Masock, A., Warren, C., and Koblanski, J. (1970): Effect of therapeutic ultrasound on tendon extensibility. Arch. Phys. Med. Rehab., 51:481-487.

101. Lehmann, J.F. (1982): Therapeutic Heat and Cold, 3rd ed. Baltimore, Williams & Wilkins, pp. xiv, 641.

102. Lehmann, J.F., deLateur, B., and Warren, C. (1967): Heating produced by ultrasound in bone and soft tissue. Arch. Phys. Med. Rehab., 48:397-401.

103. Lerman, Y., Jacubovich, R., Caner, A., and Ribak, J. (1996): Electromagnetic fields from shortwave diathermy equipment in physiotheray departments. Physiotherapy, 82:456-458.

104. Lessard, L., Scudds, R., Amendola, A., and Vaz, M. (1997): The efficacy of cryotherapy following arthroscopic knee surgery. J. Orthop. Sports Phys. Ther., 26:14-22.

105. Lewis, T. (1930): Observations upon the reactions of the vessels of the human skin to cold. Heart, 15:177-208.

106. Li, L., Scudds, R., Heck, C., and Harth, M. (1996): The efficacy of dexamethasone iontophoresis for the treatment of rheumatoid arthritic knees: A pilot study. Arthritis Care Res., 9:126-132.

107. Lide, D. (ed.). (1994): CRC Handbook of Chemistry and Physics, 74th ed. Boca Raton, FL, CRC Press.

108. Majno, G., and Joris, I. (1996): Cells, Tissues, and Disease: Principles of General Pathology. Cambridge, MA, Blackwell Scientific.

109. Mancuso, D.L., and Knight, K.L. (1992): Effects of prior physical activity on skin surface temperature response of the ankle during and after a 30-minute ice pack application. J. Athl. Train., 27:242-249.

110. Martin, C., McCallum, H., Strelley, S., and Heaton, B. (1991): Electromagnetic fields from therapeutic diathermy equipment: A review of hazards and precautions. Physiotherapy, 77:3-7.

111. Martin, S., Spindler, K., Tarter, J., et al. (2001): Cryotherapy: An effective modality for decreasing intraarticular temperature after knee arthroscopy. Am. J. Sports Med., 29:288-291.

112. Matthews, J., Fisher, B., Magee, D., and Knight, K. (2001): Lipid peroxidation and protein turnover after trauma and cold treatment in skeletal muscle of exercise-trained rats. J. Phys. Ther. Sci., 13:21-26.

113. Mayrovitz, H., Delgado, M., and Smith, J. (1997): Compression bandaging effects on lower extremity peripheral and sub-bandage skin blood perfusion. Wounds Compend. Clin. Res. Pract., 9:146-152.

114. McCulloch, J., and Boyd, V. (1992): The effects of whirlpool and the dependent position on lower extremity volume. J. Orthop. Sports Phys. Ther., 16:169-173.

115. Meeker, B. (1994): Description of the effects of whirlpool therapy on postoperative pain and surgical wound healing, Unpublished masters thesis, Louisiana State University, New Orleans, LA.

116. Meeker, B. (1998): Whirlpool therapy on postoperative pain and surgical wound healing: an exploration. Patient Educ. Couns., 33:39-48.

117. Meeusen, R., Van der Veen, P., Joos, E., et al. (1998): The influence of cold and compression on lymph flow at the ankle. Clin. J. Sports Med., 8:266-271.

118. Mendel, F., and Fish, D. (1993): New perspectives in edema control via electrical stimulation. J. Athl. Train., 28:63-64, 66-70, 72.

119. Merrick, M. (2001): Research digest: Do you diathermy? Athl. Ther. Today, 6:55-56.

120. Merrick, M. (2001): Research digest: Does 1-MHz ultrasound really work? Athl. Ther. Today, 6:48-49.

121. Merrick, M. (2000): Research digest: Does phonophoresis work? Athl. Ther. Today, 5:46-47.

122. Merrick, M. (2000): Research digest: Ultrasound and range of motion examined. Athl. Ther. Today, 5:48-49.

123. Merrick, M. (1999): Research digest: Unconventional modalities: Microcurrent. Athl. Ther. Today, 4:53-54.

124. Merrick, M. (1999): Research digest: Unconventional modalities: Therapeutic magnets. Athl. Ther. Today, 4:56-57.

125. Merrick, M. (2002): Secondary injury after musculoskeletal trauma: A review and update. J. Athl. Train., 37:209-217.

126. Merrick, M., Bernard, K., Devor, S., and Williams, J. (2003): Identical 3-MHz ultrasound treatments with different devices produce different intramuscular temperatures. J. Orthop. Sports Phys. Ther., 33:379-385.

127. Merrick, M., Jutte, L., and Smith, M. (2003): Cold modalities with different thermodynamic properties produce different surface and intramuscular temperatures. J. Athl. Train., 38:28-33.

128. Merrick, M., Knight, K., Ingersoll, C., and Potteiger, J. (1993): The effects of ice and compression wraps on intramuscular temperatures at various depths. J. Athl. Train., 28:236-245.

129. Merrick, M., Rankin, J., Andres, F., and Hinman, C. (1999): A preliminary examination of cryotherapy and secondary injury in skeletal muscle. Med. Sci. Sports Exerc., 31:1516-1521.

130. Michlovitz, S.L. (1996): Thermal Agents in Rehabilitation, 3rd ed. Philadelphia, F.A. Davis, pp. xxvi, 405.

131. Milne, S., Welch, V., Brosseau, L., et al. (2003): Transcutaneous Electrical Nerve Stimulation (TENS) for Chronic Low Back Pain. The Cochrane Library, Oxford, Update Software.

132. Misasi, S., Morin, G., Kemler, D., et al. (1995): The effect of a toe cap and bias on perceived pain during cold water immersion. J. Athl. Train., 30:49-52.

133. Mlynarczyk, J. (1984): Temperature Changes during and after Ice Pack Application of 10, 20, 30, 45, and 60 Minutes. Terre Haute, Indiana State University, Department of Physical Education.

134. Myrer, J., Draper, D., and Durrant, E. (1994): Contrast therapy and intramuscular temperature in the human leg. J. Athl. Train., 29:318-322, 376-317.

135. Myrer, J., Higgins, D., and Kaminski, T. (1999): Some concerns: "Contrast therapy does not cause fluctuations in human gastrocnemius intramuscular temperature" (J. Athl. Train. 1998; 33:336-340). J. Athl. Train., 34:231.

136. Myrer, J., Measom, G., Durrant, E., and Fellingham, G. (1997): Cold- and hot-pack contrast therapy: Subcutaneous and intramuscular temperature change. J. Athl. Train., 32:238-241.

137. Myrer, J., Measom, G., and Fellingham, G. (2000): Exercise after cryotherapy greatly enhances intramuscular rewarming. J. Athl. Train., 35:412-416.

138. Myrer, J., Measom, G., and Fellingham, G. (1998): Temperature changes in the human leg during and after two methods of cryotherapy. J. Athl. Train., 33:25-29.

139. Myrer, J., Myrer, K., Measom, G., et al. (2001): Muscle temperature is affected by overlying adipose when cryotherapy is administered. J. Athl. Train., 36:32-36.

140. Norwig, J. (1997): Injury management update. Edema control and the acutely inverted ankle sprain. Athl. Ther. Today, 2:40-41.

141. Ogiwara, S. (2001): Calf muscle pumping and rest positions during and/or after whirlpool therapy. J. Phys. Ther. Sci., 13:99-105.

142. Ohkoshi, Y., Ohkoshi, M., Nagasaki, S., et al. (1999): The effect of cryotherapy on intraarticular temperature and postoperative care after anterior cruciate ligament reconstruction. Am. J. Sports Med., 27:357-362.

143. Oldham, J., Howe, T., Petterson, T., et al. (1995): Electrotherapeutic rehabilitation of the quadriceps in elderly osteoarthritic patients: A double blind assessment of patterned neuromuscular stimulation. Clin. Rehab., 9:10-20.

144. Osiri, M., Welch, V., Brosseau, L., et al. (2003): Transcutaneous Electrical Nerve Stimulation for Knee Osteoarthritis. The Cochrane Library, Oxford, Update Software.

145. Otte, J., Merrick, M., Ingersoll, C., and Cordova, M. (2002): Subcutaneous adipose tissue thickness alters cooling time during cryotherapy. Arch. Phys. Med. Rehab., 83:1501-1505.

146. Palmer, J., and Knight, K. (1996): Ankle and thigh skin surface temperature changes with repeated ice pack application. J. Athl. Train., 31:319-323.

147. Palmieri, R., Ingersoll, C., Edwards, J., et al. (2003): Arthrogenic muscle inhibition is not present in the limb contralateral to a simulated knee joint effusion. J. Athl. Train., 38:S-35.

148. Peres, S., Draper, D., Knight, K., and Ricard, M. (2002): Pulsed shortwave diathermy and prolonged long-duration stretching increase dorsiflexion range of motion more than identical stretching without diathermy. J. Athl. Train., 37:43-50.

149. Perron, M., and Malouin, F. (1997): Acetic acid iontophoresis and ultrasound for the treatment of calcifying tendinitis of the shoulder: A randomized control trial. Arch. Phys. Med. Rehab., 78:379-384.

150. Pincivero, D., Gieck, J., and Saliba, E. (1993): Rehabilitation of a lateral ankle sprain with cryokinetics and functional progressive exercise. J. Sport Rehab., 2:200-207.

151. Prentice, W. (1999): Therapeutic Modalities in Sports Medicine, 4th ed. Boston, WCB McGraw-Hill.

152. Proctor, M., Smith, C., Farquhar, C., and Stones, R. (2003): Transcutaneous Electrical Nerve Stimulation and Acupuncture for Primary Dysmenorrhoea. The Cochrane Library, Oxford, Update Software.

153. Rimington, S., Draper, D., Durrant, E., and Fellingham, G. (1994): Temperature changes during therapeutic ultrasound in the precooled human gastrocnemius muscle. J. Athl. Train., 29:325-327, 376-327.

154. Rivers, D.A. (1995): The influence of cryotherapy and Aircast bracing on total body balance and proprioception. J. Athl. Training, 30:5-15.

155. Robertson, V., and Baker, K. (2001): A review of therapeutic ultrasound: Effectiveness studies. Phys. Ther., 81:1339-1350.

156. Robinson, V., Brosseau, L., Casimiro, L., et al. (2003): Thermotherapy for Treating Rheumatoid Arthritis. The Cochrane Library, Oxford, Update Software.

157. Rose, S., Draper, D., Schulthies, S., and Durrant, E. (1996): The stretching window part two: Rate of thermal decay in deep muscle following 1-MHz ultrasound. J. Athl. Train., 31:139-143.

158. Seib, T., Price, R., Reyes, M., and Lehmann, J. (1994): The quantitative measurement of spasticity: Effect of cutaneous electrical stimulation. Arch. Phys. Med. Rehab., 75:746-750.

159. Serwa, J., Rancourt, L., Merrick, M., et al. (2001): Effect of varying application pressures on skin surface and intramuscular temperatures during cryotherapy (Abstract). J. Athl. Train., 36:S-90.

160. Smith, J., Stevens, J., Taylor, M., and Tibbey, J. (2002): A randomized, controlled trial comparing compression bandaging and cold therapy in postoperative total knee replacement surgery. Orthop. Nurs., 21:61-66.

161. Smutok, M., Mayo, M., Gabaree, C., et al. (2002): Failure to detect dexamethasone phosphate in the local venous blood postcathodic iontophoresis in humans. J. Orthop. Sports Phys. Ther., 32:461-468.

162. Starkey, C. (1999): Therapeutic Modalities, 2nd ed. Philadelphia, F.A. Davis, p. 397.

163. Stewart, H. (1982): Ultrasound Therapy. In: Respacholi, M., and Benwell, D. (eds.), Essentials of Medical Ultrasound, Clifton, NJ, Humana Press, p. 196.

164. Streator, S., Ingersoll, C., and Knight, K. (1995): Sensory information can decrease cold-induced pain perception. J. Athl. Train., 30:293-296.

165. Taylor, K., Mendel, F., Fish, D., et al. (1997): Effect of high-voltage pulsed current and alternating current on macromolecular leakage in hamster cheek pouch microcirculation. Phys. Ther., 77:1729-1740.

166. Thieme, H., Ingersoll, C., Knight, K., and Ozmun, J. (1996): Cooling does not affect knee proprioception. J. Athl. Train., 31:8-11.

167. Thornton, R., Mendel, F., and Fish, D. (1998): Effects of electrical stimulation on edema formation in different strains of rats. Phys. Ther., 78:386-394.

168. Tsang, K., Buxton, B., Guion, W., et al. (1997): The effects of cryotherapy applied through various barriers. J. Sport Rehab., 6:343-354.

169. Uchio, Y., Ochi, M., Fujihara, A., et al. (2003): Cryotherapy influences joint laxity and position sense of the healthy knee joint. Arch. Phys. Med. Rehab., 84:131-135.

170. Van, H.G. (1997): Iontophoresis: A review of the literature. N.Z. J. Physiother., 25:16-17.

171. Varpalotai, M., and Knight, K. (1991): Pressures exerted by elastic wraps applied by beginning and advanced student athletic trainers to the ankle and the thigh with and without an ice pack. Athl. Train. JNATA, 26:246-250.

172. Wallace, M., Ridgeway, B., Jun, E., et al. (2001): Topical delivery of lidocaine in healthy volunteers by electroporation, electroincorporation, or iontophoresis: An evaluation of skin anesthesia. Reg. Anesth. Pain Med., 26:229-238.

173. Ward, A., and Shkuratova, N. (2002): Russian electrical stimulation: The early experiments. Phys. Ther., 82:1019-1030.

174. Webb, J., Williams, D., Ivory, J., et al. (1998): The use of cold compression dressings after total knee replacement: A randomized controlled trial. Orthopedics, 21:59-61.

175. Weber, M., Servedio, F., and Woodall, W. (1994): The effects of three modalities on delayed onset muscle soreness. J. Orthop. Sports Phys. Ther., 20:236-242.

176. Whitelaw, G., DeMuth, K., Demos, H., et al. (1996): The cryo/cuff versus ice and elastic wrap: postoperative care of knee arthroscopy patients. (Reprinted with permission from the American Journal of Knee Surgery, 1995;8:28-31.) Today's OR Nurse, 18:31-34.

177. Zemke, J., Andersen, J., Guion, W., et al. (1998): Intramuscular temperature responses in the human leg to two forms of cryotherapy: Ice massage and ice bag. J. Orthop. Sports Phys. Ther., 27:301-307.

CHAPTER 5

MEASUREMENT IN REHABILITATION

Gary L. Harrelson, Ed.D., ATC
Elizabeth Swann, Ph.D., ATC

CHAPTER OBJECTIVES

At the end of this chapter the reader will be able to:

- Explain and recommend various instruments and methods of measurement.
- Perform and interpret objective measurements of girth and joint motion.
- Discuss the reliability and validity of the various instruments used to measure girth and joint motion.
- Take appropriate actions to improve the reliability of girth and joint motion measurements.

Measurement has long been used to chart progress during the rehabilitation process. Therefore, it is important for all clinicians to be competent in performing and interpreting objective measurements of girth and joint motion. This chapter addresses the reliability and validity of these measurements, ensuring reliable measurements, and various techniques for performing girth and joint motion assessments.

GIRTH MEASUREMENTS

In the clinical setting, objective measurements must be obtained when decision-making is necessary for a therapeutic exercise program. A flexible tape measure can be used to measure the girth of the limb and is probably the most common clinical method to document muscle bulk and swelling. Girth assessment by use of a tape measure is also referred to as girth measurement, circumferential measurement, or anthropometric measurement. Not only is this assessment technique used before a weight-training program is implemented to assess its impact on muscle hypertrophy, but it is also used to assess muscle atrophy or joint swelling after injury or surgery and to determine the subsequent effect of a rehabilitation program on muscle hypertrophy and joint swelling. Girth measurements have been reported in the literature for documenting the effects of a rehabilitation program on muscle atrophy or hypertrophy and joint swelling[49] after injury,[12,25,60] surgery, or implementation of a rehabilitation program.[33,36,42,46]

The increase or decrease in girth measurement is thought to indicate a direct relationship between an increase or decrease in muscle strength. For example, as a muscle atrophies, the loss of strength is directly related to muscle size because the muscle fibers themselves reduce in size; the outcome, therefore, is a reduction in strength. However, there is evidence to support the absence of a direct relationship between girth measurement and muscle size.[7]

Most of the variability in obtaining girth measurements arises from use of different anatomic landmarks, tension placed on the tape measure by the clinician, and contraction of the muscle. The tension placed on the tape measure by the clinician when assessing girth does not appear to be as big an issue as was thought previously.[21,54] Box 5-1 lists recommendations to improve intra- and interclinician reliability during girth assessments.

Several investigators[21,54] have assessed the reliability of lower extremity girth measurements in young healthy patients. The data suggest that these measurements are reliable and can be reproduced with a high degree of accuracy, particularly when the same clinician takes the measurements. Measurements taken by different clinicians are not as reliable when a standard tape measure is used.[21] Also, many times clinicians use a healthy extremity to determine the amount of atrophy that may have occurred as a result of trauma. Healthy right and left lower extremities appear to have similar circumferences, which should not vary more than 1.5 cm between right and left sides.[54] Additionally, comparisons between a standard flexible tape measure and a Lufkin tape measure with a Gulick

Box 5-1

Recommendations for Improving Reliability of Girth Measurements

- The clinician should attempt to place the same amount of tension on the tape measure with each measurement.
- All clinicians should use the same anatomical landmarks when determining the site of the girth measurements.
- If possible, the clinician should take the girth measurement with the muscle contracted.
- When possible, the same clinician should take all the measurements to improve reliability.

spring-loaded end indicate that both intra- and interclinician reliability is better with the Gulick spring-loaded end versus a standard tape measure in lower extremity measurements in healthy subjects (Fig. 5-1).[21]

Although girth measurements appear to be reproducible, the validity of the measurement of thigh bulk has been questioned. Stokes and Young[50] were concerned that the tape measure was not sensitive and accurate enough for measuring the selective wasting of the quadriceps. Doxey[8] reported that detecting changes in muscle bulk in nonsurgical subjects probably requires more sensitive methods than girth measurements, such as ultrasonography or computed tomography. Furthermore, a small decrease (1%) in thigh measurement may be an indicator of a significant reduction (13%) in muscle bulk.[8] Research using ultrasonography[8,60] and computed tomography[7] has shown that muscle fiber atrophy is not adequately reflected by circumference measurements. Rather, extremity fat can mask this muscle atrophy. Thus, caution should be used in interpreting the results of girth measurements with regard to muscle strength and progression of individuals through a plan of care. In a rehabilitation setting, the clinician should keep accurate records of not only girth measurements but also the anatomical landmarks that are used to maintain consistency.

GONIOMETRY

Goniometry is the use of instruments to measure the range of motion in body joints. All clinicians should be able to competently perform and interpret objective measurements of joint motion. Initial range-of-motion measurements provide a basis for developing a treatment or therapeutic exercise plan, and repeated measurements throughout the course of rehabilitation help determine whether improvement has been made and goals achieved.

Historical Considerations

The literature on goniometry is extensive and describes many aspects of goniometric measuring. Gifford, in 1914,[15] was probably the first to have reported on goniometric devices in the United States. Historically, various instruments and methods of measurement have been described and recommended.[5,26,31,32,39,53,55,57] The most common methods of measuring range of motion are with a universal goniometer, an inclinometer, or a tape measure (Box 5-2). There are also special devices for measuring specific joint motion such as cervical and back motion, temporomandibular joint motion, and ankle motion.

Instruments for assessing joint motion are generally of two types: (1) devices of universal application (e.g., full-circle or half-circle universal goniometer), which remain the most versatile and popular (Fig. 5-2); and (2) goniometers designed to measure a single range of motion for a specific joint (Fig. 5-3). Although not as common as universal goniometers, gravity-dependent goniometers or inclinometers use the effect of gravity on pointers or fluid levels to measure joint position and motion and can either be mechanical or electronic.[35] Mechanical inclinometers are either (1) pendulum goniometers that consist of a 360° protractor with a weighted pointer hanging from the center of the protractor (Fig. 5-4A) or (2) fluid goniometers that have a fluid-filled circular chamber containing an air bubble, similar to a carpenter's level (Fig. 5-4B). There are

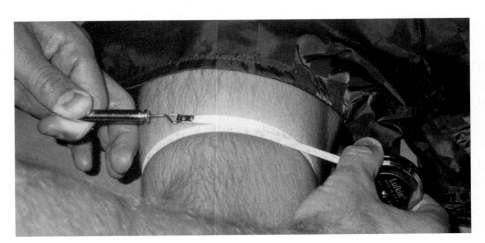

Figure 5-1. Lufkin tape measure with a Gulick spring-loaded end.

Box 5-2

Ways to Assess Joint Range of Motion

- Universal goniometer
- Joint-specific goniometer
- Inclinometer
- Tape measure
- Electrogoniometer
- Photography
- Video recording
- Radiography

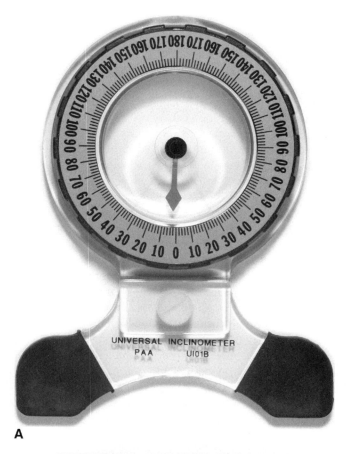

A

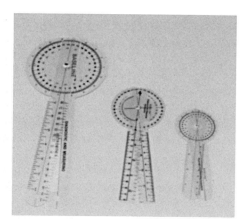

Figure 5-2. Full-circle manual universal goniometer.

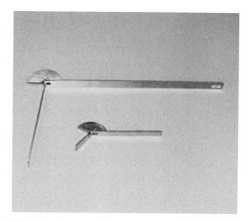

Figure 5-3. Goniometers for measuring a single joint motion.

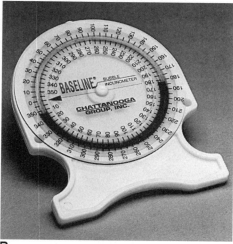

B

Figure 5-4. *A,* Universal inclinometer. (Photo courtesy of Performance Attainment Associates, St. Paul, MN.) *B,* Bubble inclinometer. (Photo courtesy of the Chattanooga Group, Chattanooga, TN.)

also electrogoniometers, which convert angular motion of the joint into an electric signal.[41] These are generally used for research purposes because of their expense and time to calibrate and attach to a patient.

As goniometry evolved, efforts were focused on standardizing methods of measurement, including developing common nomenclature and definitions of terms, clearly defining movements to be measured, and establishing normal ranges of motion. In 1965, the American Academy of Orthopaedic Surgeons published a manual of standardized methods of measuring and recording joint motion; since then, the manual has been reprinted numerous times.[2] Norkin and White[35] and Reese and Bandy[41] have also provided thorough descriptions of goniometry.

Goniometric Assessment

Anatomic Zero Position

The anatomic zero position is the starting 0° orientation for most measurements.[31] The exceptions are shoulder rotation, hip rotation, and forearm pronation-supination, in which the starting position is between the two extremes of motion. If the individual to be measured cannot assume the starting position, the position of improvisation should be noted when joint motion is recorded. Normal range of motion varies among individuals and is influenced by factors such as age and gender and whether the motion is performed actively or passively.

There are three accepted methods of recording range of motion: 0-180 system, which is the most common system used, 180-0 system, and 360° system[35,41] (Table 5-1). In the 0-180° system the neutral starting position is noted as 0°, and the degrees of joint motion are added in the direction of joint movement.[35] When a range of motion is documented, both the beginning (where the motion starts) and ending (where the motion ends) readings are reported. Motion that is beyond the anatomic zero position can be denoted with a plus (+) sign (hypermobility) and when motion is unable to reach the zero position, a minus (−) sign is used (hypomobility). Average ranges of motion for the upper and lower extremities are shown in Table 5-2.

Validity and Reliability of Goniometric Measurement

The purpose of goniometry is to measure the joint angle or range of motion.[35] It is assumed that the angle created by aligning the arms of a universal goniometer with bony landmarks truly represents the angle created by the proximal and distal bones composing the joint.[35] One infers that changes in goniometer alignment reflect changes in joint angle and represent a range of joint motion.[35] Additionally, goniometer measurements are generally compared with radiographs, which represent the "gold standard" for measurements. Several studies[1,10,16] have indicated a degree of relationship between measurements obtained with radiography and goniometry.

The reliability of goniometric joint motion measurements has been studied both within and between instruments/techniques as well as clinicians. Several reports noted that joint range of motion can be measured with good-to-excellent reliability.[9,13,16,27,28] Intratester reliability appears to be higher than intertester reliability regardless of the device used.[3,9,19,20,22,28,30,38,44,47,48] Additionally, it appears that upper extremity joint measurements are more reliable than those of the lower extremity joints,[3,38] and reliability can be less for different joints.[11,27,28,51,58] This may be due to the complexity of the joint or the difficulty in palpating anatomic landmarks.[35] Because reliability is different for each joint, the standard error of measurement can also differ for each joint. Norkin and White[35] and Reese and Bandy[41] documented the standard deviation and standard error of measurement for each joint in their books on goniometry. Boone and colleagues[3] indicated that the same individual should perform goniometric measurements when the effects of treatment are evaluated. Visual estimation is used by some clinicians to assess joint positions. Investigations assessing the accuracy and reliability of visual estimation versus goniometer measurements report the latter to be more accurate and reliable.[11,22,28,30,52,58,59]

Synthesis of the investigations evaluating the interchangeability of different types of goniometers show this is not an acceptable clinical practice.[17,40,43,45] Additionally, results of research assessing the inter- and intrareliability and validity of inclinometers and electrogoniometers vary and depend upon the technique used and the joint measured.[17,40,43,45]

Technical Considerations

The positioning of the patient should be consistent. The prone or supine position provides greater stabilization through the patient's body weight. Measurements should be acquired using passive range of motion when possible, and the body part should be uncovered for better accuracy. The goniometer is placed next to or on top of the joint whenever possible and three landmarks are used for alignment.[41] The goniometer arms are placed along the longitudinal axis of the bones of the joint after the motion has occurred. The fulcrum of the goniometer is placed over a

Table 5-1

Methods of Documenting Goniometry Readings

0-180 System	180-0 System	Full 360° Circle
Determines anatomical 0° starting point of all joints except for the forearm, which is fully supinated. Extension of a joint is recorded as 0° and as the joint flexes, motion progresses toward 180°.[41] Most common system used.	Neutral extension at each joint is recorded as 180°; movement toward flexion approaches 0°, and movement toward extension past neutral also approaches 0°.[4,41]	0° position of each joint is full flexion, neutral extension is recorded as 180°, and motions toward extension past neutral approach 360°.[41]

Table 5-2

Average Ranges of Motion for the Upper and Lower Extremities

Joint	Motion	Range of Motion (°) American Academy of Orthopaedic Surgeons	Kendall and McCreary[23]
Shoulder	Flexion	0–180	0–180
	Extension	0–60	0–45
	Abduction	0–180	0–180
	Internal rotation	0–70	0–70
	External rotation	0–90	0–90
Elbow	Flexion	0–150	0–145
Forearm	Pronation	0–80	0–90
	Supination	0–80	0–90
Wrist	Extension	0–70	0–70
	Flexion	0–80	0–80
	Radial deviation	0–20	0–20
	Ulnar deviation	0–30	0–35
Thumb			
CMC	Abduction	0–70	0–80
	Flexion	0–15	0–45
	Extension	0–20	0–45
MCP	Flexion	0–50	0–60
IP	Flexion	0–80	0–80
Digits 2 to 5			
MCP	Flexion	0–90	0–90
	Extension	0–45	
PIP	Flexion		
DIP	Extension		
Hip	Flexion	0–120	0–125
	Extension	0–30	0–10
	Abduction	0–45	0–45
	Adduction	0–30	0–10
	External rotation	0–45	0–45
	Internal rotation	0–45	0–45
Knee	Flexion	0–135	0–140
Ankle	Dorsiflexion	0–20	0–20
	Plantar flexion	0–50	0–45
	Inversion	0–35	0–35
	Eversion	0–15	0–20
Subtalar	Inversion		0–5
	Eversion	0–5	

Adapted from Norkin, C.C., and White, D.J. (1985): Measurement of Joint Motion: A Guide to Goniometry, Philadelphia, F.A. Davis.

CMC, carpometacarpal; DIP, distal interphalangeal; IP, interphalangeal; MCP, metacarpophalangeal; PIP, proximal interphalangeal.

point that is near the joint axis of rotation. Because this axis of rotation is not stationary during motion, this is the least important of the three landmarks, and emphasis is placed on proper alignment of the goniometer arms.[41]

In evaluating the joint and assessing range of motion, the clinician should view the affected joint from above and below to determine whether any additional limitations are present in the involved extremity. The opposite extremity must also be assessed to determine normal motion for that patient. Box 5-3 suggests guidelines to improve reliability of goniometry. Box 5-4 describes the principles for measuring range of motion for joints.

Special Joint Considerations

Spine

The wide range of motion available to the spine can make measurement of cervical and lumbar motions challenging.

Box 5-3

Suggested Guidelines to Improve Goniometry Reliability

- Use consistent, well-defined testing positions and anatomic landmarks to align the arms of the goniometer.[35]
- Do not interchange different types of goniometers for repeated measures from day to day on the same patient.[17,40,43,45]
- The same clinician should measure the patient from day to day if possible.[17,45]
- Use a standardized protocol for measuring joint motion.[35]
- Take repeated measurements on a subject with the same type of measurement device.[35]
- Use large universal goniometers when measuring joints with large body segments.[35]
- Inexperienced examiners should take several measurements and record the average of those measurements to improve reliability, but one measurement is usually sufficient for more experienced examiners using good technique.[35]

Note: Successive measurements are more reliable if they are taken by the same clinician rather than by different clinicians.

Box 5-4

Application Technique for Measuring Joint Range of Motion

1. The clinician places the patient in a posture that closely relates to an anatomical position.
2. It may be necessary to explain and demonstrate the procedure to the patient before the activity.
3. The clinician should take a visual estimate of the approximate range of motion that the joint will allow during active movement.
4. The clinician stabilizes the proximal segment of the joint to prevent error.
5. The landmarks are located and marked with a pen to ensure proper placement and alignment.
6. The axis of the joint is observed and the fulcrum of the goniometer is placed at this juncture. The goniometer is held 1 to 2 inches from the patient's body.
7. The stationary arm is aligned parallel to the longitudinal axis of the proximal limb segment and the appropriate anatomical landmarks.
8. After the goniometer is aligned properly, the patient is instructed to move the distal segment as far as they can go.
9. The moveable arm is aligned parallel to the longitudinal axis of the distal limb segment and the appropriate anatomical landmarks.
10. The clinician reads the goniometer.
11. It is not necessary to move the stationary arm when the measurements are repeated.
12. The clinician records and reports the data.

Many instruments are advocated for measuring motion of these areas, including tape measures, universal goniometers, and inclinometers. The use of the double inclinometer technique has also been suggested for measurement of cervical and lumbar motion.[41] Specific devices are available to measure only the cervical and lumbar spine, such as cervical range of motion (CROM) and back range of motion (BROM) devices (Performance Attainment Associates, Roseville, MN) (Figs. 5-5 and 5-6). Lumbar and thoracolumbar motions are most commonly measured with a tape measure. Flexion and extension of the lumbar spine can be measured using the Schober technique, which has been modified over time to the modified Schober technique and the modified-modified Schober technique (Table 5-3). Specific advantages and disadvantages of each technique as well as a detailed description can be found in other sources.[35,41]

The validity and reliability of the devices and techniques for measuring spine range of motion have been investigated extensively, comparing devices/techniques and inter- and intratester reliability. There is a fair amount of disparity in the research findings, and the reader is urged to consult a more in-depth review of this literature to make an informed decision regarding the devices/techniques to incorporate into their clinical practice.[35,41]

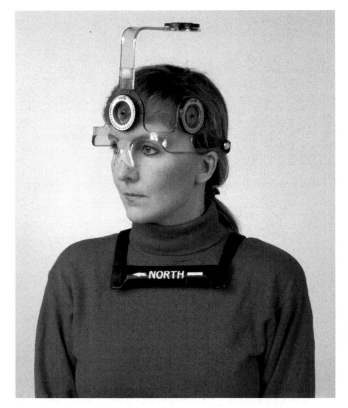

Figure 5-5. Cervical range of motion device (CROM), measuring cervical rotation. (Photo courtesy of Performance Attainment Associates, St. Paul, MN.)

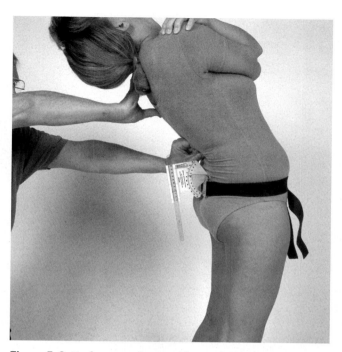

Figure 5-6. Back range of motion device (BROM), measuring lumbar flexion. (Photo courtesy of Performance Attainment Associates, St. Paul, MN.)

Scapular Position

Scapular position can have an effect on shoulder function. Thus, reliable methods of determining scapular position will allow clinicians to classify the degree of scapular abduction and the effect of therapeutic intervention(s).[34] There are two primary methods of measuring scapular abduction reported in the literature. DiVeta and associates[6] described a technique that uses a measurement from the inferior angle of the acromion to the spinous process of the third thoracic vertebra with patients standing in a relaxed position, arms at their sides. This distance is referred to as *total scapular distance*. Kibler[24] proposed what is known as the *lateral scapular slide test* (LSST) in which three measurements are made at 0, 40, and 90° of shoulder abduction. Scapular distance is measured from the inferior angle of the scapula to the T7 thoracic process.

Inter- and intratester reliability for the technique of DeVeta and associates for measuring scapular distance (abduction) is high,[6,14,18,34] as well as appearing to be a valid test for measuring scapula protraction.[18] Conversely, the data for inter- and intrareliablity for the LSST conflicts, with the only strong indication being that intratester reliability appears to be better than intertester reliability.[14,37] It appears that both techniques may be promising, but more research is needed before definite conclusions can be drawn.

Table 5-3

Schober Technique

Schober Technique	Modified Schober Technique[29]	Modified-Modified Schober Technique[56]
Two-mark method with the patient standing in a neutral standing posture: 1. Lumbosacral junction 2. 10 cm above the lumbosacral mark Patient bends forward and the increased distance between the first and second marks provides an estimate of spine flexion. Because the technique relies on stretching or distraction of the skin overlying the spine, it is also referred to as the "skin distraction method."	Introduced a third mark placed 5cm below the lumbosacral junction, along with the two marks described in the Schober technique. The rationale for this third mark was observation that during the Schober technique the skin above and below the lumbosacral junction was distracted as the patient bent forward.	Uses two landmarks: 1. Point bisecting a line that connects the two posterior superior iliac spines (PSIS) 2. A mark 15 cm superior to the PSIS landmark Rationale was the difficulty in palpating the lumbosacral junction. The PSIS are more readily palpated.

APPLICATION TECHNIQUES

Upper Extremities

SHOULDER
Flexion

Suggested Testing Position: The patient is in the anatomic supine position (Fig. 5-7).

Goniometer Alignment: The goniometer is aligned along (1) the midline of the humerus and (2) the midaxillary line of the trunk (see Fig. 5-7).

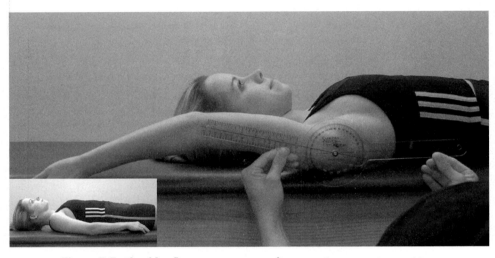

Figure 5-7. Shoulder flexion: goniometer alignment *Inset*, starting position.

Extension

Suggested Testing Position: The patient is in the anatomic prone position (Fig. 5-8).

Goniometer Alignment: The goniometer is aligned along (1) the midline of the humerus and (2) the midaxillary line of the trunk (see Fig. 5-8).

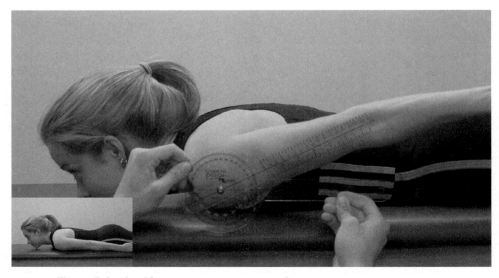

Figure 5-8. Shoulder extension: goniometer alignment *Inset*, starting position.

Abduction

Suggested Testing Position: The patient is in the anatomic supine position (Fig. 5-9), with the forearm in midposition between supination and pronation.

Goniometer Alignment: The goniometer is aligned (1) along the anterior longitudinal axis of the humerus and (2) parallel to the midline of the body (see Fig. 5-9).

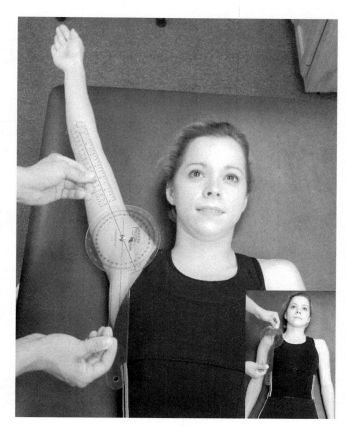

Figure 5-9. Shoulder abduction: goniometer alignment. *Inset,* starting position.

Adduction

Suggested Testing Position: The patient is in the anatomic supine position, with the forearm in midposition between supination and pronation (see Fig. 5-10).

Goniometer Alignment: The goniometer is aligned (1) along the anterior longitudinal axis of the humerus and (2) parallel to the midline of the body (Fig. 5-10).

External Rotation

Suggested Testing Position: The patient is supine, with the arm abducted to 90°, the elbow flexed to 90°, and the forearm pronated and perpendicular to the table (Fig. 5-11). A towel is placed under the humerus to bring the arm into the scapula plane.

Goniometer Alignment: The goniometer is aligned (1) along the ulna to the ulnar styloid process and (2) perpendicular to the table (see Fig. 5-11).

Continued

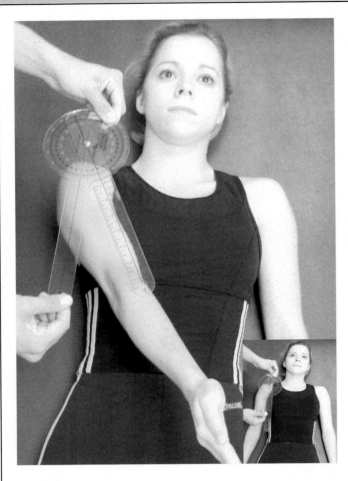

Figure 5-10. Shoulder adduction: goniometer alignment. *Inset,* starting position.

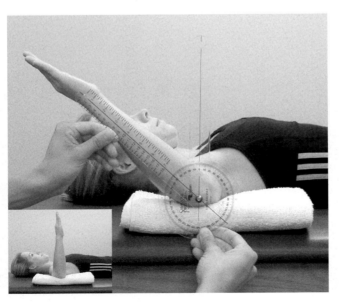

Figure 5-11. Shoulder external rotation: goniometer alignment. *Inset,* starting position.

Internal Rotation

Suggested Testing Position: The patient is supine, with the arm abducted to 90°, the elbow flexed to 90°, and the forearm pronated and perpendicular to the table (Fig. 5-12). A towel is placed under the humerus to bring the arm into the scapula plane.

Goniometer Alignment: The goniometer is aligned (1) along the ulnar styloid process and (2) perpendicular to the table (see Fig. 5-12).

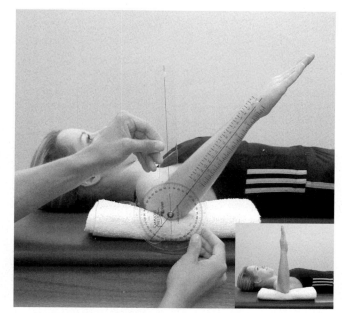

Figure 5-12. Shoulder internal rotation: goniometer alignment. *Inset,* starting position.

ELBOW
Flexion

Suggested Testing Position: The patient is in the anatomic supine position. A towel is placed under the humerus to bring the arm into the scapula plane (Fig. 5-13).

Goniometer Alignment: The goniometer is aligned along (1) the lateral midline of the humerus, humeral head to lateral condyle, and (2) the midline of the radius to the radial styloid process (see Fig. 5-13).

Extension

Suggested Testing Position: The patient is in the anatomic supine position (Fig. 5-14).

Goniometer Alignment: The goniometer is aligned along (1) the lateral midline of the humerus, humeral head to lateral condyle, and (2) the midline of the radius to the radial styloid process (see Fig. 5-14).

FOREARM
Pronation

Suggested Testing Position: The patient is seated next to the table, with the elbow flexed to 90° and the forearm midway between supination and pronation.

Continued

APPLICATION TECHNIQUES — cont'd

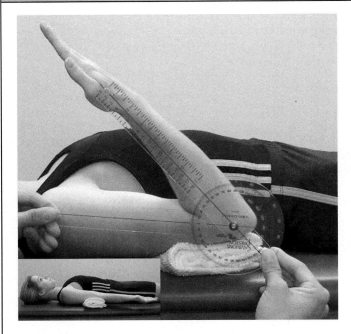

Figure 5-13. Elbow flexion: goniometer alignment. *Inset, starting position.*

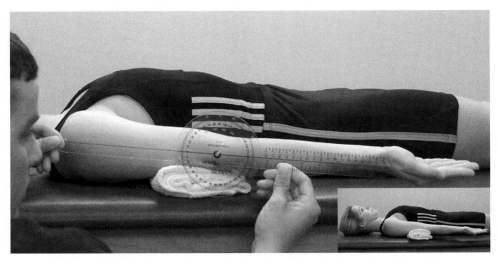

Figure 5-14. Elbow extension: goniometer alignment. *Inset, starting position.*

Goniometer Alignment:

(1) With the fingers straight, the goniometer is lined up with the line formed by the fingertips or, with the fingers flexed, lined up with the line formed by the proximal interphalangeal joints and (2) parallel to the table (Fig. 5-15).

Supination

Suggested Testing Position:

The patient is seated next to the table, with the elbow flexed to 90° and the forearm midway between supination and pronation.

Goniometer Alignment:

(1) With the fingers straight, the goniometer is lined up with the line formed by the fingertips or, with the fingers flexed, lined up with the line formed by the proximal interphalangeal joints and (2) parallel to the table (Fig. 5-16).

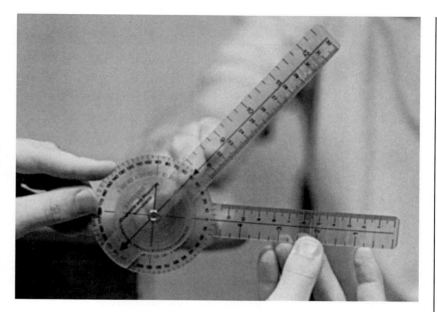

Figure 5-15. Forearm pronation: goniometer alignment.

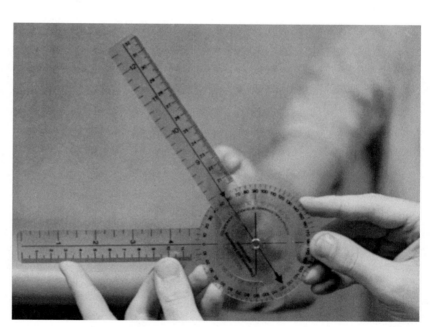

Figure 5-16. Forearm supination: goniometer alignment.

WRIST
Flexion

Suggested Testing Position: The patient is seated next to the table, with the elbow flexed to 90° and the forearm pronated (Fig. 5-17).

Goniometer Alignment: The goniometer is aligned with (1) the midline of the ulna and (2) the fifth metacarpal (see Fig. 5-17).

Continued

A P P L I C A T I O N   T E C H N I Q U E S — c o n t ' d

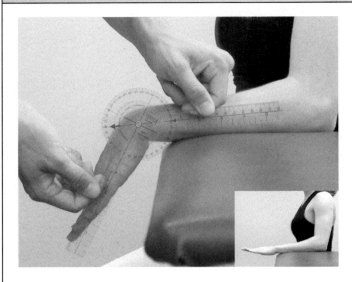

Figure 5-17. Wrist flexion: goniometer alignment. *Inset, starting position.*

Extension

Suggested Testing Position: The patient is seated next to the table, with the elbow flexed to 90° and the forearm pronated (Fig. 5-18).

Goniometer Alignment: The goniometer is aligned with (1) the midline of the ulna and (2) the fifth metacarpal (see Fig. 5-18).

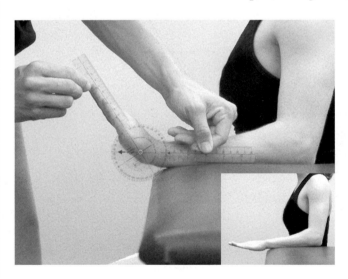

Figure 5-18. Wrist extension: goniometer alignment. *Inset, starting position.*

RADIUS AND ULNA
Radial Deviation

Suggested Testing Position: The patient is seated next to the table, with the elbow flexed to 90° and the forearm pronated.

Goniometer Alignment: The goniometer is aligned (1) over the ulnar styloid process and parallel to the third metacarpal and (2) perpendicular to the third metacarpal (Fig. 5-19).

Figure 5-19. Radial deviation: goniometer alignment.

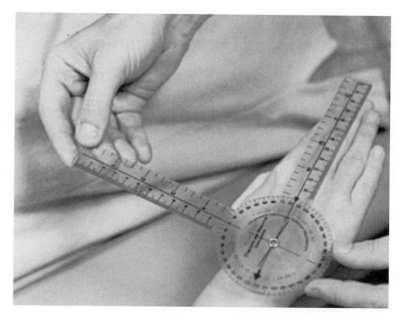

Ulnar Deviation

Suggested Testing Position: The patient is seated next to the table, with the elbow flexed to 90° and the forearm pronated.

Goniometer Alignment: The goniometer is aligned (1) over the radial styloid process parallel to the third metacarpal and (2) perpendicular to the third metacarpal (Fig. 5-20).

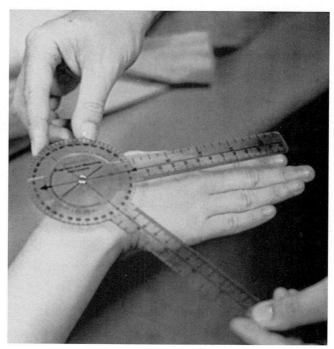

Figure 5-20. Ulnar deviation: goniometer alignment.

Continued

A P P L I C A T I O N   T E C H N I Q U E S — c o n t ' d

FINGERS
Flexion

Goniometer Alignment: The goniometer is aligned along (1) the medial side of the proximal phalanx and (2) the medial side of the distal phalanx (Fig. 5-21).

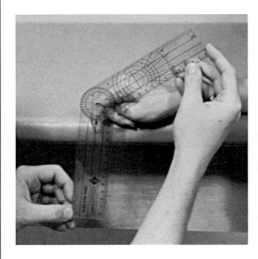

Figure 5-21. Finger flexion: goniometer alignment.

Extension

Goniometer Alignment: The goniometer is aligned along (1) the medial side of the proximal phalanx and (2) the medial side of the distal phalanx (Fig. 5-22).

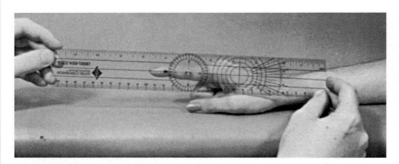

Figure 5-22. Finger extension: goniometer alignment.

LOWER EXTREMITIES
HIP

Flexion

Suggested Testing Position: The patient is in the anatomic supine position, with the knee bent to 90° when going through the motion (Fig. 5-23).

Goniometer Alignment: The goniometer is aligned (1) laterally along the long axis of the trunk and (2) on the lateral side, along the longitudinal axis of the femur, from greater trochanter to lateral femoral condyle (see Fig. 5-23).

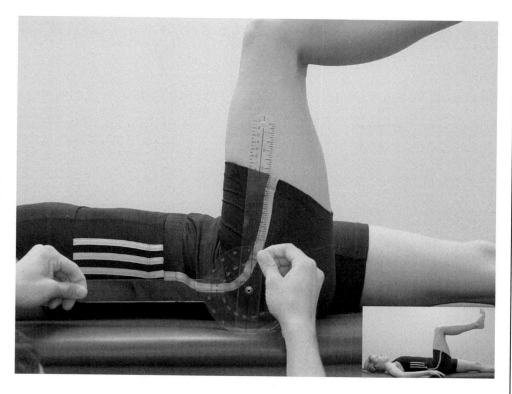

Figure 5-23. Hip flexion: goniometer alignment. *Inset, starting position.*

Extension

Suggested Testing Position: The patient is in the anatomic prone position (Fig. 5-24).

Goniometer Alignment: The goniometer is aligned (1) laterally along the long axis of the trunk and (2) on the lateral side, along the longitudinal axis of the femur, from greater trochanter to lateral femoral condyle (see Fig. 5-24).

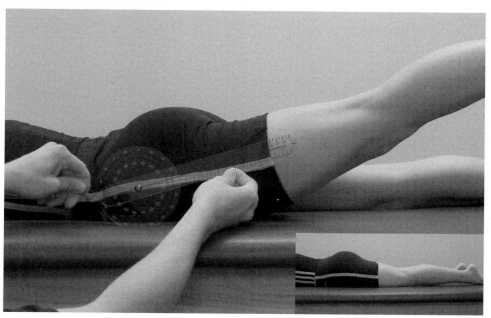
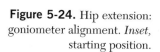

Figure 5-24. Hip extension: goniometer alignment. *Inset, starting position.*

Continued

A P P L I C A T I O N   T E C H N I Q U E S — c o n t'd

Abduction

Suggested Testing Position: The patient is in the anatomic supine position (Fig. 5-25).

Goniometer Alignment: The goniometer is aligned (1) over the two anterior superior iliac spines and (2) along the anterior thigh, from the midline of the thigh to the midline of the patella (see Fig. 5-25).

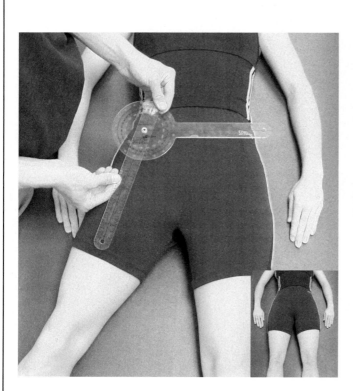

Figure 5-25. Hip abduction: goniometer alignment. *Inset, starting position.*

Adduction

Suggested Testing Position: The patient flexes the hip and knee in a supported position, with the extremity to be tested brought under the other extremity.

Goniometer Alignment: The goniometer is aligned (1) over the two anterior superior iliac spines and (2) along the anterior thigh, from the midline of the thigh to the midline of the patella (Fig. 5-26).

Internal Rotation

Suggested Testing Position: The patient is seated, with the hip flexed to 90° and the knee flexed to 90° over the edge of the table (Fig. 5-27).

Goniometer Alignment: The goniometer is aligned (1) perpendicular to the table and (2) along the midline of the anterior tibia, from the patella to midposition between the malleoli (see Fig. 5-27).

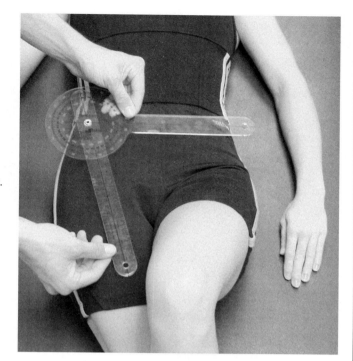

Figure 5-26. Hip adduction: goniometer alignment.

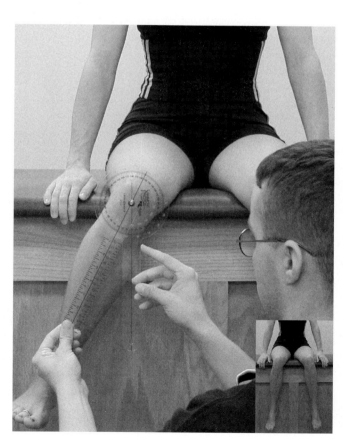

Figure 5-27. Hip internal rotation: goniometer alignment. *Inset,* starting position.

Continued

APPLICATION TECHNIQUES—cont'd

External Rotation

Suggested Testing Position: The patient is seated, with the hip flexed to 90° and the knee flexed to 90° over the edge of the table (Fig. 5-28).

Goniometer Alignment: The goniometer is aligned (1) perpendicular to the table and (2) along the midline of the anterior tibia, from the patella to midposition between the malleoli (see Fig. 5-28).

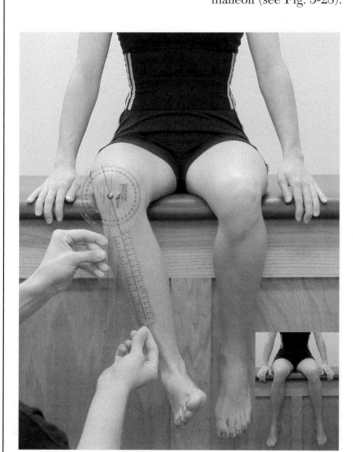

Figure 5-28. Hip external rotation: goniometer alignment. *Inset,* starting position.

KNEE
Flexion

Suggested Testing Position: The patient is in the supine position, with the hip flexed.

Goniometer Alignment: The goniometer is aligned along (1) the lateral femur, from the greater trochanter to the lateral femoral condyle and (2) the fibular head to the lateral malleolus (Fig. 5-29).

Extension

Suggested Testing Position: The patient is in the anatomic supine position.

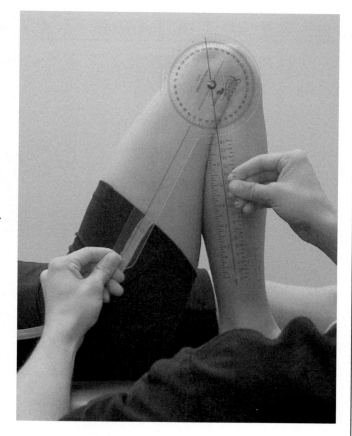

Figure 5-29. Knee flexion: goniometer alignment.

Goniometer Alignment: The goniometer is aligned along (1) the lateral femur, from the greater trochanter to the lateral femoral condyle and (2) the fibular head to the lateral malleolus (Fig. 5-30).

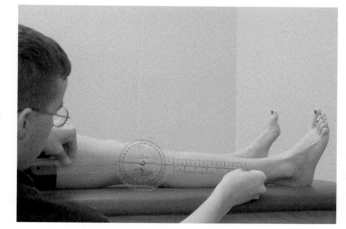

Figure 5-30. Knee extension: goniometer alignment.

ANKLE
Plantar Flexion

Suggested Testing Position: The patient is in the anatomic supine position, with the knee straight, or is seated, with the knee flexed.

Goniometer Alignment: The goniometer is aligned (1) along the midline of the fibula, fibula head to lateral malleolus, and (2) along the midline of the fifth metatarsal (Fig. 5-31).

Continued

APPLICATION TECHNIQUES — cont'd

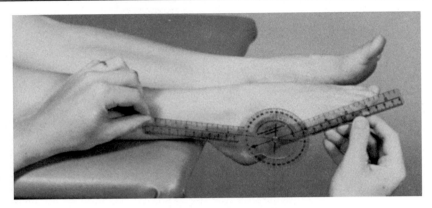

Figure 5-31. Ankle plantar flexion: goniometer alignment.

Dorsiflexion

Suggested Testing Position: The patient is in the anatomic supine position, with the knee straight, or is seated, with the knee flexed.

Goniometer Alignment: The goniometer is aligned (1) along the midline of the fibula, fibula head to lateral malleolus, and (2) along the midline of the fifth metatarsal (Fig. 5-32).

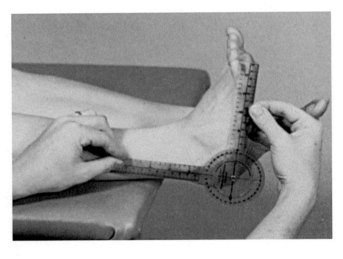

Figure 5-32. Ankle dorsiflexion: goniometer alignment.

Inversion

Suggested Testing Position: The patient is in the anatomic supine position.

Goniometer Alignment: The goniometer is aligned (1) across the two malleoli and (2) parallel to the second metatarsal (Fig. 5-33).

Eversion

Suggested Testing Position: The patient is in the anatomic supine position.

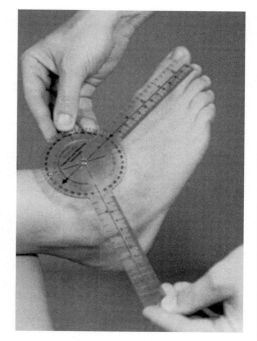

Figure 5-33. Ankle inversion: goniometer alignment.

Goniometer Alignment: The goniometer is aligned (1) across the two malleoli and (2) parallel to the second metatarsal (Fig. 5-34).

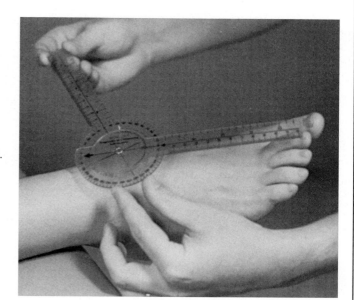

Figure 5-34. Ankle eversion: goniometer alignment.

SPINE, CERVICAL
Flexion

Suggested Testing Position: The patient is sitting in a chair with good support for the spine.

Goniometer Alignment: The goniometer is aligned (1) laterally with the fulcrum over the external ear, (2) with the stationary arm so it is perpendicular to the ground, and (3) with the moveable arm aligned with the base of the nose (Fig. 5-35). Move into flexion (see Fig. 5-35).

Continued

APPLICATION TECHNIQUES — cont'd

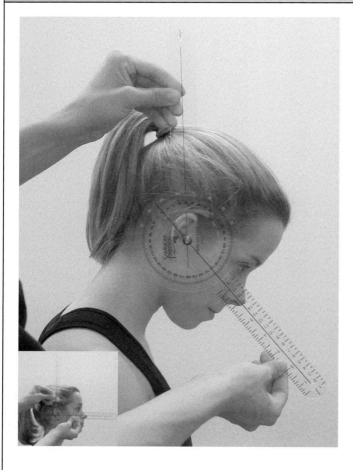

Figure 5-35. Cervical flexion: goniometer alignment. *Inset, starting position.*

Extension

Suggested Testing Position: The patient is sitting in a chair with good support for the spine.

Goniometer Alignment: The goniometer is aligned (1) laterally with the fulcrum over the external ear, (2) with the stationary arm so it is perpendicular to the ground, and (3) with the moveable arm aligned with the base of the nose (Fig. 5-36). Move into extension (see Fig. 5-36).

Lateral Flexion

Suggested Testing Position: The patient is sitting in a chair with good support for the spine.

Goniometer Alignment: The goniometer is aligned (1) with the fulcrum over the spinous process of the C7 vertebrae, (2) with the stationary arm along the spinous processes of the vertebrae, (3) and with the moveable arm along the midline of the head (Fig. 5-37). Move into lateral flexion (see Fig. 5-37).

Rotation

Suggested Testing Position: The patient is sitting in a chair with good support for the spine. The bridge of the nose is used for a point of reference.

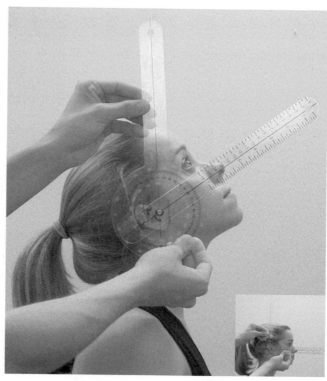

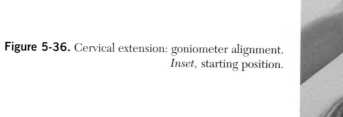

Figure 5-36. Cervical extension: goniometer alignment. *Inset,* starting position.

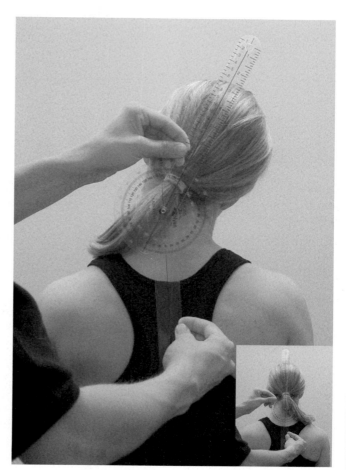

Figure 5-37. Cervical lateral flexion: goniometer alignment. *Inset,* starting position.

Continued

APPLICATION TECHNIQUES — cont'd

Goniometer Alignment: The goniometer is aligned (1) with the fulcrum over the center of the cranium, (2) with the proximal arm parallel to an imaginary lone drawn between the ears, and (3) with the distal arm aligned with the tip of the nose (Fig. 5-38). Move into rotation (see Fig. 5-38).

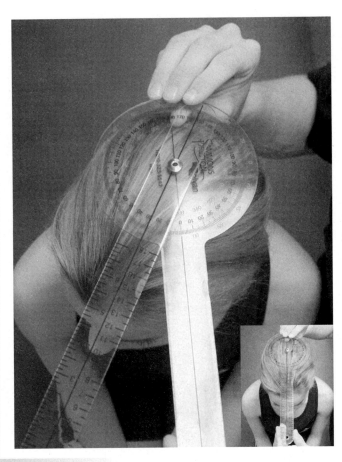

Figure 5-38. Cervical rotation: goniometer alignment. *Inset, starting position.*

SPINE, THORACOLUMBAR
Thoracicolumbar Flexion

Suggested Testing Position: The patient is in a standing position with the spine easily visualized.

Alignment: The tape measure is positioned with one end (1) at the patient's seventh cervical vertebra and the other end (2) over the first sacral vertebra (Fig. 5-39). From the starting position the patient moves into forward flexion, keeping the tape at the point of the seventh cervical vertebra fixed and allowing the tape to unwind at the sacral point (see Fig. 5-39). The difference in the initial measurement and the end point of the range of motion is the amount of thoracic and lumbar flexion that is present.

Lumbar Extension

Suggested Testing Position: The patient is in a standing position with the spine easily visualized.

Alignment: The tape measure is positioned with one end (1) beginning at the midline of the spine in line with the PSIS, while the other end (2) approximately 15 cm above base line mark. From the starting position the patient moves into extension,

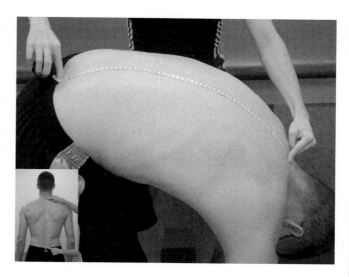

Figure 5-39. Thoracolumbar flexion: goniometer alignment. *Inset,* starting position.

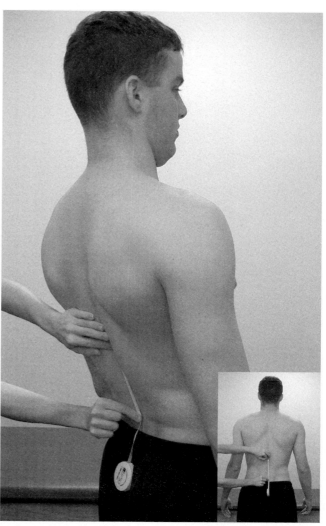

Figure 5-40. Lumbar extension: tape measure alignment. *Inset,* starting position.

Continued

APPLICATION TECHNIQUES — cont'd

keeping the tape fixed at the superior position allowing the tape to unwind at the base position (Fig. 5-40). The difference in the initial measurement and the end point of the range of motion is the amount of lumbar extension that is present.

Lumbar Lateral Flexion

Suggested Testing Position: The patient is in a standing position with the spine easily visualized.

Alignment: The tape measure is positioned with one end (1) at the patient's third finger and the other end (2) at the floor (Fig. 5-41). From this starting position a measurement is taken. The patient laterally flexes his or her trunk. Using the same landmarks, the clinician takes the measurement again (see Fig. 5-41). The difference in the initial and second measurement is the amount of lateral flexion in that direction.

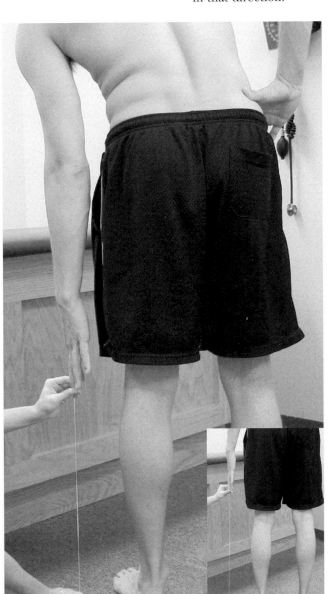

Figure 5-41. Lumbar lateral flexion: tape measure alignment.

SUMMARY

Girth

▦ The use of a standard tape measure appears to be a reliable instrument to measure girth, particularly when the same clinician makes all the measurements.

▦ There is no direct relationship between girth measurements and muscle size.

Goniometry

▦ The most common instruments used to measure joint motion are a universal goniometer, inclinometer, or tape measure.

▦ The most common system used to record joint motion is the 0-180 system.

▦ In general, goniometric measurements of joint motion are considered valid and reliable, but this varies based on the instrument, technique, and joint measured.

▦ It appears that intraclinician reliability is better than interclinician reliability; therefore, when possible, the same clinician should make all the measurements.

▦ Different types of goniometers should not be interchanged for repeated measures from day to day on the same patient.

REFERENCES

1. Ahlback, S.O., and Lindahl, O. (1964): Sagittal mobility of the hip joint. Acta Orthop. Scand., 34:310-314.
2. American Academy of Orthopaedic Surgeons. (1965): Joint Motion: Methods of Measuring and Recording. Chicago, American Academy of Orthopaedic Surgeons.
3. Boone, D.C., Azen, S.P., Linn, C.N., et al. (1978): Reliability of goniometric measurements. Phys. Ther., 58:1355-1360.
4. Clark, W.A. (1920): A system of joint measurements. J Orthop Surg, 2:687-700.
5. Clark, W.A. (1921): A protractor for measuring rotation of joint. J. Orthop. Surg., 3:154-155.
6. DiVeta, J., Walker, M.L., and Skibinski, B. (1990): Relationship between performance of selected scapular muscles and scapular abduction in standing subjects. Phys Ther, 70:470-476.
7. Doxey, G. (1987): Assessing quadriceps femoris muscle bulk with girth measurements in subjects with patellofemoral pain. J. Orthop. Sports Phys. Ther., 9:177-183.
8. Doxey, G. (1987): The association of anthropometric measurement of thigh size and B-mode ultrasound scanning of muscle thickness. J. Orthop. Sports Phys. Ther., 8:462-468.
9. Ekstaund, J., Wiktorsson, M., and Oberg, B. (1982): Lower extremity goniometric measurements: a study to determine their reliability. Arch. Phys. Med., 63:171-175.
10. Enwemeka, C.S. (1986): Radiographic verification of knee goniometry. Scand. J. Rehabil. Med., 18:47-50.
11. Fitzgerald, G.K., Wynveen, K.J., Rheault, W., and Rothschild, B. (1983): Objective assessment with establishment of normal values for lumbar spine range of motion. Phys. Ther., 62:1776-1781.
12. Fowler, P.J., and Regan, W.D. (1987): The patient with symptomatic chronic anterior cruciate ligament insufficiency. Am. J. Sports Med., 15:321-325.
13. Gajdoski, R.L., and Bohannon, R.W. (1987): Clinical measurement of range of motion: Review of goniometry emphasizing reliability and validity. Phys. Ther., 67:1867-1872.
14. Gibson, M.H., Goebel, G.V., Jordan, T.M., et al. (1995): A reliability study of measurement techniques to determine static scapular position. J. Orthop. Phys. Ther., 21:100-106.
15. Gifford, H.D. (1914): Instruments for measuring joint movements and deformities in fracture treatment. Am. J. Surg., 28:237-238.
16. Gogia, P.P., Braatz, J.H., Rose, S.J., and Norton, B. (1987): Reliability and validity of goniometric measurements of the knee. Phys. Ther., 67:192-195.
17. Goodwin, J., Clark, C., Deakes, J., et al. (1992): Clinical methods of goniometry: A comparative study. Disabil Rehabil., 14:10-15.
18. Greenfield, B., Catlin, P.A., Coats, P.W., et al. (1995): Posture in patients with shoulder overuse injuries and healthy individuals. J. Orthop. Phys. Ther., 21(5):287-295.
19. Grohmann, J.L. (1983): Comparison of two methods of goniometry. Phys. Ther., 67:192-195.
20. Hamilton, G.F., and Lachenbruch, P.A. (1969): Reliability of goniometers in assessing finger joint angle. Phys. Ther., 49:465-469.
21. Harrelson, G.L., Leaver-Dunn, D., Fincher, A.L., and Leeper, J.D. (1998): Inter- and intratester reliability of lower extremity circumference measurements. J. Sport Rehab., 7:300-306.
22. Hellebradt, F.A., Duvall, E.N., and Moore, M.L. (1949): The measurement of joint motion. Part III. Reliability of goniometry. Phys. Ther. Rev., 29:302-307.
23. Kendall, F.P., and McCreary, E.K. (1983): Muscle Testing and Function, 3rd ed. Baltimore: Williams & Wilkins.
24. Kibler, W.B. (1991): Role of the scapula in the overhead throwing motion. Contemp. Orthop., 22:525-532.
25. Kirwan, J.R., Byron, M.A., Winfield, J., et al. (1979): Circumferential measurements in the assessment of synovitis of the knee. Rheumatol. Rehab., 18:78-84.
26. Leighton, J.R. (1955): An instrument and technic for the measurement of range of joint motion. Arch. Phys. Med., 36:571-577.
27. Lovell, F.W., Rothstein, J.M., and Personius, W.J. (1989): Reliability of clinical measurement of lumbar lordosis taken with a flexible rule. Phys. Ther., 69:96-101.
28. Low, J.L. (1976): The reliability of joint measurement. Physiotherapy, 62:227-229.
29. Macrae, I.F., and Wright, V. (1969): Measurement of back movement. Ann. Rheum. Dis., 28:584-589.
30. Mayerson, N.H., and Milano, R.A. (1984): Goniometric measurement reliability in physical medicine. Arch. Phys. Med. Rehabil., 65:92-97.
31. Moore, M.L. (1949): The measurement of joint motion. Part I. Introductory review of the literature. Phys. Ther. Rev., 29:195-205.
32. Moore, M.L. (1949): The measurement of joint motion. Part II. The technic of goniometry. Phys. Ther. Rev., 29:256-264.
33. Morrissey, M.C., Brewster, C.E., Shields, C.L., and Brown, M. (1985): The effects of electrical stimulation on the quadriceps during postoperative knee immobilization. J. Sports Med., 12:40-45.

34. Neiers, L., and Worrell, T.W. (1993): Assessment of scapular position. J. Sport Rehab., 2:20-25.

35. Norkin, C.C., and White, D.J. (1995): Measurement of Joint Motion: Guide to Goniometry, 2nd ed. Philadelphia, F.A. Davis.

36. Noyes, F.R., Mangine, R.E., and Barber, S. (1987): Early knee motion after open and arthroscopic anterior cruciate ligament reconstruction. Am. J. Sports Med., 15:149-160.

37. Odom, C.J., Taylor, A.B., Hurd, C.E., and Denegar, C.R. (2001): Measurement of scapular asymmetry and assessment of shoulder dysfunction using the lateral scapular slide test: A reliability and validity study. Phys. Ther., 81:799-809.

38. Pandya, S., Florence, J.M., King, W.M., et al. (1985): Reliability of goniometric measurement in patients with Duchenne muscular dystrophy. Phys. Ther., 65:1339-1345.

39. Parker, J.S. (1929): Recording arthroflexometer. J. Bone Jt. Surg., 11:126-127.

40. Petherick, M., Rheault, W., Kimble, S., et al. (1988): Concurrent validity and intertester reliability of universal and fluid-based goniometers for active elbow range of motion. Phys. Ther., 68:966-969.

41. Reese, N.B., and Bandy, W.D. (2002): Joint Range of Motion and Muscle Length Testing. Philadelphia, W.B. Saunders.

42. Reynolds, N.L., Worrell, T.W., and Perrin, D.H. (1992): Effect of a lateral step-up exercise protocol on quadriceps isokinetic peak torque values and thigh girth. J. Orthop. Sports Phys. Ther., 15:151-155.

43. Rheault, W., Miller, M., Nothnagel, P., et al. (1988): Intertester reliability and concurrent validity of fluid-based and universal goniometers for active knee flexion. Phys. Ther., 68:1676-1678.

44. Riddle, D.L., Rothstein, J.M., and Lamb, R.L. (1987): Goniometric reliability in a clinical setting: Shoulder measurements. Phys. Ther., 67:668-673.

45. Rome, K., and Cowieson, F. (1996): A reliability study of the universal goniometer, fluid goniometer and electrogoniometer for the measurement of ankle dorsiflexion. Foot Ankle Int., 17:28-32.

46. Romero, J.A., Sanford, T.L., Schroeder, R.V., and Fahey, T.D. (1982): The effects of electrical stimulation on normal quadriceps strength and girth. Med. Sci. Sports Exerc., 14:194-197.

47. Rothstein, J.M., Miller, P.J., and Roettger, R.F. (1983): Goniometric reliability in a clinical setting: Elbow and knee measurement. Phys. Ther., 63:1611-1615.

48. Solgaard, S., Carlsen, A., Krauhoft, M., and Petersen, V.S. (1986): Reproducibility of goniometry of the wrist. Scand. J. Rehab. Med., 18:5-7.

49. Spencer, J.D., Hayes, K.C., and Alexander, I.J. (1984): Knee joint effusion and quadriceps reflex inhibition in man. Arch. Phys. Med. Rehab., 65:171-177.

50. Stokes, M., and Young, A. (1984): The contribution of reflex inhibition to arthrogenous muscle weakness. Clin. Sci., 67: 7-14.

51. Tucci, S.M., Hicks, J.E., Gross, E.G., et al. (1986): Cervical motion assessment: A new, simple and accurate method. Arch. Phys. Med. Rehab., 67:225-230.

52. Watkins, M.A., Riddle, D.L., Lamb, R.L., and Personius, W.J. (1991): Reliability of goniometric measurements and visual estimates of knee range of motion obtained in a clinical setting. Phys. Ther., 71:90-96.

53. West, C.C. (1945): Measurement of joint motion. Arch. Phys. Med., 26:414-425.

54. Whitney, S.L., Mattocks, L., Irrgang, J.J., et al. (1995): Reliability of lower extremity girth measurements and right- and left-side differences. J. Sports Rehab., 4:108-115.

55. Wiechec, F.J., and Krusen, F.H. (1939): A new method of joint measurement and a review of the literature. Am. J. Surg., 43:659-668.

56. Williams, R., Binkley, J., Bloch, R., et al. (1993): Reliability of the modified-modified Schober and double inclinometer methods for measuring lumbar flexion and extension. Phys Ther, 73:26-37.

57. Wilson, J.D., and Stasch, W.H. (1945): Photographic record of joint motion. Arch. Phys., 27:361-362.

58. Youdas, J.W., Bogard, C.L., and Suman, V.J. (1993): Reliability of goniometric measurements and visual estimates of ankle joint active range of motion obtained in a clinical setting. Arch. Phys. Med. Rehab., 74:1112-1118.

59. Youdas, J.W., Carey, J.R., and Garrett, T.R. (1991): Reliability of measurement of cervical spine range of motion: Comparison of three methods. Phys. Ther., 71:2-7.

60. Young, A., Stokes, M., and Iles, J.F. (1987): Effects of joint pathology on muscle. Clin. Orthop., 219:21-27.

CHAPTER 6

RANGE OF MOTION AND FLEXIBILITY

Jeff G. Konin, M.Ed., ATC, M.P.T.
Gary L. Harrelson, Ed.D., ATC
Deidre Leaver-Dunn, Ph.D., ATC

CHAPTER OBJECTIVES

At the end of this chapter the reader will be able to:

- Recognize and describe methods of assessing and measuring range of motion and flexibility.
- Identify principles associated with stretching of connective tissue structures.
- Explain the principles and techniques for active, active-assisted, passive, and resistive stretching.
- Identify the basic principles of proprioceptive neuromuscular facilitation and recognize its benefits for rehabilitation of athletes.
- Identify key principles, indications, and contraindications of joint mobilization.

Range of motion is the available amount of movement of a joint, whereas flexibility is the ability of soft tissue structures, such as muscle, tendon, and connective tissue, to elongate through the available range of joint motion. Whether it is undergoing therapeutic stretching during postinjury rehabilitation or during a routine flexibility program, connective tissue is the most important physical focus of range-of-motion exercises. For favorable physiologic potentials to exist, both range of motion and flexibility ranges need to be optimized. Connective tissue involved in the body's reparative process after trauma or surgery often limits normal joint motion. Therefore, understanding the biophysical factors of connective tissue is important for determining optimal ways of increasing range of motion because histologic evidence has shown that fibrosis can occur within 4 days of the onset of immobility.[98] To effectively maintain and improve range of motion and flexibility knowledge of both the related tissue structures and the various techniques utilized to facilitate extensibility of these structures is imperative.

REASONS FOR RANGE-OF-MOTION LIMITATIONS

Physiologic conditions that are associated with range of motion limitations may vary. Oftentimes, a single structural component may be the cause of a movement restriction. However, it is not uncommon to have related concurrent limitations from more than one structure. Structures that play a role in limiting one's range of motion are summarized in Box 6-1. Limitations as a result of structural involvement may be caused by a traumatic incident such as surgery or may develop over time from disuse, such as a lack of stretching. Furthermore, pain associated with disruption to tissue or as a result of joint swelling that becomes a space-occupying lesion and compresses against joint receptors and cutaneous nerves may inhibit one's ability to actively and passively generate joint movement.

STRETCHING
Biophysical Considerations
Properties of Connective Tissue

Connective tissue is composed of collagen and other fibers within a ground substance—a protein-polysaccharide complex. A thorough discussion of connective tissue composition is found in Chapter 2. Connective tissue has viscoelastic properties, defined as two components of stretch, which allow elongation of the tissue.[39,51,90,98] The viscous component permits a plastic stretch that results in permanent tissue elongation after the load is removed. Conversely, the elastic component allows an elastic stretch, a temporary elongation, with the tissue returning to its previous length once the stress is removed. Range-of-motion exercise techniques should primarily be designed to produce plastic deformation. Repetitive intervention that incorporates sustained tissue elongation with low loads of stress versus shorter duration aggressive loads may be more beneficial for clinical outcomes of obtaining plastic deformational changes.

Box 6-1

Structures and Factors Contributing to Range-of-Motion Limitations

- Joint capsule tightness
- Ligamentous adhesions
- Muscular spasm
- Muscular tightness
- Myofascial tightness
- Pain
- Joint effusion
- Bony blocks

Neurophysiology

All stretching techniques are based on the premise of the stretch reflex, which involves two muscle receptors—the Golgi tendon organ (GTO) and the muscle spindle—that are sensitive to changes in muscle length.[111] The GTO is also affected by changes in muscle tension. These receptors must be considered in the process of selecting any stretching procedure. The intrafusal muscle spindle responds to rapid stretch by initiating a reflexive contraction of the muscle being stretched.[111] If a stretch is held long enough (at least 6 seconds),[83] this protective mechanism can be negated by the action of the GTO, which can override the impulses from the muscle spindle.[111] The reflexive relaxation that results is referred to as *autogenic inhibition,* and it allows effective stretching of the muscle tissue. Additionally, an isotonic contraction of an agonist muscle causes a reflex relaxation in the antagonist muscle, allowing it to stretch. This phenomenon is referred to as *reciprocal inhibition.* Conversely, a quick stretch of the antagonist muscle will cause a contraction of the agonist muscle. For example, when the quadriceps muscle contracts, a reflexive relaxation of the hamstring muscles occurs. In other words, once a tight muscle or muscles have been identified, an isotonic contraction of its antagonist will result in relaxation of the tight muscles and an improved range of motion. Autogenic inhibition and reciprocal inhibition are two components on which proprioceptive neuromuscular facilitation (PNF) stretching is based.

Duration

The amount and duration of the applied force during performance of the stretch are some of the principal factors determining how much elastic or plastic stretch occurs with connective tissue stretching. Elastic stretch is enhanced by high-force, short-duration stretching, whereas plastic stretch results from low-force, long-duration stretching. Numerous studies representing decades of research have noted the effectiveness of prolonged stretching at low to moderate tension levels.[3,28,30,39,40,47,51,53,60,73,89,90,100,105,112,113] A precise time frame for holding a static stretch has not been determined.

Research has suggested that static stretches be held between 6 and 60 seconds,[83] with 15- to 30-second holds being most commonly advocated. Some authors have proposed that a single static stretch of 15 to 30 seconds one time each day is sufficient for most people.[93]

Temperature of Connective Tissue

Research has shown that temperature has a significant influence on the mechanical behavior of connective tissue under tensile stretch.[56-58,90,115] Because connective tissue is composed of collagen, which is resistant to stretch at normal body temperature, the effect of increased tissue temperature on stretch has been studied. Synthesis of the body of research shows that higher therapeutic temperatures at low loads produce the greatest plastic tissue elongation with the least damage. Lentell and colleagues[59] reported greater increases in range of motion of healthy shoulders after heat application.

Increased connective tissue temperature decreases connective tissue resistance to stretch and promotes increased soft tissue extensibility.[53,58] It has been reported that collagen is very pliable when heated to a range between 102° and 110°F.[56,90] The use of ultrasound before joint mobilization has proved effective in elevating deep tissue temperature and extensibility.[57] Draper and Ricard[18] demonstrated the presence of a "stretching window" after a 3 MHz ultrasound application. This window indicates that for optimal tissue elongation, stretching should be performed during ultrasound treatment or within 3.3 minutes after termination of the treatment.[18] In a follow-up study, Rose and colleagues[87] reported that after a 1 MHz ultrasound application, the deeper tissues cooled at a slower rate than did superficial tissues; thus, the stretching window was open longer for deeper structures than for superficial ones. Although superior stretching results have been reported with the application of heat before and during stretching, other studies have reported greater increases in flexibility after the application of cold packs. Brodowicz and colleagues[9] reported improved hamstring flexibility in healthy subjects after 20 minutes of hamstring stretching with an ice pack applied to the posterior thigh compared with the group that received heat or that performed stretching without application of any therapeutic agent. Kottke and colleagues[51] have also shown that a greater plastic stretch results if the tissue is allowed to cool before tension is released, whereas others[59] have reported that the use of cold during the end stages of stretching diminished the cumulative gains in flexibility that occurred after application of heat. Moreover, it appears that the use of either a superficial heat or a cold modality in conjunction with stretching results in greater improvements in flexibility than stretching alone.[9,59] It remains to be seen whether increased extensibility is the sole result of a single structure or a combination of structural changes perhaps related to musculotendinous, capsuloligamentous, or fascial tissue.

Objectivity of Range of Motion and Flexibility Assessment

Range of motion and flexibility are measured in a number of different ways. Typically, the type of tissue being assessed will dictate the method of assessment, although some methods may be used for various tissues. The primary movements that are assessed are termed as being *physiologic* or *accessory*. Physiologic movement comprises the major portion of the range and can be measured with a goniometer (see Chapter 5). Physiologic joint movements occur in the cardinal movement planes and include flexion-extension, abduction-adduction, and rotation.[81] Accessory motion, also referred to as arthrokinematics, is necessary for normal physiologic range of motion; it occurs simultaneously with physiologic motion and cannot be measured precisely.

The ability to accurately assess and measure physiologic range of motion appears to be joint dependent.[10,20,24,31,32,38,62,86,114] These findings are detailed in Chapter 5, and the reader is encouraged to be inventive in developing improved methods of measurement to enhance those that currently exist. Devices such as a sit-and-reach tool can be utilized to assess the excursion of the hamstring muscles[43,45,78] (Fig. 6-1).

Accessory range of motion is much more difficult to assess and measure because it is often measured in units of millimeters. Experience with assessing both normal and abnormal joint accessory movement plays a critical role in one's ability to accurately process such movement. Studies have shown a clear difference between the novice and expert clinician in determining accessory range of motion.[12,21,37,66] Equipment can also be used to assess joint accessory motion, such as that seen when one is measuring the amount of anterior translation of the knee as a result of an anterior cruciate ligament injury[2,26,52,71,79] (Fig. 6-2).

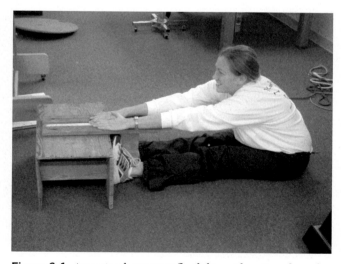

Figure 6-1. Assessing hamstring flexibility with a sit-and-reach box.

Types of Stretching Techniques

Limited joint range of motion caused by soft tissue restriction often inhibits the initiation or completion of the rehabilitative process. Conservative treatment of contractures is only moderately successful, and overly aggressive stretching may result in undesired adverse effects. Optimal stretching is achieved only when voluntary and reflex muscle resistances are overcome or eliminated, and tissue elongation is facilitated. The main types of tissue that are stretched include musculotendinous, capsuloligamentous, and myofascial.

Three types of stretching techniques are generally recognized to facilitate musculotendinous flexibility: ballistic, static, and PNF. Ballistic stretching consists of repetitive bouncing movements that stretch a muscle group. Ballistic stretching has not been advocated because forces could be applied to a muscle that exceed its extensibility or that activate the muscle spindles described previously, with resultant microtrauma to the muscle fibers.[6,92,96,99] However, it has been reported that because many physical activities involve dynamic movement, ballistic stretching should follow a static stretching routine.[41] Static stretching involves stretching a muscle to a point of discomfort and holding the stretch for a length of time, followed by a return to normal resting muscle length. PNF involves alternating muscle contractions and stretching.[49] The efficacy of all three techniques has been evaluated, and it appears that each technique has the capacity to increase flexibility, with static stretching being the safest of the three.[11,14,15,22,30,34,61,68,70,75,76,80,88,101,104,110,116] In some cases static stretching has been advocated over PNF because it is easier to teach and perform.[116] Some clinicians prefer PNF stretching because it allows for stretching to occur in functional planes of movement that more closely simulate activities. Each of the techniques should be performed with a prescribed set of repetitions with care being taken to avoid overstretching. Contraindications to general stretching are indicated in Box 6-2.

Passive and Active-Assisted Stretching Techniques

Various mechanical passive and active assisted techniques augment manual passive stretching. Methods of achieving the desired outcome are often limited only by creativity and improvisational skills. Once the soft tissue restriction has been assessed, the clinician should analyze appropriate and effective ways of carrying out the treatment and rehabilitation plan. Several methods of stretching can be used, but a clinician should be careful to consider joint positioning when assessing extensibility and use standardized and consistent approaches to most accurately reflect reliable and valid measurements.

Spray and Stretch

This technique has been described in detail by Travell and Simons.[106,107] Spraying of Fluori-Methane* or ethyl

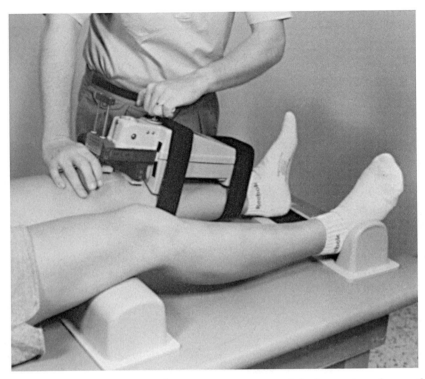

Figure 6-2. Assessment of anterior translation accessory motion of the knee using a knee arthrometer.

chloride* cools taut muscle fibers and desensitizes palpable myofascial trigger points, thereby facilitating stretching of the muscle to its full length. Passive stretch remains the central component within this technique. Concerns about usage of both vapocoolants have been documented. Travell and Simmons[106] advocated the use of Fluori-Methane spray. However, because Fluori-Methane is a chlorofluorocarbon, which destroys the ozone atmospheric layer, its use has been questioned.[108] Conversely, although ethyl chloride is not a chlorofluorocarbon, it is colder than Fluori-Methane, flammable, and explosive in a critical concentration with air and is a potent, readily-acting general anesthesic[94,106] (see Chapter 4 for additional information on vapocoolants). Ice-stroking has been advocated as an alternative to the use of vapocoolants.[42,94,106]

Prolonged Weighted Stretch

The rationale for a prolonged-duration, low-load stretch has been discussed. Figure 6-3 illustrates a method of prolonged weighted stretching for the knee using a small cuff weight placed distally on the lower leg, which serves as a gentle passive stretch for the hamstring muscle group. Similar types of stretches can be performed for the upper extremity, as seen in Figure 6-4. The key to succeeding with prolonged-duration, low-load types of stretches is to allow for muscle relaxation and gentle overpressure. If an athlete is not comfortable, he or she will contract the muscles surrounding the joint and resist the overpressure, resulting in no short-term or long-term flexibility gains.

Assistive Devices

These appliances aid in gaining and maintaining end range of motion. Assistive devices include pulleys, extremity traction,[58,90] T-bars or wands, and continuous passive range-of-motion units. Pulleys are commonly used for

---

Box 6-2

Contraindications to Stretching

- Limitation of joint motion by a bony block
- Recent fracture
- Evidence of an acute inflammatory or infectious process (heat and swelling) in or around joints
- Sharp, acute pain with joint movement or muscle elongation
- Hematoma or other indications of tissue trauma
- Contractures or shortened soft tissues providing increased joint stability in lieu of normal structural stability or muscle strength
- Contractures or shortened soft tissues forming the basis for increased functional abilities, particularly in individuals with paralysis or severe muscle weakness

Data from Kisner, C., and Colby, L. (2002): Therapeutic Exercise: Foundations and Techniques. Philadelphia, F.A. Davis.

---

*Available from Gebauer Chemical Co., Cleveland, Ohio.

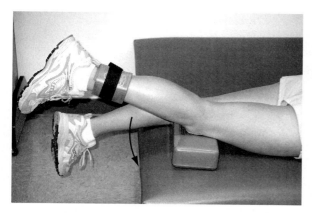

Figure 6-3. Prone low-load weighted stretch for the hamstring muscle group.

joint restriction of the shoulder (Fig. 6-5) and knee. Wands, T-bars, towels, sport sticks (Fig. 6-6), or other similar apparatus may be used for individual active assisted stretching of the upper extremities.

Continuous passive range-of-motion units are often valuable mechanical devices that can benefit various joints.[7,23,27,54,55,65,74] They can provide constant movement of a joint after surgical intervention and are most helpful because longer durations of passive movement can be implemented. Postoperatively, most continuous passive range-of-motion units are not set within a range of motion that provides for tissue stretching beyond even the slightest level of discomfort. Rather, movement is facilitated within the range of motion that currently exists, allowing the device to serve as more of a passive component to maintain range of motion and promote joint nutrition. As joint range of motion gradually increases, the controls can be adjusted to allow for movement within a larger range of motion. A passive mode can be used on other equipment, including isokinetic units, to allow a controlled passive range of motion with a pause to provide a stretch at the end range of motion (Fig. 6-7). Some clinicians, and

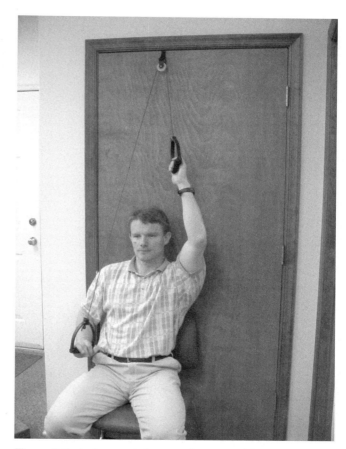

Figure 6-5. Active-assisted range of motion of the shoulder with the use of pulleys.

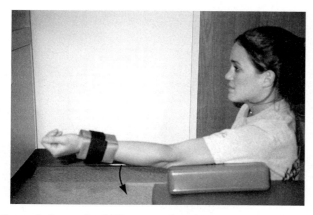

Figure 6-4. Weighted elbow stretch utilizing low-load long duration stretch.

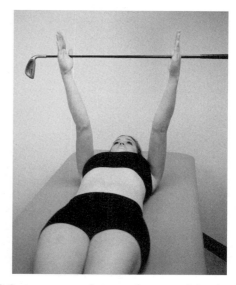

Figure 6-6. Active-assisted range of motion of the shoulder with the use of a golf club.

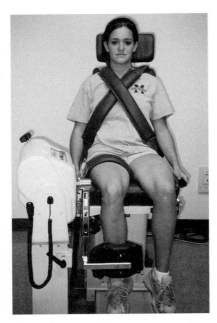

Figure 6-7. Isokinetic dynamometer unit setup in a passive mode.

patients alike do not promote the use of continuous passive range-of-motion and isokinetic units as a mechanism to maintain and gain joint range of motion for fear of the patient not being able to understand how to control the unit should any increase in pain be felt during use.

Adjustable dynamic splints can produce prolonged-duration, low-load force. The construction of these devices offers a lower progressive load that can be self-adjusted and graduated as orthotic tolerance time increases (Fig. 6-8). Dynamic splints have been used successfully in the treatment of motion restrictions of the knee and elbow.[8,39,40]

Proprioceptive Neuromuscular Facilitation Techniques

PNF can be defined as a method of promoting or hastening the response of neuromuscular mechanisms through stimulation of the mechanoreceptors.[49,109] PNF stretching techniques are based on the reduction of sensory activity through spinal reflexes to cause relaxation of the muscle to be stretched. Sherrington's principle of reciprocal inhibition demonstrates relaxation of the muscle being stretched (agonist) through voluntary concentric contraction of its opposite (antagonist) muscle.[49,70,104] Many studies[13-15,22,29,34,70,75,76,80,88,104,110] support the efficacy of PNF and show greater increases in flexibility when PNF is used rather than static or dynamic stretching techniques. Other investigations[11,61,68,101,116] have found PNF to be at least as effective as other types of stretching. Originally, PNF was described as a rehabilitation technique for those recovering from neurologic disorders,[49] but the technique has the capability of being used for various orthopedic conditions as well.[25,36,64,67,72,76,88,95,97,103]

PNF patterns can be performed in a single plane, such as flexion-extension, or in rotational and diagonal patterns that incorporate multiple planes and synergistic patterns (Table 6-1). PNF techniques generally comprise five trials of 5 seconds of passive stretching followed by a 5- to 10-second maximal voluntary contraction, as indicated

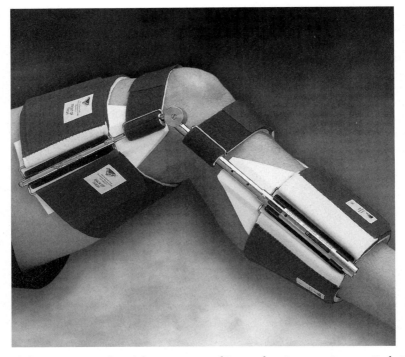

Figure 6-8. Knee Dynasplint. (Photo courtesy of Dynasplint Systems, Severna Park, MD.)

Table 6-1

Upper and Lower Diagonal PNF Patterns

| Extremity | Diagonal 1 | | Diagonal 2 | |
	Flexion	Extension	Flexion	Extension
Upper				
Scapula	Elevation	Depression	Elevation	Depression
Shoulder	Flexion	Extension	Flexion	Extension
	Adduction	Abduction	Abduction	Adduction
	External rotation	Internal rotation	External rotation	Internal rotation
Elbow	Flexion	Extension	Flexion	Extension
Forearm	Supination	Pronation	Supination	Pronation
Wrist	Radial deviation	Ulnar deviation	Radial deviation	Ulnar deviation
Fingers	Flexion	Extension	Extension	Flexion
Lower				
Pelvis	Elevation	Depression	Elevation	Depression
Hip	Flexion	Extension	Flexion	Extension
	Adduction	Abduction	Abduction	Adduction
	External rotation	Internal rotation	Internal rotation	External rotation
Knee	Flexion	Extension	Flexion	Extension
Ankle	Dorsi flexion	Plantar flexion	Dorsi flexion	Plantar flexion
Foot	Inversion	Eversion	Eversion	Inversion
Toes	Extension	Flexion	Extension	Flexion

by the technique used. The work of Cornelius and colleagues[15] showed that significant increases in systolic blood pressure occurred after three trials consisting of a protocol of 5 seconds of passive stretching, followed by a 6-second maximal voluntary antagonist contraction. Thus, caution is warranted when one works with populations who have a predisposition to cardiovascular conditions.

Contract-Relax

The contract-relax technique[34,75,76,102,109] produces increased range of motion in the agonist pattern by using consecutive isotonic contractions of the antagonist. Box 6-3 outlines how this technique is performed.

The procedure is repeated several times, followed by the athlete's moving actively through the obtained range

Box 6-3

Contract-Relax Technique

Step	Procedure
1	The body part to be stretched is moved passively into the agonist pattern until range-of-motion limitation is felt.
2	The athlete contracts isotonically into the antagonist pattern against strong manual resistance.
3	When the clinician realizes that relaxation has occurred, the body part is again moved passively into as much range of motion as possible until limitation is again felt.

(Fig. 6-9). When performing the contract-relax technique, the clinician must maintain proper stabilization to ensure that an isometric contraction occurs.

Hold-Relax

Hold-relax[14,15,49,102] is a PNF technique used to increase joint range of motion that is based on an isometric contraction of the antagonist performed against maximal resistance. This technique is performed in the same sequence as the contract-relax technique, but because no motion is allowed on isometric contraction, this is the method of choice when joint restriction is accompanied by muscle spasm and pain. The intensity of each contraction is gradually increased with each successive repetition (Fig. 6-10).

Slow Reversal Hold-Relax

The slow reversal hold-relax technique[49,109] uses reciprocal inhibition, as does the hold-relax technique. Box 6-4 outlines how this technique is performed. The technique is good for increasing range of motion when the primary limiting factor is the antagonist muscle group (Fig. 6-11).

Special Considerations for Proprioceptive Neuromuscular Facilitation

Proprioceptive neuromuscular feedback depends not only on the performance of an athlete, but also on the ability of the clinician to provide appropriate and timely verbal and tactile commands. Verbal commands such as "contract" and "relax" must be made clear and at the precise moment to enhance range-of-motion gains and minimize any associated discomfort. Hand placement by the clinician also

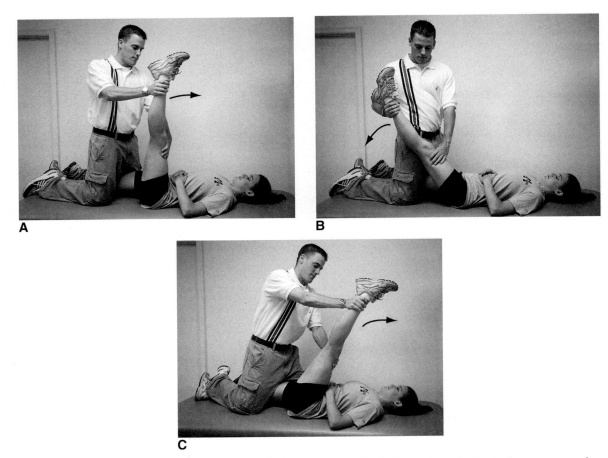

Figure 6-9. Contract-relax proprioceptive neuromuscular facilitation pattern for the hamstrings. *A*, The body part is moved passively by the clinician into the agonist pattern until limitation is felt. *B*, The athlete performs an isotonic contraction through the antagonist pattern. *C*, The clinician applies a passive stretch into the agonist pattern until limitation is felt. The procedure is repeated.

provides tactile feedback and serves to inform the athlete what direction a joint should be moving into and with how much resistance. The limitations that exist will help to dictate which PNF pattern is appropriate and how much resistance should be applied during the application of the technique.

Although specific patterns and techniques have been identified, it is also important to progress the athlete through increasing levels of difficulty if one chooses to use a PNF technique to increase range of motion and muscle strength. Figure 6-12 demonstrates an upper extremity diagonal pattern that has been modified from the traditional supine position. Although not in accordance with standard teachings of true PNF techniques, use of the PNF upper extremity diagonal "2" extension pattern in a seated position applies not only similar resistance as when it is performed supine but also requires the athlete to develop trunk control without the assistance of gravity or a table. This modification more closely resembles an individual who may be preparing to throw a baseball or football.

CLINICAL PEARL #1

Consider the activity and position when choosing PNF techniques for athletes in an attempt to closely simulate sport-specific function, proprioception, and strength gains; clear and concise verbal commands will assist with optimal performance of an athlete during PNF exercises.

JOINT MOBILIZATION
Techniques

Manual joint mobilization techniques are a form of passive range of motion used to improve joint arthrokinematics. The proper use of mobilization helps facilitate healing, reduce disability, relieve pain, and restore full range of motion.[69] The traditional approach to restoring loss of joint motion is to apply a passive sustained stretch without regard to a defined cause of motion limitation. This can result in increased stimulation of pain receptors and a reflexive contraction of muscles, which may interfere with

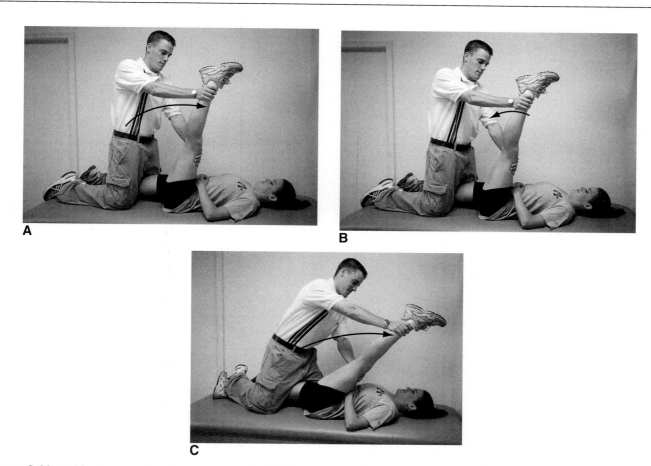

Figure 6-10. Hold-relax proprioceptive neuromuscular facilitation pattern for the hamstrings. *A,* The body part is moved passively by the clinician into the agonist pattern until limitation is felt. *B,* The athlete performs an isometric contraction into the antagonist pattern. *C,* The clinician applies a passive stretch into the agonist pattern until limitation is felt. The procedure is repeated.

attempts to increase motion.[84,85] The traditional approach is not necessarily effective if the joint restriction is related to capsuloligamentous adhesions. These adhesions need to be treated in a different manner that incorporates a stretching of the joint capsule structures, referred to as accessory motion. Table 6-2 compares physiologic

---

Box 6-4

Slow Reversal Hold-Relax Technique

Step	Procedure
1	The body part is moved actively into the agonist pattern to the point of pain-free limitation.
2	An isometric contraction is performed in the antagonist pattern for a 5- to 10-second hold.
3	The agonist muscle group actively brings the body part into a greater range of motion in the agonist pattern.
4	The process is repeated several times.

(stretching) and accessory (mobilization) movement techniques.[85]

Joint mobilization techniques emphasize accessory motion. Accessory motion occurs between the two articulating surfaces and is described by the terms *roll, glide,* and *spin.* A roll involves multiple surfaces of a moving bone coming in contact with multiple surfaces of a stationary bone. A glide involves the same surface of a moving bone coming in contact with multiple surfaces of a stationary bone. A spin involves multiple surfaces of the moving bone coming in contact with the same surface of a stationary bone. Both rolling and gliding motions occur simultaneously at some point in the range of motion[81] (Fig. 6-13).

Because accessory motion is necessary for physiologic motion to occur, an assessment to determine the cause of the restricted motion is necessary. When restriction of a joint is assessed on passive movement, determination should be made as to whether the restriction is in a capsular or noncapsular pattern. A capsular pattern is found only in synovial joints that are controlled by muscles.[4] Capsular patterns or restrictions indicate loss of mobility

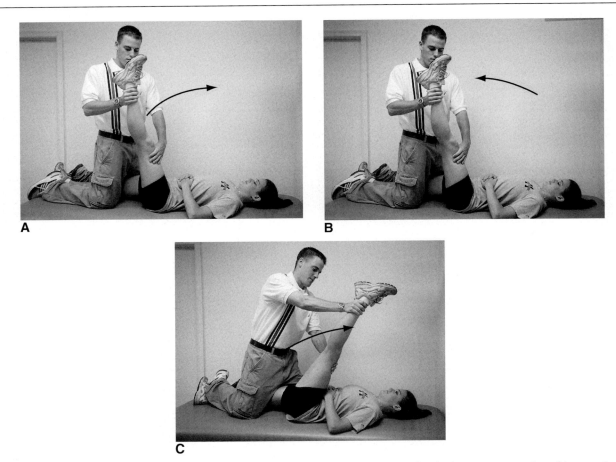

Figure 6-11. Slow reversal hold-relax proprioceptive neuromuscular facilitation pattern for the hamstrings. *A,* The athlete performs an active movement of the body part into the agonist pattern. *B,* The athlete performs an isometric contraction into the antagonist pattern. *C,* The athlete actively moves the body part further into the agonist pattern. The procedure is repeated.

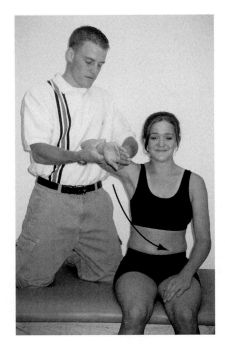

Figure 6-12. Demonstration of proprioceptive neuromuscular facilitation upper extremity diagonal "2" pattern for extension with the athlete seated.

of the entire joint capsule from fibrosis, effusion, or inflammation. Capsular and noncapsular patterns can be differentiated by noting the endfeel at the extremes of movement. The endfeels described in Table 6-3 may be normal or pathologic.[16] Joint restrictions from noncapsular patterns fall into three categories: ligament adhesions, internal derangement, and extra-articular limitations[16] (Table 6-4).

It is also important to recognize that an endfeel may be normal or abnormal depending upon where it occurs within one's range of motion. For example, as the elbow moves into full extension, the resultant end range of motion should be a bony endfeel. However, if the athlete has a loose body floating in the joint, the elbow may be limited from achieving full range of motion. Although Cyriax[16] described this as being a form of internal derangement, it will nonetheless feel like a bony endfeel to the examining clinician. Likewise, elbow flexion normally presents with the endfeel of a soft tissue approximation when no restrictions exist. However, if the elbow joint has a significant amount of swelling within it after an acute injury, the total amount of elbow flexion may be limited,

Table 6-2

Stretching Versus Mobilization

Stretching	Mobilization
Used when muscular resistance is encountered	Used when ligament or capsule resistance is encountered
Effective only at the end of the physiologic range of motion	Performed at any point in the range of motion
Limited to one direction	Can be done in any direction
Increased pain with increased range of motion	Decreased pain with increased range of motion
Used for tight muscular structures	Used for tight articular structures
Employs long lever arm techniques	Safer–employs short lever arm techniques

From Quillen, W.S., Halle, J.S., and Rouillier, L.H. (1992): Manual therapy: Mobilization of the motion-restricted shoulder. J. Sports Rehabil., 1:237-248.

yet a soft tissue approximation endfeel may continue to exist.

Physiologic Effects

Joint mobilization techniques serve to restore the accessory motions. Effects of joint mobilization include mitigating capsular restrictions and breaking adhesions, distracting impacted tissue, and providing movement and lubrication for normal articular cartilage. Pain reduction and decreased muscle tension are achieved through the stimulation of fast-conducting fibers (type A-β and A-α fibers) to block small pain fibers (type C afferent fibers) and through activation of dynamic mechanoreceptors to produce reflexive relaxation. Joint mobilization is indicated for the treatment of capsular restrictions. Contraindications and precautions are listed in Table 6-5.[4,19,110]

One of the important factors that one should consider before the application of a joint mobilization technique is the underlying history. Many capsular and ligamentous adhesions form as a result of a traumatic injury and subsequently as a result of disuse of the joint. A common example is seen in the shoulder, where a person may have a rotator cuff tear. If not treated immediately, the individual may simply opt not to use the affected arm because raising it and performing daily activities are quite painful. As healing tissue forms, the fibers are "laid down" in close approximation to each other and not with optimal elasticity (nonbiased tissue formation) because the joint is not being moved under controlled circumstances.[41] With adequate and controlled movement and stresses, the tissue would have a better chance of healing via joint nutrition and lubrication associated with movement and gentle stress applied to the healing tissue to allow for optimal growth

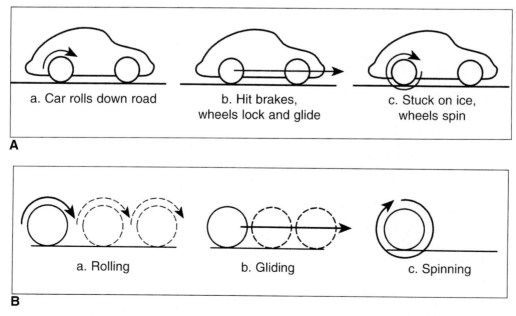

Figure 6-13. Types of accessory motion: *A*, rolling; *B*, gliding; *C*, spinning. (From Konin, J.G. [1999] *Practical Kinesiology for the Physical Therapist Assistant.* Thorofare, NJ: Slack, Inc., p. 37.)

Table 6-3

Normal and Pathologic Endfeels

Endfeel	Description and Example
Normal	
Capsular	Firm; forcing the shoulder into full external rotation
Bony	Abrupt; moving the elbow into full extension
Soft-tissue approximation	Soft; flexing the normal knee or elbow
Muscular	Rubbery; tension of tight hamstrings
Pathologic	
Adhesions and scarring	Sudden; sharp arrest in one direction
Muscle spasm	Rebound; usually accompanies pain felt at the end of restriction
Loose	Ligamentous laxity; a hypermobile joint
Boggy	Soft, mushy; joint effusion
Internal derangement	Springy; mechanical block such as a torn meniscus
Empty	No resistance to motion

Data from Cyriax, J.H. (1975): Textbook of Orthopaedic Medicine, 6th ed., Vol. 1. Diagnosis of Soft-Tissue Lesions. Baltimore, Williams & Wilkins.

and regeneration (biased tissue formation) (Fig. 6-14). With a case such as this, performance of joint mobilizations to dissemble resultant scar tissue would include added risk because the underlying pathologic condition may be affected with use of a technique that is too aggressive. This becomes a more critical factor if the underlying pathologic condition is joint instability.

Table 6-4

Joint Restrictions from Noncapsular Patterns

Type	Description
Ligament adhesions	These occur when adhesions form about a ligament after an injury and may cause pain or a restriction of mobility. Some movements will be painful, some are slightly limited, and some are pain free.
Internal derangement	Restriction in joint mobility is the result of a loose fragment within the joint. The onset is sudden, pain is localized, and movements that engage against the block are limited, whereas all others are free.
Extra-articular limitation	Loss in joint mobility results from adhesions in structures outside the joint. Movements that stress the adhesion will be limited and painful.

Table 6-5

Contraindications and Precautions for Joint Mobilization

Contraindications	Precautions
Premature stressing of surgical structures	Unexplained pain
Vascular disease	Onset of new symptoms
Hypermobility	Joint ankylosis
Advanced osteoarthritis	Protective muscle spasm
Acute inflammation	Scoliosis
Neurologic signs	Pregnancy
Infection	
Congenital bone deformities	
Fractures	
Osteoporosis	
Malignancy	
Rheumatoid arthritis	
Spondylolysis/spondylolisthesis	
Paget's disease	
Tuberculosis	
Vertebral artery insufficiency	
Spinal cord instability	

Data from Barak, T., Rosen, E.R., and Sofer, R. (1990): Basic concepts of orthopaedic manual therapy. In: Gould, J.A. (ed.): Orthopaedic and Sports Physical Therapy. St. Louis, C.V. Mosby, pp. 195-211; Prentice, W.E. (1992): Techniques of manual therapy for the knee. J. Sports Rehabil., 1:249-257; Wadsworth, C.T. (1988): Manual Examination and Treatment of The Spine and Extremities. Baltimore, Williams and Wilkins, p. 27; and Edmond, S.L. (1993): Manipulation and Mobilization. St. Louis, Mosby, pp. 8-9.

CLINICAL PEARL #2

Mobilization of any joint should be performed with extreme caution when the underlying pathologic condition is a known instability.

Fundamentals

Systems of Grading Mobilization

Systems of grading joint mobilization have been described by Maitland,[63] Kaltenborn,[46] and Paris.[77] Maitland[63] described five grades of mobilization techniques (Table 6-6). Grade I and grade II mobilizations are used primarily for treatment of pain, and grades III and IV are used for treating stiffness. It is necessary to treat pain first and stiffness second.[63]

Traction is used to separate the joint surfaces to varying degrees into an open-packed position, thus increasing the mobility of the joint.[81,82] Kaltenborn[46] proposed a system that uses traction combined with mobilization as a means of reducing pain or mobilizing hypomobile joints. All joints have some looseness that is described by

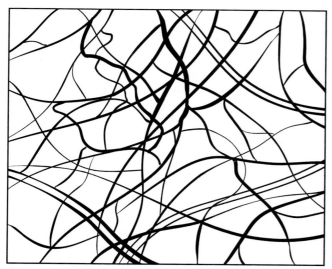

A Wound collagen, unstressed

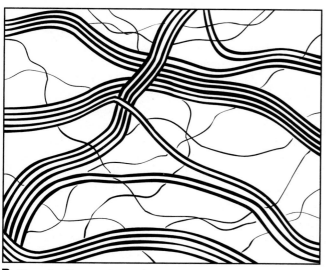

B Wound collagen, stressed

Figure 6-14. Unstressed *(A)* and stressed *(B)* wound collagen. In the wound subject to stress, collagen reorganizes with larger, more parallel aligned fibers. (From Hertling, D., and Kessler, R.M. [1996]: Management of Common Musculoskeletal Disorders: Physical Therapy Principles and Methods, 3rd ed. Philadelphia, J.B. Lippincott, p. 56.)

Kaltenborn as slack, and some degree of slack is necessary for normal joint motion. Kaltenborn's stages of traction are described in Table 6-7.[46] It has been recommended that 10-second intermittent stage I and stage II traction be used, distracting the joint surfaces up to stage III and then releasing distraction until the joint returns to its resting position.[82] Also, stage III traction should be used with mobilization glides to treat joint hypomobility.[46] Traction and translatoric gliding can be applied separately or together in various mobilization techniques (Fig. 6-15).[4]

Table 6-6
Grades of Mobilization Techniques

Grade	Description
I	This is a small-amplitude movement at the beginning of the range of motion, used when pain and spasm limit movement early in the range of motion.
II	This is a large-amplitude movement within the midrange of motion. It is used when slowly increasing pain restricts movement halfway into the range.
III	This is a large-amplitude movement up to the pathologic limit in the range of motion. It is used when pain and resistance from spasm, inert tissue tension, or tissue compression limit movement near the end of the range.
IV	This is a small-amplitude movement at the very end of the range of motion, used when resistance limits movement in the absence of pain and spasm.
V	This is a small-amplitude, quick thrust delivered at the end of the range of motion, usually accompanied by a popping sound called a manipulation.

Data from Maitland, G.D. (1977): Extremity Manipulation, 2nd ed. London, Butterworth Publishers.

Table 6-7
Kaltenborn's Stages of Traction

Stage	Description
I (piccolo)	This is traction that neutralizes pressure in the joint without actual separation of the joint surfaces. The purpose is to relieve pain by reducing griding when performing mobilization techniques. This stage is analogous to a grade I mobilization.
II (take up the slack)	This is traction that effectively separates the articulating surfaces and takes up the slack or eliminates play in the joint capsule. Stage II is used to relieve pain and is the same as a grade IV mobilization.
III (stretch)	This is traction that involves actual stretching of the soft tissue surrounding the joint for the purpose of increasing mobility in a hypomobile joint.

Data from Kaltenborn, F.M. (1980): Mobilization of the Extremity Joints: Examination and Basic Treatment Techniques. Oslo, Olaf Noris Bokhandel; and Prentice, W.E. (1992): Techniques of manual therapy for the knee. J. Sports Rehabil., 1:249-257.

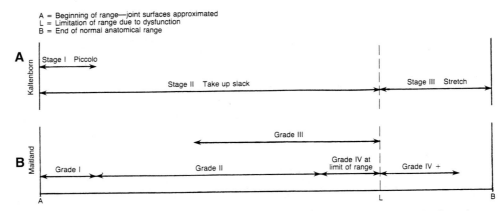

Figure 6-15. Comparison of mobilization technique applications. *A*, Kaltenborn's technique. *B*, Maitland's technique. (From Barak, T., Rosen, E.R., and Sofer, R. [1990]: Basic concepts of orthopaedic manual therapy. *In:* Gould, J.A. [ed.]: Orthopaedic and Sports Physical Therapy, 2nd ed. St. Louis, C.V. Mosby, pp. 195-211.)

CLINICAL PEARL #3

When using joint mobilization to increase tissue extensibility, often a clinician will begin with a grade appropriate for pain relief, then move to a grade to increase tissue length, and conclude with a grade of mobilization to once again provide some pain relief.

Joint Position and Force Application

Successful joint mobilization depends upon position of the joint to be mobilized, direction of the force, and magnitude of the force applied. Correct positioning of a joint is critical when one mobilizes a joint. A joint may be in either a close-packed or an open-packed position. A joint is in a close-packed position when the joint surfaces are most congruent. In a close-packed position the major ligaments are maximally taut, the intracapsular space is minimal, and the surfaces cannot be pulled apart by traction forces.[4] This position is used as a testing position but is never used for mobilization because there is no freedom of movement.[4] The maximal open-packed position is known as the resting position and is characterized by the surrounding tissues being as lax as possible and the intracapsular space being its greatest.[4] The maximal open-packed position of a joint is the optimal position for joint mobilization.[4,41,46,48,63,69] The open-packed positions of joints have been described by many[19,46,110] and are summarized in Table 6-8.

The direction of the mobilizing force depends on the contour of the joint surface of the structure to be mobilized. In most articulations, one joint surface is considered to be concave and the other convex. The concave-convex rule[63,77] takes these joint surface configurations into account and states that when the concave surface is stationary and the convex surface is mobilized, a glide of the convex segment should be in the direction opposite to the restriction of joint movement.[48,82] If the convex articular surface is stationary and the concave surface is mobi-

lized, gliding of the concave segment should be in the same direction as the restriction of joint movement (Fig. 6-16). Typical treatment of a joint may involve a series of three to six mobilizations lasting up to 30 seconds, with one to three oscillations per second.[81] General principles for applying mobilizations are summarized in Box 6-5. The grades of mobilization and stages of traction were described earlier in this chapter. Traction should be used in conjunction with mobilization techniques to treat hypomobile joints. Prentice[82] reported that grade III traction stretches the joint capsule and increases the space between the articulating surfaces, placing the joint in an open-packed position. Applying grade III and grade IV oscillations within the athlete's pain limitations should maximally improve joint mobility.[82] Some examples of commonly used joint mobilization techniques follow.

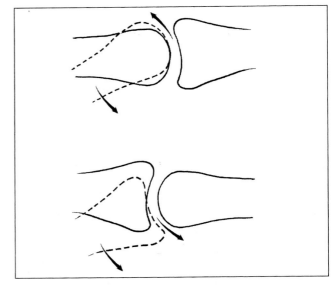

Figure 6-16. Convex-concave relationship of movement. (From Konin, J.G. [1999] Practical Kinesiology for the Physical Therapist Assistant. Thorofare, NJ, Slack, Inc., p. 37.)

Table 6-8

Open and Closed Pack Positions of Synovial Joints

Joint	Open Packed	Closed Pack
Facet	Midway between flexion and extension	Extension
TMJ	Mouth slightly open	Mouth closed with teeth clenched
Glenohumeral	55-70° abduction, 30° horizontal adduction	Maximum abduction and external rotation
Acromioclavicular	Arm resting at side	Arm abducted to 90°
Sternoclavicular	Arm resting at side	Arm maximally elevated
Humeroulnar	70° flexion, 10° supination	Full extension and supination
Humeroradial	Full extension and supination	90° elbow flexion and 5° supination
Proximal radioulnar	70° elbow flexion and 35° supination	5° supination and full extension
Distal radioulnar	10° supination	5° supination
Radiocarpal	Neutral, slight ulnar deviation	Full extension
Metacarpophalangeal	Slight flexion	Full flexion (2-5) Full extension (1)
Interphalangeal	PIP: 10° flexion DIP: 30°	Full extension
Hip	30° flexion, 30° abduction and slight external rotation	Full extension, internal rotation and abduction (ligamentous) 90° flexion, slight abduction and internal rotation (bony)
Tibiofemoral	25° flexion	Full extension
Talocrural	10° plantar flexion, midway between inversion and eversion	Maximum dorsi flexion
Subtalar	10° plantar flexion and midway between inversion and eversion	Maximum inversion
Midtarsal	10° plantar flexion and midway between pronation and supination	Maximum supination
Tarsometatarsal	Midway between pronation and supination	Maximum supination
Metatarsophalangeal	Midway between flexion and extension, abduction and adduction	Full extension
Interphalangeal	Slight flexion	Full extension

Modified from Edmond, S.L. (1993): Manipulation and Mobilization. St. Louis, Mosby.

Box 6-5

Joint Mobilization Application Principles

- Remove jewelry and rings.
- Be relaxed (both athlete and clinician).
- Always examine the contralateral side.
- Use an open-packed joint position.
- Avoid pain.
- Perform smooth, regular oscillations.
- Apply each technique for 20-60 sec.
- Repeat each technique only 4-5 times per treatment session; it is easy to overmobilize.
- Mobilize daily for pain and 2-3 times per week for restricted motion.
- Follow mobilization with active range-of-motion exercises.

APPLICATION TECHNIQUES

Upper Extremity

SHOULDER
Glenohumeral Joint Distraction

Use: This technique is effective for pain reduction.

Position: The athlete is supine, with the arm resting at the side.

Stabilization: The scapula may be stabilized with a small towel roll at the posterior aspect and with one of the clinician's hands held at the inferior aspect of the glenoid.

Procedure: The mobilizing hand or hands grasp the humerus just above the elbow. A distraction force is then applied along the long axis of the humerus. As the athlete relaxes, the arm can be gradually moved into various degrees of abduction (Fig. 6-17).

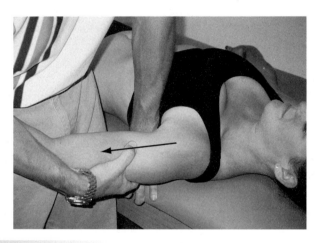

Figure 6-17. Glenohumeral joint distraction.

Glenohumeral Joint Inferior Glide

Use: This technique is effective for increasing shoulder abduction and flexion.

Position: The athlete is supine, with the shoulder in a loose-packed position.

Stabilization: The scapula may be stabilized with a small towel roll at the posterior aspect.

Procedure: The mobilizing hands grasp the proximal humerus. An inferiorly directed force is applied along the long axis of the humerus (Fig. 6-18).

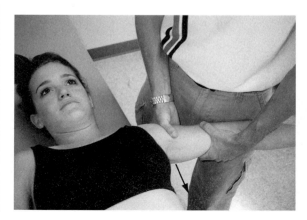

Figure 6-18. Glenohumeral joint inferior glide.

Range of Motion and Flexibility

Glenohumeral Joint Anterior Glide

Use: This technique is effective for increasing shoulder external rotation.

Position: The athlete is prone, with the shoulder in a loose-packed position.

Stabilization: The scapula is stabilized with the assistance of the table.

Procedure: The mobilizing hands grasp the proximal humerus. An anteriorly directed force is applied to the posterior aspect of the proximal humerus (Fig. 6-19).

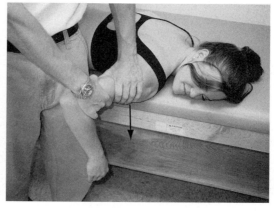

Figure 6-19. Glenohumeral joint anterior glide.

Glenohumeral Joint Posterior Glide

Use: This technique is effective for increasing shoulder internal rotation.

Position: The athlete is supine, with the shoulder in a loose-packed position.

Stabilization: The scapula may be stabilized with a small towel roll at the posterior aspect.

Procedure: The mobilizing hands grasp the proximal humerus. A posteriorly directed force is applied to the anterior proximal aspect of the humerus (Fig. 6-20).

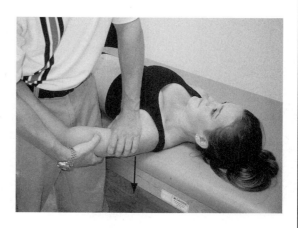

Figure 6-20. Glenohumeral joint posterior glide.

Scapulothoracic Joint Lateral Glide

Use: This technique is effective for increasing shoulder abduction and flexion.

Position: The athlete is side-lying, facing the clinician.

APPLICATION TECHNIQUES — cont'd

Stabilization: A side-lying position is maintained, without allowing the athlete to lean forward and protract the scapula.

Procedure: The medial border of the scapula is glided laterally away from the vertebral column (Fig. 6-21).

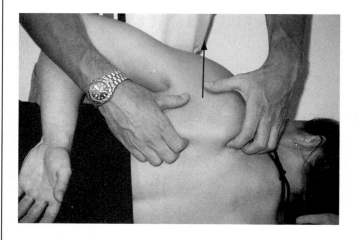

Figure 6-21. Scapulothoracic joint lateral glide.

ELBOW
Humeroulnar Joint Distraction

Use: This technique is effective for increasing elbow extension and reducing pain.

Position: The athlete is supine, with the arm by the side, elbow flexed, and forearm in neutral position.

Stabilization: The distal humerus is stabilized with one of the clinician's hands.

Procedure: The forearm is grasped by the clinician's hand and a distraction force is applied along the long axis of the forearm. A slight supination force can also be applied. The elbow may be gradually extended as movement increases (Fig. 6-22).

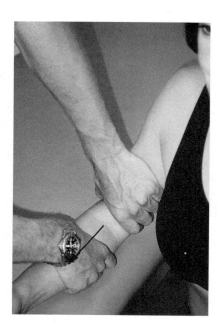

Figure 6-22. Humeroulnar joint distraction.

Proximal Radioulnar Joint Glides

Use:　　　　　This technique is effective for increasing supination and pronation.

Position:　　　The athlete is supine or sitting.

Stabilization:　The ulna is stabilized proximally by one of the clinician's hands.

Procedure:　　The radius is grasped proximally by the clinician's other hand. Posteriorly (to increase pronation) or anteriorly (to increase supination) directed force is applied perpendicular to the long axis of the forearm (Fig. 6-23).

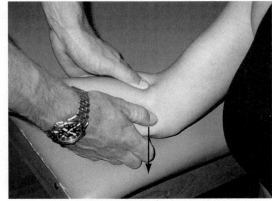

Figure 6-23. Proximal radioulnar joint glide.

WRIST
Radiocarpal Joint Distraction

Use:　　　　　This technique is effective for reducing pain.

Position:　　　The athlete is seated, with the hand hanging over the edge of the table. The forearm may be supported over a small towel roll.

Stabilization:　The forearm is stabilized at the distal radioulnar joint by one of the clinician's hands.

Procedure:　　The proximal row of carpal joints is grasped by one of the clinician's hand, and a distraction force is applied along the long axis of the forearm (Fig. 6-24).

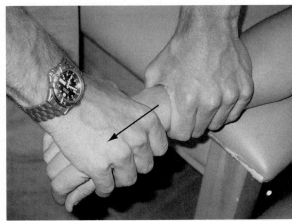

Figure 6-24. Radiocarpal joint distraction.

Continued

A P P L I C A T I O N   T E C H N I Q U E S — c o n t ' d

Dorsal and Volar Radiocarpal Joint Glides

Use: This technique is effective for increasing wrist flexion and extension.

Position: The athlete is seated, with the hand hanging over the edge of the table. The forearm may be supported over a small towel roll.

Stabilization: The forearm is stabilized at the distal radioulnar joint by one of the clinician's hands.

Procedure: The clinician grasps the proximal carpal joints and applies dorsal (to increase wrist flexion) and volar (to increase wrist extension) glides perpendicular to the long axis of the forearm (Fig. 6-25).

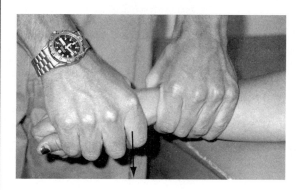

Figure 6-25. Radiocarpal joint glide.

FINGERS
Interphalangeal Joint Distraction with Volar and Dorsal Glides

Use: This technique is effective for reducing pain and increasing flexion and extension at the interphalangeal joint.

Position: The athlete is seated, with the forearm and hand in a resting position on the table.

Stabilization: The distal aspect of the proximal joint component is stabilized by the clinician's thumb and forefinger.

Procedure: The dorsal and volar sides of the proximal end of the distal joint component are grasped between the clinician's thumb and forefinger. A long axis distraction force is applied. Volar and dorsal glides can be used to increase flexion and extension, respectively (Fig. 6-26).

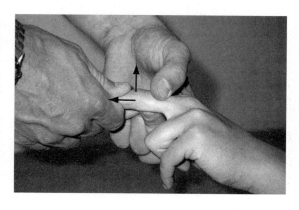

Figure 6-26. Interphalangeal joint distraction with glide.

Lower Extremity

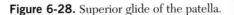

HIP
Hip Joint Posterior Glide

Use: This technique is effective for increasing hip flexion.

Position: The athlete is supine with the hip slightly flexed.

Stabilization: The pelvis is stabilized.

Procedure: The clinician grasps the proximal femur and distracts with a posteriorly directed glide perpendicular to the long arm axis of the femur (Fig. 6-27).

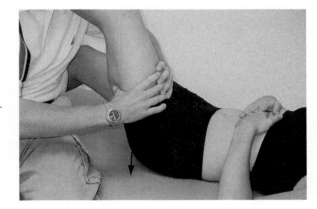

Figure 6-27. Hip joint posterior glide.

KNEE
Patellofemoral Joint Inferior and Superior Glides

Use: This technique is effective for increasing patellar mobility and facilitating knee extension or flexion.

Position: The athlete is supine with the knee slightly flexed.

Procedure: The patella is grasped between the clinician's thumbs and forefingers. A superior glide facilitates knee extension while an anterior glide facilitates knee flexion. Each should be performed for a sustained period of time to provide for adequate tissue stretch (Fig. 6-28).

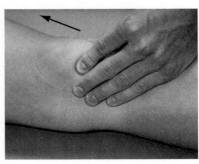

Figure 6-28. Superior glide of the patella.

Continued

APPLICATION TECHNIQUES — cont'd

Patellofemoral Joint Medial and Lateral Glides

Use: This technique is effective for increasing patellar mobility.

Position: The athlete is supine, with the knee slightly flexed.

Procedure: The clinician grasps the patella between the thumbs and forefingers of both hands. The patella is glided medially and laterally (Fig. 6-29).

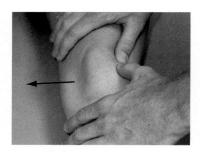

Figure 6-29. Medial glide of the patella.

Tibiofemoral Joint Anterior and Posterior Glides

Use: This technique is effective for increasing knee flexion and extension.

Position: The athlete is supine, with the knee flexed to approximately 90°.

Stabilization: The athlete's femur.

Procedure: The clinician grasps the proximal tibia with fingers interlaced in the popliteal space and applies an anteriorly directed force to facilitate extension. For increasing flexion, the clinician's thumbs are placed over the proximal tibia, and a posteriorly directed force is applied to the tibia (Fig. 6-30).

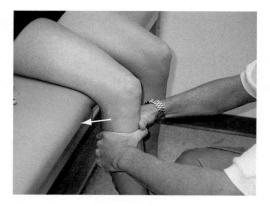

Figure 6-30. Tibiofemoral joint posterior glide.

ANKLE
Talocrural Joint Distraction

Use: This technique is effective for reducing pain.

Position: The athlete is supine, with the ankle resting in a neutral position.

Stabilization: The clinician stabilizes the distal tibia and fibula.

Procedure: The clinician grasps the rear foot and applies a distraction force parallel to the long axis of the leg (Fig. 6-31).

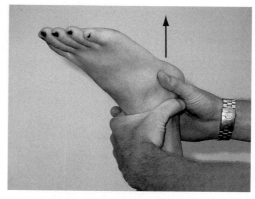

Figure 6-31. Talocrural joint distraction.

Talocrural Joint Posterior Glide

Use: This technique is effective for increasing ankle dorsiflexion.

Position: The athlete is supine, with the leg supported and the heel over the edge of the supporting surface. The ankle is in a loose-packed position.

Stabilization: The clinician stabilizes the leg by grasping the distal tibia and fibula with one hand.

Procedure: With the ankle in slight plantar flexion, the clinician's hand grasps the athlete's rear foot on the dorsal surface and applies a posteriorly directed glide to the talus (Fig. 6-32).

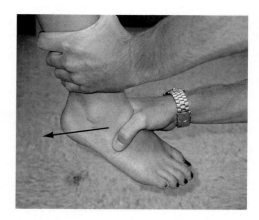

Figure 6-32. Talocrural joint posterior glide.

Talocrural Joint Anterior Glide

Use: This technique is effective for increasing plantar flexion.

Position: The athlete is prone, with the foot hanging over the edge of table. A towel may be placed under the lower leg and ankle for comfort, and the ankle is in a loose-packed position.

Continued

APPLICATION TECHNIQUES — cont'd

Stabilization: The clinician stabilizes the lower leg by grasping around the distal tibia and fibula.

Procedure: With the athlete's ankle in slight plantar flexion, the web space of the clinician's other hand is placed on the posterior aspect of the talus and calcaneus. The calcaneus is distracted, and an anteriorly directed force is applied to the calcaneus and talus (Fig. 6-33).

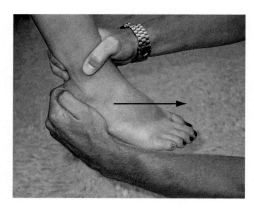

Figure 6-33. Talocrural joint anterior glide.

Metatarsophalangeal Joint Distraction and Glide

Use: This technique is effective for decreasing pain and increasing great toe flexion and extension.

Position: The athlete is supine or side-lying.

Stabilization: With one hand, the clinician stabilizes the head of the metatarsal with the thumb and index finger. With the other hand the clinician grasps the proximal phalanx of the same ray in the same manner with thumb and index finger.

Procedure: The clinician applies long axis traction to the proximal phalanx, and performs a dorsal glide (to increase toe extension) or a volar glide (to increase to flexion) perpendicular to the direction of the distraction (Fig. 6-34).

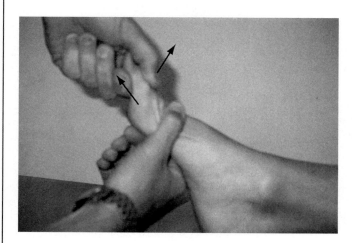

Figure 6-34. Metatarsophalangeal joint distraction and glide.

Myofascial Release Techniques

Myofascial release techniques have been anecdotally reported as being effective for relieving restrictions and increasing range of motion. These claims have not been well investigated in controlled settings. Hanten and Chandler[34] compared the effectiveness of the PNF contract-relax technique and the myofascial release leg pull technique in increasing hip flexion range of motion. Their results demonstrated significant gains in range of motion after use of both techniques, with significantly greater improvements with the contract-relax stretch compared with the leg pull.

The focus of myofacial release techniques is on the fascial system, which comprises embryologic tissue.[17] Fascial tissue is a tough connective tissue that assists the tissue it surrounds in maintaining its shape.[91] Barnes and Smith[5] believed that gentle forces applied to fascial tissue will elicit thermal changes from a vasomotor response, leading to increased blood flow. As a result, they believed that lymphatic drainage improves and optimal structural alignment was allowed to occur.

Kostopoulos and Rizopoulos[50] described the use of myofascial tissue stretching after a trigger point acupressure intervention. Others have reported successful results on restricted soft tissue injuries treated with myofascial release techniques.[1,33-35,43] Myofascial release, like all other treatment interventions, requires that the clinician have a certain level of skill and experience. Effective treatments for improved overall tissue enhancement also depend upon the subject's ability to relax and "work" with the clinician (Fig. 6-35).

CLINICAL PEARL #4

Myofascial release is a skill that requires knowledge of the body's inherent trigger points, awareness of normal versus abnormal tissue tension, and clinical practice to develop a level of expertise for successful treatment intervention.

SUMMARY

■ Range of motion and flexibility changes can be improved with repetition, frequency and consistency being key to making plastic deformation changes.

■ Plastic deformation is achieved with low-force, long duration stretching.

■ While there is no clear conclusive evidence regarding durations of stretches, one should always keep in mind the practicality of performing too many stretches for too long of a time frame, which could deter an athlete from proper technique and compliance.

■ It appears that the application of superficial heat or cold modality in conjunction with stretching results in greater improvements in flexibility than stretching alone.

■ To effectively measure progress, it is important to document on a regular basis flexibility and range of motion changes.

■ While debates regarding various stretching techniques continue to exist, ballistic stretching more closely simulates many athletic activities, and if done appropriately may not pose any greater risk of injury to an athlete than static stretching.

■ Static stretching, ballistic stretching and PNF all can improve flexibility, each with its advantages and disadvantages.

■ There is scientific evidence to suggest that PNF results in greater increases in flexibility when compared to static or dynamic stretching techniques.

■ Joint mobilization techniques are used to restore the accessory motions of spin, glide and roll and performed with the joint in the open-packed position.

■ Proprioceptive neuromuscular facilitation, joint mobilization and myofascial release are techniques that can be initiated to compliment methods of improving one's flexibility and range of motion. Each requires a sound base of anatomical knowledge combined with clinical experience before proper technique and optimal gains may be seen.

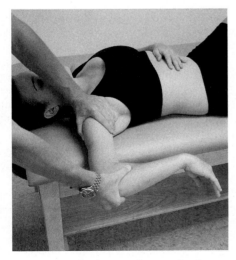

Figure 6-35. Myofascial release technique for the supraspinatus.

REFERENCES

1. Alvarez, D.J., and Rockwell, P.G. (2002): Trigger points: Diagnosis and management. Am. Fam. Phys., 15:653-660.

2. Balasch, H., Schiller, M., Friebel, H., and Hoffman, F. (1999): Evaluation of anterior knee joint instability with the Rolimeter: A test in comparison with manual assessment knee joint instability with the KT-1000 arthrometer. Knee Surg. Traumatol. Arthrosc., 7:204-208.

3. Bandy, W.D., and Irion, J.M. (1994): The effect of time on static stretch on the flexibility of the hamstring muscles. Phys. Ther., 74:845-852.

4. Barak, T., Rosen, E.R., and Sofer, R. (1990): Basic concepts of orthopaedic manual therapy. *In:* Gould, J.A. (ed.), Orthopaedic and Sports Physical Therapy. St. Louis, C.V. Mosby, pp. 195-211.

5. Barnes, J.F., and Smith, G. (1987): The body is a self-correcting mechanism. Phys. Ther. Forum, July, p. 27.

6. Beaulieu, L.A. (1981): Developing a stretching program. Phys. Sports Med., 9:59-65.

7. Beaupre, L.A., Davies, D.M., Jones, C.A., and Cintas, J.G. (2001): Exercise combined with continuous passive motion or slider board therapy compared with exercise only: A randomized controlled trial of patients following total knee arthroplasty. Phys. Ther., 81:1029-1037.

8. Bonutti, P.M., Windau, J.E., Ables, B.A., and Miller, B.G. (1994): Static progressive stretch to reestablish elbow range of motion. Clin. Orthop., 303:128-134.

9. Brodowicz, G.R., Welsh, R., and Wallis, J. (1996): Comparison of stretching with ice, stretching with heat, or stretching alone on hamstring flexibility. J. Athl. Train., 31:324-327.

10. Brosseau, L., Balmer, S., Tousignant, M., et al. (2001): Intra- and intertester reliability and criterion validity of the parallelogram and universal goniometers for measuring maximum active knee flexion and extension of patients with knee restrictions. Arch. Phys. Med. Rehabil., 82:396-402.

11. Condom, S.M., and Hutton, R.S. (1987): Soleus muscle electromyographic activity and ankle dorsiflexion range of motion during four stretching procedures. Phys. Ther., 67:24-30.

12. Cooperman, J.M., Riddle, D.L., and Rothstein, J.M. (1990): Reliability and validity of judgments of the integrity of the anterior cruciate ligament of the knee using the Lachman's test. Phys. Ther., 70:225-233.

13. Cornelius, W.L., and Craft-Hamm, K. (1988): Proprioceptive neuromuscular facilitation flexibility techniques: Acute effects on arterial blood pressure. Physician Sportsmed., 16:152-161.

14. Cornelius, W.L., Ebrahim, K., Watson, J., and Hill, D.W. (1992): The effects of cold application and modified PNF stretching techniques on hip joint flexibility in college males. Res. Q. Exerc. Sport, 63:311-314.

15. Cornelius, W.L., Jensen, R.L., and Odell, M.E. (1995): Effects of PNF stretching phases on acute arterial blood pressure. Can. J. Appl. Physiol., 20:222-229.

16. Cyriax, J.H. (1975): Textbook of Orthopaedic Medicine, Vol. I, Diagnosis of Soft Tissue Lesions, 6th ed. Baltimore, Williams & Wilkins.

17. Davis, C.M. (1997): Complimentary Therapies in Rehabilitation. Thorofare, NJ, Slack, pp. 21-47.

18. Draper, D.O., and Ricard, M.D. (1995): Rate of temperature decay in human muscle following 3 MHz ultrasound: The stretching window revealed. J. Athl. Train., 30:304-307.

19. Edmond, S.L. (1993): Manipulation and Mobilization. St. Louis, Mosby, pp. 8-9.

20. Ellis, B., Burton, A., and Goddard, J.R. (1997): Joint angle measurement: A comparative study of the reliability of goniometry and wire tracking for the hand. Clin. Rehab., 11:314-320.

21. Elveru, R.A., Rothstein, J.M., Lamb, R.L., and Riddle, D.L. (1988): Methods for taking subtalar joint measurements. A clinical report. Phys. Ther., 68:678-682.

22. Etnyre, B.R., and Abraham, L.D. (1986): Gains in range of ankle dorsiflexion using three popular stretching techniques. Am. J. Phys. Med., 65:189-196.

23. Ferrari, J., Higgins, J.P., and Williams, R.L. (2000): Intervention for treating hallux valgus (abductovalgus) and bunions. Cochrane Database Syst. Rev., 2:CD000964.

24. Gajdosik, R.L., and Bohannon, R.W. (1987): Clinical measurements of range of motion. Review of goniometry emphasizing reliability and validity. Phys. Ther., 67:1862-1872.

25. Galilee-Belfer, A. (1999): The Effect of Modified PNF Trunk Strengthening on Functional Performance in Female Rowers. Eugene, OR, University of Oregon, Microform Publications.

26. Ganko, A., Engebretson, L., and Ozer, H. (2000): The rolimeter: An new arthrometer compared with the KT-1000. Knee Surg. Sports Traumatol. Arthrosc., 8:36-39.

27. Gasper, L., Farkas, C., Szepesi, K., and Csernatomy, Z. (1997): Therapeutic value of continuous passive motion after cruciate ligament replacement. Acta Chir. Hung., 36:104-105.

28. Gillette, T.M., Holland, G.J., Vincent, W.J., and Loy, S.F. (1991): Relationship of body core temperature and warm-up to knee range of motion. J. Orthop. Sports Phys. Ther., 12:126-131.

29. Godges, J.J., MacRae, H., Longdon, C., et al. (1989): The effects of two stretching procedures on hip range of motion and gait economy. J. Orthop. Sports Phys. Ther., 11:350-357.

30. Godges, J.J., MacRae, P.G., and Engelke, K.A. (1993): Effects of exercise on hip range of motion, trunk muscle performance, and gait economy. Phys. Ther., 73:468-477.

31. Goodwin, J., Clark, C., Deakes, J., et al. (1992): Clinical methods of goniometry: A comparative study. Disabil. Rehabil., 14:10-15.

32. Groth, G.N., VanDeven, K.M., Phillips, E.C., and Ehretsman, R.L. (2001): Goniometry of the proximal and distal interphalangeal joint. Part II: Placement preferences, interrater reliability and concurrent validity. J. Hand Ther., 14:23-29.

33. Han, S.C., and Harrison, P. (1997): Myofascial pain syndrome and trigger-point management. Reg. Anesth., 22:89-101.

34. Hanten, W.P., and Chandler, S.D. (1994): Effects of myofascial release leg pull and sagittal plane isometric contract-relax techniques on passive straight leg raise angle. J. Orthop. Sports Phys. Ther., 20:138-144.

35. Hanten, W.P., Olson, S.L., Butts, N.L., and Nowicki, A.L. (2000): Effectiveness of a home program of ischemic pressure followed by sustained stretch for treatment of myofascial trigger points. Phys. Ther., 80:997-1003.

36. Havanloo, F., and Parkhotik, I. (2000): Rehabilitation process of patients with brachial plexus injury. Exerc. Soc. J. Sport Sci., 25:286.

37. Hayes, K.W., Peterson, C., and Falconer, J. (1994): An examination of Cyriax's passive motion tests with patients having osteoarthritis of the knee. Phys. Ther., 74:697-709.

38. Hayes, K., Walton, J.R., Szomor, Z.R., and Murrell, G.A. (2001): Reliability of five methods of assessing shoulder range of motion. Aust. J. Physiother. 47:289-294.

39. Hepburn, G.R. (1987): Case studies: Contracture and stiff joint management with Dynasplint. J. Orthop. Sports Phys. Ther., 8:498-504.

40. Hepburn, G.R., and Crivelli, K.J. (1984): Use of elbow Dynasplint for reduction of elbow flexion contractures: A case study. J. Orthop. Sports Phys. Ther., 5:269-274.

41. Hertling, D., and Kessler, R.M. (1996): Management of Common Musculoskeletal Disorders: Physical Therapy Principles and Methods, 3rd ed. Philadelphia, J.B. Lippincott, p. 19.

42. Houglum, P.A. (2001): Therapeutic Exercise for Athletic Injuries. Champaign, IL, Human Kinetics, p. 170.

43. Hui, S.S., and Yuen, P.Y. (2000): Validity of the modified back-saver sit-and-reach test: A comparison with other products. Med. Sci. Sports Exerc., 32:1655-1659.

44. Ingber, R. (1999): Myofascial Pain in Lumbar Dysfunction. Philadelphia, P.A. Hanley and Belfus.

45. Jones, C.J., Rikli, R.E., Max, J., and Noffal, G. (1988): The reliability and validity of a chair sit-and-reach test as a measure of hamstring flexibility in older adults. Res. Q. Exerc. Sport, 69:338-343.

46. Kaltenborn, F.M. (1980): Mobilization of the Extremity Joints, Examination and Basic Treatment Techniques. Oslo, Olaf Noris Bokhandel.

47. Kirkendall, D.T., and Garrett, W.E. (1997): Function and biomechanics of tendons. Scand. J. Med. Sci. Sports, 7:62-66.

48. Kisner, C., and Colby, L. (2002): Therapeutic Exercise: Foundations and Techniques, 4th ed. Philadelphia, F.A. Davis.

49. Knott, M., and Voss, D.E. (1968): Proprioceptive Neuromuscular Facilitation, 2nd ed. New York, Harper & Row.

50. Kostopoulos, D., and Rizopoulos, K. (2001): The Manual of Trigger Point and Myofascial Therapy. Thorofare, NJ, Slack, pp. 51-57.

51. Kottke, F.J., Pauley, D.L., and Ptak, K.A. (1966): The rationale for prolonged stretching for correction of shortening of connective tissue. Arch. Phys. Med. Rehabil., 47:345-352.

52. Kovaleski, J.E., Gurchiek, L.R., Heitman, R.J., et al. (1999): Instrumented measurement of anteroposterior and inversion-eversion laxity of the normal ankle joint complex. Foot Ankle Int., 20:808-814.

53. Laban, N.M. (1962): Collagen tissue: Implications of its response to stress in vitro. Arch. Phys. Med. Rehabil., 43:461-466.

54. Lastayo, P.C., Wright, T., Jaffe, R., and Hartzel, J. (1998): Continuous passive motion after repair of the rotator cuff: A prospective outcome study. J. Bone Joint Surg., 80:1002-1011.

55. Lau, S.K., and Chiu, K.Y. (2001): Use of continuous passive motion after total knee arthroplasty. J. Arthroplasty, 16:336-339.

56. Lehmann, J.F., and DeLateur, B.J. (1982): Therapeutic heat. In: Lehmann, J.F. (ed.), Therapeutic Heat and Cold. Baltimore, Williams & Wilkins, pp. 404-405, 428.

57. Lehmann, J.F., DeLateur, B.J., and Silverman, D.R. (1966): Selective heating effects of ultrasound in human beings. Arch. Phys. Med. Rehabil., 47:331-339.

58. Lehmann, J.F., Masock, A.J., Warren, C.G., and Koblanski, J.N. (1970): Effect of therapeutic temperatures on tendon extensibility. Arch. Phys. Med. Rehabil., 51:481-487.

59. Lentell, G., Hetherington, T., Eagan, J., and Morgan, M. (1992): The use of thermal agents to influence the effectiveness of a low-load prolonged stretch. J. Orthop. Sports Phys. Ther., 16:200-207.

60. Light, K.E., Nuzik, S., Personius, W., and Barstrom, A. (1984): Low load prolonged stretch versus high load restretch treating knee contractures. Phys. Ther., 64:330-333.

61. Lucas, R.C., and Koslow, R. (1984): Comparative study of static, dynamic, and proprioceptive neuromuscular facilitation stretching techniques on flexibility. Percept. Motor Skills, 58:615-618.

62. MacDermid, J.C., Chesworth, B.M., Patterson, S., and Roth, J.H. (1999): Intratester and intertester reliability of goniometric measurement of passive lateral shoulder rotation. J. Hand Ther., 12:187-192.

63. Maitland, G.D. (1977): Extremity Manipulation, 2nd ed. London: Butterworth Publishers.

64. McAttee, R.E. (1993): A variation of PNF stretching that's safer and more effective. Track Field Q. Rev., 93:53-54.

65. McCarthy, M.R., Yates, C.K., Anderson, M.A., and Yates-McCarthy, J.L. (1993): The effects of immediate continuous passive motion on pain during the inflammatory phase of soft tissue following anterior cruciate ligament reconstruction. J. Orthop. Sports Phys. Ther., 17:96-101.

66. McClure, P.W., Rothstein, J.M., and Riddle, D.L. (1989): Intertester reliability of clinical judgments of medial knee ligament integrity. Phys. Ther., 69:268-275.

67. McCullen, J., and Uhl, T.L. (2000): A kinetic chain approach for shoulder rehabilitation. J. Ath. Train., 35:329-337.

68. Medeiros, J.M., Smidt, G.L., Burmeister, L.F., and Soderbert, G.L. (1977): The influence of isometric exercise and passive stretch on hip joint motion. Phys. Ther., 57:518-523.

69. Mennell, J. (1964): Joint Pain. Boston, Little, Brown & Company.

70. Moore, M.A., and Hutton, R.S. (1980): Electromyographic investigation of muscle stretching technique. Med. Sci. Sports Exerc., 12:322-329.

71. Muellner, T., Bugge, W., Johansen, S., et al. (2001): Inter- and intratester comparison of the Rolimeter knee tester: Effect of tester's experience and the examination technique. Knee Surg. Sports Traumatol. Arthrosc., 9:302-306.

72. Ninos, J. (2001): PNF-self stretching techniques. J. Strength Cond., 23:28-29.

73. Noonan, T.J., Best, T.M., Seaber, A.V., and Garrett, W.E. (1994): Identification of a threshold for skeletal muscle injury. Am. J. Sports Med., 22:257-261.

74. O'Driscoll, S.W., and Giori, N.J. (2000): Continuous passive motion (CPM): Theory and principles of clinical application. J. Rehabil. Res. Dev., 37:179-188.

75. Osternig, L.R., Robertson, R., Troxel, R., and Hansen, P. (1987): Muscle activation during proprioceptive neuromuscular facilitation (PNF) stretching techniques. Am. J. Phys. Med., 66:298-307.

76. Osternig, L.R., Robertson, R.N., Troxel, R.K., and Hansen, P. (1990): Differential responses to proprioceptive neuromuscular (PNF) facilitation stretch techniques. Med. Sci. Sports Exerc., 22:106-111.

77. Paris, S.V. (1979): Extremity Dysfunction and Mobilization. Atlanta, Institute Press.

78. Patterson, P., Wiksten, D.L., Ray, L., et al. (1996): The validity and reliability of the back saver sit-and-reach test in middle school girls and boys. Res. Q. Exerc. Sport, 67:448-451.

79. Pizzari, T., Kolt, G.S., and Remedios, L. (1999): Measurement of anterior-to-posterior translation of the glenohumeral joint using the KT-1000. J. Orthop. Sports Phys. Ther., 29:602-608.

80. Prentice, W.E. (1983): A comparison of static stretching and PNF stretching for improving hip joint flexibility. Athl. Train., 18:56-59.

81. Prentice, W.E. (1992): Techniques of manual therapy for the knee. J. Sport Rehabil., 1:249-257.

82. Prentice, W.E. (1999): Mobilization and traction techniques in rehabilitation. In: Prentice, W.E. (ed.), Rehabilitation Techniques in Sports Medicine. McGraw-Hill: New York, pp. 188-197.

83. Prentice, W.E. (1999): Restoring range of motion and improving flexibility. In: Prentice, W.E. (ed.), Rehabilitation Techniques in Sports Medicine. McGraw-Hill: New York, pp. 62-72.

84. Quillen, W.S., and Gieck, J.H. (1988): Manual therapy: Mobilization of the motion-restricted knee. Athl. Train., 23:123-130.

85. Quillen, W.S., Halle, J.S., and Rouillier, L.H. (1992): Manual therapy: Mobilization of the motion-restricted shoulder. J. Sport Rehabil., 1:237-248.

86. Riddle, D.L., Rothstein, J.M., and Lamb, R.L. (1987): Goniometric reliability in a clinical setting: Shoulder measurement. Phys. Ther., 667:668-673.

87. Rose, S., Draper, D.O., Schulthies, S.S., and Durrant, E. (1996): The stretching window part two: Rate of thermal decay in deep muscle following 1-MHz ultrasound. J. Athl. Train., 31:139-143.

88. Sady, S.P., Wortman, M., and Blanke, D. (1982): Flexibility training: Ballistic, static, or proprioceptive neuromuscular facilitation? Arch. Phys. Med. Rehabil., 63:261-263.

89. Safran, M.R., Garrett, W.E., Seaber, A.V., et al. (1988): The role of warmup in muscular injury prevention. Am. J. Sports Med., 16:123-129.

90. Sapega, A.A., Quendenfeld, T.C., Moyer, R.A., and Butler, R.A. (1981): Biophysical factors in range of motion exercise. Phys. Sportsmed., 9:57-65.

91. Scott, J. (1986): Molecules that keep you in shape. New Scientist, 111:49-53.

92. Shellock, F.G., and Prentice, W.E. (1989): Warming-up and stretching for improved physical performance and prevention of sports-related injuries. Sports Med., 2:267-278.

93. Shrier, M.D., and Gossal, K. (2000): Myths and truths of stretching. Phys. Sports Med., 28:1-11.

94. Simons, D.G., Travell, J.G., and Simons, L.S. (1990): Protecting the ozone layer. Arch. Phys. Med. Rehabil., 71:64.

95. Spernoga, S.G., Uhl, T.L., Arnold, B.L., and Gansneder, B.M. (2001): Duration of maintained hamstring flexibility after a one-time, modified hold-relax stretching protocol. J. Ath. Train., 36:44-48.

96. Stamford, B. (1984): Flexibility and stretching. Phys. Sports Med., 12:171.

97. Stanley, S.N., Knappstein, A., and McNair, P.J. (1999): How long do the immediate increases in flexibility last after a PNF stretching session? Presented at the Fifth IOC World Congress on Sport Sciences, Canberra, Australia.

98. Stap, L.J., and Woodfin, P.M. (1986): Continuous passive motion in the treatment of knee flexion contracture. Phys. Ther., 66:1720-1722.

99. Stark, S.D. (1997): Stretching techniques. In: Stark, S.D. (ed.), The Stark Reality of Stretching. Richmond, BC, Stark Reality Publishing, pp. 73-80.

100. Stromberg, D., and Wiederhielm, C.A. (1969): Viscoelastic description of a collagenous tissue in simple elongation. J. Appl. Physiol., 26:857-862.

101. Sullivan, M., Dejulia, J.J., and Worrell, T.W. (1992): Effects of pelvic position and stretching method on hamstring muscle flexibility. Med. Sci. Sports Exerc., 24:1383-1389.

102. Sullivan, P.E., and Markos, P.D. (1987): Clinical Procedures in Therapeutic Exercise. Norwalk, CT, Appleton & Lange.

103. Surburg, P.R., and Schrader, J.W. (1997): Proprioceptive neuromuscular facilitation techniques in sports medicine: A reassessment. J. Athl. Train., 32:34-39.

104. Tanijawa, M.D. (1972): Comparison of the hold relax procedure in passive immobilization on increasing muscle length. Phys. Ther., 52:725-735.

105. Taylor, D.C., Dalton, J.D., Seaber, A.V., and Farrett, W.E. (1990): Viscoelastic properties of muscle-tendon units. The biomechanical effects of stretching. Am. J. Sports Med., 18:300-309.

106. Travell, J.G., and Simons, D.G. (1983): Myofascial Pain and Dysfunction: The Trigger Point Manual. Baltimore, Williams & Wilkins.

107. Travell, J.G., and Simons, D.G. (1992): Myofascial Pain and Dysfunction: The Trigger Point Manual. The Lower Extremity. Baltimore, MD: Williams & Wilkins.

108. Vallentyne, S.W., and Vallentyne, J.R. (1988): The case of the missing ozone: Are physiatrists to blame? Arch. Phys. Med. Rehabil., 69:992-993.

109. Voss, D.E., Ionta, M.K., and Myers, B.J. (1985): Proprioceptive Neuromuscular Facilitation: Patterns and Techniques, 3rd ed. Philadelphia, Harper & Row.

110. Wadsworth, C.T. (1988): Manual Examination and Treatment of the Spine and Extremities. Baltimore, MD, Williams & Wilkins, p. 27.

111. Wallin, D., Ekblon, B., Grahn, R., and Nordenborg, T. (1985): Improvement of muscle flexibility. Am. J. Sports Med., 13:263-268.

112. Warren, C.G., Lehmann, J.F., and Koblanski, J.N. (1971): Elongation of rat tail tendon: Effect of load and temperature. Arch. Phys. Med. Rehabil., 52:465-474.

113. Warren, C.G., Lehmann, J.F., and Koblanski, J.N. (1976): Heat and stress procedures: An evaluation using rat tail tendon. Arch. Phys. Med. Rehabil., 57:122-126.

114. Watkins, M.A., Riddle, D.L., Lamb, R.L., and Personius, W.J. (1991): Reliability of goniometric measurements and visual estimates of knee range of motion obtained in a clinical setting. Phys. Ther., 71:90-96.

115. Wiktorsson, M.M., Oberg, B., Ekstrand, J., and Gillquist, J. (1988): Effects of warming up, massage, and stretching and range of motion for muscle strength in the lower extremity. Am. J. Sports Med., 11:249-252.

116. Worrell, T.W., Smith, T.L., and Winegardner, J. (1994): Effect of hamstring stretching on hamstring muscle performance. J. Orthop. Sports Phys. Ther., 20:154-159.

CHAPTER 7

PRINCIPLES OF REHABILITATION

R. Barry Dale, Ph.D., P.T., ATC, C.S.C.S.
Gary L. Harrelson, Ed.D., ATC
Deidre Leaver-Dunn, Ph.D., ATC

CHAPTER OBJECTIVES

At the end of this chapter the reader will be able to:

- Differentiate between rehabilitation and physical conditioning.
- List the general goals of rehabilitation.
- Define and explain the general phases of rehabilitation and the objectives for each phase.
- Explain the influence and the importance of the neurologic system in rehabilitation.
- List and describe types of therapeutic exercise.
- List and summarize the methods of progressing resistance exercise.
- Discuss the differences between and implications for using open versus closed chain exercises.
- Discuss strategies of physical conditioning during rehabilitation.
- Explain the parameters of conditioning and rehabilitation.
- Explain the importance for function-based rehabilitation.

In this chapter we will provide an overview of the rehabilitation process and review key concepts that need attention during the development of athletic rehabilitation programs. We begin with a broad definition of rehabilitation and discuss various stages of rehabilitation. We will also review some key concepts pertaining to the neuromuscular system and motor learning. We address different types of exercises utilized in the rehabilitation process and considerations for their incorporation into rehabilitation programs. Finally, we discuss physical conditioning during rehabilitation and the various parameters pertinent to program progression. Many of the concepts are discussed briefly, and the reader will be referred to other specified sources, such as other chapters in this book.

Rehabilitation, from the Medieval Latin root word *rehabilitare*, literally means "to restore to a rank."[8]

From the aforementioned definition, rehabilitation is a broad conceptual term used to describe restoration of physical function. Physical rehabilitation reverses various physical conditions associated with injury or dysfunction.

Rehabilitation is similar to other types of physical conditioning. Essentially, various systems respond to physical stresses by undergoing adaptations that ultimately improve the functioning of the specific system (see section on conditioning later in this chapter). Rehabilitation is the process of applying stress to healing tissue in accordance with the specific stresses that it will face upon return to a specific activity. Thus, rehabilitation involves *re*conditioning injured tissue. Once the healing tissue is mature, the emphasis moves to more aggressive conditioning for the athlete to re-enter the sport.

There are many health care professionals who can potentially have an impact on physical rehabilitation (Box 7-1). It is important that all professionals play an active role in the rehabilitation process and strive to work together, because no one professional can best serve all the needs of an athlete undergoing physical rehabilitation.

Before a rehabilitation program is implemented, the rehabilitation specialist should perform and be familiar with the findings of a thorough physical examination.[158] The physical examination should rule out other pathologic conditions and reveal problems inherent with the athlete's current physical condition. Clinical decisions regarding the course of rehabilitation depend upon adequate information derived from a comprehensive clinical examination.[54] The physical examination should address joint range of motion, muscle flexibility, muscle strength, proprioception, posture, and ambulation and gait patterning, in addition to other specific criteria.[158] Thus, depending upon the findings of the evaluation, the rehabilitation program may address multiple problem areas.[98] Box 7-2 lists the key components of a physical examination.

Box 7-1

Professions Potentially Influencing Athletic Rehabilitation

- Physician
- Athletic trainer
- Physical therapist
- Nutritionist
- Registered Nurse
- Strength and conditioning specialist
- Coach
- Clergy
- Psychologist

CLINICAL PEARL #1

Effective rehabilitation occurs when health professionals use coordinated efforts based upon written and verbal communication and documentation. As appropriate, research the medical records to get the most accurate picture of an athlete's present condition. Next, make sure that you document the athlete's condition on your examination and frequently record changes in status. This helps other health care providers who may need information at a point later in the rehabilitation process.

Rehabilitation programs, whether conservative or occurring after invasive procedures, are specifically tailored to an injury or surgical intervention. No matter how specific the rehabilitation is to a particular condition, general physiologic events that occur in response to trauma must be considered (see Chapter 2). Keep in mind that the

Box 7-2

Foundation of Any Rehabilitation Program: Key Components of Physical Examination

1. History (subjective)
2. Examination of specific systems (objective)
   a. Neurologic: sensation via dermatome assessment, gross strength via myotome assessment, and reflexes
   b. Musculoskeletal: range of motion/flexibility, strength, coordination, agility, special tests, and functional performance tests
   c. Cardiopulmonary: respiratory rate, heart rate, and blood pressure
   d. Integumentary: skin condition, color, and temperature
3. Assessment
   a. Problem list, short-term goals (1 to 2 weeks), long-term goals (functional goals), rehabilitation potential
   b. Summarizes evaluation
4. Plan
   a. Specify interventions and the frequency and duration of treatment.

effectiveness of rehabilitation in the recovery period usually determines the degree and success of future athletic competition.[69] Thus, it is the clinician's role to optimize the healing environment of the injured tissue and return the athlete to competition as soon as possible without compromising the healing process. There are at least two foundational goals applicable to any rehabilitation program: (1) reverse or deter the adverse sequelae resulting from immobility or disuse and (2) facilitate tissue healing and avoid excessive stress on immature tissue. The generic goals of any rehabilitation program are listed in Box 7-3.

Incomplete rehabilitation and premature sport re-entry predispose the athlete to reinjury. Figure 7-1 illustrates the body's response to injury and the result of inadequate rehabilitation.[151]

CLINICAL PEARL #2

The cardinal rule of rehabilitation is to avoid worsening the athlete's present condition. The athlete's pain and tissue responses dictate progression through the various stages of rehabilitation.

GENERAL REHABILITATION CONSIDERATIONS

Specific problems associated with injury include swelling, pain, and muscle spasm. On a positive note, pain and swelling serve to alert the rehabilitation specialist and athlete that tissue damage is present, which facilitates clinical decision-making and the proper determination of exercise progression. However, the presence of these tissue injury by-products may also inhibit early institution of a therapeutic exercise program and cause untoward manifestations such as muscle inhibition.[34,45,70,141,151]

Peripheral Receptor Afferent Activity

Pain is something directly unseen by clinicians; we must rely upon the patient's subjective complaint and interpret it according to the nature and time frame of the injury.[40] Pain may be acute, chronic, or persistent.[19,40] Acute pain occurs soon after injury and is typically of short duration (matter of days). Acute pain is often a protective response

Box 7-3

Generic Goals of Rehabilitation

- Decrease pain
- Decrease inflammatory response to trauma
- Return of full active and pain-free range of motion
- Decrease effusion
- Return of full muscular strength, power, and endurance
- Return to full asymptomatic functional activities at the preinjury level

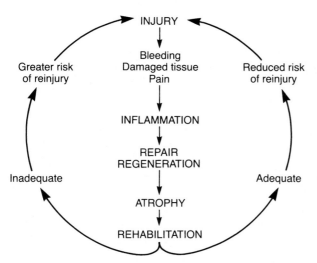

Figure 7-1. The body's response to injury and the role of rehabilitation. (From Welch, B. [1986]: The injury cycle. Sports Med. Update, 1:1.)

that alerts us that something is wrong. Chronic pain is present for at least 6 months, frequently recurs, and resists alleviation with intervention.[19] It may continue long after the original injury has healed, as a result of factors such as altered biomechanics or learned habits of guarding. In the person with chronic pain, the pain may become a dysfunction in itself.[96] Persistent pain, unlike chronic pain, generally occurs with a condition that responds to treatment over a period of time, which is variable according to condition and the individual's interpretation of pain (pain threshold).[40]

Control of existing edema (present in soft tissue outside of a joint) and prevention of further effusion (excess fluid inside a joint) are critical in the rehabilitation process for several reasons. Edema increases localized pressure that compresses sensory nerve endings, contributing to the sensation of pain. Joint effusion increases intra-articular pressure and afferent activity, which contributes to muscle inhibition.[167] In fact, even small increases of fluid in a joint (as little as 10 mL) can produce a 50% to 60% decrease in maximal voluntary contractions of the quadriceps.[34,45,70,141] (See section on arthrogenic inhibition later in this chapter.)

Rehabilitation adjuncts such as electrophysical modalities are instrumental in controlling and reducing these responses, allowing the athlete to begin early range-of-motion and strengthening exercises.[85,152,155,156,159,160] The modality itself, however, is almost never considered the only course of treatment for most athletic injuries. Only through therapeutic exercise can the injured body part or parts be returned to the preinjury level. If therapeutic exercise is not included within a rehabilitation program with therapeutic modalities, the injury cycle may continue. Why does this occur? Therapeutic modalities assist the body's response to inflammation but do little to *stress* healing

tissue. Therapeutic exercise provides specific stresses that benefit healing tissue.[5,154-156]

Additionally, exercise early in the rehabilitation process is essential to diminishing the adverse effects of disuse or immobility. Athletes can improve their physical condition by training, yet those training responses readily reverse when activity ceases or diminishes with ill effects becoming evident in as little as a few days. Unfortunately, the rate of reversal is much faster than the rate of improvement. For example, nontrained individuals can improve their cardiovascular condition by 1% per day of training yet the rate of reversal can be as high as 3% to 7% if they suddenly become totally inactive (Box 7-4).[20] Therefore, the longer an athlete is inactive, the longer it takes to return to pre-injury fitness levels.[1,11,12,20,28,66,112]

CLINICAL PEARL #3

Remove or diminish the presence of pain, edema, and joint effusion as soon as possible. These sources of afferent activity result in reflex inhibition of associated musculature, which delays the rehabilitation process.

REHABILITATION CONCEPTS
Healing Constraints

The most important factors to consider in designing a rehabilitation program are the physiologic constraints to healing. Generally, across different tissue types, tissue strength decreases after injury but as time elapses and healing occurs, tissue strength increases (Table 7-1).[67,68] The athlete's age, health, and nutritional status and the magnitude of injury are also factors influencing the rate of physiologic healing and the rehabilitation program must be structured around these constraints (see Chapter 2).

Connective tissue, present in some form or another in almost all tissue, accommodates force, or stress, in a manner described by Hooke's law and the stress-strain curve (see Box 7-5 for definitions of force terms).[68,87,163] The specific connective tissue composition and fiber arrangement determine the tissue's relative reaction to stress. For example, ligaments stretch relatively further than tendons from the same magnitude of tensile force.[163] Ligaments stretch further because of their more irregular or multidirectional arrangement of collagen fibers compared with those of tendons, which are more specialized to resist tensile force.[163]

The aforementioned stress-strain curve graphically depicts how stress affects connective tissue.[68,87,163] It is described as a sinusoidal curve with specific areas of toe, the elastic region, the plastic region, and the point of failure (Fig. 7-2).[68] The toe area is the elongation of the connective tissue up to its point of stretch, (e.g., taking up the

Box 7-4

Adverse Effects of Immobility (Unilateral Limb Suspension or Absolute Bed Rest)

1. Muscle
    a. Cross-sectional area
        i. Atrophy rates of 0.5% to 1% per day of inactivity for quadriceps
    b. Strength
        i. Decreases 0.5% to 2% per day of inactivity for plantar flexors and quadriceps
2. General deconditioning (reduced strength production and endurance capacity)
3. Structural changes of articular capsule connective tissue, causing decreased range of motion
4. Articular cartilage degeneration
5. Cardiovascular deconditioning
6. Reduced stimulus for bone mineral deposition, possibly contributing to diminished bone density

Data from Adams, G.R., Hather, B.M., and Dudley, G.A. (1994): Effect of short-term unweighting on human skeletal muscle strength and size. Aviat. Space Environ. Med., 65:116-1121; Bamman, M.M., Clarke, M.S.F., Feeback, D.L., et al. (1998): Impact of resistance exercise during bed rest on skeletal muscle sarcopenia and myosin isoform distribution. J. Appl. Physiol., 84:157-163; Bamman, M.M., Hunter, G.R., Stevens, B.R., et al. (1997): Resistance exercise prevents plantar flexor deconditioning during bed rest. Med. Sci. Sports Exerc., 29: 1462-1468; Bortz, W. (1984): The disuse syndrome. West. J. Med., 141:169; Cooper, D.L., and Fair, J. (1976): Reconditioning following athletic injuries. Phys. Sports Med., 4:125-128; Houglum, P. (1977): The modality of therapeutic exercise: Objectives and principles. Athl. Train., 12:42-45; and Noyes, F.R. (1977): Functional properties of knee ligaments and alterations induced by immobilization. Clin. Orthop., 123:210-242.

slack in the tissue).[68] The elastic point begins once the tissue stretches beyond approximately 2% of its resting length. Within the elastic region, tissue returns to its prestretch length. Permanent elongation occurs to a degree once the tissue surpasses its resting length by approximately 4%, known as the plastic region. The permanent elongation results from actual disruption of a few but not all collagen fibers present within the connective tissue. Finally, the failure point of the connective tissue results from stretch beyond 6% to 10% of the tissue's resting length.[68] Thus, excessive stress applied to tissue may result in failure of that tissue. Rehabilitation must accommodate the fragility of healing tissue because its ability to withstand tensile stresses is compromised early in rehabilitation.[67]

Table 7-1

Healing Rates for Various Tissue Types

Tissue	Time to Return to Approximately Normal Strength
Bone	12 weeks
Ligament	40-50 weeks
Muscle	6 weeks up to 6 months
Tendon	40-50 weeks

Data from Houglum, P. (1992): Soft tissue healing and its impact on rehabilitation. J. Sports Rehabil., 1:19-39; and Houglum, P. (2001): Muscle strength and endurance. In: Houglum, P. (ed.), Therapeutic Exercise for Athletic Injuries. Champaign, IL, Human Kinetics, pp. 203-265.

Stages of Rehabilitation

"Time waits for no one," and "timing is everything" are clichés that describe how dependent we are upon time. Just as in everything else, timing is crucial during recovery from injury and rehabilitation. We have already mentioned that proper intervention from the rehabilitation expert may include the use of therapeutic modalities or therapeutic

Box 7-5

Definitions of Key Terms Specific to Physical Stress

Force: something that causes or tends to cause a change in the motion or shape of tissue
Stress: generally synonymous with force; types include compression, tension, torsion, and shear
Compression: pushing or squeezing tissue together
Tension: pulling tissue apart
Torsion: twisting tissue
Shear: tearing across
Strain: deformation of tissue
Elasticity: ability for tissue to accommodate strain and return to original length
Plasticity: permanent change in tissue structure resulting from strain beyond elastic region
Failure: tissue disruption resulting from strain beyond plastic region

Data from Kreighbaum, E., and Barthels, K.M. (1996): Biomechanics: A Qualitative Approach for Studying Human Movement, 4th ed. Boston, Allyn & Bacon.

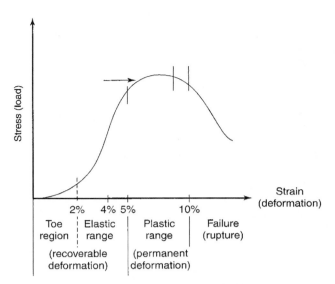

Figure 7-2. The stress-strain curve. (Modified from Houglum, P. [2001]: Muscle strength and endurance. *In:* Houglum, P. (ed.), Therapeutic Exercise for Athletic Injuries. Champaign, IL, Human Kinetics, pp. 203-265.)

exercises. However, certain intensities of therapeutic exercise and certain forms of therapeutic modalities may damage immature tissue in the early phases of rehabilitation. Damage to immature tissue incites further inflammation and prolongs the recovery process.

Rehabilitation phases are time frames that consider general healing constraints and assist the rehabilitation specialist in planning rehabilitative interventions.[82] However, it is important to recognize that there is no absolute transition from one rehabilitation phase to the next. In fact, there may be overlap between phases.[82] Furthermore, there is interindividual variability within these time constraints. Therefore, these stages or phases should not dictate rehabilitation progression but should serve as a guide for the clinician because the experience of the rehabilitation specialist is important for maneuvering through the sometimes-murky waters of rehabilitation and recovery.[68,69]

Overall, phases are progressive in nature; that is, they should build upon one another like building blocks. Once the athlete accomplishes tasks that are relatively basic, such as range of motion, he or she may progress to strengthening within the newly acquired range of motion. As healing occurs and newly formed connective tissue matures, tolerance improves for increased exercise intensity.

Phases of rehabilitation include the acute, subacute (intermediate), and chronic or return-to-sport phases.[82] Other authors describe a fourth phase, the advanced strengthening phase, which follows the subacute (intermediate) phase and precedes the return-to-sport phase.[158]

Acute Phase

The acute phase occurs from the moment that tissue sustains injury until the time that inflammation becomes controlled. Generally, the acute phase of soft tissue healing lasts 4 to 6 days postinjury.[82] The goals of the acute phase of rehabilitation are to diminish pain, control inflammation, and begin the restoration of joint range of motion, muscle flexibility and strength, and proprioception in a pain-free fashion.[158]

Rest, ice, compression, and elevation are necessary to combat pain and swelling in the acute injury state. Rest is the primary weapon used to manage inflammation during the first 24 hours after injury.[82] Therapeutic modalities, especially cryotherapy and electrophysical agents, play a crucial role in controlling the inflammation process and the athlete's pain early in rehabilitation. Cryotherapy helps prevent secondary hypoxic injury and helps control hemorrhage and edema. Application of external pressure to the injury site helps to control the amount of soft tissue edema. Compression wraps should be applied in a distal to proximal direction, with a decreasing pressure gradient. Stockinettes are excellent for compression and can be applied and removed easily by the athlete. Elevation assists the lymphatic system in moving any extracellular tissue fluid away from the injury site. Passive- and active-assistive movements, when indicated, are beneficial to assist proper healing of soft tissue.[82,113] Motion stresses immature collagen, which assists its fiber alignment along lines of stress while preventing excessive adhesion development. Table 7-2 summarizes treatment considerations during the acute stage of soft tissue healing.

Advancement from the acute stage into the intermediate phase begins when the effects of cryotherapy have plateaued, which is manifested with the stabilization of edema, the relative restoration of pain free range of motion, and the removal of hyperemia.[55] Another way to view the criteria for progression into the subacute or intermediate phase is the relative reduction of inflammation, which is evidenced by the diminution of its five classic indicators: redness (rubor), heat (calor), pain (dolor), swelling (tumor), and loss of function (functio laesa). Once pain and inflammation are under control, emphasis shifts to restoring function, because diminished pain does not imply that the restoration of function has occurred.[27]

Subacute (Intermediate) Phase

As mentioned earlier, the subacute phase of soft tissue resolution begins as the effects of inflammation decrease.[55] In this phase the healing connective tissue is still immature and relatively fragile; therefore, therapeutic exercises used during this phase should be gentle and cause no pain. This phase is transitional for active movement. Also, tissue may revert back into the acute stage if it is overstressed and inflammation recurs.[169] However, an appropriate amount of stress is necessary in this phase to avoid understressing

Table 7-2

Rehabilitation during the Acute Phase of Soft Tissue Healing

Goals	Treatment
1. Control inflammation	Rest and protect injured area, cryotherapy, compression, and elevation, gentle (grade I) pain-free mobilization of affected joint
2. Minimize deleterious effects of immobilization	Passive motion within limits of pain, isometric muscle setting, electrical stimulation, axial loading for early proprioception
3. Reduce joint effusion	Pain-free, active range of motion as tolerated; medical intervention (joint aspiration) if necessary
4. Maintain condition of noninjured areas	Activity as tolerated of nonaffected extremities

Data from Kisner, C., and Colby, L.A. (2002): Therapeutic Exercise: Foundations and Techniques, 4th ed. Philadelphia, F.A. Davis.

tissue. Inadequate stress of soft tissue diminishes its mobility, which not only delays the restoration of range of motion but also potentially results in more severe consequences, such as formation of adhesions.[31]

Joint range of motion should dramatically improve in the subacute stage, allowing the rehabilitation specialist to progress the rehabilitation program with flexibility training and strengthening exercises.[82] Joint range of motion forms the basis for physical performance and its improvement is paramount for successful rehabilitation.[82] To improve joint range of motion, specific joint motion must occur progressively and be in the form of accessory or physiologic movements (see section on therapeutic exercise later in this chapter and Chapter 6). Strengthening should also occur progressively in a rehabilitation program during the subacute stage. A few methods that serve to progress strength training include the low-resistance, high-repetition method, the DeLorme and Watkins regimen, the Oxford technique, and daily adjustable progressive resistive exercise philosophies (see section on progressive resistive exercise later in this chapter).[37,38,84] As range of motion and

strength improve, coordination and agility activities begin to increase as rehabilitation progresses.

Coordination and agility are important for normal functioning, whether it is functional activities or performance-specific actions of a particular sport. Normal movement requires complex neuromuscular coordination between similar and or opposing muscle groups. Movement patterns are smoother and more fluid-like when there is coordination between muscle groups. The subacute (intermediate) stage plays a role in reestablishing neuromuscular control via progression of proprioceptive exercises (see Chapter 8).

The ultimate goal of the subacute stage is to prepare the athlete for more complex activities that occur in the return-to-sport phase. Table 7-3 summarizes treatment considerations during the subacute stage of soft tissue healing.

The Chronic or Return-to-Sport Phase

The culmination of the earlier phases should provide the athlete with full range of motion and strength of the

Table 7-3

Rehabilitation during the Subacute Phase of Soft Tissue Healing, from Days 4-21 of Recovery from Injury

Goals	Treatment
1. Continue to control inflammation	Protect area with prophylactic devices if necessary; gradually increase amount of joint movement; continuously monitor tissue response to exercise progression and adjust intensity/duration accordingly.
2. Progressively increase mobility	Progress from passive to more active ROM; gradually increase intensity of tissue stretch for tight structures.
3. Progressively strengthen muscles	Progress from isometric to active ROM without resistance, gradually increase amount of resistance; progress to isotonic exercise as joint integrity/kinematics allow.
4. Continue to maintain condition of non-injured areas	Progressively strengthen and or recondition noninjured areas with increased intensity/duration of activity as healing tissue allows.

Data from Kisner, C., and Colby, L.A. (2002): Therapeutic Exercise: Foundations and Techniques, 4th ed. Philadelphia, F.A. Davis.
ROM, range of motion.

affected extremity. Connective tissue by this time has improved tensile strength, primarily because the orientations of its fibers are better suited to withstand tensile stress.[75] The intensity of the strengthening exercises increases in this phase. Agility, coordination, and plyometric activities are now being performed at a more intense level to prepare the athlete for demands of specific activities within his or her particular sport. Table 7-4 summarizes treatment considerations during the chronic or return-to-sport stage of soft-tissue healing.

Neurologic Considerations

The neurologic system transmits information, recognizes and interprets the information, and then formulates a response, if necessary.[59] Afferent impulses travel from the body to the central nervous system (brain and spinal cord), delivering information about the body or environment whereas efferent impulses carry impulses to effector organs or muscles to carry out a specific response.[59] We will review key concepts of neurologic physiology, particularly afferent activity, because of its crucial role in rehabilitation. We begin with a review of peripheral receptors and finish the discussion with a review of concepts of motor learning and voluntary neuromuscular activation.

Peripheral Receptors

Sherrington[126] identified and categorized afferent receptors into three groups according to location: articular, deep (muscle-tendon related), and superficial (cutaneous). We turn our attention to the joint receptors, which have profound effects associated with neuromuscular function.

Peripheral Receptors: Joints

In 1863, Hilton described the innervation of joints by articular branches of nerves supplying the muscles of each articulation (Hilton's law).[64] Sherrington[126] was the first to note the presence of receptors in the pericapsular structures. He coined the term *proprioception* to include all neural input originating from the joints, muscles, tendons, and associated deep tissues.[126]

Articular receptors are located within the joint capsule, ligaments, and any other joint structures within the body.[72,76,111,122] The human joint capsule has been studied extensively and contains four very distinct types of nerve endings: Ruffini's corpuscles, Golgi receptors (also present within the Golgi tendon organ), Pacinian corpuscles, and free nerve endings[51,60,123] (Table 7-5).

Arthrogenic Inhibition

Afferent activity from arthrogenous receptors contributes to the manifestation of arthrogenic inhibition of an affected muscle group. Afferent activity may occur as a result of increased articular pressure or from the transmission of pain signals.[34,45,70,141] Joint trauma often causes fluid to collect inside the joint (effusion), which increases intra-articular pressure. Increased intra-articular pressure subsequently causes the joint capsule to stretch, which activates afferent joint receptors. Joint pain may occur with or without joint effusion and typically is associated with an increased firing rate of free nerve endings. Joint receptor afferents integrate with an inhibitory interneuron at the spinal cord. The interneuron releases an inhibitory neurotransmitter in response to increased activity from the

---

Table 7-4

Rehabilitation during the Chronic Phase of Soft Tissue Healing, from 21 Days up to 12 Months Following Injury

Goals	Treatment
1. Decrease pain from adhesions	Appropriate modalities where indicated; mechanical stretching of affected structures
2. Increase extensibility of other structures	Passive stretches, joint mobilizations, cross–soft tissue friction massage, flexibility exercises
3. Progress strengthening of affected and supporting musculature	Isotonic and isokinetics where indicated and supporting musculature
4. Progress proprioception, coordination and agility	Balance activities; surface modification

Data from Kisner, C., and Colby, L.A. (2002): Therapeutic Exercise: Foundations and Techniques, 4th ed. Philadelphia, F.A. Davis.

Table 7-5

Nerve Endings Found in the Human Joint Capsule

Nerve Ending	Characteristics
Ruffini's corpuscles	Sensitive to stretching of the joint capsule.
Golgi receptors	Intraligamentous and become active when the ligaments are stressed at the extremes of joint movement.
Pacinian corpuscles	Sensitive to high-frequency vibration.
Free nerve endings	Sensitive to mechanical stress.

Data from Gardner, E. (1948): The innervation of the knee joint. Anat. Rec., 101:109-130; Halata, F., Rettig, T., and Schulze, W. (1985): The ultrastructure of sensory nerve endings in the human knee joint capsule. Anat. Embryol., 172:265-275; and Schutte, M.J., Dabezies, E.J., and Zimny, M.L. (1987): Neural anatomy of the human anterior cruciate ligament. J. Bone Joint Surg. [Am.], 69:243-247.

joint afferents. Ultimately, this diminishes the activity of motor neurons supplying muscles that act upon the affected joint (Fig. 7-3). Diminished motor unit activity results in atrophy and weakness, most commonly seen in the quadriceps and shoulder after surgery or gross articular trauma.[34,45,70,141] The body intends to protect the associated joint by "shutting down" the associated musculature, but the resulting atrophy and weakness prolong recovery time unless the rehabilitation specialist takes proper steps to minimize and reverse the adverse effects of arthrogenic inhibition.

Neuromuscular Considerations

The motor cortex does not think in terms of specific motor unit activation, rather our bodies attempt to achieve a specified movement by activating certain muscles and or muscle groups.[14,15] Movements often require complicated neuromuscular coordination, which we learn over time through experience or practice.[94] However, injury often causes temporary loss of the ability to activate specific muscles or muscle groups.[14,15,34,45,70,141] Measures that directly improve volitional motor control and motor unit activation while concomitantly decreasing arthrogenic inhibition by controlling joint effusion and pain are essential to rehabilitation. Physical training in conjunction with motor learning principles assists the process of muscle reactivation and motor skill reacquisition.[39,52,53,86]

More complicated movement patterns associated with functional and sport-specific activities are not possible until muscle inhibition is reduced or removed.[14,15,34,45,70,141] Furthermore, complex sport-specific activities in the advanced stages of rehabilitation ensure that the athlete

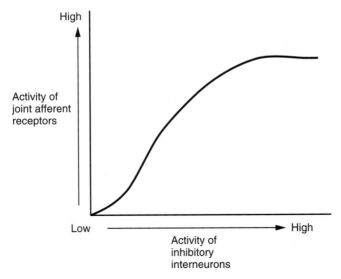

Figure 7-3. Increased activity of joint afferent nerve fibers due to pain or joint effusion concomitantly increases the activity of inhibitory interneurons. Increased activity of inhibitory interneurons contributes to muscle inhibition.

reacquires motor skills inherent to his or her particular sport.

Many rehabilitation professionals often unknowingly use motor learning concepts in one capacity or another during athletic rehabilitation. Whether the athlete is acutely recovering from surgical reconstruction or is in the final return-to-sport phase, it is imperative that the rehabilitation specialist uses instructions, verbal or visual feedback, and practice conditions that match the learning needs of the athlete.[94] It is beyond the scope of this brief synopsis on motor learning to cover all theories and issues related to this important topic and the reader is referred to other sources for more information.[43,44,65,88,94,120,136] Rather, we present key concepts pertinent to teaching athletes movement patterns related to therapeutic exercise, which should ultimately prepare them to return to their sport. Nonetheless, before discussing some of those concepts, we briefly review two major theories concerning motor learning: the three-stage model and the two-stage model.

The Three-Stage Model

In 1967, Paul Fitts and Michael Posner presented a classic motor learning theory, known as the three-stage model.[47] The three-stage model consists of the cognitive, associative, and autonomous stages[39,47,94] (Table 7-6).

The cognitive stage requires a great deal of attention from the athlete because he or she must focus on cognitively oriented problems.[47,109,120] In this stage, athletes generally must put forth conscious effort to either learn new movements or reacquire movements previously mastered. During rehabilitation, the athlete's neurologic system must "relearn" how to accomplish a given task as the appropriate movement patterns are selected and proper muscle groups are recruited to perform the task. Oftentimes the athlete may be fearful of using the involved extremity and the apprehension to do so invokes cognitive activity on the task at hand. The athlete commits numerous errors while performing the task but begins to get a "feel" for the activity with repetition and feedback.[47,136] Thus, the rehabilitation specialist plays an important role in this stage by providing appropriate extrinsic feedback.[82,94] As the practice level of the athlete increases within this phase, he or she begins to obtain a sense of correct and incorrect or safe and unsafe movements within the exercise or activity.[136]

Cognitive activity changes somewhat in the associative stage as the athlete begins to associate certain environmental cues with the performance of the movements.[47,94] The athlete performs the task with fewer errors and refines the movement; in fact, Fitts and Posner refer to the associative stage as the *refining stage*.[47] The timing and distance of the movement are examples of how the athlete refines the activity or exercise, which begins to decrease performance variability. Coordination of muscle activity

Table 7-6				
Comparison of the Three- and Two-Stage Motor Learning Models				

Three-Stage Model		Two-Stage Model	
Stage	**Characteristics**	**Stage**	**Characteristics**
Cognitive	Athlete puts forth conscious effort to either learn new movements or reacquire movements previously mastered.	"Getting the idea"	The correct movement pattern is selected according to various regulatory conditions such as distance, size, and shape of the object.
Associative	Athlete begins to associate certain environmental cues with the performance of movements.	Fixation and diversification	Fixation implies that the athlete performs the movement in a nonchanging environment.
Autonomous stage	Activity becomes automatic, requiring very little cognitive processing for proper performance.		Diversification refers to a changing environment, requiring the athlete to make modifications to the skill for proper performance.

improves, which produces more efficient movements. Feedback is still important in the associative stage, but the athlete depends less upon it for proper performance. The athlete begins to detect errors independently and make corrections to the performance.[47,136] Additionally, as the practice level increases within this stage, the athlete may explore modifications of the movement, such as environmental variation.[47,120]

Finally, the athlete reaches the autonomous stage whereby the activity becomes automatic, requiring very little cognitive processing for proper performance.[47] This allows the athlete to incorporate the activity into more complex exercises or to concentrate on other simultaneous tasks.[39,47,94] Performance variability decreases tremendously, and the athlete consistently performs the task well in this stage. However, many healthy noninjured athletes may never even reach this level of learning; therefore, it is rarely accomplished during rehabilitation because of the amount of practice time required to achieve it.[94] Nonetheless, the minimal goal of rehabilitation is to return the athlete to preinjury levels of motor functioning.

An important concept to consider is that athletes move in a continuum across the three stages.[94] Consistent practice over time with the activity moves the athlete from the cognitive stage into the associative stage and finally into the autonomous stage. It may be difficult for the rehabilitation professional to determine exactly what stage an athlete is in at any given moment, especially because there is overlap to a degree across the continuum.[94]

The Two-Stage Model

Another motor learning theoretical model, the two-stage model, was described by Gentile in 1972 and 1987 (Table 7-6).[52,53] The two-stage model occurs with the learner moving from "getting the idea" in the first stage into fixation and diversification in the second stage.[52,53,94] For the athlete to "get the idea" in the first stage, the correct movement pattern must be selected according to various regulatory conditions (environmental mandates). Regulatory conditions *regulate* performance based upon certain variables: distance, speed, and the weight, size, and shape of the object.[52,53] The term *nonregulatory conditions* pertains to environmental qualities that do not affect the movement strategy, such as whether the person uses a broomstick or a T-bar for active-assisted shoulder range-of-motion exercises. As practice continues in the first stage, skill improvement occurs, which gradually moves the athlete into the second stage.[52,53]

Fixation and diversification occur in the second stage. Briefly, fixation implies that the athlete refines the movement in a closed (nonchanging) environment while diversification occurs in an open or changing environment, which requires the athlete to make modifications to the skill for proper performance.[52,53,94]

Applying Principles of Motor Learning to Rehabilitation

Before injury, athletes attain advanced motor learning skills necessary to accomplish complex motor tasks. However, with injury, the athlete is unable (due to reflex inhibition) or unwilling (because of pain or guarding) to use an affected extremity, and motor skills become repressed. Motor learning principles assist the rehabilitation professional to properly reintroduce the movement patterns to the athlete. The two primary motor learning principles to consider during rehabilitation are the amount and type of practice and the amount and type of feedback available to the athlete.[94,109]

Practice

Practicing the activity or movement is perhaps the most important factor for the learning process.[88,94,120] The athlete should deliberately and purposefully practice to achieve optimal motor learning results.[44] Additionally, the type of practice is also important to consider. Systematic manipulation of practice may assist the motor learning process, especially practice condition variability in the later stages of rehabilitation.[105,164] The types of practice include mental and physical; whole versus part; and random, blocked, and random-blocked[82,107,120,164] (Table 7-7).

Physical practice implies that the athlete physically performs an exercise or activity during the rehabilitation process, whereas mental practice indicates that athlete uses mental images to rehearse the movement.[94,97,101,120,166] *Mental imagery* and *visualization* are two common terms used to describe the cognitive processes that occur during mental practice.[50] Often, the rehabilitation specialist focuses more on the physical performance of an exercise and overlooks the potential benefits of using mental practice to achieve motor learning outcomes. Research in this area documents the effect of mental practice upon physical performance.[43,50,97,101,166] An example of an athlete using mental practice is as follows: during rehabilitation an athlete recovering from a shoulder injury performs a unilateral active range-of-motion exercise with the unaffected extremity and before performing the exercise with the affected shoulder, the athlete uses mental practice to rehearse the movement. The mental practice before actual performance with the affected upper extremity prepares the athlete by allowing him or her to gauge the requirements necessary for the movement. The specific preparation offered by mental practice relies upon some type of movement experience; in this case it was from the unaffected shoulder.

Whole practice implies that the athlete performs the entire task from start to finish, whereas part-practice occurs when the exercise is divided into different segments or phases.[107] Complicated movement tasks and activities occurring in early phases of rehabilitation are usually divided into smaller, less complex activities for the athlete to practice.[107] When the athlete masters the smaller tasks, activity progression occurs by adding the smaller tasks together to ultimately form the larger and more complex movement pattern.[107] For example, an athlete "relearns" how to voluntarily activate the quadriceps after knee surgery by first performing and mastering the basic quadriceps setting exercise. As muscle control improves, the athlete builds upon the basic quadriceps setting exercise by lifting the lower extremity into a straight leg raise exercise. Straight leg raises require the isometric activity of quadriceps-setting to maintain knee extension during the dynamic activity of hip flexion. In this simplified example, quadriceps-setting exercises could be considered "part-practice" whereas the straight leg raises would be "whole practice."

As rehabilitation progresses, the athlete should be able to perform the newly acquired or reacquired task under more functional or sport-specific conditions because clinical situations often do not match those in real life.[56,105,161] The ability to perform the skill under different conditions, or practice variability, enforces motor skill retention and allows the athlete to "generalize" the skill to new conditions.[56,105,161,164] Examples of varying practice include alternating the surface, implementing distractions, and adding secondary tasks such as an athlete progressing from stationary balance activities on one foot to throwing and catching a ball while balancing on one foot.[105]

Practice variability leads us to a brief definition of random, blocked, and random-blocked practice. Essentially, blocked practice implies that the practice or exercise conditions remain constant or unchanging.[164] Blocked practice is beneficial for performance enhancement during early phases of rehabilitation.[82] However, blocked practice is not necessarily best for motor skill retention.[164] Random practice requires the rehabilitation specialist to randomly alternate practice conditions, thereby introducing variability into the performance.[164] Random practice, because of the inherent practice variability, leads to better retention of a motor skill.[82,120,164] Random-blocked practice implies that qualities of random and blocked practice both prevail within an exercise session.[82] Typically, in random-blocked practice, an exercise or activity is performed for more than one repetition before new conditions are implemented. This allows the athlete to correct errors before making adjustments to new practice conditions.[82] An example of random-blocked practice is having an athlete perform a task for two repetitions, followed by an adjustment to the conditions of the exercise, and then having the athlete perform the activity with the new practice conditions.

Feedback

Feedback, information that an athlete receives during or after movement execution, is perhaps the second most important factor affecting motor learning.[82,94,120,162]

Table 7-7

Types of Practice

Type	Characteristics
Physical	Athlete physically performs an exercise or activity.
Mental	Athlete uses mental images to rehearse the movement.
Whole	Athlete performs the entire task from start to finish.
Part	Exercise is divided into different segments or phases.
Blocked	Practice or exercise conditions remain constant or unchanging.
Random	Practice or exercise conditions are randomly alternated, thereby introducing variability into the performance.
Random-blocked	Qualities of random and blocked practice both prevail within an exercise session.

Although there are many different types of feedback, we present only several specific types of feedback relevant to physical rehabilitation. The major types of feedback are intrinsic and extrinsic[82,94,162] (Table 7-8).

Intrinsic feedback is the information acquired by the athlete's own sensory system.[94,120] The senses most commonly used to acquire information during physical movement are the visual, proprioceptive, and auditory sensory systems.[94,108,114,120,150]

Vision provides a large amount of information to the human nervous system about movement and allows for corrective actions to occur during exercise performance. We rely on our vision for many tasks, whether performing an activity of daily living or an activity specific to a given sport.[94,150] We use vision to aim and reach for objects, both in static and dynamic environments and during complex motor activities that involve walking, running, and jumping.[150] Because of vision's role in providing feedback during and after exercise performance, the rehabilitation specialist should incorporate visual stimuli into rehabilitation exercises. Visual targets on a wall, which correspond to a targeted range of motion during active-assisted shoulder exercise, are an example of visual stimuli that allow the athlete to make adjustments during movement.

Proprioception offers the second greatest amount of information about movements during exercise.[114] Our discussion of proprioceptive feedback is brief because Chapter 8 is devoted entirely to proprioception. We rely on proprioceptive feedback during motor learning to develop a "feel" for the exercise, which improves muscle activation during the movement.[108,114] An example would be having the athlete perform an exercise bilaterally and instructing him or her to concentrate on how each extremity feels during the movement. The athlete should understand that the goal is to attempt to have the involved side work or "feel" like the uninvolved extremity during the movement. This is accomplished by the athlete's attempting to activate the function of the involved extremity similarly to that of the uninvolved extremity by using

proprioceptive discernment, or feedback, of the motor activation discrepancy between the extremities.[108,114] Proprioceptive feedback also has an impact on spatial accuracy and the timing of motor commands.[13,94] However, proprioceptors may incur damage from soft tissue injury, which diminishes their ability to transmit afferent information. Activities designed to restore and retrain proprioception in previously injured tissues are outlined in Chapter 8.

Auditory feedback is simply sound information associated with a movement or physical performance. Auditory feedback associated with rehabilitation is usually not intrinsic; that is, we do not rely upon sound to gather information about our movements unless it comes from another source, which is technically extrinsic feedback. A biofeedback apparatus that interprets and then converts physiologic information into auditory information during an exercise is an example of auditory information assembled from an extrinsic source.[128]

Extrinsic feedback is information about the performance of an exercise that occurs from a source other than the athlete.[94,120] This extrinsic information is processed by the same intrinsic sensory systems of the athlete mentioned earlier for auditory feedback. When deciding whether feedback information is intrinsic or extrinsic to the athlete, it is important to remember who or what is providing the actual information about the performance and not necessarily what sensory registers of the athlete acquire the information. For example, an athlete uses his or her vision to observe the rehabilitation professional providing an initial introductory demonstration. Similarly, having the athlete observe his or her reflection in a mirror integrates visual information of the activity. In both these cases, the demonstration of the exercise and the use of the mirror, information about the movement originated from an external source. We may not always have a demonstration or a mirror to use when we perform a given task.

The rehabilitation specialist or a sophisticated apparatus may provide extrinsic information about physical

Table 7-8

Types of Feedback

Intrinsic	Extrinsic
Information is acquired by the athlete's own sensory system.	Information about the performance of an exercise that occurs from a source other than the athlete.
Usually the visual, proprioception, and auditory sensory systems are involved.	This information can come from the clinician or a piece of equipment.
	Two types of extrinsic feedback:
	Knowledge of performance (KP) provides information on movement characteristics that lead to a certain outcome.
	Knowledge of results (KR) provides information relating the outcome of the exercise performance to the goal for a particular exercise.

performance at different time points of exercise execution.[92,128] Extrinsic feedback supplied during an activity is known as *concurrent augmented feedback,* whereas information occurring after the performance of an activity is *terminal augmented feedback.*[94]

There are two primary types of extrinsic feedback. These are known as *knowledge of performance (KP)* and *knowledge of results (KR).*[65,94,162]

KP provides the athlete with information about the movement characteristics that lead to a certain outcome, making it pertinent to physical rehabilitation.[94] KP is especially useful in identifying patterns of substitution or compensation during movements. There are two types of KP—verbal and visual. Verbal KP includes descriptive and prescriptive varieties.[94] Descriptive verbal KP merely identifies the error within the exercise performance, whereas prescriptive KP identifies the error and then prescribes the remedy to correct the error.[94] Visual KP implies that the rehabilitation professional uses a visual display to provide information about the performance. The rehabilitation specialist typically acquires information about the performance and then passes along the information in some sort of visual display to the athlete. Another source of visual information during performance may arise from biofeedback equipment. Heart rate and electromyographic traces are two common types of biofeedback used in rehabilitation settings.[92,94,128]

In providing KP, the rehabilitation specialist must use some type of performance analysis to acquire information about the exercise. The analysis can be either quantitative or qualitative.[87] For quantitative analysis certain characteristics of the performance are quantified; this requires equipment such as high-speed cameras, motion analysis software packages, force platforms, and research quality electromyographic equipment.[87] For qualitative analysis the qualities of the movement are simply described, which is usually sufficient during rehabilitation.[87] Rehabilitation professionals must at least possess the ability to qualitatively analyze the movement patterns associated with performance of an exercise to provide this type of feedback. Videotaped rehabilitation sessions also allow for qualitative analysis, which the rehabilitation professional may use as an educational tool to provide the athlete with KP.[94] In later stages of rehabilitation, such as when an athlete begins sport-specific activities, quantitative analysis of an activity may be more appropriate.

KR provides information relating the outcome of exercise performance to the goal for a particular exercise.[65,162] For example, the rehabilitation specialist provides an athlete with the knowledge of an amount of knee flexion achieved during a rehabilitation session and relates it to the rehabilitation goal for knee flexion. However, Winstein[162] defined KR feedback as the "augmented extrinsic information about task success provided to the performer." She continued by stating that the information

serves as a basis for error correction on the next trial and thus can be used to achieve more effective performance as practice continues. Several variables of KR are important to consider when one uses it as a tool to enhance motor learning during rehabilitation: the form utilized (e.g., verbal or visual), the precision or amount of information contained in KR, and the frequency or schedule of the KR.[65,162] The precision or amount of information contained in the KR influences the number of performance errors: specifically, the greater the precision of the KR, the lesser the amount of performance error. There is perhaps a ceiling effect with the amount of precision, and the optimal levels necessary to improve performance may depend upon the type of performer (i.e., novice versus elite performers). Research demonstrates that the frequency of the KR influences the acquisition and retention of a task.[65] Specifically, KR presented after every trial produces better acquisition of a skill whereas KR presented after several trials actually produces better learning over time.[65] KR presented after every trial leads the athlete to become sensory dependent upon the externally presented information for improving performance and ignore information available from intrinsic acquisition systems.[65] Performance decrements occur when KR is removed as a source of feedback after the athlete becomes dependent upon extrinsic feedback.[65,162]

Basic Strategies for Implementing Concepts of Motor Learning in Rehabilitation

Learning is not directly observable; rather, the effects of learning are manifest in certain behaviors or performance characteristics. According to Kisner and Colby,[82] there are several specific instructional strategies available to the rehabilitation specialist that maximize patient learning during exercise instruction. First, select an environment that allows the athlete to pay attention to your instructions.[82] If it is not feasible or possible to interact one on one with the athlete without distractions, it may be necessary to schedule rehabilitation sessions at times when there are relatively fewer distractions or interruptions. Use clear and concise verbal instructions followed by a proper demonstration of the exercise or activity.[82] The athlete should follow the demonstration with a performance of his or her own while the rehabilitation professional guides movements and provides feedback of the performance both during (KP) and after (KR) the exercise.[82] As exercises and activities become more complicated throughout the progression of rehabilitation, it may be useful to break down complex movements into simple ones. The athlete may then synthesize simple movements into more complex movements.[82]

Crossover Training Effect

A well-documented phenomenon, the crossover training effect or crossover education, associates improved muscle activation of an affected or unexercised extremity with physical exercise of the unaffected extremity.[73,134,135] Physical performance indices such as strength, power, speed, endurance, and range of motion may improve with crossover education.[73,106,134,135] An intriguing characteristic of the crossover effect is that it not only occurs in normal, unaffected extremities, but also in extremities affected by immobilization, orthopedic surgery, and stroke.[134,135] Crossover training may occur in occupationally imbedded tasks as well[106] with the untrained extremity improving in movement speed and accuracy as a result of training the contralateral limb.

Clinical Implications

Knowledge of the crossover effect offers several advantages for physical rehabilitation:

1. It prevents deconditioning of the unaffected extremity,
2. It augments early exercise efforts of affected extremity, and
3. It is useful with conditions that contraindicate movement of the affected extremity[135] (e.g., it is beneficial for early postoperative rehabilitation of an extremity after surgical repair of muscles, tendons, or both).[106]

According to the work of Stromberg[134] and others, the major benefit of using the crossover phenomenon resides in strength gains. Strength gains attributed to the crossover effect range from 30% to 50%,[134,135] although others report more modest improvements.[73] Nonetheless, any gain in muscle strength is advantageous for an affected extremity undergoing a rehabilitation program, especially when exercise of the affected side is contraindicated.

Using both extremities simultaneously at low levels (submaximal) of force intensity also promotes neuromuscular facilitation.[9,10] Simultaneous bilateral activation of the affected and unaffected extremities has implications for rehabilitation, because the patient is able to "feel" the difference between the affected and unaffected muscle groups while also benefiting from the effects of crossover training. The patient's ability to detect differences between simultaneous bilateral muscle activation is a proprioceptive feedback mechanism, which increases motor learning and control.[94]

As rehabilitation progresses and force intensity increases, specific training considerations may contraindicate simultaneous bilateral activities to a degree. De-emphasizing bilateral actions later in rehabilitation may be necessary if the sport of interest requires maximal power of unilateral muscle activation, mainly because higher intensities of resistance during bilateral homologous limbs may actually inhibit relative force production.[9] Beutler and associates[17] recently found that muscle activation relatively increased when the affected extremity was exercised alone, compared with when both extremities were exercised together during closed kinetic chain exercises, which is in agreement with data on the bilateral deficit phenomenon.[9,33]

TYPES OF THERAPEUTIC EXERCISE

Therapeutic exercise is physical activity prescribed to restore or favorably alter specific functions in an individual after injury. These specific physical functions include joint range of motion, soft tissue flexibility, muscle strength and power, and neuromuscular coordination and balance. Figure 7-4 classifies the various therapeutic exercises that a clinician can incorporate into a therapeutic rehabilitation program.

Joint Range of Motion Exercise

Passive Exercise

Passive exercise is carried out by the application of an external force, with minimal participation of muscle action by the injured athlete (Fig. 7-5). Passive exercise may be forced or nonforced. Nonforced exercises are those used to help maintain normal joint motion and are usually kept within a painless range of motion, such as grade I joint mobilizations.[82,102] Conversely, forced passive exercises generally produce movement beyond the limits of available range of motion and are associated with some discomfort to the individual. Forced passive exercises are rarely indicated and should only be performed by experienced clinicians.

The goal of passive exercise techniques is to restore accessory and physiologic joint motions. Accessory motions are necessary for physiologic motions to occur, yet accessory motions do not occur under volitional control of the athlete.[31] Accessory motion (spins, rolls, and glides) restoration occurs with mobilization and manipulation techniques implemented by the clinician[82] (see Chapter 6). Passive restoration of physiologic motion is usually performed for the injured athlete by the clinician or a mechanical appliance such as a continuous passive motion unit or isokinetic dynamometer set in the passive mode.

Active Exercise

Active and active-assistive exercises are beneficial for moving the associated joint, regaining neuromuscular control of an affected extremity, and allowing the patient to have control over the exercise.[82] Active exercise requires muscle activity, at least to some degree, during joint movement. In all cases, the athlete may not have complete neuromuscular control of the extremity, in which case some type of assistance may facilitate the performance of the activity. Active and active-assistive exercises are usually safe, unless a muscle or tendon has been repaired, in which case active range of motion is initially contraindicated.[82]

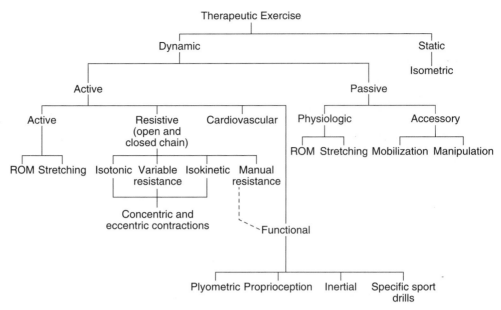

Figure 7-4. Classification of therapeutic exercise. ROM, range of motion. (Modified from Irrgang, J.J. [1995]: Rehabilitation. *In:* Fu, F.H., and Stone, D. [eds.], Sports Injuries: Mechanisms, Prevention, Treatment. Baltimore, Williams & Wilkins.)

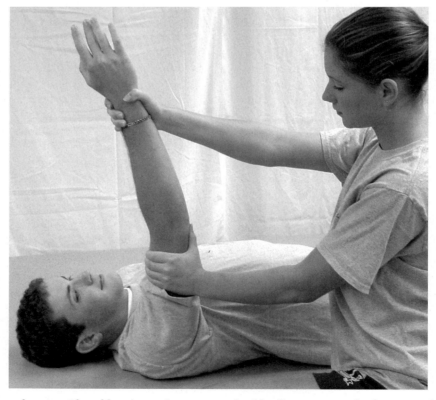

Figure 7-5. Passive range of motion: The athlete (supine) moves into shoulder flexion as a result of an external force (applied by a clinician).

Therapeutic Exercise for Neuromuscular Strength/Endurance

Essentially, there is a natural progression into resistive exercise as the athlete moves from early range-of-motion and flexibility exercises into active range of motion against gravity without assistance. Once the athlete has noncompensatory active range of motion, we add resistance to the active range of motion to further strengthen the musculature involved.

Houglum[66] described this natural rate of strength progression for individuals in a rehabilitation program. In the initial phase there is a relatively rapid improvement in strength, followed by a second phase, in which there is slowing or tapering of the improvement rate, and a third (final) phase, consisting of a progression toward a plateau state in which minimal or no improvement in strength occurs (Fig. 7-6).

Muscular strength and endurance increase with progressive resistive exercise (PRE), as long as it occurs in an orderly and progressive manner. PRE permits an ever-increasing overload to be applied to the musculature, which allows bones, ligaments, tendons, and muscles to adapt to the applied stress. This philosophy is based on the principle of specific adaptation to imposed demands (see section on conditioning later in this chapter),[124,144] which implies that the body responds to a given demand with a specific and predictable adaptation.[124,160] Stated another way, specific adaptation requires that a specific demand be imposed.[84] With rehabilitation, it is important that overload not be applied too quickly to avoid further damage to the healing tissue.

Rehabilitative strength training may involve static (isometric) or dynamic exercise. Types of dynamic resistance exercise include isotonic, isokinetic, and inertial. Box 7-6 summarizes factors related to muscle force production.

Static Exercise

Static exercises, or isometric actions, occur without joint movement. The activated muscle groups maintain a fixed length because the tension generated is equal to the resistance encountered.[98] Because strength gains generally occur within 20° above and below the specific angle in which the isometric exercise occurs, it is important for the athlete to perform the exercise at multiple joint angles.[147] For example, to strengthen elbow flexors throughout the full 150° of available motion, sets should be done at 20°, 60°, 100°, and 140° of elbow flexion. Generally, the muscle should remain under tension for 3 to 10 seconds.[147]

The clinician should ensure that the athlete does not strain during the holding period of the isometric action, particularly as the intensity of the action increases. Straining instinctively causes one to "hold one's breath," also known as the Valsalva maneuver, which is associated with momentary increases in arterial blood pressure.[46,93] For most athletes, this may not be a concern because the intensity of their normal weight training bout far exceeds that of a rehabilitation program, but individuals suffering from hypertension may incur an adverse sequela when blood pressure rises to dangerous levels.[46,93]

CLINICAL PEARL #4

Have the athlete count out loud during isometric actions to relatively attenuate increases in blood pressure associated with isometric actions. Blood pressure may still increase, but not to the extent that occurs during a Valsalva maneuver.

Dynamic Exercise

Dynamic exercise implies that movement occurs. Most types of dynamic exercise include isotonic, variable-resistance, manual, and isokinetic (accommodating variable-resistance) movements.[100] Additionally, dynamic exercise may be more functional in nature, some examples of which are plyometric, proprioceptive, and inertial exercises and sport-specific drills. Almost all dynamic exercises include concentric and eccentric movement phases.

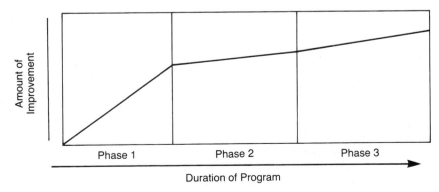

Figure 7-6. Typical progression during a rehabilitation program. (Adapted from Houglum, P. [1977]: The modality of therapeutic exercise: Objectives and principles. Athl. Train. J. Natl. Athl. Train. Assoc., 12:43.)

Box 7-6

Factors Affecting Muscle Force Production

- Muscle fiber type
- Length-tension relationship
- Number of motor units activated
- Firing frequency
- Muscle temperature
- Elastic energy of muscle and the type of muscle action
- Force-velocity relationship
- Size of muscle fibers (cross-sectional area)
- Decreased activity of inhibitory reflexes
- Angle of pull during muscle action

Data from Kreighbaum, E., and Barthels, K.M. (1996): Biomechanics: A Qualitative Approach for Studying Human Movement, 4th ed. Boston, Allyn & Bacon.

Concentric and Eccentric Actions

As mentioned earlier, the two types of muscle actions that occur during dynamic training are (1) concentric actions, in which a shortening of muscle fibers results in a decrease in the angle of the associated joint and (2) eccentric, in which the muscle resists lengthening so that the joint angle increases during the action.[82,98] Concentric and eccentric actions are also referred to as positive and negative work, respectively.[35] Concentric contractions generally function to accelerate a limb; for example, the shoulder internal rotators accelerate the arm during the acceleration phase of throwing. Conversely, eccentric actions generally function to decelerate a limb and provide shock absorption; for example, the shoulder external rotators decelerate the shoulder during the follow-through phase of throwing.[77] Another interesting difference between concentric and eccentric muscle actions is their relative capabilities for force production. A maximum eccentric action may generate forces 14% to 50% greater than a maximal concentric contraction of the same group.[35] How is this possible? There are at least two reasons: (1) the energy-consuming mechanical work of sliding actin and myosin together has already been done, we now only have to allow the actin and myosin to "pull apart," which takes less energy; and (2) we derive some energy from the elongation of the elastic (parallel and series) components of muscle.[68,87] Training studies clearly demonstrate an association with eccentric actions and muscle hypertrophy and strength increases compared with concentric only actions. In fact, it is advisable for individuals to employ both concentric and eccentric actions to maximize benefits derived from strength training.[115]

Besides force production advantages, another benefit of eccentric exercise is its positive effects for tendonitis and overuse syndromes.[4,142] Alfredson and colleagues[4] utilized heavy eccentric training during rehabilitation of Achilles tendonitis in recreational runners (ERR). After

12 weeks, the ERR group exhibited increased plantar flexor strength and were able to return to their running regimens compared with a conventional treatment group (rest, nonsteroidal medication, shoe orthotics, and physical modalities), who were not able to return to running and many of whom ultimately underwent surgery.[4] Eccentric training may directly improve the integrity of the musculotendinous structures by inducing hypertrophy and increased tensile strength or by lengthening the muscle-tendon unit, which induces relatively less strain during active motion.[4,129] It is conceivable that eccentric training may elicit its therapeutic effects by both of the proposed mechanisms. Nonetheless, rehabilitation using eccentric actions is effective for restoring strength and function in tendinitis, as long as progression is slow.

A major reason to progress eccentric exercise slowly is its association with delayed-onset muscle soreness (DOMS).[26,36,149] DOMS is defined as muscular pain or discomfort presenting 1 to 5 days after unusual muscular exertion.[77] The syndrome of DOMS also includes joint swelling[26] and weakness.[26,36,149] The weakness associated with DOMS may continue after cessation of pain.[26] The onset and degree of DOMS are inversely proportional to the intensity of eccentric exercise and generally occur in individuals unaccustomed to eccentric exercise.[77] Therefore, eccentric activities should be progressed gradually in the rehabilitation setting.

CLINICAL PEARL #5

Eccentric actions may be emphasized by having the athlete perform the activity with both extremities (bilateral) during the concentric phase but then use only the affected extremity (unilateral) during the eccentric phase.

Isotonic Exercise

Isotonic exercise is perhaps the most common type of dynamic exercise. With isotonic exercise, the actual muscle length changes as an external force causes a change in joint angle.[87] In pure isotonic exercise, the resistance remains constant, whereas the velocity of movement depends upon the load, known as the force-velocity relationship.[87] Eccentric and concentric phases occur during isotonic exercise. There are two inherent disadvantages of isotonic exercise: (1) the weight is fixed and does not adjust to the variation in force expression present during speed work or at various ranges of motion; and (2) the momentum of weight propulsion diminishes the strength required at the extremes of joint motion. This type of exercise is readily available in the form of exercises performed with ankle weights, free weights, and weight machines (Fig. 7-7).

Variable-Resistance Exercise

Production of muscle force is less at extreme joint range of motion (e.g., the muscle is too short or excessively exercise machines are commonly used in rehabilitation and fitness settings. The machines commonly have adjustments that allow proper joint alignment (the joint axis of rotation should always be in alignment with the machine's axis of rotation) and range-of-motion limiters, which are beneficial for some types of rehabilitation.

Manual Resistance

Manual resistance is a variation of accommodating variable-resistance exercise. The clinician provides the resistance with this mode of exercise and can modify the resistance and speed during the exercise as the athlete's fatigue is recognized (Fig. 7-9). This exercise mode is applicable to an extent during all rehabilitation phases because it is capable of producing movement patterns that cannot be duplicated on machines (e.g., proprioceptive neuromuscular facilitation diagonals).

Isokinetic Exercise

Isokinetic exercise, or accommodating variable-resistance exercise, is performed at a set speed, with resistance matching the input of force at that speed. As the force input changes, the resistance changes to match the input, but the speed remains constant. Application of the athlete's own muscular resistance is met with a proportional amount of resistance throughout a range of motion. Isokinetic machines may be set to offer concentric-concentric,

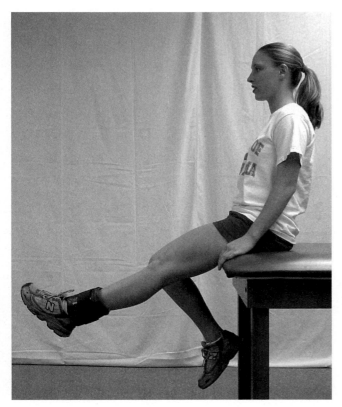

Figure 7-7. Long-arc knee extensions. Isotonic exercise in which the resistance remains constant and the velocity is inversely proportional to the load.

lengthened). Variable-resistance exercise machines address the relative force decrements throughout the range of motion by a cam that varies the resistance to match normal force decrements during resisted exercise.[147] The cam varies the resistance by changing the length of the machine's lever arm of the weight being lifted (Fig. 7-8). Variable-resistance

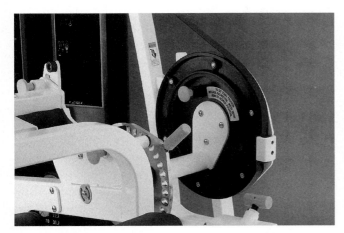

Figure 7-8. Variable resistance exercise. This is possible because of a specialized cam. (Photo courtesy of Cybex International, Medway, MA.

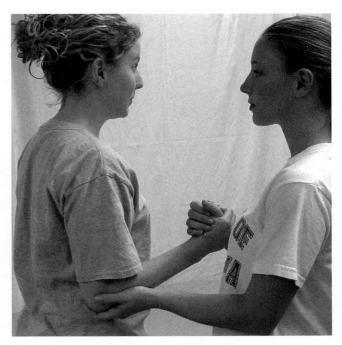

Figure 7-9. Manual resistance of isotonic elbow flexion. Note how the athlete's elbow (darker shirt) is stabilized by the clinician as resistance is applied distally at the hand (may also be modified to provide resistance at a more proximal location to protect the wrist and hand joints of the athlete, if necessary).

concentric-eccentric, or eccentric-eccentric actions at various velocities (Fig. 7-10). Chapter 9 provides an in-depth discussion of isokinetics.

Inertial Exercise

Inertial loading, compared with other forms of dynamic exercise, is a relatively novel mode of exercise.[3] This mode of exercise simulates the momentum and velocity changes of functional activity through the reciprocal acceleration and deceleration of a variable mass[140] (Fig. 7-11). Albert[2] described the type of loading that the impulse machine produces as "horizontal, sub-maximal, gravity eliminated plyometrics."

PROGRESSION OF RESISTANCE EXERCISE

Before an athlete begins a PRE program, he or she must have functional range of motion.[67] The theory behind resistance exercise is to apply an overload to increase muscular strength and, at the same time, to maintain the integrity of the tissues of concern and not impede the healing process. There are several progression philosophies discussed in the literature. These include the low-resistance, high-repetition method, the DeLorme and Watkins regimen, the Oxford technique, the daily adjustable progressive resistance exercise (DAPRE) methods, and the Sanders program.

The Low-Resistance, High-Repetition Method

Before 1945, the traditional method of strength training during rehabilitation actually stressed muscle endurance more so than strength.[100] Even today, the low-resistance,

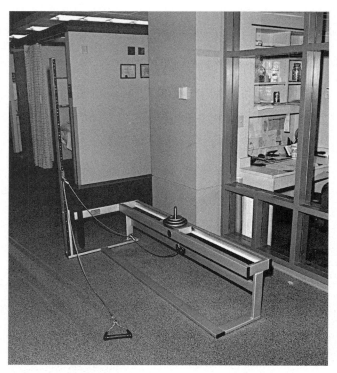

Figure 7-11. Impulse machine (EMA, Inc., Newnan, GA) for inertial exercise.

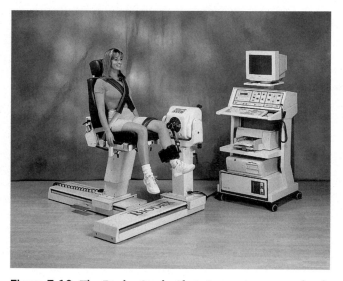

Figure 7-10. The Biodex Single Chair System is an example of isokinetic (accommodating variable-resistance) equipment. The resistance changes to match the input, but the speed remains constant. (Courtesy of Biodex, Shirley, NY.)

high-repetition technique may be the best regimen for athletes with injuries of insidious onset and during the early postoperative period.[18] Resistance exercise of high resistance or intensity could potentially cause a breakdown of the supporting structures and only exacerbate the condition. Use of smaller weights and submaximal intensities provides a therapeutic effect that stimulates blood flow, diminishes tissue breakdown, and promotes local muscle endurance.[16,18,104]

The PRE program outlined here can be carried out early in rehabilitation using the low-resistance, high-repetition concept (Table 7-9). Early rehabilitation begins with an active range of motion of two or three sets of 10 repetitions (even up to 20 or 30 repetitions), progressing to five sets of 10 repetitions (up to 50 repetitions), as tolerated. When the athlete can perform 50 repetitions without stopping and without overcompensation of other muscle groups or joint actions, 1 pound of weight may be added and the number of repetitions is reduced to three sets of 10 or 30 repetitions. The cycle repeats when the athlete reaches 50 repetitions and as another pound of weight is added the repetitions are reduced to 10 to 30. The athlete progresses through the PRE program as tolerated, with emphasis placed on proper lifting technique. All exercises should be performed smoothly, with a pause at the terminal position. The athlete must also concentrate on lowering the weight in a controlled fashion.

Table 7-9

Low-Resistance, High-Repetition Progression

Week	Sun	Mon	Tues	Day Wed	Thurs	Fri	Sat
1			Surgery Injury	30 rep	40 rep	50 rep	30 rep@1 lb
2	40 rep@1 lb	50 rep@1 lb	30 rep@2 lb	40 rep@2 lb	50 rep@2 lb	30 rep@3 lb	40 rep@3 lb
3	50 rep@3 lb	30 rep@4 lb	40 rep@4 lb	50 rep@4 lb	30 rep@5 lb	40 rep@5 lb	50 rep@5 lb
•	etc.						
•							
•							
•							

rep, repetitions.

Houglum[68] outlined a program utilizing a resistance that the athlete safely controls for 6 to 15 repetitions for two sets. That resistance is continued until the athlete successfully performs three sets of 2 to 25 repetitions each. At this point, resistance increases and the number of repetitions decreases accordingly. As the athlete progresses into later stages of rehabilitation and the healing tissue is capable of tolerating increased stress, other more intense models of progression could be used such as those of DeLorme and Watkins or Knight.

The DeLorme and Watkins Program

DeLorme[37] first introduced the concept of PRE in 1945 as a challenge to the traditional concept of low-resistance, high-repetition exercise.[100] The rationale for using PRE is that it creates a condition in which an individual muscle or muscles must work against an ever-increasing resistance in subsequent sets.[63]

DeLorme's[37] concept of PRE was based on the amount of weight that could be carried through a full range of motion for 10 repetitions. DeLorme[37] referred to this as heavy-resistance exercise because the weights used were heavy compared with those used in previous strengthening methods, and an all-out effort was necessary to lift them. This mode of PRE, however, is generally not applicable to athletes in early postoperative stages. Table 7-10 outlines the DeLorme and Watkins program.[38]

The Oxford Technique

The Oxford technique, developed by Zinovieff,[168] also incorporates relatively heavy resistance after the determination of a 10 repetition maximum (RM). However, unlike the DeLorme and Watkins regimen, the Oxford technique decrease exercise intensity with each new set to accommodate fatiguing muscle (Table 7-11).[168] Zinovieff suggested this modification after observing that most patients were excessively fatigued during the final set of repetitions with the DeLorme and Watkins technique.

The Daily Adjustable Progressive Resistance Exercise Technique

Knight's technique[83] of DAPRE, along with other modifications of DeLorme's PRE concept,[66,83,121,168] uses the same basic principles of PRE. According to Knight,[83] the DAPRE technique allows for individual differences in the rate at which a person regains strength in the muscle and provides an objective method for increasing resistance in accordance with strength increases. The key to the program is that athletes perform as many full repetitions as they can in the third and fourth sets.[83] These numbers of repetitions are then used to determine the amount of weight that is added or removed to the working weight for the fourth set in the current bout and the first set of the

Table 7-10

The DeLorme and Watkins Progressive Resistive Exercise Program

1. First set of 10 repetitions: use one half of 10 RM
2. Second set of 10 repetitions: use three fourths of 10 RM
3. Third set of 10 repetitions: use full 10 RM

Modified from DeLorme, T.L., and Watkins, A. (1948): Techniques of progressive resistance exercise. Arch. Phys. Med., 29:263-268.
RM, repetition maximum.

Table 7-11

The Oxford Technique of Progressive Resistance Exercise

Set	Amount of Resistance (Intensity)	Repetitions (Duration)
1	50% of 10 RM	10
2	75% of 10 RM	10
3	100% of 10 RM	10

From Zinovieff, A.N. (1951): Heavy resistance exercise: The Oxford technique. Br. J. Phys. Med., 14:129-132.
RM, repetition maximum.

next session. The working weight is estimated for the initial reconditioning session. A good estimate would result in five to seven repetitions during the third set. More repetitions are performed if the estimate is low, and fewer are performed if it is too high.

During the first and second sets, the athlete performs 10 repetitions against one half of the estimated working weight and six repetitions against three quarters of the working weight (Tables 7-12 and 7-13). These sets warm up and educate the muscles and neuromuscular structures involved.

Emphasis during the third and fourth sets is on the athlete's performing the greatest number of full repetitions possible. The full working weight is used in the third set, and the athlete performs as many repetitions as possible. The number of full repetitions performed in the third set is used to determine the adjusted working weight for the fourth set, and the number of full repetitions performed in the fourth set is used to determine the working weight for the next day.

The Sanders Program

Athletes tolerate higher intensities in advanced stages of rehabilitation, which is addressed in the Sanders program of resistance exercise progression.[119] The beginning resistance intensity varies according to the athlete's body weight and the particular exercise (e.g., leg extension, squats, or bench press). The athlete exercises at high intensities (100% of 2 to 5 RM) for three sessions per week. Table 7-14 summarizes the Sanders program.

NEUROMUSCULAR COORDINATION AND PROPRIOCEPTION

In a comprehensive rehabilitation program the clinician must not overlook the component of neuromuscular

Table 7-12

Daily Adjustable Progressive Resistance Exercise

Set	Portion of Working Weight Used	Number of Repetitions
1	One half	10
2	Three fourths	6
3*	Full	Maximum
4†	Adjusted	Maximum

From Knight, K.L. (1985): Guidelines for rehabilitation of sports injuries. Clin. Sports Med., 4:413.
*The number of repetitions performed during the third set is used to determine the adjusted working weight for the fourth set according to the guidelines in Table 7-13.
†The number of repetitions performed during the fourth set is used to determine the adjusted working weight for the next day according to the guidelines in Table 7-13.

Table 7-13

General Guidelines for Adjustment of Working Weight

Number of Repetitions Performed during Set	Adjustment of Working Weight Fourth Set°	Next Day†
0-2	Decrease by 5-10 lb and perform the set over	
3-4	Decrease by 0-5 lb	Keep the same
5-7	Keep the same	Increase by 5-10 lb
8-12	Increase by 5-10 lb	Increase by 5-15 lb
13+	Increase by 10-15 lb	Increase by 10-20 lb

From Knight, K.L. (1985): Guidelines for rehabilitation of sports injuries. Clin. Sports Med., 4:414.
*The number of repetitions performed during the third set is used to determine the adjusted working weight for the fourth set according to the guidelines in Table 7-12.
†The number of repetitions performed during the fourth set is used to determine the adjusted working weight for the next day according to the guidelines in Table 7-12.

control that is necessary for joint stability. The healing of static or dynamic restraints and the strengthening of the appropriate muscles do not prepare a joint for sudden position changes that occur during sport-specific activities.[62,71] To adequately address this phenomenon, the clinician must be familiar with the structures contributing to proprioception, as well as the process by which articular sensations contribute to functional stability.

When joint sensation is described, the terms *proprioception* and *kinesthesia* are often erroneously interchanged. Proprioception describes the awareness of posture, movement, and changes in equilibrium and the knowledge of position, weight, and resistance of objects in relation to the body.[137] Kinesthesia, however, refers to the ability to perceive the extent, direction, or weight of movement.[137] These two definitions are combined into a comprehensive, operational definition: "Proprioception is considered a specialized variation of the sensory modality

Table 7-14

The Sanders Program of Progressing Resistance Exercise

Determining the initial resistance load (median starting points) for 10 repetitions:
  Universal leg extension: 15% of body weight
  Universal leg press: 50% of body weight
  Barbell squat: 45% of body weight
  Barbell bench press: 30% of body weight

Adapted from Sanders, M. (1990): Weight training and conditioning. In: Sanders, B. (ed.), Sports Physical Therapy. Norwalk, CT, Appleton & Lange, pp. 239-250.

of touch and encompasses the sensations of joint movement (kinesthesia) and joint position (joint position sense)."[91] As Lephart and others describe, both conscious and unconscious proprioception are essential for proper joint function in sports and other daily tasks as well as for reflex stabilization.[58,89,132] These articular sensations are the direct focus of proprioceptive rehabilitation and are crucial for efficient, noninjurious movement. Figures 7-12 and 7-13 provide examples of exercises used for proprioceptive training for the lower and upper extremities, respectively. Chapter 8 provides more detailed information concerning proprioception.

Improving neuromuscular coordination builds upon foundations of range of motion, strengthening, and proprioception. Athletic coordination, often an innate skill that is difficult to teach or coach, may be enhanced with training.[147] Most physical tasks require actions of multiple joints and

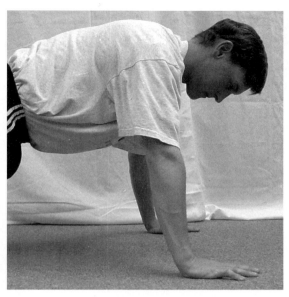

Figure 7-13. Closed kinetic chain exercise for the upper extremities. The push-up position incorporates joint compression and facilitates joint stability.

muscle groups; as the complexity of the task increases, so must the coordination between the working muscle groups. Generally, complex tasks are composed of multiple smaller tasks. The athlete must be able to unconsciously carry out these tasks while concentrating his or her mental attention on the outcome of the performance and using feedback to modify performance as necessary.[94] The physical act of practicing a given task increases the skill level at which it is performed and its automaticity (see section on motor learning earlier in this chapter).[94]

NEUROMUSCULAR POWER
Plyometrics

Plyometrics are drills or exercises that aim to link strength and speed of movement to produce an explosive-reactive type of muscle response.[24,25,153,154] The purpose of plyometric training is to heighten the excitability of the neurologic receptors for improved reactivity of the neuromuscular system.[143,159] By means of an eccentric muscle action, the muscle is fully stretched immediately preceding the concentric contraction. The greater the stretch placed on the muscle from its resting length immediately before the concentric contraction, the greater the load the muscle can lift or overcome. Thus, plyometrics have been referred to as "stretch-shortening" drills or "reactive neuromuscular" training.[159] Wilk and colleagues[159] described the three phases of a plyometric exercise (Table 7-15).

Plyometrics should be implemented in the later stages of rehabilitation and should mimic a sport-specific skill. Plyometrics should also be used judiciously because of the relative stress placed upon involved tissue. The clinician

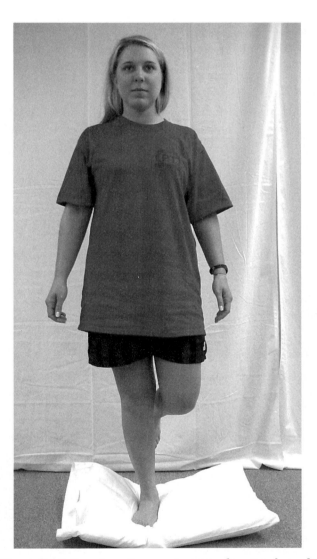

Figure 7-12. Proprioceptive exercise in standing: "stork stand." This athlete is standing on a pillow, which increases the difficulty of exercise compared with standing on a firm surface.

Table 7-15

Three Phases of Plyometric Exercises

Phase	Characteristics
Eccentric	This is the preloading period in which the muscle spindle is prestretched prior to activation.
Amortization	This is the time between the eccentric contraction and initiation of a concentric force. The rate of the stretch is more critical than the duration of the stretch. Therefore, the more quickly an athlete can overcome the yielding eccentric force and produce a concentric force, the more powerful the response.
Concentric	This is a summation of the eccentric and amortization phases, with the product being an enhanced concentric contraction.

should remember that both postexercise soreness and delayed-onset muscle soreness are by-products of this type of exercise.

Absolute contraindications for plyometrics include acute recovery from surgery, gross instability, pain, and a state of unconditioning. Chapter 11 is devoted to plyometric exercise and the reader is referred to it for a more in-depth discussion of the topic.

CLINICAL PEARL #6

Plyometrics are a form of exercise that trains muscles to produce power. Power production also increases when the athlete performs repetitions at the same relative resistance (intensity) but with higher velocities. A metronome may be used to keep the athlete on a faster "pace" while performing repetitions within a set.

Kinetic Chain

The term *kinematic chain* was introduced by Reuleaux[118] in 1875 to refer to a mechanical system of links in engineering. In engineering, a kinematic chain is usually a closed system of links joined together so that if any free link is moved on a fixed link, all the other links move in a predictable pattern. Steindler[130] first suggested the terms *open kinetic chain (OKC)* and *closed kinetic chain (CKC)*. He defined a kinetic chain in the human body as a combination of successively arranged joints that constitutes a complex motor unit.[130]

Steindler[131] described an OKC as being characterized by the distal segment terminating freely in space, whereas in a CKC the distal segment of the joint is fixed and meets with considerable external resistance, which prohibits or restrains its free motion. Initially, CKC exercise (CKCE)

was characterized by the distal segment being fixed, with the body weight being supported by the extremity, which was associated with considerable external resistance (see Fig. 7-13). Open kinetic chain exercise (OKCE) was characterized by the distal segment not being fixed, body weight not being supported, and the affected muscles working against relatively less external resistance. As researchers have examined CKCE and OKCE, the basic characteristics have expanded (Table 7-16).

Most of the research regarding CKCE has targeted the lower extremity, specifically the knee joint. With regard to the effect of CKCE on the knee, most investigations have examined anterior tibial displacement and the resultant stresses placed on the anterior cruciate ligament. The advantages of CKCE over OKCE have been well reported in the literature and include a decrease in shear forces, stimulation of proprioceptors, enhancement of joint stability, allowance for more functional patterns of movement, and greater specificity for athletic activities.[21,22,57,61,127,148,157,165]

Although the characterization of CKCE and OKCE has broadened, there is some debate about the application of lower extremity CKCE principles to the upper extremity. The upper extremity has unique anatomic, biomechanical, and functional features, especially the shoulder, which makes applying the traditional definitions of OKCE and CKCE difficult.[157] Wilk and colleagues state the following[157]:

The conditions that apply to the lower extremity such as weight-bearing forces, which create a closed kinetic chain effect, do not routinely occur in the upper extremity. However, due to the unique anatomical configuration of the glenohumeral joint, whereas the stabilizing muscles contract producing a joint compression force that stabilizes the joint

Table 7-16

Characteristics of Closed Kinetic Chain Exercise Versus Open Kinetic Chain Exercise

Closed Kinetic Chain Exercise	Open Kinetic Chain Exercise
Large resistance and low acceleration forces	Large acceleration and low resistance forces
Greater compressive forces	Distraction and rotatory forces
Joint congruity	Promotion of a stable base
Decreased shear	Joint mechanoreceptor deformation
Stimulation of proprioceptors	Concentric acceleration and eccentric deceleration
Enhanced dynamic stabilization	Assimilation of function

Data from Lephart, S.M., and Henry, T.J. (1995): Functional rehabilitation for the upper and lower extremity. Orthop. Clin. North Am., 26:579-592.

much to the same effect as closed kinetic chain exercise for the lower extremity. It is for this reason we believe that the principle of closed kinetic chain exercise as explained for the lower extremity may not apply for upper extremity exercises. Rather, we suggest specific terminology for the upper extremity exercise program under specific conditions, such as weight bearing or axial compression.

Because of incongruities between the lower and upper extremities, some authors[42,90] have recommended different classification systems for describing OKCE and CKCE for the upper extremity. Dillman and colleagues[42] proposed three classifications for OKCE and CKCE for the upper extremity based on mechanics. Their system takes into account the boundary condition and the external load encountered at the distal segment. The boundary condition of the distal segment may be either fixed or moveable, and an external load may or may not exist at the distal link. Thus, the categories include a fixed boundary with an external load, a moveable boundary with an external load, and a moveable boundary with no external load (MNL). The terms *fixed boundary with an external load* and *moveable boundary with no external load* correspond to the extremes of CKC and OKC exercises, respectively, and *moveable boundary with an external load* refers to the "gray" region between these two extremes. These authors suggest that the confusing terms OKC and CKC be eliminated and that the biomechanics, load, and muscular response of the exercises be utilized.

Lephart and Henry[90] proposed a functional classification system for upper extremity rehabilitation with the objective of restoring functional stability of the shoulder by reestablishing neuromuscular control for overhead activities. This system addresses three areas of the shoulder complex: scapulothoracic stabilization, glenohumeral stabilization, and humeral control. The functional classification system considers boundary and load and also the direction in which the load is applied. Table 7-17 summarizes the functional classification system.

There appears to be agreement that the traditional classification system for OKC and CKC exercises, which considers the fixation of the distal segment, the body weight, and the external resistance, is not adequate for describing exercises for the upper extremities. Nonetheless, both open- and closed-chain exercises have characteristics that are important in restoring strength and neuromuscular control to an injured upper extremity, and both should be incorporated into an upper extremity rehabilitation program.[90,116,157]

Physical Conditioning and Rehabilitation

General Considerations

Within the context of rehabilitation and conditioning, several considerations affect the quality of exercise performance and the outcome of the program. These

considerations include a general to specific exercise progression and the specific order of exercise.

Exercises should progress from general (simple) to specific (complex).[7] This consideration applies to initial conditioning programs as well as to rehabilitation programs because untrained or healing tissue may not tolerate the stress inherent to some types of specific exercises. Specific exercises are usually better tolerated as tissue integrity improves, which usually occurs in more advanced phases of rehabilitation. The concept of generalized adaptation relies upon the premise that a bout of physical exercise affects more than one physiologic system simultaneously.[100] For instance, cardiovascular exercise specifically stresses the heart, lungs, and circulatory systems and improves local muscle endurance in the extremities performing the mode of exercise. Even though the exercise bout specifically targets cardiovascular and muscular endurance, relative muscular force production also improves compared with previous force production capability.[100]

Another consideration that optimizes the outcomes of exercise is the specific order of exercises.[125] To minimize the deleterious effects of fatigue, higher intensity exercises using larger muscle groups and multiple joints should be performed early in the exercise session.[7,125] Thus, exercises that use lower intensities and that stress single joints and or smaller muscle groups are best performed at the end of the bout.

Physical conditioning and comprehensive athletic rehabilitation both stress multiple physiologic systems that influence athletic performance. These systems include the cardiovascular, neurologic, thermoregulatory, and musculoskeletal systems. The efficiency of operation of these systems is improved, which results in improved functioning and sport performance. The following discussion emphasizes the cardiovascular and neuromuscular systems.

Stresses to the aforementioned systems can be adjusted from one or more conditioning parameters. These parameters include intensity, duration, frequency, specificity, and exercise progression. Incorporating knowledge of the various conditioning parameters allows for systematic physiologic stress manipulation.

Conditioning during Rehabilitation

A very challenging aspect of rehabilitation for the clinician is providing the athlete with a form of physical stress to noninjured extremities, especially the cardiovascular system, to minimize the deleterious effects of a relative decrease in activity.[32] Sport-specific activities are most desirable as long as there are no contraindications for including them during rehabilitation. Principles of generality and specificity are important to consider with physical conditioning during rehabilitation.

Cardiovascular fitness should be addressed, if possible, throughout the various rehabilitation phases. General adaptations occur within the cardiovascular system, due to

Table 7-17

Summary of Upper Extremity Functional Classification System

Classification	Characteristics	Examples
Fixed boundary: external, axial load	Considerable load, slow velocity NM reaction: active or reactive MM action: coactivation, acceleration, deceleration Coactivation of force couples Joint compression Minimal shear forces Promotion of dynamic stability	Axial loading in tripod position Slide board Unstable platform
Moveable boundary: external, axial load	Considerable load, variable velocity MM action: coactivation, acceleration, deceleration Coactivation of force couples Promotion of dynamic stability Activation of prime movers Minimal shear forces	Closed-chain protraction/retraction on an isokinetic dynamometer Traditional bench press Rhythmic stabilization activities
Moveable boundary: external, axial load	Variable load, functional speeds NM reaction: active or reactive MM action: coactivation, acceleration, deceleration Stability of scapular and glenohumeral base Activation of prime movers Functional point kinematics Functional motor patterns	Isokinetics in functional diagonal patterns Multiaxial machine Resistance tubing exercise Proprioceptive neuromuscular facilitation exercise
Moveable boundary: no load	Negligible load, variable velocity NM reaction: active or passive MM action: coactivation, acceleration, perceptual Activation of muscles: proximal to distal Low muscle activation without resistance Functional significance	Joint sensibility training: active and passive

From Lephart, S.M., and Henry, T.J. (1996): The physiological basis for open and closed kinetic chain rehabilitation for the upper extremity. J. Sports Rehabil., 5:77.
MM, muscular; NM, neuromuscular.

participation in nonspecific aerobic activity. For example, an athlete with a lower extremity injury may not be able to participate in running or cycle ergometry with the lower extremities but may be able to participate in aerobic activities with the upper extremities. General adaptations are useful in early phases of rehabilitation because they allow injured tissue to recover from the mechanisms causing injury. General conditioning is beneficial up to a point; altogether it is rather unsatisfactory for returning the athlete to a given sport because the adaptations may not be sufficiently specific to the demands of the sport.

Specific conditioning, according to the demands of an athlete's sport, is relatively more stressful because it integrates the previously injured tissue into the activity or exercise. Therefore, sport-specific conditioning usually takes place later in the rehabilitation program because healing tissue needs to reach a maturation level that is able to withstand the specific stresses incurred of a specific sport.

Prehabilitation

Prehabilitation, or prehab, describes one of two possible scenarios: (1) preventive conditioning based upon findings from a preparticipation examination[49,81] or (2) rehabilitation after an injury requiring surgical intervention, which better prepares the patient for postsurgical rehabilitation. Although clinicians are quite familiar with the benefits of both types of prehabilitation, there are relatively few scientific data to substantiate its practice.

Prophylactic Prehabilitation

Prehabilitation may mean that athletes continue with maintenance exercises/activities to prevent or avoid injury or reinjury. An example of this concept is a healthy baseball pitcher who incorporates specific rotator cuff exercises into his off-season workout regimen. It is beneficial to screen athletes during the preseason, (e.g., with a preparticipation examination [PPE]), to reveal a predisposition to injury.

A PPE routinely evaluates flexibility, strength, power, and endurance of athletes during the preseason because vulnerability in these areas may predispose the athlete to injury.[78,80,99,110] Equally important, the rehabilitation specialist must understand the inherent demands of various sports to be able to provide a sound preventive conditioning program.[81] Together with the PPE, the prehabilitation program targets specific areas of vulnerability and addresses sport-specific requirements in an attempt to prevent injury occurrence.[23,79] Thus, in this context, prehabilitation is a type of conditioning program used to seek physiologic adaptations to increase neuromuscular activity and coordination, bone and joint integrity, metabolic capacity, recovery mechanisms, and joint stability force couples.[79] Generally, improvements in these areas will also correlate with improvements in physical performance, which is the typical goal of most regular conditioning programs.

Prehabilitation Preceding Surgery

Prehabilitation also refers to specific exercises and patient education before surgery. This is thought to result in a decrease in morbidity and a reduction in the relative loss of muscular strength and endurance postoperatively. It is also beneficial because the individual has an understanding of what to expect in addition to beginning the postoperative period with a higher level of conditioning.

Patient education plays an integral role in prehabilitation and rehabilitation programs. The preoperative and postoperative education of the athlete is often taken for granted, and the surgical procedure, extent of damage, prognosis, and rehabilitation course are often not discussed with the athlete. Therefore, it is important to educate the athlete about the initial rehabilitation program and what is expected of him or her in the early phases of rehabilitation; to perform gait training; to take baseline measurements, if indicated and tolerated by the athlete; and to fit any orthotic appliances that are to be used in the early postoperative phases. The athlete should also be informed about the surgical procedure to be performed, the prognosis after surgery, any potential complications, and precautions and limitations after surgery. The importance of rehabilitation, its function, and its approximate duration should also be discussed. Finally, it is beneficial for the clinician to involve athletes in goal setting, to allow them to have input into their rehabilitation program, and to be sure they understand early rehabilitation restrictions and realize the consequences of noncompliance with rehabilitation.[82]

A long period of prehab is usually not necessary for the conditioned athlete. In the deconditioned athlete or individual, the initiation of a therapeutic exercise program 4 to 6 weeks before surgical intervention is preferable. Generally, the program focuses on regaining range of motion and on therapeutic exercises that do not exacerbate symptoms or further damage the injured area.

PARAMETERS OF CONDITIONING AND REHABILITATION

The functional capability developed by the athlete coincides with the progression of conditioning attained during the rehabilitation period. The progression of rehabilitation and conditioning depends upon the systematic manipulation of the following parameters: intensity, duration, frequency, specificity (such as the mode of exercise) and the speed of the movement, and finally, the amount of rest and recovery within or between rehabilitation sessions. The clinician adjusts these parameters to ensure that the athlete continues to improve his or her state of physical conditioning.

Intensity

The goal of the rehabilitation program is to overload not overwhelm.[41] Generally, exercise intensity is less at the onset of rehabilitation and increases as the tissue becomes stronger. Higher intensities are demanding to the tissues and systems involved during physical activity. Thus, the rehabilitation professional modulates exercise intensity according to the injury time frame. Also, intensity is inversely related to the duration of activity. As intensity increases, duration decreases and vice versa.

Strengthening Muscle and Connective Tissue

Muscle and connective tissue must be subjected to a load greater than that of the usual stresses of daily activity to induce hypertrophy and strengthening. Resistance training is the mode of exercise most often used to elicit these adaptive responses of muscle and connective tissue.[6,7] Increasing resistance linearly increases the intensity of the exercise bout. Generally speaking, the number of repetitions performed in each exercise set decreases as the intensity of the repetitions increases.[145,147]

Resistance training programs designed for strength gains call for intensities ranging from 35% to 80% of 1 RM, depending upon the training status of the individual.[48,145] The intensity advocated to increase strength in healthy adults corresponds with resistance intensities allowing 8 to 12 repetitions.[7] However, rehabilitation intensity must also accommodate healing tissue to avoid reactive inflammation.[41] Rehabilitation programs incorporating resistance exercise must begin with relatively less weight to accommodate the fragility of healing tissue. The lower weight and higher repetitions improve local muscular endurance to a greater extent than muscular strength, but after the program is underway, an increase in exercise intensity (higher weight and lower number of repetitions) increases the rate of strength gain.[7]

Cardiovascular Condition

Cardiovascular condition improves when the intensity of the exercise bout is equal to 60% to 90% of the maximum heart rate for trained individuals and 35% to 45% for relatively untrained individuals.[6] Barring contraindications from affected limb impairment, athletes should exercise at intensities appropriate to maintain cardiovascular condition during rehabilitation.

Duration

The duration of an exercise bout, or rehabilitation session, pertains to the time that an athlete spends in an exercise or rehabilitation session. Similar yet technically different, the duration of exercise is the amount of time the athlete spends performing a specific mode of exercise. This includes the number of repetitions and the time spent performing the repetition during a resistance-training bout. As previously discussed, duration inversely interacts with the intensity of the exercise bout. Generally, duration increases as intensity decreases and vice versa.

Exercise duration necessary to improve cardiovascular conditioning during continuous exercise generally ranges from 20 to 60 minutes.[6] This is adjusted according to the intensity of the exercise bout, which is influenced by the integrity of healing tissue. It may be necessary for the athlete to perform several bouts of shorter duration (approximately 10 minutes) early in the rehabilitation program and gradually increase duration as tolerated.[6]

The duration of the entire rehabilitation program relates to how long it will take the athlete to return to full (100%) activity. Obviously, one of the major factors affecting duration of rehabilitation programs is the individual healing rates of the injured tissue, which vary with the specific tissue type (see Table 7-1 and Chapter 2). Other factors affecting the duration of the rehabilitation program include the athlete's compliance, the number of incidences exacerbating inflammation, and the severity of tissue reinjury.

Frequency

Frequency refers to the number of exercise bouts within a given period of time (usually per day or week). Frequency is interdependent upon intensity and duration of exercise.[6] Recovery time, or the time between exercise bouts, increases concomitantly with increases in intensity and duration. Therefore, exercise performed more often must be of an appropriate intensity to allow adequate recovery.[146]

Muscle strengthening responds best at 2 to 4 days per week of resistance training in healthy individuals.[7] The training status of the individual largely determines the frequency of the bouts; less trained individuals need less frequent sessions to see improvement whereas highly trained individuals have a better response with more frequent sessions.[7] However, this principle applies mostly to healthy individuals capable of sustaining intensities not yet tolerated by individuals undergoing rehabilitation.

Dickinson and Bennett[41] reported that exercise performed twice daily in the early phases of rehabilitation yields a greater improvement in strength than exercise performed once per day. When the athlete is in the early phases of rehabilitation, an exercise routine can be implemented twice daily (Fig. 7-6).[66] With the use of this concept, the athlete's performance should be monitored, and a reduction in exercise may be needed occasionally. As the athlete's condition improves and comes closer to the final goal, a once-daily exercise program should be sufficient. This usually corresponds to a change in the PRE schedule toward increased resistance, lower repetitions, and advancement toward functional activities. The reduction in routine should be instituted for two reasons: it helps minimize the athlete's chances of becoming bored and discontented with the program, and no reports have noted that exercising isotonically during advanced phases more than once a day produces any significant physical benefits.[66] When the athlete returns to participation he or she can advance to a once- or twice-weekly program for maintenance. It is important that the athlete continue a rehabilitation maintenance program during the season, particularly if the regular weight-room regimen does not specifically address the appropriate muscle groups or necessary movements.

The frequency advocated for improving cardiovascular function varies according to the training level, or functional capacity, of the individual. Frequencies range from 1 to 2 times per day for low-intensity and short-duration exercise up to 3 to 5 times per week for higher-intensity or long-duration exercise.[6,7]

Speed and Specificity

Speed or velocity refers to the rate at which the exercise is performed. The exercises should be performed in a slow and deliberate manner, with emphasis placed on concentric and eccentric contractions. The athlete should pause at the end of the exercise and should exercise through the full range of motion that is allowed, avoiding jerky movements.

In the late stages of rehabilitation, the exercise speed should be varied. Traditional PRE exercises are performed at a rate of about 60° per second, a speed that is not functional for attempts to return athletes to their sports.[30] For example, a pitcher's throwing arm travels at approximately 7000° per second.[90] Thus, the continuation of a PRE program as the only tool in restoring this baseball pitcher to function does not prepare him or her for the great demands placed on the throwing arm on return to competition. As Costill and associates[29] have noted, it is important to vary the type and speed of the exercise. Surgical tubing can be used to implement a high-speed regimen to produce a concentric or eccentric synergist pattern, and isokinetic units at the highest speeds on the spectrum can also be used.

There is a specific response to the type of exercise performed.[124,147] As previously discussed, the exercise program must be tailored to meet the specific needs of the individual. Activities or exercises that simulate part of the athlete's activity are ideal for this aspect of rehabilitation and ultimately, the athlete should progressively perform sport-specific activities.[103] For example, a baseball pitcher should progressively return to throwing using a progressive throwing program.[156,158] Thus, the mode of exercise is important to consider, especially during late phases of rehabilitation.

Rest and Recovery

The body needs time to recover from the stresses encountered during exercise. Relative recovery occurs in the rest periods between exercise sets. Recovery also occurs between exercise sessions within the same day or between sessions on multiple days of the week.

Longer periods of rest between exercises allow the anaerobic system to recharge.[138,146] Longer periods of rest are periods of time greater than the amount of time spent during an activity, usually 3 to 20 times than that spent during exercise.[133] This allows the athlete to better tolerate exercise performance at high intensities. Coincidentally, it improves anaerobic performance, both in expressions of cardiovascular performance and muscle force production.[138,146]

Shorter rest periods between exercises, equal to 0.5 to 2 times that spent during the exercise bout, do not allow the anaerobic system to recharge, causing the oxidative system to fuel the activity.[133,146] Thus, improvements in aerobic capability and endurance occur with the incorporation of shorter rest periods.

Interval training is an effective conditioning tool that manipulates work-to-rest ratios. Almost any type of repetitive exercise regimen may be manipulated to follow principles of interval training. This includes cardiovascular activities, progressive resistive exercise, and plyometrics.

FUNCTION BASED REHABILITATION

If the rehabilitated athlete cannot perform activities specific to his or her sport upon the completion of the rehabilitation program, it does not matter if the athlete regains normal range of motion and strength, agility, and power. The rehabilitation program would have failed if this were to happen; in fact, although we may have resolved many different problems inherent to the injury, technically we did not rehabilitate the athlete based upon our earlier definition of rehabilitation.

Initial considerations for implementation of a functional progression program revolve around the physical parameters of the athlete's intended activity. This involves an analysis of the demands of specific athletic endeavors, which are assessed for difficulty and complexity of response. The tasks are then placed on a continuum of difficulty with respect to the athlete's status. Overlaps occasionally occur as a particular task is accomplished but still remains in the athlete's program for solidification as the next task is begun. Because there is a motor learning component to performing a specific motor skill, rehabilitation should include activity specific to the athlete's sport.[94] Care should be taken to ensure the blending of task progressions with specific restrictions concerning the nature of the pathologic condition.[74,90,95,117,139]

SUMMARY

- Rehabilitation and physical conditioning are similar processes that evoke physiologic adaptation.
- The goals of rehabilitation are to (1) reverse and or prevent adverse sequelae resulting from immobility or disuse and (2) facilitate tissue healing and avoid excessive stress on immature tissue.
- The general phases of rehabilitation include the acute, subacute (intermediate), and chronic (return-to-sport) phases.
- The neurological system affects rehabilitation in a number of ways. Protective reflexes such as arthrogenic inhibition involuntarily diminish muscular activity. Therefore, the clinician should recognize arthrogenic inhibition as a threat to timely rehabilitation and treat the manifestations of pain, edema, and effusion as potential harbingers of impending muscle inhibition. Furthermore, the clinician should incorporate motor learning and facilitory techniques, such as cross-over education, to maximize recovery rates following injury.
- The types of therapeutic exercise employed during rehabilitation include range of motion, strengthening, proprioceptive, and plyometric.
- Therapeutic exercises may be open- or closed-chain activities during rehabilitation.
- Methods of progressive resistance exercise include the low-resistance, high-repetition method, the DeLorme and Watkins regimen, the Oxford technique, the daily adjustable progressive resistance exercise methods, and the Sanders program.

- Physical conditioning may occur as prehabilitation, which is preventive in nature, or may occur to nonaffected extremities/physiologic systems as an adjunct during rehabilitation.
- Parameters of conditioning and rehabilitation include the intensity, duration, frequency, specificity and the mode of exercise, and the speed of the movement.

REFERENCES

1. Adams, G.R., Hather, B.M., and Dudley, G.A. (1994): Effect of short-term unweighting on human skeletal muscle strength and size. Aviat. Space Environ. Med., 65:116-1121.
2. Albert, M. (1991): Inertial training concepts. *In:* Albert, M. (ed.): Eccentric Muscle Training in Sports and Orthopaedics. New York, Churchill Livingston, pp. 75-97.
3. Albert, M., Hillegas, E., and Spiegel, P. (1994): Muscle torque changes caused by inertial exercise training. J. Orthop. Sports Phys. Ther., 20:254-261.
4. Alfredson, H., Pietila, T., Jonsson, P., and Lorentzon, R. (1998): Heavy-load eccentric calf muscle training for the treatment of chronic Achilles tendinosis. Am. J. Sports Med., 26:360-366.
5. Allman, F.L. (1985): Rehabilitative exercises in sports medicine. Instr. Course Lect., 34:389-392.
6. American College of Sports Medicine. (1995): General principles of exercise prescription. *In:* ACSM's Guidelines for Exercise Testing and Prescription, 5th ed. Baltimore, Williams & Wilkins, pp. 153-176.
7. American College of Sports Medicine. (2002): Position stand: Progression models in resistance training for healthy adults. Med. Sci. Sports Exerc., 34:364-380.
8. American Heritage College Dictionary. (2000): 3rd ed. Boston, Houghton Mifflin, p. 1150.
9. Archontides, C., and J.A. Fazey. (1993): Inter-limb interactions and constraints in the expression of maximum force: A review, some implications, and suggested underlying mechanisms. J. Sports Sci., 11:145-158.
10. Asanuma, H., and Okuda, O. (1962): Effects of transcallosal volleys on pyramidal tract cell activity of cat. J. Neurophysiol., 25:198-208.
11. Bamman, M.M., Clarke, M.S.F., Feeback, D.L., et al. (1998): Impact of resistance exercise during bed rest on skeletal muscle sarcopenia and myosin isoform distribution. J. Appl. Physiol., 84:157-163.
12. Bamman, M.M., Hunter, G.R., Stevens, B.R., et al. (1997): Resistance exercise prevents plantar flexor deconditioning during bed rest. Med. Sci. Sports Exerc., 29: 1462-1468.
13. Bard, C., Paillard, J., Lajoie, Y., et al. (1992): Role of afferent information in the timing of motor commands: A comparative study with a deafferented patient. Neuropsychologica, 30:201-206.
14. Basmajian, J.V. (1970): Re-education of the vastus medialis: A misconception. Arch. Phys. Med. Rehabil., 51:245-247.
15. Basmajian, J.V. (1977): Motor learning and control: A working hypothesis. Arch. Phys. Med. Rehabil., 58:38-41.
16. Berger, R.A. (1982): Applied Exercise Physiology. Philadelphia, Lea & Febiger.
17. Beutler, A.I., Cooper, L.W., Kirkendall, D.T., and Garrett, W.E. (2002): Electromyographic analysis of single-leg, closed chain exercises: Implications for rehabilitation after anterior cruciate ligament reconstruction. J. Athl. Train., 37:13-18.
18. Blackburn, T.A. (1987): Rehabilitation of the shoulder and elbow after arthroscopy. Clin. Sports Med., 6:587-588.
19. Bonica, J. (1990): The Management of Pain. Philadelphia, Lea & Febiger.
20. Bortz, W. (1984): The disuse syndrome. West. J. Med., 141:169.
21. Bunton, E.E., Pitney, W.A., Kane, A.W., et al. (1993): The role of limb torque, muscle action and proprioception during closed kinetic chain rehabilitation of the lower extremity. J. Athl. Train., 28:10-20.
22. Bynum, E.B., Barrack, R.L., and Alexander, A.H. (1995): Open versus closed chain kinetic exercise after anterior cruciate ligament reconstruction. Am. J. Sports Med., 23:401-406.
23. Chandler, T.J., and Kibler, W.B. (1993): Muscle training in injury prevention. *In:* Renstrom, P. (ed.), Sports Injuries: Basic Principles and Care. Oxford, Blackwell, pp. 252-261.
24. Chu, D.A. (1984): Plyometric exercise. Natl. Strength Cond. Assoc. J., 6:56-62.
25. Chu, D.A. (1992): Jumping into Plyometrics. Champaign, IL, Human Kinetics.
26. Cleak, M.J., and Eston, R.G. (1992): Muscle soreness, swelling, stiffness, and strength loss after intense eccentric exercise. Br. J. Sports Med., 26:267-272.
27. Cole A.J., and Herring, S.A.(1997): Lumbar spine pain: Rehabilitation and return to play. *In:* Sallis, R.E., and Massimino, F. (eds.), ACSM's Essentials of Sports Medicine. St. Louis, Mosby, pp. 396-402.
28. Cooper, D.L., and Fair, J. (1976): Reconditioning following athletic injuries. Phys. Sports Med., 4:125-128.
29. Costill, D.L., Fink, W.J., and Habansky, A.J. (1971): Muscle rehabilitation after knee surgery. Phys. Sports Med., 5:71-77.
30. Coyle, E.F., Feiring, D.C., Rotkis, T.C., et al. (1981): Specificity of power improvements through slow and fast isokinetic training. J Appl. Physiol., 51:1437-1442.
31. Cyriax, J. (1982): Textbook of Orthopedic Medicine, Vol.1, Diagnosis of Soft Tissue Lesions, 8th ed. London, Bailliere and Tindall.
32. Dale, R.B., Childress, R., and Riewald, S. (2002): Conditioning during rehabilitation of swimming injuries. *In:* Bourdreau, C., Riewald, S., Sokolovas, G., and Tuffey, S. (eds.), The Science in the Science and Art of Coaching. Colorado Springs, CO, USA Swimming Sport Science.
33. Dale, R.B, Sirikul, B., and Bishop, P.A. (2001): Bilateral indices of knee extensors and flexors in males and females at 1 and 10 RM. J. Athl. Train., 36:S-86.
34. de Andrade, J.R., Grant, C., and Dixon, A.S. (1965): Joint distension and reflex inhibition in the knee. J. Bone Joint Surg. [Am.], 47:313-322.
35. Dean, E. (1988): Physiology and therapeutic implication of negative work. Phys. Ther., 68:233-237.
36. Dedrick, M.E., and Clarkson, P.M. (1990): The effects of eccentric exercise on motor performance in young and older women. Eur. J. Appl. Physiol., 60:183-186.
37. DeLorme, T.L. (1945): Restoration of muscle power by heavy resistance exercise. J. Bone Joint Surg., 27:645-667.
38. DeLorme, T.L., and Watkins, A. (1948): Techniques of progressive resistance exercise. Arch. Phys. Med., 29:263-268.

39. Dennis, J.K., and McKeough, D.M. (1999): Mobility. *In:* May, B.J. (ed.), Home Health and Rehabilitation—Concepts of Care, 2nd ed. Philadelphia, F.A. Davis, pp. 121-123.

40. Dickerman, J. (1992): The use of pain profiles in clinical practice. Fam. Pract. Recertif., 14:35-44.

41. Dickinson, A., and Bennett, K. (1985): Therapeutic exercise. Clin. Sports Med., 4:417-429.

42. Dillman, C.J., Murray, T.A., and Hintermeister, R.A. (1994): Biomechanical differences of open and closed chain exercises with respect to the shoulder. J. Sports Rehabil., 3:228-238.

43. Doheny, M.O. (1993): Mental practice: An alternative approach to teaching motor skills. J. Nurs. Educ., 32:260-264.

44. Ericcsson, K.A., Krampe, R., and Tesch-Romer, C. (1993): The role of deliberate practice in the acquisition of expert performance. Psychol. Rev., 100:363-406.

45. Fahere, H., Rentsch, H.U., and Gerber, N.J. (1988): Knee effusion and reflex inhibition of the quadriceps. J. Bone Joint Surg. [Br.], 70:635-638.

46. Fardy, P. (1981): Isometric exercise and the cardiovascular system. Phys. Sportsmed., 9:43.

47. Fitts, P.M., and Posner, M.I. (1967): Human Performance. Belmont, CA, Brooks/Cole.

48. Fleck, S.J., and Kraemer, W.J. (1987): Designing Resistance Training Programs. Champaign, IL, Human Kinetics.

49. Friedman, M.J., and Nichaolas, J.A. (1984): Conditioning and Rehabilitation. *In:* Scott, W.N., Nisonson, B., and Nichaolas, J.A. (eds.), Principles of Sports Medicine. Baltimore, Williams & Wilkins, pp. 396-402.

50. Gabriele, T., Hall, C.R., and Lee, T.D. (1989): Cognition in motor learning: Imagery effects on contextual interference. Hum. Mov. Sci., 8:227-245.

51. Gardner, E. (1948): The innervation of the knee joint. Anat. Rec., 101:109-130.

52. Gentile, A.M. (1972): A working model of skill acquisition with application to teaching. Quest Monogr., 17:3-23.

53. Gentile, A.M. (1987): Skill acquisition: Action, movement, and the neuromotor processes. *In:* Carr, J.H., Shepherd, R.B., Gordon, J., et al. (eds.), Movement Science: Foundations for Physical Therapy in Rehabilitation. Rockville, MD, Aspen, pp. 93-154.

54. Giallonardo, L. (2001): Clinical decision making in rehabilitation. *In:* Prentice, W.E., and Voight, M.I. (eds.), Techniques in Musculoskeletal Rehabilitation. New York, McGraw-Hill.

55. Gieck, J.H., and Saliba, E.N. (1988): The athletic trainer and rehabilitation. *In:* The Injured Athlete, 2nd ed. Philadelphia, J.B. Lippincott, pp. 165-239.

56. Gouvier, W.D. (1987): Assessment and treatment of cognitive deficits in brain-damaged individuals. Behav. Modif., 11:312-328.

57. Graham, V.L., Gehlsen, G.M., and Edwards, J.A. (1993): Electromyographic evaluation of closed and open kinetic chain knee rehabilitation exercises. Athl. Train., 28:23-30.

58. Gross, M.T. (1987): Effects of recurrent lateral ankle sprains on active and passive judgments of joint position. Phys. Ther., 67:1505-1509.

59. Guyton, A.C. (1991): Basic Neuroscience: Anatomy and Physiology, 2nd ed. Philadelphia, W.B. Saunders.

60. Halata, F., Rettig, T., and Schulze, W. (1985): The ultrastructure of sensory nerve endings in the human knee joint capsule. Anat. Embryol., 172:265-275.

61. Harter, R.A. (1996): Clinical rationale for closed kinetic chain activities in functional testing and rehabilitation of ankle pathologies. J. Sports Rehabil., 5:13-24.

62. Harter, R.A., Osternig, L.O., and Singer, K.M. (1992): Knee joint proprioception following anterior cruciate ligament reconstruction. J. Sports Rehabil., 1:103-110.

63. Hellebrandt, F.A. (1951): Physiological bases of progressive resistance exercise. *In:* DeLorme, T.L., and Watkins, A.L. (eds.), Progressive Resistance Exercise. New York, Appleton-Century-Crofts.

64. Hilton, J. (1863): On the Influence of Mechanical and Physiological Rest in the Treatment of Accidents and Surgical Diseases, and the Diagnostic Value of Pain: A Course of Lectures. London, Bell and Daldy.

65. Hobbel, S.L., and Rose, D.J. (1993): The relative effectiveness of three forms of visual knowledge of results on peak torque output. J. Orthop. Sports Phys. Ther., 18: 601-608.

66. Houglum, P. (1977): The modality of therapeutic exercise: Objectives and principles. Athl. Train., 12:42-45.

67. Houglum, P. (1992): Soft tissue healing and its impact on rehabilitation. J. Sports Rehabil., 1:19-39.

68. Houglum, P. (2001): Muscle strength and endurance. *In:* Houglum, P. (ed.), Therapeutic Exercise for Athletic Injuries. Champaign, IL, Human Kinetics, pp. 203-265.

69. Hughston, J.C. (1980): Knee surgery: A philosophy. Am. Phys. Ther., 60:1611-1614.

70. Iles, J.F., Stokes, M., and Young, A. (1990): Reflex actions of knee joint afferents during contraction of the human quadriceps. Clin. Physiol., 10:489-500.

71. Irrgang, J.J. (1995): Rehabilitation. *In:* Fu, F.H., and Stone, D. (eds.), Sports Injuries: Mechanisms, Prevention, Treatment. Baltimore, Williams & Wilkins.

72. Jimmy, M.L. (1988): Mechanoreceptors in articular tissues. Am. J. Anat., 182:16-32.

73. Kannus, P., Alosa, D., Cook, L., et al. (1992): Effect of one-legged exercise on the strength, power and endurance of the contralateral leg. A randomized, controlled study using isometric and concentric isokinetic training. Eur. J. Appl. Physiol. Occup. Physiol., 6:117-126.

74. Kegerreis, S. (1983): The construction and implementation of functional progressions as a component of athletic rehabilitation. J. Orthop. Sports Phys. Ther., 5:14-19.

75. Kellett J., (1986): Acute soft tissue injuries—A review of the literature. Med. Sci. Sports Exerc., 18:489-500.

76. Kennedy, J.C., Alexander, I.J., and Hayes, K.C. (1982): Nerve supply of the human knee and its functional importance. Am. J. Sports Med., 10:329-335.

77. Keskula, D.R. (1996): Clinical implications of eccentric exercise in sports medicine. J. Sports Rehabil., 5:321-329.

78. Kibler, W.B., and Chandler, T.J. (1993): Preparticipation evaluations. *In:* Renstrom, P. (ed.), Sports Injuries: Basic Principles of Prevention and Care. Oxford, Blackwell, pp. 223-241.

79. Kibler, W.B., and Chandler, T.J. (1994): Sport-specific conditioning. Am. J. Sports Med., 22:424-432.

80. Kibler, W.B., Chandler, T.J., and Uhl, T.L. (1989): A musculoskeletal approach to the preparticipation physical examination. Am. J. Sports Med. 17:525-531.

81. Kibler, W.B., and Safran, M.R. (2000): Pediatric and adolescent sports injuries. Clin. Sports Med., 19:781-792.

82. Kisner, C., and Colby, L.A. (2002): Therapeutic Exercise: Foundations and Techniques, 4th ed. Philadephia, F.A. Davis.

83. Knight, K.L. (1979): Rehabilitating chondromalacia patellae. Physician Sportsmed., 7:147-148.

84. Knight, K.L. (1985): Guidelines for rehabilitation of sports injuries. Clin. Sports Med., 4:405-416.

85. Knight, K.L. (1995): Cryotherapy in Sports Injury Management. Champaign, IL, Human Kinetics, p. 11.

86. Kraemer, W.J. (1994): General adaptations to resistance and endurance training programs. In: Baechle, T.R. (ed.), Essentials of Strengthening and Conditioning. Champaign, IL, Human Kinetics, pp. 127-150.

87. Kreighbaum, E., and Barthels, K.M. (1996): Biomechanics: A Qualitative Approach for Studying Human Movement, 4th ed. Boston, Allyn & Bacon.

88. Lee, T.D., Swanson, L.R., and Hall, A.L. (1991): What is repeated in a repetition? Effects of practice conditions on motor skill acquisition. Phys Ther., 71:150-156.

89. Lephart, S.M., and Henry, T.J. (1995): Functional rehabilitation for the upper and lower extremity. Orthop. Clin. North Am., 26:579-592.

90. Lephart, S.M., and Henry, T.J. (1996): The physiological basis for open and closed kinetic chain rehabilitation for the upper extremity. J. Sports Rehabil., 5:77.

91. Lephart, S.M., Kocher, M.S., Fu, F.H., et al. (1992): Proprioception following anterior cruciate ligament reconstruction. J. Sports Rehabil., 1:188-196.

92. Levitt, R., Deisinger, J.A., Remondet, W.J., et al. (1995): EMG feedback-assisted postoperative rehabilitation of minor arthroscopic knee surgeries. J. Sports Med. Phys. Fitness, 35:218-223.

93. MacDougal, J., McKelvie, R.S., Moroz, D.E., et al. (1992): Factors affecting blood pressure during heavy weight lifting and static contractions. J. Appl. Physiol., 73:1590-1597.

94. Magill, R.A. (1998): Motor Learning: Concepts and Applications, 5th ed. Boston, McGraw-Hill.

95. Mandelbaum, B.R., Myerson, M.S., and Forster, R. (1995): Achilles tendon rupture: A new method of repair, early range of motion, and functional rehabilitation. Am. J. Sports Med., 23:392-395.

96. Mannheimer, J.S., and Lampe, G.N. (1984): Clinical Transcutaneous Electrical Nerve Stimulation. Philadelphia, F.A. Davis.

97. Maring, J.R. (1990): Effects of mental practice on rate of skill acquisition. Phys Ther., 70:165-172.

98. Marino, M. (1986): Current concepts of rehabilitation in sports medicine: Research and clinical interrelationship. In: Nicholas, J.A., and Hershman, E.D. (eds.), The Lower Extremity in Sports Medicine. St. Louis, C.V. Mosby, pp. 126-128.

99. Matsen, F.A., Harryman, D.T., and Sidles, J.A. (1991): Mechanics of glenohumeral instability. Clin. Sports Med., 10:783-788.

100. McArdle, W.D., Katch, F.I., and Katch, V.L. (2001): Muscular strength: Training muscles to become stronger. In: McArdle, W.D., Katch, F.I., and Katch, V.L., (eds.), Exercise Physiology: Energy, Nutrition, and Human Performance, 5th ed. Baltimore, Williams & Wilkins, pp. 501-547.

101. McBride, E., and Rothstein, A. (1979): Mental and physical practice and the learning and retention of open and closed motor skills. Percept. Mot. Skills, 49:359-365.

102. McCarthy, M.R., Yates, C.K., Anderson, M.A., et al. (1993): The effects of immediate continuous passive motion on pain during the inflammatory phase of soft tissue healing following anterior cruciate ligament reconstruction. J. Orthop. Sports Phys. Ther., 17:96-101.

103. Morrissey, M.C., Harman, E.A., and Johnson, M.J. (1995): Resistance training modes: Specificity and effectiveness. Med. Sci. Sports Exerc., 27:648-660.

104. Moss, C.L., and Grimmer, S. (1993): Strength and contractile adaptations in the human triceps surae after isotonic exercise. J. Sports Rehabil., 2:104-114.

105. Mulder, T. (1991): A process-oriented model of human motor behavior: Toward a theory-based rehabilitation approach. Phys Ther., 71:157-164.

106. Nagel, M.J., and Rice, M.S. (2001): Cross-transfer effects in the upper extremity during an occupationally embedded exercise. Am. J. Occup. Ther., 55:317-323.

107. Naylor, J., and Briggs, G. (1963): Effects of task complexity and task organization on the relative efficiency of part and whole training methods. J. Exp. Psychol., 65:217-244.

108. Newell, K.M., Sparrow, W.A., and Quinn, J.T. (1985): Kinetic information feedback for learning isometric tasks. J. Hum. Mov. Studies, 11:113-123.

109. Nicholson, D.E. (1997): Teaching psychomotor skills. In: Shepard, K.F., and Jensen, G.M. (eds.), Handbook of Teaching for Physical Therapists. Boston, Butterworth-Heinemann, p. 271.

110. Noble, R.M., Linder, M., Janssen, E., et al. (1997): Prehabilitation exercises for the lower extremities. Strength Cond., 19:25-33.

111. Norkin, C., and Levangie, P. (2001): Joint Structure and Function: A Comprehensive Analysis, 3rd ed. Philadelphia, F.A. Davis.

112. Noyes, F.R. (1977): Functional properties of knee ligaments and alterations induced by immobilization. Clin. Orthop., 123:210-242.

113. Noyes, F.R., Mangine, R.E., and Barber, S. (1987): Early knee motion after open and arthroscopic anterior cruciate ligament reconstruction. Am. J. Sports Med., 15:149-160.

114. Nyland, J., Brosky, T., Currier, D., et al. (1994): Review of the afferent neural system of the knee and its contribution to motor learning. J. Orthop. Sports Phys. Ther., 19:2-11.

115. O'Hagan, F.T., Sale, D.G., MacDougall, J.D., and Garner, S.H. (1995): Comparative effectiveness of accommodating and weight resistance training modes. Med. Sci. Sports Exerc., 27: 1210-1219

116. Prentice, W.E. (2001): Open versus closed kinetic chain exercise in rehabilitation. In: Prentice, W.E., and Voight, M.I. (eds.), Techniques in Musculoskeletal Rehabilitation. New York, McGraw-Hill, pp. 179-195.

117. Reider, B., Sathy, M.R., Talkington, J., et al. (1993): Treatment of isolated medial collateral ligament injuries in athletes with early functional rehabilitation. Am. J. Sports Med., 22:470-477.

118. Reuleaux, F. (1875): Theoretische Kinematic: Grundigeiner Theorie des Maschinenwessens [The Kinematic Theory of Machinery: Outline of a Theory of Machines]. Braunschweig, I.F., Vieweg und Sohn. Kennedy, L.E., (trans.). London, Macmillan.

119. Sanders, M. (1990): Weight training and conditioning. In: Sanders, B. (ed.), Sports Physical Therapy. Norwalk, CT, Appleton & Lange, pp. 239-250.

120. Schmidt R.A., and Lee, T.D. (1999): Motor control and Learning: A Behavioral Emphasis, 3rd ed. Champaign, IL, Human Kinetics.

121. Schram, D.A., and Bennett, R.L. (1951): Underwater resistance exercise. Arch. Phys. Med., 32:222-226.

122. Schultz, R.A., Miller, D.C., and Kerr, C.S. (1984): Mechanoreceptors in human cruciate ligament: A histological study. J. Bone Joint Surg. [Am.], 69:1072-1076.

123. Schutte, M.J., Dabezies, E.J., and Zimny, M.L. (1987): Neural anatomy of the human anterior cruciate ligament. J. Bone Joint Surg. [Am.], 69:243-247.

124. Selye, H. (1978): The Stress of Life, rev. ed. New York, McGraw-Hill.

125. Sforzo, G.A., and Touey, P.R. (1996): Manipulating exercise order affects muscular performance during a resistance exercise training session. J. Strength Cond. Res. 10:20-24.

126. Sherrington, C.S. (1906): On the proprioceptive system, especially in its reflex aspects. Brain, 29:467-479.

127. Snyder-Mackler, L. (1996): Scientific rationale and physiological basis for the use of closed kinetic chain exercise in the lower extremity. J. Sports Rehabil., 5:2-12.

128. Sprenger, C.K., Carlson, K., and Wessman, H.C. (1979): Application of electromyographical biofeedback following medial meniscectomy. Phys Ther. 59:167-169.

129. Stanish, W.D., Rubinovich, R.M., and Curwin, S. (1986): Eccentric exercise in chronic tendonitis. Clin. Orthop. 208:65-68.

130. Steindler, A. (1955): Kinesiology of the Human Body. Springfield, IL, Charles C Thomas.

131. Steindler, A. (1970): Kinesiology of the Human Body under Normal and Pathological Conditions. Springfield, IL, Charles C Thomas.

132. Stone, J.A., Partin, N.B., Lueken, J.S., et al. (1994): Upper extremity proprioceptive training. J. Athl. Train., 29:15-18.

133. Stone, M.H., and Conley, M.S. (1994): Bioenergetics. In: Baechle, T.R. (ed.), Essentials of Strengthening and Conditioning. Champaign, IL, Human Kinetics, pp. 67-85.

134. Stromberg, B.V. (1986): Contralateral therapy in upper extremity rehabilitation. Am. J. Phys. Med., 65:135-143.

135. Stromberg, B.V. (1988): Influence of cross-education training in postoperative hand therapy. South. Med. J., 81:989-991.

136. Sullivan, S.B., and Schmidtz, T.J. (1988): Strategies to improve motor control. In: Sullivan, S.B., and Schmidtz, T.J., (eds.), Physical Rehabilitation: Assessment and Treatment, 2nd ed. Philadelphia, F.A Davis, pp. 269-274.

137. Taber's Cyclopedic Medical Dictionary. (1993): 17th ed. Philadelphia, F.A. Davis.

138. Tesch, P., and Larson, L. (1982): Muscle hypertrophy in body builders. Eur. J. Appl. Physiol., 49:301-306.

139. Tippett, S.R., and Voight, M.L. (1995): Functional Progressions for Sports Rehabilitation. Champaign, IL, Human Kinetics, pp. 3-18.

140. Tracy, J.E., Obuchi, S., and Johnson, B. (1995): Kinematic and electromyographic analysis of elbow flexion during inertial exercise. J. Athl. Train., 30:254-258.

141. Tsang, K.K.W., Hertel, J., Denegar, C.R., et al. (2002): The effects of induced effusion of the ankle on EMG activity of the lower leg muscles. J. Athl. Train., 37:S-25.

142. Uhl, T.L., and Madaleno, J.A. (2001): Rehabilitation concepts and supportive devices for overuse injuries of the upper extremities. Clin. Sports Med., 20:621-639.

143. Voight, M.L, and Draovitch, P. (1991): Plyometrics. In: Albert, M. (ed.), Eccentric Muscle Training in Sports and Orthopaedics. New York, Churchill Livingstone, pp. 45-73.

144. Wallis, E.L., and Logan, G.A. (1964): Figure Improvement and Body Composition Through Exercise. Englewood Cliffs, NJ, Prentice-Hall.

145. Wathen, D. (1994): Load assignment. In: Baechle, T.R. (ed.), Essentials of Strengthening and Conditioning. Champaign, IL, Human Kinetics, pp. 435-446.

146. Wathen, D. (1994): Rest periods. In: Baechle, T.R. (ed.), Essentials of Strengthening and Conditioning. Champaign, IL, Human Kinetics, pp. 447-450.

147. Wathen, D., and Roll, F. (1994): Training methods and modes. In: Baechle, T.R. (ed.), Essentials of Strengthening and Conditioning. Champaign, IL, Human Kinetics, pp. 403-415.

148. Wawrzyniak, J., Tracy, J., and Catizone, P. (1996): Effect of closed chain exercise on quadriceps femoris peak torque and functional performance. J. Athl. Train., 31:335-345.

149. Weber, M.D., Servedio, F.J., and Woodall, W.R. (1994): Effect of three modalities on delayed onset muscle soreness. J. Orthop. Sports Phys. Ther., 20:236-242.

150. Weir, P.L., and Leavitt, J.L. (1990): The effects of model's skill level and model's knowledge of results on the performance of a dart throwing task. Hum. Mov. Sci. 9:369-383.

151. Welch, B. (1986): The injury cycle. Sports Med. Update, 1:1.

152. Wigerstad-Lossing, I., Grimby, G., and Jonsson, T. (1988): Effects of electrical muscle stimulation combined with voluntary contractions after knee ligament surgery. Med. Sci. Sports Exerc., 20:93-98.

153. Wilk, K.E. (1990): Plyometrics for the upper extremity. In: Advances on Shoulder and Knee Symposium. Cincinnati, OH, Cincinnati Sportsmedicine and Deaconess Hospital.

154. Wilk, K.E., and Andrews, J.R. (1993): Current concepts in the treatment of anterior cruciate ligament disruption. J. Orthop. Sports Phys. Ther., 15:279-293.

155. Wilk, K.E., and Arrigo, C. (1993): Current concepts in the rehabilitation of the athletic shoulder. J. Orthop. Sports Phys. Ther., 18:365-378.

156. Wilk, K.E., Arrigo, C., and Andrews, J.R. (1993): Rehabilitation of the elbow in the throwing athlete. J. Orthop. Sports Phys. Ther., 17:305-317.

157. Wilk, K.E., Arrigo, C.A., and Andrews, J.R. (1996): Closed and open kinetic chain exercise for the upper extremity. J. Sports Rehabil., 5:88-102.

158. Wilk, K.E., Meister, K., and Andrews, J.R. (2002): Current concepts in the rehabilitation of the overhead throwing athlete. Am. J. Sports Med., 30:136-151.

159. Wilk, K.E., Voight, M.L., Keirns, M.A., et al. (1993): Stretch-shortening drills for the upper extremities: Theory and clinical application. J. Orthop. Sports Phys. Ther., 17:225-239.

160. Wilmore, J.H. (1976): Athletic Training and Physical Fitness. Boston, Allyn & Bacon.

161. Wilson, B. (1989): Models of cognitive rehabilitation. In: Wood, R.L., and Eames, P. (eds.), Models of Brain Injury. London, Chapman & Hall, pp. 117-142.

162. Winstein, C.J. (1991): Knowledge of results and motor learning-implications for physical therapy. Phys Ther. 71:140-149.

163. Woo, S. (1986): Biomechanics of tendons and ligaments. In: Fund, Y.C. (ed.), Frontiers in Biomechanics. New York, Schmid-Schonbein, pp. 180-195.

164. Wrisberg, C.A., and Liu, Z. (1991): The effect of contextual variety on the practice, retention, and transfer of an applied motor skill. Res. Q. Exerc. Sport, 62:406-411.

165. Yack, H.J., Collins, C.E., and Whieldon, T.J. (1993): Comparison of closed and open kinetic chain exercise in the anterior cruciate ligament-deficient knee. Am. J. Sports Med., 21:49-54.

166. Yoo, E., Park E., and Chung, B. (2001): Mental practice effect on line-tracing accuracy in persons with hemiparetic stroke: A preliminary study. Arch. Phys. Med. Rehabil., 82:1213-1218.

167. Young, A. (1993): Current issues in arthrogenous inhibition. Ann. Rheumatol. Dis., 52:829-834.

168. Zinovieff, A.N. (1951): Heavy resistance exercise: The Oxford technique. Br. J. Phys. Med., 14:129-132.

169. Zohn, D., and Mennell, J. (1976): Musculoskeletal Pain: Principles of Physical Diagnosis and Physical Treatment. Boston, Little, Brown.

CHAPTER 8

PROPRIOCEPTION AND NEUROMUSCULAR CONTROL

Todd S. Ellenbecker, M.S., P.T., S.C.S., O.C.S., C.S.C.S.
Jake Bleacher, M.S., P.T., C.S.C.S.

CHAPTER OBJECTIVES

At the end of this chapter the reader will be able to:

- Define proprioception, kinesthesia, and other related aspects using terminology consistent with expanded classical definitions contained in this chapter.
- Identify the different types and functions of mechanoreceptors in the upper and lower extremities.
- List and describe clinical measurements for proprioception and kinesthesia in the upper and lower extremities.
- Identify factors that affect diminished proprioception and the effects of injury and disuse and aging on neuromuscular control and joint stability in the upper and lower extremities.
- Design and implement progressive proprioception training programs that meet the functional demands of the patient and are appropriate for the patient's level of skill and recovery when returning from an upper or lower extremity injury.

Human beings are unique in their capacity to propel themselves through their environment in an upright posture. This is achieved through a complex interaction of lower limb muscle activity coordinated by the central nervous system (CNS). To maintain balance and postural control we rely on sensory information from the periphery from our visual, vestibular, and somatosensory systems. The nervous system integrates this peripheral afferent information to maintain postural control during stance.

The control of locomotion, including walking or running, occurs through complex neural pathways in the spinal cord called central pattern generators or limb controllers. These motor programs for locomotion are automatic but are modulated by the CNS through feedback and feedforward mechanisms. The feedforward mecha-nism operates on the premise of initiating a motor response in anticipation of a load or activity, which will disrupt the integrity of a joint, and gauges the response from previous experiences. In contrast, the feedback system operates directly in response to a potentially destabilizing event, using a normal reference point to monitor the necessary muscle activity to restore homeostasis.[107]

Both feedback and feedforward systems rely on the processing of afferent information from the periphery at different levels of the CNS (spinal cord, brain stem and cerebellum, and cerebral cortex) with the end result being coordinated muscle activity during movement to maintain joint stability.[107] The motor response varies depending on joint position, force type, direction of force, and which higher center predominates with information processing.

Segmental spinal reflexes involve the processing of afferent input between peripheral receptors in the muscle spindle and Golgi tendon organs at the musculotendinous junction with the efferent output of the α motor neurons in the ventral horn of the spinal cord. On the most basic level the monosynaptic reflexes produce excitatory or inhibitory efferent motor response to the stimulus received from the periphery. Along with the physiologic properties of the muscle itself (length/tension curve) these peripheral receptors potentially assist with modulating muscle stiffness with muscle tension varying based on the amount of afferent input.[107]

Afferent information received in the cortical area of the brain from peripheral mechanoreceptors produces voluntary motor response to potential disturbances in functional joint stability. The latency of the response is usually greater than 120 msec and longer sometimes, depending on the amount of information in the environment being processed. In addition to the response to an environmental stimulus, the potential exists for a theorized motor program operating under the assumption that the individual components of performing skilled movements, such as swinging a bat, that require sequential steps would be difficult to enact successfully without having a

189

preprogrammed set of instructions to optimize efficiency, speed, and coordinated muscle activity.[59]

The function of the cerebellum and brain stem is to integrate peripheral feedback from the environment with the motor commands from the cerebral cortex to enable humans to perform skilled and coordinated movement. The action of these neural centers allows for necessary adjustments to carry out an intended motor skill with precision and efficiency.[59]

DEFINITIONS

A review of the orthopaedic and musculoskeletal rehabilitation literature identifies many different versions of definitions for the terms associated with joint proprioception and neuromuscular control. In *Goetz's Textbook of Clinical Neurology,* proprioception is defined as any postural, positional, or kinetic information provided to the CNS by sensory receptors in muscles, tendons, joints, or skin.[40] Other texts define proprioception as "awareness of the position and movements of our limbs, fingers, and toes derived from receptors in the muscles, tendons and joints."[1] Sherrington's classical definition of proprioception is "afferent information arising from the proprioceptive field, and identified mechanoreceptors or proprioceptors as being the source of the origination or this afferent information."[87]

These original definitions of the term *proprioception* continue to be used today; however a more advanced definition of the sensory functions that encompass human proprioceptive function is clearly needed. In a classic monograph entitled *Physiologie des Muskelsinnes,* Goldsheider[42] proposed that muscle sense be divided into four distinct and separate sensory functions. These functions were described as sensation of passive movements, sensation of active movements, sensation of position, and appreciation or sensation of heaviness and resistance. These original classifications or definitions have been expanded upon to decrease confusion. The sensation of passive movements is considered to be a product of sensations induced by external forces, which result in a change in limb position with noncontracting muscles. The sensation of active movement (or *kinesthesia* as it is now better known) encompasses the appreciation of change in position of a limb with contracting muscles. The appreciation

of the position of a limb in space has been termed *stagnosia,* and, lastly in the presence of tension, the appreciation of force applied during a voluntary contraction has been termed *dynamaesthesia.*[84] Although these expanded definitions found in the classic literature provide additional information about human proprioception, adaptations of these classic definitions have been suggested and will be used for the purposes of this chapter (Table 8-1).

AFFERENT NEUROBIOLOGY OF THE JOINT

Early discussions of afferent proprioceptive function of the human joint included investigations into the role of joint- and muscle-based afferent receptors in human active and passive movement and joint position detection.[84] Goldsheider, in 1898, proposed that sensation of passive movements was solely the product of joint-based receptors. This view is still widely accepted today for passive movements.[42,84]

The view up until the 1970s about sensory feedback of active human movements was that, once voluntary movement was initiated by the cerebral cortex, only low-level control was presented by the receptors in the muscles and tendons. This sensory information from the muscles and tendons yielded information to the spinal cord and some subcortical extrapyramidal parts of the brain such as the cerebellum, but played no contributing role in conscious sensation, which remained in the province of the joint receptors.[84] In the early 1970s, however, important research by Goodwin and colleagues[43] and Eklund[27] independently demonstrated the important role that muscular receptors play in contributing to sensations of active movement qualitatively. This section of the chapter will focus on both the joint- and muscle-based afferent receptors to allow the clinician a more complete understanding of the sources of afferent information in the human body. This will later lead to a greater understanding of how specific treatment strategies can be used clinically to improve proprioceptive and neuromuscular function in both upper and lower extremity rehabilitation.

Afferent Mechanoreceptor Classification

Mechanoreceptors are sensory neurons or peripheral afferents located with joint capsular tissues, ligaments,

---

Table 8-1

Definitions of Proprioception and Associated Functions in Humans

Proprioception: Afferent information including joint position sense, kinesthesia, and sensation of resistance
Joint position sense: The ability to recognize joint position in space
Kinesthesia: The ability to appreciate and recognize joint movement or motion
Sensation of resistance: The ability to appreciate and recognize force generated within a joint
Neuromuscular control: appropriate efferent responses to afferent proprioceptive input

tendons, muscle, and skin.[44,108] Deformation or stimulation of the tissues in which the mechanoreceptors lie produces a gated release of sodium, eliciting an action potential.[70] Four primary types of afferent mechanoreceptors have been classified and are commonly present in noncontractile capsular and ligamentous structures in human joints (Table 8-2).

Type I articular receptors are traditionally globular or ovoid corpuscles with a very thin capsule. They are numerous in the capsular tissues in all the limb joints, as well as the apophyseal joints of the vertebral column. Wyke[108] reported that the population of type I receptors appears to be more dense in proximal joints than in distal joints. Type I receptors are typically located in the superficial layers of the joint capsule.

Physiologically, type I receptors are low-threshold, slowly adapting mechanoreceptors. A proportion of the type I receptors are always active in every joint position.[108] The resting discharge of the type I receptors allows the body to know where the limb is placed and receive constant output on limb position in virtually any joint position. The type I receptor is categorized as both a static and dynamic mechanoreceptor,[108] whose discharge pattern signals static joint position, intra-articular pressure changes, and the direction, amplitude, and velocity of joint movements.

Type II mechanoreceptors are elongated, conical corpuscles with thick multilaminated connective tissue capsules. These type II corpuscles are present in the fibrous capsules of all joints but are reported to be present in greater number in distal joints than in proximal joints.[107] Type II corpuscles are located in the deeper layers of the fibrous joint capsule, particularly at the border between the fibrous capsule and the subsynovial fibroadipose tissue, often alongside articular blood vessels. Type II mechanoreceptors are low-threshold, rapidly adapting receptors and are reported to be entirely inactive in immobile joints.[108] These receptors become activated for very brief moments (1 second or less), at the onset of joint movement. The type II receptor is considered to be a dynamic mechanoreceptor whose brief, high-velocity discharges signal joint acceleration and deceleration with both active and passive joint movements.

The type I and type II mechanoreceptors described in the preceding paragraphs are the primary receptors located in the joint capsule. Type III receptors are primarily confined to the joint ligamentous structures. These type III receptors are found in both intrinsic and extrinsic ligamentous structures[108] and are similar in nature to the Golgi tendon organs found in tendons, which will be discussed in later sections of this chapter. Type III receptors are predominantly found in the superficial surfaces of the joint ligaments, near their bony attachments. Research delineating the type III mechanoreceptor classifies this receptor as a high-threshold, slowly adapting structure, again similar in nature to the Golgi tendon organ. These type III receptors are completely inactive in immobile joints and only become active or stimulated toward the extreme ends of joint ranges of motion where the ligamentous structures become taut. When considerable stress is generated in the joint ligaments, the type III receptor will become actively stimulated. Wyke[109] also reported that the type III receptors become activated with longitudinal traction to the limbs; the receptors remain activated centripitally at a high velocity only if extreme joint displacement or joint traction is maintained.

The final joint receptor to be discussed in this section is the type IV receptor. These receptors are noncorpuscular, unlike type I, II, and III receptors and are represented by plexuses of small unmyelinated nerve fibers or free nerve endings. Type IV receptors are typically distributed throughout the fibrous joint capsule, adjacent periosteum, and articular fat pads. The type IV receptor represents the pain receptor system or articular tissues and is entirely inactive in normal circumstances. Marked mechanical deformation or chemical irritation such as exposure of the nerve endings to agents such as histamine, bradykinin, and

Table 8-2

Mechanoreceptor Classification in the Human Body

Type	Location	Threshold	Response	Active
I	Superficial joint capsule Limbs and vertebrae Greater density proximal joints	Low	Slow adapting	Always Static/dynamic
II	Deeper layers of joint capsule Greater density distal joints	Low	Rapidly adapting	Dynamic only
III	Superficial surface of joint Ligament	High	Slowly adapting	Dynamic end range movements Joint traction
IV	Joint capsule, adjacent periosteum Articular fat pads			Not active in normal circumstances

other inflammatory exudates produced by damaged or necrosing tissues can stimulate activation of the type IV receptor.[71,108,109]

AFFERENT MECHANORECEPTORS IN THE LOWER EXTREMITY

The distribution of afferent articular nerves in synovial joints consists of medium and large myelinated fibers innervating the small end organs or mechanoreceptors throughout joint tissue. These nerves comprise approximately 55% of total articular nerves, with the remaining 45% consisting of small unmyelinated fibers, which transmit nociception or pain sensation.[108]

Type I or Ruffini receptors located in the superficial layers of the joint capsule are low-threshold, slow-adapting mechanoreceptors. These receptors respond to changing mechanical stresses and are always active because of the gradient pressure difference in the joint capsule. They undergo deformation with natural movement owing to their location in the superficial joint capsule. In the limbs, type I receptors are found to be more densely distributed in the proximal joints of the hip and are not as prevalent in the distal joints of the ankle.[108] Ruffini receptors have also been found in the meniscofemoral, cruciate, and collateral ligaments of the knee.[59]

Type II or Pacinian receptors are located in the deep layers of the joint capsule, the meniscofemoral, cruciate, and collateral ligaments of the knee. In addition, type II receptors are located in the intra-articular and extra-articular fat pads of all synovial joints. These Pacinian receptors are more prevalent in distal joints such as the ankle and are less densely distributed in proximal joints such as the hip. They function as rapidly adapting, low-threshold receptors, which respond to acceleration, deceleration, and passive joint movement but are silent during inactivity and joint movements at constant velocities.[59]

Type III or Golgi tendon organ–like endings are predominantly found in intra-articular and extra-articular joint ligaments including the collateral ligaments and cruciate ligaments in the knee.[108] These receptors have also been identified in the menisci of the knee.[59] Type III Golgi tendon organ–like endings are structurally identical to the Golgi tendon organ receptors, and function as slowly adapting, high-threshold receptors with a function similar to that of the Golgi tendon organs found in tendons.

Type IV free nerve endings function as the pain receptor or nociception system in synovial joints. These type IV receptor nerve endings are found throughout the joints of the extremities in the fibrous capsule and adjacent periosteum, articular fat pads and are the most prevalent receptor type in the knee menisci. They are completely inactive in normal situations and are activated by marked mechanical deformation or chemical stimuli resulting from an inflammatory response.[59]

AFFERENT JOINT RECEPTORS IN THE UPPER EXTREMITY

The classification system mentioned earlier for the four primary types of mechanoreceptors found in human non-contractile capsular and ligamentous tissues described by Wyke[108,109] provides generalized information about the location of these receptors in the human body. Vangsness and associates[98] studied the neural histology of the human shoulder joint, including the glenohumeral ligaments, labrum, and subacromial bursa. They found two types of mechanoreceptors and free nerve endings in the glenohumeral joint capsular ligaments. Two types of slowly adapting Ruffini end organs and rapidly adapting Pacinian corpuscles were identified in the superior, middle, and inferior glenohumeral ligaments. The most common mechanoreceptor was the classic Ruffini end organ in the glenohumeral joint capsular ligaments. Pacinian corpuscles were less abundant overall, however, Kikuchi[53] and Shimoda[88] reported that the type II Pacinian corpuscles were more commonly found in the human glenohumeral joint capsular ligaments than in the human knee. Analysis of the coracoclavicular and acromioclavicular ligaments showed equal distribution of type I and II mechanoreceptors. Morisawa and colleagues[70] identified types I, II, III, and IV mechanoreceptors in human coracoacromial ligaments. These reviews show how the glenohumeral joint capsular ligaments aid in the provision of afferent proprioceptive input by their inherent distributions of both type I Ruffini mechanoreceptors along with the more rapidly adapting Pacinian receptors. A rapidly adapting receptor such as the Pacinian receptor can identify changes in tension in the joint capsular ligaments, but quickly decreases its input once the tension becomes constant.[98] In this way, the type II receptor has the ability to monitor acceleration and deceleration of the tension of a ligament.

Several authors have also studied the labrum and subacromial bursa. Vangsness and associates[98] reported that no evidence was found for mechanoreceptors in the glenoid labrum; however, free nerve endings were noted in the fibrocartilage tissue in the peripheral half. The subacromial bursa was found to have diffuse, yet copious, free nerve endings, with no evidence of larger, more complex mechanoreceptors. Ide and co-workers[47] also studied subacromial bursa, taken from three cadavers, and found a copious supply of free nerve endings, most of which were found on the roof side of the subacromial arch, which is exposed to impingement type stresses. Unlike the study by Vangsness and associates,[98] Ide and co-workers[47] did find evidence of both Ruffini and Pacinian mechanoreceptors in the subacromial bursa. Their findings suggested that the subacromial bursa receives both nociceptive and proprioceptive stimuli and may play a role in regulation of shoulder movement. Further research into the exact distribution of these important structures in the human shoulder is indicated to give clinicians further information and to enhance the understanding of proprioceptive function of the shoulder.

AFFERENT RECEPTORS OF CONTRACTILE STRUCTURES IN THE UPPER EXTREMITY

In addition to the afferent structures found in the non-contractile tissues of the human shoulder (joint capsule, subacromial bursa, and intrinsic and extrinsic ligaments), significant contributions to the regulation of human movement and proprioceptive feedback are obtained from receptors located in contractile structures.

Two of the primary mechanisms for afferent feedback from the muscle tendon unit are the muscle spindle and the Golgi tendon organ.[71,75] Research classifying muscle spindles has traditionally grouped intrafusal muscle fibers into two groups based on the type of afferent projections.[6,75] These two groups consist of nuclear bag and nuclear chain fibers. Nuclear chain fibers project from large afferent axons.[6,75] Nuclear bag fibers are innervated by γ_1 (dynamic) motor neurons and are more sensitive to the rate of muscle length change, such as that which occurs during a rapid stretch of a muscle during an eccentric contraction or passive stretch.[75] Intrafusal nuclear chain fibers are innervated by γ_2 (static) motor neurons and are more sensitive to static muscle length. The combination of the nuclear chain and nuclear bag fibers allows the afferent communication from the muscle tendon unit to remain sensitive over a wide range of motion (ROM), during both reflex and voluntary activation (Table 8-3).

Muscle spindles provide much of the primary information for motor learning, including muscle length and joint position. Upper levels of the CNS can bias the sensitivity of muscle spindle input and sampling.[75] Muscle spindles do not occur in similar densities in all muscles in the human

body. Spindle density probably is related to muscle function, with greater densities of muscle spindles being reported in muscles that initiate and control fine movements or maintain posture. Muscles that cross the front of the shoulder, such as the pectoralis major and biceps, have a very high number of muscle spindles per unit of muscle weight.[100] Muscles with attachment to the coracoid, such as the biceps, pectoralis minor and coracobrachialis also have high spindle densities. Lower spindle densities have been reported for the rotator cuff muscle tendon units, with the subscapularis and infraspinatus having greater densities than the supraspinatus and teres minor.[100] This lower rotator cuff spindle density probably suggests synergistic mechanoreceptor activation with the scapulothoracic musculature with glenohumeral joint movement.[48,75] This coupled or shared mechanoreceptor activation is an example of kinetic link or proximal to distal sequencing that occurs with predictable or programmed movement patterns in the human body.[67] This kinetic link activation concept is further demonstrated by the deltoid/rotator cuff force couple[48] and other important biomechanical features of the human glenohumeral joint and will be discussed later in this chapter.

The second major aspect of musculotendinous afferent activity is the Golgi tendon organ. These tendonous mechanoreceptors are present in the human shoulder and respond to tension generated with muscular contraction.[71,75] The activation of the Golgi tendon organs relays afferent feedback about muscle tension and joint position. Additionally, as a protective mechanism, activation of the tension-sensitive Golgi tendon organ produces a protective mechanism, which causes relaxation of the agonist muscle that is undergoing tension, with simultaneous stimulation of antagonistic musculature.

CLINICAL ASSESSMENT OF PROPRIOCEPTION IN THE LOWER EXTREMITY

The two primary tests measuring proprioception and kinesthetic awareness in the knee joint are threshold to detection of passive motion (TTDPM) for movement sense and reproduction of angular position for joint position sense. The TTDPM test has been more standardized in the literature.[57,59,79] The method described by Barrack and colleagues[8] and Skinner and associates[89] involves placing the subject in a seated position with the leg hanging freely over the seat, suspended by a motorized pulley system in 90° of flexion (Fig. 8-1). Tactile, visual, and auditory cues are eliminated with the use of custom-fitted Jobst air splints and wearing of a blindfold. Initiation of movement into either flexion or extension proceeds at a rate of angular deflection of 0.5°/sec. When subjects initially detect movement to occur, they engage a control switch to indicate the test leg has been moved.[89]

Testing for joint position sense involves passive movement of the extremity to a specified angle by the clinician

Table 8-3

Characteristics of the Muscle Spindle

Type	Fiber Length	Motor Axon Type	Function
Nuclear bag	7-8 mm long	Medium size	Stimulation of larger motor fibers increases tension in the bag
Nuclear chain	4-5 mm long	Small	Stimulation of the smaller motor fibers reduces tension on the bag

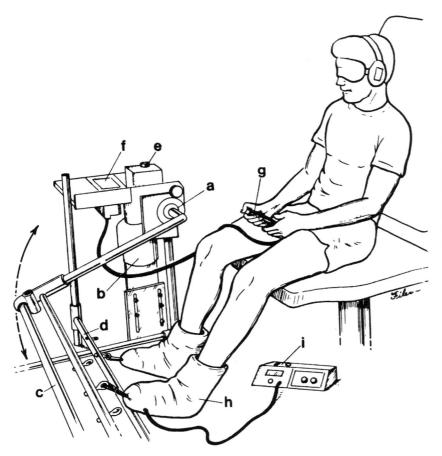

Figure 8-1. Proprioceptive testing device. a, Rotational transducer; b, motor; c, moving arm; d, stationary arm; e, control panel; f, digital microprocessor; g, hand-held disengage switch; h, pneumatic compression boot; and i, pneumatic compression device. Threshold to detection of passive movement is assessed by measuring the angular displacement until the subject senses motion in the knee. (From Lephart, S.M., Kocher, M.S., Fu, F.H., et al. [1992]: Proprioception following anterior cruciate ligament reconstruction. J. Sports Rehabil., 1:188-196.)

Table 8-4
Factors Effecting Joint Proprioception

Fatigue	Immobility
Injury	Surgery
Disuse	Ligamentous laxity
Aging	Arthritis

and holding the position for several seconds, with passive return of the extremity to the reference starting position. The patient is then asked to actively move the extremity to the specified angle without visual input. The difference between the actual and replicated angle can be calculated as either an absolute or a real angular error. With absolute error only the magnitude of the error is used and whether the subject over- or underestimates knee position is not considered. Real error calculations, however, consider both the magnitude and direction of the error and can be used to determine whether a subject over- or underestimates the reference angle.[13] Barrack and co-workers[9] demonstrated through studies on proprioception that there is a high degree of symmetry with joint position sense between extremities that show no evidence of pathologic conditions.

There are essentially no standard protocols for measuring joint position sense or for joint replication tests, and so many variations exist, including the apparatus used for angular measurement, starting reference angle, active or passive reproduction, and open chain (seated) versus closed chain (standing).[37] Lattanzio and associates[57] and Marks and Quinney[66] used closed chain weight-bearing joint replications and reported high degrees of accuracy. Their results may be due to the fact that there is greater proprioceptive input in the standing weight-bearing position in which multiple joints are being loaded.

Single-limb postural stability tests have also been used for measuring the amount of sway measured in those individuals with complaints of ankle instability. Tropp and colleagues[97] developed such a test for measuring ankle instability, which has been used with variations throughout the years. Using a force platform, individuals stood for 60 seconds with measurement of the instantaneous center of pressure along a graph; the magnitude of sway was compared with that of the uninvolved side.

Single-leg hop tests are often used for assessing stability in patients with knee or ankle pathologic conditions. Variations of the test include single-leg or triple-leg hop tests for distance, the crossover hop test, and the timed hop test. The relationship of hop tests to functional parameters such as instability, proprioception, and leg strength has been inconclusive in studies to date.

ASSESSMENT OF PROPRIOCEPTION AND NEUROMUSCULAR CONTROL IN THE UPPER EXTREMITY WITH SPECIFIC REFERENCE TO THE HUMAN SHOULDER

Determining which patients require particular emphasis in rehabilitation to restore proprioception and neuromuscular control requires the use of clinical assessment techniques. In this section techniques used in research investigations, as well as in clinical applications, to allow the clinician to perform a detailed evaluation will be reviewed.

Primary Measures of Proprioception and Neuromuscular Control for the Shoulder

Evaluation of proprioception and neuromuscular control in the human shoulder encompasses both afferent and efferent neural function, as well as the resulting muscular activation patterns.[71] Proprioception for the purposes of this and many other articles, texts, and chapters[15,59,71] consists of three major submodalities: kinesthesia, joint position sense, and sensation of resistance. Separate techniques can be used to assess each of these aspects of proprioception.

Measurement of Kinesthesia

The assessment of glenohumeral joint kinesthesia has been performed using a test called the *threshold to detection of passive motion*. This test assesses the subject's or patient's ability to detect a passive movement occurring typically at very slow angular velocities.[59,71,93] Elaborate testing devices have been used in several studies that have reported on TTDPM, such as an instrumented (motorized) shoulder wheel[93] and other devices such as the one

used by the University of Pittsburgh whose characteristics are described next (Fig. 8-2).[59] Extensive research[59,62,71] using the TTDPM test has resulted in selection and recommendation of slow angular velocities (0.5 to 2°/sec) to enhance reliability of data acquisition. In addition to the device used, blindfolds, earphones, and a pneumatic cuff are recommended to eliminate cues from the visual, auditory, and tactile realm. This ensures that only joint kinesthesia is being assessed and not simply visual or auditory responses to perceived movement.

Physiologically, the TTDPM test is designed to selectively stimulate the Ruffini or Golgi-type mechanoreceptors in the articular structures being tested. Testing is typically performed for internal and external rotation of the glenohumeral joint in varying positions of elevation in the scapular and coronal planes. Testing in the literature has been done at mid-range and end-range positions of glenohumeral rotation.[59,62,71] As stated earlier, TTDPM in the human shoulder was measured by Blaiser and co-workers,[15] and passive motion was found to be enhanced (smaller amount of movement before detection) at or near the end-range external rotation compared with mid-range external rotation or internal rotation.

Normative data on 40 healthy college-aged individuals using the TTDPM test were reported by Warner and associates[101] from both neutral rotational starting positions and 30° of humeral rotations at 90° of glenohumeral joint abduction. They found an average of 1.5° to 2.2° for all testing conditions, with no significant difference measured between the dominant or preferred hand relative to the nondominant extremity.[102] Allegrucci and colleagues[2] measured shoulder kinesthesia in healthy athletes who performed unilateral upper extremity sports, such as baseball, tennis, or volleyball. The TTDPM test was performed

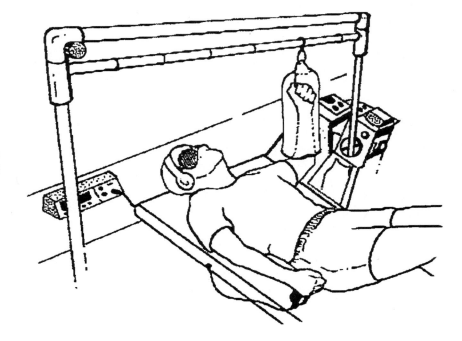

Figure 8-2. Upper extremity proprioceptive testing device. (From Pollack, R. [2000]: Role of shoulder stabilization relative to restoration of neuromuscular control and joint kinematics *In*: Lephart, S.M., and Fu, F.H. (eds.), Proprioception and Neuromuscular Control. Champaign, IL: Human Kinetics.)

with the shoulder in 90° of abduction at both 0 and 75° of external rotation and compared bilaterally. Results showed that the athletes had greater difficulty in detecting passive motion in the dominant extremity compared with the non-dominant extremity. Consistent with earlier research,[15] Allegrucci and colleagues[2] measured greater sensitivity to passive movement with the shoulder in 75° of external rotation bilaterally compared with the more neutral condition. The findings in this study suggested that athletes in unilaterally dominant upper extremity sports may have a proprioceptive deficit on the dominant arm that may interfere with optimal afferent feedback regarding joint position.[2] This finding provides a rationale for proprioceptive upper extremity training in athletes from this population.

Measurement of Joint Position Sense

Joint position sense measures the ability of the subject to appreciate where the extremity is oriented in space. Testing procedures to assess joint position sense are called *joint angular replication* tests. These tests typically place the extremity in a particular position to allow the subject to appreciate the spatial orientation of the extremity. After this period of joint positioning, the subject's extremity is returned to a starting position. The subject then reapproximates the position initially selected as closely as possible, without any visual, auditory, or tactile cues. Researchers have used both active[19,59,62,71,99] and passive[99] angular replication tests in assessment of the glenohumeral joint. Various apparatus have been used to facilitate the accuracy of joint angular replication testing. Voight and associates[99] used an isokinetic dynamometer with 90° of abduction and elbow flexion, with standard isokinetic stabilization, to perform active angular joint replication testing using a fatigue paradigm. They also used the passive mode of the isokinetic dynamometer set at (2°/sec) to perform passive joint angular replication testing. Various authors[49,59,92] have used complex three-dimensional spatial tracking devices to quantify arm position, using multiple positions of active joint angular replication testing.

In the most clinically applicable research study on active joint angular reproduction, Davies and Hoffman[19] tested subjects in a seated position using an electronic digital inclinometer (EDI).* Reference angles were chosen in several ranges and verified with the EDI, with subsequent active angular replication by the patient and verification of extremity position with the EDI. Angles chosen were >90° and <90° of flexion and abduction, external rotation >45° and <45°, and internal rotation >45° and <45°. Normative data developed by Davies and Hoffman for 100 male subjects without shoulder pathologic conditions show the average of the seven measurements to be 2.7°.[19] This represents the average difference between the seven reference angles and the actual matched angles by the subjects over the seven measurements.

Regardless of testing methodology, the active joint angular position replication tests primarily involve the stimulation of both joint and muscle receptors and provide a thorough assessment of afferent pathways of the human shoulder.[59,71]

Assessment of Neuromuscular Control of the Shoulder

Several methods have been used by clinicians and researchers to assess neuromuscular control of the shoulder. Widespread use of electromyographic (EMG) studies to measure muscular activity during shoulder rehabilitative exercise,[5,14,69,96] functional movement patterns such as the throwing motion[21] and tennis serve and groundstrokes,[82] and abnormal muscular activity patterns during planar motions[55,65,68] and functional activities[39] is reported in the scientific and clinical literature. Most of these studies comparing muscular activity expressed the contribution or activity of the muscle, based on the amount of muscle activity relative to the maximal activity assessed via a maximal isolated manual muscle test (MMT). This is commonly referred to as %MMT or %MVC (maximum voluntary contraction) and allows comparison and expression of the relative activity of human muscle activity during activities of daily living (ADL) and sport-specific movement patterns.[21, 82]

Muscular Strength Testing

Another important aspect of assessing neuromuscular control is the measurement of muscular strength. Methods such as manual muscle testing and the use of hand-held dynamometers and isokinetic apparatus have been used extensively for documentation of both upper and lower extremity strength. Further discussion is beyond the scope of this chapter; however, the reader is referred to Chapter 9.

Closed Kinetic Chain Upper Extremity Testing

Closed chain upper extremity tests are also used to assess neuromuscular control of the shoulder. Although widespread use of closed chain training techniques has been reported in the physical medicine and rehabilitation literature,[28,29,32,105,106] currently existing evaluation methods to properly assess closed chain function of the upper extremity are limited.

One of the gold standards in physical education for gross assessment of upper extremity strength has been the push-up. This test has been used to generate sport-specific normative data in normal populations,[32,83] but it is not typically considered appropriate for use in patients with shoulder dysfunction. Positional demands placed upon the anterior capsule and increased joint loading limit the effectiveness of this test in musculoskeletal rehabilitation. Modification of the push-up has been reported, and the modified push-up has been used clinically as an acceptable

---

*Available from Cybex, Inc. (Medway, MA)

alternative to assess closed chain function in the upper extremities.

Davies developed the closed kinetic chain (CKC) upper extremity stability test in an attempt to provide a test to assess the functional ability of the upper extremity more accurately.[30,32,41] The test is initiated in the starting position of a standard push-up for males and modified (off knees) push-up for females. Two strips of tape are placed parallel to each other, 3 feet apart on the floor. The subject or patient then moves both hands back and forth, touching each line alternatively as many times as possible in 15 seconds. Each touch of the line is counted and tallied to generate the CKC upper extremity stability test score. Normative results have been established, with males averaging 18.5 touches in 15 seconds and females averaging 20.5 touches. The CKC upper extremity stability test has been subjected to a test-retest reliability test, with an intraclass correlation coefficient generated at 0.927, indicating high clinical reliability between sessions with this examination method.[41]

EFFECTS OF AGING, INSTABILITY, AND INJURY ON LOWER EXTREMITY PROPRIOCEPTION

The effects of age and injury have been correlated with diminished proprioception sense.[81] Studies[50,90] have shown decreased proprioceptive acuity in older adults with testing, suggesting that this decreased capacity for movement sense results in higher incidences of falling and joint degeneration in this population. In addition, it has been found that with regular physical activity, the age-related decline in proprioception can be lessened through dampening of the effect on disuse atrophy of the neuromuscular system.[59] In addition to age-related deficits, injuries sustained to the lower extremity joints through repetitive microtrauma or a single traumatic event can create an environment in which degenerative changes to the joint occur with a disruption in the neuromuscular response. With the presence of pain and inflammation in a joint there is an inhibitory effect on neuromuscular activation with decreased mechanoreceptor afference.[12] Hurley and Newham[46] and Sharma and Pai[86] demonstrated arthrogenous muscle inhibition in patients with degenerative arthritis. This inability to achieve full voluntary muscle contraction may lead to continued overload to the joints through the loss of dynamic control and force attenuation.

The loss of capsuloligamentous stability has been shown to cause proprioceptive deficits due to inadequate activation of the mechanoreceptors resulting in delayed muscle reaction latencies. Barrack and colleagues[7] found decreased proprioception in a group of ballet dancers and attributed this clinical loss of proprioception to the hyperlaxity found in the ligamentous restraints in this population. It is theorized that without adequate tension in the capsuloligamentous restraints, there is insufficient stimulation of the mechanoreceptors used for proprioception, resulting in

decreased motor control. A study by Garn and Newton[38] also showed that individuals suffering from chronic ankle instability have diminished proprioception with threshold to passive plantar flexion. A similar study by Lentell and associates[58] tested subjects with chronic lateral ankle instability who demonstrated a decreased passive movement sense, using the uninvolved ankle as the control. Subjects in this study demonstrated no evidence of everter strength contributing to functional instability. Therefore, the chronic instability was a result of the loss of mechanoreceptor function from ligamentous laxity resulting in a delayed muscular reflex. Lephart and Fu[59] and Nawoczenski and co-workers[74] confirmed this decreased muscular stabilization in a study involving subjects with ankle instability. The results of their studies supported this loss of motor control, with a delay in the onset latency in the peroneal muscles when subjected to sudden inversion stresses.

Effects of Knee Injury on Proprioception

Degenerative arthritis in the knee causes pain, inflammation, and muscular inhibition, resulting in decreased functional performance with gait and weight-bearing activities.[59] Combined with pain and altered muscle activity, the inadequate ligamentous tension resulting from narrowing of the joint space contributes to the interruption of afferent signals for proprioception and neuromuscular control. The goal of joint replacement surgery is to restore function through resurfacing joint surfaces, retensioning soft tissue structures, and ultimately restoring dynamic stability. Research performed by Warren and colleagues[103] and Barrett and associates[10] suggested that joint replacement surgery may actually improve joint position sense with subjects showing significant improvements in position sense 6 months postoperatively. Furthermore, correlations have been made between improved functional outcomes and gait parameters and proprioceptive scores, suggesting that a relationship between restoration of proprioception and improved functional outcomes exists.

Results of studies to date on the selection of joint prosthesis and the effects of retaining versus sacrificing the posterior cruciate ligament (PCL) on proprioception have been inconclusive. However, it has been theorized that by restoring joint integrity and retensioning of soft tissue structures, retention of the PCL will enhance dynamic joint stability through preservation of the neural reflexive pathway.[4,10,25]

Studies in the literature consistently have demonstrated decreases in proprioception sense and altered muscle patterns after rupture of the anterior cruciate ligament (ACL).[13,59,107] With loss of stability of the ACL, alterations in muscle activity and reflex patterns occur, primarily with the ACL-hamstring reflex. Measuring the ACL-hamstring reflex in patients with ACL rupture, Beard and co-workers[11] showed significant reflex latency delays, which were directly correlated with functional instability. Using EMG studies, Limbird and co-workers[63] showed variations in muscle activation patterns with increased hamstring activation and concomitant decreased quadriceps activity with joint loading during gait. Andriacchi and Birac[3] had similar findings with patients performing normal activities of ambulation, stair climbing, and jogging. With the loss of stability and neural sensory input, many individuals experience functional disability with normal ADL.

EFFECTS OF SHOULDER PATHOLOGIC CONDITIONS ON PROPRIOCEPTION AND NEUROMUSCULAR CONTROL

In this section the normal afferent neurobiology of the joint and peri-articular structures will be reviewed, examples of how proprioception and neuromuscular control are affected in pathologic conditions of shoulder will be provided. Examples of both glenohumeral joint instability and rotator cuff pathologic conditions will be reviewed, as well as dysfunction of the scapulothoracic joint.

Effects of Glenohumeral Joint Instability on Proprioception

Several studies have been performed that address the influence of glenohumeral joint instability on proprioception. One of the most common clinical maladies addressed by clinicians is anterior glenohumeral joint instability. Speer and associates[95] studied the effects of a simulated Bankart lesion in cadavers. Coupled anterior/posterior translations were assessed in the presence of sequentially applied loads of 50 N in anterior, posterior, superior, and inferior directions. The effects of a simulated Bankart lesion were small (maximum of 3.4 mm) increases in anterior and inferior translations of the humeral head relative to the glenoid in all positions of elevation and in posterior translation at 90° of elevation only.[95] The relevance of this article to this current discussion on proprioception is that Speer and associates[95] concluded that detachment of the anterior inferior labrum from the glenoid (Bankart lesion) alone does not create large enough increases in humeral head translation to allow for anterior glenohumeral joint dislocation. They indicate that permanent stretching or elongation of the inferior glenohumeral ligament may also occur and be necessary to produce a full dislocation of the glenohumeral joint. This elongation or permanent stretching of the ligamentous structures may lead to alterations of the intrinsic tensile relationships of the glenohumeral joint capsule and capsular ligaments. The authors concluded that capsular elongation may be responsible for the high incidence of anterior reconstructions that fail to address anterior glenohumeral joint instability and do not fully restore normal capsular tension of the anterior structures.

Blaiser and co-workers[15] examined the proprioceptive ability of subjects without known shoulder pathologic conditions and compared them with individuals with clinically determined generalized joint laxity. Individuals with greater glenohumeral joint laxity were found to have less sensitive proprioception, compared with those who had less glenohumeral joint laxity. The authors found enhanced proprioception at or near the end range of external rotation, when the anterior capsular structures have greater internal tension. They concluded that decreased joint angular reposition sense is one characteristic in individuals with increased glenohumeral joint laxity.

Smith and Brunolli[93] examined kinesthesia after glenohumeral joint dislocation in 8 subjects and compared their inherent joint position sense with that of 10 normal subjects using an instrumented modification of a shoulder wheel. Their results indicated a significant decrease in joint awareness in the involved shoulders after shoulder dislocation compared with all uninvolved shoulders tested in the study.

Lephart and co-workers[62] studied glenohumeral joint proprioception in 90 subjects in three experimental groups. One group consisted of 40 normal college-aged shoulders, another group consisted of 30 patients with anterior instability, and the third group included 20 subjects who had surgical reconstruction for shoulder instability. No significant difference was found between extremities (dominant versus nondominant) in the normal subject's proprioceptive ability; however, subjects with anterior instability showed significant differences between the normal and unstable shoulder. Finally, Lephart and co-workers[62] found no significant difference for the operated extremity compared with the uninjured extremity after reconstructive surgery. This study was performed at least 6 months after subjects had open or arthroscopic repair for chronic, recurrent shoulder anterior instability. The authors concluded that these results provide evidence, consistent with the studies mentioned earlier, for partial deafferentation leading to proprioceptive deficits when the capsuloligamentous structures are damaged. Reconstructive surgery in this experiment appeared to restore normal joint proprioception 6 months or more after the surgical procedure.

Effects of Glenohumeral Joint Instability on Neuromuscular Control

Lephart and Fu[59] defined neuromuscular control as the unconscious efferent response to an afferent signal concerning dynamic joint stability. Several studies highlighting changes in neuromuscular control issues in subjects with glenohumeral joint instability have been published. Glousman and colleagues,[39] using an indwelling EMG electrode, studied the muscular activity patterns of normal healthy baseball pitchers and compared them to throwers with anterior glenohumeral joint instability. Results of the study showed marked increases in muscular activation of the supraspinatus and biceps muscle, as well as selective increases in the infraspinatus muscle during the early cocking and follow-through phases.[39] Also of interest was the finding of decreased muscular activation of the pectoralis major, lateral, subscapularis, and serratus anterior muscles in the throwing athletes with anterior glenohumeral joint instability. This study showed neuromuscular compensations in the group with glenohumeral joint instability, evidenced by the increased activation of primary dynamic stabilizers. Inhibition of the serratus anterior in the group with anterior instability may decrease scapular stability and jeopardize joint congruity further, through improper scapulothoracic muscle sequencing.

McMahon and co-workers[68] tested normal shoulders and those with anterior instability, and monitored them via indwelling EMG muscular activation patterns. Planar motions of flexion, abduction, and scapular plane elevation (scaption) were studied in 30° increments. Significant decreases in serratus anterior muscle activity were measured in all three planar motions in the group of subjects with anterior glenohumeral joint instability. None of the other muscles—rotator cuff, deltoid, or scapular—showed a significant difference with testing during standard planar movement patterns. This study clearly shows the importance of the scapulothoracic musculature and dynamic stabilization during both aggressive overhead and common ADL-type movement patterns.

Finally, Kronberg and associates[55] compared shoulder muscle activity between patients with generalized joint laxity and normal control subjects, using intramuscular electrodes. Increased subscapularis muscular activity was measured during internal rotation in the subjects with increased glenohumeral joint laxity, as well as increased middle and anterior deltoid activity during abduction and flexion. These studies clearly show the increased demand required in the dynamic stabilizers in the presence of joint laxity and glenohumeral joint instability. Application of the resistive exercise progressions and utilization of the kinetic chain exercise series listed later in this chapter have these research-based rationales and can directly enhance neuromuscular control of the shoulder complex.

Effects of Rotator Cuff Dysfunction on Neuromuscular Control in the Shoulder

Research similar to that discussed in the preceding section measuring the muscular activation patterns in patients with rotator cuff impingement has been published. Ludewig and Cook[65] studied 52 male construction workers, of whom 26 had unilateral shoulder impingement, and 26 had no symptoms of impingement or other shoulder pathologic condition. Similar to subjects in the previously discussed research studies on glenohumeral joint instability, subjects with unilateral impingement demonstrated a decrease in serratus anterior muscle activation during active elevation of the arm compared with normal, uninjured subjects.[65] Additionally, increases in upper and lower trapezius muscle activity were also measured in the subjects with unilateral

impingement. This altered neuromuscular control mechanism also resulted in abnormal scapular posturing, consisting of decreased upward rotation with elevation, increased anterior tipping, and increased medial rotation. These scapular modifications are thought to be contributing factors to rotator cuff impingement and demonstrate the importance of optimal and coordinated muscular control of the scapulothoracic and glenohumeral joints.

EFFECTS OF FATIGUE ON LOWER EXTREMITY PROPRIOCEPTION

Muscle fatigue reduces the force-generating capacity of the neuromuscular system, which essentially leads to increased laxity in the knee joint.[91] Skinner and colleagues[89] found an increase in laxity of the ACL measured with a KT-1000* arthrometer after a fatigue protocol. Similarly, Weisman and co-workers[104] found increased laxity in the medial collateral ligament in athletes at a university after participation in various sporting activities. Furthermore, studies in the literature[56,57,89] have shown a decrease in the sensitivity of muscle receptors to fatigue conditions. The consequences of decreased proprioception sense from fatigue can be deleterious because of the possibility of sustaining injuries under these conditions when higher-level activities are performed. Skinner and colleagues[89] studied the effects of fatigue on joint position sense and knee angle reproduction in a group of healthy, highly trained male recruits in the Special Forces division of the Navy. Subjects underwent an interval running program followed by isokinetic measurement of knee extension and flexion. Fatigue was determined through a percentage decrement in work output measured from pretraining to post-training on an isokinetic device. The authors concluded that after fatigue measures, there was a significant change with decreased angular replication tests, but no significant changes with threshold of movement sense. They determined that the loss of muscle receptor efficiency from fatigue played a key role in angular replication errors. The authors concluded that the dual role of afferent input by the receptors in the contractile and noncontractile elements of the knee is important for proprioception sense.

Lattanzio and associates[57] conducted a study involving healthy male and female subjects performing three different cycling protocols (ramp, continuous, and interval training) at a percentage of their $\dot{V}o_2$ max. In this study, methods for threshold to detection of movement were similar, but angular replications were performed with subjects in the standing weight-bearing position instead of the seated open chain protocol used in the study of Skinner and colleagues. Results of the study of Lattanzio and associates[57] were similar to those of Skinner and colleagues, with statistically significant decrements in male subjects for joint replication

---

*Available from Medmetric Corporation, San Diego, California.

after the three different fatigue protocols. Female subjects similarly showed significant differences for joint replication after the continuous and interval programs but not with the ramp protocol for joint angular replication. The conclusions drawn by the authors in this study were that anatomical gender differences possibly accounted for the variation in response to fatigue with proprioception.

Finally, Barrack and co-workers[9] and Barrett and associates[10] studied the effects of total knee replacement on knee joint proprioception. This research paradigm is of particular interest, because insertion of the total knee joint prosthesis results in the removal of most joint receptors in the human knee. Both groups of investigators found no significant loss of proprioception in the operated extremity with the total knee replacement compared with the contralateral extremity 6 months postoperatively. These groups of authors both concluded that their research again pointed to the important role the muscle-based mechanoreceptors play in knee joint proprioception.

EFFECTS OF MUSCULAR FATIGUE ON UPPER EXTREMITY PROPRIOCEPTION AND NEUROMUSCULAR CONTROL

The role of specific afferent receptors in the human body has been examined using different methods to better understand the role of joint and muscular afferents. Provins[81] reported a decrease in the ability to detect passive motion of the finger when digital nerves containing both joint and cutaneous afferents were blocked by local anesthesia. He concluded that both types of afferent feedback may be equally important when joint proprioception is analyzed.

Zuckerman and associates[110] used lidocaine injections into the subacromial space and glenohumeral joint to assess proprioception in young and old male subjects. They found no adverse effects from the injection of lidocaine in either location, proposing that compensatory extracapsular feedback ensured intact proprioception after injection. No differences in joint position sense and TTDPM testing were noted between the dominant and nondominant extremity; however, a decline in proprioception with age was measured for the young (aged 20 to 30 years) and older (aged 50 to 70 years) subjects.

Several studies have been performed using the human shoulder to investigate the effect of muscular fatigue on various indices of joint proprioception and neuromuscular control. Carpenter and co-workers[16] tested subjects using a TTDPM test with the shoulder in 90° of abduction and 90° of external rotation. After an isokinetic fatigue protocol, subjects' detection of passive motion was marred or decreased by 171% for internal rotation and 179% for external rotation. In pre-exercise testing, Carpenter and co-workers found increased sensitivity moving into external rotation compared with internal rotation but no difference between the dominant and nondominant extremity.[16]

These authors concluded that the effect of muscular fatigue on joint proprioception may play a role in injury and decrease athletic performance.

Voight and associates[99] tested subjects using an active and passive joint angular replication protocol, after isokinetically induced muscular fatigue of the glenohumeral joint internal and external rotators. No significant difference in shoulder joint angular replication was found between the dominant and nondominant extremity. Significant decreases in accuracy were noted after muscular fatigue in both the active and passive joint angular replication tests. Pederson and colleagues[78] tested the ability of healthy subjects to discriminate movement velocity of the glenohumeral joint in the transverse plane. Results of their study showed that subjects had a decrement in the discrimination of movement velocity after a hard isokinetic horizontal flexion/extension exercise fatigue protocol compared with a light exercise condition.

Finally, Myers and associates[72] used an active angular replication test and neuromuscular control test to examine the effects of muscle fatigue in normal shoulders. A concentric isokinetic internal and external rotation fatigue protocol was used. Fatigue of the internal and external rotators of the shoulder decreased subjects' accuracy in detecting both mid-range and end-range absolute angular error but did not have a negative effect on neuromuscular control in a bilaterally assessed unilateral closed chain stability–type test measuring postural sway velocity.

The consistent finding of a proprioceptive decrement after muscular fatigue in these studies has led researchers to emphasize the importance of the muscle-based receptors. The use of active joint angular positioning tests has been reported to stimulate both joint and muscle mechanoreceptors and is considered to be a more functional assessment of afferent pathways.[59,71,72] The exact mechanism by which muscle-based proprioception is affected is not entirely clear or known. Muscle fatigue is thought to desensitize the muscle spindle threshold, leading to decrements in both joint position sense and neuromuscular control. Djupsjobacka and co-workers[22-24] reported alterations of muscle spindle output in the presence of lactic acid, potassium chloride, arachidonic acid, and bradykinin. Intramuscular concentrations of these substances are altered during muscular exertion and fatigue. This consistent relationship has provided further rationale and support for the improvement of muscular endurance of the dynamic stabilizers of the glenohumeral joint. This topic will be covered in detail in the application section of this chapter.

EFFECTS OF TRAINING ON PROPRIOCEPTION IN THE LOWER EXTREMITY

Some studies in the literature have investigated the notion of injury prevention and improving neuromuscular stabilization through proprioceptive training. In a prospective study by Cerulli and colleagues[17] 600 semiprofessional and amateur soccer players were followed for three seasons to determine the frequency of ACL injury among players who underwent a progressive proprioceptive training program and a control group who performed only traditional strengthening exercises. Results showed significant differences between the experimental and control groups, with the proprioception training group sustaining fewer lesions to the ACL than the control group who performed traditional strengthening exercises.

Osborne and associates[76] studied the effects of ankle disk training in eight individuals who sustained an inversion ankle sprain within the preceding 1½ years, and who had not received any formal rehabilitation. Subjects performed 15-minutes of daily training on a disk with the involved leg in an 8-week training program. After completion of the 8-week training program, subjects were tested for onset latencies with surface EMG electrodes on the muscles of the ankle influencing stability to measure the motor response to a simulated inversion sprain on a platform. Results showed significant improvements in anterior tibialis latency times in both the trained and untrained control ankles.

A similar study by Eils and Rosenbaum[26] showed significant improvements in muscle reaction times and patterns of muscle co-activation in 30 subjects with chronic ankle sprains. The subjects performed a multistation proprioceptive exercise program including 12 stations using various devices once weekly for 6 weeks. The frequency of once per week and the types of exercises were chosen for their ability to be implemented easily into a rehabilitation program. The exercises included a Biodex balance system*, inversion boards, mini-trampoline, and ankle disk. The subjects performing the exercises showed significant improvement over the control group for position sense and reported subjective improvements with functional stability.

Fitzgerald and colleagues[37] conducted a study in subjects with ACL deficiencies who performed traditional lower extremity strengthening exercises compared with subjects who performed traditional rehabilitation along with perturbation training. The perturbation program consisted of progressive exercises using rocker boards and roller boards, with advancement to the next phase after successful completion of the task without evidence of instability or pain. After the training program, the perturbation group was found to have significantly greater success with subjective reports of stability during completion of higher level activities than the traditional training group.

Beard and associates[11] conducted a similar study, but used hamstring reflex latencies and the Lyshom rating scale for measuring functional outcomes. They concluded that the group who underwent perturbation training had improved functional outcomes for knee stability while performing ADL.

CLINICAL APPLICATION: TECHNIQUES TO IMPROVE LOWER EXTREMITY PROPRIOCEPTION AND NEUROMUSCULAR CONTROL

Lower extremity injuries occur often in competitive and recreational sports. These injuries sometimes are caused by physical contact with another individual, but usually are caused by a noncontact injury, in which the external forces in the environment exceed the internal forces of the body.[17] Some of the more common injuries involve damage to the ligamentous and cartilaginous components in the knee and ankle. The injuries that do not involve another person occur when the player or individual attempts to suddenly change the rate of speed or course of direction or an obstacle in the external environment causes overload to static joint restraints. The questions that have received recent attention in the literature are the degree to which these injuries can be prevented, and, once an individual is injured, ways in which recurrent injuries to an existing compromised system can be prevented through dynamic neuromuscular stabilization.[61]

For a patient with an ACL deficiency, neuromuscular training is achieved through coordinated muscle activation in response to controlled perturbation forces being imparted to the joint. One strategy for dynamic stabilization is co-contraction of opposing muscle groups to essentially stabilize the knee in a rigid posture. This strategy may be successful for simple tasks, but with higher-level activities such as sporting activities, stabilization is achieved through selective motor recruitment that is task dependent. A force feedback mechanism has been discussed, in which stability is achieved through varied patterns of muscle recruitment depending on the situational needs of the task.[59,107] This theory acknowledges that different patterns of movement require varied muscular stabilization, depending on the direction, speed, and amount of force occurring at the joint.

At the University of Delaware, Snyder-Mackler and co-workers[36,107] designed a rehabilitation program based on the premise of achieving dynamic muscular stabilization during normal and higher-level skills through neuromuscular perturbation training. They use the term *copers* for individuals who successfully perform varied high-level activities without experiencing functional instability. For copers, the muscular strategies used for joint stability allow for normal joint movement while deleterious compressive and shear forces at the joint are minimized. The term given to individuals who are unsuccessful in maintaining joint stability during lower extremity weight-bearing tasks is *non-copers*. In the group of non-copers, a co-contraction stiffening strategy is utilized with all tasks, which results in inefficient movement strategies and functional instability.

---

*Available from Biodex, Shirley, New York.

Furthermore, with this inadequate coping mechanism, progressive deterioration to joint surfaces and capsuloligamentous restraints occurs due to excessive shear and compressive forces at the joint.[59,107]

The faculty at the University of Delaware have designed a program utilizing the guidelines of Fitzgerald and colleagues for implementing a neuromuscular training program for patients with ACL deficiency in an attempt to restore functional stability during higher-level sporting activities. In selection of individuals for the program, certain criteria must be met to assure successful outcome of the training.

The program is designed to identify individuals who would be successful rehabilitation candidates through a screening process. Criteria include isolated injury to the ACL, infrequent episodes of instability (<1), a passing score on functional hop tests, and a passing percentage with two subjective rating scales for functional knee impairments. Before a stabilization program is initiated, the early focus of rehabilitation is to decrease joint effusion, restore ROM, and increase quadriceps and hamstring strength to allow stabilization through muscle recruitment.[107] When these goals have been met, an advanced neuromuscular training program can be initiated. The program is progressive in nature and is designed for specificity of sport or activity.

The program consists of 10 treatment sessions at a frequency of two to three times a week and is progressive in nature with three phases of implementation (early phase: sessions 1 to 4; middle phase: sessions 5 to 7; and late phase: sessions 8 to 10). Progression of the program is based on the symptomatic patient response (i.e., increased effusion or pain), which is used as a guideline, and the ability of the patient to perform successful motor strategies to the perturbation force, which includes no episodes of falling or instability. All three phases include the use of rocker boards, roller boards, and platforms with the introduction to sport-specific agility drills in the middle to later stages.

In the early phase perturbation training, patients are subjected to perturbation forces on all three devices in slow predictable directions with the use of verbal cues as necessary for onset and direction of the forces. Initially the directions of the applied forces are in the anterior/posterior and medial/lateral directions with progression to diagonal and rotational planes. The clinical implication of this phase thus involves the application of progressive variable perturbation forces in multiple directions (sagittal, transverse, and frontal planes) in a controlled manner to retrain the nervous system in a number of applications or situational needs while avoiding the use of rigid co-contraction strategies.[59]

The middle phases of training continue with perturbation training and require successful adaptive strategies in phase one. Variations in the parameters of training including predictability, speed, amplitude, intensity, and direction of force are advanced, with the implementation of light sport-specific drills while the individual is wearing a functional knee brace. In the last phase of treatment, sport-specific movements are emphasized with the use of agility drills. Initially, training begins in straight planes and then moves to variable direction drills such as cutting and changing direction on command. The drills are initially performed at 50% and progress to 100% in the later stages. Examples of some of the agility drills are side shuffles, shuttle running, and cutting maneuvers at 45° and 90° angles. With no evidence of instability, patients then perform sport-specific activities while they receive perturbations on roller boards and platforms to simulate the competitive demands of the sporting environment. Before returning to full athletic competition, the athletes are required to pass a post-treatment ACL screening using measures similar to those used during prescreening for acceptance into the program.[59]

GUIDELINES FOR IMPLEMENTING LOWER EXTREMITY PROPRIOCEPTION TRAINING

Regardless of whether surgery or conservative care is chosen to restore stability and function to a degenerative or unstable joint, rehabilitation is crucial for restoring neuromuscular control or dynamic stability to a compromised joint. The loss of neuromuscular control results from damage to the mechanoreceptors within the capsuloligamentous structures of the joint and the interruption of the afferent sensory pathways that play a crucial role in producing smooth, coordinated movement.[59]

Several considerations are important when a rehabilitation program is designed to restore proprioception and dynamic stability. In selecting exercises for training, the focus on restoring function to the individual should remain at the forefront. Exercises chosen should then focus on an individual's deficits in strength, ROM, and balance and most importantly on the individual's ability to meet the demands of stability while performing daily or sporting activities.

Traditionally a combination of open and closed kinetic chain exercises have been utilized in rehabilitation. Open chain exercises have been defined as movements in which the distal segment is free to move in space, and closed chain movements occur where the distal segment is fixed or meets considerable resistance.[34] Recently, emphasis on the use of close chain exercises has predominated because they are thought to more closely resemble the functional demands placed on the lower extremity during a variety of activities. Other advantages of closed chain exercises are the simultaneous movement of multiple joints requiring co-contraction of opposing muscle groups to control joint movement. Closed chain exercises can also reduce shear forces across joint surfaces due to the stability of joint-through-joint compression forces and co-contraction of opposing muscle groups. The advantage of open chain exercises is the ability to isolate targeted muscle groups for strengthening.

In a study by Snyder-Mackler and colleagues,[92] isolated open chain quadriceps strengthening was found to be superior to closed kinetic chain exercises for improving quadriceps function in patients after ACL surgery because the involvement of other muscle groups in performing the closed chain exercises did not isolate the quadriceps as effectively. In fact, most functional activities, such as ambulation, utilize a combination of both open and closed kinetic chain muscle activation patterns and therefore both should be incorporated in the design of a successful program.

In the early stages of rehabilitation, the development of an exercise program should identify deficits in ROM, strength, and joint effusion and progression should not exceed the rate of natural healing or limitations in the involved structures. Any number of exercises will elicit proprioception training based on the fact that deformation of the joint mechanoreceptors occurs with active, active assisted, and passive movements providing sensory input to improve neural mechanisms.[59] Performing ROM exercises on an immobilized joint and weight shifting early after an ankle sprain or surgery on the ACL are examples of early forms of proprioception training.

When sufficient healing has taken place in the subacute stages of recovery, the initiation of resistance exercises for building muscular strength and endurance will enable sufficient muscle recruitment patterns for dynamic stabilization for advanced forms of training. Proprioception training in this stage may involve two-legged stance exercises on an unstable surface such as the Biodex stability balance system (Fig. 8-3), which can be advanced to a functional squatting movement pattern. The exercise progression can include single-leg stance (Fig. 8-4) and single-leg stance with partial squatting on the machine with the benefit of a visual cursor to assess weight distribution to avoid compensatory patterns.

Other exercises that are beneficial for proprioception are the use of rocker boards for directional perturbations for selective muscle recruitment patterns in a variety of planes of movement. These training techniques can be advanced to sport-specific activities such as tossing a ball against a trampoline, while manual perturbations are applied to the board (Fig. 8-5). Movement patterns such as a straight plane or multidirectional lunge are also useful for selective motor recruitment in functional or sport-related activities (Figs. 8-6 and 8-7). These patterns can be performed on balance pads or exercise mats to enhance motor control through maintaining balance while performing initially slow and then more rapid movements beyond the base of support (Fig. 8-8).

The goal of proprioception training is to reestablish stability or dynamic neuromuscular control and should

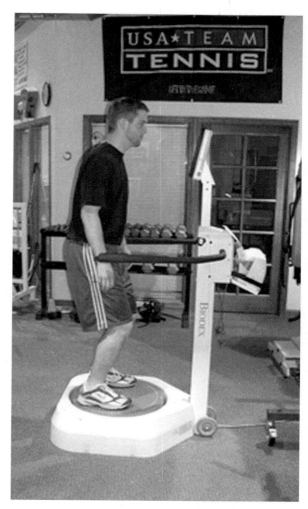

Figure 8-3. Incorporating functional movements such as the squat on the Biodex balance system.

emphasize a return to functional or sport-specific activity. In the later stages of training, exercise should focus on restoring and ideally optimizing the adaptive neuromuscular response to situational needs. If stabilization training has yielded the appropriate muscular response toward the final stages of rehabilitation, more advanced exercises to perform sport-specific drills should be incorporated. Exercises on a Fitter board° or Slideboard can be performed to challenge the patient with higher-velocity movements while performing sport-specific drills, utilizing full body movement patterns on a yielding surface (Figs. 8-9 and 8-10). Agility drills including progressively quicker directional changes while pivoting on the involved extremity should be incorporated in the final stages of rehabilitation for athletes who perform such maneuvers in the competitive arena.

°Available from Fitter International, Calgary, Alberta, Canada.

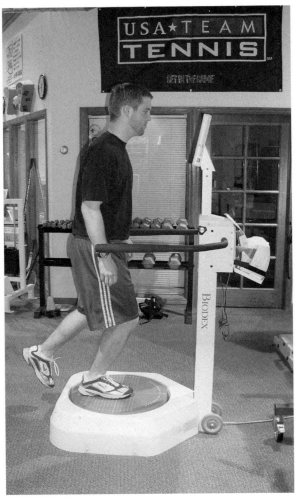

Figure 8-4. Single-leg balance on Biodex balance system. The level of difficulty is progressed by decreasing the stability of the platform or removing visual cues by having the patient close his or her eyes.

CLINICAL APPLICATION: TECHNIQUES TO IMPROVE PROPRIOCEPTION AND NEUROMUSCULAR CONTROL OF THE UPPER EXTREMITY WITH SPECIFIC REFERENCE TO THE SHOULDER

Application of the basic science information on proprioception and neuromuscular control of the shoulder to clinical practice allows clinicians to most appropriately provide stability to the glenohumeral joint and optimize shoulder girdle arthrokinematics. Several areas will be covered in this section, including the use of closed kinetic chain and joint approximation exercises, joint oscillation exercises, postoperative interventions, and techniques to improve muscular endurance of the rotator cuff and scapular musculature.

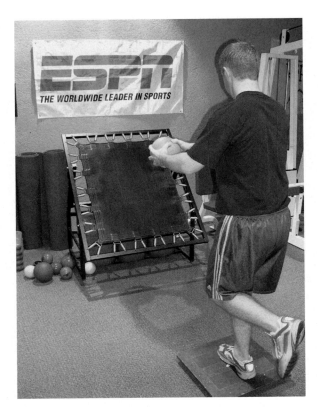

Figure 8-5. Chest pass with a weighted ball incorporates plyometric exercises with proprioceptive exercise, increasing the difficulty by manual perturbations of the rocker board while patient throws and catches the ball.

Closed Kinetic Chain (Joint Approximation) Exercises

The use of exercises that produce approximation of the glenohumeral joint and are characterized by a fixed distal aspect of the extremity are typically referred to as joint approximation or closed kinetic chain upper extremity exercises. The approximation of the joint surfaces and multiple joint loading inherent in closed kinetic chain exercise are reported to increase mechanoreceptor stimulation[59,77] and produce muscular co-contraction. The presence of muscular co-contraction around the human shoulder is particularly beneficial because of the important role the musculature surrounding the scapulothoracic joint plays in stabilizing and controlling movement of the shoulder.[51,52]

Significantly less EMG research has been published on upper extremity closed chain exercise compared with that for upper extremity open kinetic chain exercise. Moesley and co-workers[69] published a comprehensive analysis of the scapular muscles during traditional rehabilitation exercises. Two closed chain upper extremity exercises were included in their analysis. These exercises were the push-up with a "plus" and the press-up. The push-up with a plus includes maximal protraction of the scapula during the end of the ascent phase of a modified push-up and produces very high levels of serratus anterior muscle activity. The

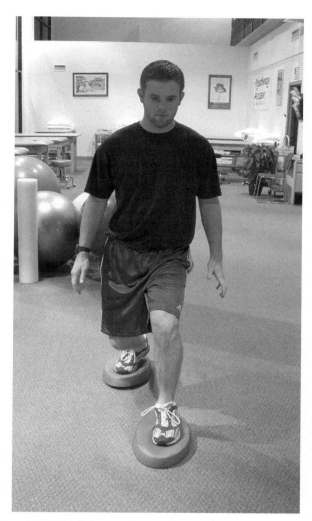

Figure 8-6. Combination of proximal pelvic control with lower extremity proprioception with the patient performing lunges on Thera-Band balance pads.

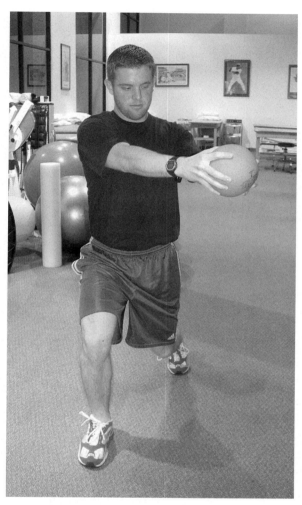

Figure 8-7. A lunge being performed with rotation of the torso while a weighted ball is held outside the base of support for integration of upper and lower extremity movement pattern.

press-up exercise did not elicit high levels of muscular activity in the trapezius or serratus, but instead elicited high activation levels in the pectoralis minor. Decker and associates[20] confirmed the importance of the plus position for serratus anterior activation and concluded that exercises emphasizing scapular upward rotation and accentuated protraction produce the highest levels of muscular activity in the serratus anterior.

Kibler and colleagues[52] published EMG research on a series of very low-level closed chain exercises for the upper extremity. These exercises included weight-bearing upper extremity weight shifts and rocker board or biomechanical ankle platform system exercises with the upper extremity. Muscle activation levels with these exercises were very low in the rotator cuff, deltoid, and scapular muscles; however, low levels of activity were present in virtually all of these muscles during these activities. This indicates that high degrees of co-activation and co-contraction are inherent in this type of exercise.

Recent research has demonstrated the important role that joint compression plays in glenohumeral joint closed kinetic chain exercise. Warner and co-workers[101] studied the effects of applying a 5-, 25-, and 50-pound compressive force to cadaveric shoulder specimens. These amounts of compression resulted in decreases in anterior humeral head translation in neutral elevation from 11 to 2 mm with 5 and 25 pounds of compressive force and from 21.5 to 1.4 mm at 45° of abduction, respectively. This study portrays the potential benefit of a compressive load in the provision of glenohumeral joint stability points out the important application that closed kinetic chain exercises may have to enhance neuromuscular control for patients with glenohumeral joint instability.

Application of closed kinetic chain exercises clinically is facilitated through a thorough review of glenohumeral joint anatomy. It is imperative that the clinician realize the osseous relationship of the glenohumeral joint. The human glenoid is oriented slightly inferiorly with the arm held at

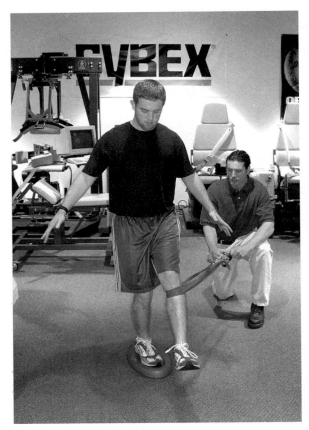

Figure 8-8. Single-leg balance on Thera-Band balance pads while opposite extremity movements are resisted beyond the base of support in functional planes.

the side and tilted anteriorly 30° from the coronal plane of the body.[80,85] This anterior version of the scapula is aligned with 30° of retrotorsion of the humeral head, with optimal bony congruity occurring with the arm placed in the scapular plane.[85] Understanding these important relationships will guide the clinician in shoulder positioning and ROM selection during joint approximation exercise with the arm placed in the scapular plane.[85]

Limited research exists for closed kinetic chain upper extremity training. Lephart and associates[60] used five neuromuscular control exercises that emphasized joint positioning, joint approximation and compression, and muscular co-contraction in one experimental group, in addition to traditional open kinetic chain shoulder rehabilitation exercises in patients with glenohumeral joint instability. They found significant improvements in kinesthetic ability, scapular slide testing, and isokinetically documented protraction and retraction strength in the group that performed these neuromuscular control exercises during rehabilitation.

Application of these concepts for the patient with rotator cuff dysfunction and glenohumeral joint instability is pictured in Figures 8-11 to 8-15. Guidelines for the time-based sets of exercise are patient dependent, with the ability of the patient to maintain the desired scapulothoracic stabilization being a governing factor. Careful monitoring

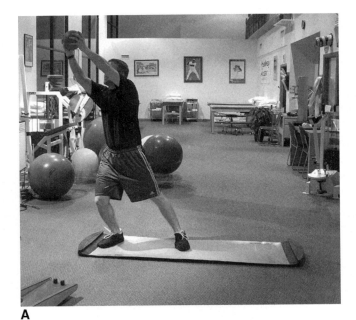

A

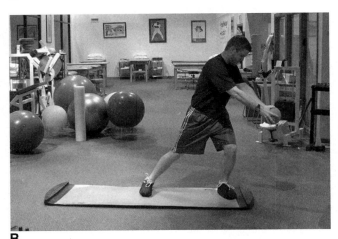

B

Figure 8-9. Dynamic balance on a Slideboard, incorporating upper body movements with resistance in proprioceptive neuromuscular facilitation patterns. *A,* Reaching high. *B,* Reaching low.

of the medial and inferior borders of the scapula is important to ensure proper neuromuscular control and avoid development of undesired motor patterning.[51] Sets of exercises of up to 30 or 45 seconds are desired in later stages of rehabilitation.

Joint Oscillation Exercises

Rehabilitative exercises using joint oscillation have increased in popularity in recent years. Appliances such as the Bodyblade,° Boing,† and resistance bar‡ have

---

°Available from Hymanson Inc, Playa Del Rey, California.
†Available from OPTP, Minneapolis, Minnesota.
‡Available from Hygenic Corp, Akron, Ohio.

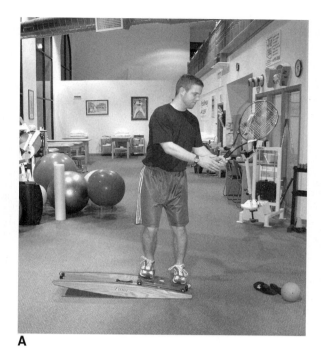

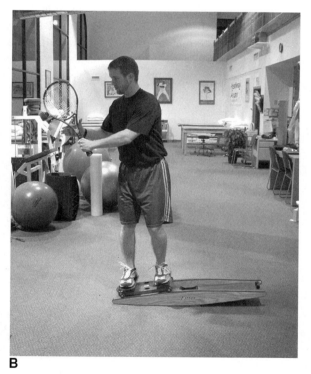

Figure 8-10. Dynamic balance on a Fitter board, with sport-specific drills such as the ground stroke in tennis. *A,* Forehand. *B,* Backhand.

facilitated the use of joint oscillation exercises. Rapid oscillation of these devices coupled with external loads such as light weights, manual resistance, and TheraTubing‡ can provide additional emphasis on particular muscle groups during these exercises. Figures 8-16 to 8-19 show exercises

‡Available from Hygenic Corp, Akron, Ohio.

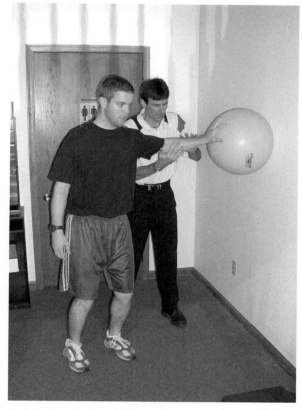

Figure 8-11. Closed chain wall scapular plane rhythmic stabilization. The patient's arm is placed on a medicine ball or small exercise ball in varying degrees of abduction in the scapular plane. The clinician performs rhythmic stabilization with the patient remaining as stable as possible over the ball, varying the position of hand contacts progressing further toward the patient's hand to increase the intensity of the exercise.

using oscillatory devices or manual contacts that require the rotator cuff and scapular musculature to respond to external cues induced via the oscillation and stretch imparted during the exercise. The ability of these time-based exercises to promote local muscular endurance is increased by manipulation of set duration and rest cycles.[54] Progression to the external rotation oscillation exercise in Figure 8-17 using the 90° abducted scapular plane position is followed as rehabilitation progresses to more closely approximate the glenohumeral and scapulothoracic positions inherent in overhead sport-specific movement patterns.[35] Figure 8-20 shows the push-up with a plus exercise. Care is used with this exercise to protect the shoulder complex by only descending approximately one-half the distance of a standard push-up and then maximally protracting the scapula on the ascent phase to increase activity of the serratus anterior muscle.[69]

Recently Holt and associates[45] investigated four different positions of exercise using the Bodyblade and its effect on infraspinatus muscle activity. These four positions

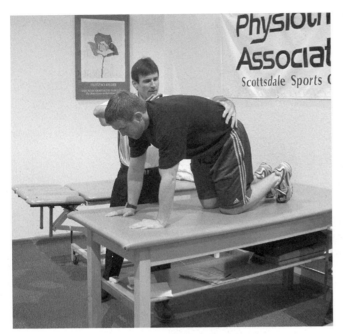

Figure 8-12. Quadruped rhythmic stabilization exercise progression with instruction to maintain scapular protraction or the "plus" position during repeated multidirectional challenges.

included (1) standing with the glenohumeral joint in neutral abduction/adduction position for internal and external rotation, (2) side-lying position with the glenohumeral joint in neutral abduction/adduction for internal and external rotation (Fig. 8-17), (3) 90° of glenohumeral joint scapular plane elevation with stabilization, and (4) 90° of

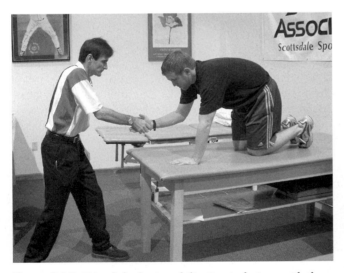

Figure 8-13. Triped rhythmic stabilization technique with the involved extremity in the closed chain position and maintenance of the "plus" position to increase serratus anterior muscle activation. The clinician alternately provides multidirectional challenges to the non–weight-bearing limb as the patient attempts to isometrically hold the pictured position.

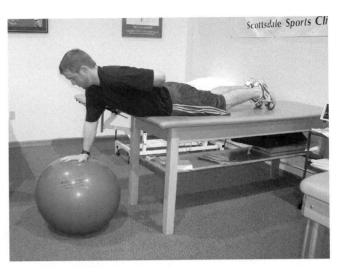

Figure 8-14. Unilateral prone exercise ball stabilization exercise. The degree of support is progressively decreased, increasing the challenge to the patient by sliding the patient in a cephalad direction.

scapular plane elevation with the unsupported arm. Results of a repeated measures analysis of variance showed that the side-lying internal/external rotation oscillatory pattern elicited the highest levels of infraspinatus muscle activation.[45] Further research such as this is needed to guide clinicians in the use of oscillatory type exercise.

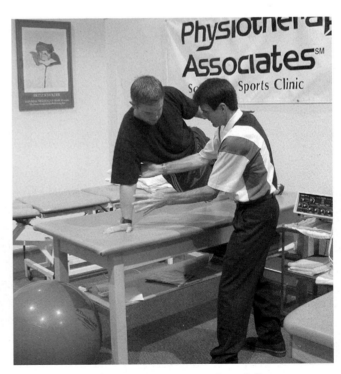

Figure 8-15. High-level unilateral scapular stabilization exercise with the patient in a closed chain unilateral scapular plane stance position with rhythmic stabilization superimposed on the upper extremity to increase the exercise challenge.

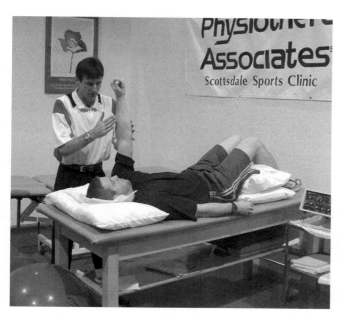

Figure 8-16. Supine modified rhythmic stabilization technique performed in 90° of shoulder flexion with scapular protraction.

Muscular Endurance Exercise

Exercises to increase endurance and fatigue resistance of the rotator cuff and scapular musculature would have a direct effect on improving performance and enhancing proprioception and neuromuscular control. All of the exercises described in this chapter can be used to promote local muscular endurance by increasing the work duration and decreasing the rest periods of the exercise format. Exercises utilizing sets of 15 to 20 repetitions and 15 to 20 repetition maximum loading schemes are geared for improving local muscular endurance.[54] Current practices in orthopedic and sports physical therapy usually include exercises with this type of prescription or recommendation.[28,105] The use and integration of joint oscillation, joint approximation or closed chain, plyometric,

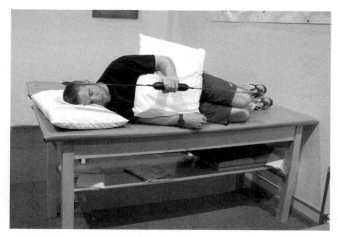

Figure 8-17. Side-lying glenohumeral rotational oscillation exercise using the Bodyblade.

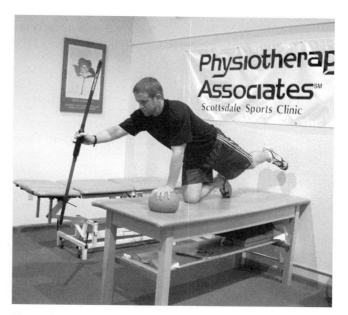

Figure 8-18. Biped closed kinetic chain using the Bodyblade to provide joint oscillation in the non–weight-bearing upper extremity and a medicine ball to decrease surface stability of the closed chain upper extremity. Alteration of scapular position can be instituted with this exercise based on the intended goal of muscular activation.

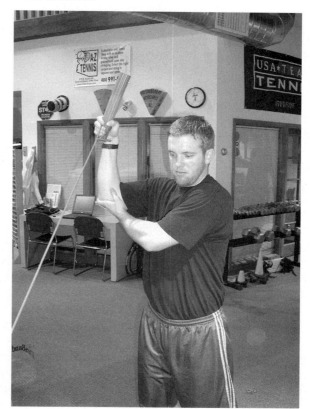

Figure 8-19. "Statue of Liberty" external rotation oscillation exercise using Thera-band elastic resistance and a resistance bar for oscillation. The scapular plane position in 90° of elevation is used with the contralateral extremity providing support to decrease the role of the deltoid in actively holding the exercising extremity in the 90° position.

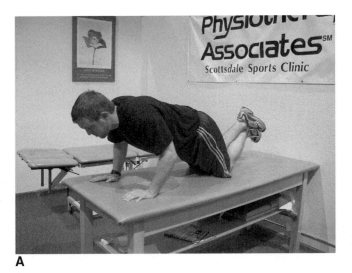 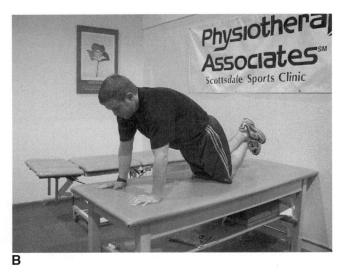

A   **B**

Figure 8-20. Push-up with a plus with maximal protraction of the scapula eliciting higher levels of serratus anterior activity. *A,* Starting position. *B,* End position of movement.

and isotonic and isokinetic training of targeted muscles or muscle groups have clear benefits and research-oriented rationales outlined in this chapter and other sources.[28,30,54,71,105]

One additional study performed by Ellenbecker and Roetert[34] specifically evaluated the relative muscular fatigue of the rotator cuff with isokinetic testing. Seventy-two elite junior tennis players underwent isokinetic fatigue testing consisting of 20 reciprocal concentric contractions of internal and external rotation with 90° of glenohumeral joint abduction. Results showed significantly different fatigue responses between the internal and external rotators. Analysis of the relative fatigue ratio, which compares the work performed in the second half of the testing protocol with the work performed in the first half, showed that the internal rotators fatigued to a level of only 83%. The external rotators, however, fatigued to level of 69% over the 20 testing repetitions.[34] This study demonstrated a greater relative degree of muscular fatigue in the external rotators, even in healthy trained subjects, and provides an important rationale for the inclusion of copious amounts of endurance-oriented training of the external rotators in patients with rotator cuff dysfunction or glenohumeral joint instability.

Chen and colleagues[18] demonstrated the effects of muscular fatigue on glenohumeral joint kinematics. Subjects were studied radiographically, as they elevated their shoulders before and after a series of rehabilitation exercises that produced substantial levels of muscular fatigue in the shoulder. They found significantly greater amounts of superiorly directed humeral head translation documented radiographically with arm elevation after fatigue. This study shows the important role the rotator cuff plays in maintaining glenohumeral joint congruity and stabilizing the humeral head within the glenoid.[18] Repeated attempts to enhance muscular endurance based on these studies, as well as on earlier

literature citations linking muscular fatigue of the glenohumeral rotators to decrements in proprioception, are clinically indicated.

Postoperative Applications

Use of treatment techniques to enhance proprioception and neuromuscular control are indicated in the shoulder after surgery. Current methods of addressing glenohumeral joint instability include capsular plication and application of thermal energy to produce capsular shortening, which create changes in capsular length and may acutely alter glenohumeral joint proprioception.[64,75] Myers and co-workers[73] measured joint position sense, kinesthesia, and shoulder function in patients who underwent thermal capsular shrinkage for glenohumeral joint instability. No significant differences were found in active and passive angular reproduction of joint position sense 6 to 24 months postoperatively. The acute effects of thermal capsular shrinkage on glenohumeral joint proprioception are not completely understood; however, this study shows that a full return of proprioceptive function is expected after rehabilitation.

Early postoperative proprioceptive training consists of passive angular joint repositioning in available ROMs with elimination of visual cues. Replication of either the contralateral extremity position or repeated movements can be done passively initially and then be progressed to active angular joint position replication as patient status and tissue healing allows. Early application of joint approximation exercises and rhythmic stabilization exercises described earlier in this chapter are also beneficial in the early progression after rotator cuff repair and open and arthroscopic stabilization.[33]

Neuromuscular control is the result of the efferent response to the afferent signals generated through the sensory system. Proprioception plays a critical role with this feedback system. When injury or disruption to the proprioceptive pathways occurs, there is potential for not only inefficient motor responses but also greater risk for injury especially in the area of athletics in which overcoming resistance from opposing players is coupled with environmental obstacles in an often fast-paced arena. In preparing athletes for competition, the clinician should consider the effects of fatigue and disuse on proprioception and also their potential impact when designing a comprehensive training or rehabilitation program.

Utilization of the clinically oriented exercise progressions highlighted in this chapter including techniques such as joint approximation, joint oscillation, and local muscular endurance applications provides the framework for objectively based rehabilitation programs using the scientific concepts reviewed in this chapter.

SUMMARY

Introduction

- More is known about proprioception in the lower extremity than in the upper extremity.
- To maintain balance and postural control we rely on sensory information from the periphery as well as from our visual, vestibular, and somatosensory systems.
- Feedforward and feedback mechanisms are responsible for initiating a motor response in anticipation of a stimulus.

Afferent Mechanoreceptor Classification

- Mechanoreceptors are sensory neurons or peripheral afferents located with joint capsular tissues, ligaments, tendons, muscle, and skin.
- There are four primary types of afferent mechanoreceptors that are commonly present in noncontractile capsular and ligamentous structures in human joints; these are types I, II, III, and IV.
- Type I and II mechanoreceptors are the primary receptors located in the joint capsule.
- The lower extremity contains types I, II, III, and IV mechanoreceptors, whereas the glenohumeral joint appears to have all four types, which are structure dependent. Types I and II predominate in the glenohumeral joint.
- The primary mechanisms for afferent feedback from the muscle tendon unit are the muscle spindle and the Golgi tendon organ.

Clinical Assessment of Proprioception in the Lower Extremity

- The two primary tests measuring proprioception and kinesthetic awareness in the knee and glenohumeral joint are threshold to detection of passive motion for movement sense and reproduction of angular position for measuring joint position sense.
- There are essentially no standard protocols for measuring joint position sense or for joint replication tests.

Assessment of Proprioception and Neuromuscular Control in the Upper Extremity

- There is evidence to suggest that athletes performing unilaterally dominant upper extremity movements, such as those involved in baseball, tennis or volleyball, may have a proprioceptive deficit on the dominant arm that may interfere with optimal afferent feedback regarding joint position.
- Active joint angular position replication tests primarily involve the stimulation of both joint and muscle receptors and provide a thorough assessment of afferent pathways of the human shoulder.
- Neuromuscular control of the shoulder can be assessed with electromyography, functional movement patterns, abnormal muscular activity patterns during planar motion, functional activities, muscular strength, and closed kinetic chain upper extremity tests.
- Evaluation methods to assess closed chain function of the upper extremity are limited. Those that have been used include the push-up and the closed kinetic chain stability test.

Effects of Aging, Instability, and Injury on Lower Extremity Proprioception

- Age and injury result in diminished proprioception sense.
- The loss of capsuloligamentous stability causes proprioceptive deficits due to inadequate activation of the mechanoreceptors resulting in delayed muscle reaction latencies.
- There is evidence to suggest that a total knee replacement results in improved proprioception scores although the effects of sacrificing or retaining the posterior cruciate ligament are inconclusive.
- There is a decrease in proprioception sense and altered muscle patterns after rupture of the anterior cruciate ligament.

Effects of Shoulder Pathologic Conditions on Proprioception and Neuromuscular Control

- Damage to the capsuloligamentous structures of the shoulder leads to deficits in proprioception.
- Glenohumeral joint instability and rotator cuff dysfunction result in changes in neuromuscular control patterns.

Effects of Fatigue on Lower Extremity Proprioception

■ Muscle fatigue reduces the force-generating capacity of the neuromuscular system, which essentially leads to increased laxity in the knee joint.

■ There is evidence to show a decrease in the sensitivity of muscle receptors to fatigue conditions. The consequences of decreased proprioception sense from fatigue can be deleterious because of the possibility of sustaining injuries under these conditions while higher-level activities are performed.

Effects of Muscular Fatigue on Upper Extremity Proprioception and Neuromuscular Control

■ Evidence suggests that the effect of muscular fatigue on joint proprioception may play a role in injury and decrease athletic performance.

■ The consistent finding of a proprioceptive decrement after muscular fatigue has led researchers to emphasize the importance of the muscle-based receptors.

Effects of Training on Proprioception in the Lower Extremity

■ It appears that proprioception can be enhanced through a proprioception training program.

Techniques to Improve Lower Extremity Proprioception and Neuromuscular Control

■ Different patterns of movement require varied muscular stabilization, depending on the direction, speed, and amount of force occurring at the joint.

■ Progression of proprioception and neuromuscular control training during the early and middle phases of training consists of moving along a continuum that modifies predictability, speed, amplitude, intensity, and direction of force.

Guidelines for Implementing Lower Extremity Proprioception Training

■ When one selects exercises for restoring proprioception and dynamic stability the focus on restoring function to the individual should remain at the forefront. Exercises chosen should then focus on an individual's deficits in strength, ROM, and balance and most importantly on the individual's ability to meet the demands of stability while performing daily or sporting activities.

■ Any number of exercises will elicit proprioception training based on the fact that deformation of the joint mechanoreceptors occurs with active, active assisted, and passive movements providing sensory input to improve neural mechanisms.

■ The goal of proprioception training is to reestablish stability or dynamic neuromuscular control and should emphasize a return to functional or sport-specific activity.

Techniques to Improve Proprioception and Neuromuscular Control of the Upper Extremity

■ The approximation of the joint surfaces and multiple joint loading inherent to closed kinetic chain exercise are reported to increase mechanoreceptor stimulation and produce muscular co-contraction.

■ Patients with rotator cuff dysfunction or glenohumeral joint instability are progressed on a continuum of difficulty with the patient's ability to maintain the desired scapulothoracic stabilization being a governing factor. Careful monitoring of the medial and inferior boarders of the scapula are important, to ensure proper neuromuscular control and to avoid development of undesired motor patterning.

■ Exercises to increase endurance and fatigue resistance of the rotator cuff and scapular musculature have a direct effect on improving performance and enhancing proprioception and neuromuscular control.

■ Exercises utilizing sets of 15 to 20 repetitions and using 15 to 20 repetition maximum loading schemes are geared for improving local muscular endurance.

REFERENCES

1. Adams, R.D., Victor, M., and Ropper, A.H. (1997): Principles of Neurology, 6th ed. New York, McGraw-Hill Health Professions Division.
2. Allegrucci, M., Whitney, S.L., Lephart, S.M., et al. (1995): Shoulder kinesthesia in healthy unilateral athletes participating in upper extremity sports. J. Orthop. Sports. Phys. Ther., 21:220-226.
3. Andriacchi, T.P., and Birac, D. (1993): Functional testing in the anterior cruciate ligament-deficient knee. Clin. Orthop., 288:40-47.
4. Andriacchi, T.P., and Galante, J.O. (1988): Retensioning of the posterior cruciate ligament in total knee arthroplasty. J. Arthroplasty, S13-S19.
5. Ballantyne, B.T., O'Hare, S.J., Paschall, J.L., et al. (1993): Electromyographic activity of selected shoulder muscles in commonly used therapeutic exercises. Phys. Ther., 73:668-682.
6. Barker, D., Banks, R.W., Harker, D.W. et al. (1976): Studies of the histochemistry, ultrastructure, motor innervation, and regeneration of mammalian intrafusal muscle fibers. Exp. Brain Res., 44:67-88.
7. Barrack, R.L., Skinner, H.B., Brunet, M.E., and Cook, S.D. (1983): Joint laxity and proprioception in the knee. Phys. Sports Med., 11:130-135.
8. Barrack, R.L., Skinner, H.B., and Buckley, S.L. (1989): Proprioception in the anterior cruciate-deficient knee. Am. J. Sports Med., 17:1-6.
9. Barrack, R.L., Skinner, H.B., Cook, S.D., et al. (1983): Effect of articular disease and total knee arthroplasty on knee joint-position sense. J. Neurophysiol., 50:684-687.

10. Barrett, D.S., Cobb, A.G., and Bently, G. (1991): Joint proprioception in normal osteoarthritic and replaced knees. J. Bone Joint Surg., 73B:53-56.

11. Beard, D.J., Dodd, C.F., Trundle, H.R., and Simpson, A.W. (1994): Proprioception enhancement for anterior cruciate ligament deficiency. J. Bone Joint Surg., 76B:654-659.

12. Beard, D.J., Kyberd, P.J., Ferguson, C.M., et al. (1993): Proprioception after rupture of the anterior cruciate ligament. J. Bone Joint Surg., 73B:311-315.

13. Beynnon, B.D., Good, L., and Risberg, M.A. (2002): The effect of bracing on proprioception of knees with anterior cruciate ligament injury. J. Orthop. Sports Phys. Ther., 32(1):11-23.

14. Blackburn, T.A., McLeod, W.D., White, B., et al. (1990): EMG analysis of posterior rotator cuff exercises. Athl. Train., 25:40-45.

15. Blaiser, R.B., Carpenter, J.E., and Huston, L.J. (1994): Shoulder proprioception: Effect of joint laxity, joint position, and direction of motion. Orthop. Rev., 23:45-50.

16. Carpenter, J.E., Blaiser, R.B., and Pellizon, G.G. (1998): The effects of muscle fatigue on shoulder joint position sense. Am. J. Sports Med., 26:262-265.

17. Cerulli, G., Benoit, D.L., Caraffa, A., et al. (2001): Proprioceptive training and prevention of anterior cruciate ligament injuries in soccer. J. Orthop. Sports Phys. Ther., 31:655-661.

18. Chen, S.K., Simonion, P.T., Wickiewicz, T.L., and Warren, R.F. (1999): Radiographic evaluation of glenohumeral kinematics: A muscle fatigue model. J. Shoulder Elbow Surg., 8:49-52.

19. Davies, G.J., and Hoffman, S.D. (1993): Neuromuscular testing and rehabilitation of the shoulder complex. J. Orthop. Sports Phys. Ther., 18:449-457.

20. Decker, M.J., Hintermeister, R.A., Faber, K.J., and Hawkins, R.J. (1999): Serratus anterior muscle activity during selected rehabilitation exercises. Am. J. Sports Med., 27:784-791.

21. DiGiovine, N.M., Jobe, F.W., Pink, M., et al. (1994): An electromyographic analysis of the upper extremity in pitching. J. Shoulder Elbow Surg., 1:15-25.

22. Djupsjobacka, M., Johansson, H., and Bergenheim, M. (1994): Influences on the gamma muscle spindle system from muscle afferents stimulated by increased intramuscular concentrations of arachidonic acid. Brain Res., 663:293-302.

23. Djupsjobacka, M., Johansson, H., Bergenheim, M., et al. (1995): Influences on the gamma muscle spindle system from muscle afferents stimulated by increased intramuscular concentrations of bradykinin and 5-HT. Neurosci. Res., 22:325-333.

24. Djupsjobacka, M., Johansson, H., Bergenheim, et al. (1995): Influences on the gamma muscle spindle system from contralateral muscle afferents stimulated by KCl and lactic acid. Neurosci. Res., 21:301-309.

25. Dorr, L.D., Ochsner, J.L., Growley, J., and Perry J. (1988): Functional comparisons of posterior cruciate retained versus sacrificed in total knee arthroplasty. Clin. Orthop., 236: 36-43.

26. Eils, E., and Dieter, R. (2001): A multi-station proprioceptive exercise program in patients with ankle instability. Med. Sci. Sports Exer., 33:1991-1998.

27. Eklund, G. (1972): Position sense and state of contraction: the effects of vibration. J. Neurol. Neurosurg. Psychiatry, 35:606-611.

28. Ellenbecker, T.S. (1995): Rehabilitation of shoulder and elbow injuries in tennis players. Clin. Sports Med., 14:87-110.

29. Ellenbecker, T.S., and Cappel, K. (2000): Clinical application of closed kinetic chain exercises in the upper extremities. Orthop. Phys. Ther. Clin. North Am., 9:231-245.

30. Ellenbecker, T.S., and Davies, G.J. (2000): The application of isokinetics in testing and rehabilitation of the shoulder complex. J. Athl. Train., 35:338-350.

31. Ellenbecker, T.S., and Davies, G.J. (2001): Closed Kinetic Chain Exercise. Champaign IL, Human Kinetics.

32. Ellenbecker, T.S., Manske, R., and Davies, G.J. (2000): Closed kinetic chain testing techniques of the upper extremities. Orthop. Phys. Ther. Clin. North Am., 9:219-245.

33. Ellenbecker, T.S., and Mattalino, A.J. (1999): Glenohumeral joint range of motion and rotator cuff strength following arthroscopic anterior stabilization with thermal capsulorraphy. J. Orthop. Sports Phys. Ther., 29:160-167.

34. Ellenbecker, T.S., and Roetert, E.P. (1999): Testing isokinetic muscular fatigue of shoulder internal and external rotation in elite junior tennis players. J. Orthop. Sports Phys. Ther., 29:275-281.

35. Elliot, B., Marsh, T., and Blanksby, B. (1986): A three dimensional cinematographic analysis of the tennis serve. Int. J. Sport Biomech., 2:260-271.

36. Fitzgerals, G.K., Axe, M.J., and Snyder-Mackler, L. (2000): The efficacy of perturbation training in nonoperative anterior cruciate ligament rehabilitation programs for physically active individuals. Phys. Ther., 80:128-140.

37. Friden, T., Roberts, M., Ageberg, E., et al. (2001): Review of knee proprioception and the relation to extremity function after an anterior cruciate ligament rupture. J. Orthop. Sports Phys. Ther., 31:568-576.

38. Garn, S. N., and Newton, R. A., (1988): Kinesthetic awareness in subjects with multiple ankle sprains. Phys. Ther. 68(11):1667-1671.

39. Glousman, R., Jobe, F., Tibone, J., et al. (1988): Dynamic electromyographic analysis of the throwing shoulder with glenohumeral instability. J. Bone Joint Surg., 70-A:220-226.

40. Goetz, C.G. (1999): Textbook of Clinical Neurology, 1st ed., Philadelphia, W.B. Saunders.

41. Goldbeck, T.G., and Davies, G.J. (2000): Test-retest reliability of the closed kinetic chain upper extremity stability test: A clinical field test. J. Sport Rehab., 9:35-45.

42. Goldscheider, A.: Gesammelte Abhandlungen. II. Physiologie des Muskelsinnes. Leipzig, Barth.

43. Goodwin, G.M., McCloskey, D.I., and Matthews, P.B.C. (1972): The contribution of muscle afferents to kinesthesia shown by vibration induced illusions of movement and by the effects of paralyzing joint afferents. Brain, 95:705-748.

44. Grigg, P. (1994): Peripheral mechanisms in proprioception. J. Sport Rehab., 3:2-17.

45. Holt, S., O'Brien, M., Davies, G.J., et al. (2000): An investigation of shoulder muscle electrical activity during bodyblade exercises. Presented at Wisconsin State Physical Therapy Association Spring Meeting.

46. Hurley, M.V., and Newham, D.J. (1993): The influence of arthrogenous muscle inhibition on quadriceps rehabilitation of patients with early, unilateral osteoarthritic knees. Br. J. Rheumatol., 32:127-131.

47. Ide, K., Shirai, Y., Ito, H., et al. (1996): Sensory nerve supply in the human subacromial bursa. J. Shoulder Elbow Surg., 5:371-382.

48. Inman, V.T., Saunders, J.B., and Abbot, L.C. (1994): Observations on the function of the shoulder joint. J. Bone Joint Surg., 26:1-30.

49. Jerosch, J.G. (2000): Effects of shoulder instability on joint proprioception. *In:* Lephart, S.M., and Fu, F.H. (eds), Proprioception and Neuromuscular Control in Joint Stability. Champaign, II, Human Kinetics.

50. Kaplan, F.S., Nixon, J.E., Reitz, M., et al. (1985): Age-related changes in joint proprioception and sensation of joint position. Acta Orthop. Scand., 56:72-74.

51. Kibler, W.B. (1998): The role of the scapula in athletic shoulder function. Am. J. Sports Med. 26:325-337.

52. Kibler, W.B., Livingstone, B., and Bruce, R. (20xx): Current concepts in shoulder rehabilitation. *In:* Advances in Operative Orthopaedics. St. Louis, Mosby-Year Book, Vol. 3, pp, 249-297.

53. Kikuchi, T. (1968): Histological studies on the sensory innervation of the shoulder joint. J. Iwate Med. Assoc., 20:554-567.

54. Kraemer, W.J., and Fleck, S.J. (2003): Designing Resistance Training Programs, 3rd ed. Champaign, IL, Human Kinetics.

55. Kronberg, M., Brostrom, L.A., and Nemeth, G. (1991): Differences in shoulder muscle activity between patients with generalized joint laxity and normal controls. Clin. Orthop., 209:181-192.

56. Lattanzio, P.J., and Petrella, R.J. (1998): Knee proprioception: A review of mechanisms, measurements, and implications of muscular fatigue. Orthopedics 21:463-470.

57. Lattanzio, P.J., Petrella, R.J., and Sproule, J.R., et al. (1997): Effects of fatigue on knee proprioception. Clin. J. Sports Med., 7:22-27.

58. Lentell, G.G., Baas, B., Lopez, D., et al. (1995): The contributions of proprioceptive deficit, muscle function, and anatomic laxity to functional instability of the ankle. J. Orthop. Sports Phys. Ther., 21:206-215.

59. Lephart, S.M., and Fu, F.H. (2000): Proprioception and Neuromuscular Control in Joint Stability. Champaign, IL, Human Kinetics.

60. Lephart, S.M., Henry, T.J., Riemann, B.L., et al. (1998): The effects of neuromuscular control exercises on functional stability in the unstable shoulder. J. Athl. Trai., 33:S15.

61. Lephart, S.M., Pincivero, D.M., Giraldo, J.L., and Fu, F.H. (1997): The role of proprioception in the management and rehabilitation of athletic injuries. Am. J. Sports Med., 25:130-137.

62. Lephart, S.M., Warner, J.J.P., Borsa, P.A., and Fu, F.H. (1994): Proprioception of the shoulder joint in healthy, unstable, and surgically repaired shoulders. J. Shoulder Elbow Surg., 3:371-380.

63. Limbird, T.J., Shiavir, R., Frazer, M., and Borra, H. (1988): EMG profiles of knee joint musculature during walking: Changes induced by anterior cruciate ligament deficiency. J. Orthop. Res., 6:630-638.

64. Lu, Y., Hayashi, K., Edwards, R.B., et al, (2000): The effect of monopolar radiofrequency treatment pattern on joint capsular healing. In vitro and in vivo studies using an ovine model. Am. J. Sports Med., 28:711-719.

65. Ludewig, P.M., and Cook, T.M. (2000): Alterations in shoulder kinematics and associated muscle activity in people with symptoms of shoulder impingement. Phys. Ther., 80:276-291.

66. Marks, R., and Quinney, H.A. (1993): Effect of fatiguing maximal isokinetic quadriceps contractions on ability to estimate knee position. Percept. Mot. Skills, 77:1195-2002.

67. Marshall, R.N., and Elliot, B.C. (2000): Long-axis rotation: The missing link in proximal to distal segmental sequencing. J. Sports Sci., 18:247-254.

68. McMahon, P.J., Jobe, F.W., Pink, M.M., et al. (1996): Comparative electromyographic analysis of shoulder muscles during planar motions: Anterior glenohumeral instability versus normal. J. Shoulder Elbow Surg., 5:118-123.

69. Moesley, J.B., Jobe, F.W., and Pink, M. (1992): EMG analysis of the scapular muscles during a shoulder rehabilitation program. Am. J. Sports Med., 20:128-134.

70. Morisawa, Y., Kawakami, T., Uermura, H., et al. (1994): Mechanoreceptors in the coraco-acromial ligament. A study of the aging process. J. Shoulder Elbow Surg., 3:S45.

71. Myers, J.B., and Lephart, S.M. (2000): The role of the sensorimotor system in the athletic shoulder. J. Athl. Train., 35:351-363.

72. Myers, J.B., Guskiewicz, K.M., Schneider, R.A., et al. (1999): Proprioception and neuromuscular control of the shoulder after muscle fatigue. J Athl. Train., 34:362-367.

73. Myers, J.B., Lephart, S.M., Riemann, B.L., et al. (2000): Evaluation of shoulder proprioception following thermal capsulorrahy. Med. Sci. Sports Exer., 32:S123.

74. Nawoczenski, D.A., Owen, G., Ecker, B., et al. (1985): Objective evaluation of peroneal response to sudden inversion stress. J. Orthop. Sports Phys. Ther., 25:107-109.

75. Nyland, J, A., Caborn, D.N.M., and Johnson, D.L. (1998): The human glenohumeral joint: A proprioceptive and stability aliance. Knee Sur. Sports Traumatol. Arthrosc., 6:50-61.

76. Osborne, M.D., Chou, L.S., Laskowski, E.R., et al. (2001): The effect of ankle disk training on muscle reaction time in subjects with a history of ankle sprain. Am. J. Sports Med., 29:627-632.

77. Palmitier, R.A., An, K.N., Scott, S.G., et al. (1991): Kinetic chain exercise in knee rehabilitation. Sports Med., 11:402-413.

78. Pederson, J., Jonn, J., Hellstrom, F., et al. (1999): Localized muscle fatigue decreases the acuity of the movement sense in the human shoulder. Med. Sci. Sports Exer., 31:1047-1052.

79. Pincivero, D.M., and Coelho, A.J. (2001): Proprioceptive measures warrant scrutiny. Biomechanics, 3:77-86.

80. Poppen, N.K., and Walker, P.S. (1976): Normal and abnormal motion of the shoulder. J. Bone Joint Surg., 58:195-201.

81. Provins, K.A. (1958): The effect of peripheral nerve block on the appreciation and execution of finger movements. J. Physiol., 143:55-67.

82. Rhu, K.N., McCormick, J., Jobe, F.W., et al. (1988): An electromyographic analysis of shoulder function in tennis players. Am. J. Sports Med., 16:481-485.

83. Roetert, E.P., and Ellenbecker, T.S. (1998): Complete Conditioning for Tennis. Champaign, IL, Human Kinetics.

84. Roland, P.E., and Ladegaard-Pedersen, H. (1977): A quantitative analysis of sensations of tension and of kinesthesia in man: Evidence for a peripherally originating muscular sense and for a sense of effort. Brain, 100:671-692.

85. Saha, A.K. (1983): Mechanism of shoulder movements and a plea for the recognition of "zero-position" of glenohumeral joint. Clin. Orthop., 173:3-10.

86. Sharma, L., and Yi-Chung, P. (1997): Impaired proprioception and osteoarthritis. Curr. Opin. Rheumatol., 9:253-258.

87. Sherrington, C. (1906): The Integrative Action of the Nervous System. New York, Scribner's Son.

88. Shimoda, F. (1955): Innervation, especially sensory innervation of the knee joint and motor organs around it in early stage of human embryo. Arch. Histol. (Jpn.), 9:91-108.

89. Skinner, H.B., Wyatt, M.P., Hodgdon, J.A., et al. (1986): Effect of fatigue on joint position sense of the knee. J. Orthop. Res., 4:112-118.

90. Skinner, H.B., Barrack, R.L., and Cook, S.D. (1984): Age related decline in proprioception. Clin. Orthop., 184: 208-211.

91. Skinner, H.B., Wyatt, M.P., Stone, M.L., et al. (1986): Exercise related knee joint laxity. Am. J. Sports Med., 14: 30-34.

92. Slobounov, S.M., Poole, S.T., Simon, R.F., et al. (1999): The efficacy of modern technology to improve healthy and injured shoulder joint position sense. J. Sport Rehab., 8:10-23.

93. Smith, R.L., and Brunolli, J. (1989): Shoulder kinesthesia after anterior glenohumeral joint dislocation. Phys. Ther., 69:106-112.

94. Snyder-Mackler, L.A., Delitto, S.L., and Straka, S.W. (1995): Strength of the quadriceps femoris muscle and functional recovery after reconstruction of the anterior cruciate ligament. J. Bone Joint Surg., 77:1166-1173.

95. Speer, K.P., Deng, X., Borrero, S., Torzilli, P.A., et al. (1994): Biomechanical evaluation of a simulated Bankart lesion. J. Bone Joint Surg., 76-A:1819-1826.

96. Townsend, H., Jobe, F.W., Pink, M., et al. (1991): Electromyographic analysis of the glenohumeral muscles during a baseball rehabilitation program. Am. J. Sports Med., 19:264-272.

97. Tropp, H., Ekstrand, J., and Gillquist, J. (1984): Factors affecting stabilometry recordings of single limb stance. Am. J. Sports Med., 12:185-188.

98. Vangsness, C.T., Ennis, M., Taylor, J.G., et al. (1995): Neural anatomy of the glenohumeral ligaments, labrum, and subacromial bursa. Arthroscopy, 11:180-184.

99. Voight, M.L., Hardin, J.A., Blackburn, T.A., et al. (1996): The effects of muscle fatigue on and the relationship of arm dominance to shoulder proprioception. J. Orthop. Sports Phys. Ther., 23:348-352.

100. Voss, H. (1971): Tabelle der absoluten und relativen Muskelspindelzahlen der menschlichen Skelettmuskulatur. Anat. Anz., 129:562-572.

101. Warner, J.J.P., Bowen, M.K., Deng, X., et al. (1999): Effect of joint compression on inferior stability of the glenohumeral joint. J. Shoulder Elbow Surg., 8:31-36.

102. Warner, J.J.P., Lephart, S., and Fu, F.H. (1996): Role of proprioception in pathoetiology of shoulder instability. Clin. Orthop., 330:35-39.

103. Warren, P.J., Olankun, T.K., Cobb, A.G., and Bentley, G. (1993): Proprioception after knee arthroplasty: The influence of prosthetic design. Clin. Orthop., 297:182-187.

104. Weisman, G., Pope, M.H., Hohnson, R.J. (1980): Cyclic loading in knee ligament injuries. Am. J. Sports Med., 8:24-30.

105. Wilk, K.E, and Arrigo, C. (1993): Current concepts in the rehabilitation of the athletic shoulder. J. Orthop. Sports Phys. Ther., 18:365-378.

106. Wilk, K.E., Arrigo, C.A., and Andrews, J.R. (1996): Closed and open kinetic chain exercises for the upper extremity. J. Sport Rehab., 5:88-102.

107. Williams, G.N., Chmielewski, T., Rudolph, K.S., Buchanan, T.S., et al. (2001): Dynamic knee stability: Current theory and implications for clinical scientists. J. Orthop. Sports Phys. Ther., 31(10):546-566.

108. Wyke, B. (1972): Articular neurology—A review. Physiotherapy, 58:94-99.

109. Wyke, B.D. (1967): The neurology of joints. Ann. R. Coll. Surg. Engl., 41:25.

110. Zuckerman, J.D., Gallagher, M.A., Lehman, C., et al. (1999): Normal shoulder proprioception and the effect of lidocaine injection. J. Shoulder Elbow Surg., 8:11-16.

CHAPTER 9

APPLICATION OF ISOKINETICS IN TESTING AND REHABILITATION

George J. Davies, M.Ed., P.T., S.C.S, ATC, C.S.C.S.

Todd S. Ellenbecker, M.S., P.T., S.C.S, O.C.S.C.S.C.S.

CHAPTER OBJECTIVES

At the end of this chapter the reader will be able to:

- Define the terminology used with isokinetics.
- Apply general guidelines regarding the application of isokinetic testing.
- Explain the specific applications of isokinetic assessment of muscular power in the upper extremities.
- Implement the application of isokinetics as part of rehabilitation programs.
- Explain the scientific and clinical rationale for the use of isokinetics in evaluation and rehabilitation of sports injuries.

Isokinetics plays a significant role in evaluation and rehabilitation of injured athletes. The utilization of isokinetics has changed as the interest in isokinetics has varied over the past 25 years. Isokinetics was developed in the 1960s and was increasingly used during the 1970s. However, research on this subject was minimal and the potential uses and applications of isokinetics were not clearly understood. In the 1980s the field of isokinetics came into its own, with increasing popularity and, most importantly, with an increasing body of knowledge through numerous publications that supported the appropriate use of isokinetics in the testing and rehabilitation of athletes. During this period, isokinetics was increasingly used in many different areas and with many different applications. The first book dedicated solely to isokinetics was published in the early 1980s[27]; it provided an overview of the testing and application of isokinetics using a combination of published research and empirically based clinical experiences. However, in the 1990s, there was a trend away from the utilization of isokinetics as part of the total evaluation and rehabilitation process. Despite extensive publications on isokinetics (more than 2000 published articles on the utilization and efficacy of isokinetics, an entire journal dedicated to the art and science of isokinetics [*Isokinetics and Exercise Science*], and four books dedicated exclusively to isokinetics[19,27,42,117]), many practicing clinicians have discontinued using isokinetics on the grounds that it is not functional. Although admittedly most athletes do not sit and flex and extend their knees as a functional activity, there is a high correlation between isokinetic testing of the knee and functional testing. Unfortunately, many clinicians are disregarding the extensive documentation of isokinetics in the evaluation and treatment of athletes and are embracing closed kinetic chain (CKC) exercises as a panacea without significant documentation of efficacy. We do not advocate that only isokinetics should be used or that CKC exercises should not be used; we would, however, like to emphasize the need for an integrated approach that uses many modes of testing and rehabilitation.

OVERVIEW AND TERMINOLOGY

There are numerous modes of exercise that can be utilized in the evaluation and rehabilitation of athletes. These include isometrics, isotonics, plyometrics, isoacceleration, isodeceleration, and isokinetics.

The concept of isokinetic exercise was introduced by James Perrine in the late 1960s, and it proved to be a revolution in exercise training and rehabilitation. Instead of the traditional exercises that were performed at variable speeds against a constant weight or resistance, Perrine developed the concept of isokinetics, which involves a dynamic preset fixed speed with resistance that is totally accommodating throughout the range of motion (ROM). Since the inception of isokinetics, this form of testing and exercise has become increasingly popular in clinical, athletic, and research settings, with the first article describing isokinetic exercise being published in 1967.[74] Since then, numerous articles and research presentations have documented the use of isokinetics for objective testing or for training.

Isokinetics means that exercise is performed at a fixed velocity (ranging from 1° per second to approximately

1000° per second), with an accommodating resistance. Accommodating resistance means that isokinetic exercise is the only way to dynamically load a muscle to its maximum capability through every point throughout the ROM. Therefore, the resistance varies to exactly match the force applied by the athlete at every point in the ROM. This is important because, as the joint goes through the ROM, the amount of torque that can be produced varies because of the Blix curve (musculotendinous length-to-tension ratio) and because of the physiologic length-to-tension ratio changes that occur in the muscle-tendon unit and in biomechanical skeletal leverage. The advantages and limitations of isokinetics are listed in Box 9-1.

Open Kinetic Chain

An open kinetic chain (OKC) assessment or rehabilitation exercise is considered to be an activity in which the distal component of the extremity is not fixed but is free in space.[47] It is questionable whether many exercises are pure OKC, CKC, or combinations of the two. Nevertheless, an operational definition of an OKC test or exercise, within the limitations of this chapter, is one in which the distal end of the extremity is free and not fixed to an object. One of the best examples of the OKC pattern is performance of a knee flexion-to-extension pattern while sitting. This OKC pattern will serve as the model to describe OKC exercises.

Closed Kinetic Chain

A CKC assessment or rehabilitation exercise is considered to be an activity in which the distal component of the extremity is fixed.[47] The fixed end may be either stationary or moveable.[47] An example of a CKC exercise in which the distal end is stationary is a squat exercise in which the foot is fixed to the ground. An example of a CKC exercise in which the distal end is moveable is exercise on a leg press system in which the athlete's body is stationary and there is a moveable footplate.

The terms OKC and CKC will be used often throughout this chapter in describing both testing and rehabilitation applications of isokinetic exercise.

ISOKINETIC TESTING

In this section we will briefly describe some general guidelines and principles of isokinetic testing. For more detailed information, the reader is referred to *A Compendium of Isokinetics in Clinical Usage and Rehabilitation Techniques.*[28]

The purposes of isokinetic testing are several: to obtain objective records, to screen athletes, to establish a database, to quantify objective information, to obtain objective serial reassessments, to develop normative data, to

correlate isokinetic torque curves with pathologic conditions, and to use the shape of the curve to individualize the rehabilitation program to a specific athlete's needs.

Isokinetic assessment allows the clinician to objectively assess muscular performance in a way that is both safe and reliable.[154] It produces objective criteria for the clinician and provides reproducible data for assessing and monitoring an athlete's status. Isokinetic testing has been demonstrated to be reliable and valid.[8,28,53,56,64,79,81,100,103-105,116,120,132,137,139,146,153]

Absolute and relative contraindications for testing and using isokinetics in rehabilitation must be established, as with any methodology in medicine. Examples of such contraindications are soft tissue healing constraints, pain, limited ROM, effusion, joint instability, acute strains and sprains, and, occasionally, subacute conditions.

A standard test protocol should be established, which will enhance the reliability of the testing. There are numerous considerations, which include the following: (1) educating the athlete regarding the particular requirements of the test, (2) testing the uninvolved side first to establish a baseline and to demonstrate the requirements so that the athlete's apprehension is decreased, (3) providing appropriate warm-ups at each speed, (4) having consistent verbal commands for instructions to the athlete, (5) having a consistent protocol for testing different joints, (6) having properly calibrated equipment, and (7) providing proper stabilization. A standard orthopedic testing protocol should be followed during isokinetic testing.[28] Box 9-2 provides such an example.

Isokinetic testing allows for a variety of testing protocols ranging from power to endurance tests (see Davies[28] for a detailed description of the various isokinetic testing protocols). Our primary recommendation is to perform velocity spectrum testing so that the test will assess the muscle's capabilities at different speeds, thus simulating various activities. Often, deficits in a muscle's performance may show up at one speed and not at others. For example, athletes with a patellofemoral problem often have more power deficits at slow speeds, whereas after various surgical procedures of the knee, athletes will have fast-velocity deficits.

ISOKINETIC DATA AND ANALYSIS

One of the advantages of isokinetic testing is that it provides numerous objective parameters which can be used to evaluate and analyze an athlete's performance. Various isokinetic testing data that are frequently used to analyze an athlete's performance are peak torque, time rate of torque development, acceleration, deceleration, ROM, total work, average power, and shape of the torque curves.[28] After these data are collected from the tests and analyzed to determine specific deficits and limitations of the athlete, the results need to be interpreted using the criteria in Box 9-3.[28]

Box 9-1

Advantages and Limitations of Isokinetics

Advantages

- Efficiency: It is the only way to load a dynamically contacting muscle to its maximum capability at all points throughout the ROM.
- Safety: An individual will never meet more resistance than he or she can handle, because the resistance is equal to the force applied.
- Accommodating resistance: Accommodating resistance occurs, which is predicated on changes in the musculotendinous length-to-tension ratio, changes in the skeletal leverage (biomechanics), fatigue, and pain.
- Decreased joint compressive forces at higher speeds: This is an empiric clinical observation that one of us (G.J.D.) has made in more than 25 years of using isokinetics in testing and rehabilitation of athletes. This occurs because often an athlete exercises at a slow speed and pain develops; however, if the athlete exercises at a faster velocity, pain does not develop. Furthermore, at faster speeds, there is less time to develop force, and the torque decreases with concentric isokinetics according to the force-velocity curve.
- Physiologic overflow through the velocity spectrum: When an athlete exercises at a particular speed, there is a specificity response, with the greatest power gains occurring at the speed of training; however, a concomitant increase in power gain occurs at other speeds as well. The majority of studies demonstrate that this phenomenon occurs at the slower speeds, although some research demonstrates an overflow in both directions from the training speed.
- Velocity spectrum training: Because of the various velocities at which functional and sporting activities are performed, the ability to train at various functional velocities is important, because of the specificity of training. It is important to train the muscles neurophysiologically to develop a normal motor recruitment pattern of neural contraction of the muscle.
- Minimal postexercise soreness with concentric isokinetic contractions
- Validity of the equipment
- Reliability of the equipment
- Reproducibility of physiologic testing (reliability)
- Development of muscle recruitment quickness (time rate of torque development)
- Objective documentation of testing
- Computer feedback provided so an athlete can train at submaximal or maximal levels

Limitations

- Isolated joint/muscle testing
- Nonfunctional patterns of movement
- Limited velocities to replicate the actual speeds of sports performance
- Increased compressive forces at slower speeds
- Increased tibial translation at slow speeds without proximal pad placement

Data from Davies, G.J. (1992): A Compendium of Isokinetics in Clinical Usage and Rehabilitation Techniques. 4th ed. Onalaska, WI, S & S Publishers.

Box 9-2

Orthopedic Testing Protocol

- Educate the athlete: The athlete must first be informed and educated about the purpose, procedures, and requirements of the testing.
- Test the uninvolved side first: The uninvolved side is tested first to establish a baseline and to decrease the athlete's apprehension before the involved extremity is tested.
- Perform warm-ups: The athlete should perform several submaximal gradient warm-ups and at least one maximal warm-up before each test. The submaximal warm-ups (25%, 50%, and 75%) prepare the extremity for the test and allow the athlete to get a feel for the machine. The maximal effort is performed to create a positive learning transfer from a maximal warm-up to a maximal testing effort. This procedure improves the reliability of the testing sequence.[28,100]
- Give consistent verbal commands: These should be standardized and remain the same throughout the testing sequence to improve test-retest reliability.
- Use standardized test protocols: The recommended testing protocols for each joint have been described in detail. The specific anatomic position and stabilization guidelines, ROM, speed, and other considerations have been described.[28]
- Test at different speeds: We recommend the use of a velocity spectrum testing protocol. Velocity spectrum testing refers to testing at slow (0° per second to 60° per second), intermediate (60° per second to 180° per second), fast (180° per second to 300° per second), and functional (300° per second to 1000° per second) contractile velocities. Performing three to five test repetitions at each speed and 20 to 30 repetitions at a fast speed (240° per second or 300° per second) for an endurance test is recommended.

Box 9-3

Criteria for Interpreting Isokinetic Tests Results

- Bilateral comparison: Comparing the involved to the uninvolved extremity is probably the most common evaluation. Bilateral differences of 10% to 15% are considered to represent significant asymmetry. However, this single parameter by itself has limitations.
- Unilateral ratios: Comparing the relationship between the agonist and the antagonist muscles may identify particular weaknesses in certain muscle groups. This parameter is particularly important to assess with velocity spectrum testing, because the percentage relationships of the muscles change with changing speeds in many muscle groups. (Percentage relationship means that the unilateral ratio of antagonistic muscle torque is a certain percentage of agonist muscle torque. This percentage of torque production of the antagonist to the agonist muscle changes through the velocity spectrum.)
- Torque-to-body weight relationship: Comparing the torques to the body weight adds another dimension in interpreting test results. Often, even though bilateral symmetry and normal unilateral ratios are present, the torque-to-body weight relationship is altered.
- Total leg strength: Nicholas and colleagues,[109] Gleim and associates,[57] and Boltz and Davies[13] have published articles on the importance of considering the entire kinetic chain concept of total leg strength.
- Comparison to normative data: Although the use of normative data is controversial, if properly used relative to a specific population of athletes, it can provide guidelines for testing or rehabilitation.

RATIONALE AND NEED FOR ISOKINETIC TESTING AND REHABILITATION

Although the purpose of this chapter is to describe the rationale and need for isokinetic rehabilitation, a few comments about why CKC exercises should be used instead of just OKC exercises are necessary. Many articles have described the rationale for using CKC exercises,[6,14,20,23,36,41,59,66,76,110,112,122] particularly in rehabilitating athletes with anterior cruciate ligament (ACL) reconstructions.[2,37,40,60,68,69,72,83,91,92,94-99,107,110,121,124,128-130] However, Crandall and co-workers[24] performed a meta-analysis of 1167 articles on the treatment of athletes with ACL injuries published between 1966 and 1993 and found that only five articles (and three of these articles included data on the same athletes) met the criteria for meta-analysis of prospective, randomized, controlled, experimental clinical trials. Consequently, many of the articles that are commonly thought of as "definitive treatment articles" are simply descriptive studies. Therefore, although the benefits of using CKC exercises in rehabilitation have been described quite extensively, few scientifically based,

prospective, randomized, controlled, experimental clinical trials[17,35,133] document the efficacy of CKC exercises. The reader is referred to a text that outlines these research studies and the application of CKC exercise as a complement to the material presented here on OKC isokinetic training and testing.[47]

The rationale for the use of CKC exercise only is thus founded not on scientific studies that have documented its efficacy, but more on unverified empiric observations and descriptive studies.[25]

RATIONALE FOR OPEN KINETIC CHAIN ISOKINETIC ASSESSMENT

Despite the many disadvantages described for OKC assessment, there are still several reasons why OKC exercises should be incorporated in both assessment and rehabilitation. These are listed in Box 9-4.

The primary purpose for performing OKC isokinetic assessment is the need to test specific muscle groups of a pathologic joint in isolation. Although the muscles do not work in an isolated fashion, a deficit, or "weak link," in a kinetic chain will never be identified unless specific isolated OKC isokinetic testing is performed. Furthermore, on serial retesting, one will not know how the athlete is progressing and if and when the athlete meets the parameters for discharge. Examples of the importance of performing isolated testing of the kinetic chain to identify specific dysfunctions have been offered by several authors including Nicholas and colleagues[109] and Gleim and associates.[57]

Nicholas and colleagues[109] performed total leg strength isokinetic testing and developed a composite lower extremity score. They evaluated several groups of athletes with various pathologic conditions and determined that certain characteristic patterns of muscle weakness could be correlated with the specific pathologic syndromes. In ankle and foot problems, knee ligamentous instabilities, intra-articular defects, and patellofemoral dysfunctions, there was an irrefutable deficit in total leg strength ($p < 0.01$). For example, athletes with ankle and foot problems have statistically significant weaknesses of the ipsilateral hip abductors and adductors. Furthermore, there was a trend toward ipsilateral weakness of the quadriceps and hamstring muscles, although these trends are not statistically significant.

Gleim and associates[57] also determined that the total percent deficit in the injured leg was the one value that was most informative. Typically, when a single muscle group is compared bilaterally, values that fall within 10% are empirically determined to be normal. Because the total leg strength composite score is more sensitive and minimizes the variability, Gleim and associates[57] suggested that even a 5% difference in bilateral comparison is significant.

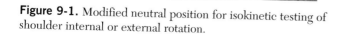

Figure 9-1. Modified neutral position for isokinetic testing of shoulder internal or external rotation.

are for the heavy emphasis on strength development and assessment in rehabilitation. Additional research has identified the IR and ER movement pattern as the preferred testing pattern in athletes with rotator cuff tendinosis.[75]

This study supports the use of isokinetic muscle testing because of the correlation with basic lower extremity functional measures. Further development of the concept

1000° per second) currently available on commercial isokinetic dynamometers provides specificity for testing the upper extremity by allowing the clinician to assess muscu

Table 9-6

Unilateral External Rotation/Internal Rotation Ratios in Professional Baseball Pitchers

Speed	Dominant Arm	Nondominant Arm
180°/sec		
Torque	65	64
300°/sec		
Torque	61	70
210°/sec		
Torque	64	74
Work	61	66
300°/sec		
Torque	65	72
Work	62	70

Data from Wilk, K.E., Andrews, J.R., Arrigo, C.A., et al. (1993): The strength characteristics of internal and external rotator muscles in professional baseball pitchers. Am. J. Sports Med., 21:61–66, and Ellenbecker, T.S., and Mattalino, A.J. (1997): Concentric isokinetic shoulder internal and external rotation strength in professional baseball pitchers. J. Orthop. Sports Phys. Ther., 25:323–328.

skilled adult tennis players.[43] Normative data need to be developed further to define strength more clearly in these upper extremity patterns. Body position and gravity compensation are, again, key factors affecting proper interpretation of data.

Scapulothoracic Testing (Protraction-Retraction)

In addition to the supraspinatus-deltoid force couple, the serratus anterior-trapezius force couple is of critical importance for a thorough evaluation of upper extremity strength. Gross manual muscle testing and screening that attempts to identify scapular winging are commonly utilized in the clinical evaluation of the shoulder complex. Davies and Hoffman[33] published normative data on 250 shoulders for isokinetic protraction-retraction testing. An approximately 1:1 relationship of protraction-retraction strength was reported. Testing and training the serratus anterior, trapezius, and rhomboid musculature enhance scapular stabilization and strengthen the primary musculature involved in the scapulohumeral rhythm. Emphasis on the promotion of proximal stability to enhance distal mobility is a concept used and recognized by nearly all disciplines of rehabilitative medicine.[135]

Concentric versus Eccentric Considerations

The availability of eccentric dynamic strength assessment has made a significant impact, primarily in research investigations. The extrapolation of research-oriented isokinetic principles to patient populations has been a gradual process. Eccentric testing in the upper extremity is clearly indicated on the basis of the prevalence of functionally

specific eccentric work. Maximal eccentric functional contractions of the posterior rotator cuff during the follow-through phase of the throwing motion and tennis serve provide a rationale for eccentric testing and training in rehabilitation and preventive conditioning.[80] Kennedy and co-workers[85] found mode-specific differences between the concentric and eccentric strength characteristics of the rotator cuff. Further research on eccentric muscular training is necessary before widespread use of eccentric isokinetics can be applied to patient populations.

The basic characteristics of eccentric isokinetic testing, such as greater force production compared with concentric contractions at the same velocity, have been reported for the internal and external rotators.[31,48,106] This enhanced force generation is generally explained by the contribution of the series elastic (noncontractile) elements of the muscle-tendon unit in eccentric conditions. An increase in post-exercise muscle soreness, particularly of latent onset, is a common occurrence after periods of eccentric work. Therefore, eccentric testing would not be the mode of choice during early inflammatory stages of an overuse injury.[32] Many clinicians recommend the use of dynamic concentric testing before they perform an eccentric test. Both concentric and eccentric isokinetic training of the rotator cuff have produced objective concentric and eccentric strength improvements in elite tennis players.[48,106]

RELATIONSHIP OF ISOKINETIC TESTING TO FUNCTIONAL PERFORMANCE

Dynamic muscular strength assessment is used to evaluate the underlying strength and balance of strength in specific muscle groups. This information is used to determine the specific anatomic structure that requires strengthening, as well as to demonstrate the efficacy of treatment procedures. Isokinetic testing of the shoulder internal and external rotators has been used as one parameter for demonstrating the functional outcome after rotator cuff repair in select patient populations.[58,119,142,143] An additional purpose for isokinetic testing is to determine the relationship of muscular strength to functional performance. Several groups have tested upper extremity muscle groups and have correlated their respective levels of strength to sport-specific functional tests. Pedegana and colleagues[115] found a statistical relationship between elbow extension, wrist flexion, shoulder extension-flexion, and ER strength measured isokinetically and throwing speed in professional pitchers. Bartlett and associates,[11] in a similar study, found that shoulder adduction correlated with throwing speed. These studies are in contrast to those of Pawlowski and Perrin,[114] who did not find a significant relationship in throwing velocity.

Ellenbecker and associates[48] determined that 6 weeks of concentric isokinetic training of the rotator cuff resulted in a statistically significant improvement in serving velocity in collegiate tennis players. Mont and co-workers,[106] in a similar study, found serving velocity improvements after both concentric and eccentric IR and ER training. A direct statistical relationship between isokinetically measured upper extremity strength and tennis serve velocity was not obtained by Ellenbecker,[43] despite earlier studies showing increases in serving velocity after isokinetic training. The complex biomechanical sequence of segmental velocities and the interrelationship of the kinetic chain link with the lower extremities and trunk make delineation and identification of a direct relationship between an isolated structure and a complex functional activity difficult. Isokinetic testing can provide a reliable, dynamic measurement of isolated joint motions and muscular contributions to assist the clinician in the assessment of underlying muscular strength and strength balance. The integration of isokinetic testing with a thorough, objective clinical evaluation allows the clinician to provide optimal rehabilitation both after overuse injuries and after surgery.

APPLICATION OF ISOKINETICS IN DESIGNING REHABILITATION PROGRAMS

Many types of exercise programs are in widespread use for rehabilitating injured athletes. This section focuses on resistive rehabilitation programs, as well as on the specific progression of resistive exercise recommended during rehabilitation. The resistive rehabilitation programs vary from isometric, concentric, and eccentric isotonics to concentric and eccentric isokinetics to isoacceleration and isodeceleration programs. The scientific and clinical rationale for progression through a resistive exercise rehabilitation program is described, including the specific progression and inclusion of isokinetic exercise in the clinical rehabilitation of upper extremity overuse injuries.

Patient Progression Criteria

Several important concepts predicate the progression through the resistive exercise program. These include athlete status, signs and symptoms, time after surgery, and soft tissue healing constraints. The athlete's progression through the various levels of the resistive exercise program is determined by continual charting and assessment of subjective and objective evaluative criteria (Table 9-7). This resistive exercise progression continuum[28] is based on the concept of a trial treatment. If any adverse changes occur, the rehabilitation program continues at the previous level of intensity of repetitions, sets, or duration without the athlete's progressing to the next level of the exercise progression continuum.

If, however, an athlete performs the trial treatment without any negative effects, then the athlete progresses

Table 9-7

Commonly Used Subjective and Objective Criteria for Patient Progress in a Rehabilitation Program

Subjective Criteria (Symptoms)	Objective Criteria (Signs)
Pain	Anthropometric measurements
Stiffness	Goniometric measurements
Changes in function	Palpable cutaneous temperature changes
	Redness
	Manual muscle testing
	Isokinetic testing
	Kinesthetic testing
	Functional performance testing
	KT-1000 testing

From Davies, G.J. (1992): A Compendium of Isokinetics in Clinical Usage and Rehabilitation Techniques, 4th ed. Onalaska, WI, S & S Publishers.

gradually to the next higher level in the exercise continuum. An athlete may enter the exercise rehabilitation continuum at any stage, depending on the results of the initial evaluation. Furthermore, an athlete may also progress through several stages from one treatment session to the next, depending primarily on his or her response. Before the athlete begins the actual resistive exercise portion of the rehabilitation program, various warm-up exercises and mobilization-stretching exercises are appropriate.

Resistive Exercise Progression Continuum

The rehabilitation program is designed along a progression continuum. The program begins with the safest exercises and progresses to the more stressful exercises. These are illustrated in Figure 9-2 and Table 9-8.

Multiple-Angle Isometrics

The exercise rehabilitation program typically begins with multiple-angle isometrics that are performed at a submaximal intensity level. The isometrics are performed approximately every 20° through the ROM that is indicated, based on the athlete's safe and comfortable ROM demonstrated during examination. The rationale for using this particular exercise is the presence of a 20° physiologic overflow with the application of isometrics[28] (Fig. 9-3). Therefore, as an example (Fig. 9-4), if the athlete presents with a painful arc syndrome, which is common in a shoulder with a rotator cuff pathologic condition, the isometrics can be applied every 20° through the ROM, and the athlete will still obtain a concomitant strengthening effect

STAGES:

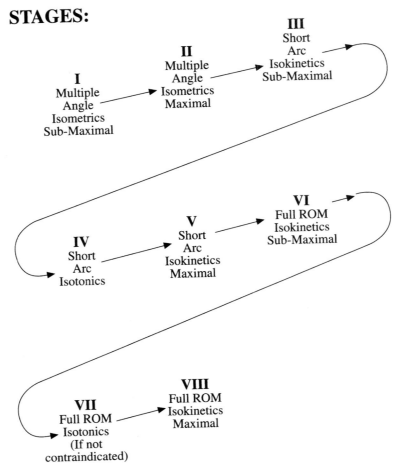

Figure 9-2. Stages of Davies' resistive exercise progression continuum. (From Davies, G.J. [1992]: A Compendium of Isokinetics in Clinical Usage and Rehabilitation Techniques, 4th ed. Onalaska, WI, S & S Publishers.)

throughout the entire ROM without increasing the symptomatic area. The painful arc that is typical in athletes with rotator cuff pathologic conditions occurs between 85° and 135° of elevation, at which point peak forces against the undersurface of the acromion occur.[90] Performing isometric exercise around the painful arc during the rehabilitation process is a prime example of applying isometrics early in rehabilitation of the shoulder after overuse injury or after surgery.

The next consideration with isometric exercise is that the athlete uses the rule of tens: 10-second contractions, 10-second rest, 10 repetitions, and so on. The athlete is usually taught to perform the isometrics in the following sequence: (1) take 2 seconds to gradually build up the desired tension, whether working at a submaximal or maximal intensity level; (2) hold the desired tension of the isometric contraction for 6 seconds, which is the optimum duration for an isometric contraction[7]; and (3) gradually relax, releasing the tension in the muscle over the last 2 seconds (Fig. 9-5). This sequence allows for a controlled build-up and easing of the contraction with an optimum 6-second isometric contraction.

Gradient Increase and Decrease in Force Production

Gradient increase and decrease in muscle force production are concepts that athletes have taught us over the years. As an example, if an athlete has effusion or pain in a joint and performs a muscle contraction, pain is often created. This is usually the result of capsular distention from the internal pressure of the effusion. The submaximal muscle contraction places external pressure on the capsule, which is highly innervated,[123] and subsequently increases the pain. However, with a gradient increase in the muscle contraction to the desired intensity (submaximal or maximal), an accommodation is often created that either eliminates or minimizes pain. At the completion of the 6-second isometric contraction, the gradient decrease in the muscle contraction is performed. Again, when an effusion is present and the athlete suddenly releases the

Table 9-8

Davies' Resistive Exercise Progression Continuum

Percentage of Exercise Effort	Exercise Program
100%	Submaximal multiple-angle isometrics
	Subjective/objective assessment and plan (SOAP)
	Trial treatment (TT) of maximal multiple-angle isometrics
50%/50%	Submaximal multiple-angle isometrics + maximal multiple-angle isometrics
	SOAP
100%	Maximal multiple-angle isometrics
	SOAP
	TT of submaximal short-arc isokinetics
50%/50%	Maximal multiple-angle isometrics + submaximal short-arc isokinetics
	SOAP
100%	Submaximal short-arc isokinetics
	SOAP
	TT of maximal short-arc isokinetics or short-arc isotonics
	SOAP
50%/50%	Submaximal short-arc isokinetics + maximal short-arc isokinetics
	SOAP
100%	Maximal short-arc isokinetics
	SOAP
	TT of submaximal full range-of-motion isokinetics
	SOAP
50%/50%	Maximal short-arc isokinetics + submaximal full ROM isokinetics
	SOAP
100%	Submaximal full ROM isokinetics
	SOAP
	TT of maximal full ROM isokinetics
	SOAP (Full ROM isotonics here, if not contraindicated)
50%/50%	Submaximal full ROM isokinetics + maximal full ROM isokinetics
	SOAP
100%	Maximal full ROM isokinetics
	SOAP

From Davies, G.J. (1992): A Compendium of Isokinetics in Clinical Usage and Rehabilitation Techniques, 4th ed. Onalaska, WI, S & S Publishers.

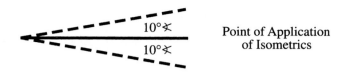

20° ⩶ Physiologic Overflow

Figure 9-3. Isometric exercises and physiologic overflow through the range of motion. (From Davies, G.J. [1992]: A Compendium of Isokinetics in Clinical Usage and Rehabilitation Techniques, 4th ed. Onalaska, WI, S & S Publishers.)

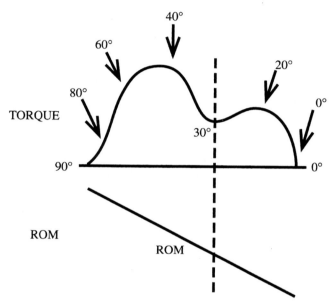

Figure 9-4. Application of isometric exercises through the range of motion with a "painful" deformation. Isometrics are applied every 20° through the range of motion. Note particularly the application of isometrics on each side of "painful" deformation. (From Davies, G.J. [1992]: A Compendium of Isokinetics in Clinical Usage and Rehabilitation Techniques, 4th ed. Onalaska, WI, S & S Publishers.)

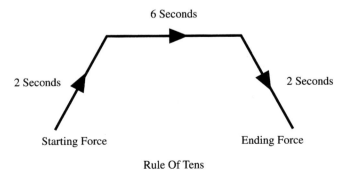

Rule Of Tens

Figure 9-5. Isometric contraction applied by the rule of tens. (From Davies, G.J. [1992]: A Compendium of Isokinetics in Clinical Usage and Rehabilitation Techniques, 4th ed. Onalaska, WI, S & S Publishers.)

contraction, pain results. This is perhaps due to a rebound type of phenomenon, because the effusion in the joint pushes the capsule out, and the muscular contraction that was pushing in against the capsule and compressing it causes an "equalizing" of the pressure. At the release of the muscular contraction, the external pressure is relieved; therefore, the internal pressure causes a rebound phenomenon, stretching the capsule and creating the discomfort. If the athlete gradually releases the muscle contraction, and some type of accommodation occurs, it either eliminates or minimizes the pain.

Determining Submaximal Exercise Intensity

Submaximal exercise intensity can be distinguished from maximal exercise intensity in various ways. If a submaximal exercise is being applied, it can be determined by using the symptom-limited submaximal exercises (exercises performed at less than maximum efforts that do not cause pain) or a musculoskeletal rating of perceived exertion for submaximal effort. Furthermore, the distinction must be made between "good" and "bad" pain after exercise. "Good" pain refers to the transient acute exercise-bout pain that is due to lactic acid accumulation, pH changes in the muscle, and an ischemic response. However, "bad" pain is pain that occurs at the site of the actual injury or at the muscle-tendon unit of injury. An example of this pain classification used in shoulder rehabilitation would be posteriorly oriented discomfort or pain over the infraspinous fossa after an external rotation exercise ("good" pain) versus anteriorly directed pain over the greater tuberosity or biceps long head tendon ("bad" pain).

Guidelines for Pain during Exercise

The following are guidelines that we use during the rehabilitation program: (1) If no pain is present at the start of an exercise bout, but it develops after the exercise, that particular exercise is stopped, and modifications to the exercise are made. (2) If pain is present at the start of the exercise and the pain increases, that exercise is terminated. (3) If pain is present at the start of an exercise and the pain plateaus, the athlete continues the exercise program.

Trial Treatment

When a rehabilitation program includes the progression of the athlete through a resistive exercise continuum, a key element is how to determine the progression from one stage to the next in the continuum. One of the keys to this progression is the use of a trial treatment. The trial treatment essentially consists of the athlete's performing one set from the next stage in the exercise progression continuum that was illustrated in Figure 9-2. After the athlete completes the exercise program at one level of the exercise progression continuum, he or she performs a trial of the next stage of treatment. The athlete's signs and symptoms

are then evaluated at the conclusion of that particular treatment session as well as at the next scheduled visit, at which time the athlete's condition is reevaluated, and a decision is made on the basis of the athlete's signs and symptoms. If these have stayed the same or improved, the athlete can progress to the next level of exercise because the trial treatment has demonstrated that the athlete's muscle-tendon unit or joint is ready for the higher exercise intensity. Any negative sequelae such as increased pain or effusion in the joint are an indication that the joint or muscle is not ready for progression, and, consequently, the athlete continues to work at the same level of intensity. Further physical therapy is performed to decrease the irritability of the joint or muscle-tendon unit, and during the next visit, the trial treatment is once again attempted to determine whether the athlete's injury can tolerate the progression.

Submaximal Exercise: Fiber Recruitment

Several exercise modes can be performed at a submaximal level to enhance selective fiber recruitment. Preferential muscle fiber recruitment is predicated on the intensity of the muscle contraction to recruit either slow-twitch or fast-twitch A or fast-twitch B fibers. It is generally accepted that during voluntary contractions of human muscle there is orderly recruitment of motor units according to the size principle.[71] In mixed muscle containing both slow-twitch and fast-twitch fibers, this implies that the involvement of the slow-twitch fibers is obligatory, regardless of the power and velocity being generated with fast-twitch A and fast-twitch B muscle fibers that are recruited once higher intensities are generated.[61] Figure 9-6 summarizes this preferential muscular recruitment. The slow-twitch motor units have relatively low contraction velocities and long contraction times that require only low levels of stimulus to contract. In contrast, the fast-twitch motor units require a very high intensity stimulus to contract and have very short contraction times. The preferential recruitment of muscle fibers is an important concept for the clinician to understand relative to the manipulation of submaximal and maximal exercise intensities with rehabilitative exercise. Submaximal exercise can stimulate the slow-twitch muscle fibers and allow athletes to exercise at lower, pain-free intensities early in the rehabilitation process, with a progression to higher exercise intensities later in rehabilitation, preferentially stimulating the fast-twitch fibers.

Short-Arc Exercises

The athlete next progresses from static isometric exercises to more dynamic exercise. The dynamic exercises start with short-arc exercises and the ROM within symptom and soft tissue healing constraints. Short-arc exercises are often started using submaximal isokinetics (Fig. 9-7) because of the accommodating resistance inherent in submaximal isokinetic exercise that makes it safe for the athlete's healing

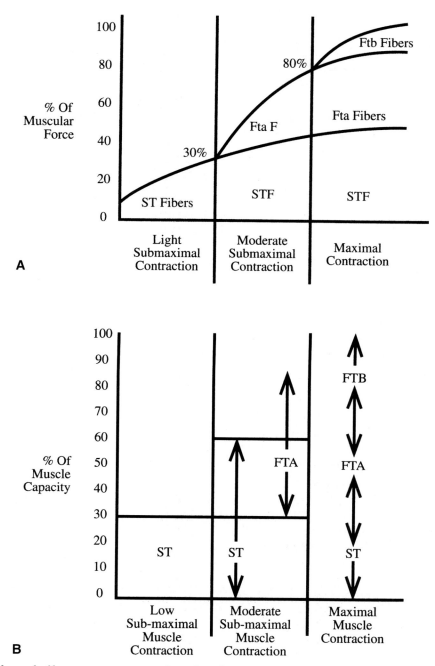

Figure 9-6. Preferential muscle fiber recruitment is predicated on the intensity of the muscle contraction. STF, slow-twitch fiber; FTA or Fta, fast-twitch A; FTB or Ftb, fast-twitch B. (From Davies, G.J. [1992]: A Compendium of Isokinetics in Clinical Usage and Rehabilitation Techniques, 4th ed. Onalaska, WI, S & S Publishers.)

tissues. With short-arc isokinetics, speeds ranging from 60° per second to 180° per second are utilized (Fig. 9-8). The athlete works with what is called a velocity spectrum rehabilitation protocol (VSRP). When the athlete is performing short-arc isokinetics, slower contractile velocities (60° per second to 180° per second) are chosen because of the acceleration and deceleration response (Fig. 9-9). Isokinetic exercise contains three major components, as

identified in Figure 9-9: acceleration, deceleration, and load range. Acceleration is the portion of the ROM in which the athlete's limb is accelerating to "catch" the preset angular velocity; deceleration is the portion of the ROM in which the athlete's limb is slowing before cessation of that repetition; and the load range is the actual portion of the ROM in which the preset angular velocity is met by the athlete, and a true isokinetic load is imparted to

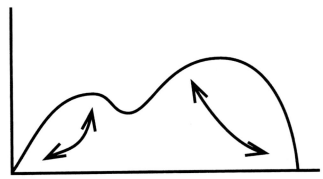

Figure 9-7. Short-arc isokinetic exercises being applied at different points in the range of motion. If an isokinetic torque curve has a deformity in the range of motion as illustrated, short-arc isokinetic exercises can be applied to each side of the deformity. (From Davies, G.J. [1992]: A Compendium of Isokinetics in Clinical Usage and Rehabilitation Techniques, 4th ed. Onalaska, WI, S & S Publishers.)

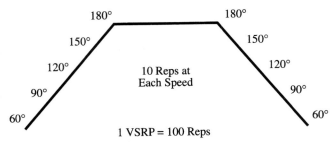

Figure 9-8. Short-arc isokinetic velocity spectrum rehabilitation protocol (VSRP) performed at intermediate contractile velocities. Reps, repetitions. (From Davies, G.J. [1992]: A Compendium of Isokinetics in Clinical Usage and Rehabilitation Techniques, 4th ed. Onalaska, WI, S & S Publishers.)

the athlete. Load range is inversely related to isokinetic speed. A larger load range is found at slower contractile velocities, with a statistically shorter load range at faster contractile velocities.[15]

Consequently, the athlete's available ROM must be evaluated to determine the optimal ROM for exercise. With short-arc isokinetic exercise, there is a physiologic overflow of approximately 30° through the ROM (Fig. 9-10). Therefore, when an athlete with a rotator cuff pathologic condition is exercising, an abbreviated ROM in internal-external rotation can be utilized in the pain-free range, with overflow into the painful ROM, without actually placing the injured structures into that movement range. Another example of isokinetic exercise for the upper extremities would be the limitation of external ROM to 90° during isokinetic training, even though the demands on the athletic shoulder in overhead activities exceed the 90° ER. Limiting the ER to 90° protects the anterior capsular structures of the shoulder, with physiologic overflow improving strength at ranges of ER exceeded during training.

In addition to ROM, the speed selected with isokinetic exercise is also of vital importance in a VSRP. The speeds in the protocol are designed so that the athlete will exercise 30° per second through the velocity spectrum. The reason for using an interval of 30° per second in the velocity spectrum is the physiologic overflow with respect to speed that has been identified with isokinetic research (Fig. 9-11).[18,89,102]

Rest Intervals

When the athlete is performing either submaximal or maximal short-arc isokinetics using a VSRP, the rest interval between each set of 10 training repetitions may be as long as 90 seconds.[4] However, this is not a viable clinical rest time because it takes too much time to complete the exercise session. Consequently, rest intervals are often applied on a symptom-limited basis. If the athlete does complete a total VSRP, a rest period of 3 minutes after the completion of the VSRP has been shown to be an effective rest interval[5] (Fig. 9-12). Additional research provides guidance for rest interval selection with isotonic and isokinetic exercise in rehabilitation. According to Fleck,[55] 50% of the adenosine triphosphate and creatine phosphate is restored in

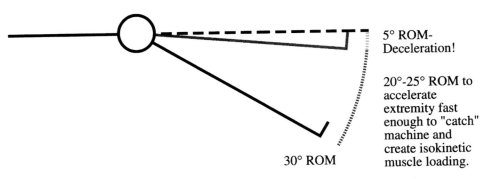

Figure 9-9. Acceleration and deceleration range of motion (ROM) with short-arc isokinetic exercise. (From Davies, G.J. [1992]: A Compendium of Isokinetics in Clinical Usage and Rehabilitation Techniques, 4th ed. Onalaska, WI, S & S Publishers.)

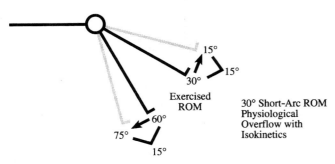

Figure 9-10. Thirty-degree short-arc range of motion (ROM) overflow with isokinetics. (From Davies, G.J. [1992]: A Compendium of Isokinetics in Clinical Usage and Rehabilitation Techniques, 4th ed. Onalaska, WI, S & S Publishers.)

20 seconds after an acute bout of muscular work. Seventy-five percent and 87% of the intramuscular stores are replenished in 40 and 60 seconds, respectively. Knowledge of the phosphagen replenishment schedule allows clinicians to make scientifically based decisions on the amount of rest needed or desired after periods of muscular work. Another factor in determining the optimum rest intervals with isotonic and isokinetic training is specificity. For example, during rehabilitation of the shoulder of a tennis player, a high-repetition format is used to improve local muscular endurance. Rest cycles are limited to 25 to 30 seconds because that is the time allotted during tennis play for rest between points. Applying activity or sport-specific muscular work rest cycles is an important consideration during rehabilitation.

When isotonic exercises are applied, they are implemented between isokinetic submaximal and maximal exercises (see Fig. 9-2). The reason is that isotonic muscle loading loads a muscle only at its weakest point in the ROM. Figure 9-13 demonstrates the effects of isotonic muscle loading through the ROM. Consequently, when isotonic muscle exercise is performed through the ROM, a combination of maximal and submaximal loading occurs, whereas with isokinetics, submaximal exercises can be performed throughout the ROM, or maximal intensity loading of the muscle is maximal throughout the ROM, because of the accommodating resistance phenomena inherent with isokinetic exercise.

Full Range-of-Motion Exercises

The athlete next progresses to full ROM isokinetic exercise beginning with submaximal exercises and then progressing to maximal intensity (Fig. 9-14). Straight planar movements are used initially to protect the injured plane of movement. Faster contractile velocities are also used from 180° up to the maximum capabilities of the isokinetic dynamometer. There are numerous reasons for using the faster isokinetic speeds: physiologic overflow to slower speeds, specificity response, motor learning response, and decreased joint compressive forces.[28] Joint compressive forces are decreased, based on Bernoulli's principle that at faster speeds, there is a decreased surface pressure on the articular surface because of the synovial fluid interface.[10] This is probably due to the interfacing of the hydrodynamic pattern of the articular cartilage and the synovial fluid movement. Another consideration is the positioning of the athlete to use the length-tension curve of the muscle. With isokinetic exercise, the athlete's position is often modified to bias the respective muscles, for example, to stretch them to facilitate contraction or to place them in a shortened position if that is the functional position. Obviously, of greatest importance is the attempt to replicate the ultimate functional performance position of the individual.

Isoacceleration and Deceleration

Because functional activities are primarily accelerative and decelerative movement patterns, it is important to try to replicate these patterns when one performs different types of rehabilitation activities. Also, because of the functional activities involved with various sports, such as the deceleration phase of tennis or baseball that is applied to the posterior rotator cuff or to the forearm or biceps muscles, the potential use of eccentric exercise may also be important.

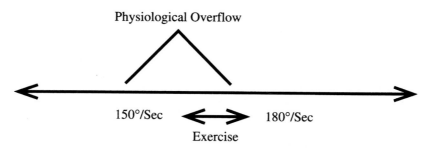

Figure 9-11. Thirty degrees per second physiologic overflow through the velocity spectrum. (From Davies, G.J. [1992]: A Compendium of Isokinetics in Clinical Usage and Rehabilitation Techniques, 4th ed. Onalaska, WI, S & S Publishers.)

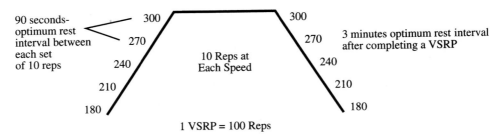

Figure 9-12. Optimum rest intervals. Reps, repetitions; VSRP, velocity spectrum rehabilitation protocol. (From Davies, G.J. [1992]: A Compendium of Isokinetics in Clinical Usage and Rehabilitation Techniques, 4th ed. Onalaska, WI, S & S Publishers.)

There are few studies that demonstrate the efficacy of performing eccentric exercise or eccentric isokinetic rehabilitation programs at this time.[48] Ellenbecker and associates[48] reported concentric strength improvement in IR and ER after 6 weeks of eccentric isokinetic training of the internal and external rotators in elite tennis players. Mont and co-workers[106] found both concentric and eccentric strength improvements with eccentric isokinetic training of the rotator cuff in elite tennis players. Despite the lack of research on eccentric exercise training, particularly in athletes, specific application of eccentric exercise programs to the posterior rotator cuff, quadriceps, and other important muscle-tendon units that must perform extensive eccentric work may be indicated. Empirically, we support the integration and application of eccentric isokinetics as part of the whole rehabilitation program.

OUTCOMES RESEARCH

The evolution of rehabilitation modes over the past few decades can best be described as follows:

1970s: Functional rehabilitation
1980s: OKC assessment and rehabilitation (with emphasis on isokinetics)
1990s: CKC rehabilitation

2000: Integrated assessment and rehabilitation that include both OKC and CKC

Bynum and associates[17] published the results of the first prospective, randomized study comparing OKC and CKC exercises. With respect to the parameters listed, their conclusions indicate the following about the CKC exercises:

1. Lower mean KT-1000 arthrometer side-to-side differences (KT-20, $p = 0.057$, not significant; KT-Max, $p = 0.018$, significant)
2. Less patellofemoral pain ($p = 0.48$, not significant)
3. Patients generally more satisfied with the end result ($p = 0.36$, not significant)
4. Patients returned to activities of daily living sooner than expected ($p = 0.007$, significant)
5. Patients returned to sports sooner than expected ($p = 0.118$, not significant)

The authors stated: "As a result of this study, we now use the CKC protocol *exclusively* after anterior cruciate ligament reconstruction."[17] Surprisingly, Bynum and associates[17] came to several conclusions for data that were not statistically significant and probably not clinically significant either. Yet they based their entire protocol exclusively on these findings.

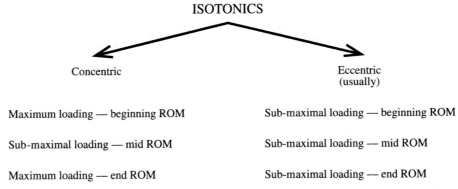

Figure 9-13. Concentric and eccentric isotonic muscle loading and submaximal and maximal loading through the range of motion (ROM). (From Davies, G.J. [1992]: A Compendium of Isokinetics in Clinical Usage and Rehabilitation Techniques, 4th ed. Onalaska, WI, S & S Publishers.)

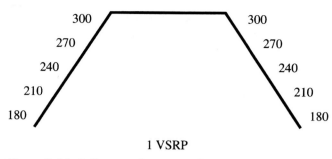

Figure 9-14. Full range-of-motion isokinetic velocity spectrum rehabilitation protocol (VSRP) performed at fast contractile velocities. (From Davies, G.J. [1992]: A Compendium of Isokinetics in Clinical Usage and Rehabilitation Techniques, 4th ed. Onalaska, WI, S & S Publishers.)

CKC exercises have almost replaced OKC exercises in the rehabilitation of athletes after an ACL reconstruction. As indicated earlier, this change is not founded on solid experimental or clinical studies, with limited published prospective, randomized, experimental studies to prove the efficacy of CKC exercises.[53] In contrast, the literature on OKC isokinetics and OKC isotonics is extensive, but most clinicians have ignored past successes with OKC exercises and have chosen to use CKC exercises without documentation.[91]

Snyder-Mackler and colleagues[133] described prospective, randomized clinical trials and the effects of intensive CKC rehabilitation programs and different types of electrical stimulation on athletes with ACL reconstructions. These researchers had previously demonstrated that the strength of the quadriceps femoris muscle correlates well with the function of the knee during the stance phase of gait. In their later study,[133] after an intensive CKC rehabilitation program, they reported a residual weakness in the quadriceps that produced alterations in the normal gait function of these athletes. The authors concluded that CKC exercise alone does not provide an adequate stimulus to the quadriceps femoris to permit more normal knee function in the stance phase of gait in most athletes soon after ACL reconstruction. They suggested that the judicious application of OKC exercises for the quadriceps femoris muscle (with the knee in a position that does not stress the graft) improves the strength of this muscle and the functional outcome after reconstruction of the ACL.

Isokinetic assessment and treatment techniques are only one part of the evaluation and rehabilitation process. The diversity in assessment and rehabilitation is tremendous, as illustrated by the fact that after ACL reconstruction, some athletes return to sports after 12 weeks, and others return after 12 months. Therefore, we strongly encourage clinicians to use an integrated approach to assessment and rehabilitation, to review the literature critically, and to contribute to the advancement of the art and science of sports medicine by performing research and sharing results through peer-reviewed publications.

SUMMARY
Overview and Terminology

- The concept of isokinetic exercise was developed by James Perrine in the late 1960s.
- Isokinetics refers to exercise that is performed at a fixed velocity, with an accommodating resistance. Accommodating resistance means that the resistance varies to exactly match the force applied by the athlete at every point in the ROM; thus, the muscle is loaded to its maximum capability through every point throughout the ROM.
- Isokinetic exercise contains three major components: acceleration, deceleration, and load range.

Isokinetic Testing

- Isokinetic assessment allows the clinician to objectively assess muscular performance in a way that is both safe and reliable.
- Contraindications for testing and using isokinetics include soft-tissue healing constraints, pain, limited ROM, effusion, joint instability, acute strains and sprains, and occasionally, subacute conditions.
- A standard test protocol should be used, which will enhance the reliability of testing.
- Isokinetic testing allows for a variety of testing protocols ranging from power to endurance tests. Use of velocity spectrum testing is recommended so that the test will assess the muscle's capabilities at different speeds, thus simulating various activities.
- Isokinetic testing provides numerous objective parameters that can be used to evaluate and analyze an athlete's performance.
- Differentiation of agonist and antagonist muscular strength balance using manual techniques is not as reliable as using an isokinetic apparatus.
- With isokinetic testing the assessment of the strength of an extremity relative to the contralateral side forms the basis for data interpretation.
- It is necessary to perform isolated testing of specific muscle groups usually affected by certain pathologic changes. If the component parts of the kinetic chain are not measured, the weak link will not be identified or adequately rehabilitated, which will affect the entire chain.

CKC versus OKC Isokinetic Assessment and Rehabilitation

- The benefits of using CKC exercises in rehabilitation have been described quite extensively; however, few scientifically based, prospective, randomized, controlled, experimental clinical trials document the efficacy of CKC exercises.

- The primary purpose of performing OKC isokinetic assessment is the need to test specific muscle groups of a pathologic joint in isolation. Although the muscles do not work in an isolated fashion, a deficit, or "weak link," in a kinetic chain will never be identified unless specific isolated OKC isokinetic testing is performed.
- Evidence suggests that there is a correlation between OKC isokinetic testing with CKC functional performance as well as with sport-specific functional tests.

Use of Isokinetics in Upper Extremity Testing and Rehabilitation

- One rationale for using isokinetics in upper extremity testing and rehabilitation is that the upper extremities function almost exclusively in an OKC format.
- Initial testing and rehabilitation of the shoulder should be done using the modified base position before progressing to the 90°-abducted position.
- The 90°-abducted position for isokinetic strength assessment is more specific for assessing the muscular functions required for overhead activities.
- Research has identified the IR and ER movement patterns as the preferred testing patterns in athletes with rotator cuff tendinosis.
- In some athletic populations there is significantly greater IR then ER strength in the dominant arm, which produces significant changes in agonist-antagonist muscular balance.
- Alteration of ER-to-IR ratio has been reported in athletes with glenohumeral joint instability and impingement.
- Eccentric testing in the upper extremity is clearly indicated on the basis of the prevalence of functionally specific eccentric work.

Use of Isokinetics in Rehabilitation Programs

- The athlete should progress from static isometric exercises to more dynamic exercise.
- Isometrics are performed at approximately every 20° through the ROM that is indicated. The rationale for 20° is the physiologic overflow that occurs with isometrics.
- Performing isometric exercise around the painful arc during the rehabilitation process is an example of applying isometrics early in the rehabilitation process.
- It is recommended that isometrics be performed using the rule of tens: 10-second contractions, 10-second rest, 10 repetitions, and so on.
- The 10-second contraction should be performed with a 2-second gradual build-up to the desired tension, which should be held for 6 seconds with gradual relaxation for 2 seconds. This technique can also result in

a decrease in pain that can result from a muscle contraction around an injury area.

- When an athlete progresses through a progressive resistive program trial, treatments can be used to determine if the athlete is ready to advance to a next stage of an exercise progression continuum.
- Submaximal exercise can stimulate the slow-twitch muscle fibers and allow athletes to exercise at lower, pain-free intensities early in the rehabilitation process, with a progression to higher exercise intensities later in rehabilitation, preferentially stimulating the fast-twitch fibers.
- Dynamic exercises begin with short-arc exercises and are within the ROM that consider symptom and soft tissue healing constraints.
- Short-arc exercises are often started using submaximal isokinetics.
- With short-arc isokinetics, speeds ranging from 60° per second to 180° per second are utilized.
- With short-arc isokinetic exercise, there is a physiologic overflow of approximately 30° through the ROM.
- The speed selected with isokinetic exercise is of vital importance in a VSRP. The speeds in the protocol are designed so that the athlete will exercise 30° per second through the velocity spectrum. The reason for using an interval of 30° per second in the velocity spectrum is the physiologic overflow with respect to speed that has been identified with isokinetic research.
- With full ROM exercises, straight planar movements are used initially to protect the injured plane of movement. Faster contractile velocities are also used from 180° per second up to the maximum capabilities of the isokinetic dynamometer.
- Despite the lack of research on eccentric exercise training, particularly in athletes, specific application of eccentric exercise programs to the posterior rotator cuff, quadriceps, and other important muscle-tendon units that must perform extensive eccentric work may be indicated.

REFERENCES

1. Alderink, G.J., and Kluck, D.J. (1986): Isokinetic shoulder strength in high schools and college pitchers. J. Orthop. Sports Phys. Ther., 7:163-172.
2. Anderson, A.F., and Lipscomb, A.B. (1989): Analysis of rehabilitation techniques after anterior cruciate reconstruction. Am. J. Sports Med., 17:154-160.
3. Anderson, M.A., Gieck, J.H., Perrin, D., et al. (1991): The relationship among isometric, isotonic and isokinetic concentric and eccentric quadriceps and hamstring force and three components of athletic performance. J. Orthop. Sports Phys. Ther., 14:114-120.
4. Ariki, P., Davies, G.J., Siweart, M., et al. (1985): Rest interval between isokinetic velocity spectrum rehabilitation speeds. Phys. Ther., 65:735-736.

5. Ariki, P., Davies, G.J., Siweart, M., et al. (1985): Rest interval between isokinetic velocity spectrum rehabilitation sets. Phys. Ther., 65:733-734.

6. Arms, S.W., Pope, M.H., Johnson, R.J., et al. (1984): The biomechanics of anterior cruciate ligament rehabilitation and reconstruction. Am. J. Sports Med., 12:8-18.

7. Astrand, P., and Rodahl, K. (1977): Textbook of Work Physiology. New York, McGraw-Hill.

8. Barbee, J., and Landis, D. (1984): Reliability of Cybex computer measures. Phys. Ther., 68:737.

9. Barber, S.D., Noyes, F.R., Mangine, R.E., et al. (1990): Quantitative assessment of functional limitations in normal and anterior cruciate ligament deficient knees. Clin. Orthop., 225:204-214.

10. Barnam, J.N. (1978): Mechanical Kinesiology. St. Louis, C.V. Mosby.

11. Bartlett, L.R., Browne, A.O., Morrey, B.F., and An, K.N. (1994): Glenohumeral muscle force and moment mechanics in a position of shoulder instability. J. Biomech., 23:405-415.

12. Basset, R.W., Browne, A.O., Morrey, B.F., and An, K.N. (1994): Glenohumeral muscle force and moment mechanics in a position of shoulder instability. J. Biomech., 23:405-415.

13. Boltz, S., and Davies, G.J. (1984): Leg length differences and correlation with total leg strength. J. Orthop. Sports Phys. Ther., 6:23-29.

14. Brask, B., Lueke, R.H., and Soderberg, G.L. (1984): Electromyographical analysis of selected muscles during the lateral step-up exercise. Phys. Ther., 64:324-329.

15. Brown, L.E., Whitehurse, M., Findley, B.W., et al. (1995): Isokinetic load range during shoulder rotation exercise in elite male junior tennis players. J. Strength Cond. Res., 9:160-164.

16. Brown, L.P., Neihues, S.L., Harrah, A., et al. (1988): Upper extremity range of motion and isokinetic strength of the internal and external shoulder rotators in major league baseball players. Am. J. Sports Med., 16:577-585.

17. Bynum, E.B., Barrack, R.L., and Alexander, A.H. (1995): Open versus closed chain kinetic exercises after anterior cruciate ligament reconstruction: A prospective randomized study. Am. J. Sports Med., 23:401-406.

18. Caizzo, V.J., et al. (1980): Alterations in the in-vivo force-velocity. Med. Sci. Sports Exerc., 12:134.

19. Chan, K.M., and Maffulli, N. (1966): Principles and Practice of Isokinetics in Sports Medicine and Rehabilitation. Hong Kong, Williams & Wilkins.

20. Chandler, T.J., Wilson, G.D., and Store, M.H. (1989): The effects of the squat exercise on knee stability. Med. Sci. Sports Exerc., 21:299-303.

21. Chandler, T.J., Kibler, W.B., Stracener, E.C., et al. (1992): Shoulder strength, power, and endurance in college tennis players. Am. J. Sports Med., 20:455-458.

22. Cook, E.E., Gray, V.L., Savinor-Nogue, E., et al. (1987): Shoulder antagonistic strength ratios: A comparison between college-level baseball pitchers. J. Orthop. Sports Phys. Ther., 8:451-461.

23. Cook, T.M., Zimmerman, C.L., Lux, K.M., et al. (1992): EMG comparison of lateral step-up and stepping machine exercise. J. Orthop. Sports Phys. Ther., 16:108-113.

24. Crandall, D., Richmond, J., Lau, J., et al. (1994): A meta-analysis of the treatment of the anterior cruciate ligament.

Presented at the American Orthopedic Society of Sports Medicine, Palm Desert, CA.

25. Crowell, J.R. (1987): College football: To brace or not to brace (Editorial). J. Bone Joint Surg. [Am.], 69:1.

26. Daniels, L., and Worthingham, C. (1986): Muscle Testing: Techniques of Manual Examination. 5th ed. Philadelphia, W.B. Saunders.

27. Davies, G.J. (1984): A Compendium of Isokinetics in Clinical Usage and Rehabilitation Techniques. La Crosse, WI, S & S Publishers.

28. Davies, G.J. (1992): A Compendium of Isokinetics in Clinical Usage and Rehabilitation Techniques. 4th ed. Onalaska, WI, S & S Publishers.

29. Davies, G.J. (1995): The need for critical thinking in rehabilitation. J. Sports Rehab., 4:1-22.

30. Davies, G.J. (1995): Descriptive study comparing OKC vs. CKC isokinetic testing of the lower extremity in 200 patients with selected knee pathologies. Presented at the World Confederation of Physical Therapy.

31. Davies, G.J., and Ellenbecker, T.S. (1992): Eccentric isokinetics. Orthop. Phys. Ther. Clin. North Am., 1:297-336.

32. Davies, G.J., and Ellenbecker, T.S. (1993): Total arm strength rehabilitation for shoulder and elbow overuse injuries. In: Timm, K.E. (ed.). Orthopaedic Physical Therapy Home Study Course. Orthopaedic Section, American Physical Therapy Association.

33. Davies, G.J., and Hoffman, S.D. (1993): Neuromuscular testing and rehabilitation of the shoulder complex. J. Orthop. Sports Phys. Ther., 18:449-458.

34. Davies, G.J., and Malone, T. (1995): Proprioception, open and closed kinetic chain exercises and application to assessment and rehabilitation. Presented at the American Orthopaedic Society of Sports Medicine, Toronto, ON, Canada.

35. Davies, G.J., and Romeyn, R.L. (1992 to present): Prospective, randomized single blind study comparing closed kinetic chain versus open and closed kinetic chain integrated rehabilitation programs of patients with ACL autograft infrapatellar tendon reconstructions. Research in progress.

36. DeCarlo, M., Porter, D.A., Gehlsen, G., et al. (1992): Electromyographic and cinematographic analysis of the lower extremity during closed and open kinetic chain exercise. Isokin. Exerc. Sci., 2:24-29.

37. DeCarlo, M., Shelbourne, K.D., McCarroll, J.R., et al. (1992): Traditional versus accelerated rehabilitation following ACL reconstruction: A one-year follow-up. J. Orthop. Sports Phys. Ther., 15:309-316.

38. Dillman, C.J. (1991): The upper extremity in tennis and throwing athletes. Presented at the United States Tennis Association Meeting, Tucson, AZ.

39. Dillman, C.J., Fleisig, G.S., and Andrews, J.R. (1993): Biomechanics of pitching with emphasis upon shoulder kinematics. J. Orthop. Sports Phys. Ther., 18:402-408.

40. Draganich, L.F., Jaeger, R.J., and Kralj, A.R. (1989): Coactivation of the hamstrings and quadriceps during extension of the knee. J. Bone Joint Surg. [Am.], 71:1075-1081.

41. Draganich, L.F., and Vahey, J.W. (1990): An in vitro study of anterior cruciate ligament strain induced by quadriceps and hamstring forces. J. Orthop. Res., 8:57-63.

42. Dvir, Z. (1993): Isokinetic Exercise and Assessment. Champaign, IL, Human Kinetics.

43. Ellenbecker, T.S. (1991): A total arm strength isokinetic profile of highly skilled tennis players. Isokin. Exerc. Sci., 1:9-21.

44. Ellenbecker, T.S. (1992): Shoulder internal and external rotation strength and range of motion of highly skilled junior tennis players. Isokin. Exerc. Sci., 2:1-8.

45. Ellenbecker, T.S. (1994): Muscular strength relationship between normal grade manual muscle testing and isokinetic measurement of the shoulder internal and external rotators. J. Orthop. Sports Phys. Ther., 1:72.

46. Ellenbecker, T.S., and Derscheid, G.L. (1988): Rehabilitation of overuse injuries in the shoulder. Clin. Sports Med., 8:583-604.

47. Ellenbecker, T.S., and Davies, G.J. (2000): Closed Kinetic Chain Exercise. Champaign, IL, Human Kinetics.

48. Ellenbecker, T.S., Davies, G.J., and Rowinski, M.J. (1988): Concentric versus eccentric isokinetic strengthening of the rotator cuff: Objective data versus functional test. Am. J. Sports Med., 16:64-69.

49. Ellenbecker, T.S., Dehart, R.L., and Boeckmann, R. (1992): Isokinetic shoulder strength of the rotator cuff in professional baseball pitchers. Phys. Ther., 72:S81.

50. Ellenbecker, T.S., Feiring, D.C., Dehart, R.L., and Rich, M. (1992): Isokinetic shoulder strength: Coronal versus scapular plane testing in upper extremity unilateral dominant athletes. Phys. Ther., 72:S80-S81.

51. Ellenbecker, T.S., and Mattalino, A.J. (1997): Concentric isokinetic shoulder internal and external rotation strength in professional baseball pitchers. J. Orthop. Sports Phys. Ther., 25:323-328.

52. Elliot, B., March, T., and Blanksby, B. (1986): A three dimensional cinematographic analysis of the tennis serve. Int. J. Sport Biomech., 2:260-271.

53. Farrell, M., and Richards, J.G. (1986): Analysis of the reliability and validity of the kinetic communicator exercise device. Med. Sci. Sports Exerc., 18:44.

54. Feiring, D.C., and Ellenbecker, T.S. (1995): Open versus closed chain isokinetic testing with ACL reconstructed patients. Med. Sci. Sports Exerc., 17:S106.

55. Fleck, S. (1983): Interval training: Physiological bases. J. Strength Cond. Res., 5:4-7.

56. Francis, K., and Hoobler, T. (1987): Comparison of peak torque values of the knee flexor and extensor muscle groups using the Cybex II and Lido 2.0 isokinetic dynamometers. J. Orthop. Sports Phys. Ther., 8:480-483.

57. Gleim, G.W., Nicholas, J.A., and Webb, J.N. (1978): Isokinetic evaluation following leg injuries. Physician Sportsmed., 6:74-82.

58. Gore, D.R., Murray, M.P., Sepic, S.B., and Gardner, G.M. (1986): Shoulder muscle strength and range of motion following surgical repair of full thickness rotator cuff tears. J. Bone Joint Surg. [Am.], 68:266-272.

59. Graham, V.L., Gehlsen, G.M., and Edwards, J.A. (1993): Electromyographic evaluation of closed and open kinetic chain knee rehabilitation exercises. J. Athl. Train., 28:23-30.

60. Grana, W.A., and Muse, G. (1988): The effect of exercise on laxity in the anterior cruciate ligament deficient knee. Am. J. Sports Med., 16:586-588.

61. Green, H.J. (1986): Muscle power: Fibre type, recruitment, metabolism and fatigue. In: Jones, N.L., McCartney, N., and McCoas, A.J. (eds.), Human Muscle Power. Champaign, IL, Human Kinetics.

62. Greenberger, H.B., and Paterno, M.V. (1994): Comparison of an isokinetic strength test and functional performance test in the assessment of lower extremity function. J. Orthop. Sports Phys. Ther., 19:61.

63. Greenfield, B.H., Donatelli, R., Wooden, M.J., and Wilkes, J. (1990): Isokinetic evaluation of shoulder rotational strength between the plane of the scapula and the frontal plane. Am. J. Sports Med., 18:124-128.

64. Griffin, J.W. (1985): Differences in elbow flexion torque measure concentrically, eccentrically, and isometrically. Phys. Ther., 67:1205.

65. Grood, E.S., Suntay, W.J., Noyes, F.R., et al. (1984): Biomechanics of the knee-extension exercise. J. Bone Joint Surg. [Am.], 66:725-734.

66. Gryzlo, S.M., Pateck, R.M., Pink, M., et al. (1989): Effects of position and speed on eccentric and concentric isokinetic testing of the shoulder rotators. J. Orthop. Sports Phys. Ther., 11:64-69.

67. Hageman, P.A., Mason, D.K., Rydlund, K.W., et al. (1989): Effects of position and speed on eccentric and concentric isokinetic testing of the shoulder rotators. J. Orthop. Sports Phys. Ther., 11:64-69.

68. Harter, R.A., Osternig, L.R., Singer, K.M., et al. (1988): Long-term evaluation of knee stability and function following surgical reconstruction for anterior cruciate ligament insufficiency. Am. J. Sports Med., 16:434-443.

69. Hefzy, M.S., Grood, E.S., and Noyes, F.R. (1989): Factors affecting the region of most isometric femoral attachments. Part II. The anterior cruciate ligament. Am. J. Sports Med., 17:208-216.

70. Hellwig, E.V., Perrin, D.H., Tis, L.L., and Shenk, B.S. (1991): Effect of gravity correction on shoulder external/internal rotator reciprocal muscle group ratios. J. Natl. Athl. Trainers Assoc., 26:154.

71. Henneman, E., Somjen, G., and Carpenter, D.O. (1965): Functional significance of cell size in spinal motorneurons. J. Neurophysiol., 28:560-580.

72. Henning, C.E., Lynch, M.A., and Glick, K.R. (1985): An in-vivo strain gauge study of elongation of the anterior cruciate ligament. Am. J. Sports Med., 13:22-26.

73. Hinton, R.Y. (1988): Isokinetic evaluation of shoulder rotational strength in high school baseball pitchers. Am. J. Sports Med., 16:274-279.

74. Hislop, H.J., and Perrine, J.J. (1967): The isokinetic concept of exercise. Phys. Ther., 47:114-117.

75. Holm, I., Brox, J.I., Ludvigsen, P., and Steen, H. (1996): External rotation-best isokinetic movement pattern for evaluation of muscle function in rotator tendinosis. A prospective study with a 2-year follow up. Isokin. Exerc. Sci., 5:121-125.

76. Hsieh, H., and Walker, P.S. (1976): Stabilizing mechanisms of the loaded and unloaded knee joint. J. Bone Joint Surg. [Am.], 58:87-93.

77. Inman, V.T., Saunders, J.B., De, C.M., and Abbot, L.C. (1944): Observations of the function of the shoulder joint. J. Bone Joint Surg. [Am.], 26:1-30.

78. Ivey, F.M., Calhoun, J.H., Rusche, K., et al. (1984): Normal values for isokinetic testing of shoulder strength. Med. Sci. Sports Exerc., 16:127.

79. Jackson, A.L., Highgenboten, C., Meske, N., et al. (1987): Univariate and multivariate analysis of the reliablity of the kinetic communicator. Med. Sci. Sports Exerc., 19(Suppl.):23.

80. Jobe, F.W., Tibone, J.E., Perry, J., et al. (1983): An EMG analysis of the shoulder in throwing and pitching. A preliminary report. Am. J. Sports Med., 11:3-5.

81. Johnson, J., and Siegel, D. (1978): Reliability of an isokinetic movement of the knee extensors. Res. Q., 49:88.

82. Jurist, K.A., and Otis, J.C. (1985): Anteroposterior tibiofemoral displacements during isometric extension efforts. Am. J. Sports Med., 13:254-258.

83. Kannus, P.M., Jarvinen, M., Johnson, R., et al. (1992): Function of the quadriceps and hamstring muscles in knees with chronic partial deficiency of the ACL. Am. J. Sports Med., 20:162-168.

84. Kendall, F.D., and McCreary, E.K. (1983): Muscle Testing and Function, 3rd ed. Baltimore, Williams & Wilkins.

85. Kennedy, K., Altcheck, D.W., and Glick, I.V. (1993): Concentric and eccentric isokinetic rotator cuff ratios in skilled tennis players. Isokin. Exerc. Sci., 3:155-159.

86. Knight, K.L. (1979): Knee rehabilitation by the daily adjustable progressive resistive exercise technique. Am. J. Sports Med., 7:336.

87. Knight, K.L. (1985): Quadriceps strengthening with DAPRE technique: Case studies with neurological implications. Med. Sci. Sports Exerc., 17:636.

88. Kronberg, M., Nemeth, F., and Brostrom, L.A. (1990): Muscle activity and coordination in the normal shoulder: An electromyographic study. Clin. Orthop., 257:76-85.

89. Lesmes, G.R., Costill, D.L., Coycle, E.F., and Fine, W.J. (1978): Muscle strengthening and power changes during maximal isokinetic training. Med. Sci. Sports Exerc., 10:266-269.

90. Lucas, D.B. (1973): Biomechanics of the shoulder joint. Arch. Surg., 107:425.

91. Lutz, G.E., Palmitier, R.A., An, K.N., et al. (1991): Closed kinetic chain exercises for athletes after reconstruction of the anterior cruciate ligament. Med. Sci. Sports Exerc., 23:413.

92. Lutz, G.E., Palmitier, R.A., An, K.N., et al. (1993): Comparison of tibiofemoral joint forces during open kinetic chain and closed kinetic chain exercises. J. Bone Joint Surg. [Am.], 75:732-739.

93. Maitland, M.E., Lowe, R., and Stewart, S. (1993): Does Cybex testing increase knee laxity after anterior cruciate ligament reconstructions? Am. J. Sports Med., 21:690-695.

94. Maltry, J.A., Noble, P.C., Woods, G.W., et al. (1989): External stabilization of the anterior cruciate ligament deficient knee during rehabilitation. Am. J. Sports Med., 17:550-554.

95. Markolf, K.L., Barger, W.L., Shoemaker, S.C., et al. (1981): Role of joint load in knee stability. J. Bone Joint Surg. [Am.], 63:579-585.

96. Markolf, K.L., Gorek, J.F., Kabo, J.M., et al. (1990): Direct measurement of resultant forces in the anterior cruciate ligament. J. Bone Joint Surg. [Am.], 72:557-567.

97. Markolf, K.L., Graff-Radford, A., and Amstutz, H.C. (1978): In-vivo knee stability. J. Bone Joint Surg. [Am.], 60:664-674.

98. Markolf, K.L., Kochan, A., and Amstutz, H.C. (1984): Measurement of knee stiffness and laxity in patients with documented absence of anterior cruciate ligament. J. Bone Joint Surg. [Am.], 66:242-253.

99. Markolf, K.L., Mensch, J.S., and Amstutz, H.C. (1976): Stiffness and laxity of the knee. The contributions of the supporting structures. J. Bone Joint Surg. [Am.], 58:583-594.

100. Mawdsley, R.H., and Knapik, J.J. (1982): Comparison of isokinetic measurements with test repetitions. Phys. Ther., 62:169.

101. Meister, K., and Andrews, J.R. (1993): Classification and treatment of rotator cuff injuries in the overhand athlete. J. Orthop. Sports Phys. Ther., 18:413-421.

102. Moffroid, M., et al. (1970): Specificity of speed of exercise. Phys. Ther., 50:1693-1699.

103. Moffroid, M., Whipple, R., Hofkosh, J., et al. (1969): A study of isokinetic exercise. Phys. Ther., 49:735.

104. Molnar, G.E., and Alexander, J. (1973): Objective, quantitative muscle testing in children: A pilot study. Arch. Phys. Med. Rehab., 54:225-228.

105. Molnar, G.E., Alexander, J., and Gudfeld, N. (1979): Reliability of quantitative strength measurements in children. Arch. Phys. Med. Rehab., 60:218.

106. Mont, M.A., Choen, D.B., Campbell, K.R., et al. (1994): Isokinetic concentric versus eccentric training of the shoulder rotators with functional evaluation of performance enhancement in elite tennis players. Am. J. Sports Med., 22:513-517.

107. More, R.C., Karras, B.T., Neiman, R., et al. (1993): Hamstrings: An anterior cruciate ligament protagonist. An in vitro study. Am. J. Sports Med., 21:231-237.

108. Nicholas, J.A., Sapega, A., Kraus, H., and Webb, J.N. (1978): Factors influencing manual muscle tests in physical therapy. J. Bone Joint Surg. [Am.], 60:186.

109. Nicholas, J.A., Strizak, A.M., and Veras, G. (1976): A study of thigh muscle weakness in different pathological states of the lower extremity. Am. J. Sports Med., 4:241-248.

110. Ohkoski, Y., and Yasada, K. (1989): Biomechanical analysis of shear force exerted to anterior cruciate ligament during half squat exercise. Orthop. Trans., 13:310.

111. Ohkoski, Y., Yasuda, K., Kaneda, K., et al. (1991): Biomechanical analysis of rehabilitation in the standing position. Am. J. Sports Med., 19:605-610.

112. Palmitier, R.A., An, K.N., Scott, S.G., et al. (1991): Kinetic chain exercise in knee rehabilitation. Sports Med., 11:402-413.

113. Patel, R.R., Hurwitz, D.E., Bush-Joseph, C.A., et al. (2003): Comparison of clinical and dynamic knee function in patients with anterior cruciate ligament deficiency. Am. J. Sports Med., 31:68-74.

114. Pawlowski, D., and Perrin, D.H. (1989): Relationship between shoulder and elbow isokinetic peak torque, torque acceleration energy, average power, and total work and throwing velocity in intercollegiate pitchers. Athl. Train., 24:129-132.

115. Pedegana, L.R., Elsner, R.C., Roberts, D., et al. (1982): The relationship of upper extremity strength to throwing speed. Am. J. Sports Med., 10:352-354.

116. Perrin, D.H. (1986): Reliability of isokinetic measures. Athl. Train., 23:319.

117. Perrin, D.H. (1993): Isokinetic Exercise and Assessment. Champaign, IL, Human Kinetics.

118. Quincy, R., Davies, G.J., Kolbeck, K., et al. Isokinetic exercise: The effects of training specificity on shoulder power. J. Sports Rehab., in press.

119. Rabin, S.J., and Post, M.P. (1990): A comparative study of clinical muscle testing and Cybex evaluation after shoulder operations. Clin. Orthop., 258:147-156.

120. Reitz, C.L., Rowinski, M.J., and Davies, G.J. (1988): Comparison of Cybex II and Kin-Com reliability of the measures of peak torque, work and power at three speeds. Phys. Ther., 69:782.

121. Renstrom, P., Arms, S.W., Stanwyck, T.S., et al. (1986): Strain within the anterior cruciate ligament during hamstring and quadriceps activity. Am. J. Sports Med., 14:83-87.

122. Reynolds, N.L., Worrell, T.W., and Perrin, D.H. (1992): Effects of a lateral step-up exercise protocol on quadriceps isokinetic peak torque values and thigh girth. J. Orthop. Sports Phys. Ther., 15:151-155.

123. Rowinski, M.J. (1985): Afferent neurobiology of the joint. In: Davies, G.J., and Gould, J.A. (eds.), Orthopaedic and Sports Physical Therapy. St. Louis, C.V. Mosby.

124. Sachs, R.A., Daniel, D.M., Stone, M.L., et al. (1989): Patellofemoral problems after anterior cruciate ligament reconstruction. Am. J. Sports Med., 17:760-764.

125. Saha, A.K. (1971): Dynamic stability of the glenohumeral joint. Acta Orthop. Scand., 42:491-505.

126. Shaffer, S.W., Payne, E.D., Gabbard, L.R., et al. (1994): Relationship between isokinetic and functional tests of the quadriceps. J. Orthop. Sports Phys. Ther., 19:55.

127. Shapiro, R., and Steine, R.L. (1992): Shoulder rotation velocities. Technical Report submitted to the Lexington Clinic, Lexington, KY.

128. Shelbourne, K.D., and Nitz, P. (1990): Accelerated rehabilitation after anterior cruciate ligament rehabilitation. Am. J. Sports Med., 18:292-299.

129. Shoemaker, S.C., and Markolf, K.L. (1982): In-vivo rotatory knee stability. J. Bone Joint Surg. [Am.], 64:208-216.

130. Shoemaker, S.C., and Markolf, K.L. (1985): Effects of joint load on the stiffness and laxity of ligament-deficient knees. J. Bone Joint Surg. [Am.], 67:136-146.

131. Smith, M.J., and Melton, P. (1981): Isokinetic versus isotonic variable-resistance training. Am. J. Sports Med., 9:275-279.

132. Snow, D.J., and Johnson, K. (1988): Reliability of two velocity controlled tests for the measurement of peak torque of the knee flexors during resisted muscle shortening and resisted muscle lengthening. Phys. Ther., 68:781.

133. Snyder-Mackler, L., Delitto, A., Bailey, S.L., et al. (1995): Strength of the quadriceps femoris muscle and functional recovery after reconstruction of the anterior cruciate ligament. J. Bone Joint Surg. [Am.], 77:1166-1173.

134. Soderberg, G.J., and Blaschak, M.J. (1987): Shoulder internal and external rotation peak torque production through a velocity spectrum in differing positions. J. Orthop. Sports Phys. Ther., 8:518-524.

135. Sullivan, E.P., Markos, P.D., and Minor, M.D. (1982): An Integrated Approach to Therapeutic Exercise: Theory and Clinical Application. Reston, VA, Reston Publishing.

136. Tegner, Y., Lysholm, J., Lysholm, M., et al. (1986): A performance test to monitor rehabilitation and evaluate anterior cruciate ligament injuries. Am. J. Sports Med., 14:156-159.

137. Thorstensson, A., Grimby, G., and Karlsson, J. (1976): Force-velocity relations and fiber composition in human knee extensor muscles. J. Appl. Physiol., 40:12.

138. Timm, K.E. (1988): Post-surgical knee rehabilitation: A five year study of four methods and 5,381 patients. Am. J. Sports Med., 16:463-468.

139. Timm, K.E. (1988): Reliability of Cybex 340 and MERAC isokinetic measures of peak torque, total work, and average power at five test speeds. Phys. Ther., 69:782.

140. Vangheluwe, B., and Hebbelinck, K.M. (1986): Muscle actions and ground reaction forces in tennis. Int. J. Sport Biomech., 2:88-99.

141. Wakin, K.G., Clarke, H.H., Elkins, E.C., and Martin, G.M. (1950): Relationship between body position and application of muscle power to movements of joints. Arch. Phys. Med. Rehab., 31:81-89.

142. Walker, S.W., Couch, W.H., Boester, G.A., and Sprowl, D.W. (1987): Isokinetic strength of the shoulder after repair of a torn rotator cuff. J. Bone Joint Surg. [Am.], 69:1041-1044.

143. Walmsley, R.P., and Hartsell, H. (1992): Shoulder strength following surgical rotator cuff repair: A comparative analysis using isokinetic testing. J. Orthop. Sports Phys. Ther., 15:215-222.

144. Walmsley, R.P., and Szybbo, C. (1987): A comparative study of the torque generated by the shoulder internal and external rotator muscles in different positions and at varying speeds. J. Orthop. Sports Phys. Ther., 9:217-222.

145. Warner, J.P., Micheli, L.J., Arslanian, L.E., et al. (1990): Patterns of flexibility, laxity and strength in normal shoulders and shoulders with instability and impingement. Am. J. Sports Med., 18:366-375.

146. Wessel, J., Mattison, G., Luongo, F., et al. (1988): Reliability of eccentric and concentric measurements. Phys. Ther., 68:782.

147. Wiklander, J., and Lysholm, J. (1987): Simple tests for surveying muscle strength and muscle stiffness in sportsmen. Int. J. Sports Med., 8:50-54.

148. Wilk, K.E., and Andrews, J.R. (1993): The effects of pad placement and angular velocity on tibial displacement during isokinetic exercise. J. Orthop. Sports Phys. Ther., 17:23-30.

149. Wilk, K.E., Andrews, J.R., Arrigo, C.A., et al. (1993): The strength characteristics of internal and external rotator muscles in professional baseball pitchers. Am. J. Sports Med., 21:61-66.

150. Wilk, K.E., and Arrigo, C.A. (1993): Current concepts in the rehabilitation of the athletic shoulder. J. Orthop. Sports Phys. Ther., 18:365-378.

151. Wilk, K.E., Arrigo, C.A., and Andrews, J.R. (1991): Standardized isokinetic testing protocol for the throwing shoulder: The throwers series. Isokin. Exerc. Sci., 1:63-71.

152. Wilk, K.E., Arrigo, C.A., and Andrews, J.R. (1992): Isokinetic testing of the shoulder abductors and adductors: Windowed vs. nonwindowed data collection. J. Orthop. Sports Phys. Ther., 15:107-112.

153. Wilk, K.E., and Johnson, R.E. (1988): The reliability of the Biodex B-200. Phys. Ther., 68:792.

154. Wilk, K.E., Romaniello, W.T., Soscia, S.M., et al. (1994): The relationship between subjective knee scores, isokinetic (OKC) testing and functional testing in the ACL reconstructed knee. J. Orthop. Sports Phys. Ther., 20:60-73.

155. Wilk, K.E., Voight, M.L., Keirns, M.A., et al. (1993): Stretch-shortening drills for the upper extremities: Theory and clinical application. J. Orthop. Sports Phys. Ther., 17:225-239.

FUNCTIONAL TRAINING AND ADVANCED REHABILITATION

Michael L. Voight, P.T., D.H.S.C., O.C.S., S.C.S., ATC
Barb Hoogenboom, P.T., M.H.S., S.C.S., ATC
Turner A. Blackburn, P.T., M.Ed., ATC
Gray Cook, P.T., M.S., O.C.S.

CHAPTER OBJECTIVES

At the end of this chapter the reader will be able to:

- Define and discuss the importance of proprioception in the neuromuscular control process.
- Define and discuss the different levels of central nervous system motor control and the neural pathways responsible for the transmission of afferent and efferent information at each level.
- Apply a systematic functional evaluation designed to provoke symptoms.
- Demonstrate consistency between functional and clinical testing information (combinatorial power).
- Apply a three-step model designed to promote the practical systematic thinking required for the effective therapeutic exercise prescription and progression.
- Define and discuss the objectives of the functional neuromuscular rehabilitation program.
- Develop a rehabilitation program that utilizes various exercise techniques for development of neuromuscular control.

FUNCTION AND FUNCTIONAL REHABILITATION

The basic goal in rehabilitation is to restore and enhance function within the environment and to perform the specific activities of daily living (ADL). The entire rehabilitation process should be focused on improving the functional status of the patient. The concept of functional training is not new nor is it limited to function related to sport. By definition, *function* means having a purpose or duty. Therefore, *functional* can be defined as performing a practical or intended function or duty. Function should be considered as a spectrum because ADLs encompass many different tasks for many different people. What is functional to one person may not be functional to another. It is widely accepted that to perform a specific activity better, one must practice that activity. Therefore, the functional exercise progression for return to ADL can best be defined as breaking the specific activities down into a hierarchy and then performing them in a sequence that allows for the acquisition or reacquisition of that skill. It is important to note that although people develop differing levels of skill, function, and motor control there are fundamental tasks that are common to nearly all individuals (barring pathologic conditions and disability). Lifestyle, habits, injury, and other factors can erode fundamental components of movement without obvious alterations in higher-level function and skill. Ongoing higher-level function is a testament to the compensatory power of the neurologic system. Imperfect function and skill create stress in other body systems. Fundamental elements can first be observed during the developmental progression of posture and motor control. The sequence of the developmental progression can also give insight to the original acquisition of skill. The ability to assess the retention or loss of fundamental movement patterns is therefore a way to enhance rehabilitation. The rehabilitation process starts with a two-part appraisal that creates perspective by viewing both ends of the functional spectrum:

- The current level of function (ADL, work, and sport/recreation) relative to the patient's needs and goals.
- The ability to demonstrate the fundamental movement patterns that represent the foundation of function and basic motor control.

Objectives of Functional Rehabilitation

The overall objective of the functional exercise program is to return the patient to his or her preinjury level as quickly and as safely as possible. Specific training activities are designed to restore both dynamic joint stability and ADL skills.[3] To accomplish this objective, a basic tenet of exercise physiology is used. The S.A.I.D. (specific *a*daptations to *i*mposed *d*emands) principle states that the body will adapt to stress and strain placed upon it.[46] Athletes cannot succeed if they have not been prepared to meet all of the demands of their specific activity.[46] Reactive neuromuscular training (RNT) helps to bridge the gap from traditional rehabilitation via proprioceptive and balance training to promote a more functional return to activity.[46] The S.A.I.D. principle provides constructive stress, and RNT creates opportunities for input and integration. The main objective of the RNT program is to facilitate the unconscious process of interpreting and integrating the peripheral sensations received by the central nervous system (CNS) into appropriate motor responses. This approach is enhanced by the unique clinical focus on pathologic orthopedic and neurologic states and their functional representation. This special focus forces the clinician to consider evaluation of human movement as a complex multisystem interaction and the logical starting point for exercise prescription. Exercise prescription choices must continually represent the specialized training of the clinician through a consistent and centralized focus on human function and consideration of the fundamentals that make function possible. Exercise used at any given therapeutic level must refine movement, not simply create general exertion with the hope of increased movement tolerance.[17] Moore and Durstine state; "Unfortunately, exercise training to optimize functional capacity has not been well studied in the context of most chronic diseases or disabilities. As a result, many exercise professionals have used clinical experience to develop their own methods for prescribing exercise."[1] Experience, self-critique, and specialization produce seasoned clinicians with intuitive evaluation abilities and exercise innovations that are sometimes difficult to follow and even harder to ascertain; however, common characteristics do exist. The clinical expert uses *parallel* (simultaneous) consideration of all factors influencing functional movement. RNT as a treatment philosophy is inclusive and adaptable with the ability to address a variety of clinical situations. There also is an understanding that a clinical philosophy is designed to serve, not to be served. The treatment design demonstrates specific attention to the parts (clinical measurements and isolated details) with continual consideration of the whole (restoration of function).[17] Moore and Durstine follow their previous statement by acknowledging that "Experience is an acceptable way to guide exercise management, but a systematic approach would be better."[1]

The Three-Phase Model for Exercise Prescription

The purpose of this chapter is to demonstrate a three-step model designed to promote the practical systematic

thinking required for effective therapeutic exercise prescription and progression at each phase of rehabilitation.[17] The approach will be a *serial* (consecutive) step-by-step method that will, with practice and experience, lead to *parallel* thinking and multilevel problem solving. The intended purpose of this method is to reduce arbitrary trial and error exercise attempts and protocol-based thinking. It will give the novice clinician a framework that will guide but not confine clinical exercise prescription. It will provide experienced clinicians with a system to observe their particular strengths and weaknesses in exercise dosage and design. Inexperienced and experienced clinicians alike will develop practical insight by applying the model and observing the interaction of the systems that produce human movement. The focus is specifically geared to orthopedic rehabilitation and the clinical problem-solving strategies used to develop an exercise prescription through an outcome-based goal setting process. All considerations for therapeutic exercise prescription will give equal importance to conventional orthopedic exercise standards (biomechanical and physiologic parameters) and neurophysiologic strategies (motor learning, proprioceptive feedback, and synergistic recruitment principles). This three-phase model (Box 10-1) will create a mechanism that will necessitate interaction between orthopedic exercise approaches and optimal neurophysiologic techniques. It includes a four-principle foundation that demonstrates the hierarchy and interaction of the founding concepts utilized in rehabilitation (both orthopedic and neurologic). For all practical purposes, these four categories help demonstrate the efficient and effective continuity necessary for formulation of a treatment plan and prompt the clinician to maintain an inclusive, open-minded clinical approach.

This chapter is written with the clinic-based practitioner in mind. It will help the clinician formulate an exercise philosophy. Some clinicians will discover reasons for success that were intuitive and therefore hard to communicate to other professionals. Others will discover a missing step in the therapeutic exercise design process. Much of the confusion and frustration encountered by the rehabilitation specialist is due to the vast variety of treatment options afforded by ever improving technology and accessibility to emerging research evidence. To effectively utilize the wealth of current information and that which the future has yet to bestow, the clinician must adopt an operational framework or personal philosophy about therapeutic exercise. If a clinical

Box 10-1

Three-Phase Rehabilitation Model

Phase	Description
1	Proprioception and kinesthesia
2	Dynamic stability
3	Reactive neuromuscular control

exercise philosophy is based on technology, equipment, or protocols, the scope of problem solving is strictly confined. It would continually change because no universal standard or gauge exists. However, a philosophy based solely on the structure and function of the human body will keep the focus (Box 10-2) uncorrupted and centralized. Technologic developments can only enhance exercise effectiveness as long as the technology, system, or protocol remains true to a holistic functional standard. Known functional standards should serve as governing factors that improve the clinical consistency of the clinician and rehabilitation team for pre-scription and progression of training methods. The four principles for exercise prescription are based on human movement and the systems upon which it is constructed (Box 10-2). The intention of these four distinct categories is to break down and reconstruct the factors that influence functional movement and to stimulate inductive reasoning, deductive reasoning, and the critical thinking needed to develop a therapeutic exercise progression. Hopefully, these factors will serve the intended purpose of organization and clarity, thereby giving due respect to the many insightful clinicians who have provided the foundation and substance for the construction of this practical framework.[17]

PROPRIOCEPTION, RECEPTORS, AND NEUROMUSCULAR CONTROL

Success in skilled performance depends upon how effectively an individual detects, perceives, and uses relevant sensory information. Knowing exactly where our limbs are in space and how much muscular effort is required to perform a particular action is critical for successful performance of all activities requiring intricate coordination of the various body parts. Fortunately, information about the position and movement of various body parts is available from the peripheral receptors located in and around the articular structures and surrounding the musculature.

Joints: Support and Sensory Function

Around the normal healthy joint, both static and dynamic stabilizers provide support. The role of the capsuloliga-

---

Box 10-2

Four Principles for Exercise Prescription

- Functional evaluation and assessment in relationship to dysfunction (disability) and impairment.
- Identification and management of motor control.
- Identification and management of osteokinematic and arthrokinematic limitations.
- Identification of current movement patterns followed by facilitation and integration of synergistic movement patterns.

---

mentous tissues in the dynamic restraint of the joint has been well established in the literature.[4,5,14,25,29-34,58] Although the primary role of these structures is mechanical in nature by provision of structural support and stabilization to the joint, the capsuloligamentous tissues also play an important sensory role by detecting joint position and motion.[20,24,25,56] Sensory afferent feedback from the receptors in the capsuloligamentous structures projects directly to the reflex and cortical pathways, thereby mediating reactive muscle activity for dynamic restraint.[4,5,24,25,40] The efferent motor response that ensues from the sensory information is called *neuromuscular control.* Sensory information is sent to the CNS to be processed, and appropriate motor strategies are executed.

Physiology of Proprioception

Sherrington[56] first described the term *proprioception* in the early 1900s when he noted the presence of receptors in the joint capsular structures that were primarily reflexive in nature. Since that time, mechanoreceptors have been morphohistologically identified about the articular structures in both animal and human models. In addition, the well-described muscle spindle and Golgi tendon organs are powerful mechanoreceptors. Mechanoreceptors are specialized end organs that function as biologic transducers that can convert the mechanical energy of physical deformation (elongation, compression, and pressure) into action nerve potentials yielding proprioceptive information.[30] Although receptor discharge varies according to the intensity of the distortion, mechanoreceptors can also be described based upon their discharge rates. Quickly adapting receptors cease discharging shortly after the onset of a stimulus whereas slowly adapting receptors continue to discharge while the stimulus is present.[15,25,30] Around the healthy joint, quick adapting receptors are responsible for providing conscious and unconscious kinesthetic sensations in response to joint movement or acceleration whereas slow adapting mechanoreceptors provide continuous feedback and thus proprioceptive information relative to joint position[15,30,43] (see Chapter 8 for examples of quick and slow adapting receptors).

Once stimulated, mechanoreceptors are able to adapt. With constant stimulation, the frequency of the neural impulses decreases. The functional implication is that mechanoreceptors detect change and rates of change, as opposed to steady-state conditions.[53] This input is then analyzed in the CNS for joint position and movement.[80] The status of the musculoskeletal structures is sent to the CNS so that information about static versus dynamic conditions, equilibrium versus disequilibrium, or biomechanical stress and strain relations can be evaluated.[71,73] Once processed and evaluated, this proprioceptive information becomes capable of influencing muscle tone, motor execution programs, and cognitive somatic perceptions or kinesthetic awareness.[49] Proprioceptive information also protects the joint from damage caused by movement exceeding the normal physiologic range of motion and helps to determine the appropriate balance of synergistic and antagonistic forces. All of this information helps to generate a somatosensory image within the CNS. Therefore, the soft tissues surrounding a joint serve a double purpose: they provide biomechanical support to the bony partners making up the joint, keeping them in relative anatomical alignment, and, through an extensive afferent neurologic network, they provide valuable proprioceptive information.

CENTRAL NERVOUS SYSTEM: MOTOR CONTROL INTEGRATION

The CNS response falls under three categories or levels of motor control: spinal reflexes, brainstem processing, and cognitive cerebral cortex program planning. The goal of the rehabilitation process is to retrain the altered afferent pathways to enhance the neuromuscular control system. To accomplish this goal, the objective of the rehabilitation program should be to hyperstimulate the joint and muscle receptors to encourage maximal afferent discharge to the respective CNS levels.[13,43,64,68,69]

First Level Response: Muscle

When faced with an unexpected load, the first reflexive muscle response is a burst of electromyographic (EMG) activity that occurs between 30 and 50 msec. The afferent fibers of both the muscle spindle and the Golgi tendon organ mechanoreceptors synapse with the spinal interneurons and produce a reflexive facilitation or inhibition of the motor neurons.[64,69,74] The monosynaptic stretch reflex is one of the most rapid reflexes underlying limb control. The stretch reflex occurs at an unconscious level and is not affected by outside factors. These responses can occur simultaneously to control limb position and posture. Because they can occur at the same time, are in parallel, are subconscious, and do not have cortical interference, they do not require attention and are thus automatic.

At this level of motor control, activities to encourage short-loop reflex joint stabilization should dominate.[13,43,58,69] These activities are characterized by sudden alterations in joint position that require reflex muscle stabilization. With sudden alterations or perturbations, both the articular and muscular mechanoreceptors will be stimulated for the production reflex stabilization. Rhythmic stabilization exercises encourage monosynaptic co-contraction of the musculature, thereby producing a dynamic neuromuscular stabilization.[60] These exercises serve to build a foundation for dynamic stability.

Second Level Response: Brainstem

The second level of motor control interaction is at the level of the brainstem.[11,64,73] At this level, afferent mechanoreceptors interact with the vestibular system and visual input from the eyes to control or facilitate postural stability and equilibrium of the body.[13,43,64,68,73] Afferent mechanoreceptor input also works in concert with the muscle spindle complex by inhibiting antagonistic muscle activity under conditions of rapid lengthening and periarticular distortion, both of which accompany postural disruption.[49,69] In conditions of disequilibrium where simultaneous neural input exists, a neural pattern is generated that affects the muscular stabilizers, thereby returning equilibrium to the body's center of gravity.[64] Therefore, balance is influenced by the same peripheral afferent mechanism that mediates joint proprioception and is at least partially dependent upon an individual's inherent ability to integrate joint position sense with neuromuscular control.[62]

CLINICAL PEARL #1

Balance activities, both with and without visual input, will enhance motor function at the brainstem level.[11,64]

It is important that these activities remain specific to the types of activities or skills that will be required of the athlete upon return to sport.[52] Static balance activities should be used as a precursor to more dynamic skill activity.[52] Static balance skills can be initiated when the individual is able to bear weight on the lower extremity. The general progression of static balance activities is to move from bilateral to unilateral and from eyes open to eyes closed.[43,52,64,75,76] With balance training, it is important to remember that sensory systems respond to environmental manipulation. To stimulate or facilitate the proprioceptive system, vision must be disadvantaged, which can be accomplished in several ways (Box 10-3).

Third Level Response: Central Nervous System/Cognitive

The appreciation of joint position at the highest or cognitive level needs to be included in the RNT program. These types of activities are initiated on the cognitive level and

Box 10-3

Ways to Disadvantage Vision to Stimulate the Proprioceptive System

- Remove vision with either the eyes closed or blindfolded.
- Destabilize vision by demanding hand and eye movements (ball toss) or moving the visual surround.
- Confuse vision with unstable visual cues that disagree with the proprioceptive and vestibular inputs (sway referencing).

include programming motor commands for voluntary movement. The repetitions of these movements will maximally stimulate the conversion of conscious programming to unconscious programming.[13,43,64,65,68,73] The term for this type of training is *the forced-use paradigm*. By making a task significantly more difficult or asking for multiple tasks, we bombard the CNS with input. The CNS attempts to sort and process this overload information by opening additional neural pathways. When the individual goes back to a basic task of ADL, the task becomes easier. This information can then be stored as a central command and ultimately performed without continuous reference to the conscious as a *triggered response*.[13,43,64,67,68] As with all training the single greatest obstacle to motor learning is the conscious mind. We must get the conscious mind out of the act!

Closed-Loop, Open-Loop, and Feed Forward Integration

Why is a coordinated motor response important? When an unexpected load is placed upon a joint, ligamentous damage occurs between 70 and 90 msec unless an appropriate response ensues.[8,51,81] Therefore, reactive muscle activity must occur that provides sufficient magnitude in the 40- to 80-msec timeframe after loading begins to protect the capsuloligamentous structures. The closed-loop system of CNS integration may not be fast enough to produce a response to increase muscle stiffness. There is simply no time for the system to process the information and feedback about the condition. Failure of the dynamic restraint system to control abnormal forces will expose the static structures to excessive forces. In this case, the open-loop system of anticipation becomes more important in producing the desired response. Preparatory muscle activity in anticipation of joint loading can influence the reactive muscle activation patterns. Anticipatory activation increases the sensitivity of the muscle spindles, thereby allowing the unexpected perturbations to be detected more quickly.[22]

Very quick movements are completed before feedback can be used to produce an action to alter the course of movement. Therefore, if the movement is fast enough, a mechanism like a motor program would have to be used to control the entire action, with the movement being carried out without any feedback. Fortunately, the open-loop control system allows the motor control system to organize an entire action ahead of time. For this to occur, previous knowledge needs to be preprogrammed into the primary sensory cortex (Box 10-4).

In the open-loop system, a program that sets up some kind of neural mechanism or network that is preprogrammed organizes movement in advance. A classic example of this occurs in the body as postural adjustments are made before the intended movement. When an individual raises his or her arm up into forward flexion, the first

---

Box 10-4

Preprogrammed Information Needed for an Open-Loop System to Work

- The particular muscles that are needed to produce an action
- The order in which these muscles need to be activated
- The relative forces of the various muscle contractions
- The relative timing and sequencing of these actions
- The duration of the respective contractions

---

muscle groups to fire are not even in the shoulder girdle region. The first muscles to contract are those in the lower back and legs (approximately 80 msec passes before noticeable activity occurs in the shoulder) to provide a stable base for movement.[9] Because the shoulder muscles are linked to the rest of the body, their contraction affects posture. If no preparatory compensations in posture were made, raising the arm would shift the center of gravity forward causing a slight loss of balance. The feed forward motor control system takes care of this potential problem by preprogramming the appropriate postural modification first, rather than requiring the body to make adjustments after the arm begins to move.

Lee[42] demonstrated that these preparatory postural adjustments are not independent from the arm movement but rather are a part of the total motor pattern. When the arm movements are organized, the motor instructions are preprogrammed to adjust posture first and then move the arm. Therefore, arm movement and postural control are not separate events but rather are different parts of an integrated action that raises the arm while maintaining balance. Lee showed that these EMG preparatory postural adjustments disappear when the individual leans against some type of support before raising the arm. The motor control system recognizes that advance preparation of postural control is not needed when the body is supported against the wall.

It is important to remember that most motor tasks are a complex blend of both open- and closed-loop operations. Therefore, both types of control are often at work simultaneously. Both feedforward and feedback neuromuscular control can enhance dynamic stability if the sensory and motor pathways are frequently stimulated.[43] Each time a signal passes through a sequence of synapses, the synapses become more capable of transmitting the same signal.[34,36] When these pathways are "facilitated" regularly, memory of that signal is created and can be recalled to program future movements.[34,54]

Conclusion: Relationship to Rehabilitation

A rehabilitation program that addresses the need for restoring normal joint stability and proprioception cannot be constructed until one has a total appreciation of both the mechanical and sensory functions of the articular structures.[13] Knowledge of the basic physiology of how these muscular and joint mechanoreceptors work together in the production of smooth controlled coordinated motion is critical in developing a rehabilitation training program. This is because the role of the joint musculature extends well beyond absolute strength and the capacity to resist fatigue. With simple restoration of mechanical restraints or strengthening of the associated muscles the smooth coordinated neuromuscular controlling mechanisms required for joint stability are neglected.[13] The complexity of joint motion necessitates synergy and synchrony of muscle firing patterns, thereby permitting proper joint stabilization, especially during sudden changes in joint position, which is common in functional activities. Understanding of these relationships and functional implications will allow the clinician greater variability and success in returning patients safely back to their playing environment

FOUR PRINCIPLES FOR THERAPEUTIC EXERCISE

We propose four principles for therapeutic exercise prescription, which will be described as the four "P's" within this section. These principles serve to guide decisions for therapeutic exercise choices, progressions, and termination of interventions. The application of these four principles in the appropriate sequence will allow the clinician to understand a starting point, a consistent progression, and the end point for each exercise prescription. This sequence is achieved by utilizing functional activities and fundamental movement patterns as goals. By proceeding in this fashion, the clinician will have the ability to evaluate the whole before the parts and then discuss the parts as they apply. Table 10-1 lists and describes the four principles for therapeutic exercise prescription.

CLINICAL PEARL #2

The true art of rehabilitation is to understand the whole of synergistic functional movement and the therapeutic techniques that will have the greatest positive effect on that movement in the least amount of time.

The Four P's

The four P's represent the four principles: purpose, posture, position, and pattern (Table 10-2). They serve as quick reminders of the hierarchy, interaction, and application of each principle. The questions of what, when, where, and how for functional movement assessment and exercise prescription are answered in the appropriate order (Table 10-2).

Purpose

The word *purpose* is simply a cue to be used both during the evaluation process and the exercise prescription process to keep the clinician intently focused on the greatest single limiting factor of function (Table 10-2). The primary questions to ask for this principle appear in Box 10-5. It is not uncommon for the clinician to attempt

Table 10-1

Four Principles for Therapeutic Exercise Prescription

Principle	Description
Functional evaluation and assessment in relationship to dysfunction (disability) and impairment	The evaluation must identify a functional problem or limitation resulting in a functional diagnosis. The observation of whole movement patterns tempered with practical knowledge of key stress points and common compensatory patterns will improve evaluation efficiency.
Identification and management of motor control	Rehabilitation can be greatly advanced by understanding functional milestones and fundamental movements such as those demonstrated during the positions and postures paramount to growth and development. These milestones serve as key representations of functional mobility and control as well as play a role in the initial setup and design of the exercise program.
Identification and management of osteokinematic and arthrokinematic limitations	The skills and techniques of orthopedic manual therapy are beneficial in identification of specific arthrokinematic restrictions that would limit movement or impede the motor learning process. Management of myofascial as well as capsular structures will improve osteokinematic movement as well as allow for balanced muscle tone between the agonist and antagonist. This will also help the clinician understand the dynamics of the impairment.
Identification of current movement patterns followed by facilitation and integration of synergistic movement patterns	Once restrictions and limitations are managed and gross motion is restored, the application of proprioceptive neuromuscular facilitation–type patterning will further improve neuromuscular function and control. The consideration of synergistic movement is the final step in the restoration of function by focusing on coordination, timing, and motor learning.

Table 10-2

Memory Cues and Primary Questions Associated with the Four Principles for Therapeutic Exercise Prescription

Principle	Memory Cue	Memory Cue Definition	Primary Questions
Functional evaluation and assessment	PURPOSE	Used both during the evaluation process and the exercise prescription process to keep the clinician intently focused on the greatest single limiting factor of function	1. "*What* functional activity is limited?" 2. "*What* does the limitation appear to be—a mobility problem or a stability problem?" 3. "*What* is the dysfunction or disability?" 4. "*What* fundamental movement is limited?" 5. "*What* is the impairment?"
Identification of motor control	POSTURE	Helps the clinician to remember to consider a more holistic approach to exercise prescription	1. "*When* in the development sequence is the impairment obvious?" 2. "*When* do the substitutions and compensations occur?" 3. "*When* in the developmental sequence does the patient demonstrate success?" 4. "*When* in the developmental sequence does the patient experience difficulty?" 5. "*When* is the best possible starting point for exercise with respect to posture?"
Identification of osteokinematic and arthrokinematic limitations	POSITION	Describes not only the location of the anatomic structure (joint, muscle group, ligament, etc.) where impairment has been identified but also the positions (with respect to movement and load) that the greatest and least limitations occur	1. "*Where* is the impairment located?" 2. "*Where* among the structures (myofascial or articular) does the impairment have its greatest effect?" 3. "*Where* in the ROM does the impairment affect position the greatest?" 4. "*Where* is the most beneficial position for the exercise?"
Integration of synergistic movement patterns	PATTERN	Cues the clinician to continually consider the functional movements of the human body that occur in unified patterns that occupy three-dimensional space and cross three planes (frontal, sagittal, and transverse)	1. "*How* is the movement pattern different upon bilateral comparison?" 2. "*How* can synergistic movement, coordination, recruitment and timing be facilitated?" 3. "*How* will this affect the movement limitation?" 4. "*How* will this affect function?"

to resolve multiple problems with the initial exercise prescription. However, the practice of identifying the single greatest limiting factor will reduce frustration and also not overwhelm the patient. There may be other factors that have been identified in the evaluation; however, a major limiting factor or a single weak link should stand out and be the focus of the initial therapeutic exercise intervention. Alterations in the limiting factor may produce positive changes elsewhere, which can be identified and considered before the next exercise progression.

The functional evaluation process should take on three distinct layers or levels (Table 10-3). Each of the three levels should involve qualitative observations followed by quantitative documentation when possible. Normative data are helpful, but bilateral comparison is also effective and demonstrates the functional problem to the patient at each level. Many patients think the problem is simply symptomatic and structural in nature and have no example of dysfunction outside of pain with movement. Moffroid and Zimny suggest that, "Muscle strength of the right and left sides is more similar in the proximal muscles whereas

Box 10-5

Primary Questions for Purpose

1. "*What* functional activity is limited?"
2. "*What* does the limitation appear to be—a mobility problem or a stability problem?"
3. "*What* is the dysfunction or disability?"
4. "*What* fundamental movement is limited?"
5. "*What* is the impairment?"

Table 10-3

Three Levels of Functional Evaluation

Level	Name	Description
I	Functional activity assessment	Combined movements common to the patient's lifestyle and occupation are reproduced. They usually fit the definition of general or specific skill.
II	Functional or fundamental movement assessment	The clinician takes what is learned through the observation of functional movements and breaks those movements down to the static and transitional postures seen in the normal developmental sequence.
III	Specific clinical measurement	Clinical measurements are used to identify and quantify specific problems that contribute to limitation of motion or limitation of control.

we accept a 10% to 15% difference in strength of the distal muscles.... With joint flexibility, we accept a 5% difference between goniometric measurements of the right and left sides."[55]

The functional activity assessment is a reproduction of combined movements common to the patient's lifestyle and occupation. These movements usually fit the definition of general or specific skill. The clinician must have the patient demonstrate a variety of positions and not just positions that correspond to symptom reproduction.[18] Static postural assessment is included as well as assessment of dynamic activity. The quality of control and movement is assessed. Specific measurement of bilateral differences is difficult, but demonstration and observation is helpful for the patient. The clinician should note the positions and activities that provoke symptoms as well as the activities that illustrate poor body mechanics, poor alignment, right-left asymmetries, and inappropriate weight shifting. When the clinician has observed gross movement quality, it may be necessary to also quantify movement performance. Repetition of the activity for endurance evaluation, symptom reproduction, or rapidly declining quality will create a functional baseline for bilateral comparison and documentation.

Next is the functional or fundamental movement assessment. The clinician must take what is learned through the observation of functional movements and break those movements down to the static and transitional postures seen in the normal developmental sequence. This breakdown will reduce activities to the many underlying mobilizing and stabilizing actions and reactions that constitute the functional activity. More simply stated, the activity is broken down into a sequence of primary movements that can be observed independently. It must be noted that these movements still involve multiple joints and muscles.[18] Individual joint and muscle group assessment will be performed during clinical measurements. Martin notes, "The developmental sequence has provided the most consistent base for almost all approaches used by physical therapists."[55] This is a powerful statement and, because true qualitative measurements of normal movement in adult populations are limited, the clinician must look for universal movement similarities. Changes in fundamental movements can effect significant and prompt changes in function and therefore must be considered functional as well. Because the movement patterns of most adults are habitual and specific and therefore are not representative of a full or optimal movement spectrum, the clinician must first consider the nonspecific basic movement patterns common to all individuals during growth and development. The developmental sequence is predictable and universal in the first 2 years of life.[61] There are individual differences in rate and quality of the progression. The differences are minimal compared with variations seen in the adult population with their many habits, occupations, and lifestyles. In addition to diverse movement patterns, the adult population has the consequential complicating factor of previous medical and injury history. Each medical problem and injury has had some degree of influence on activity and movement. Thus, evaluation of functional activities alone may hide many uneconomical movement patterns, compensations, and asymmetries that when integrated into functional activities are not readily obvious to the clinician. By using the fundamental movements of the developmental progression, the clinician can view mobility and static and dynamic stability problems in a more isolated setting. Although enormous variations of functional movement quality and quantity exist between specific adult patient populations, most individuals have the developmental sequence in common.[61] The movements used in normal motor development are the building blocks of skill and function.[61] Many of these building blocks can be lost while the skill is maintained or retained at some level (although rarely optimal). We will refer to these movement building blocks as *fundamental movements* and consider them as precursors to higher function. Bilateral comparison is helpful when the clinician identifies qualitative differences between right and left sides. These movements (like functional activities) can be compared quantitatively as well.

Lastly, clinical measurements will be used to identify specific problems. Clinical measurements should be used to identify and quantify specific problems that contribute to limitation of motion or limitation of control. Clinical measurements will first classify a patient through qualitative assessment. The parameters that define that classification must then be quantified to reveal impairment. These classifications are called hypermobility and hypomobility and help to create treatment guides considering the functional status, anatomical structures, and severity of symptoms. The clinician should not proceed into exercise prescription without proper identification of one of these general categories. The success or failure of a particular exercise treatment regimen probably depends more on this classification than on the choice of exercise technique or protocol.

Once the appropriate clinical classification is produced, specific quantitative measurements will define the level of involvement within the classification and set a baseline for exercise treatment. Periodic reassessments may identify a different major limiting factor or weak link that may require reclassification followed by specific measurement. The new problem or limitation would then be inserted as the purpose for a new exercise intervention. A simple diagram (Fig. 10-1) will help the clinician separate the different levels of function so that intervention and purpose will always be at the appropriate level and assist with clinical decision making relative to exercise prescription.[23]

Posture

Posture is a word to help the clinician consider a more holistic approach to exercise prescription (see Table 10-2).

The primary questions to ask for this principle appear in Box 10-6. Janda[38] stated an interesting point when discussing posture and the muscles responsible for its maintenance. Most discussions on posture and postural musculature generally refer to erect standing. However "..., erect standing position is so well balanced that little or no activity is necessary to maintain it."[38] Therefore, "basic human posture should be derived from the principle movement pattern, namely gait. Since we stand on one leg for most of the time during walking, the stance on one leg should be considered to be the typical posture in man; the postural muscles are those which maintain this posture." Janda reported the ratio of single- to double-leg stance in gait to be 85% to 15%. "The muscles which maintain erect posture in standing on one leg are exactly those which show a striking tendency to get tight."[66] Infants and toddlers use tonic holding before normal motor development and maturation produces abilities for the use of co-contraction as a means of effective support. "Tonic holding is the ability of tonic postural muscles to maintain a contraction in their shortened range against gravitational or manual resistance."[10] The adult orthopedic patient may revert to some level of tonic holding after injury or in the presence of pain and altered proprioception. Likewise, adults who have habitual postures and limited activity may adopt tonic holding for some postures. Just as Janda uses single-leg stance to observe postural function with greater specificity than the more conventional double-leg erect standing, the developmental progression can offer greater

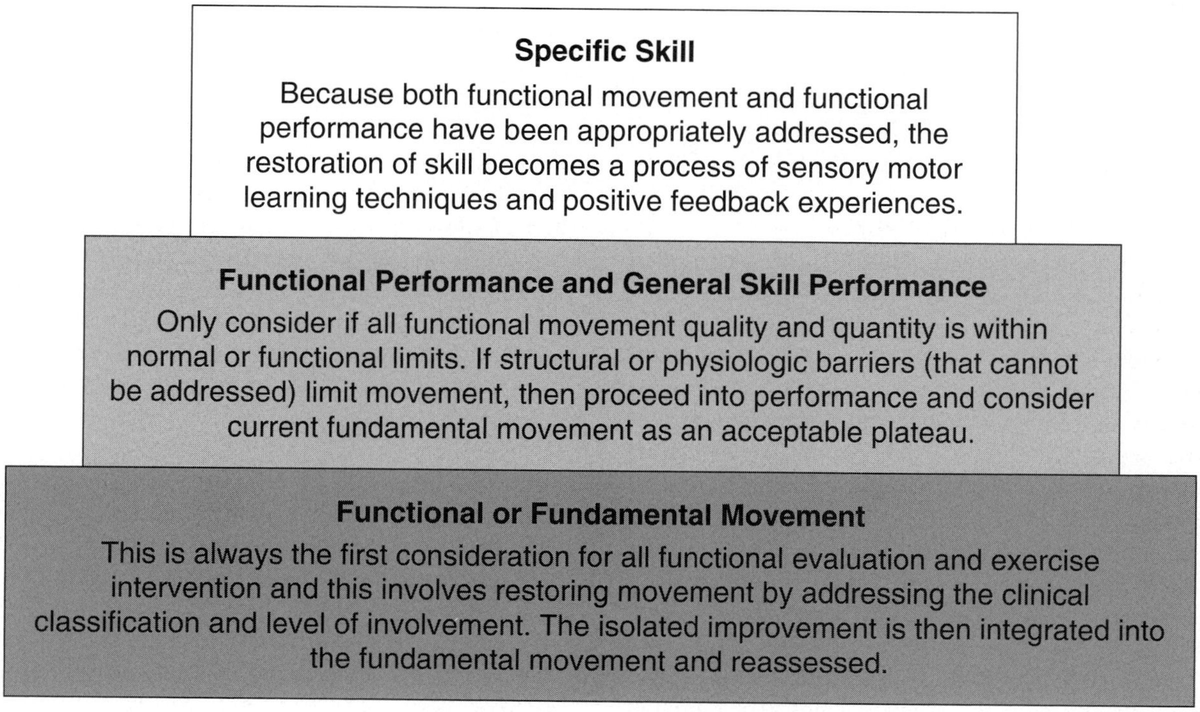

Specific Skill

Because both functional movement and functional performance have been appropriately addressed, the restoration of skill becomes a process of sensory motor learning techniques and positive feedback experiences.

Functional Performance and General Skill Performance

Only consider if all functional movement quality and quantity is within normal or functional limits. If structural or physiologic barriers (that cannot be addressed) limit movement, then proceed into performance and consider current fundamental movement as an acceptable plateau.

Functional or Fundamental Movement

This is always the first consideration for all functional evaluation and exercise intervention and this involves restoring movement by addressing the clinical classification and level of involvement. The isolated improvement is then integrated into the fundamental movement and reassessed.

Figure 10-1. Different levels of function.

Box 10-6

Primary Questions for Posture

1. "*When* in the development sequence is the impairment obvious?"
2. "*When* do the substitutions and compensations occur?"
3. "*When* in the developmental sequence does the patient demonstrate success?"
4. "*When* in the developmental sequence does the patient experience difficulty?"
5. "*When* is the best possible starting point for exercise with respect to posture?"

understanding by examination of the precursors of single-leg stance.[16] As stated earlier, fundamental movements are basic representations of mobility, stability, and dynamic stability and include the transitional postures used in growth and development. This approach will help the clinician consider how the mobility or stability problem, which was isolated in the evaluation, has been (temporarily) integrated by substitution and compensation of other body parts. The clinician must remember that motor learning is a survival mechanism. The principles that the clinician will use in rehabilitation to produce motor learning have already been activated by the functional response to the impairment. Necessity or affinity, repetition, and reinforcement have been used to avoid pain or produce alternative movements since the onset of symptoms. Therefore, a new motor program has been activated to manage the impairment and produce some level of function that is usually viewed as dysfunction. It should be considered a natural and appropriate response of the body reacting to limitation or symptoms. The body will sacrifice movement quality to maintain a degree of movement quantity. Considering this, two distinct needs are presented.

Posture for Protection and Inhibition

The clinician must restrict or inhibit the inappropriate motor program. In the case of a control or stability problem, the patient must have some form of support, protection, or facilitation. Otherwise, the inappropriate program will take over in an attempt to protect and respond to the postural demand. Although most adult patients function at the necessary skill level, upon evaluation many qualitative problems are noted. Inappropriate joint loading and locking, poor tonic responses, or even tonic holding can be observed with simple activities. Some joint movements are used excessively whereas other joint movements are unconsciously avoided. Many primary stability problems exist in the presence of underlying secondary mobility problems. Moreover, in some patients the mobility problem precedes the stability problem. This is a common explanation for microtraumatic and overuse injuries. It is

also why bilateral comparison and assessment of proximal and distal structures are mandatory in the evaluative process. For a mobility problem, a joint is not used appropriately because of weakness or restriction. The primary mobility problem may be the result of compromised stability elsewhere. Motor programs have been created to allow the patient to push on in the presence of the mobility or stability problem. The problems can be managed by mechanical consideration of the mobility and stability status of the patient in the fundamental postures.

For primary stability problems mechanical support or other assistance must be provided. This can be done simply by a reduction of partial or complete stress, which may include non–weight bearing or partial weight bearing of the spine and extremities or temporary bracing. If the stability problem is only in a particular range of movement then that movement must be managed. If there is an underlying mobility problem, then it must be managed and temporarily taken out of the initial exercise movement. The alteration of posture can effectively limit complete or partial motion with little need for active control by the patient. The patient must be trained to deal with the stability problem independently of the mobility problem or at a great mechanical advantage to avoid compensation. The secondary mobility problem, once managed, should be reintroduced in a nonstressful manner so the previous compensatory pattern is not activated.

Manual articular and soft tissue techniques, when appropriate, can be used for the primary mobility problem, followed by movement to integrate any improved range and benefit from more appropriate tone. If the mobility limitation seems to be the result of weakness, make sure that the proximal structures have the requisite amount of stability before strengthening. Then proceed with strengthening or endurance activities with a focus on recruitment, relaxation, timing, coordination, and reproducibility. Note that the word *resistance* was not used initially. Resistance is not synonymous with strengthening and is only one of many techniques used to improve functional movement in early movement reeducation. However, the following sections on position and pattern will address resistance in greater detail. Use posture to mechanically block or restrict substitution of stronger segments and improve quality at the segment being exercised.

Posture for Recruitment and Facilitation

The clinician must facilitate or stimulate the correct motor program, coordination, and sequence of movement. Although verbal and visual feedback is helpful through demonstration and cueing, kinesthetic feedback is paramount to motor learning.[72] Correct body position or posture will improve feedback. Posture and movement that occur early in the developmental sequence require a less complex motor task and activate a more basic motor program. This will create positive feedback and reinforcement and mark the point (posture) at which appropriate and inappropriate actions and reactions meet. From this point, the clinician can manipulate frequency, intensity, and duration or advance to a more difficult posture in the appropriate sequence.

The clinician must also consider developmental biomechanics that divides the movement ability into two categories—internal forces and external forces. *Internal forces* include the center of gravity, base of support, and line of gravity. *External forces* include gravity, inertia of the body segment, and ground reaction. Considering these, the clinician should evaluate the patient's abilities in the same manner by first observing management of the mass of the body over the particular base provided by the posture. Then the clinician progresses the patient toward more external stresses such as inertia, gravity, and ground reaction forces. This interaction will require various degrees of acceleration production, deceleration control, anticipatory weight shifting, and increased proprioception. Resistance and movement can stress static and dynamic postures, but the clinician should also understand that resistance and movement could be used to refine movement and stimulate appropriate reactions.[72] Postures must be chosen to reduce compensation and allow the patient to exercise below the level at which the impairment hinders movement or control. This is easily accomplished by creating "self-limiting" exercises.[17] These exercises require passive or active "locking" by limiting movement of the area the patient will most likely use to substitute or "cheat" with during exercise.

To review, posture identifies the fundamental movements used in growth and development. These movements serve as steps toward skill that are also helpful in the presence of skill when quality is questionable. Figs. 10-2 through 10-5 illustrate a few examples of these types of movements.

By following this natural sequence of movement, the clinician can observe where a mobility or stability problem will first limit the quality of a whole movement pattern. A patient with a mild knee sprain or even a total knee replacement may demonstrate segmental rolling to one

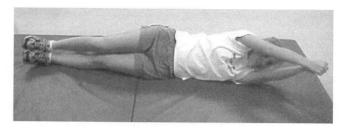

Figure 10-3. Rolling to prone.

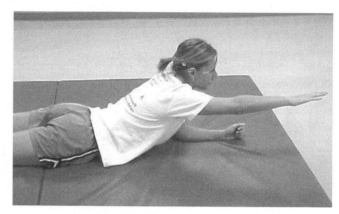

Figure 10-4. Prone on elbows with reaching.

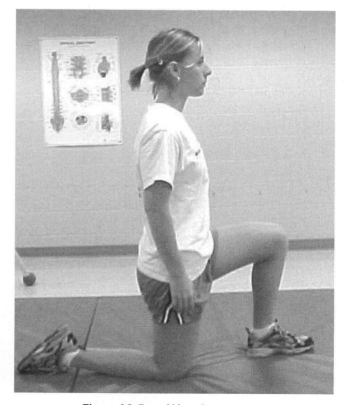

Figure 10-5. Half-kneeling position.

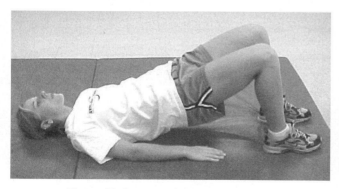

Figure 10-2. Supine bridging movement.

side but "log roll" to the other simply to avoid using a flexion adduction medial rotation movement pattern with the involved lower extremity. The clinician has now identified where success and failure meet in the developmental sequence. The knee problem creates a dynamic stability problem in the developmental sequence long before partial or full weight bearing is an issue. It therefore must be addressed at that level. The patient is provided with an example of how limited knee mobility can greatly affect movement patterns (such as rolling) that seem to require little of the knee. However, by restoring the bilateral segmental rolling function, many gait problems will be affected with measurable qualitative and quantitative observations. By use of a postural progression, the earliest level of functional limitation can be easily identified and incorporated into the exercise program. Limitations can also be placed on the posture and movement (the self-limiting concept) to limit postural compensation and focus.

CLINICAL PEARL #3

The clinician must define postural levels of success and failure to identify the postural level at which therapeutic exercise intervention should start. Otherwise, the clinician could potentially prescribe exercise at a postural level at which the patient creates significant amounts of inappropriate compensation and substitution during exercise.

Position

The word *position* describes not only the location of the anatomic structure (e.g., joint, muscle group, or ligament) at which impairment has been identified but also the positions (with respect to movement and load) at which the greatest and least limitations occur (Table 10-2). The limitations can be either reduced strength and control or restricted movement. The primary questions to ask for this principle appear in Box 10-7. Orthopedic manual assessment of joints and muscles in various functional positions will demonstrate the influence of the impairment and symptoms throughout the range of movement. The clinician will identify various deficits. Each will be qualified or quantified through assessment and objective testing and then addressed through the appropriate dosage and positioning for exercise.

Box 10-7

Primary Questions for Position

1. "*Where* is the impairment located?"
2. "*Where* among the structures (myofascial or articular) does the impairment have its greatest effect?"
3. "*Where* in the range of motion does the impairment affect position the greatest?"
4. "*Where* is the most beneficial position for the exercise?"

Purpose is the obvious reason for exercise intervention whereas posture describes the orientation of the body in space. Position refers to the specific mobilizing or stabilizing segment. For the "single-leg bridge" (Fig. 10-6), the hip is moving toward extension. If range of motion were broken down into thirds, this would only involve the extension third of movement. The flexion third and middle third of movement are not needed because no impairment was identified in those respective ranges. Not only was the hip in extension, but also the knee was in flexion. This is important because the hamstring muscle will try to assist hip extension in the end range of movement when gluteal strength is not optimal. However, the hamstrings cannot assist hip extension to any significant degree because of "active insufficiency." Likewise, the lumbar extensors cannot assist the extension pattern due to the passive stretch placed upon them via maximal passive hip flexion. The hip extension proprioception is now void of any inappropriate patterning or compensation from the hamstrings or spinal erectors through the positional use of active and passive insufficiency.[39]

Qualitative measures will provide specific information about exercise start position, finish position, movement speed and direction, open and closed chain considerations and the need for cueing and feedback. Close observation of osteokinematic and arthrokinematic relationships for movement and bilateral comparison is the obvious starting point. Specific identification of the structure and position represent mobility observed by selective tension (active, passive, and resisted movements), and endfeel of the joint structures would provide specific information about the mechanical nature of limitations and symptoms.[21] Assessment of positional static and dynamic control will describe stability limitations and provide a more specific starting point for exercise.

Quantitative measures will reveal a degree of deficit, which can be recorded in the form of a percentage through bilateral comparison and compared with normative data

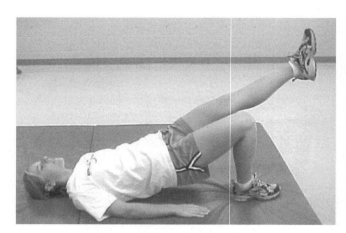

Figure 10-6. Single-leg bridge.

when possible. Range of motion, strength, endurance, and recovery time should be considered along with many other (quantitative) clinical parameters to describe isolated or positional function. This will provide clear communication and specific documentation for goals as well as a tracking device for treatment effectiveness, information that will help define the baseline for initial exercise considerations. As stated earlier, any limitation in mobility or stability will require a bilateral comparison as well as clearing of the joints above and below. The proximal and distal structures must also be compared with their contralateral counterparts. This central point of physical examination is often overlooked. Cyriax[21] noted, "Positive signs must always be balanced by corroborative negative signs. If a lesion appears to lie at or near one joint, this region must be examined for signs identifying its site. It is equally essential for the adjacent joints and the structures around them to be examined so that, by contrast, their normality can be established. These negative findings then reinforce the positive findings emanating elsewhere; then only can the diagnosis be regarded and established."

After position and movement options have been established, a trial exercise session should be used to observe and quantify performance before exercise prescription. Variables including intensity and duration can be used to establish strength or endurance baselines. Bilateral comparison should be used to document a performance deficit, which is also recorded as a percentage. A maximum repetition test (with or without resistance) to fatigue, onset of symptoms, or loss of exercise quality is a common example. This will allow close tracking of home exercise compliance and help establish a rate of improvement. If all other factors are addressed, the rate of improvement should be quite large. This is the benefit of correct dosage for prescription of exercise position and appropriate workload. Most of the significant improvement is not due to training volume, tissue metabolism, or muscle hypertrophy but to the efficient adaptive response of *neural factors.*[2] These factors can include motor recruitment efficiency, improved timing, increased proprioceptive awareness, improved agonist/antagonist coordination, appropriate phasic and tonic response to activity, task familiarity, and motor learning as well as to psychologic factors. Usually greater deficits are associated with more drastic improvement. Treatments should be geared to stimulate these changes whenever possible.

Pattern

The primary questions to ask for this pattern principle appear in Box 10-8. The word *pattern* will serve as a cue to the clinician to continually consider the functional movements of the human body occurring in unified patterns that occupy three-dimensional space and cross three planes (frontal, sagittal, and transverse)[17] (see Table 10-2). Sometimes this is not easily ascertained by observing the

---

Box 10-8

Primary Questions for Pattern

1. "*How* is the movement pattern different upon bilateral comparison?"
2. "*How* can synergistic movement, coordination, recruitment, and timing be facilitated?"
3. "*How* will this affect the movement limitation?"
4. "*How* will this affect function?"

---

design and usage of fixed axis exercise equipment and the movement patterns suggested in some rehabilitation protocols. The basic patterns of proprioceptive neuromuscular facilitation (PNF), for both the extremities and the spine, are excellent examples of how the brain groups movement. Muscles of the trunk and extremities are recruited in the most advantageous sequence (proprioception) to create movement (mobility) or control (stability) movement. Not only does this provide efficient and economical function but also it effectively protects the respective joints and muscles from undue stress and strain. Voss and associates[77] clearly and eloquently state this: "The mass movement patterns of facilitation are spiral and diagonal in character and closely resemble the movements used in sports and work activities. The spiral and diagonal character is in keeping with the spiral rotatory characteristics of the skeletal system of bones and joints and the ligamentous structures. This type of motion is also in harmony with the topographical alignment of the muscles from origin to insertion and with the structural characteristics of the individual muscles." When a structure within the sequence is limited by impairment, the entire pattern is limited in some way. The clinician should document the limited pattern as well as the isolated segment causing the pattern to be limited. The isolated segment is usually identified in the evaluation process and outlined in the "position" considerations. The resultant effect on one or more movement patterns must also be investigated. A review of the basic PNF patterns can be beneficial to the rehabilitation specialist. Once a structure is evaluated, look at the basic PNF patterns involving that structure. Multiple patterns can be limited in some way, but usually one pattern in particular will demonstrate significantly reduced function. Obviously, poor function in a muscle group or joint can limit the strength, endurance, and range of motion of an entire PNF pattern to some degree. However, the clinician must not simply view reduced PNF pattern function as an output problem. It should be equally viewed as an input problem. When muscle and joint functions are not optimal, mechanoreceptor and muscle spindle functions are not optimal. This can create an input or proprioceptive problem and greatly distort joint position and muscle tension information, which distorts initial information (before movement is initiated) as well as feedback (once movement is in progress). Therefore, the clinician cannot only consider functional output. Altered proprioception, if not properly identified and outlined, can unintentionally become part of the recommended exercises and therefore be reinforced. The clinician must focus on synergistic and integrated function at all levels of rehabilitation. The orthopedic outpatient cannot afford to have a problem simply isolated three times a week for 30 minutes only to reintegrate the same problem at a subconscious level during necessary daily activities throughout the remaining week. PNF style movement pattern exercise can often be taught as easily as an isolated movement and will produce a significantly greater benefit. Therapeutic exercise is no longer limited by sets as repetitions of the same activity. Successive intervals of increasing difficulty (although not physically stressful) building on the accomplishment of an earlier task will reinforce one level of function and continually be a challenge for the next. A simple movement set focused on isolation of a problem can be quickly followed by a pattern that will improve integration. The integration can be followed by a familiar fundamental movement or functional activity that may reduce the amount of conscious and deliberate movement and give the clinician a chance to observe subcortical control of mobility and stability as well as appropriate use of phasic and tonic responses.

CLINICAL PEARL #4

By continuously considering the pattern options as well as pattern limitations, the clinician will be able to refine the exercise prescription and reduce unnecessary supplemental movements that could easily be incorporated into pattern-based exercise.

Direction, speed, and amount of resistance (or assistance) will be used to produce more refined patterns. Manual resistance, weighted cable or elastic resistance, weight-shifting activities, and even proprioceptive taping can improve recruitment and facilitate coordination. The clinician should refrain from initially discussing specific structural control such as "pelvic tilting" or "scapular retraction." Instead, the clinician should use posture and position to set the initial movement and design proprioceptive feedback to produce a more normal pattern whenever possible.

REESTABLISHING PROPRIOCEPTION AND NEUROMUSCULAR CONTROL

Although the concept and value of proprioceptive mechanoreceptors have been documented in the literature, treatment techniques focused on improving their function generally have not been incorporated into the overall rehabilitation program. The neurosensory function

of the capsuloligamentous structures has taken a back seat to the mechanical structural role. This is mainly due to the lack of information about how mechanoreceptors contribute to the specific functional activities and how they can be specifically activated.[26,28]

Effects of Injury on the Proprioceptive System

After injury to the capsuloligamentous structures, it is thought that a partial deafferentation of the joint occurs as the mechanoreceptors become disrupted. This partial deafferentation may be due to either direct or indirect injury. Direct trauma effects would include disruption of the joint capsule or ligaments, whereas post-traumatic joint effusion or hemarthrosis[40] illustrate indirect effects.

Whether from a direct or indirect cause, the resultant partial deafferentation alters the afferent information into the CNS and therefore the resulting reflex pathways to the dynamic stabilizing structures. These pathways are required by both the feedforward and feedback motor control systems to dynamically stabilize the joint. A disruption in the proprioceptive pathway will result in an alteration of position and kinesthesia.[6,59] Barrett[7] showed an increase in the threshold to detection of passive motion in a majority of patients with anterior cruciate ligament (ACL) rupture and functional instability. Corrigan and co-workers,[19] who also found diminished proprioception after ACL rupture, confirmed this finding. Diminished proprioceptive sensitivity has also been shown to cause giving way of or episodes of instability in the ACL-deficient knee.[12] Therefore, injury to the capsuloligamentous structures not only reduces the mechanical stability of the joint but also diminishes the capability of the dynamic neuromuscular restraint system. Therefore, any aberration in joint motion and position sense will affect both the feedforward and feedback neuromuscular control systems. Without adequate anticipatory muscle activity, the static structures may be exposed to insult unless the reactive muscle activity can be initiated to contribute to dynamic restraint.

Restoration of Proprioception and Prevention of Reinjury

Although it has been demonstrated that a proprioceptive deficit occurs after knee injury, both kinesthetic awareness and reposition sense can be at least partially restored with surgery and rehabilitation. A number of studies have examined proprioception after ACL reconstruction. Barrett[7] measured proprioception after autogenous graft repair and found that the proprioception was better than that of the average patient with an ACL deficiency but still significantly worse than the proprioception in the normal knee. He further noted that patients' satisfaction was more closely correlated with their proprioception than with their clinical score.[7] Harter and associates[35] could not demonstrate a significant difference in the reproduction of passive positioning between the operative and nonoperative knee at an average of 3 years after ACL reconstruction. Kinesthesia has been reported to be restored after surgery as detected by the threshold to the detection of passive motion in the midrange of motion.[6] A longer threshold to the detection of passive motion was observed in the knee with a reconstructed ACL compared with the contralateral uninvolved knee when tested at the end range of motion.[6] Lephart and colleagues[44] found similar results in patients after either arthroscopically assisted patellar-tendon autograft or allograft ACL reconstruction. The importance of incorporating a proprioceptive element in any comprehensive rehabilitation program is justified based upon the results of these studies.

Methods to improve proprioception after injury or surgery could improve function and decrease the risk for reinjury. Ihara and Nakayama[37] demonstrated a reduction in the neuromuscular lag time with dynamic joint control after a 3-week training period on an unstable board. The maintenance of equilibrium and improvement in reaction to sudden perturbations on the unstable board improved the neuromuscular coordination. This phenomenon was first reported by Freeman and Wyke first in 1967[23] when they reported that proprioceptive deficits could be reduced with training on an unstable surface. They found that proprioceptive training through stabilometry, or training on an unstable surface, significantly reduced the episodes of giving way after ankle sprains. Tropp and associates[66] confirmed the work of Freeman and Wyke by demonstrating that the results of stabilometry could be improved with coordination training on an unstable board.

Relationship of Proprioception to Function

Barrett[7] demonstrated the relationship between proprioception and function. His study suggested that limb function relied more on proprioceptive input than on strength during activity. Blackburn and Voight[11] also found a high correlation between diminished kinesthesia with the single-leg hop test.[11] The single-leg hop test was chosen for its integrative measure of neuromuscular control because a high degree of proprioceptive sensibility and functional ability is required to successfully propel the body forward and land safely on the limb. Giove and co-workers[27] reported a higher success rate in returning athletes to competitive sports through adequate hamstring rehabilitation. Tibone and associates[63] and Ihara and Nakayama[37] found that simple hamstring strengthening alone was not adequate; it was necessary to obtain voluntary or reflex-level control on knee instability for return to functional activities. Walla and associates[78] found that 95% of patients were able to successfully avoid surgery after ACL injury when they were able to achieve "reflex-level" hamstring control. Ihara and Nakayama[37] found that the reflex arc between stressing the ACL and hamstring contraction

could be shortened with training. With the use of unstable boards, the researchers were able to successfully decrease the reaction time. Because afferent input is altered after joint injury, proprioceptive sensitivity to retrain these altered afferent pathways is critical for shortening of the time lag of muscular reaction to counteract the excessive strain on the passive structures and guard against injury.

Restoration of Efficient Motor Control

How do we modify afferent/efferent characteristics? The mechanoreceptors in and around the respective joints offer information about the change of position, motion, and loading of the joint to the CNS, which in turn stimulates the muscles around the joint to function.[37] If a time lag exists in the neuromuscular reaction, injury may occur. The shorter the time lag, the less stress to the ligaments and other soft tissue structures around the joint. Therefore, the foundation of neuromuscular control is to facilitate the integration of peripheral sensations relative to joint position and then process this information into an effective efferent motor response. The main objective of the rehabilitation program for neuromuscular control is to develop or reestablish the afferent and efferent characteristics around the joint that are essential for dynamic restraint.[43]

There are several different afferent and efferent characteristics that contribute to the efficient regulation of motor control. As discussed earlier, these characteristics include the sensitivity of the mechanoreceptors and facilitation of the afferent neural pathways, enhancement of muscle stiffness, and the production of reflex muscle activation. The specific rehabilitation techniques must also take into consideration the levels of CNS integration. For the rehabilitation program to be complete, each of the three levels must be addressed to produce dynamic stability. The plasticity of the neuromuscular system permits rapid adaptations during the rehabilitation program that enhance preparatory and reactive activity.[8,36,37,43,44,82]

CLINICAL PEARL #5

Specific rehabilitation techniques that produce adaptations to enhance the efficiency of neuromuscular techniques include balance training, biofeedback training, reflex facilitation through reactive training, and eccentric and high-repetition/low-load exercises.[43]

THE THREE-PHASE REHABILITATION MODEL

The following is a three-phase model designed to progressively retrain the neuromuscular system for complex functions of sport and ADL (Box 10-9). The model phases are successively more demanding and provide sequential training toward the objective of reestablishment of neuromuscular control. This three-phase model has also been

Box 10-9

Three-Phase Rehabilitation Model

Phase	Description	Objective
1	Restore static stability through proprioception and kinesthesia	Restoration of proprioception
2	Restore dynamic stability	Encourage preparatory agonist-antagonist co-contraction
3	Restore reactive neuromuscular control	Initiate reflex muscular stabilization

described as *reactive neuromuscular training*. Ideally, the phases should be followed in order and should use the four rehabilitation considerations mentioned earlier (the four P's) at each phase. Application of the four P's at each phase is crucial to place successive demands on the athlete during rehabilitation.

Phase One: Restore Static Stability Through Proprioception and Kinesthesia

Functional neuromuscular rehabilitation activities are designed to restore both functional stability about the joint and enhance motor control skills. The RNT program is centered on stimulation of both the peripheral and central reflex pathways to the skeletal muscles. The first objective that should be addressed in the RNT program is the restoration of proprioception. Reliable kinesthetic and proprioceptive information provides the foundation on which dynamic stability and motor control is based. It has already been established that altered afferent information into the CNS can alter the feedforward and feedback motor control systems. Therefore, the first objective of the RNT program is to restore the neurosensory properties of the damaged structures while at the same time enhancing the sensitivity of the secondary peripheral afferents.[44]

To facilitate appropriate kinesthetic and proprioceptive information into the CNS, joint reposition exercises should be used to provide maximal stimulation of the peripheral mechanoreceptors. The use of closed kinetic chain activities creates axial loads that maximally stimulate the articular mechanoreceptors via the increase in compressive forces.[16,30] The use of closed chain exercises not only enhances joint congruency and neurosensory feedback, but also minimizes the shearing stresses about the joint.[70] At the same time, the muscle receptors are facilitated by both the change in length and tension.[16,30] The objective is to induce unanticipated perturbations, thereby stimulating reflex stabilization. The persistent use of these pathways will decease the response time when an unanticipated joint load is present.[47] In addition to weight-bearing exercises, active and passive joint repositioning exercises can be utilized to enhance the conscious appreciation of proprioception. Rhythmic stabilization exercises can be included early in the RNT program to enhance neuromuscular coordina-

tion in response to unexpected joint translation. The intensity of the exercises can be manipulated by increasing either the weight loaded across the joint or the size of the perturbation (Tables 10-4 and 10-5). The addition of a compressive sleeve, wrap, or taping about the joint can also provide additional proprioceptive information by stimulating the cutaneous mechanoreceptors.[7,43,45,48] Figs. 10-7 through 10-10 provide examples of exercises that can be begun in this phase.

Phase Two: Restore Dynamic Stability

The second objective of the RNT program is to encourage preparatory agonist-antagonist co-contraction. Efficient co-activation of the musculature restores the normal force couples that are necessary to balance joint forces and increase joint congruency, thereby reducing the loads imparted onto the static structures.[43] The cornerstone of rehabilitation during this phase is postural stability training. Environmental conditions are manipulated to produce a sensory response (Box 10-10). The use of unstable surfaces allows the clinician to utilize positions of compromise to produce maximal afferent input into the spinal cord, thereby producing a reflex response. Dynamic co-activation of the muscles about the joint to produce a stabilizing force requires both the feedforward and feedback motor control systems. To facilitate these pathways, the joint must be placed into positions of compromise for the patient to develop reactive stabilizing strategies. Although it was once believed that the speed of the stretch reflexes could not be directly enhanced, efforts to do so have been successful in human and animal studies. This has significant implications for reestablishing the reactive capability of the dynamic restraint system. Reducing the electromechanical delay between joint loading and the protective muscle activation can increase dynamic stability. In the controlled clinical environment, positions of vulnerability can be used safely (Tables 10-4 and 10-5). Figs. 10-11 and 10-12 provide examples of exercises that can be implemented in this phase.

Proprioceptive training for functionally unstable joints has been documented in the literature after injury.[37,57,65,66] Tropp and associates[66] and Wester and colleagues[79]

Table 10-4

Upper Extremity Neuromuscular Exercises

Phase I: Proprioception and Kinesthesia Phase	Phase II: Dynamic Stabilization Phase	Phase III: Reactive Neuromuscular Control Phase
Goals	**Goals**	**Goals**
Normalize motion	Enhance dynamic functional stability	Improve reactive neuromuscular abilities
Restore proprioception and kinesthesia	Reestablish neuromuscular control	Enhance dynamic stability
Establish muscular balance	Restore muscular balance	Improve power and endurance
Diminish pain and inflammation	Maintain normalized motion	Gradual return to activities/throwing
Stability Exercises	**Stability Exercises**	**Stability Exercises**
Joint repositioning	PNF D2 Flex/Ext	PNF D2 Flex/Ext
Movement awareness	Supine	RS with T-band
RS	Side-lying	Perturbation RS
RI	Seated	Perturbation RS—eyes closed
SRH	Standing	90/90°
PNF D2 Flex/Ext	PNF D2 Flex/Ext at end range	ER at end range RS
PNF D2 Flex/Ext RS, SRH, RI	90/90° ER at end range	ER conc/ecc
Side-lying RS, SRH, RI	Scapular strengthening	ER conc/ecc RS
Weight bearing (axial compression)	Scapular PNF—RS, SRH	ER/IR conc/ecc
Weight-bearing RS, RI	ER/IR at 90° abduction—eyes closed	ER/IR conc/ecc RS
Standing-leaning on hands	PNF D2 Flex/Ext.—eyes closed	Eyes closed
Quadruped position	Balance beam	Standing on one leg
Tripod position	PNF D2 Flex/Ext—balance beam	Reactive plyoballs
Biped position	Slide board—side to side	Push ups on unstable surface
Axial compression with ball on wall	Slide board push-ups	UE plyometrics
OTIS	Axial compression—side to side	Two-handed overhead throw
	Axial compression—unstable surfaces	Side-to-side overhead throw
	Plyometrics—two hand (light and easy)	One-hand baseball throw
	Two-hand chest throw	Endurance
	Two-hand underhand throw	Wall dribble
		Wall baseball throw
		Axial compression circles
		Axial compression—side/side
		Sports-specific
		Underweighted throwing
		Overweighted throwing
		Oscillating devices
		BOING
		Body Blade

PNF, proprioceptive neuromuscular facilitation; Flex, flexion; Ext, extension; RS, rhythmic stabilization; RI, reciprocal isometrics; SRH, slow reversal hold; ER, external rotation; IR, internal rotation; conc, concentric; ecc, eccentric; UE, upper extremity; OTIS, oscillating techniques for isometric stabilization.

reported that ankle disk training significantly reduced the incidence of ankle sprain. Concerning the mechanism of effects, Tropp and associates[66] suggested that unstable surface training reduced the proprioceptive deficit. Sheth and co-workers[57] demonstrated changes with healthy adults in the patterns of contractions on the inversion and eversion musculature before and after training on an unstable surface. They concluded that the changes would be supported by the concept of reciprocal Ia inhibition via the mechanoreceptors in the muscles. Konradsen and

Ravin[41] also suggested from their work that the afferent input from the calf musculature was responsible for dynamic protection against sudden ankle inversion stress. Pinstaar and associates[50] reported that postural sway was restored after 8 weeks of ankle disk training when performed three to five times a week. Tropp and Odenrick also showed that postural control improved after 6 weeks of training when performed 15 minutes per day.[67] Bernier and Perrin,[10] whose program consisted of balance exercises progressing from simple to complex sessions (3 times

Table 10-5

Lower Extremity Neuromuscular Exercises

Phase I: Proprioception and Kinesthesia Phase	Phase II: Dynamic Stabilization Phase	Phase III: Reactive Neuromuscular Control Phase
Goals	**Goals**	**Goals**
Normalize motion	Enhance dynamic functional stability	Improve reactive neuromuscular abilities
Restore proprioception and kinesthesia	Reestablish neuromuscular control	Enhance dynamic stability
Establish muscular balance	Restore muscular balance	Improve power and endurance
Diminish pain and inflammation	Maintain normalized motion	Gradual return to activities, running, jumping, cutting
Develop static control and posture		
Stability Exercises	**Stability Exercises**	**Stability Exercises**
Bilateral to unilateral	Oscillating techniques for isometric stabilization (OTIS)	Squats
Eyes open to eyes closed	AWS	Assisted
	PWS	AWS
Stable to unstable surfaces	MWS	PWS
Level surfaces	LWS	MWS
Foam pad	Chops/lifts	LWS
Controlled to uncontrolled	ITIS	
PNF	PACE	Chops/lifts
Rhythmic stabilization	PNF	Lunges (front and lateral)
Rhythmic isometrics	Rhythmic stabilization	AWS
Slow reversal hold	Rhythmic isometrics	PWS
	Slow reversal hold	MWS
	Stable to unstable surface	LWS
	Rocker board	Stationary walking with unidirectional
	Wobble board	WS
	BAPS	Stationary running
	Balance beam	PWS
	Foam rollers	MWS
	Dyna-disc	LWS
		AWS
		Mountain climber
		CKC side-to-side
		Fitter
		Slide board
		Plyometrics
		Jumps in place
		Standing jumps
		Bounding
		Multiple hops and bounds
		Hops with rotation
		Bounds with rotation
		Resisted lateral bounds
		Box jumps
		Depth jumps
		Multidirectional training
		Lunges
		Rock wall
		Clock drill
		Step-to's
		Four-square
		Agility training

AWS, anterior weight shift; PWS, posterior weight shift; MWS, medial weight shift; LWS, lateral weight shift; PNF, proprioceptive neuromuscular facilitation; ITIS, impulse techniques for isometric stabilization; PACE, Partial Arc Controlled Exercise; WS, weight shift; BAPS, biomechanical ankle platform system; CKC, closed chain kinetic.

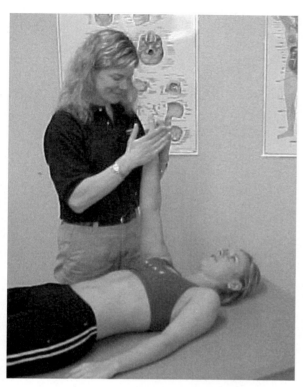

Figure 10-7. Rhythmic stabilization.

a week for 10 minutes) also found that postural sway was improved after 6 weeks of training. Although there were some differences in each of these training programs, the postural control improved after 6 to 8 weeks of proprioceptive training for subjects with functional instability of the ankle.

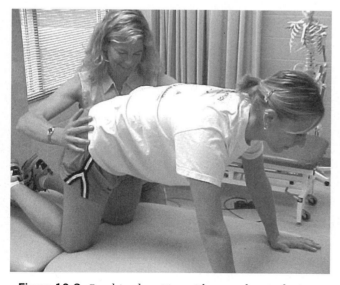

Figure 10-8. Quadriped position with manual perturbations.

Phase Three: Restore Reactive Neuromuscular Control

Dynamic reactive neuromuscular control activities should be initiated into the overall rehabilitation program after adequate healing and dynamic stability has been achieved. The key objective is to initiate reflex muscular stabilization.

The progression to these activities is predicated on the athlete satisfactorily completing the activities that are considered prerequisites for the activity being considered. With this in mind, the progression of activities must be goal oriented and specific to the tasks that will be expected of the athlete.

The general progression for activities to develop dynamic reactive neuromuscular control is from slow-speed to fast-speed activities, from low-force to high-force activities, and from controlled to uncontrolled activities. Initially these exercises should evoke a balance reaction or weight shift in the lower extremities and ultimately progress to a movement pattern. A sudden alteration in joint position either by the clinician or self-induced by the athlete may decrease the response time and serve to develop reactive strategies to unexpected events. These reactions can be as simple as a static control with little or no visible movement or a complex as a dynamic plyometric response requiring explosive acceleration, deceleration, or change in direction. The exercises will allow the clinician to challenge the patient using visual and/or proprioceptive input via tubing (oscillating techniques for isometric stabilization) and other devices (e.g., medicine balls, foam rolls, or visual obstacles). Although these exercises will improve physiologic parameters, they are specifically designed to facilitate neuromuscular reactions. Therefore, the clinician must be concerned with the kinesthetic input and quality of the movement patterns rather than the particular number of sets and repetitions. When fatigue occurs, motor control becomes poor and all training effects are lost. Therefore, during the exercise progression, all aspects of normal function should be observed. These include isometric, concentric, and eccentric muscle control; articular loading and unloading; balance control during weight shifting and direction changes; controlled acceleration and deceleration; and demonstration of both conscious and unconscious control (Tables 10-4 and 10-5). Figs. 10-13 through 10-15 are examples of exercises that can be implemented in this phase.

When dynamic stability and reflex stabilization have been achieved, the focus of the neuromuscular rehabilitation program is to restore ADL and sport-specific skills. Make sure that the exercise program is specific to the patient's needs. The most important factor to consider during the rehabilitation of patients is that they should be performing functional activities that simulate their ADL requirements. This rule applies not only to the specific joints involved, but also the speed and amplitude of movement required in ADL. Exercise and training drills should

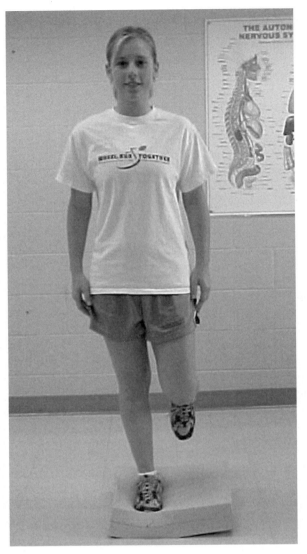

Figure 10-9. Single-limb balance on unstable (foam) base.

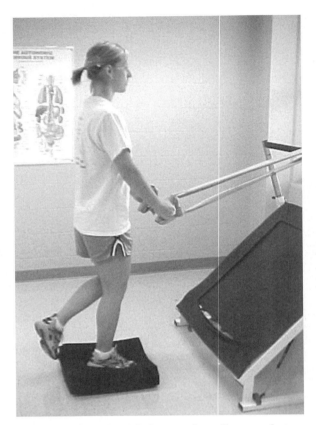

Figure 10-10. Single-limb balance with oscillating techniques for isometric stabilization (OTIS).

be incorporated into the program that will refine the physiologic parameters that are required for the return to preinjury levels of function. The progression should be from straight plane to multiplane movement patterns. ADL movement does not occur along a single joint or plane of movement. Therefore, exercise for the kinetic

chain must involve all three planes simultaneously. Emphasis in the RNT program must be placed upon a progression from simple to complex neuromotor patterns that are specific to the demands placed upon the patient during function. The function progression breaks an activity down into its component parts so that they can be performed in a sequence that allows for the acquisition or reacquisition of the activity. Basic conditioning and skill acquisition must be acquired before advanced conditioning and skill acquisition. The training program should begin with simple activities, such as walking/running, and then progress to highly complex motor skills requiring refined neuromuscular mechanisms including proprioceptive and kinesthetic awareness that provides reflex joint stabilization. Make sure to include a significant amount of "controlled chaos" in the program. Unexpected activities with ADL are by nature unstable. The more patients rehearse in this type of environment, the better they will react under unrehearsed conditions. The final and most important consideration of this phase is to make the rehabilitation program fun. The first three letters of functional are *FUN*. If the program is not fun, then compliance will suffer and so will the results.

Box 10-10

Balance Variables That Can Be Manipulated in the Dynamic Stability Phase to Produce a Sensory Response

- Bilateral to unilateral stance
- Eyes open to eyes closed
- Stable to unstable surfaces

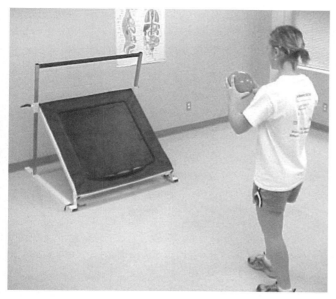

Figure 10-11. Plyoback, two-handed upper extremity chest pass.

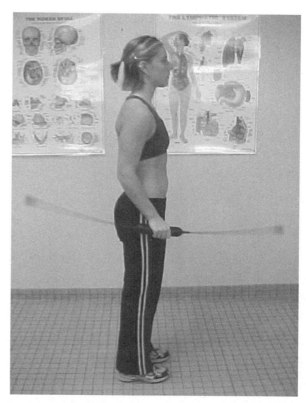

Figure 10-13. Dynamic training; Body Blade low position.

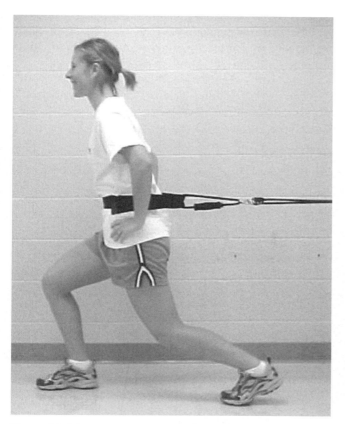

Figure 10-12. Lunging movement, forward with sport cord resistance.

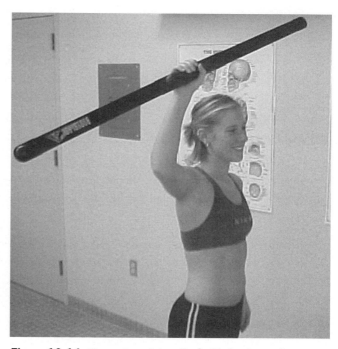

Figure 10-14. Dynamic training; Body Blade elevated position.

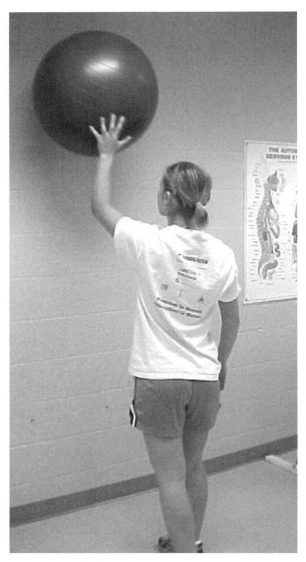

Figure 10-15. Elevated wall dribble.

SUMMARY

■ There has been increased attention devoted to the development of balance, proprioception, and neuromuscular control in the rehabilitation and reconditioning of athletes after injury.

■ It is believed that injury results in altered somatosensory input that influences neuromuscular control.

■ If static and dynamic balance and neuromuscular control are not re-established after injury, then the patient will be susceptible to recurrent injury and his or her performance may decline.

■ The three-phase model for reactive neuromuscular training may be an excellent method to assist athletes in regaining optimal neuromuscular performance and high-level function after injury or surgery.

■ The three-phase model consists of restoring static stability through proprioception and kinesthesia, dynamic stability, and reactive neuromuscular control.

■ Current information has been synthesized to produce a new perspective for therapeutic exercise decisions. This new perspective was specifically designed to improve treatment efficiency and effectiveness and have a focus on function.

■ The four principles of purpose, posture, position, and pattern assist problem solving by providing a framework that categorizes clinical information in a hierarchy.

■ The four principles serve as quick reminders of the hierarchy, interaction, and application for each therapeutic exercise prescription principle. The questions of what, when, where, and how for functional movement assessment and exercise prescription are answered in the appropriate order.

■ Functional evaluation and assessment = *purpose*.

■ Identification of motor control = *posture*.

■ Identification of osteokinematic and arthrokinematic limitations = *position*.

■ Integration of synergistic movement patterns = *pattern*.

■ The clinician should always ask: Does the program make sense? If it does not make sense, then it is probably not functional and therefore not optimally effective.

■ Clinical wisdom is the result of experience and *applied knowledge*. Intense familiarity and practical observation improve *application*. To be of benefit, available *knowledge* must be organized and tempered by an objective and inclusive framework. Hopefully this framework will provide a starting point to better organize and apply each clinician's knowledge and experience of functional exercise prescription.

REFERENCES

1. American College of Sports Medicine. (1997): Exercise Management for Persons with Chronic Diseases and Disabilities. Champaign, IL, Human Kinetics.
2. Baechle, T.R. (1994): Essentials of Strength Training and Conditioning. Champaign, IL, Human Kinetics.
3. Barnett, M., Ross, D., Schmidt, R., and Todd, B. (1973): Motor skills learning and the specificity of training principle. Res. Q., 44:440-447.
4. Barrack, R.L., Lund, P.J., and Skinner, H.B. (1994): Knee joint proprioception revisited. J. Sport. Rehab., 3:18-42.
5. Barrack, R.L., and Skinner, H.B. (1990). The sensory function of knee ligaments. *In:* Daniel, D., et al. (eds.), Knee Ligaments: Structure, Function, Injury, and Repair. New York, Raven Press.
6. Barrack, R.L., Skinner, H.B., and Buckley, S.L. (1989): Proprioception in the anterior cruciate deficient knee. Am. J. Sports Med., 17:1-6.
7. Barrett, D.S. (1991): Proprioception and function after anterior cruciate reconstruction. J. Bone Joint Surg., 3B:833-837.
8. Beard, D.J., Dodd, C.F., Trundle, H.R., et al. (1993): Proprioception after rupture of the ACL: An objective indication of the need for surgery? J. Bone Joint Surg., 75B:311.

9. Belen'kii, V.Y., Gurfinkle, V.S., and Pal'tsev, Y.I. (1967): Elements of control of voluntary movements. Biofizika, 12:135-141.

10. Bernier, J.N., and Perrin, D.H. (1998): Effect of coordination training on proprioception of the functionally unstable ankle. J. Orthop. Sports Phys. Ther., 27:264-275.

11. Blackburn, T.A., and Voight, M.L. (1995): Single leg stance: Development of a reliable testing procedure. In: Proceedings of the 12th International Congress of the World Confederation for Physical Therapy, Washington, DC.

12. Borsa, P.A., Lephart, S.M., Irrgang, J.J., et al. (1997): The effects of joint position and direction of joint motion on proprioceptive sensibility in anterior cruciate ligament deficient athletes. Am. J. Sports Med., 25:336-340.

13. Borsa, P.A., Lephart, S.M., Kocher, M.S., and Lephart, S.P. (1994): Functional assessment and rehabilitation of shoulder proprioception for glenohumeral instability. J. Sports Rehab., 3:84-104.

14. Ciccotti, M.R., Kerlan, R., Perry, J., and Pink, M. (1994): An electromyographic analysis of the knee during functional activities: I. The normal profile. Am. J. Sports Med., 22:645-650.

15. Clark, F.J., and Burgess, P.R. (1975): Slowly adapting receptors in cat knee joint: Can they signal joint angle? J. Neurophysiol. 38:1448-1463.

16. Clark, F.J., Burgess, R.C., Chapin, J.W., and Lipscomb, W.T. (1985): Role of intramuscular receptors in the awareness of limb position. J. Neurophysiol. 54:1529-1540.

17. Cook, G. (1997): The Four P's (Exercise Prescription): Functional Exercise Training Course Manual. Greeley, CO, North American Sports Medicine Institute, Advances in Clinical Education, Nashville, T.N.

18. Cook, G., and Fields, K. (1997): Functional Training for the Torso. National Strength and Conditioning Association, pp. 14-19. Colorado Springs, CO

19. Corrigan, J.P., Cashman, W.F., and Brady, M.P. (1992): Proprioception in the cruciate deficient knee. J. Bone Joint Surg., 74B: 247-250.

20. Cross, M.J., and McCloskey, D.I. (1973): Position sense following surgical removal of joints in man. Brain Res., 55:443-445.

21. Cyriax, J. (1982): Textbook of Orthopedic Medicine, Vol. I, Diagnosis of Soft Tissue Lesions, 8th ed. London, Bailliere Tindall.

22. Dunn, T.G., Gillig, S.E., Ponser, E.S., and Weil, N. (1986): The learning process in biofeedback: Is it feed-forward or feedback? Biofeedback Self Regul., 11:143-155.

23. Freeman, M.A.R., and Wyke, B., (1966): Articular contributions to limb reflexes. Br. J. Surg., 53:61-69.

24. Freeman, M.A.R., and Wyke, B. (1967): Articular reflexes of the ankle joint. An electromyographic study of normal and abnormal influences of ankle-joint mechanoreceptors upon reflex activity in leg muscles. Br. J. Surg., 54:990-1001.

25. Functional Movement Service Manual. (1998): Danville, VA, Athletic Testing Services.

26. Gandevia, S.C., and McCloskey, D.I. (1976): Joint sense, muscle sense and their contribution as position sense, measured at the distal interphalangeal joint of the middle finger. J. Physiol., 260:387-407.

27. Giove, T.P., Miller, S.J., Kent, B.E., et al. (1983): Non-operative treatment of the torn anterior cruciate ligament. J. Bone Joint Surg,. 65A:184-192.

28. Glenncross, D., and Thornton, E. (1981): Position sense following joint injury. Am. J. Sports Med., 21:23-27.

29. Grigg, P. (1976): Response of joint afferent neurons in cat medial articular nerve to active and passive movements of the knee. Brain Res., 118:482-485.

30. Grigg, P. (1994): Peripheral neural mechanisms in proprioception. J. Sport Rehab. 3:1-17.

31. Grigg, P., Finerman, G.A., and Riley, L.H. (1973): Joint position sense after total hip replacement. J. Bone Joint Surg., 55:1016-1025.

32. Grigg, P., and Hoffman, A.H. (1984): Ruffini mechanoreceptors in isolated joint capsule. Reflexes correlated with strain energy density. Somatosensory Res., 2:149-162.

33. Grigg, P., and Hoffman, A.H. (1982): Properties of Ruffini afferents revealed by stress analysis of isolated sections of cat knee capsule. J. Neurophysiol., 47:41-54.

34. Guyton, A.C. (1991): Textbook of Medical Physiology, 6th ed. Philadelphia: W.B. Saunders.

35. Harter, R.A., Osternig, L.R., Singer, S.L., et al. (1988): Long-term evaluation of knee stability and function following surgical reconstruction for anterior cruciate ligament insufficiency. Am. J. Sports Med., 16:434-442.

36. Hodgson, J.A., Roy, R.R., DeLeon, R., et al. (1994): Can the mammalian lumbar spinal cord learn a motor task? Med. Sci. Sports. Exerc., 26:1491-1497.

37. Ihara, H., and Nakayama, A. (1986): Dynamic joint control training for knee ligament injuries. Am. J. Sports Med., 14:309-315.

38. Janda, V. (1987): Muscles and motor control in low back pain: Assessment and management. In: Twomey, L. (ed.), Physical Therapy of the Low Back. New York, Churchill-Livingston, pp. 253-278.

39. Kendall, F.P., McCreary, K.E., and Provance, P.G. (1993): Muscle Testing and Function, 4th ed. Baltimore, Williams & Wilkins.

40. Kennedy, J.C., Alexander, I.J., and Hayes, K.C. (1982): Nerve supply to the human knee and its functional importance. Am. J. Sports Med., 10:329-335.

41. Konradsen, L., and Ravin, J.B. (1991): Prolonged peroneal reaction time in ankle instability. Int. J Sports Med., 12:290-292.

42. Lee, W.A. (1980): Anticipatory control of postural and task muscles during rapid arm flexion. J. Motor Behav., 12:185-196.

43. Lephart, S. (1994): Reestablishing proprioception, kinesthesia, joint position sense and neuromuscular control in rehab. In: Prentice, W.E. (ed.), Rehabilitation Techniques in Sports Medicine, 2nd ed. St. Louis, Mosby.

44. Lephart, S.M., Pincivero, D.M., Giraldo, J.L., and Fu, F. (1997): The role of proprioception in the management and rehabilitation of athletic injuries. Am. J. Sports Med., 25:130-137.

45. Matsusaka, N., Yokoyama, S., Tsurusaki, T., et al. (2001): Effect of ankle disk training combined with tactile stimulation to the leg and foot in functional instability of the ankle. Am. J. Sport Med., 29:25-30.

46. McNair, P.J., and Marshall, R.N. (1994): Landing characteristics in subjects with normal and anterior cruciate ligament deficient knee joints. Arch. Phys. Med., 75:584-589.

47. Ognibene, J., McMahon, K., Harris, M., et al. (2000): Effects of unilateral proprioceptive perturbation training on postural sway and joint reaction times of healthy subjects. In: Proceedings of the National Athletic Training Association Annual Meeting. Champaign, IL, Human Kinetics.

48. Perlau, R.C., Frank, C., and Fick, G. (1995): The effects of elastic bandages on human knee proprioception in the uninjured population. Am. J. Sports Med., 23:251-255.

49. Phillips, C.G., Powell, T.S., and Wiesendanger, M. (1971): Protection from low threshold muscle afferents of hand and forearm area 3A of Babson's cortex. J. Physiol., 217:419-446.

50. Pinstaar, A., Brynhildsen, J., and Tropp, H. (1996): Postural corrections after standardized perturbations of single limb stance: Effect of training and orthotic devices in patients with ankle instability. Br. J Sports Med., 30:151-155.

51. Pope, M.H., Johnson, D.W., Brown, D.W., and Tighe, C. (1972): The role of the musculature in injuries to the medial collateral ligament. J. Bone Joint Surg., 61A: 398-402.

52. Rine, R.M., Voight, M.L., Laporta, L., and Mancini, R. (1994): A paradigm to evaluate ankle instability using postural sway measures (Abstract). Phys. Ther., 74:S72.

53. Schulte, M.J., and Happel, L.T. (1990): Joint innervation in injury. Clin. Sports Med., 9:511-517.

54. Schmidt, R.A. (1988): Motor Control and Learning. Champaign, IL, Human Kinetics.

55. Scully, R., and Barnes, M. (1989): Physical Therapy. Philadelphia, J.B. Lippincott.

56. Sherrington, C.S. (1911): The Interactive Action of the Nervous System. New Haven, CT, Yale University Press.

57. Sheth, P., Yu, B., Laskowski, E.R., et al. (1997): Ankle disk training influences reaction times of selected muscles in a simulated ankle sprain. Am. J. Sports Med., 25:538-543.

58. Skinner, H.B., Barrack, R.L., Cook, S.D., and Haddad, R.J. (1984): Joint position sense in total knee arthroplasty. J. Orthop. Res., 1:276-283.

59. Skinner, H.B., Wyatt, M.P., Hodgdon, J.A., et al. (1986): Effect of fatigue on joint position sense of the knee. J. Orthop. Res., 4:112-118.

60. Small, C., Waters, C.L., and Voight, M.L. (1994): Comparison of two methods for measuring hamstring reaction time using the Kin-Com isokinetic dynamometer. J. Orthop. Sports Phys. Ther., 19:335-340.

61. Sullivan, P.E., Markos, P.D., and Minor, M.D. (1982): An Integrated Approach to Therapeutic Exercise: Theory and Clinical Application. Reston, VA: Reston Publishing.

62. Swanik, C.B., Lephart, S.M., Giannantonio, F.P., and Fu, F. (1997): Reestablishing proprioception and neuromuscular control in the ACL-injured athlete. J Sport Rehab., 6:183-206.

63. Tibone, J.E., Antich, T.J., Funton, G.S., et al. (1986): Functional analysis of anterior cruciate ligament instability. Am. J. Sports Med., 14:276-284.

64. Tippett, S., and Voight, M.L. (1995): Functional Progressions for Sports Rehabilitation. Champaign, IL, Human Kinetics.

65. Tropp, H., Askling, C., and Gillquist, J. (1985): Prevention of ankle sprains. Am. J. Sports Med., 13:259-262.

66. Tropp, H., Ekstrand, J., and Gillquist, J. (1984): Factors affecting stabilometry recordings of single leg stance. Am. J. Sports Med., 12:185-188.

67. Tropp, H., and Odenrick, P. (1988): Postural control in single limb stance. J. Orthop. Res., 6:833-839.

68. Voight, M.L. (1990): Functional exercise training. Presented at the 1990 National Athletic Training Association Annual Conference, Indianapolis.

69. Voight, M.L. (1994): Proprioceptive concerns in rehabilitation. In: Proceedings of the XXVth FIMS World Congress of Sports Medicine, Athens, Greece. The International Federation of Sports Medicine, Athens, Greece.

70. Voight, M.L., Bell, S., and Rhodes, D. (1992): Instrumented testing of tibial translation during a positive Lachman's test and selected closed-chain activities in anterior cruciate deficient knees. J. Orthop. Sports Phys. Ther., 15:49.

71. Voight, M.L., Blackburn, T.A., and Hardin, J.A., et al. (1996): The effects of muscle fatigue on the relationship of arm dominance to shoulder proprioception. J. Orthop. Sports Phys. Ther., 23:348-352.

72. Voight, M.L., and Cook, G. (1996): Clinical application of closed kinetic chain exercise. J. Sport Rehabil., 5:25-44.

73. Voight, M.L., Cook, G., and Blackburn, T.A. (1997): Functional lower quarter exercise through reactive neuromuscular training. In: Bandy, W.E. (ed): Current Trends for the Rehabilitation of the Athlete. Lacrosse, WI, SPTS Home Study Course.

74. Voight, M.L., and Draovitch, P. (1991): Plyometric training. In: Muscle Training in Sports and Orthopaedics. New York, Churchill Livingstone.

75. Voight, M.L., Rine, R.M., Apfel, P., et al. (1993): The effects of leg dominance and AFO on static and dynamic balance abilities (Abstract). Phys. Ther., 73:S51.

76. Voight, M.L., Rine, R.M., Briese, K., and Powell, C. (1993): Comparison of sway in double versus single leg stance in unimpaired adults (Abstract). Phys. Ther., 73:S51.

77. Voss, D.E., Ionta, M.K., and Myers, B.J. (1985): Proprioceptive Neuromuscular Facilitation: Patterns and Techniques, 3rd ed. Philadelphia, Harper & Row.

78. Walla, D.J., Albright, J.P., McAuley, E., et al. (1985): Hamstring control and the unstable anterior cruciate ligament-deficient knee. Am. J. Sports Med., 13:34-39.

79. Wester, J.U., Jespersen, S.M., Nielsen, K.D., et al. (1996): Wobble board training after partial sprains of the lateral ligaments of the ankle: A prospective randomized study. J. Orthop. Sports Phys. Ther., 23:332-336.

80. Willis, W.D., and Grossman, R.G. (1981): Medical Neurobiology, 3rd ed. St. Louis, C.V. Mosby.

81. Wojtys, E., and Huston, L. (1994): Neuromuscular performance in normal and anterior cruciate ligament-deficient lower extremities. Am. J. Sports Med., 22:89-104.

82. Wojtys, E., Huston, L.J., Taylor, P.D., and Bastian, S.D. (1996): Neuromuscular adaptations in isokinetic, isotonic, and agility training programs. Am. J. Sports Med., 24:187-192.

CHAPTER 11

PLYOMETRIC TRAINING AND DRILLS

Timothy F. Tyler, M.S., P.T., ATC
Anthony Cuoco, D.P.T., M.S., C.S.C.S.

CHAPTER OBJECTIVES

At the end of this chapter the reader will be able to:

■ Explain the fundamental basis of plyometric training, its origins, and its applications.

■ Describe the neuromuscular physiologic processes involved in the stretch-shortening cycle and how it applies to plyometrics.

■ Describe the important clinical considerations surrounding the appropriate use of plyometrics in the orthopedic and sports medicine rehabilitation setting.

■ Describe and apply important fundamentals for use of plyometrics as a rehabilitation tool, including pretraining assessment and application of exercise prescription principles and injury prevention.

■ Design a basic plyometric training program at low-, medium-, and high-intensity levels.

■ Use a variety of upper and lower extremity plyometric exercises as a part of the rehabilitation process.

Speed and strength are integral components of sport found in varying degrees in virtually all athletic movements. Simply put, the combination of speed and strength is power. For many years coaches and athletes have sought to improve power to enhance performance. Recently, rehabilitation specialists have implemented techniques to improve power to optimize postsurgical and postinjury outcomes. Throughout this century and no doubt long before, jumping, bounding, and hopping exercises have been used in various ways to enhance athletic performance. In recent years this distinct method of training for power or explosiveness has been termed *plyometrics*. Plyometrics is a form of strength training designed to develop explosive power for athletics.[1] Plyometric exercises stress the rapid generation of force, primarily during the "eccentric" (lengthening) phase of muscle action, and speeding the transition between the eccentric and concentric (shortening) phases. This increases the ability of a muscle to sustain a load throughout its range of motion, allowing an athlete to translate strength into power more efficiently.[9,12]

Although the actual term *plyometrics* is new, this particular form of training has been in existence for quite some time. Translated from its Latin origins, it literally means "measurable increases," although there may be some speculation about the effectiveness of this particular form of training to translate into improved functional performance outcomes.[34] It is thought of as the missing link between weight training (strength) and athletic performance (power), with particular emphasis on the speed of activity. Plyometric training was first developed in the Soviet Union for its intense, and very effective, athletic development program, during the 1960s. It came to the attention of the West during the 1970s and by about 1980 had become a valuable tool in major athletic programs. The term was first applied in 1975 by American track and field coach Fred Wilt to describe the training methods used for Eastern European athletes at the time, which supposedly were the reason for differences between the performances of Eastern and Western athletes. During the 1980s, Donald Chu published the first articles on plyometric training methods in this country, and he has been a leader in this area ever since.[20] In the early 1990s, George Davies and Kevin Wilk introduced plyometrics into rehabilitation programs.

In the early years of plyometric training most plyometric drills focused on developing jumping ability. More recently, there are some that develop lateral movement qualities and others that improve upper body power, but plyometrics seem to have been focused traditionally on enhancing lower body power. In the past 10 years, plyometrics have not only been used in the lower extremity for strength and conditioning but also in the upper extremity as a rehabilitation tool and as part of injury prevention programs.

GENERAL THEORY

The premise behind plyometric training is that the maximum force that a muscle can develop is attained during a rapid eccentric contraction. However, it should be recognized that muscles seldom perform one type of contraction in isolation during athletic movements. When a concentric contraction occurs (muscle shortens) immediately after an eccentric contraction (muscle lengthens) then the force generated can be dramatically increased. If a muscle is stretched, much of the energy required to stretch it is lost as heat, but some of this energy can be stored by the elastic components of the muscle. This stored energy is available to the muscle only during a subsequent contraction. It is important to realize that this energy boost is lost if the eccentric contraction is not followed immediately by a concentric effort. To express this greater force the muscle must contract within the shortest time possible. This whole process is usually called the stretch-shortening cycle and is the underlying mechanism of plyometric training.

CLINICAL RELEVANCY

The goal of the final phase of rehabilitation when the use of plyometrics is appropriate is specificity of training. This means that the movement the patient performs in training should match, as closely as possible, the movements encountered during competition without jeopardizing the patient's health status. If the patient is a basketball player practicing for rebounding or a volleyball player interested in increasing vertical jump height, then drop jumping or box jumping may be the right exercise.[22] However, if the patient is a quarterback at 6 months after a thermal shrinkage procedure who is trying to increase throwing velocity, then upper body plyometrics are far more appropriate.[70]

Plyometric training may not be appropriate for all patients in the clinic. It is great for increasing power. For instance, one study showed that plyometric training significantly improved vertical jump performance in elite volleyball players.[37] However, plyometric training is generally not a favored choice of exercise for increasing muscle mass or muscular endurance. Therefore, plyometric training is not appropriate for muscles that are predominately type I muscle fibers and act as stabilizers. In fact, unless the athlete participates in a sport that requires explosive movements (i.e., volleyball, sprinting, basketball, high jump, or others), there is no compelling reason to introduce plyometrics into his or her rehabilitation program.

APPLIED ANATOMY/PHYSIOLOGY AND BIOMECHANICS OF PLYOMETRICS

Similar to other modes of therapeutic exercise, safe and effective interventions using plyometrics require that clinicians be familiar with applied neuromuscular physiologic principles. The use of plyometrics as a training method is primarily based on two fundamental dynamic qualities of muscle tissue: elasticity and contractility. The capacity of working muscles to generate greater (or maximal) force in a minimal amount of time depends on these tissue qualities along with neuromuscular control, strength, and flexibility. In fact, most of the early physiologic research relevant to plyometrics was described as a muscle action called the *stretch-shortening cycle (SSC)*.[20] Currently, the SSC is the physiologic theory that forms the basis of plyometrics.

Stretch-Shortening Cycle

The SSC can be defined as a phenomenon whereby the natural pattern of lengthening of active muscle produces energy that is stored in the musculotendinous unit for later use in a subsequent shortening or concentric contraction of the SSC. It is this eccentric-concentric coupling that forms the basis of the SSC. In an often-referenced study, Cavagna[18] established that there is an enhanced concentric muscle performance in an SSC compared with that in a pure concentric-only action. In practical terms, plyometrics involves high-velocity eccentric contraction or pre-stretching of a muscle before an immediate reciprocal concentric contraction of that same muscle (group). The eccentric contraction stores energy that can be utilized to maximize the amount of power produced during the concentric contraction of that muscle or muscle group.[16,61,63] This storage of elastic energy in the musculotendinous tissues contributes to the increased force produced in the subsequent concentric contraction phase and increased efficiency of movement.[36,62,68] There is an intrinsic stiffness to the muscles and tendons that resists stretch and then reciprocates with a muscle contraction stimulated by the stretch reflex loop.[16,72] Although an oversimplification, this phenomenon can be visualized as the action of a spring. Biomechanically, one can relate SSC to the simple action of a person attempting to improve his or her vertical leap by instinctively performing a partial squat before jumping in place. The simple act of walking or running utilizes the SSC with each stride that begins with the loading response through an eccentric contraction of the quadriceps, soleus, and gastrocnemius muscles followed by a concentric push-off action. Hence, the SSC of plyometric exercise is a natural motion, given the mechanical properties of the musculoskeletal system. Although the SSC has been studied by many investigators, there is general agreement that several important factors of the neuromuscular anatomy and physiology should be considered, i.e., serial elastic components of muscles and tendons, proprioception and gross musculotendinous architecture. The eccentric-concentric coupling of the SSC stimulates the proprioceptors of the muscle spindle, Golgi-tendon organs (GTOs), and ligament receptors to facilitate recruitment of the motor units required to maximize the concentric power generated during plyometric activity (Box 11-1).

Box 11-1

Important Factors in Neuromuscular Anatomy and Physiology[17,43,68]

- Serial elastic and histologic components of muscle and tendons, i.e., myosin and actin sliding filaments/cross bridge attachments, sarcomeres, fiber types, and metabolic properties
- Proprioception mediated through muscle spindles and Golgi-tendon organs and their contribution to stretch (or myotonic) reflex loops
- Gross musculotendinous architecture

Skeletal Muscle Histological Considerations

Histologically, the level of the fascicles is a fundamental component of the serial elasticity of muscle. Although much research has been conducted on the dynamics of the SSC at the histologic level, the behavior of human skeletal muscles during SSC exercises has not been directly investigated in vivo. It has been well documented in the literature that activated muscle stretched before shortening performs more forcefully.[18] However, the exact mechanisms that mediate the stretch-enhanced performance have been a source of controversy. Kubo and colleagues examined fascicle length and tendon structure changes in humans during SSC exercises for the gastrocnemius muscle at both fast and slow speeds using real-time ultrasonography. They found that both fascicle and tendon structures were lengthened at the dorsiflexion phase and shortened at the plantar flexion phase.[45] The stretching ability depends on many factors, but the rate and magnitude of the stretch applied contribute to how much force a muscle can generate.

Although perhaps not as critical in terms of the stretching dynamics, the fiber types utilized for plyometrics are worth reviewing. It is well documented that type II, or fast twitch fibers, are capable of generating more force than type I, or slow twitch fibers. This is primarily a function of the increased cross-sectional area, larger motor units, and high glycolytic capacities associated with type II fibers.[25,49,53,59] The amount of force necessary during the eccentric and subsequent explosive concentric phases of SSC exercise necessitates the recruitment of type II fibers. It should also be noted that type II fibers are also readily fatigable. Although a detailed discussion of the metabolic properties of muscle fiber types is beyond the scope of this chapter, it is important for the clinician to be aware of the metabolic systems that contribute to optimal performance of muscle tissues during plyometric exercise. Type II fibers are classified further into at least two basic types: type IIa and type IIb. Fast-twitch type IIb fibers are those that rely primarily on the phosphate and glycolytic energy systems and are termed fast glycolytic fibers. Type IIa fibers are more like a hybrid between the slow oxidative type I fibers and the type IIb fibers and are termed fast glycolytic-oxidative fibers.[25,49,53,59] Plyometric exercise should focus on the adaptation of these fibers to overload with anaerobic training, while still taking into consideration those type IIa fibers that use both oxidative and glycolytic energy systems. Both the force generation and endurance qualities necessary in functional athletic activity require that the athlete develop both classes of type II fibers.

Neuromuscular Physiology: Muscle Spindles and Golgi-Tendon Organs

The muscle spindles function primarily as stretch receptors, observed clinically in the performance of standard reflex testing, e.g., the knee jerk. When the quadriceps tendon is tapped with the reflex hammer, the muscle spindles are stimulated, causing an immediate concentric contraction of the quadriceps muscle group. This minimal latency time between the quick stretch and subsequent contraction is mediated at the level of the spinal cord as a monosynaptic reflex. Muscle spindles are sensitive to velocity changes and are innervated by type 1a nerve fibers. These afferent nerve fibers conduct the impulse directly to the spinal cord, where they are immediately conducted via interneurons to α motor neurons, which stimulate muscle contraction. The brain is not involved in this spinal reflex loop, contributing to the speed at which the stretch-contraction cycle occurs.[41,76]

Muscle spindles are located within extrafusal (skeletal) muscle fibers and comprise connective tissue that surrounds intrafusal fibers in a capsular structure. The muscle spindles are innervated by myelinated afferent nerve fibers, which enter the capsule of and spiral around the intrafusal fibers. Based on the architecture of the muscle spindle, stretching of the skeletal (extrafusal) fibers also stretches the intrafusal fibers. This stretch increases the firing rate of the afferent fibers innervating the intrafusal fibers, thus "loading" the muscle spindle. When the stretch is released or lessened the firing rate diminishes. There are both primary and secondary afferent fibers, and these fibers contribute to the ability of the spindle to detect small changes in length. Thus, the muscle spindle is sensitive to changes in muscle length as well as to the speed and magnitude of the stretch.[41]

Although the muscle spindle reacts to stretch, it does not simply "turn off" when the muscle is no longer stretched, because the fibers continue to send messages when the muscle has begun to concentrically contract and shorten. The CNS regulates the loading through γ motor neurons, which modulate the spindle activity, thereby making the transitions from stretch to contraction smoother.[41] This modulation contributes to muscle tone and, thus, to the intrinsic stiffness of the muscle. Therefore, the muscle tends to act as a spring, enabling the SSC to produce force with precision.

Although the muscle spindle is sensitive to stretch, the GTOs provide complementary information to the CNS about muscle activity. Specifically, length and degree of tension are monitored by the GTOs. GTOs are encapsulated collagen structures typically located at the musculotendinous junction. Each GTO is innervated by nerve fibers that wrap around the collagen bundles. As the collagen bundles are stretched, they straighten and the nerve fibers fire more rapidly. GTOs are sensitive to small changes in muscle tension. Because the GTOs surrounds collagen and not extrafusal muscle fibers, they are not as sensitive to stretch because the collagen is a stiffer molecular structure than muscle fiber. Thus, most of the stretch is absorbed by the muscle fibers and the muscle spindles. This makes the GTO more sensitive to active muscle contraction that stresses the musculotendinous junction to a greater degree.[41]

Gross Musculotendinous Structure

On a more gross anatomical and clinical level, the muscle and tendon resist stretch as force increases. Muscle stiffness can be defined as the change in force over the change in muscle length. This inherent stiffness is the resistance to stretch by the fibers of the active muscle and tendons before the changes in activation modulated by the muscle spindles and GTO described earlier occur. Benn and associates[10] described this property of stiffness as stretch work utilized in the completion of the SSC. Several authors have studied the relationship between SSC performance and muscle stiffness. Goslow and colleagues[31] found that cat tendons with a high degree of stiffness may transfer energy more rapidly to attached muscles, resulting in earlier activation of the stretch reflex, and, thus, more rapid contraction of the muscle. Wilson and co-workers[72] concluded that, in humans, a stiffer musculotendinous unit may result in an increased rate of concentric contraction and a more rapid transmission of forces to the working limbs. In another study these authors concluded that decreased musculotendinous stiffness actually enhanced SSC performance in a bench press exercise because more elastic energy could be stored in a less stiff musculotendinous unit. Other studies have concluded that increased musculotendinous stiffness may be more important than the ability to store more elastic energy in terms of enhancing SSC performance in activities such as sprinting.[10] Given these equivocal results, the principle of specificity in terms of mode and the muscles involved may be important distinctions in determining the optimal musculotendinous stiffness.

To this point, one can see that the histologic structure of muscle and tendons can both enhance and hinder movement and force-generating capacity. Although the inherent elastic components of the musculotendinous unit can store energy for use in generating force and powerful movement, there may be gross structural aspects that limit the ability of a muscle to maximize the SSC. Neural factors and recruitment of fibers as well as the metabolic capacities of muscle and the appropriate exercise conditioning all have an impact on performance.

Brownstein and Bronner[17] formulated three types of musculotendinous units. Their theory centers around gross muscle structure (i.e., length of the muscles and tendons). The first musculotendinous unit type comprises muscles with long fascicles and relatively short tendons, such as the gluteus maximus. This type of muscle is usually located proximally and tends to be large in size. These muscles are typically powerful movers with a large muscle fiber cross-sectional area. They are capable of moving the limb through a wide range of motion and can absorb a significant amount of energy. For the gluteus maximus, stepping off of a box and into a squat position smoothly is partially a function of the eccentric contracting (lengthening) of the gluteal muscles.

Muscles with long, thick, inelastic tendons are the second class of musculotendinous units. An example of this type would be the gastrocnemius. These muscles are also located proximally. The tendons have a high degree of stiffness and provide strong control of the distal segment.

Muscles such as the tibialis anterior have short fascicles and long, slender tendons. This third type of musculotendinous unit can store large amounts of elastic energy when stretched rapidly, because they are less stiff. These muscles shorten very little and are more efficient on the length-tension and force-velocity curves. These tend to have more slow-twitch, highly oxidative fibers and are therefore metabolically efficient.

Fundamentals of Plyometrics

Plyometrics are an inherent part of the functional aspects of athletic movement. The primary basis of plyometrics is to utilize the neurophysiologic components described earlier to combine speed and strength. Plyometrics have been described as stretch shortening drills or reactive neuromuscular training. There are basically three phases of a plyometric exercise.

The *preloading, setting,* or *eccentric phase* refers to the early moments in the movement in which the muscle spindles are loaded and stretched during an eccentric contraction, such as stepping from a box onto the ground and squatting as one lands to absorb the ground reaction forces. This is when the storing of elastic energy takes place. The time interval for this phase depends on how much stretch facilitation is desired for the subsequent phases. For rehabilitation, this phase will most likely be dictated by the range of motion and amount of shock absorption the athlete's body is capable of withstanding or the amount of eccentric loading the agonist musculature and passive restraints (e.g., ligaments) can tolerate.

The *amortization phase* refers to the time between the end of the eccentric contraction and the initiation of the concentric, explosive reaction force that accelerates the body or working limb in the desired direction. This phase should be as short as possible, because with a long interval there is the risk of losing much of the elastic energy as heat within the muscle.[21] The successful performance of a plyometric drill depends on the ability of the musculotendinous unit to effectively absorb and exploit the stored elastic energy. The rapid stretching (eccentric loading) must be immediately followed by a rapid, explosive concentric contraction to maximize the force generated. The quicker an athlete can overcome the yielding eccentric force and produce a concentric contraction, the more power he or she can produce. The *concentric phase* represents the cumulative effect of the eccentric and amortization phases through a powerful concentric contraction[2,69] (Box 11-2).

CLINICAL CONSIDERATIONS FOR PLYOMETRICS

Although all athletes may not necessarily need to produce explosive strength to excel at a given sport, most athletes undergoing rehabilitation need to regain strength and proprioception after an injury. Although plyometrics have been traditionally used in a realm of sports that require strength, speed, and power, such as sprinting and other track and field events, all competitive athletes may be able to reduce the risk of future injury by maximizing their dynamic restraint system. Joint stability depends on both passive and dynamic restraint structures. Passive structures, such as the arthrokinematics of articulating surfaces, ligaments, joint capsule, and menisci, provide support to the musculoskeletal components. The dynamic restraints that provide joint stability include the muscles and neural controls associated with movement. It is often the passive restraints that are damaged in sports and daily activities involving high-velocity movements and perturbations to dynamic balance.[40,74] Unfortunately, although the healing of passive restraints can be addressed through physical therapy, these structures are not easily modified by active conservative treatment on the part of the athlete, because the healing process is more passive (modalities, passive range of motion and manual therapy). Thus, protective and rehabilitation efforts have focused primarily on modifying the dynamic neuromuscular elements, including joint capsule mechanoreceptors. To this end, proprioceptive training, active range of motion, flexibility, and strengthening interventions are typically utilized, empowering the patient to maximize the ability of the dynamic restraints to contribute to stability and injury prevention. Any displacement that occurs too quickly for reflex reactions to protect a joint requires that the mechanical properties of the musculotendinous unit resist the displacement. Active muscle response to any perturbation that might compromise joint stability is thus an important consideration in rehabilitation for prevention and athletic performance.

Generally, plyometrics involve ballistic and repetitive movements. Although these exercises and drills are designed to optimize the SSC and improve athletic performance, clinicians need to be cautious in deciding when a patient is ready for safe and effective use of plyometrics. Specifically, a patient must have achieved a certain level of range of motion, strength and flexibility before undertaking plyometric exercises. The evaluation process should always consider the treatment goals established for a given patient at the onset of therapy (Box 11-3).

Applications in Rehabilitation

Plyometrics are also widely used in a less intense manner in the rehabilitation of many athletic injuries. In addition

---

Box 11-2

Summary of Plyometric Phases

Eccentric phase	Preloading or setting period	Muscle spindles "loaded" via stretch/eccentric contraction of agonists
Amortization phase	Interval between eccentric and concentric muscle contraction	Should be short as to utilize elastic energy stored in stretched muscle-tendon complex
Concentric phase	Concentric muscle contraction of agonists	Maximal power generation with explosive movement

---

Box 11-3

Neuromuscular Assessment before Initiating Plyometrics[26]

- Resolution of pain enough to participate in higher level exercises and activities
- No inflammation or joint effusion
- Patient has regained normal range of motion versus the uninvolved side
- Normal joint alignment and mobility
- Soft tissue flexibility, including both contractile and noncontractile structures, within normal limits
- Adequate strength for full weight bearing activity if lower extremity or strength for functional use of the upper extremity
- Normal reflexes
- Normal motor control

to increasing conditioning, they also increase or facilitate functional motor patterns, reflexes, and proprioception, all of which are crucial in the attempt to return an athlete to competition. It is important to take into consideration the phase of rehabilitation and status of the healing tissue when one implements plyometrics in a patient's program (Box 11-4).

Recently the use of lower extremity plyometrics has received attention as a possible aid in the prevention of noncontact anterior cruciate ligament (ACL) injuries. Although limited research has been done in this area, plyometrics may turn out to be a crucial component in the reduction of ACL injuries in females. A growing body of evidence is linking ACL injuries to poor neuromuscular control in the injured athletes. It is possible that some athletes may have poor technique in jumping, landing, stopping, and or turning, which may lead to injury. Neuromuscular control must be developed in all three planes of motion—frontal, sagittal, and transverse—to decrease the stress on the ACL and move it to the muscles and tendons. Proper plyometric training can decrease the force and torque placed on the knee. Proper technique increases the load placed on the muscles and tendons and removes it from the joint and ligaments. The principles of plyometric training—functional motor patterns, reflexes, and proprioception—are instrumental in the prevention of knee injuries. These same principles can be applied to an upper extremity that is functionally unstable and has lost position sense.

In fact, Hewett and colleagues[38] examined the effects of a plyometric training program on landing mechanics and leg strength in female athletes involved in jumping sports. The plyometric program was designed to decrease landing forces by helping the athletes improve neuromuscular control over the lower extremity during landing. It was also designed to increase vertical jump height. The authors reported that peak landing forces during a volleyball block jump decreased by 22%. Horizontal forces acting upon the knee during landing were reduced by approximately 50%. Hamstring-quadriceps peak torque strength ratios increased 26% on the nondominant leg and 13% on the dominant leg. Hamstring power increased 44% on the dominant leg and 21% on the nondominant leg. The mean vertical jump increased by 10% overall. This study is the first to link the preventative aspect of

plyometrics and therapeutic exercise. It suggests that a properly performed plyometric training protocol may help prevent knee injury in female athletes involved in jumping sports, such as volleyball, by increasing knee stabilization during landing and teaching athletes muscular control. Plyometrics may also help correct torque imbalances between the hamstrings and quadriceps and can help increase vertical jump height.

Although the jumping aspect of plyometric training is important for conditioning, it is the landing of each jump that is important in the theoretical prevention of knee injuries. The technique on landing is crucial to avoid a knee going into hyperextension and external rotation, the point of no return. A key concept is that the athlete should land softly and quietly while using the knees and hips as shock absorbers. Another is that the shoulders should be over the knees when the athlete lands. During plyometric training the athlete should be constantly reminded to land softly. Another key concept for prevention of ACL injury is that hyperextension should be avoided during all activities such as turning, landing, stopping, cutting, or slowing down. The final suggestion for injury prevention is for the athlete to "stick" and hold the landing. This is accomplished when balance is maintained for 5 to 6 seconds after landing, and no additional steps are taken. There should be no foot movement after landing. Recently, the effect of this type of neuromuscular training on the incidence of knee injury in female athletes was prospectively evaluated. Hewett and colleagues[37] monitored two groups of female athletes, one trained before sports participation and the other untrained, and a group of untrained male athletes throughout the high school soccer, volleyball, and basketball seasons. Weekly reports included the number of practice and competition exposures and mechanism of injury. There were 14 serious knee injuries in the 1263 athletes tracked through the study. Ten of 463 untrained female athletes sustained serious knee injuries (8 noncontact), 2 of 366 trained female athletes sustained serious knee injuries (0 noncontact), and 2 of 434 male athletes sustained serious knee injuries (1 noncontact). Untrained female athletes had a 3.6 times higher incidence of knee injury than trained female athletes and 4.8 times higher incidence than male athletes. The incidence of knee injury in trained female athletes was not significantly different from that in untrained male athletes. A significant difference was seen in the incidence of noncontact injuries between the female groups. In this prospective study a decreased incidence of knee injury was demonstrated in female athletes after a specific plyometric training program (Box 11-5).

Unfortunately, there has been a minimal amount of reliable scientific research conducted on plyometrics in rehabilitation, and little information is available on the physiologic basis, training effectiveness, or even the establishment of standard guidelines for plyometric rehabilitation. Most of the information provided in books is written

---

Box 11-4

Proposed Beneficial Effects of Plyometrics

- Improved proprioception during dynamic movement
- Improved speed-strength and power
- Improved reaction time
- Increased bone mineral density

Box 11-5

Plyometric Concepts for the Prevention of Knee Injuries in Females

- "Stick" the landing.
- Hold the landing for 5 seconds.
- Land softly.
- Land quietly.
- Keep the shoulders over the knees when landing.
- Avoid hyperextension during all activities.

by physical therapists with little knowledge of the efficacy of plyometrics. Nevertheless, as clinicians we must combine our knowledge of basic science and outcomes of plyometrics in healthy subjects to optimize our results in the patient population.

Even among healthy athletes, previous training level and ability are key components in determining if an individual is ready to tolerate plyometrics. Although we will discuss prerequisites in more detail, it is generally believed that an individual should have a reasonable amount of flexibility, strength, and agility before starting a plyometric training program. Although perhaps not as important as for other exercise modes used in the athletic training room or clinic, it is critical that specific assessment and testing be conducted before use of plyometrics. Plyometrics are demanding physically and require that the individual concentrate on controlling movements.

According to some authors, the risk of injury from plyometrics is low.[15] However, there are few studies that have actually addressed injury rates from plyometric training among healthy individuals. Although there are no studies of injury rates among patients undergoing rehabilitation and using plyometrics, there is a significant body of work studying fatigue and muscle damage in healthy subjects after SSC exercise.

Gollhofer and associates[30] found that repeated SSC muscle activity induces fatigue effects associated with a decrease in neural input to the muscle and reduced overall muscle performance. It has been suggested that during SSC exercise fatigue, the repeated stretch loads might reduce the reflex contribution to the SSC.[55] Avela and Komi[5] studied a group of experienced endurance runners and concluded that fatiguing SSC exercise reduced stretch-reflex sensitivity, which was associated with decreased muscle stiffness. They postulated that this would impair the athlete's ability to utilize the stored elastic energy in the muscle-tendon complex.

Lower extremity plyometric exercises are particularly of concern for injury to feet, ankles, shins, knees, hips, and the lower back area. As is the case during most athletic events, injuries are more likely when an individual is fatigued, typically toward the end of an event or exercise session. Sprained ankles and knee injuries are commonly

associated with a lack of control due to excessive fatigue.[21] Inadequate conditioning, no warm-up, poor-quality athletic shoes, inappropriate surfaces for plyometrics, and low levels of skill all predispose an athlete to injury.[2] Borkowski[15] reported that a preseason plyometric training program among collegiate volleyball players did not cause injuries but actually significantly reduced in-season muscle soreness. Thus, it is clear that proper assessment and testing of athletes before a plyometric program is started and diligent application of the exercise prescription principles of frequency, duration, and intensity are extremely important.

Basic Pretraining Testing

In addition to the physical assessments and strength guidelines mentioned previously, there are several basic static and dynamic tests to determine a patient's ability to begin a plyometric training program. Voight and Tippett[67] proposed that an individual be able to perform a 30-second one-leg stance with eyes open and closed before starting a plyometric program. Involved versus uninvolved legs should be compared. Voight and Draovitch[66] recommended that the stork balance test be performed for 30 seconds and that a single-leg half-squat also be evaluated before any jumping plyometric exercises are begun.

The clinician should be creative in utilizing functional testing to determine whether or not a patient is prepared to begin a plyometric program. Vertical jumps in place and horizontal long jumps on a shock-absorbing surface are two simple tests that may provide feedback about a patient's status. Any pain or observed instability during these tests may provide clues to the patient's tolerance for plyometrics. Having the patient perform step-ups and step-downs from progressively increasing heights will also provide some indication of the patient's tolerance. Lateral shuffle and carioca (crossover) drills also provide the clinician with ways of testing whether an affected lower limb is prepared to handle plyometrics. Obviously, jogging and running activities should also be performed to further assess the ability of the affected limb to bear full body weight.

Before incorporating any high-intensity, or shock, plyometric drills such as box jumps or in-depth jumps, the reader is encouraged to consult sources to determine the height of the box that should be used for an individual's ability.[20]

Strength and Conditioning Level

In terms of strength, it is generally accepted that a patient should have a sufficient strength training base. When plyometrics are used for rehabilitation, a great deal of subjective clinical judgment is necessary on the part of the clinician. The reason for this is the fact that there is a lack of evidence in the literature to support any guidelines for rehabilitation using plyometrics. As mentioned earlier, plyometrics have been used for some time in strength and conditioning programs for healthy athletes. Indeed, there is consensus that plyometric training principles are beneficial for healthy athletes, although there is much room for subjective judgment in terms of how these drills and exercises should progress. Although plyometrics can be a form of functional training for rehabilitation, the ballistic nature of most of these exercises makes them inappropriate for the early stages of rehabilitation. One major disadvantage of plyometric training is that joint excursion cannot be controlled because of the nature of the activity.

Although it is not necessary nor suggested that strength training programs focus solely on eccentric contractions, it is important that eccentric strength be established before a plyometric training program is begun, especially for the injured athlete. Studies[28,52,56] have shown that there is increased force production during eccentric contractions, allowing the tolerance of higher loads and preferential recruitment of fast twitch fibers; in addition, high eccentric loads may reduce neural inhibition and may lead to greater concentric force generation. During most athletic pursuits as well as activities of daily living, movement in the opposite direction, an eccentric motion, precedes movement in the intended direction. In most movements, the eccentric contraction is responsible for decelerating the moving limb. Similarly, the eccentric phase of the plyometric exercise absorbs the energy by decelerating the limb and allows the storing of elastic energy. Thus, the clinician should incorporate eccentric work during repetitions of various therapeutic and functional exercises. Emphasis on the eccentric phase of the motion just before the concentric work more closely matches true human movement patterns.

No discussion of strength would be complete without mention of the need for establishing a strength base using closed kinetic chain exercises before a plyometric exercises program is begun. Indeed, practically all plyometric exercises are of the closed-chain variety, like the functional movements they mimic. In the case of jumping and landing, the entire kinetic chain, from ankles through knees and hips as well as vertebral column, needs to absorb full body weight and maintain stability. The muscle synergies and neuromuscular coordination required for smooth landing and subsequent explosive movement during athletic activity and plyometrics are better served by enhancing closed-chain strength.

Chu and Cordier[21] recommended the power squat test as a good closed-chain exercise to determine whether a patient has an adequate strength base for lower extremity plyometrics. The exercise is performed with 60% of the person's body weight. Five squat repetitions are done in 5 seconds, and the depth should be to knee flexion close to 90° for each repetition. If the patient cannot perform the

exercise in the allotted time with proper technique, the clinician should continue to emphasize strength training and hold off the plyometric program. For strength training to improve vertical leap performance, Weiss and colleagues[69] concluded that training programs to enhance moderately fast squatting power may improve performance as long as body weight, especially body fat, is not increased. In a related finding, McBride and associates[48] concluded that training with light-load jump squats resulted in increased movement velocity capabilities and that velocity-specific changes in muscle activity may play a role in this adaptation. The guidelines are not as clear for the upper extremity. Anecdotally, we recommend that the patient have full range of motion, rotator cuff strength at least 75% as strong as that of the uninvolved extremity, and grade four of five for the prime movers on a manual muscle test.

For shock- and high-intensity lower extremity plyometrics, it is recommended that a healthy athlete have enough leg and hip strength to be able to perform a squat with 1.5 to 2.5 times the athlete's body weight. For high-intensity upper extremity plyometrics, it has been suggested that an athlete be able to perform five clap push-ups in a row. Alternatively, athletes weighing more than 115 kg should be able to bench press their own body weight. Those weighing less than 75 kg should be capable of bench pressing 1.5 times their body weight, whereas those between these weight guidelines should use gradations of the guidelines.[2] Clearly, this requirement is not necessary for plyometrics performed in early and middle stages of rehabilitation, but it underscores the diligence that is important in evaluating a patient before initiation of plyometrics. By definition, plyometric training involves maximal voluntary contractions. Therefore, plyometrics should be incorporated during the end stages of rehabilitation, when the clinician is preparing an athlete for return to play or for any patient to achieve maximal functional capacity.

The focus on making sure that a patient has the strength foundation necessary to engage in plyometrics should not overshadow the need for proper endurance and conditioning. Although not an endurance activity per se, a plyometric training session does require a measure of glycolytic endurance, because anaerobic or strength/power exercise is more likely to increase lactic acid levels in the muscle, which decreases the pH of the muscle. The process of removing lactic acid and metabolites from the muscle tissue, i.e., recovery, is an oxidative process. Thus, an athlete should have a reasonable measure of endurance to safely avoid fatigue and risk for injury during a plyometric training session. A plyometric program uses successive sets/repetitions and rest periods, but as the duration of the routine increases (e.g., to 15 to 30 minutes) the athlete will encounter fatigue. Similar to what occurs during an athletic event, there is a need for anaerobic endurance. Specifically, the athlete encounters short bouts of explosive anaerobic activity, with short rests, and then must continue to attempt to achieve that performance level for several minutes or even hours. Take as an example a tennis match or a basketball or football game. The same explosive movements are required at the end of the match or game as are necessary in the beginning of the competition. Gollhofer and associates[30] found that there was reduced electromyographic (EMG) activity during the eccentric phase of SSC exercise fatigue in healthy subjects. Similarly, Nicol and colleagues[55] concluded that there was a smaller EMG response of calf muscles to passive stretch after submaximal SSC exercise. Strojnik and Komi[60] also found that fatiguing submaximal SSC exercise on a sledge jump apparatus decreased the contractile characteristics of the quadriceps femoris muscle.

Anthropometrics, Age, Gender, and Previous Injury Considerations

Simply because a patient is an athlete does not mean that his or her rehabilitation program should progress to high-intensity plyometrics. Generally, high-intensity drills may not be appropriate for larger athletes (>90 kg).[2] This is especially true if the athlete's body fat level is high. A football lineman, for example, may be at increased risk, especially because his role in competition does not require jumping and leaping movements as much as does the role of a running back or wide receiver. By the same token, an endurance athlete with a low body fat level but low muscle mass might also be at risk for injury with high-impact plyometric exercises. Ugarkovic and co-workers[65] studied anthropometric and strength variables as predictors of jumping performance in elite junior basketball players and concluded that these measures alone are not the best predictors to assess movement performance in homogeneous groups of athletes. They suggest that these factors and especially sport specific movements and power be used in a comprehensive evaluation.

Nonetheless, body structure and body fat measures and particularly structural abnormalities and previous injuries must be considered. Vertebral abnormalities, as well as problems with knees, hips, and ankles are of special concern for lower extremity drills. Previous shoulder, elbow, wrist, and cervical or thoracic injuries should be considered for upper extremity plyometrics.

Younger athletes (aged 12 to 16) can engage in low- to medium-intensity plyometrics, although it is critical that they have the strength and coordination to tolerate these drills safely without incurring injuries to the epiphyseal (growth) plates of bones and overuse injuries to tendons. High-intensity (shock) plyometrics such as box jumps are generally not recommended for adolescents. Although sequential age should be considered in terms of maturity, each child should be evaluated for their maturity in terms of strength, flexibility, balance, and coordination.

Weight-bearing exercise of high load intensity is known to have osteogenic effects.[35,47] Children who participate in activities associated with higher loads have been shown to exhibit higher bone mass than children who participate in activities with lower loads.[32] Witzke and Snow[73] investigated the effects of 9 months of plyometric jump training on bone mineral content, performance, and balance in adolescent girls. They found that moderate- to high-intensity plyometric training improved trochanteric bone mineral content, leg strength, and balance in these adolescent girls.

Regarding gender differences, Aura and Komi[4] found that female subjects better utilized the prestretch phase of SSC at low-intensity levels, whereas men showed greater potentiation of elastic energy at higher prestretch levels. However, males exhibited higher work due to elasticity. They suggested that there may be fundamental differences in neuromuscular function between males and females.

Warm-Up, Stretching, and Flexibility

The importance of sufficient warm-up and stretching before one engages in any athletic activity is well documented in the literature.[3,8,14,23,25,29,33,39,75] Especially for the lower extremity when whole body movements will be employed, a general warm-up should raise heart rate, increase muscle and soft tissue temperatures, decrease viscosity of synovial fluid, and increase overall body temperature enough to generate mild perspiration. The warm-up and stretching should be activity specific, incorporating the dynamic movements associated with that activity. Although research does not support the contention, there is some evidence that stretching may decrease the potential for injury.[2] However, there is evidence that stretching consistently and regularly will significantly improve flexibility.[8] Assuming that there are no joint structures limiting range of motion, improved flexibility through stretching of muscles and soft tissues should aid in the safe performance of demanding plyometric exercises.

Although static stretching is important in the performance of plyometrics, some ballistic stretching is probably warranted. Plyometric activity is ballistic by definition so ballistic stretching specific to the activity to be performed should be helpful. Additionally, proprioceptive neuromuscular facilitation stretching may be an appropriate adjunct to flexibility improvement as well. Detailed discussion of stretching and flexibility is beyond the scope of this chapter, and the reader is encouraged to review Chapter 6 on this subject.

Proprioception

Proprioception describes the awareness of posture, movement, and changes in equilibrium and the knowledge of position, weight, and resistance of objects in relation to the body. Kinesthesia is also important, representing the ability to perceive the extent, direction, and weight of movement.[64] Conscious and unconscious perception of these circumstances is critical in the safe and effective return of the athlete to competition. Several studies have shown that in jump performances the leg extensor muscles are activated before the feet contact the ground both in humans[50] and animals.[27] Komi and associates[43] described this phenomenon as the preactivation or preinnervation phase. Melvill Jones and Watt[50] suggested that this preactivation is mediated by higher CNS processes before the person lands and that the correct timing and sequence of the (eccentric) contractions to absorb the forces have been learned from previous experience. According to Avela and co-workers,[6] many studies have confirmed this theory, and a clear relationship exists between the duration and amount of preactivation and the height drop as a result of the person's jumping. Komi and associates[42] showed that preactivation increases with increasing running speed. Despite these studies, there is evidence that the vestibular and visual systems also play a role in this process.[6] Finally, it has been shown that the preactivation phase is important in preparing the muscle to resist high impact forces and in preparing for the subsequent push-off after contact.[46] These studies suggest that plyometric training and the motor learning that takes place from repetitive practice can play a critical role in developing proprioception. The speed-strength components of the drills should better prepare a patient to handle these circumstances in the functional activity.

Joint stability depends partially on proper neuromuscular control. Presumably the clinician has addressed proprioception during the intervention leading up to initiation of a plyometric training program. Nonetheless, the plyometric program should be viewed as a higher level extension of this component in rehabilitation for a patient achieving a return to maximal functional status. It should be noted that the healing and strengthening of static and dynamic restraints do not necessarily prepare a patient for the demands of athletic endeavors. Indeed, the unanticipated changes in joint positions encountered during athletic events are something that the athlete must be prepared to tolerate. Plyometric training is the next logical step in properly preparing the athlete for return to play. Although running and changing direction are important aspects of proprioception, these conditions in the athletic training room or clinic do not adequately mimic the functional requirements during competition or even practice drills. Besier and colleagues[11] studied anticipatory effects on knee joint loading during running and cutting maneuvers. They concluded that performance of cutting maneuvers without preplanning may increase the risk of noncontact knee ligament injury. The authors suggested that training should involve drills that familiarize athletes with making unanticipated changes in direction and that

plyometrics should be included as well as helping athletes focus on visual cues to increase time available to preplan a movement.

PROGRAMMING AND IMPLEMENTATION
Exercise Surface and Environmental Considerations

Depending on the rehabilitation location, it is likely that only low-level plyometrics will be conducted in the clinical setting. Jumps in place, hops, bounds, and in-depth jumps should be performed on yielding surfaces such as hardwood or spring-loaded flooring. Bounds and hops can be performed outside on level, well-groomed grassy surfaces or artificial turf. Rubberized indoor and outdoor tracks may also be safe surfaces. The typical flooring in an athletic training room or clinic, even if carpeted, is not appropriate for lower extremity plyometrics that involve full body weight. Wrestling or gymnastics mats may also be a good choice, especially for full body weight landings. However, these surfaces should not be so soft or cushioned that they jeopardize the athlete's ability to land safely without spraining a knee or ankle. In addition, it is preferable that the athlete perform the plyometric exercises on a surface similar or specific to a given sport/activity.

Although trampolines or excessively thick exercise mats might seem like appropriate surfaces for lower extremity plyometrics, they might actually extend the amortization phase and reduce the efficient use of the stretch reflex for the SSC. Again, these surfaces are also not specific to the surface on which the athlete will be competing.

Obviously the amount of space needed for the lower extremity is a function of the type of plyometric drills being performed. Some drills may require as much as 100 m, although most bounding and running drills only require about 30 m of straightaway.[2,20,21] If plyometric exercises are performed indoors, ceilings must be high enough to accommodate vertical leaps and in-depth jumps even though a small floor surface area is needed.

Equipment

The flooring or playing surface is probably the most important "equipment" needed for plyometric training. Similarly, the footwear worn by the patient/athlete is very important. Footwear should provide good cushion and also sturdy support. A standard cross-training shoe is probably best suited for performance of lower extremity plyometric exercises, especially if lateral movements will be included. Running shoes are typically not a good choice for plyometric training, because the sole is generally more narrow and affords minimal lateral support for the ankles. A basketball or tennis shoe might also be a good choice, because these typically provide good support for lateral activities as well as changes in direction and stop/go activity.

Solid boxes have always been a staple of lower extremity plyometric training. The top or landing surfaces of the boxes should be covered with solid rubber, nonslip covers. Typically, these boxes are constructed of ¾-inch plywood or pressboard (pulp) wood. The boxes can vary from 6 to 24 inches or more in height. Plastic cones, hurdles, and physioballs are also useful pieces of equipment. Plyometric or weighted balls are very useful for both upper extremity, core, and lower extremity training. A slide board and strength/jumping/plyometric shoes are also useful pieces of equipment. Kraemer and colleagues[44] recently studied the effects of one type of strength shoe and concluded that sprint and plyometric training with the shoe along with weight training significantly increased vertical jump height in young, healthy men who were experienced with both resistance and plyometric training.

Warm-Up and Cool-Down

Similar to any other exercise session or higher level therapy regimen, proper warm-up and stretching are important components for a safer and more effective and efficient plyometric training session. Especially for lower extremity plyometric exercises, a comprehensive warm-up routine might include the following:

- Jogging for 5 to 10 minutes raises heart rate, increases respiration, and raises body temperature (especially for soft tissue and synovial fluid viscosity).
- All appropriate muscle groups, both primary agonists, antagonists, and stabilizer muscles (e.g., quadriceps, hip flexors, gluteals, hamstrings, and triceps surae as well as internal/external hip rotators, peroneals, tibialis anterior, and lumbar spine), should be stretched for 5 to 10 minutes. Stretch positions that mimic the specific plyometric movements are also helpful. Proprioceptive neuromuscular facilitation stretching with the assistance of a partner or clinician might also be indicated at this time.
- Low intensity strides, jumping, and bounding (or whatever drills will be performed) better prepare the neuromuscular units to be primed for the activity; *controlled* ballistic stretching might also be indicated here.
- After the plyometric routine has been completed, a 3- to 5-minute walk or light stationary bike ride for cool-down is warranted. Postworkout stretching for 3 to 5 minutes is also indicated.

Frequency

As for principles of traditional exercise, frequency is defined as the number of times per week that plyometric exercises are performed. Typically, one to three sessions are held each week. However, the frequency is primarily a function of the intensity and duration of the workouts, and hence, the amount of recovery that a patient needs between workouts. The frequency and intensity of other conditioning activities such as formal sport practice sessions, strength training, and aerobic activity must also be considered in designing the plyometric training program. For example, the clinician may choose to have a patient perform low-intensity plyometric exercises three times a week while in the athletic training room or clinic. As the patient's condition improves, the sessions would become more intense and last longer (duration) but only take place twice per week. The clinician would also consider how much strength training and aerobic activity the patient is performing each week.

For healthy athletes, off-season and in-season plyometric programming varies according to the demands of other conditioning, especially practice sessions and actual competition. For most sports, off-season plyometric routines are performed twice per week. Track and field athletes may perform two to three times per week. In-season, one session per week is appropriate for most sports, whereas track and field athletes may maintain the two or three per week schedule. Regardless of the frequency used, it is recommended that plyometric drills for a given muscle group(s) and joint complex not be performed on 2 consecutive days.[2]

Intensity

Intensity is simply the amount of stress that is placed on the patient during a training session. In cardiovascular exercise, intensity can be indicated by the training heart rate, the percentage of maximum oxygen consumption, or a rating of perceived exertion.[3] In strength training and anaerobic sports, intensity is typically measured in terms of the amount of resistance, speed, or weights used for a given routine. The amount of work performed in a given time period, or power, may also be used to describe intensity in any type of exercise.

For plyometrics, intensity can mean the amount of stress placed on muscles, joints, and connective tissue or the complexity and amount of work necessary to complete the exercise.[2,21] The intensity of plyometric drills is typically classified as low, medium, or high. As a general rule in any exercise prescription, volume decreases as intensity increases. However, in an effort to improve conditioning and endurance, early stages of plyometric exercises (or any exercise) can involve increases in both volume and intensity. When high-intensity levels are reached by the athlete, volume should decrease. The intensity of plyometric drills for the lower extremities has been related to foot contacts, direction of jump, speed, jump height, and body weight (Box 11-6).

Generally speaking, two-feet/two-legged jumps are less intense than one-foot/one-legged varieties. Raising box

Box 11-6

Factors That Determine Intensity of Lower Extremity Plyometric Exercises

- One versus two feet contact with surface
- Vertical versus horizontal direction of jump
- Horizontal speed
- Height to which center of gravity is raised

jump and hurdle heights, increasing resistance of elastic bands for the upper extremity, increasing vertical leap height and horizontal distance, using a heavier plyometric (medicine) ball, and increasing the number of hurdles are all examples of manipulating intensity. Chu and Cordier[21] and others have classified the types of plyometric exercises into groups according to increasing intensity; however, there are low- and high-intensity variations of each type of drill. For instance, although in-place jumps are generally a lower-intensity activity, a single-leg power vertical jump in place is a high-intensity variation. Similarly, lateral hops over a 6-inch hurdle are of lesser intensity than when the drill is performed using a 12- or 18-inch hurdle.

Classification of Plyometric Drills

There are basic categories of plyometric movements. A jump is defined as a movement that concludes with a two-foot landing. Examples of vertical jumps in place are tuck, pike, squat, and power jumps. A standing jump is a maximal effort jump that is horizontal, vertical, or lateral in direction.[2]

A hop is a movement that is initiated and is completed with a one-foot or two-foot landing. Hops are not maximal effort jumps and are repeated for a specific time or distance. Compared with maximal distance or vertical jumps that are used to train for explosive power, hops are typically focused on speed and agility as well. Short-response hops are usually performed for 10 repetitions or less, whereas a long-response hop would be completed for 30 m or more.[2]

Bounds represent a series of movements whereby the athlete lands on alternating feet. These are typically measured for long-response (> 60 m), but may be short-response (25 to 60 m).[2] High-intensity plyometric exercises such as in-depth and box jumps are sometimes referred to as "shock" response. These are typically performed repetitively, in sets of 5 to 10 repetitions each, depending on the individual's ability. Rarely will any high-intensity plyometric drills be performed in the rehabilitation setting. However, many of the higher-intensity drills can be modified for use in the athletic training room or clinic. For example, jumps from a 6-inch step would be a low-intensity variation of a high-intensity box jump.

The listing in Box 11-7 is a sample of some low-, medium-, and high-intensity plyometric drills. The reader is encouraged to consult the referenced sources for a more complete presentation of the many exercises and drills for both the upper and lower extremities.[2,13,20,21]

Generally speaking, low-intensity drills will be performed in the athletic training room or clinic. These might include in-place jumps, standing jumps, low-intensity/short-distance hops and low-height box jumps. Chu and Cordier[21] recommended that low-intensity depth jumps, known as "jump or drop downs," be performed in the athletic training room or clinic to improve eccentric strength. The patient simply steps off (does not jump) and lands on the ground without rebounding with a jump. In other words, this amounts to performing the first two phases of the SSC, i.e., preloading/eccentric and amortization, although the amortization phase is purposely too long, and the elastic energy is being lost as heat in the musculotendinous unit. As the patient's condition improves, he or she progresses to completing the concentric phase while attempting to decrease the amortization phase and increase the height or distance achieved by the concentric phase jump.

Volume

The volume of plyometric drills is a key component in that it is inherently related to intensity and stress to which bones, articular cartilage, ligaments, muscles, and tendons

Box 11-7

Categories of Plyometric Drills by Intensity with Examples

Low intensity	*Lower extremity:* squat jump, split squat jump, ankle bounces, lateral hurdle/cone jump
	Upper extremity: medicine ball chest pass, underhand medicine ball throw, overhead throw
Medium intensity	*Lower extremity:* pike jump, lateral hops, double and single leg pike jump, double leg tuck jump, standing triple jump, zigzag cone hops, double leg hop, alternate leg bounds, combination bound
	Upper extremity: medicine ball push-up, standing or kneeling side throw, backward throw
High intensity	*Lower extremity:* in-depth jumps, box-jumps, single leg vertical power jump, single leg tuck jump
	Upper extremity: drop push-up, medicine ball push-up

are exposed. This is an especially important factor for avoidance of overuse injury in a patient who has progressed well in rehabilitation. Specifically, this patient has reached all goals for range of motion, strength, and flexibility in the athletic training room or clinic and has begun to tolerate plyometric drills at some level. Although he or she may be prepared to tolerate both low- and medium-intensity plyometric drills, the patient's ability to tolerate the repetitive stresses from volume may not be evident until an overuse injury, such as patellar tendonitis, has developed. Thus, it is critical that rehabilitation specialists be cautious in the progression of a plyometric training program.

Volume in plyometrics is typically expressed as the number of foot contacts or throws of the medicine ball; the distance jumped can also represent volume. Volume is also an expression of the amount of work performed. The analog of volume in weight training is the product of the number of repetitions times the number of sets performed; repetitions and sets are appropriate terminology for most upper body plyometric exercises. Foot contacts are defined as the number of times a foot, or both feet together, make contact with the surface during each workout session.

As always, the status of the patient/athlete dictates how much volume (and intensity, duration, and recovery) is appropriate. Table 11-1 provides general recommendations for volume and intensity in a plyometric training session.[2,20,21]

Duration

Duration implies how long an exercise session lasts. Although on the surface this would seem appropriate only for cardiovascular conditioning, it is useful for plyometric sessions as well. It is true that volume and intensity will ultimately determine the duration of a session; however, duration is an excellent indicator of the patient's conditioning level. Specifically, if the patient's plyometric sessions are taking 30 minutes instead of the 20 minutes

planned, then the clinician should examine the recovery times between exercises. For example, perhaps the patient needs 5 minutes of rest between drills when you had planned on allowing only 2 to 3 minutes. This could be an indication that the current program is too intense for the patient, that the patient needs to do more cardiovascular conditioning work or that the patient is not anaerobically fit enough to tolerate this level of training volume or intensity.

Traditionally, plyometric sessions are geared for healthy athletes with adequate strength training backgrounds and good motor skills. Thus, the sessions are intense and focus on powerful, speed-strength movements. Accordingly, sessions are usually 15 to 30 minutes long. For the athlete undergoing rehabilitation, this can still be a useful plyometric session duration. However, the duration could be lengthened to accommodate the need for lower-intensity exercise and longer recovery periods. Duration is a programming variable that is highly specific to the status of the patient and the goals established during the rehabilitation process.

Recovery

Because plyometric drills involve maximum efforts on the part of the patient, recovery is extremely important. Recovery can include both rest between repetitions, sets, or drills within a given exercise session or the amount of rest a patient needs between actual sessions (in days). As mentioned previously for intensity, volume, and duration, recovery between drills during the session is an important factor in dictating the metabolic intensity of a workout. There is a threshold of anaerobic or glycolytic endurance that an athlete needs to be able to tolerate a full plyometric training session. Generally speaking, the more intense a workout is, the more rest the athlete needs between sets, exercises, or drills during a particular training session. As the athlete gets fatigued during the session, he or she will perceive the plyometric drills to be more intense or difficult. Fatigue also increases the risk for injury. It is very

Table 11-1

Recommended Volumes and Intensity for Each Plyometric Training Session Based on Patient Status and Plyometric Experience

Patient/Athlete	Number of Contacts	Intensity	Suggestions
Patient in orthopedic/sports medicine outpatient clinic	30	Low	Increase number of contacts before increasing intensity; 10% increase in contacts when 30 tolerated
Beginner	80-100	Low → medium	Primarily low, increase to medium during mid-workout when not fatigued
Intermediate	100-120	Low → medium → high	Attempt high when not fatigued
Advanced	120-140	Low → medium → high	Primarily medium and high

important that recovery periods during the session are appropriate for the conditioning and skill level of the athlete as well as the prescribed volume/intensity of the program. One of the primary reasons for this is that plyometric drills are for developing functional speed-strength, not for improving conditioning. And as mentioned previously, type II fibers are more easily fatigued, despite their force-generating capacity for plyometrics. Nonetheless, it is important to match the level of conditioning accompanying these drills to the specific metabolic demands of the sport. For example, a hurdler must be conditioned anaerobically enough to complete hurdles over a 10- to 30-second interval. A basketball player must be conditioned well enough to jump repetitively as well as run, cut, and leap intermittently over the course of several minutes at a time. High-intensity drills such as in-depth jumps and box jumps require 5 to 10 seconds of recovery between repetitions and 2 to 3 minutes between sets.[2]

As mentioned previously, muscle groups and joint complexes should not be subjected to plyometric drills on consecutive days. Two to 4 days between plyometric workouts is a general guideline, but this is mostly dictated by intensity and the status of the patient.[2,21] It is assumed that the athlete is performing strength and conditioning workouts on other days. An athlete may be able to perform some strength and endurance training on the same day as the plyometric workout, but use of body parts should be alternated. For example, one might perform upper body strength training on the same day that lower body plyometric exercises are performed. Alternatively, one might do a light-intensity endurance workout as part of the warm-up or cool-down on a plyometric training day.

According to Chu and Cordier,[21] the work-to-rest ratio should be 1:5 to 1:10 to be certain that the intensity and proper execution of the movement are preserved. Thus, a 10-second repetition of jumps should be followed by 50 to 100 seconds of rest before the next repetition is begun. If the set is composed of 10 repetitions this would yield about 100 seconds of actual work for the set and 500 to 1000 seconds of rest would need to be included in the set. Stone and Bryant, as cited in Chu and Cordier,[21] suggested that about 1 to 5 minutes of rest is needed between plyometric exercises, depending on the intensity and volume of the workout. Metabolically, high-intensity plyometrics utilize the phosphagen and anaerobic energy systems, depending on the duration of a given drill. Recovery periods that are too short for adequate recovery limit the athlete's ability to develop phosphagen and anaerobic metabolic systems.

In contrast, as stated earlier, a basic level of endurance is needed to perform plyometric exercises and to perform in a given sport or activity. In the early stages of rehabilitation it is often necessary to incorporate an endurance component within the plyometric training program. In this case, the rest period needs to be shorter, because the activity needs to also tax the aerobic or oxidative metabolic

processes of the muscle. The clinician can monitor aerobic intensity via the training heart rate. It is well documented that training at 60% maximum heart rate is a minimum level of intensity to generate aerobic improvements.[3] In practical terms, this would indicate the need for a work-to-rest ratio of 1:1 or 1:4 to stress the oxidative and fast glycolysis systems.[2]

In summary, if it has been determined that the patient is capable of tolerating maximal power exercise, then longer rest periods can be implemented. To improve anaerobic power, more rest is needed. During earlier stages of rehabilitation, it is probably more appropriate to utilize low- to medium-intensity plyometrics with longer intervals of recovery. Despite the fact that plyometrics have been traditionally reserved for healthy athletes attempting to maximize power and speed-strength, there is a place in the clinical setting for low-level plyometrics that stress both the oxidative and glycolytic systems as a precursor to more aggressive plyometrics as the patient's condition improves. Indeed, low-intensity plyometrics can be focused on improving the patient's eccentric strength, coordination, and agility; promoting normal myotatic reflexes; and restoring functional ability.[21]

Muscle Fatigue, Muscle Damage, and Plyometrics

Plyometrics incorporate a significant amount of eccentric muscle activity, and unaccustomed eccentric anaerobic exercise has been associated with an immediate decrease in tension-generating capacity, a shift in optimum muscle length, and changes in excitation-contraction coupling.[51] Eccentric resistance exercise has also been associated with increased delayed-onset muscle soreness, muscle tenderness, and weakness in healthy individuals.[54,57,58]

Exercise-induced muscle damage and injury have been studied by many investigators.[7,19,42,46,54] Kyrolainen and colleagues[46] studied muscle damage after strenuous SSC exercise in power and endurance groups of athletes who performed 400 jumps and found elevated serum levels of creatine kinase, myoglobin, and carbonic anhydrase. Levels of these blood proteins are often measured as an indication of skeletal muscle damage. Even among these athletic groups, the authors observed differences in physiologic responses between endurance and power athletes that they attributed to differences in muscle fiber type distribution, differences in recruitment order of motor units, or differences in response to power-type strength exercises. Again, the importance of closely monitoring the volume, intensity, duration, and recovery time of plyometric training programs cannot be overemphasized.

Progression of Plyometric Exercise Training

Plyometric sessions can be progressed by manipulating the variables mentioned earlier: intensity, volume, duration, and frequency. Patients begin with low-intensity lower extremity drills and are progressed to medium- and high-intensity exercises only when they have regained enough strength, range of motion, and joint integrity and have mastered basic plyometric movements. Chu and Cordier[21] recommended that patients spend 12 to 18 weeks performing low- and medium-intensity plyometric drills. Two-legged drills are a good starting point for lower extremity plyometrics, with progression to single-leg jumps and hops. A progression of lower extremity exercises is presented in Figures 11-1 to 11-12.

For the upper extremity, two-arm throws with a light ball are a good starting point. Cordaso and co-workers[24] used EMG recordings to determine the muscle activity during the two-arm plyometric ball throw in 10 healthy males. In the cocking phase, the upper trapezius, pectoralis major, and anterior deltoid muscles showed high activity (>40% to 60% maximum manual test) and the rotator cuff muscles had moderate activity (>20% to 40%). In the acceleration phase, five of the muscles demonstrated high levels of activity (>40% to 60%), and the upper trapezius and lower subscapularis muscles had very high levels of activity (>60%). Analysis of the deceleration phase revealed high activity in the upper trapezius muscle and moderate activity in all other muscles except the pectoralis major. These findings support the use of medicine ball training as a bridge between static resistive training and dynamic throwing in the rehabilitation process. The athlete is progressed from two-arm throws to one-arm throws. The cocking motion of throwing places a stretch on the shoulder muscles and is followed by a concentric contraction, incorporating the SSC into this type of plyometric training. A progression of upper extremity exercises is shown in Figures 11-13 to 11-20.

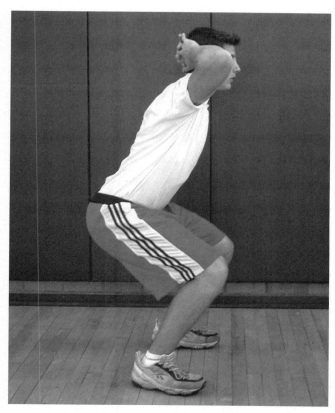

Figure 11-1. Squat jump (low intensity). With feet shoulder-width apart, the athlete begins by squatting down to approximately 90° knee flexion while simultaneously maintaining lumbar lordosis with weight equally distributed on heels and forefeet; hands should be behind the head with fingers interlocked. With no arm movement, the athlete performs a maximal vertical jump, and upon landing, immediately repeats the squat and jumps again. One set of 5 to 10 repetitions is performed. The amortization phase is slightly longer for this exercise to absorb landing until skill and strength improve.

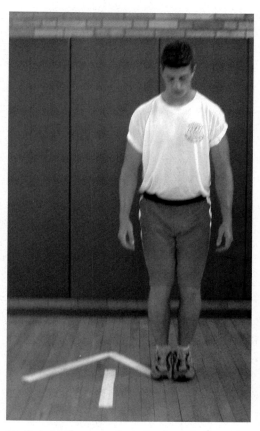

Figure 11-2. Ankle bounces (low intensity). With feet 6 to 10 inches apart, the athlete jumps in the shape of a V, then laterally, and forward/backward. Ten jumps in each direction should be performed for a total of 30 repetitions in 60 seconds; reduce the time allotted to increase agility and speed.

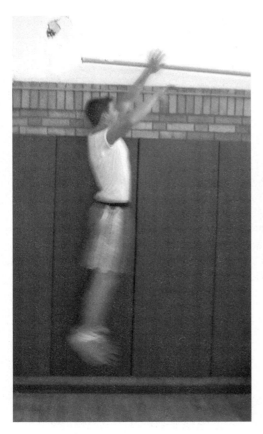

Figure 11-3. Standing jump and reach (low to medium intensity). Standing close to a target on the wall or near an object suspended overhead and feet shoulder-width apart, the athlete performs a half-squat, using double-arm action (extension → flexion) and jumps to maximal height while reaching with one hand for the target each time. Upon landing, the athlete repeats the slight squat and jumps without taking any steps before jumping. The amortization time is slightly longer for beginners; progress to reducing amortization time. Three sets of 5 to 10 repetitions are performed.

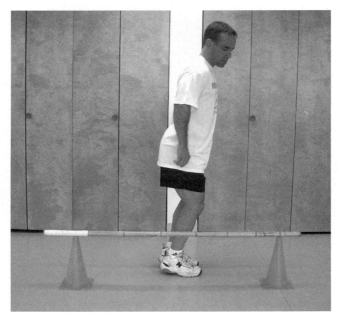

Figure 11-4. Lateral hurdle hops (low to medium intensity). Using a short cone or low 6- to 8-inch hurdle and keeping the feet together, the athlete jumps laterally over the hurdle as quickly as possible and repeats in the opposite direction. Most of the work should come from ankle action, but natural flexion of knees and hips should be used to clear the hurdle. Three sets of 10 to 15 repetitions are performed.

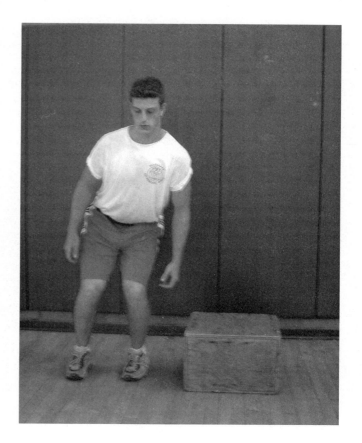

Figure 11-5. Thirty-second lateral box drill (low to medium intensity). Standing next to a 4- to 8-inch box or step with feet shoulder-width apart, the athlete jumps laterally with both feet onto the box, then off to the ground on the opposite side, and continues without stopping for 15 to 30 seconds. Ankles, knees, and hips should be used to absorb landings. Progress to reducing amortization time or increasing the height of the step/box to increase intensity.

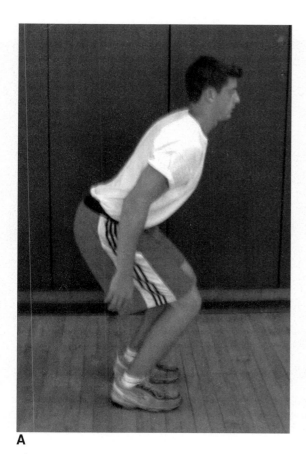

A

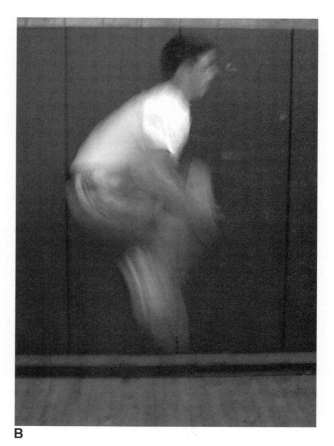

B

Figure 11-6. Double-leg tuck jump (medium intensity). Standing with feet shoulder-width apart, the athlete performs a half-squat with double-arm action, then immediately explodes vertically while pulling both knees to the chest, grasping both knees with both hands and quickly releasing as descent begins. Spending minimal time on the ground, the athlete repeats the sequence. One set of 10 repetitions is performed.

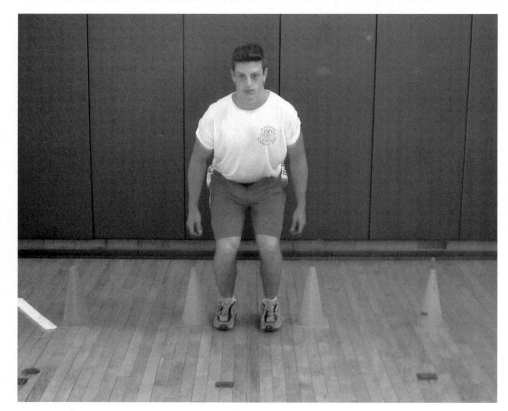

Figure 11-7. Lateral cone hops (medium intensity). Three to five cones or other obstacles are placed in a straight line, about 3 feet apart, depending on the ability and height of the athlete. Standing with feet shoulder-width apart at the end of the row of cones, the athlete jumps laterally down the row of cones, landing on both feet. At the end of the row the athlete changes directions and returns, spending minimal time on the ground. Three sets of 5 to 10 repetitions are performed (1 repetition = 1 lap, return to start position).

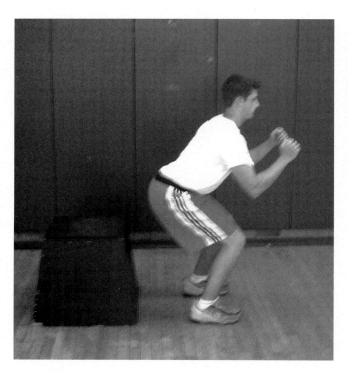

Figure 11-8. Jump from box (medium intensity). Standing on top of a 6- to 18-inch box with feet shoulder-width apart, the athlete squats slightly and jumps slightly from the box onto the floor, concentrating on absorbing landing forces and "sticking" the landing with no loss of balance or sway. A vertical jump from the box should NOT be performed; the jump direction is more horizontal than vertical. One set of 10 repetitions is performed.

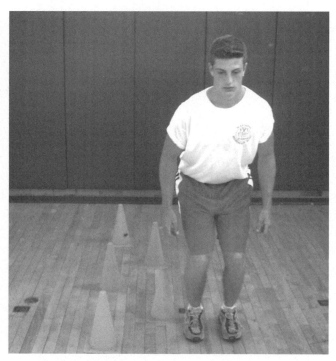

Figure 11-9. Double-leg zigzag cone hops (medium to high intensity). Five to 10 cones or similar obstacles are placed in a zigzag pattern about 20 to 30 inches apart. The athlete hops diagonally over each cone, spending minimal time on the ground between each cone while changing direction. The athlete should get as much vertical leap as possible and attempt to "hang" in the air to clear each cone with shoulders maintained perpendicularly to an imaginary straight line between the cones. One set of 5 to 10 repetitions is performed (1 repetition equals one trip down the row of cones).

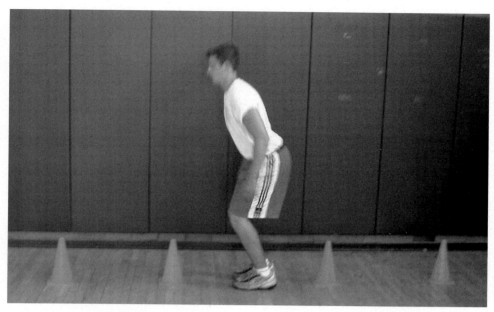

Figure 11-10. Hurdle jumps (medium to high intensity). Three to five hurdles are placed in a row. With feet shoulder-width apart, the athlete begins with a half-squat with double-arm action and leaps over hurdles consecutively, bringing the knees high and spending minimal time on the ground with each jump. Five to 10 repetitions are performed (1 repetition equals one trip down the row of hurdles).

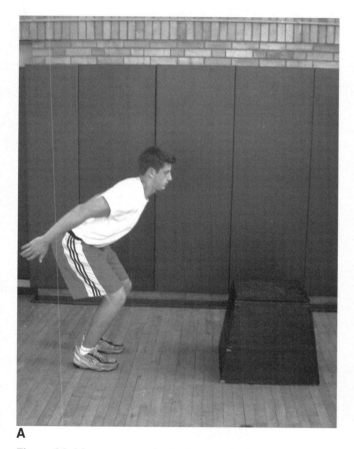

A

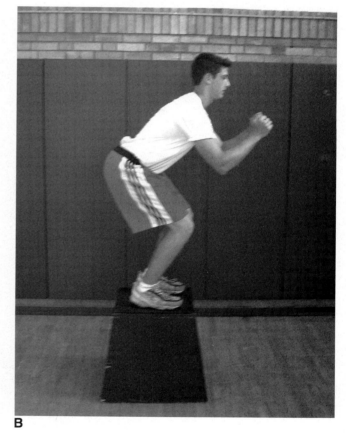

B

Figure 11-11. Box jumps (high intensity). Standing on the ground with feet shoulder-width apart about 2 feet in front of a box, the athlete performs a slight squat with double-arm action and jumps explosively forward and vertically onto the box. After a brief landing on the box top, the athlete jumps vertically and horizontally onto the ground. If multiple boxes are available, the athlete immediately jumps to the next box of equal height; if only one box is used, the athlete turns around and repeats. Two sets of 5 to 10 repetitions are performed.

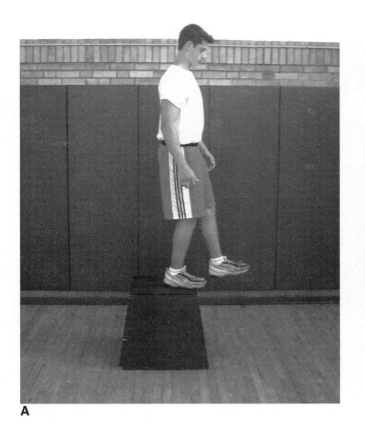

A

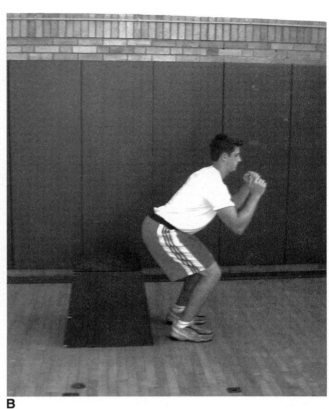

B

Figure 11-12. In-depth jumps (high intensity). The athlete starts by standing at the edge of the top of the box with feet shoulder-width apart and then steps (NOT jumps) off the box, landing on the balls of the feet to absorb the landing, but minimizes time on the ground and immediately jumps vertically or horizontally explosively, using double-arm action. One set of 5 to 10 repetitions is performed.

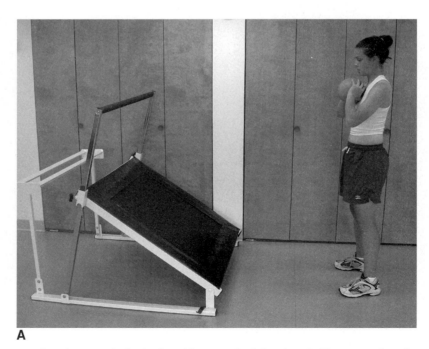

A

Figure 11-13. Chest pass. Standing facing a plyoback, the athlete uses both hands to hold a 3-pound medicine ball against the chest and pushes the ball away from the chest into the plyoback, allowing the ball to return to the starting position as he or she catches it.

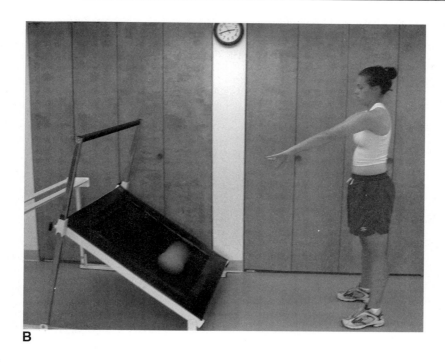

Figure 11-13. cont'd.

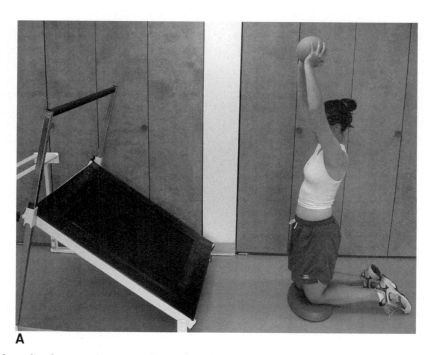

Figure 11-14. Two-hand overhead soccer throw. Standing or kneeling facing a plyoback, the athlete holds a 3- to 5-pound medicine ball in both hands, raises the ball overhead, and then throws it into the plyoback. The athlete catches the ball overhead as it rebounds.

Continued

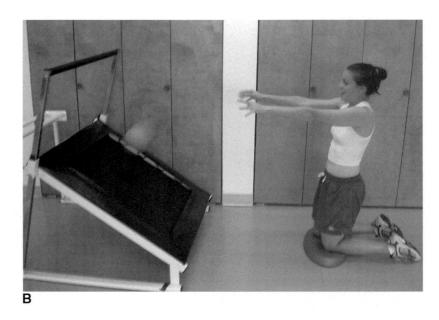

B

Figure 11-14. cont'd.

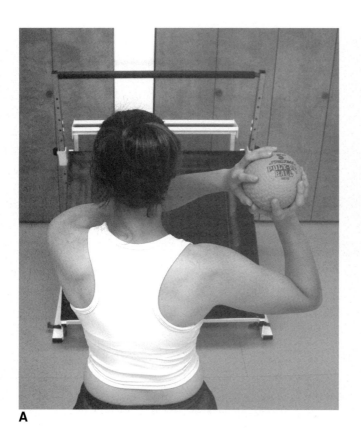

A

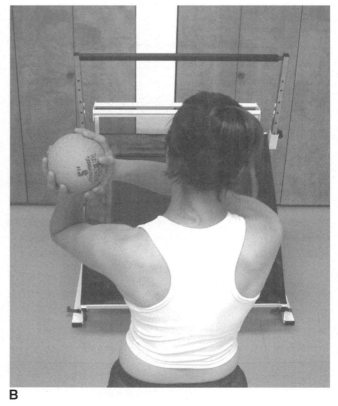

B

Figure 11-15. Two-hand side-to-side throw. Standing facing a plyoback, the athlete holds a 3- to 5-pound medicine ball with both hands, positioned over one shoulder, throws the ball into the plyoback, then catches it with both hands over the opposite shoulder, and continues by alternating sides. This exercise can also be used to train the rotation of the hips and trunk by allowing the body to rotate slightly as the ball is caught.

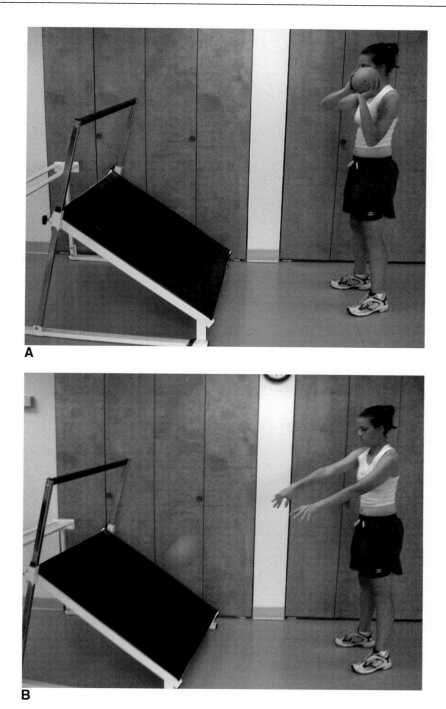

Figure 11-16. Two-hand side throw. Standing sideways in front of a plyoback, the athlete holds a small medicine ball in both hands, brings the ball over one shoulder, then throws it in a side arm fashion into the plyoback, and catches the ball, allowing the body to turn slightly.

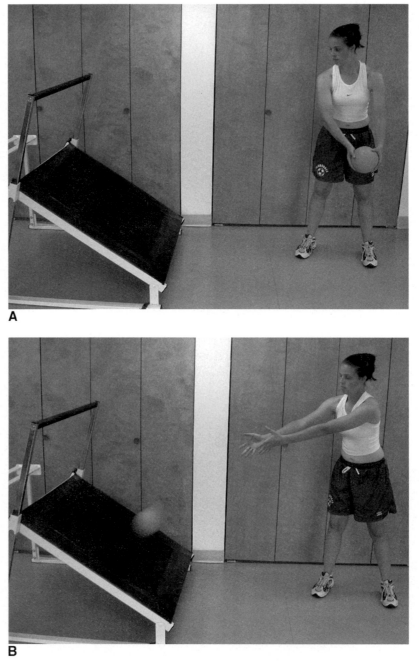

A

B

Figure 11-17. Two-hand underhand throw. Standing sideways in front of a plyoback, the athlete holds a medicine ball with both hands in front below waist level, brings the ball over to one side, throws it in an underhand fashion against the plyoback, catches the ball, and then throws it again.

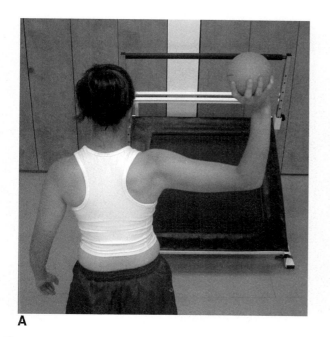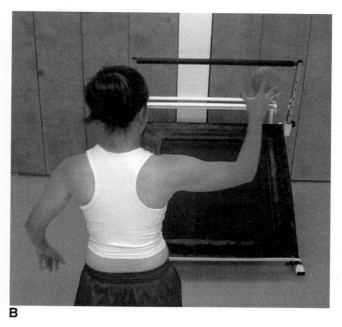

A   **B**

Figure 11-18. Baseball toss at 90/90. Standing facing a plyoback with the arm at a 90° angle away from the body with the elbow bent to 90° (cocking position), the athlete holds a 2-pound medicine ball, forcefully throws the ball into the plyoback, and then catches it as it rebounds, maintaining the same position of the arm and elbow. This exercise can also be used to train the legs and trunk to accelerate the arm by stepping out as the ball is thrown.

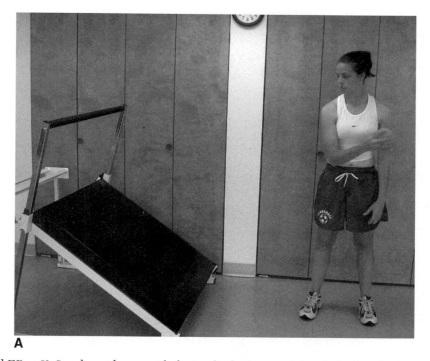

A

Figure 11-19. Backhand ER at 0°. Standing sideways with the involved side toward the plyoback and a 1- to 3-pound medicine ball in the involved hand and keeping the upper arm against the body with the elbow bent to 90°, the athlete rotates the arm toward the chest, forcefully rotates out, throwing the ball into the plyoback, and tries to catch the ball as it rebounds with the palm toward the body and the upper arm close to the side.

Continued

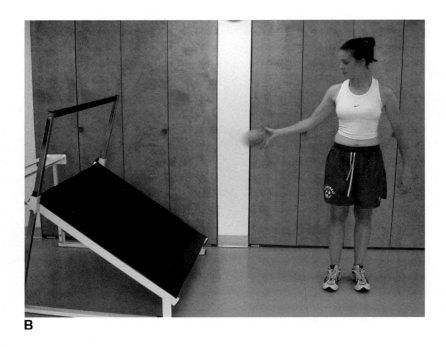

B

Figure 11-19, cont'd.

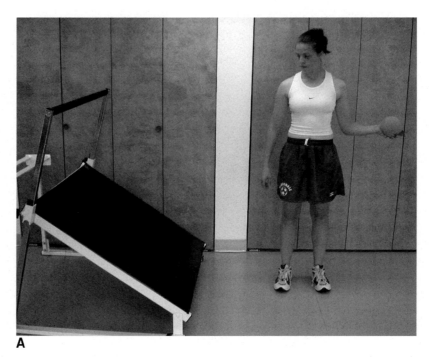

A

Figure 11-20. Backhand IR at 0°. Standing sideways with the uninvolved side nearest the plyoback and a 1- to 3-pound medicine ball in the involved hand and keeping the upper arm of the involved side close to the body with the elbow bent at 90°, the athlete allows the arm to rotate out, forcefully throws the ball into the plyoback, and catch the ball while maintaining the upper arm against the body.

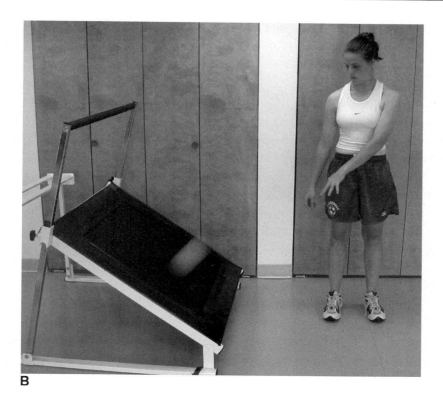

B

Figure 11-20, cont'd.

SUMMARY

- Plyometrics are based on the theory of the SSC, whereby the active lengthening (eccentric contraction) of the agonist muscle produces energy that is stored in the musculotendinous unit to be subsequently used in a more powerful and efficient concentric contraction. This eccentric-concentric coupling forms the basis of the SSC.

- There are three neuromuscular anatomical/physiologic areas important in understanding the biomechanics of plyometrics: (1) the serial elastic and histologic components of muscles and tendons, i.e., sarcomeres, fiber types, sliding filaments, and metabolic properties; (2) proprioception mediated through muscle spindles and GTOs and their contribution to the stretch reflex; and (3) gross muscle-tendon complex architecture.

- The three phases of the SSC and plyometric exercise are the eccentric phase, amortization phase, and concentric phase. The eccentric phase is the loading of the muscle spindle during the eccentric contraction and storage of elastic energy. The amortization phase is the transition from eccentric to concentric muscle activity; this phase should be as short as possible to minimize the loss of elastic energy as heat in the muscle. The explosive concentric contraction is the final phase.

- Patients must be thoroughly evaluated before they participate in a rehabilitation program with plyometrics,

and goals established at the beginning of treatment should be considered. Generally, the patient must have no joint effusion or inflammation, normal range of motion, normal joint alignment and mobility, soft tissue integrity and flexibility, adequate strength both eccentrically and concentrically, normal reflexes, normal coordination, and no pain during exercise.

- Strength and conditioning are of utmost importance for safe and effective plyometric training. Muscle performance tests via exercise as well as functional tests of strength should be administered before the clinician initiates plyometrics.

- Adequate warm-up and a variety of stretching exercises are warranted before plyometric training. These should include a full body warm-up for 5 to 10 minutes followed by static stretching and movements that mimic the drills to be performed. Controlled ballistic stretching and proprioceptive neuromuscular facilitation stretching are also useful adjuncts.

- When a plyometric training program is initiated, a shock-absorbing surface and sturdy cross-training shoes are critical for safe performance of lower extremity drills. Equipment is generally simple and can include rubber-padded wooden boxes, hurdles, cones, medicine balls, physioballs, and special strength shoes.

- Frequency, intensity, volume, and duration components of exercise prescription are extremely important. By definition, plyometrics require maximal effort, so manipulating these components for effective and safe training sessions is important to reduce the risk of overuse injury and overtraining. Volume is generally reflected in the total number of foot contacts during a given session. Intensity is mostly related to two-feet versus one-foot contacts, vertical and horizontal distances jumped, speed, height of jump, body weight, and any added resistance applied. Frequency is simply the number of training sessions per week, and duration is the length of the workout session.

■ For lower extremity plyometric exercises, two-feet contacts are generally less intense than one-foot contacts. Plyometric exercises are typically classified into low-, medium- and high-intensity categories. The individual exercises include jumps, hops, and bounds for the lower extremity. Upper extremity plyometric exercises often use a medicine ball and include weight-bearing push-up type exercises.

■ Recovery is a critical element of plyometric programming. As a general rule of thumb, plyometric workouts should only be conducted a maximum of two or three times per week. Track and field sports are traditionally more likely to utilize plyometric sessions more than twice per week. Major muscle groups should never be targeted in plyometric workouts on successive days. Although strength and endurance training can be performed concurrently with plyometrics in a comprehensive rehabilitation program, it is important to mix and match training sessions to prevent overuse and other injuries. For example, performing upper body strength training on the same day as lower extremity plyometrics would be a possible option.

■ Overall, high-intensity plyometrics will rarely be used in athletic training rooms and clinics during rehabilitation. Rather, low- and medium-intensity drills will most likely be used. Patients in outpatient clinics will mostly be limited to low-intensity drills and roughly 30 contacts per workout to begin the program, while working to a volume of 80 to 100 contacts per workout.

■ The clinician is encouraged to use his or her creativity to customize plyometric programming to achieve the best functional outcomes for patients.

REFERENCES

1. Adams, K., O'Shea, J.P., O'Shea, K.L., and Climstein, M. (1992): The effect of 6 weeks of squat, plyometric and squat-plyometric training on power production. J. Appl. Sport Sci. Res., 6:36-41.

2. Allerheiligen, W.B. (1994): Speed development and plyometric training. In: Baechle, T.R. (ed.), Essentials of Strength and Conditioning, 2nd ed., Champaign, IL, Human Kinetics, pp. 314-344.

3. American College of Sports Medicine. (2000): ACSM's Guidelines for Exercise Testing and Prescription, 6th ed. Philadelphia, Lippincott Williams & Wilkins, p. 141.

4. Aura, O., and Komi, P.V. (1986): The mechanical efficiency of locomotion in men and women with special emphasis on stretch-shortening cycle exercises. Eur. J. Appl. Physiol., 55:37-43.

5. Avela, J., Santos, P.M., and Komi, P.V. (1996): Effects of differently induced stretch loads on neuromuscular control in drop jump exercise. Eur. J. Appl. Physiol., 72:553-562.

6. Avela, J., and Komi, P.V. (1998): Interaction between muscle stiffness and stretch reflex sensitivity after long-term stretch-shortening cycle exercise. Muscle Nerve, 21:1224-1227.

7. Balnave, C.D., and Thompson, M.W. (1993): Effect of training on eccentric exercise-induced muscle damage. J. Appl. Physiol., 75:1545-1551.

8. Bandy, W.D., and Irion, J.M. (1994): The effect of time on static stretch on the flexibility of the hamstring muscles. Phys. Ther., 74:845-852.

9. Bauer, T., Thayer, R.E., and Baras, G. (1990): Comparison of training modalities for power development in the lower extremity. J. Appl. Sport Sci. Res., 4:115-121.

10. Benn, C., Forman, K., Mathewson, D., et al. (1998): The effects of serial stretch loading on stretch work and stretch-shorten cycle performance in the knee musculature. J. Orthop. Sports Phys. Ther., 27:412-422.

11. Besier, T.F., Lloyd, D.G., Cochrane, J.L., et al. (2001): External loading of the knee joint during running and cutting maneuvers. Med. Sci. Sports Exerc., 33:1168-1175.

12. Blakey, J.B., and Southard, D. (1987): The combined effects of weight training and plyometrics on dynamic leg strength and leg power. J. Appl. Sports Sci. Res. 1:14-16.

13. Bompa, T.O. (1999): Periodization Training for Sports. Champaign, IL, Human Kinetics.

14. Bonutti, P.M., Windau, J.E., Ables, B.A., et al. (1994): Static progressive stretch to reestablish elbow range of motion. Clin. Orthop., June:128-134.

15. Borkowski, J. (1990): Prevention of preseason muscle soreness: Plyometric exercise. Athl. Train., 25:122.

16. Bosco, C., Tihanyi, J., Komi, P.V., et al. (1982): Store and recoil of elastic energy in slow and fast types of human skeletal muscles. Acta. Physiol. Scand., 116:343-349.

17. Brownstein, B., and Bronner, S. (1997): Functional Movement. New York, Churchill Livingstone.

18. Cavagna, G.A. (1977): Storage and utilization of elastic energy in skeletal muscle. Exer. Sports Sci. Rev., 5:89-129.

19. Clarkson, P.M., Nosaka, K., and Braun, B. (1992): Muscle function after exercise-induced muscle damage and rapid adaptation. Med. Sci. Sports Exerc., 24:512-520.

20. Chu, D.A. (1992): Understanding plyometrics. In: Chu, D.A.: Jumping into Plyometrics. Champaign, IL, Lesiure Press, pp. 1-4.

21. Chu, D.A., and Cordier, D.J. (1998): Plyometrics—Specific applications in orthopedics. In: Orthopaedic Physical Therapy Home Study Course 98-A, Strength and Conditioning Applications in Orthopaedics. Orthopaedic Section, APTA, Inc., LaCrosse, WI.

22. Clutch, D., Wilton, M., McGown, C., and Bryce, G.R. (1983): The effect of depths jumps and weight training on leg strength and vertical jump. Res. Q., 54:1-10.

23. Condon, S.N., and Hutton, R.S. (1987): Soleus muscle electromyographic activity and ankle dorsiflexion range of motion during four stretching procedures. Phys. Ther., 67:24.

24. Cordaso, F.A., Wolfe, I.N., Wootten, M.E., and Bigliani, L.U. (1996): An electromyographic analysis of the shoulder during

a medicine ball rehabilitation program. Am. J. Sports Med., 34: 386-392.

25. Costill, D.L., and Wilmore, J.H. (1994): Physiology of Sport and Exercise. Champaign, IL, Human Kinetics.

26. Dryek, D.A. (1994): Assessment and treatment planning strategies for musculoskeletal deficits. In: O'Sullivan, S.B., and Schmitz, T.J. (ed.), Physical Rehabilitation: Assessment and Treatment, 3rd ed. Philadelphia, F.A. Davis, pp. 1-4.

27. Dyhre-Poulsen, P., and Laursen, A.M. (1984): Programmed electromyographic activity and negative incremental muscle stiffness on monkeys jumping downward. J. Physiol., 350:121-136.

28. Enoka, R.M. (1996): Eccentric contractions require unique activation strategies by the nervous system. J. Appl. Physiol., 81:2339-2346.

29. Godges, J.J., Engelke, K.A., Faehling, C.J., et al. (1989): The effects of two stretching procedures on hip range of motion and gait economy. J. Orthop. Sports Phys. Ther., 10:350-356.

30. Gollhofer, A., Komi, P.V., Fujitsuka, N., et al. (1987): Fatigue during stretch-shortening cycle exercises. II. Changes in neuromuscular activation patterns of human skeletal muscle. Int. J. Sports Med., 8:38-47.

31. Goslow, G.E., Reinking, R.M., and Stuart, D.G. (1973): The cat step cycle: Hind limb joint angles and muscle lengths during unrestrained locomotion. J. Morphol., 141:1-42.

32. Grimston, S.K., Willows, N.D., and Hanley, D.A. (1993): Mechanical loading regime and its relationship to BMD in children. Med. Sci. Sports Exerc., 25:1203-1210.

33. Halbertsma, J.P., van Bolhuis, A.I., and Goecken, L.N. (1996): Sport stretching: effect on passive muscle stiffness of short hamstrings. Arch. Phys. Med. Rehabil., 77:688-692.

34. Heiderscheit, B.C., McLean, K.P., Davies, G.J. (1996): The effects of isokinetic vs. plyometric training on the shoulder internal rotators. J. Orthop. Sports Phys. Ther., 23:125-133.

35. Heinonen, A., Oja, P., Kannus, P., et al. (1995): BMD of female athletes representing sports with different loading characteristics of the skeleton. Bone, 17:197-203.

36. Helgeson, K., and Gajdosik, R. (1993): The stretch-shortening cycle of the quadriceps femoris muscle group measured by isokinetic dynamometry. J. Orthop. Sports Phys. Ther., 17:17-23.

37. Hewett, T.E., Stroupe, A.L., Naunce, T.A., and Noyes, F.R. (1996): Plyometric training in female athletes. Decreased impact forces and increased hamstring torques. Am. J. Sports Med., 24:765-773.

38. Hewett, T.E., Lindenfeld, T.N., Riccobene, J.V., and Noyes, F.R. (1999): The effect of neuromuscular training on the incidence of knee injury in female athletes. A prospective study. Am. J. Sports Med., 27:699-706.

39. Hlasney, J. (1988): Effect of flexibility exercises on muscle strength. Phys. Ther. Forum, 7:3, 15.

40. Huston, L.J., and Wojtys, E.M. (1996): Neuromuscular performance characteristics in elite female athletes. Am. J. Sports Med., 24:427-436.

41. Kandel, E.R., Schwartz, J.H., and Jessel, T.M. (1995): Essentials of Neural Science and Behavior. Stamford, CT, Appleton & Lange.

42. Komi, P.V., Gollhofer, A., Schmidtbleicher, D., et al. (1987): Interaction between man and shoe in running: Considerations for a more comprehensive measurement approach. Int. J. Sports Med., 8:196-202.

43. Komi, P.V. (2000): Stretch-shortening cycle: A powerful model to study normal and fatigued muscle. J. Biomech., 33:1197-1206.

44. Kraemer, W.J., Ratamess, N.A., Volek, J.S., et al. (2000): The effect of the Meridian shoe on vertical jump and sprint performances following short-term combined plyometric/sprint and resistance training. J. Strength Cond. Res., 14:228-238.

45. Kubo, K., Kanehisa, H., Takeshita, D., et al. (2000): In vivo dynamics of human medial gastrocnemius muscle-tendon complex during stretch-shortening cycle exercise. Acta. Physiol. Scand., 170:127-135.

46. Kyrolainen, H., Takala, T.E.S., and Komi, P.V. (1998): Muscle damage induced by stretch-shortening cycle exercise. Med. Sci. Sports Exerc., 30(3):415-420.

47. Lanyon, L.E. (1987): Functional strain in bone tissue as the objective and controlling stimulus for adaptive bone remodeling. J. Biomech., 20:1083-1095.

48. McBride, J.M., Triplett-McBride, T., and Davie, A., et al. (2002): The effect of heavy-vs. light-load jump squats on the development of strength, power and speed. J. Strength Cond. Res., 16(1):75-82.

49. McCall, G.E., Byrnes, W.C., Dickinson, B.A., et al. (1996): Muscle fiber hypertrophy, hyperplasia and capillary density in college men after resistance training. J. Appl. Physiol., 81: 2004-2012.

50. Melvill Jones, G., and Watt, D. (1971): Observation on control of jumping and hopping movements in man. J. Physiol., 219:709-727.

51. Morgan, D.L., and Allen, D.G. (1999): Early events in stretch-induced muscle damage. J. Appl. Physiol., 87:2007-2015.

52. Nardone, A., Romano, C., and Schieppetti, M. (1989): Selective recruitment of high-threshold human motor units during voluntary isotonic lengthening of active muscles. J. Physiol. (Lond.), 409:451-471.

53. Narici, M.V., Roi, G.S., Landoni, L., et al. (1989): Changes in force, cross-sectional area and neural activation during strength training and detraining of the human quadriceps. Eur. J. Appl. Physiol., 59: 310-319.

54. Newham, D.J., Jones, D.A., and Clarkson, P.M. (1987): Repeated high-force eccentric exercise: Effects on muscle pain and damage. J. Appl. Physiol., 63:1381-1386.

55. Nicol, C., Komi, P.V., Horita, T., et al. (1996): Reduced stretch reflex sensitivity after exhaustive stretch-shortening cycle (SSC) exercise. Eur. J. Appl. Physiol., 72:401-409.

56. Sale, D.G. (1988): Neural adaptation to resistance training. Med. Sci. Sports Exerc., 20:S135-S145.

57. Saxton, J.M., and Donnelly, A.E. (1996): Length-specific impairment of skeletal muscle contractile function after eccentric muscle actions in man. Clin. Sci. (Colch.), 90:119-125.

58. Smith, L.L. (1991): Acute inflammation: The underlying mechanism in delayed-onset muscle soreness? Med. Sci. Sports Sci., 23:542-551.

59. Staron, R.S., Hikida, R.S., Hagerman, F.C., et al. (1984): Human skeletal muscle fiber type adaptability to various workloads. J. Histochem. Cytochem., 32:146-152.

60. Strojnik, V., and Komi, P.V. (2000): Fatigue after submaximal intensive stretch-shortening cycle exercise. Med. Sci. Sports Exerc., 32:1314-1319.

61. Sugi, H., and Tsuchiya, T. (1981): Enhancement of mechanical performance in frog muscle fibers after quick increases in load. J. Physiol., 319:239-252.

62. Svantesson, U., Ernstoff, B., Bergh, P., et al. (1991): Use of a Kin-Com dynamometer to study the stretch-shortening cycle during plantar flexion. Eur. J. Appl. Physiol., 62:415-419.

63. Svantesson, U., Grimby, G., and Thomee, R. (1994): Potentiation of concentric plantar flexion torque following eccentric and isometric muscle actions. Acta Physiol. Scand., 152:287-293.

64. Taber's Cyclopedic Medical Dictionary. (1993): 17th ed. Philadelphia, F.A. Davis.

65. Ugarkovic, D., Matavulj, D., Kukolj, M., and Jaric, S. (2002): Standard anthropometric, body composition, and strength variables as predictors of jumping performance in elite junior athletes. J. Strength Cond. Res., 16:227-230.

66. Voight, M.L., and Draovitch, P. (1991): Plyometrics. In: Albert. M. (ed.), Eccentric Muscle Training in Sports and Orthopaedics. New York, Churchill Livingstone, p. 45.

67. Voight, M., and Tippett, S. (1994): Plyometric exercise in rehabilitation. In: Prentice, W.E. (ed.), Rehabilitation Techniques in Sports Medicine, 2nd ed., St. Louis, Mosby, pp. 88-97.

68. Walshe, A.D., Wilson, G.J., and Ettema, G.J.C. (1998): Stretch-shorten cycle compared with isometric preload: Contributions to enhanced muscular performance. J. Appl. Physiol., 84:97-106.

69. Weiss, L.W., Fry, C., and Relyea, G.E. (2002): Explosive strength deficit as a predictor of vertical jumping performance. J. Strength Cond. Res., 16:83-86.

70. Wilk, K.E., Voight, M.L., Keirns, M.A., et al. (1993): Stretch shortening drills for the upper extremities: Theory and clinical application. J. Orthop. Sports Phys. Ther., 17:305-317.

71. Wilson, G.J., Elliot, B.C., and Wood, G.A. (1992): Stretch-shorten cycle performance through flexibility training. Med. Sci. Sports Exerc., 24:116-123.

72. Wilson, G.J., Murphy, A.J., and Pryor, J.F. (1994): Musculotendinous stiffness: Its relationship to eccentric, isometric, and concentric performance. J. Appl. Physiol., 76:2714-2719.

73. Witzke, K.A., and Snow, C.M. (2000): Effects of plyometric jump training on bone mass in adolescent girls. Med. Sci. Sports Exerc., 32:1051-1057.

74. Wojtys, E.M., Wylie, B.B., and Huston, L.J. (1996): The effects of muscle fatigue on neuromuscular function and anterior tibial translation in healthy knees. Am. J. Sports Med., 24(5):615-621.

75. Worrell, T.W., Smith, T.L., and Winegardner, J. (1994): Effect of hamstring stretching on hamstring muscle performance. J. Orthop. Sports Phys. Ther., 20:154-159.

76. Young, P.A., and Young, P.H. (1997): Basic Clinical Neuroanatomy. Philadelphia, PA, Williams & Wilkins.

CHAPTER 12

AQUATIC REHABILITATION

Jill M. Thein-Nissenbaum, M.P.T., S.C.S., ATC

CHAPTER OBJECTIVES

At the end of this chapter the reader will be able to:

■ Explain and summarize the physical properties of water, including buoyancy, hydrostatic pressure, viscosity, and fluid dynamics.

■ Summarize the effects of immersion on weight bearing and appropriately apply weight-bearing guidelines in a clinical situation.

■ Explain the physiologic responses of water immersion.

■ Compare and contrast the physiologic response to exercise on land and in water.

■ Summarize and apply recommended guidelines for cardiovascular conditioning on land and in water.

■ Design a comprehensive aquatic-based rehabilitation program for an athlete utilizing the principles of stretching, strengthening, balance, and aerobic conditioning.

Aquatic therapy, historically known as hydrotherapy, is the utilization of water as a therapeutic modality and dates back many centuries. It has been used throughout history to treat diseases and for recreation. Although it has been commonly used in Europe, aquatic-based rehabilitation was not used in the United States until the early 1900s.[28] Today, aquatic rehabilitation is a blend of many different approaches, including the Bad Ragaz ring method (Switzerland)[21] and the Halliwick method (United Kingdom).[32] Although once viewed as a tool to be used exclusively in the early stages of rehabilitation, aquatic-based rehabilitation has evolved considerably. It is now used throughout the rehabilitation process and serves as a component of prevention and wellness programs.

The purpose of this chapter is to discuss aquatic-based rehabilitation and training for the athlete. The physical properties of water will be reviewed, and current research on aquatic-based cardiovascular conditioning programs will be discussed. Extremity and core body strengthening exercises will be presented, as will balance and coordination exercises. Lastly, recommendations for the transition from aquatic-based programs to resumption of competitive sports will be made, and sample training programs will be suggested.

PHYSICAL PROPERTIES OF WATER
Buoyancy and Specific Gravity

Archimedes' principle states that when a body is wholly or partially immersed in a fluid at rest, it will experience an upward thrust equal to the weight of the fluid that was displaced. *Buoyancy* is the upward thrust acting in the opposite direction of gravity; it is related to the specific gravity of the immersed object.[8] *Specific gravity* is the ratio of the mass of one substance to the mass of the same value of water.[8] Therefore, by definition, the specific gravity of water is 1.00, and any body with a specific gravity of less than 1.00 will float. The average values for the human body range from 0.97 to 0.95, causing most humans to float.[15] However, lean individuals may have difficulty floating because of their body composition. Fat mass has a density of 0.90, whereas lean body mass, such as muscle, connective tissue, bone, and organs, has a relative density of 1.10.[13] Depending upon the athlete's body composition, he or she may rest slightly below the water's surface, or the extremities may sink while the trunk remains at the surface. This is of particular importance in treating the athlete who may be very lean. Buoyant equipment may be necessary on the trunk or at various points along the limb to maintain the athlete's buoyancy in the pool.

Buoyancy may be used in rehabilitation in a variety of ways. Buoyancy-assisted exercises are movements toward the surface of the water. These exercises are commonly used to increase mobility and range of motion.[24] Buoyancy-supported exercises are movements that are perpendicular to the upward thrust of buoyancy and parallel to the bottom of the pool. Typically, the limb will float just below the surface of the water, but this depends upon the limb's density. When buoyancy-supported exercises are performed, buoyancy neither assists nor impedes the movement; it is similar to active range of motion on land.

Lastly, buoyancy-resisted exercises directly oppose the upward thrust of buoyancy and are similar to resisted exercises on land. Buoyancy-related movements and sample exercises are summarized in Table 12-1.

CLINICAL PEARL #1

Because athletes are oftentimes very lean, they may have difficulty maintaining buoyancy. To properly position the athlete in the water, the clinician may need to strategically place buoyant equipment along the athlete's limbs and/or trunk.

Hydrostatic Pressure

Pascal's law of hydrostatic pressure states that at any given depth, the pressure from the liquid is exerted equally on all surfaces of the immersed object.[4,8] As the depth of the liquid increases, so does the hydrostatic pressure. Water exerts a pressure of 22.4 mm Hg/foot of water depth. In water at a depth of 4 feet, the force due to hydrostatic

pressure is 89.6 mm Hg, which is slightly greater than diastolic pressure.[7] Thus, hydrostatic pressure may be used in rehabilitation to control effusion in an injured extremity while allowing the athlete to exercise. Hydrostatic pressure is also responsible for the cardiovascular changes seen with immersion and has a significant impact on exercise training parameters.

CLINICAL PEARL #2

In general, in water greater than 4 feet in depth, hydrostatic pressure will exceed the athlete's diastolic pressure. Therefore, hydrostatic pressure may allow the athlete with an ankle injury to exercise acutely without increasing effusion.

Viscosity

Viscosity is defined as the friction occurring between individual molecules in a liquid, causing resistance to flow.[8] Resistance occurs as the molecules adhere to the surface of the moving object. Thus, viscosity is only noticeable when there is motion through the liquid. Because of viscosity, there is resistance to all fast movements in the water, even in a buoyancy-assisted direction.

Fluid Dynamics

Two different types of water flow exist: laminar flow and turbulent flow. Laminar flow is the smooth, streamlined flow of water molecules. It has the least amount of resistance because the water molecules are all traveling at the same speed and in the same direction. In contrast, turbulent flow is interrupted flow, such as when laminar flow encounters an object causing water molecules to rebound in all directions. As an object moves through water, resistance is created from pressure. Positive pressure exists in front of a moving object and impedes movement. The area immediately behind a moving object, the wake, is an area of low pressure and can hold the object back. This drag force created behind the object produces the majority of resistance to movement.[15]

The shape of the object moving the water effects drag. A tapered, streamlined object will produce minimal disruption of flow, whereas an unstreamlined object will create rapid disruption of flow, causing turbulence.[36] For example, forward walking is more resistive than walking sideways (Fig. 12-1).

Muscle contraction type is an important consideration when one is designing a resistance program based upon viscosity. Exercises performed against the water's resistance almost always elicit concentric muscle contractions. Consider performance of shoulder internal and external rotation at 0° abduction; the movements elicit concentric contractions of the rotator cuff muscles in a reciprocal fashion. It is possible to elicit eccentric muscle contrac-

Table 12-1

Buoyancy-Related Movements and Sample Exercises

Movement	Examples
Buoyancy-assisted (PROM, AAROM)	Standing shoulder abduction to 90°
	Standing knee extension from 90° of flexion (with the hip in 90° of flexion)
	Standing knee flexion (from full extension with the hip in neutral)
Buoyancy-supported (AROM)	Trunk lateral flexion (in supine position with flotation device supporting the body)
	Standing shoulder horizontal adduction
	Hip abduction (in supine position with flotation device supporting the body)
Buoyancy-resisted (RROM)	Standing elbow extension (with the shoulder in neutral)
	Standing knee extension (from a flexed position with the hip in neutral)
	Shoulder flexion from 0 to 90° (in prone position with flotation device supporting the body and a snorkel as needed)*

*Note: Shoulder flexion from 90 to 180° in prone would be a buoyancy assisted movement.
PROM, passive range of motion; AAROM, active-assisted range of motion; AROM, assisted range of motion; RROM, resistive range of motion.

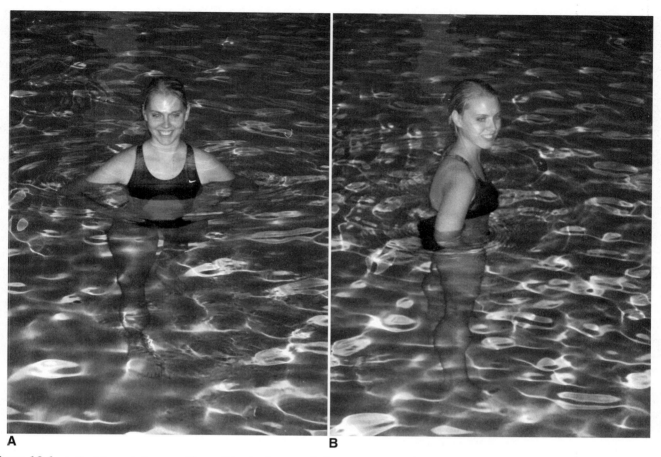

Figure 12-1. *A,* Resistance is increased by walking in the sagittal plane owing to increased surface area (thereby creating turbulent flow). *B,* Resistance in decreased by walking in the frontal plane owing to decreased surface area.

tions in three different ways: using large pieces of buoyant equipment, performing the exercises in shallow water, and using a current. For example, an eccentric contraction of the hip extensors can be achieved when hip flexion from 0 to 90° is performed if a large flotation device is placed on the ankle (Fig. 12-2). Additionally, lower extremity contractions can be achieved if the water is shallow enough to minimize the effects of buoyancy. For instance, lunges in hip-deep water can elicit eccentric quadriceps muscle contractions. Lastly, eccentric contractions can be generated with the use of a current, as with the Swim Ex or Hydro Track. For example, eccentric contractions of the right infraspinatus/teres minor can be accomplished by having the athlete stand with his or her right side toward the current. The athlete can achieve an eccentric contraction by holding a piece of equipment that increases surface area while allowing the shoulder to go from external rotation (in 0° abduction) to internal rotation in a controlled fashion. Box 12-1 summarizes the various techniques used to achieve eccentric contractions in the pool.

Resistance in the water can be modified three ways. First, resistance is affected by speed of movement. The drag force is proportional to the velocity of movement: the faster the movement, the greater the drag force and resistance to movement.[7] For example, standing knee flexion and extension at 45°/sec will not be as challenging as performing the same movement at 120°/sec. Second, the frontal surface area of the object is directly proportional to the drag force produced and may be used to alter resistance. For instance, shoulder internal and external rotation with the forearms pronated creates less drag than performance of the same exercise with the forearm in neutral position (Fig. 12-3). Lastly, the flow of the water is another factor that affects resistance.[4] Turbulent water flow increases the friction between molecules and therefore increases resistance to movement. This is the theory behind a competitive swimmer's preference of racing through "still" water; there is less resistance than in non-turbulent water, making it easier for the athletes to "pull" themselves through the water. All of these factors and their effects on movement must be taken into consideration when one designs a rehabilitation program for the athlete. Table 12-2 summarizes methods to alter resistance in the pool.

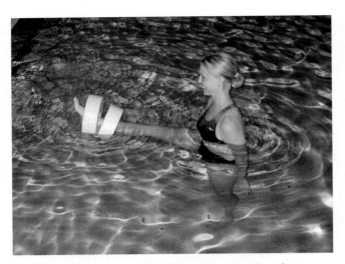

Figure 12-2. Eccentric contraction of the gluteals and hamstrings can be achieved by using buoyant equipment.

Box 12-1

Methods of Producing Eccentric Contractions in the Pool

- Utilization of large pieces of buoyant equipment
- Performance of lower extremity exercises in shallow (waist deep) water
- Utilization of a current, such as Swim Ex or Hydro Track

CLINICAL PEARL #3

Resistance can be increased three ways: by increasing the speed of movement, by increasing the frontal surface area

of the object, and by performing exercises in turbulent (versus "still" water). The clinician must choose the most appropriate progression based upon the athlete's functional needs.

Effect of Depth of Immersion on Weight Bearing

Because of buoyancy, the depth of water affects weight bearing. This is an important issue when one designs a rehabilitation program, specifically for the lower extremities, if weight bearing may be a concern. Many factors, including body composition and the water's depth, affect weight-bearing status. General weight-bearing percentages for male and females are listed in Table 12-3. These numbers reflect static weight bearing; increasing the activity level to a fast walk can increase weight-bearing by as much as 76%.[26] Thus, two options to progress lower extremity weight-bearing exist: decreasing the depth of the water and increasing the amount of impact at any given depth.

PHYSIOLOGIC RESPONSES TO AQUATIC EXERCISE
Physiologic Responses of Water Immersion

Physiologic changes occur when a person is immersed in water, both at rest and during exercise. It is imperative that the clinician be aware of these changes to modify rehabilitation programs appropriately. Changes that occur at rest during water immersion are the result of hydrostatic pressure. Most importantly, a cephalad redistribution of blood flow of approximately 0.7 liter occurs.[2,6] Of the 0.7 liter redistributed proximally, one third of the blood is redistributed to the heart and two thirds to the pulmonary arterial circulation.[6] Because of the increase in blood volume,

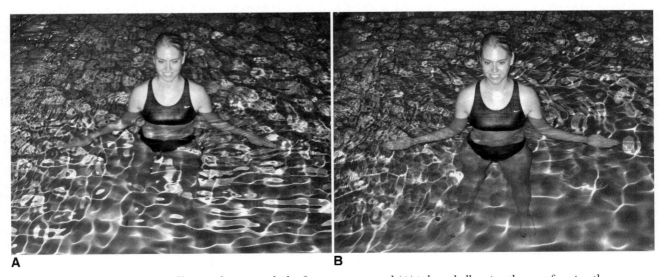

A   **B**

Figure 12-3. Performing rotator cuff strengthening with the forearms pronated (*A*) is less challenging than performing the same exercises with the forearms in neutral (*B*).

Table 12-2
Strategies to Alter Resistance in the Pool

Methods to Alter Resistance	Effect
Speed of movement	An ↑ in speed will cause an ↑ in the amount of resistance
	A ↓ in speed will cause a ↓ in the amount of resistance
Object surface area	An ↑ in surface area will cause an ↑ in the amount of resistance
	A ↓ in surface area will cause a ↓ in the amount of resistance
Water flow	Turbulent flow will ↑ the amount of resistance
	Streamlined flow will ↓ the amount of resistance

Table 12-4
Summary of Cardiovascular Responses that Occur at Rest

Measure	Response
Right atrial venous pressure	Increase (8-12 mm Hg)
Heart blood volume	Increase (180-250 ml)
Cardiac output	Increase (25% +)
Stroke volume	Increase (25% +)
Central venous pressure	Increase
Heart rate	Remains the same or decreases slightly
Systemic blood pressure	Remains the same or increases slightly

From Thein, J.M., and Brody, L.T. (1998): Aquatic-based rehabilitation and training for the elite athlete. J. Orthop. Sports Phys. Ther., 27: 32-41.

the heart distends and myocardial wall tension increases, resulting in a Frank-Starling reflex and a subsequent increase in stroke volume (SV) by approximately 35%.[2,5,6,16,19,29,34] Diuresis and hormonal changes have also been observed with sustained periods of water immersion (Table 12-4).[17,18,22,25,30]

Immersion and Response to Exercise

Several studies have been conducted to determine whether cardiovascular training can be effectively performed in the water. Byrne and colleagues[10] compared heart rate (HR), SV, and cardiac output (Q) when 20 subjects walked at 2 and 3 mph on a dry land treadmill and an underwater treadmill. Underwater treadmill walking resulted in greater Q and SV at both speeds. When oxygen consumption levels were matched, subjects in the underwater treadmill session had a significantly lower HR and higher SV. The authors concluded that HR may be a poor indicator of aquatic exercise intensity.[10]

Table 12-3
Static Weight Bearing Percentages for Males and Females

Anatomical Landmark	Weight-Bearing Percentages	
	Males	Females
Seventh cervical vertebrae	8	8
Xiphoid process	35	28
Anterior superior iliac spine	54	47

Data from Harrison, R.A., and Bulstrode, S. (1987): Percentage weight-bearing during partial immersion in the hydrotherapy pool. Physiother. Pract., 3:60.

Cassady and Nielsen[11] evaluated the oxygen consumption ($\dot{V}O_2$) and percentage of age-predicted maximal heart rate (%APMHR) response of 40 subjects performing upper and lower extremity calisthenics on land and in water. The $\dot{V}O_2$ responses were greater during water exercise whereas the %APMHR values were higher during land calisthenics. The authors concluded that both water and land calisthenics are appropriate modes of exercise for healthy persons with low physical work capabilities.[11]

Davidson and McNaughton[14] performed a study to determine the effects of deep-water running (DWR) and road running (RR) on the $\dot{V}O_{2max}$ of 10 untrained females. A pretest $\dot{V}O_{2max}$ value was obtained for subjects in either the DWR or RR group before training 3 times per week for 4 weeks in either the DWR or RR group. At 10 weeks, another $\dot{V}O_{2max}$ value was obtained, and the subjects then rested for 10 weeks. They were then retested and undertook the opposite program. The authors found no differences in the $\dot{V}O_{2max}$ values between groups and concluded that both DWR and RR can improve cardiovascular fitness in young, sedentary women.[14]

Robertson and co-workers[35] compared HRs during DWR and shallow-water running (SWR) at the same rate of perceived exertion (RPE). Forty-two subjects performed both DWR and SWR at the RPE of 15. A significant difference of 10 bpm between mean DWR (145 bpm) and mean SWR (155 bpm) was found. The authors concluded that clinicians should not prescribe SWR at HRs obtained from DWR exercise.[35] This study highlights the issue of immersion and exercise. Although DWR has been extensively studied, the HR response of SWR has not. Based on the results of this study, a DWR HR prescribed for SWR may not be effective in improving oxygen consumption.

To determine whether a water running program could maintain aerobic performance, Wilbur and associates[40] studied 16 trained male runners. The runners were assigned to either treadmill running (R) or water running (WR) and trained 5 times per week for 6 weeks for either 30 minutes at 90% to 100% $\dot{V}o_{2max}$ or 60 minutes at 70% to 75% $\dot{V}o_{2max}$. Results showed no intra- or intergroup differences. The authors concluded that DWR may be an effective alternative to land running to maintain aerobic performance.[40]

An important consideration in DWR is the skill of the athlete. Several studies have found the relationship between HR-$\dot{V}o_2$ and RPE to be skill dependent.[9,37] Subjects who were less skilled used upper extremity movements to maintain an upright position in the water, which increased their HR and RPE. Thus, the clinician should thoroughly instruct the athlete in the technique and allow a period of familiarization before utilizing DWR to maintain or improve oxygen consumption. It is recommended that training HR be established in the pool instead of attempting to apply land-based HRs to pool exercise.[41] In general, HRs during deep-water exercise will be approximately 17 bpm lower than those for comparable exercise on land.[33] Based upon the study by Robertson and co-workers,[35] SWR HRs will be approximately 7 bpm lower than those on land.

Effects of Water Temperature

Water temperature can have a profound effect on the cardiovascular response to exercise. Avellini and colleagues[3] studied three groups of males; one group exercised on land and one group each exercised in 32°C or 20°C water, respectively. Maximal oxygen consumption was tested before and after the training period, and the results showed that the water groups exercised at a lower HR for a prescribed $\dot{V}o_{2max}$ level than the land group. The authors hypothesized that the lower water temperature caused vasoconstriction in the periphery to decrease heat loss, forcing blood centrally, enhancing venous return, and increasing SV. The authors concluded that training in cold water enhanced SV and decreased HR, increasing exercise efficiency.[3]

On the other hand, exercising in warm water can increase cardiovascular demands above those of exercise alone. Choukroun and Varene[12] studied the effects of water temperature on the cardiovascular systems of resting subjects immersed to the neck in 25, 34, and 40°C water while measuring cardiovascular demands. Cardiac output increased significantly at 40°C.[12] In a similar study, Gleim and Nicholas[23] studied the effects of water temperature on individuals exercising in waist deep water. The authors found that exercise in 36°C water affects the relationship of HR to $\dot{V}o_2$ and suggested that water temperature can add a significant thermal load to the cardio-

vascular system.[23] Owing to the potential for heat illness, the recommended temperature for intense training of the athlete is between 26 and 28°C to prevent any heat-related complications.

REHABILITATION

Because of the unique properties of water, aquatic rehabilitation offers advantages over land-based rehabilitation. It is imperative that the clinician apply aquatic principles appropriately when designing a rehabilitation program for the injured athlete. Buoyancy decreases weight bearing and joint compressive forces, which may be an important consideration with lower extremity rehabilitation. Buoyancy also allows exercises to be progressed from assisted to supported to resisted by simply changing the position of the athlete in the water. Resistance due to viscosity is encountered in all directions of movement, and resistance can be modified by adjusting the lever arm, speed of movement, and turbulence of the water. Because resistance increases as the speed of movement increases, water provides an accommodating resistance to exercise, making rehabilitation programs safe for the injured athlete.

Water is also an ideal environment for cardiovascular conditioning. Training can be performed as non–weight bearing, potentially allowing the athlete to begin conditioning sooner. For instance, the athlete with a lower extremity injury (e.g., an inversion ankle sprain) may perform DWR without the deleterious effects of increased edema due to hydrostatic pressure. The athlete may also perform sport-specific rehabilitation exercises in deep water, mimicking the weight-bearing activity. As the athlete's condition improves, he or she can move to shallow water to increase weight bearing. Increasing the speed of a weight-bearing activity in shallow water will also provide progressive loading.[27]

Similar to those of land-based programs, the principles of tissue healing and exercise progression must be considered when one designs an aquatic-based rehabilitation program for the athlete. Based upon impairments, functional limitations, and disabilities identified in the examination, a program can be created with the athlete's goals in mind. The stages of healing must be taken into account to prevent delayed healing and further injury. Cardiovascular conditioning should be addressed as soon as possible to prevent deconditioning. Stretching and exercises to increase range of motion may be started when indicated, and strengthening, gait training, and increased weight bearing are initiated and progressed as tolerated with respect to tissue healing constraints. The later phases of aquatic rehabilitation involve specific cardiovascular conditioning drills combined with functional movement patterns, balance, impact loading, plyometrics, and sport-specific drills. An aquatic-based program can also be used to add variety to a maintenance program.

Cardiovascular Conditioning

Cardiovascular conditioning is a key component of a comprehensive rehabilitation program. With proper utilization of a pool, the athlete can maintain or improve cardiovascular function while an injured area is rested. This is particularly useful for the athlete with a lower extremity injury, which may have weight-bearing or impact restrictions.

An appropriate warm-up and cool-down are fundamental components of the rehabilitation program. These activities should be performed in the water and may include walking, jogging, bicycling motions, or calisthenics; stretching should complement the warm-up and cool-down sessions. Many different cardiovascular activities may be performed. Depending upon the stage of rehabilitation, the clinician may have the athlete rest the affected area or may choose to challenge muscles specific to the sport or activity. For example, a basketball player with a knee injury may perform deep-water cross-country skiing (possibly with a knee immobilizer in place to minimize knee motion) in the acute stage of rehabilitation. In the later phases of rehabilitation, SWR with impact may be appropriate. Both running and cross-country skiing may be performed in shallow or deep water, and the athlete may be tethered to the side of the pool in either depth. When teaching these techniques, the clinician should encourage proper form. The athlete is encouraged to maintain an upright posture and to avoid excessive lean, which mimics a swimming stroke. Running involves a small amount of range of motion of the upper extremity, but requires hip and knee flexion in the lower extremity. On the other hand, cross-country skiing requires a large amount of hip and shoulder flexion and extension. Techniques may be modified to protect an injured area.

After basic cardiovascular conditioning techniques have been mastered, advanced techniques such as vertical kicking may be incorporated, if indicated. Vertical kicking may be performed with or without fins and should be initiated with a small flutter kick. The athlete may initially require a flotation vest. The athlete may progress to a dolphin kick, especially if dynamic lumbar stabilization is indicated. Ideally, kicking should be performed without upper extremity assistance, with the arms held behind the back or out of the water (Fig. 12-4).

Flotation vests may be used when the athlete is initially instructed in a technique or if safety is a concern. When possible, the flotation device should be discontinued to increase the difficulty of the workout. When a belt or vest is selected, the device needs to be assessed for its primary location of flotation or buoyancy. To maintain the athlete in a vertical position, a vest or belt that provides flotation uniformly around the entire circumference of the belt is recommended.

The fundamental guidelines for cardiovascular training should be at the core of program design. A period of 25 minutes, 5 times per week or more is recommended as

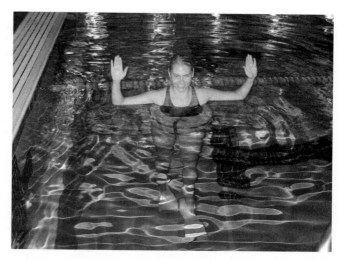

Figure 12-4. Vertical kicking using fins and a flotation vest with the arms out of the water.

a minimum; some athletes may need a longer training period, depending upon the season and sport. The intensity and duration should mimic the athlete's particular sport. Ankle floats, arm paddles, gloves and fins will increase the lever arm and resistance, and discontinuing use of the flotation vest will also make the activity more challenging. The athlete may increase speed to further increase resistance.

Like land-based exercise, the program should be as sport specific as possible. For example, the marathon runner might perform low-intensity, long-duration running and cross-country skiing, maintaining the workload at 70% to 80% maximal oxygen consumption. In contrast, the volleyball player can perform interval jumping drills, working near peak oxygen consumption, with intermittent jogging and shuffling drills for recovery. Likewise, a football lineman may perform shallow water sprints with a resistive board for 6- to 10-second intervals, with light jogging during recovery, to replicate the demands of his sport (Fig. 12-5). A number of stations or a variety of exercises performed within a single session can alleviate boredom and ensure that the workout is well-rounded.

Stretching

Mobility may be impaired after an injury or surgery, or impaired mobility can result from the pain of overuse injuries such as tendonitis. This impaired mobility may present as altered biomechanics, and a goal of rehabilitation may be to restore normal osteokinematics and joint arthrokinematics. The pool is an ideal medium for improvement of mobility in the upper extremity. Because the upward movement of the glenohumeral joint is assisted by buoyancy, the athlete may discover that normal shoulder movement patterns occur earlier in the pool than

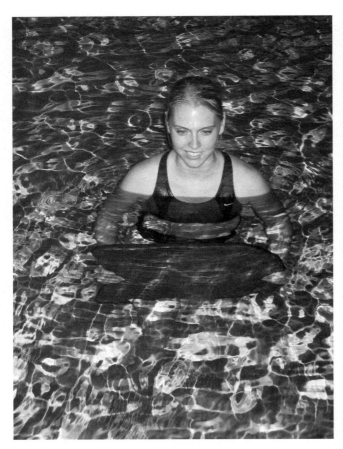

Figure 12-5. Lineman drills using increased surface area will make the exercise functional and challenging.

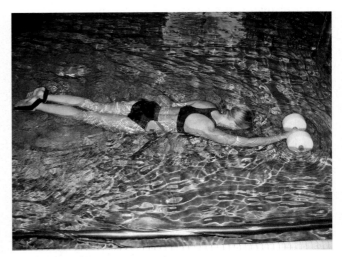

Figure 12-6. Buoyancy-assisted glenohumeral flexion greater than 90° can be achieved by having the athlete prone in the water. Use of a snorkel and mask will permit the athlete to maintain the stretch. The athlete may need cuing to maintain the spine in neutral alignment through buoyant equipment placed under the abdomen.

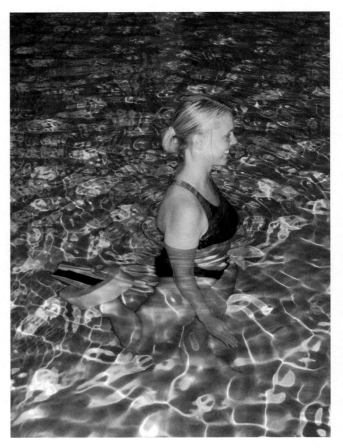

Figure 12-7. Buoyancy-assisted stretching of the quadriceps muscle. The athlete may require verbal cuing to maintain the pelvis in neutral or in a slight posterior tilt to provide optimal lengthening of the rectus femoris.

on land. This upward movement is similar to active-assistive range of motion on dry land, but instead of having the limb supported by a pulley or wand, the buoyancy of the water now supports the extremity. Accordingly, the athlete can position himself or herself in a sport-specific position, resulting in the restoration of familiar muscle length-tension relationships in the upper extremity and trunk. Buoyant equipment may assist the movement initially and may be discontinued as active and resistive range of motion exercises are initiated (Fig. 12-6).

Lower extremity stretching can also be successfully performed in the pool. Large muscle groups, such as the hamstrings, gluteals, and quadriceps may be stretched in a buoyancy-assisted fashion. Functional positions and length-tension relationships can be restored sooner in the pool than on land (Figs. 12-7 to 12-9).

A warm water pool (32 to 35°C) provides a relaxing environment, which may allow for increased soft tissue extensibility. The duration of the stretch can vary; however, to promote tissue elongation and permanent structural changes, a low-intensity, long-duration (20 to 30 seconds) stretch is most beneficial.[31] Stretching should be performed as indicated throughout the rehabilitation process.

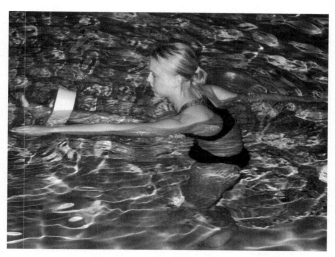

Figure 12-8. Functional stretching for a track athlete who competes as a hurdler. With the use of buoyancy equipment, the athlete is able to maintain a prolonged stretch of the hamstrings in a functional position.

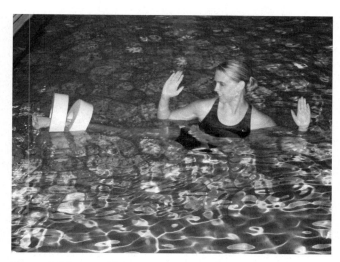

Figure 12-9. An athlete participating in martial arts may find a prolonged stretch of the hip adductors in a functional position beneficial. Buoyant equipment may be placed anywhere along the affected extremity.

Resistance Training and Functional Progression

Upper Extremity

Restoration of strength is crucial for any athlete, and strength training is a large component of any rehabilitation program. The clinician may prescribe a comprehensive aquatic strengthening program for the athlete by utilizing equipment and implementing the basic principles of aquatics. The program should be as sport specific as possible, and the intensity, duration, and type of muscular contraction the athlete will incur in their particular sport should be considered.

The viscosity of the water provides resistance, and exercises consist of isometric or dynamic contractions. Isometric contractions require the athlete to stabilize against the movement of the water, whereas dynamic exercises produce either a concentric or eccentric muscle contraction. The type of contraction required by the exercise should reflect the type of contraction needed during sport. For example, resisted walking with the arms in various positions will generate isometric contractions of the scapular stabilizers (Fig. 12-10). Dynamic contractions in the pool typically consist of reciprocal concentric contractions, which is different from what occurs on land. Weight machines and free weights elicit a concentric contraction followed by an eccentric contraction of the same muscle group (as the weight is lowered against gravity). In the pool, the athlete typically performs a concentric contraction of the agonist followed by a concentric contraction of the antagonist, as mentioned earlier. Eccentric contractions can be performed using various methods; the clinician should design a program specific to the individual (see Box 12-1).

Shoulder-strengthening exercises that are performed on land can be performed in the pool. Examples include glenohumeral flexion/extension and abduction/adduction from 0 to 90° in shoulder-deep water, horizontal abduction/adduction, elbow flexion and extension, and shoulder internal and external rotation. In addition, diagonal patterns such as those utilized in proprioceptive neuromuscular facilitation may be used. As with stretching activities, resistive exercise can be performed only through a partial range of motion (if indicated). Another consideration for upper extremity strengthening is that the mechanics are different for some water exercises compared with their land-based counterparts. For example, in the water, shoulder horizontal abduction and adduction performed at 90° abduction are resisted in the transverse plane but supported in the sagittal plane. That is, the athlete no longer has to hold the arm abducted against gravity while performing the horizontal component of the exercise. The clinician must be cognizant of these changes to appropriately utilize the principles of aquatics (Figs. 12-11 and 12-12).

Overhead activity can be performed in the pool. Resistive tubing may be used in the pool just as it is on land. Although there may not be much additional benefit to performing this type of exercise in the pool, it can be incorporated as part of a total training program that is to be performed in one location. In addition, the water will provide additional resistance to the trunk and core. For example, an athlete may practice the motion of a tennis serve while standing in waist-deep water and using resistive bands. The water is providing core body resistance while the band resists arm movement (Fig. 12-13). Secondly, exercise may be performed in the supine position, in the prone position using a snorkel, or with the athlete standing forward flexed in shallow water with the face turned and out of the water. A wide range of resistive and

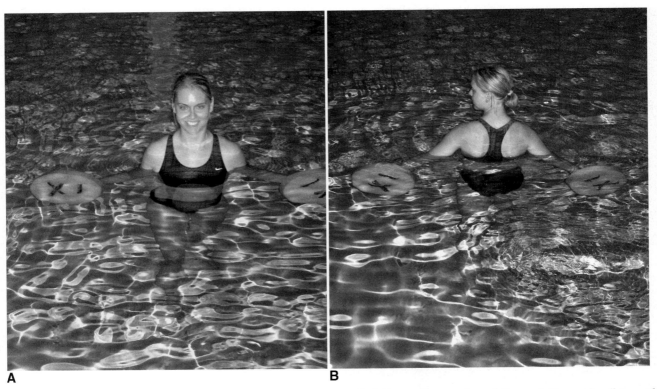

Figure 12-10. Walking with the upper extremities in various positions will challenge the scapular stabilizers. *A,* Forward walking with the arms in the scapular plane. *B,* Backward walking with the arms in 60° of abduction. The scapular stabilizers must isometrically contract to maintain the scapula in proper position.

stabilization activities can be performed in these positions. For example, in the supine position with the arms abducted 90°, rapid alternating movements of shoulder internal and external rotation can be performed (Fig. 12-14). Similarly, the athlete may perform rapid alternating shoulder flexion and extension with the arms abducted to 150° (Fig. 12-15). Both exercises are effective for athletes with symptomatic shoulder hypermobility, because they require muscular cocontraction for stabilization. Athletes should perform sport-specific repetitions and sets, such as sets of 30 to 50 repetitions to fatigue.

Upper extremity closed kinetic chain exercises are beneficial for athletes whose sports require such activities, such as gymnasts and wrestlers, and may be performed in the pool. Dips at the side of the pool, which utilize triceps, deltoids, and scapular stabilizers, may be performed more easily due to the buoyancy-assisted upward movement of the body. Buoyancy assisted pull-ups can be performed with an overhead railing or ladder. Overhead push-pull in the buoyancy-supported supine or prone position may be specific to the athlete's sport (Fig. 12-16).

Upper extremity impact may be introduced in the pool. Wall push-ups with impact can be performed safely, because viscosity will slow the body's movement through water. The athlete may start in chest deep water and progress by moving to more shallow water and by standing farther away from the wall.

When the athlete performs open chain upper extremity training, surface area will be increased substantially with equipment such as gloves, paddles, and resistive bells. Resistive boards may also be used and held under water in front of the athlete, performing a push-pull motion for scapular protraction/retraction to strengthen rhomboid, trapezius, and serratus anterior muscles. The clinician must remember that a small increase in surface area will translate into a significant increase in resistance in the upper extremity. Other equipment, specific to the athlete's sport, should be utilized throughout the rehabilitation process. For example, a baseball player may use an old bat to mimic the swinging motion, whereas the tennis player may practice forehand and backhand strokes with an old racket.

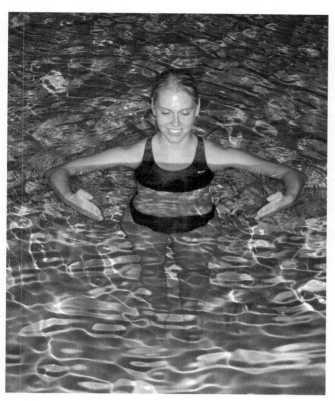

Figure 12-11. Buoyancy-supported elbow flexion and extension. Buoyancy does not affect the movement in this position; resistance can be increased by increasing speed and surface area.

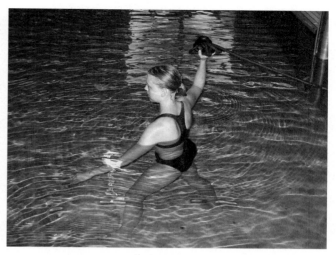

Figure 12-13. Performance of sport-specific drills, such as a tennis serve, can be done in the pool using resistive bands. The water will offer additional resistance to the trunk and core body. The clinician must be certain that the line of pull of the resistive band is similar to the resistance experienced during sport.

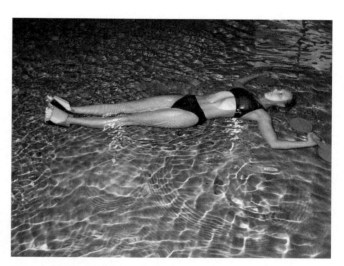

Figure 12-14. Rapid alternating movements elicit co-contraction of the glenohumeral musculature, enhancing stability. This is a functional position for an overhead throwing athlete.

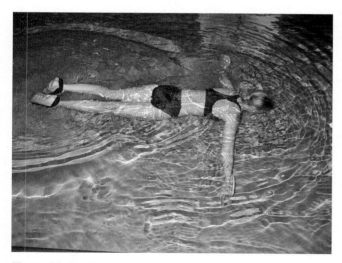

Figure 12-12. Prone supraspinatus strengthening in the scapular plane. The paddles increase the surface area, making the exercise more challenging.

Lower Extremity

The lower extremity functions in both the open and closed chain during activities of daily living and sporting activities. Thus, it is imperative the athlete's rehabilitation program consist of both open and closed chain types of exercises. Lower extremity strengthening exercises can be performed completely non–weight bearing in the open chain. Examples include hip flexion/extension and abduction/adduction and knee flexion/extension. More advanced activities, such as

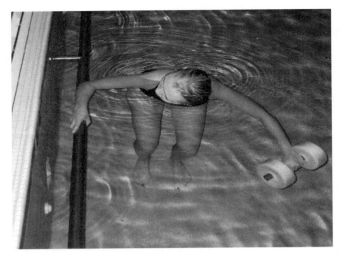

Figure 12-15. Eccentric contractions are achieved by utilization of buoyant equipment. With the athlete in the prone position with the arm overhead, the buoyant equipment forces the glenohumeral joint into increased flexion; the athlete is required to eccentrically control the movement. This can be followed by a concentric contraction of the same muscle group. When performed rapidly, this exercise requires stabilization at the glenohumeral joint and is beneficial for volleyball players, particularly outside hitters.

vertical kicking, are especially effective for increasing lower extremity muscle endurance (see Fig. 12-4). Another excellent lower extremity endurance exercise is kicking in the prone or supine position with fins. These exercises require concentric contractions at the hip and isometric contractions at the knee. Having an athlete sit on a flotation device while he or she performs repetitive knee flexion and extension with or without fins is a very fatiguing open chain quadriceps and hamstring exercise, which is beneficial for those involved in kicking sports such as football and soccer. This activity also requires trunk stabilization, because the athlete is sitting on a dynamic surface (Fig. 12-17). Fins, which increase surface area, or ankle cuffs, which increase buoyancy, are effective means to increase resistance in an open chain. Resistive boots can increase the resistance as much as fourfold, and exercises using boots are useful in sports requiring explosive power such as figure skating and gymnastics.[20,38]

To strengthen the quadriceps and gluteals in a closed kinetic chain, exercises such as lunges, step-downs, and squats should be incorporated. Owing to buoyancy, the quadriceps eccentric work with most aquatic exercise is decreased relative to that seen with comparable land-based

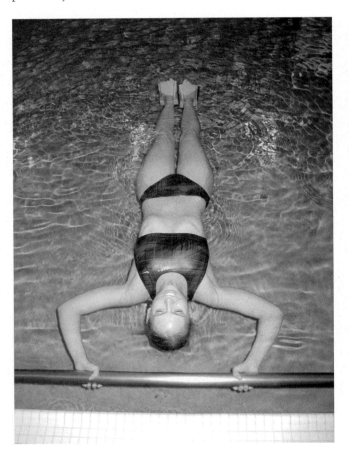

Figure 12-16. Buoyancy-supported overhead closed kinetic chain activities can be performed with the athlete holding on to the edge of the pool or to a railing.

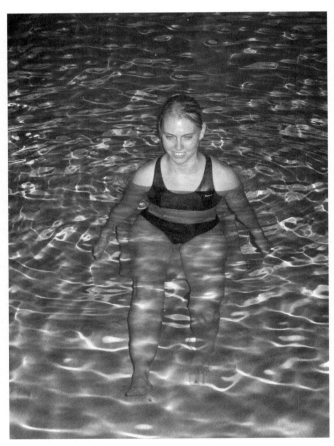

Figure 12-17. Seated open chain knee flexion and extension exercises challenge lower extremity endurance and core body strength.

exercise. Floating squats, in which the athlete stands on a flotation board and pushes down, require coordination and eccentric control. This drill can also be performed in the standing position with only one leg on the board (Fig. 12-18).

Lower extremity balance and proprioception are important to any athlete, and a well-designed rehabilitation program should address all balance impairments. Balance is controlled by sensory input, central processing, and neuromuscular responses.[39] Proprioception is defined as position sense that orients the body or specific body parts to space or other objects.[1] Balance and proprioception may be addressed in a water-based program. Any self-perturbation activity, such as hip flexion/extension and circumduction in waist-deep water while standing on the injured leg, will challenge balance. Other examples include single-leg balance on the injured leg while the center of gravity is altered by moving the upper extremity, as in a push-pull motion with a kickboard, or rotation of the upper extremity while using water paddles as resistance. Increasing knee flexion on the weight-bearing leg will increase the challenge to these muscles. Additionally, the athlete may close his or her eyes, relying more heavily on neuromuscular rather than visual input (Fig. 12-19).

If impact is required for return to sport, jumping and hopping drills may be introduced in the pool. The viscosity of the water allows jumping drills to be introduced while impact is minimized. Athletes in sports that require explosive push-offs such as track and baseball as well as athletes in jumping sports will benefit from jumping drills. Appropriate landing techniques, in which the athlete works on bent knee landings and "sticking" the landings should be emphasized. Two-footed jumping in the sagittal plane is progressed to single-leg hopping and eventually to hopping with 90° turns (Fig. 12-20). These drills are beneficial for figure skaters, gymnasts, and volleyball, soccer, and basketball players for whom jumping and turning are essential skills. The athlete may jump from different heights as well (Fig. 12-21). Tethered push-offs and tethered side-to-side jumping are also useful jumping drills, as are bounding and leaping drills (Fig. 12-22). All impact drills may be made more challenging by having the athlete close his or her eyes, by decreasing the depth of the water, by progressing to single-leg jumps, and by incorporating upper extremity activities, such as shooting a basketball or playing catch while performing the activity. Shock-absorptive shoes may be necessary for these activities.

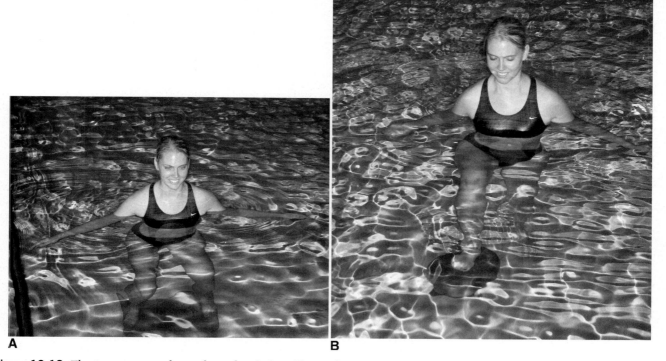

Figure 12-18. Floating squats can be performed with the athlete utilizing a flotation board. *A,* Double-leg squats. *B,* Single-leg squats.

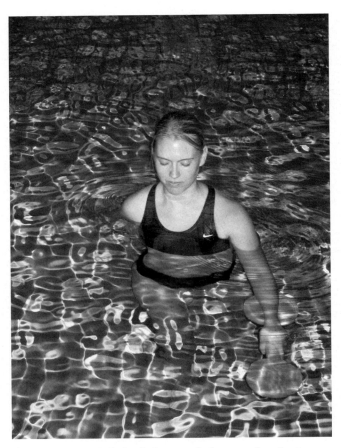

Figure 12-19. Single-leg balance with the eyes closed using upper extremity self-perturbation. The arms are moving rapidly in a reciprocal fashion.

CLINICAL PEARL #4

The pool is an excellent environment to introduce impact loading and landing techniques into the rehabilitation program. Because of buoyancy, eccentric contractions are minimized with landings and closed kinetic chain activities.

Core Body Strengthening

Core body strength and postural control are critical for any athlete. Baseball players must be able to transfer kinetic energy from the lower extremity to the arm via their trunk musculature. The soccer player must be able to twist and rotate at the trunk while kicking or passing the soccer ball. The pole vaulter must be able to stabilize the trunk and lower extremity while rotating the body around the shoulder to clear the bar. Core body strength can be easily addressed in the pool and core body strength training makes a nice addition to a rehabilitation program in the area of maintenance and prevention. Because any move-

ment of an extremity in the water must be counter-balanced by a stabilizing force in the trunk, most extremity exercises also train the core body. For example, standing leg kicks in a sagittal plane require both single-leg balance and core strength to avoid displacement by the movement of the leg against the water. Similarly, bilateral shoulder flexion and extension cause posterior and anterior displacement of the body, respectively, which must be countered by the rectus abdominus and trunk extensor muscles. Alternating shoulder flexion and extension challenges the internal and external oblique muscles as they stabilize the rotational forces created by the arm motion (Fig. 12-23).

The previous examples require the core body to perform as a static stabilizer; however, in most sporting activities, the trunk musculature performs as a dynamic stabilizer. Thus, dynamic exercises specific to the trunk are a crucial part of any athlete's rehabilitation program. For example, leg lifts at the side of the pool may be included in the rehabilitation program. Straight leg lifting will focus on the rectus abdominus, while lifting side-to-side in a V fashion will primarily work the oblique muscles. If the athlete is unable to maintain proper form with the knees extended, he or she may shorten the lever arm by flexing the knees. Eccentric work of the abdominal muscles may be performed with a buoyant ball by doing trunk flexion/extension and slowly allowing the ball to return to the surface of the water (Fig. 12-24). Sport-specific exercises such as trunk rotations with the arms abducted may benefit the soccer player, golfer, or quarterback, who require a lot of rotation for their sport (Fig. 12-25). Resisted water walking/jogging with kickboards may be helpful to the football lineman. Figure skaters as well as long and triple jumpers may increase core body strength via pike jumping.

Return to Sport

Although aquatic-based programs may be made very sport specific for the injured athlete, many athletes have difficulty mentally if they cannot train specifically for their particular sport. The biggest mistake made by most athletes is returning too quickly after injury, thereby failing to allow adequate recovery time. An extensive, intense rehabilitation program that incorporates aquatics and challenges the athlete will allow him or her to train and condition while providing adequate recovery time. Some injuries, such as stress fractures, and postoperative rehabilitation may have specific guidelines for return to sport and impact activities. Others, including overuse injuries, are often symptom limited. Thus, the clinician must rely on subjective input and the athlete's response to functional testing to determine readiness to return to sport. Regardless of the injury, gradual return to sport and impact activities is crucial to prevent reinjury.

Before resuming land activities, the athlete should be put through a battery of sport-specific tests to assess

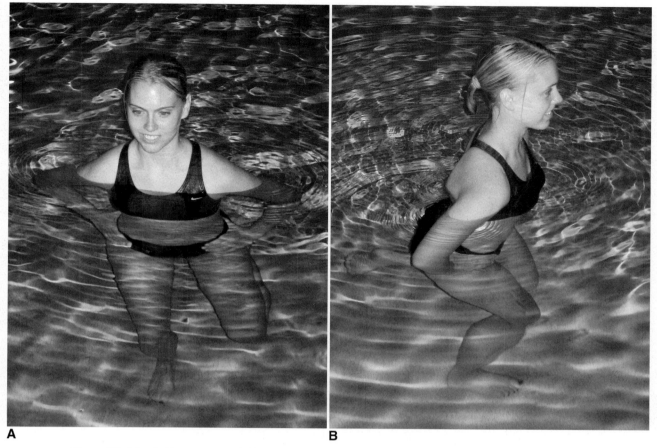

Figure 12-20. Shallow water single-leg hopping drills with 90° turns. *A*, Start position. *B*, End position.

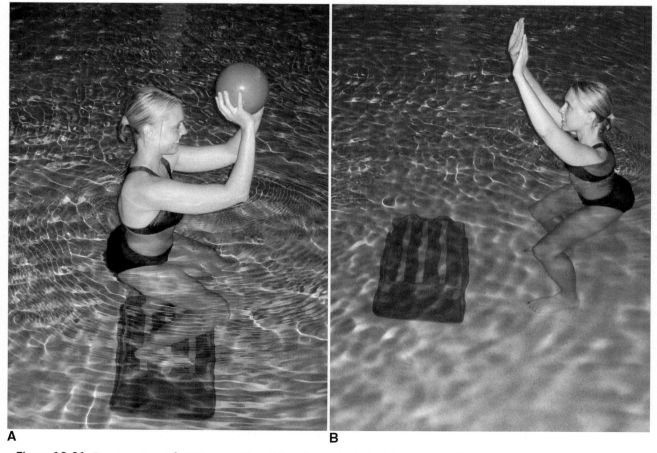

Figure 12-21. Box jumping with 180° turns. The athlete shoots the ball while turning 180°. *A*, Start position. *B*, End position.

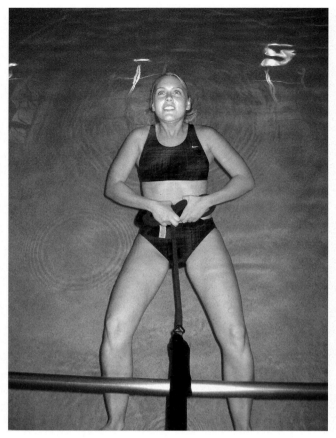

Figure 12-22. Tethered push-offs using a sport cord as resistance can be performed in a buoyancy-supported position.

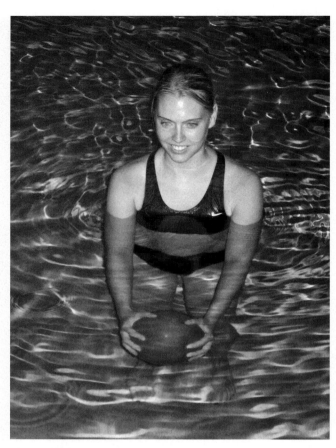

Figure 12-24. Eccentric abdominal muscle strengthening with a buoyant ball. This exercise may be performed in the sagittal plane to focus on the rectus abdominus or with trunk rotation to incorporate the oblique muscles.

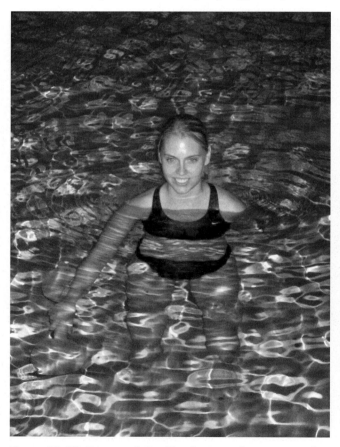

Figure 12-23. Reciprocal shoulder flexion and extension with paddles requires isometric stabilization via the internal and external obliques.

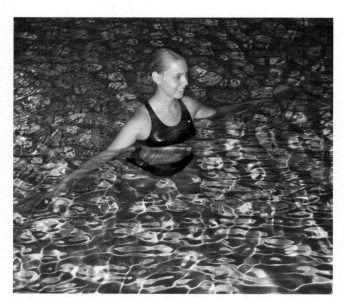

Figure 12-25. Trunk rotation with the arms abducted and paddles to increase surface area is a beneficial exercise for the athlete who requires rotation for his or her particular sport.

readiness. An athlete with a lower extremity or spine injury may be assessed by observing response to activities in the shallow water. Athletes should be able to complete any testing with proper form and without a significant increase in pain, muscle soreness, or swelling. Once the athlete tolerates the battery of tests, he or she may start a land-based program, which may or may not include impact, depending upon the response to shallow water impact. The athlete may perform their water-based program on alternate days. Ideally, the athlete should increase the time on land slowly, with no increase in pain, altered biomechanics, or significant muscle soreness. Land-based programs may continue to be complemented by pool programs indefinitely. Oftentimes, even upon returning to preinjury status, athletes may enjoy continuing to train in the pool 1 to 2 times per week for variety and to give their extremities a much needed break, especially from impact. Sample training programs for various athletes are included in Tables 12-5 to 12-7.

SUMMARY

Principles of Aquatics

Buoyancy

- Buoyancy can be used as assisted (passive range of motion and active-assisted range of motion), supported (active range of motion), or resisted (resistive range of motion).

Specific Gravity

- Athletes who are very lean may require flotation devices around their trunk or limbs to remain at the surface of the water.

Hydrostatic Pressure

- Hydrostatic pressure may be used to control effusion in the lower extremity.

Table 12-5

Sample Training Program for a Gymnast

Area of Focus	Activity
Upper extremity training	Standing shoulder horizontal abduction/adduction
	Standing shoulder proprioceptive neuromuscular facilitation D_1 and D_2 to 90° flexion
	Standing rows
	Standing wall push-ups with impact (double and single arm)
	Supine rapid shoulder internal/external rotation at 90° abduction
	Supine overhead push-pull
	Prone rapid shoulder flexion/extension at 135° abduction
	Elbow flexion and extension
Lower extremity training	Standing shallow water lunge jumps
	Vertical kicking with fins
	Seated knee flexion/extension sprints with fins
	Standing buoyancy resisted knee extension
	Seated buoyancy resisted knee flexion
	Standing hip adduction/abduction
Core training	Pike jumps
	Tuck jumps
	Side-to-side hops
	Leg lifts
	Ball push-downs
	Trunk rotations with paddles
Balance training	Eyes closed hip flexion/extension
	Eyes closed hip abduction/adduction, circumduction
	Leaping and bounding in all directions with single-leg landings (cannot use arms)
	Single-leg hopping with 90° and 180° turns
Cardiovascular training	½ mile swim
	Deep water running and cross-country skiing
	Tethered shallow water sprints (10 seconds with jogging for recovery)

Table 12-6

Sample Training Program for a Football Lineman with a History of Low Back Pain

Area of Focus	Activity
Cardiovascular training	Shallow water interval sprints 1:2 work:rest intervals (15-second interval)
Stabilization	Single-leg balance with shoulder horizontal abduction/adduction with paddles Single-leg balance with shoulder flexion/extension with paddles Kicking with fins sitting on a flotation device while passing a football Standing trunk twists with paddles Floating squats without arm support
Core training	Pike lifts at pool side Knee tucks with rotation at pool side Straddle jumps Lunge jumps
Sport specific	Standing explosive 10-second plow pushes forward and back Direction change sprinting drill Frontal and sagittal plane jump drills on aqua step Coordination drills over pool lines (such as carioca)

Table 12-7

Sample Training Program for a Basketball Player

Area of Focus	Activity

Upper extremity training	Shoulder:
	   Prone overhead flexion/extension with paddles, small movements
	   Standing abduction/adduction with gloves
	   Standing kickboard plows (scapular protraction/retraction)
	   Prone overhead wall push-ups
	   Standing wall push-ups
	Elbow:
	   Flexion/extension with gloves

Lower extremity training	Resisted hip flexion/extension, abduction/adduction and circumduction Floating squats Resisted double-/single-leg jumping (all planes, tethered to side of pool) Scissors jumping Shallow water lunges Buoyancy resisted hip extension
Core training	Tuck jumps Leg lifts in deep water with trunk supported by flotation device Interval shallow water plow running (forward/backward) Ball push-downs
Balance training	Eyes closed single-leg box jumping with holding landing pose Eyes closed double-leg jumping with 90, and 180° turns Single-leg stance with trunk rotations with paddles
Combination drills	Tuck jumps with rotation Straddle/split jumps Vertical kicking without flotation vest Sprint kickboard laps (supine and prone)
Cardiovascular training	Shallow water running, back-pedaling and shuffling with tuck jumping intervals ¾ mile swim with fins Deep-water cross-country skiing

Viscosity

- Viscosity causes resistance to movement by adhering to the surface of the moving object.

Fluid Dynamics

- The pressure immediately behind a moving object, the wake, produces the majority of resistance to movement.

Weight Bearing

- Static weight-bearing percentages change significantly (by as much as 76%) with impact.

Physiologic Responses to Aquatic Exercise

Physiologic Responses of Water Immersion

- Numerous changes occur to the body when it is submersed in the water, including a cephalad shift in blood flow, an increase in heart blood volume, and increased cardiac output and stroke volume.

Immersion and Response to Exercise

- The pool can be successfully used to maintain and/or improve aerobic conditioning.
- Heart rate in the pool differs from heart rate on land (an average of 17 bpm lower in deep water running and 7 bpm lower in shallow water running).

Water Temperature

- The temperature of the water can have a significant effect on heart rate response; intense training of the athlete should be in water that is between 26 and 28°C.

Rehabilitation

Cardiovascular Conditioning

- Aerobic conditioning is a critical component of any rehabilitation program and can successfully be performed in the pool.
- The clinician should monitor technique if the athlete is a novice.

Stretching

- The athlete may be able to achieve optimal length-tension relationships in the pool to allow for prolonged stretching due to buoyancy.
- Buoyant equipment and lever arms should be used as necessary to maintain appropriate positioning.

Resistance Training and Functional Progression

- Resistance training can be successfully performed in the pool with buoyancy resisted movements.
- Training can be progressed by increasing speed of movement and surface area.

- Impact loading can be introduced in the pool before the athlete is ready for impact on land.
- The activity should be made as sport specific as possible with utilization of sport-specific equipment, such as tennis rackets, basketballs, and baseball bats.

Core Body Strengthening

- All movements of the extremities require static stabilization of the trunk via the core body musculature.
- Dynamic strength is required in most, if not all, sports and can be easily addressed in the pool.

Return to Sport

- As on land, the late phases of the aquatic-based rehabilitation program should be as sport specific as possible.
- The pool provides a medium for maintenance programs.

REFERENCES

1. Anderson, M.A., and Foreman, T.L. (1996): Return to competition: Functional rehabilitation. *In:* Zachazewski, J.E., Magee, D.J., and Quillen, W.S. (eds), Athletic Injuries and Rehabilitation, 1st ed. Philadelphia, W.B. Saunders, p 229.
2. Arborelius, M., Jr., Balldin, U.I., Lilja, B., et al. (1972): Hemodynamic changes in man during immersion with the head above water. Aerosp. Med., 43:592-598.
3. Avellini, B.A., Shapiro, Y., and Pandolf, K.B. (1983): Cardio-respiratory physical training in water and on land. Eur. J. Appl. Physiol., 50:255-263.
4. Bates, A., and Hanson, N. (1996): Aquatic Exercise Therapy, 1st ed. Philadelphia, W.B. Saunders.
5. Begin, R., Epstein, M., Sackner, M.A., et al. (1976): Effects of water immersion to the neck on pulmonary circulation and tissue volume in man. J. Appl. Physiol., 40:293-299.
6. Becker, B.E. (1994): The biologic aspects of hydrotherapy. J. Back Musculoskel. Rehab., 4:255.
7. Becker, B.E. (1997): Aquatic physics. *In:* Ruoti, R.G., Morris, D.M., and Cole, A.J. (eds.), Aquatic Rehabilitation, 1st ed. Philadelphia, Lippincott Williams & Wilkins, p 15.
8. Beiser, A. (1978): Physics, 2nd ed. Menlo Park, CA, Benjamin/Cummings.
9. Bishop, P.A., Frazier, S., Smith, J., et al. (1989): Physiologic responses to treadmill and water running. Phys Sportsmed., 17:87.
10. Byrne, H.K., Craig, J.N., and Willmore, J.H. (1996): A comparison of the effects of underwater treadmill walking to dry land treadmill walking on oxygen consumption, heart rate, and cardiac output. J. Aquatic Phys. Ther., 4:4.
11. Cassady, S.L., and Nielsen, D.H. (1992): Cardiorespiratory responses of healthy subjects to calisthenics performed on land versus in water. Phys Ther., 72:532-539.
12. Choukroun, M.L., and Varene, P. (1990): Adjustments in oxygen transport during head-out immersion in water at different temperatures. J. Appl. Physiol., 68:1475-1480.
13. Cunningham, J. (1994): Historical review of aquatics and physical therapy. Orthop. Phys. Ther. Clin. North Am., 2:83.

14. Davidson, K., and McNaughton, L. (2000): Deep water running and road running training improve VO_{2max} in untrained women. J. Strength Cond. Res., 14:191.

15. Davis, B., and Harrison, R.A. (1993): Hydrotherapy in Practice, 1st ed. New York, Random House.

16. Echt, M., Lange, L., and Gauer, O.H. (1974): Changes of peripheral venous tone and central transmural venous pressure during immersion in a thermo-neutral bath. Pfluegers Arch., 352: 211-217.

17. Epstein, M. (1978): Renal effects of head-out water immersion in man: Implications for an understanding of volume homeostasis. Physiol. Rev., 58:529-581.

18. Epstein, M., Preston, S., and Weitzman, R.E. (1981): Isoosmotic central blood volume expansion suppresses plasma arginine vasopressin in normal man. J. Clin. Endocrinol. Metab., 52: 256-262.

19. Farhi, L.E., and Linnarsson, D. (1977): Cardiopulmonary readjustments during graded immersion in water at 35°C. Respir. Physiol., 30:35-50.

20. Frey, L.A., and Smidt, G.L. (1996): Underwater forces produced by the Hydro-Tone bell. J. Orthop. Sports Phys. Ther., 23: 267.

21. Garrett, G. (1997): Bad Ragaz ring method. In: Ruoti, R.G., Morris, D.M., and Cole, A.J. (eds.), Aquatic Rehabilitation, 1st ed. Philadelphia, Lippincott Williams & Wilkins, p 289.

22. Gauer, O.H., and Henry, J.P. (1976): Neurohormonal control of plasma volume. In: Guyton, A.C., and Cowley, A.W. (eds.), Cardiovascular Physiology II, Baltimore, University Park Press, vol IX, p 145.

23. Gleim, G.W., and Nicholas, J.A. (1989): Metabolic costs and heart rate responses to treadmill walking in water at different depths and temperatures. Am. J. Sports Med., 17:248-252.

24. Golland, A. (1981): Basic hydrotherapy. Physiotherapy, 67: 258-262.

25. Greenleaf, J.E., Shvartz, E., and Keil, L.C. (1981): Hemodilution, vasopressin suppression, and diuresis during water immersion in man. Aviat. Space Environ. Med., 52:329-336.

26. Harrison, R.A., and Bulstrode, S. (1987): Percentage weight-bearing during partial immersion in the hydrotherapy pool. Physiother. Pract., 3:60.

27. Harrison, R.A., Hillman, M., and Bulstrode, S. (1992): Loading of the lower limb when walking partially immersed. Physiotherapy, 78:164.

28. Irion, J.M. (1997): Historical overview of aquatic rehabilitation. In: Ruoti, R.G., Morris, D.M., and Cole, A.J. (eds.), Aquatic Rehabilitation, 1st ed. Philadelphia, Lippincott Williams & Wilkins, p 3.

29. Lange, L., Lange, S., Echt, M., et al. (1974): Heart volume in relation to body posture and immersion in a thermoneutral bath. A roentgenometric study. Pfluegers Arch., 352:219-226.

30. Lin, Y.C. (1984): Circulatory findings during immersion and breath-hold dives in humans. Undersea Biomed Res., 11: 123-138.

31. Malone, T.R., Garrett, W.E., and Zachazewski, J.E. (1996): Muscle deformation, injury, repair. In: Zachazewski, J.E., Magee, D.J., and Quillen, W.S. (eds), Athletic Injuries and Rehabilitation, 1st ed. Philadelphia, WB Saunders, p.71.

32. Martin, J. (1981): The Halliwick method. Physiotherapy, 67: 288-291.

33. McArdle, W.D., Katch, F.I., and Katch, V.L. (1991): Exercise Physiology: Energy, Nutrition, and Human Performance, 3rd ed. Philadelphia, Lea & Febiger.

34. Risch, W.D., Koubenec, H.J., Beckmann, U., et al. (1978): The effect of graded immersion on heart volume, central venous pressure, pulmonary blood distribution, and heart rate in man. Pfluegers Arch., 374:115-118.

35. Robertson, J.M., Brewster, E.A., and Factora, K.I. (2001): Comparison of heart rates during water running in deep water and shallow water at the same rating of perceived exertion. J. Aquatic Phys. Ther., 9:21.

36. Skinner, A.T., and Thompson, A.M. (1983): Duffield's Exercise in Water. London, Bailliere Tindall.

37. Svedenhag, J., and Seger, J. (1992): Running on land and in water: Comparative exercise physiology. Med. Sci. Sports Exerc., 24:1155-1160.

38. Visnic, M.A. (1994): Aquatic physical therapy comes of age. Aquatic Phys. Ther. Rep., 1:6.

39. Wegener, L., Kisner, C., and Nichols, D. (1997): Static and dynamic balance responses in persons with bilateral knee osteoarthritis. J. Orthop. Sports Phys. Ther., 25:13-18.

40. Wilbur, R.L., Moffatt, R.J., Scott, B.E., et al. (1996): Influence of water run training on the maintenance of aerobic performance. Med. Sci. Sports Exerc., 28:1056-1062.

41. Wilder, R.P., Brennan, D., and Schotte, D.E. (1993): A standard measure for exercise prescription for aqua running. Am. J. Sports Med., 21:45-48.

CHAPTER 13

REHABILITATION CONSIDERATIONS FOR THE FEMALE ATHLETE

Terese Chmielewski, Ph.D., P.T., S.C.S.
Reed Ferber, Ph.D., C.A.T.(C.), ATC

CHAPTER OBJECTIVES

At the end of this chapter the reader will be able to:

- Explain the biomechanical and neuromuscular factors that may predispose females to lower extremity injury.
- Relate biomechanical and neuromuscular factors to lower extremity injuries more commonly experienced by females.
- Describe specific neuromuscular rehabilitation interventions than can be used with female athletes.

Women have become more involved in both recreational and competitive sports since the enactment of Title IX and are therefore receiving more attention in the sports medicine literature. Recent studies suggest that some lower extremity injuries are encountered more often by female athletes. Most impressive is the two to eight times increased risk of noncontact anterior cruciate ligament (ACL) tears in females compared with male basketball and soccer players.[3,21,31] Women runners are also reported to sustain twice as many overall lower extremity injuries compared with their male counterparts.[37] In addition, studies indicate that female runners are twice as likely to develop stress fractures[54,57] and patellofemoral dysfunction than male runners.[2,15] The injury patterns in women may be a consequence of structural, mechanical, or neuromuscular factors or some combination of these.

Rehabilitation programs for the injured female athlete, in addition to resolving impairments, should include therapeutic exercises to alter the factors that may have led to injury. Although it may not be possible to alter structure, normalization of mechanical and neuromuscular problems is necessary to decrease the possibility of reinjury. In this chapter, an overview of structural, biomechanical, and neuromuscular factors that may predispose females to injury and a summary of gender differences in movement will be given, followed by descriptions of specific rehabilitation programs and techniques that may be useful in minimizing the influence of these factors.

GENDER DIFFERENCES
Structural Differences

Several differences in lower extremity structure have been noted between males and females (Fig. 13-1). Compared with men, women exhibit greater amounts of static external knee rotation alignment[77] and greater active internal hip rotation,[64] which may result in greater rotational motion and work at both the hip and knee. In addition, women have been shown to exhibit a greater interacetabular distance[36] and increased hip width when normalized to femoral length than men.[27] Greater pelvic width and increased external knee rotation have been suggested to contribute to greater amounts of standing genu valgum alignment in women than in men[28,77] (see Fig. 13-1). In addition, the structural combination of increased hip adduction, femoral anteversion, and genu valgum may explain, in part, the well-documented larger Q angle in women than in men[1,27,42,75] (Fig. 13-2).

A more valgus knee position has been suggested to increase frontal plane motion at the knee and increase the risk of lower extremity overuse injuries.[12,34,49] Cowan and colleagues[12] found that subjects with a Q angle of more than 15° had a significantly increased risk of overuse injury and that the risk of lower extremity stress fractures was significantly higher among participants with the most valgus knee positions.[12] An increased knee valgus angle also increases the Q angle, which is thought to lead to patellofemoral disorders (see Fig. 13-2). Mizuno and colleagues[51] investigated the relationship between Q angle and patellofemoral kinematics. Through a manipulation of the Q angle in vitro, these authors reported that a larger Q angle may lead to greater lateral patellar contact forces and increase the potential for patellofemoral pain

315

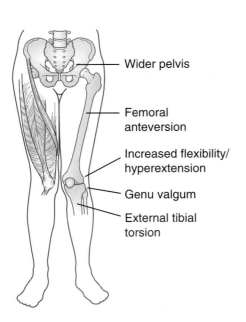

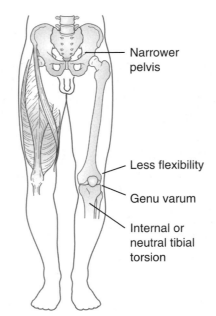

Figure 13-1. Structural differences between men and women. Women (*left*) typically exhibit a wider pelvis, femoral anteversion, greater tibial external rotation, and genu valgum. (From Ireland, M.L., and Hutchinson, M.R. (1995): Women. *In:* Griffin, L.Y. (ed.), Rehabilitation of the Injured Knee. St. Louis, Mosby, p. 298.)

syndrome and lateral patellar dislocations. In support of this hypothesis, runners with patellofemoral pain were found to exhibit a significantly greater Q angle than those of a group of healthy control subjects.[49]

CLINICAL PEARL #1

Gender differences in lower extremity structure include increased pelvic and hip width, static knee external rotation, genu valgum, and Q angle and decreased intercondylar notch size in females.

Intercondylar notch size and shape (Fig. 13-3) has been suggested as a potential contributor to the greater

incidence of ACL injury in women.[20,61] It has been suggested that women have a narrower notch width than men, and some investigators have reported that this contributes to a smaller and potentially weaker ACL.[20,61] Lund-Hanssen and associates[44] found that women with a narrow notch width were six times more likely to rupture their ACL than women with larger notch widths. However, more recent work has suggested that there are no differences in intercondylar notch width between males and females.[33,69] Ireland and co-workers[33] performed a retrospective investigation and measured the notch width of male and females with and without ACL injuries and reported that smaller notch widths were associated with previous ACL injury regardless of gender or notch shape.

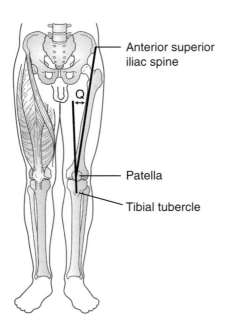

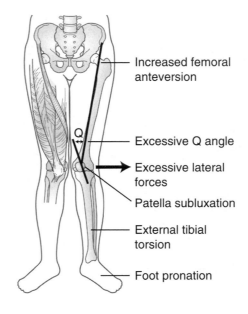

Figure 13-2. Gender differences in Q angle. Women (*right*) exhibit greater Q angle, increased external tibial torsion, and femoral anteversion. The combination of these structural differences can lead to increased lateral patellar compressive forces and patellar subluxation. (From Ireland, M.L., and Hutchinson, M.R. (1995): Women. *In:* Griffin, L.Y. (ed.), Rehabilitation of the Injured Knee. St. Louis, Mosby, p. 299.)

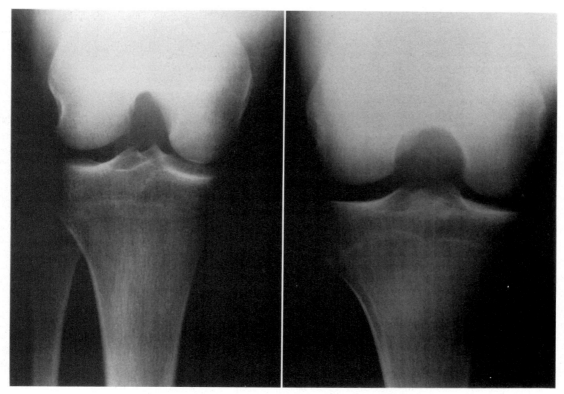

Figure 13-3. Radiographs of the intercondylar notch from a male *(right)* and female *(left)*. Note that the shape and size of the female's notch is markedly smaller and narrower than that of the male. (From Ireland, M.L., and Hutchinson, M.R. (1995): Women. *In:* Griffin, L.Y. (ed.), Rehabilitation of the Injured Knee. St. Louis, Mosby, p. 301.)

Thus, further investigation is warranted to better determine the influence of femoral intercondylar notch width and shape in the incidence of ACL injury.

Differences in Mechanics

It is believed that structural differences may lead to different movement patterns, which in turn place women at risk for injury compared with their male counterparts. Although relatively few studies have been performed in the area of gender differences in lower extremity mechanics during functional tasks, the studies that have been conducted show that females may perform some tasks differently from males. The following section will address each of these activities with respect to possible gender-related differences.

Landing

Landing from a jump results in forces between 3 and 14 times body weight that must be attenuated by the lower extremity.[16] One of the most common noncontact mechanisms of lower extremity injury is landing from a jump, and it has been reported that women are more likely to injure themselves during sports that involve jumping and landing than men.[17] Huston and colleagues[29] studied the landing

patterns of males and females and reported that females land with less knee flexion than men and thus experience greater ground reaction force vertical loading rates. Specifically, women experienced a 9% increase in loading rate per unit of body weight compared with men.[29] Lephart and associates[40] found that females land in less knee flexion, and greater femoral internal and tibial external rotation than males. The decreased amount of knee flexion exhibited by females may reduce their ability to attenuate impact forces experienced during landing. Furthermore, because ACL strain has been found to be greatest when the knee is near or at full extension, the extended knee position during landing may predispose female athletes to greater ACL strain.[6]

CLINICAL PEARL #2

Females do not flex their knee as much as males during running and when landing from a jump.

CLINICAL PEARL #3

Females experience a higher ground reaction force and have increased femoral rotation motion during landing.

Running

Gender differences during running have received little attention in the scientific literature, but the studies that have been conducted show that women have different running mechanics than men. Similar to the results of the landing studies, women tend to run with less knee flexion.[46] Women also exhibit a significantly greater knee valgus angle throughout stance than men and demonstrate a significantly greater peak hip adduction and hip internal rotation angle than men, which may be the result of a greater Q angle.[46] Hip frontal and transverse plane negative work is greater in women than in men, which suggests that the muscles controlling hip adduction and internal rotation are under greater eccentric loading while running. These gender differences in running mechanics may lend insight into the greater incidence of specific lower extremity injuries, such as patellofemoral pain, seen in women than in men.

Greater femoral internal rotation and tibial external rotation exhibited by female runners may also place them in a biomechanical dilemma with respect to the patellofemoral joint. Tiberio[70] suggested that excessive femoral internal rotation might result in malalignment of the patellofemoral joint and lead to anterior knee pain. It has also been suggested that abnormal tibial rotation results in a subsequent interruption of the normal tibiofemoral rotational relationship and an alteration in normal patellofemoral mechanics.[34] The increased femoral internal rotation observed in female athletes, coupled with the increased tibial external rotation position, may result in a greater Q angle, thereby increasing the risk of patellofemoral disorders in females.

CLINICAL PEARL #4

The hip adduction and hip internal rotation angles and the frontal and transverse plane work are greater in females than in males during running.

Cutting

Another common noncontact mechanism of injury is performance of a cutting maneuver while running. It has been suggested that when the knee approaches a valgus position, the load experienced by the ACL may be five times greater than that when the knee is aligned in the frontal plane.[5] Women tend to exhibit less knee flexion and greater knee valgus during side-cutting and cross-cutting tasks,[46] which, in turn, may place the knee in a position in which significant ACL strain can occur. No differences were found between males and females in knee rotation during cutting; however, females exhibit greater intertrial variability in femoral rotation patterns.[47] This amount of variability was most strongly influenced by level of experience, with less experienced female athletes exhibiting

greater knee rotation variability. Thus, it may be possible to train female athletes to exhibit specific lower extremity movement patterns that do not predispose them to lower extremity injury or reinjury.

CLINICAL PEARL #5

During cutting maneuvers, females exhibit greater genu valgum and show a dependence of knee rotation variability on the level of experience with performing cutting.

Neuromuscular Differences

Stiffness

A potential contributor to the greater incidence of lower extremity injury in females than in males is the gender difference in joint stability from active muscle stiffness. Stiffness has been defined as the resistance exerted by the soft tissue structures in response to a force that may result in joint stress, and active joint stiffness can be modulated through voluntary muscle contraction.[73] In addition, it has been suggested that individuals who are less able to voluntarily contract their muscles in response to an external force or perturbation may be more likely to sustain an injury. Wojtys and co-workers[73] used a dynamic stress test to measure anterior tibial translation and simultaneous muscular response to an externally applied stress. It was reported that muscle co-contraction significantly decreased anterior tibial translation in both men and women. However, men exhibited significantly greater stiffness than women suggesting that women demonstrated a reduced ability to actively protect the knee in response to an anteriorly applied force. Other studies measuring active muscle stiffness of males and females during isometric knee flexion and extension contractions and during functional hopping tasks have been conducted.[22,23] During either task, females demonstrated reduced active muscle stiffness compared with males.[22,23] Thus, it is possible that reduced active muscle stiffness may lead to reduced joint stability and may predispose females to lower extremity joint injury.

Neuromuscular Response

Considerable attention has been focused on how the muscles surrounding the knee joint react during joint loading and to unexpected perturbations. This area of research is particularly important because failure of the ACL occurs when large mechanical loads exceed the capacity of the stabilizing ligaments.[58,67] In addition, whereas the ACL provides a significant static restraint to anterior tibial translation, active muscle recruitment can assist the ACL to maintain joint stability and prevent injury.[58] Thus, gender-related differences in muscle activation in response to joint loading and unexpected perturbations may shed light on the gender bias of lower extremity injury. Previous work by

Huston and Wojtys[30] indicated that female athletes initially used their quadriceps muscles for knee stabilization in response to anterior tibial translation, whereas female nonathletes and males initially relied on their hamstring muscles. In addition, female athletes took significantly longer to generate maximum hamstring muscle torque during isokinetic testing than males.[30] However, other studies have reported no differences in the timing of muscle recruitment between men and women when exposed to a lower extremity standing perturbation.[63] Thus, it is unclear whether or not gender-related differences in muscle recruitment exist, and the artificial nature of the unexpected perturbations may limit the ability to generalize the results to possible neuromuscular differences sport-specific tasks.

Only two studies that looked at gender differences in muscle recruitment during functional activities such as running and landing have been conducted. Females have been found to exhibit reduced hamstring and greater quadriceps electromyographic activity during running, side-cutting, and cross-cutting tasks.[46] These muscle recruitment patterns, in combination with less knee flexion and greater loading rates exhibited by female athletes, certainly increase the potential for ACL strain. The combination of these muscle activation patterns may produce excessive strain on the ACL. In addition, it has been reported that females exhibit hamstring muscle onsets less coincident with anterior tibial shear forces during landings, thereby increasing the potential for ACL injury.[13]

CLINICAL PEARL #6

Neuromuscular responses that may predispose females to injury include a decrease in knee stiffness, a reliance on quadriceps contraction for knee stabilization after an applied perturbation, and greater quadriceps activity in the performance of running and cutting.

Hormonal influence

Although not a structural difference, the most obvious differences between males and females are those in reproductive hormones and the menstrual cycle exhibited by women. The menstrual cycle ranges from 24 to 35 days, averaging 28 days, and can be broken down into three phases with varying levels of reproductive hormones within each stage. The first phase is the menstrual phase (days 1 to 5) and is marked by low estrogen and progesterone levels. The follicular phase (days 6 to 13) is marked by rising levels of estrogen and leads to ovulation, which occurs immediately after a surge in estrogen. Finally, the luteal phase lasts approximately 14 days during which progesterone is the dominant hormone, but estrogen also increases to approximately one half the value of the late follicular phase surge.[25]

The physiologic link between surges in estrogen levels and ACL laxity has been the topic of recent research because some studies have identified estrogen receptors on the human ACL.[43] Thus, it has been suggested that, based on in vitro data, higher rates of ACL injury in women may be due to decreased fibroblastic proliferation and decreased procollagen synthesis in the human ACL caused by increases in estrogen concentration.[78] Whether or not increasing levels of estrogen cause females to have a greater risk for ACL injury remains debatable.

Few studies have investigated the effect of the menstrual cycle on ACL injury. In a prospective study, Myklebust and associates[52] reported that 14 women suffered injury in the late follicular or menstrual phases in a group of 17 female team handball players with ACL injuries. Wojtys and colleagues[74] also attempted to determine the menstrual phase in which ACL injury occurred using a retrospective approach up to 3 months postinjury. These authors reported a significantly higher frequency of ACL injury than expected during the late follicular phase and a significantly lower frequency of ACL injury than expected in the early follicular phase. However, the phase of the menstrual cycle was self-reported in these investigations and not confirmed by direct hormone measurements. More recently, Slauterback and co-workers[65] studied the relationship between ACL injury and serum estrogen levels in women within 48 hours after ACL injury. These authors stated that a significant number of ACL injuries occurred on days 1 and 2 of the menses when estrogen levels were lowest. Thus, it remains unclear whether or not reproductive hormones influence ACL injury.

CLINICAL PEARL #7

The presence of estrogen receptors on the ACL and the prevalence of ACL injuries in certain phases of the menstrual cycle may indicate a link between hormones and injury in female athletes.

Summary

Many differences exist between males and females, and the differences appear to influence injury patterns in females. Females have a different structural alignment of the lower extremities, and the alignment may predispose them to specific injuries. The structural alignment also has the potential to influence mechanics, further predisposing females to specific injuries. Although there is relatively little information available regarding gender differences during functional, sport-specific activities, it appears that females may perform tasks differently, regardless of their alignment, and the manner in which they perform these tasks may make them susceptible to injury. Two areas receiving greater attention in recent years are the influence of neuromuscular responses and hormones on injuries in female athletes. Further research is warranted to determine the magnitude of their influence.

REHABILITATION INTERVENTIONS

The majority of rehabilitation programs developed specifically for female athletes have been designed to decrease the risk of ACL injury. Although these programs have been designed with injury prevention in mind, the principles behind these programs can be implemented into postinjury rehabilitation for females as a means to prevent future injury. This section will present specific exercises, along with published programs, that can be implemented into rehabilitation for the injured female athlete.

Core Stability Training

Core stability training is gaining popularity in rehabilitation as clinicians become more aware of the influence of weakness in the "core" of the body on lower extremity mechanics and performance. The lumbar, pelvis, and hip region together are considered to be the core of the body and are collectively called the *lumbopelvic-hip complex* (LPHC). Optimal core function involves both trunk mobility and stability. When the core is functioning efficiently, advantageous length/tension relationships are maintained, allowing the athlete to produce strong movements in the extremities.[11]

Core stability may also be important in allowing an athlete to maintain the center of gravity over the base of support.[59]

Core stability training may be particularly important for the female athlete because weakness in the core could alter posture, exacerbating factors that are believed to contribute to injury. For example, weakness of the hip abductors and external rotators could result in greater hip adduction and femoral internal rotation, which could contribute to increased knee valgus and thus possibly result in patellofemoral injury. In addition, weakness of the gluteus musculature has been hypothesized to cause tightness in the tensor fasciae latae and a more erect hip and trunk, which could result in greater loads across the knee.[11,71] To create a comprehensive core stability training program, the practitioner must first understand the functional anatomy of the core.

CLINICAL PEARL #8

A weak core can result in inefficient movements and altered postures which can lead to injury.

There are many muscles in the core region important for postural alignment and dynamic postural equilibrium during activities.[11,55] A summary of these muscles and their functions is found in Table 13-1. In the lumbar region, the main muscles include the transversospinalis group, erector

Table 13-1

Muscles of the Core and Their Function in Providing Core Stability

Muscle Group	Muscle	Function
Lumbar spine	Transversospinalis group	Intersegmental stabilization
		Proprioceptive feedback
	Erector spinae	Intersegmental stabilization
		Back extension
	Quadratus lumborum	Frontal plane stabilization
	Latissimus dorsi	Dynamic stabilization
Abdominal muscles	Rectus abdominus	Trunk flexion
	External oblique	Lateral trunk flexion
		Contralateral rotation
	Internal oblique	Lateral trunk flexion
		Ipsilateral rotation
	Transverse abdominus	Increased abdominal pressure
		Dynamic stabilization
Hip muscles	Gluteus maximus	Hip extension
		Femoral external rotation
		Stabilize SI joint
	Gluteus medius	Frontal plane stabilization
		Femoral external rotation
		Femoral abduction
	Psoas major	Hip flexion
		Trunk extension

From Clark, M.A., Fater, D., and Reuteman, P. (2000): Core (trunk) stabilization and its importance for closed kinetic chain rehabilitation. Orthop. Phys. Ther. Clin. North Am., 9:119-135.

spinae, quadratus lumborum, and latissimus dorsi. The transversospinalis group is mainly responsible for LPHC dynamic stabilization during movement and plays a very small role in producing movement. In addition, the transversospinalis muscles have been found to contain two to six times the number of muscle spindles compared with other muscles, thus providing a significant amount of proprioceptive feedback to the central nervous system.[55] The erector spinae muscles contract to produce trunk extension and also serve to provide dynamic intersegmental stabilization whereas the quadratus lumborum muscles provide for frontal plane stabilization along with the gluteus medius and tensor fasciae latae muscle.

CLINICAL PEARL #9

The initial difficulty of exercises in core stability training should be adapted to the level of proficiency of the patients

The abdominal muscles include rectus abdominus, external oblique, internal oblique, and transverse abdominus.[55] Although the rectus abdominus is mainly responsible for trunk flexion, the internal and external oblique muscles produce lateral trunk flexion. In addition, the internal and external oblique muscles produce ipsilateral and contralateral trunk rotation, respectively. The transverse abdominus is perhaps the most important of the abdominal muscles because contraction of this muscle dramatically increases intra-abdominal pressure and provides the greatest degree of LPHC stability during dynamic movement. In addition, it has been reported that contraction of the transverse abdominus, similar to the multifidus muscle of the transversospinalis group, precedes initiation of limb movement.[14]

The core hip muscles are primarily the gluteus maximus, gluteus medius, and psoas major.[55] The gluteus maximus contracts to produce hip extension and external rotation and provides dynamic stability to the sacroiliac joint during movment.[55] The gluteus medius muscle provides frontal plane stabilization and causes femoral abduction and external rotation, and the psoas major muscle produces hip flexion and assists in trunk extension.[55]

Various rehabilitation interventions are specifically designed for improving core stability. Most notably are Pilates, Swiss ball, and medicine ball exercises. Regardless of the specific exercise initiated for core stabilization training, several principles should be followed in developing a core stability training program to produce the best outcome. First, the training program should be systematic and in each phase of training, specific goals should be met.[11] Second, the program should be progressive.[11] This includes a progression from straight plane to multiplane movements, from isometric to concentric and eccentric contractions, from slow to fast movements, from nonre-

sisted to resisted movements, from no limb movement to the addition of limb movement, and from lying down positions to standing. Finally, the program should be functional.[11] Isolated movements may be proficient for targeting specific muscles, but the gains may not carry over into functional movement.

CLINICAL PEARL #10

Exercises should only be progressed when the patient is able to maintain spinal stability and a normal breathing pattern

In the initial phases of core stability training, the focus should be to increase the base level of strength and endurance in muscles of the core region. Slow, controlled, isometric movements may be necessary initially, depending on the starting level of strength and control in the patient. Pelvic tilting and isometric transversus abdominus exercises are very basic exercises that may be prescribed. The isometric transversus abdominus exercise requires the athlete to draw the navel in by contracting the muscles and hold the contraction with a normal breathing pattern and without global muscle activation.[35] When the athlete is able to perform these exercises correctly and can maintain a normal breathing pattern during the exercises, the difficulty may be progressed as noted earlier. Exercises that may be prescribed include leg slides, prone arm or leg raises, abdominal crunches on a Swiss ball, or a bicycle exercise (Fig. 13-4). It is imperative that the athlete maintains spinal stabilization during each exercise, and if the athlete cannot, the exercise difficulty should be decreased. Next, resistance should be added to further increase muscular strength, and the duration of the exercises should be increased to enhance muscular endurance. Potential exercises in this phase include crunches with a ball toss into a rebounder or trunk rotation with a medicine ball (Fig. 13-5). Finally, exercises that closely mimic movements during the athlete's sport should be incorporated into training

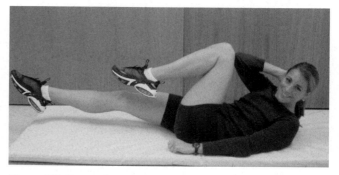

Figure 13-4. Bicycle exercise for core stability training. When properly performed, the pelvis should not move as leg movements are alternated.

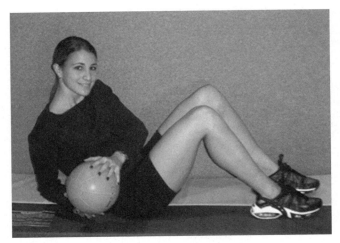

Figure 13-5. Side-to-side rotation with a medicine ball. The pelvis and low-back position should remain stable as the upper body is rotated from side to side.

(Fig. 13-6) or sports activities should be performed with an emphasis on maintaining core stability.

Jump or Plyometric Training

Studies that document gender differences in landing provide support for including jump or plyometric training in rehabilitation programs for female athletes. A 6-week training program developed by Hewett and associates[26] includes jump training in addition to stretching and strengthening exercises (Table 13-2). After participating in the training program, female athletes had decreased knee abduction and adduction moments, predictors of peak landing forces, and lower peak vertical ground reaction forces compared to males.[26] A prospective investigation using a similar program demonstrated that less knee injuries were experienced by female athletes who had participated in the training program than in untrained female athletes.[26] The Prevent Injury and Enhance Performance (PEP) program was modeled after the program of Hewett and associates[26] but was designed specifically for female soccer players.[60] The program includes a series of stretching, strengthening, agility training, and jumping exercises (Table 13-3). Preliminary results, reported as an abstract at the 2002 American Academy of Orthopaedic Surgeons Annual Meeting, showed 88% fewer ACL injuries in female soccer players who participated in this program than in untrained female soccer players. Another program, the Frappier Acceleration Sports Training Program,° combines graded incline treadmill running with plyometric jump training. Female high school soccer players who participated in the 7-week program had a significantly reduced incidence of injuries to their lower extremities than untrained athletes.[24] Although each of the above programs includes

---

°Available from Frappier Acceleration, Fargo, North Dakota.

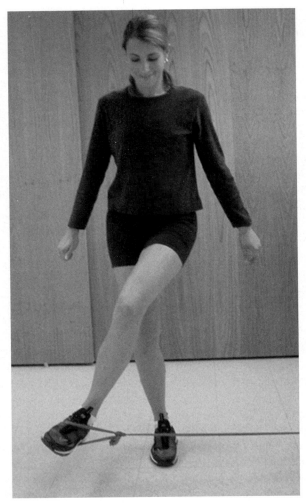

Figure 13-6. Soccer kicking is performed with resistance from a Theraband attached to the leg. The athlete is instructed to maintain stability through the trunk as the kicking motion is performed.

components other than jump training, jump training is a critical component. The combined results of these reports support jump training as a means for normalizing mechanical differences and preventing future knee injury.

CLINICAL PEARL #11

Jump training can be used to decrease forces on the knee and normalize lower limb alignment when landing

Instruction by clinicians can be used to increase the effectiveness of jump training. Patients should be instructed to land on the balls of the feet, as opposed to flat-footed, and with a flexed knee. Verbally instructing subjects to land on the balls of their feet and with flexed knees has been found to be effective in decreasing impact landing forces.[26,50] Instructing subjects to use the sound made at impact as a guide to decreasing impact forces has

Table 13-2

Jump Training Program

Exercise	Repetitions/Time	
Phase I		
Wall jumps	20 seconds	25 seconds
Tuck jumps	20 seconds	25 seconds
Broad jumps stick land	5 repetitions	10 repetitions
Squat jumps	10 seconds	15 seconds
Double leg cone jumps (side to side, back to front)	30 seconds each	30 seconds each
180° jumps	20 seconds	25 seconds
Bounding in place	20 seconds	25 seconds
Phase II		
Wall jumps	30 seconds	30 seconds
Tuck jumps	30 seconds	30 seconds
Jump, jump, jump, vertical jump	5 repetitions	8 repetitions
Squat jumps	20 seconds	20 seconds
Bounding for distance	1 run	2 runs
Double leg cone jumps	30 seconds each	30 seconds each
Scissor jump	30 seconds	30 seconds
Hop, hop, stick	5 repetitions/leg	5 repetitions/leg
Phase III		
Wall jumps	30 seconds	30 seconds
Step, jump up, down, vertical		
Mattress jumps (side to side, back to front)	30 seconds	30 seconds
Single-leg jumps distance	5 repetitions/leg	5 repetitions/leg
Squat jumps	25 seconds	25 seconds
Jump into bounding	3 runs	3 runs
Single-leg hop, hop, stick	5 repetitions/leg	5 repetitions/leg

Adapted from Hewett, T.E. (2002). Neuromuscular and hormonal factors associated with knee injuries in female athletes. Strategies for intervention. Sports Med., 28:313-327.

Table 13-3

PEP (Prevent Injury, Enhance Performance) Program

Warm-up	Stretching	Strengthening	Plyometrics	Agility Exercises
Jogging	Calf	Walking lunges	Lateral, forward, and backward hops over cones	Backward and forward shuttle runs
Shuttle run from side to side	Quadriceps	Russian hamstring exercise	Single-leg hops over cones	Diagonal runs
Backward running	Hamstring	Single-toe raises	Vertical jumps combined with heading the ball	Bounding runs with knees up toward chest
	Inner thigh		Scissors jumps	
	Hip flexor			

Adapted from: Roniger, L.R. (2002): Training improves ACL outcomes in female athletes. Biomechanics, January, pp. 51-57.

also been found to be effective.[48,56] Clinicians should also cue patients on alignment, such as avoiding increased knee valgus when landing (Fig. 13-7). An ability to maintain alignment may also indicate a need for core stability training.

CLINICAL PEARL #12

Verbal feedback by clinicians can enhance jump training technique

Balance Training

Balance training is implemented into many postinjury rehabilitation programs as a mechanism for improving proprioception, or joint awareness, after injury. Decreased proprioception has been found after injuries such as ACL rupture and ankle sprain[7,19,39] and is attributed to altered mechanoreceptor afferent input after injury.[41] Because

reflex pathways, including those that are responsible for postural sway, depend on afferent input, the loss of afferent input or altered afferent input after injury can also influence postural sway.[76] Increased sway during single-leg standing has been found in subjects with ACL deficiency, ACL reconstruction, and lateral ankle sprains.[10,38,45,62] Sensory input achieved during balance training may restore neuromuscular pathways.

A variety of therapeutic exercise techniques can be categorized under balance training. Some exercises primarily involve the maintenance of balance without applied disturbance, for example, single-leg standing exercises on an unstable board (Fig. 13-8). Other exercises involve the maintenance of balance in response to an applied postural disturbance (Fig. 13-9). These exercises may not be equivalent; however, research is needed to determine whether these exercises produce similar outcomes.

There is conflicting research on the ability of training with unstable boards to prevent lower extremity injury;

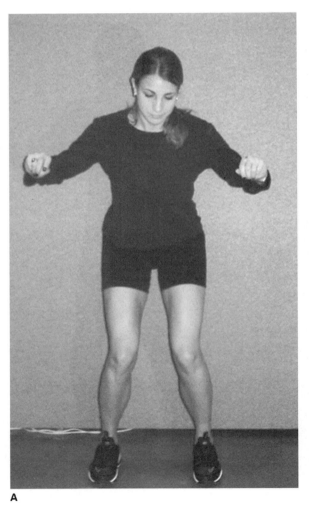

A

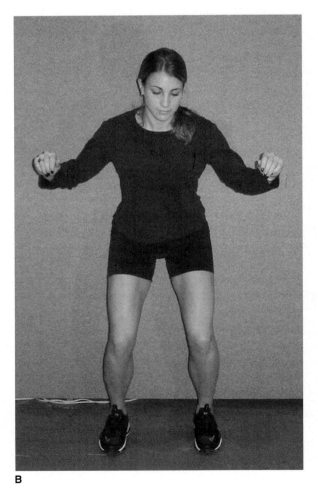

B

Figure 13-7. (A) Improper knee alignment during jump training. (B) The athlete should be instructed to maintain a knee position that is over the feet when landing.

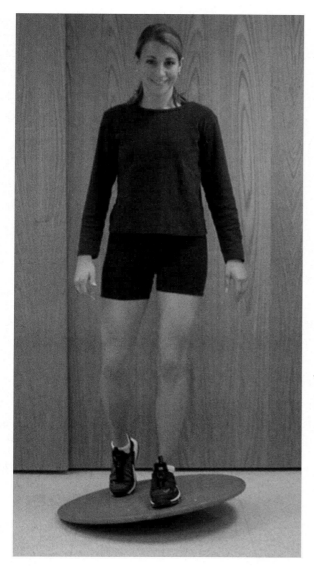

Figure 13-8. Unilateral standing balance on an unstable board.

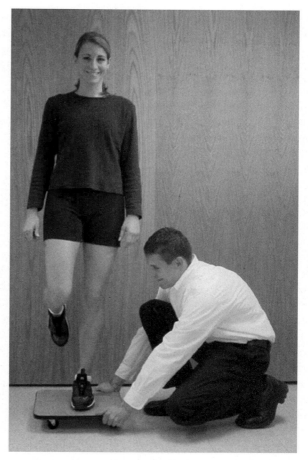

Figure 13-9. A perturbation training technique. The athlete stands in a unilateral stance on a rolling board and attempts to maintain balance as the therapist applies a disturbance to the rolling board.

however, some positive adaptations can be made for muscular reflexes. Male soccer players who performed single-leg standing and step-up exercises on wobble boards for 20 minutes per day during preseason training had fewer ACL injuries than untrained players,[8] and female handball players who used an ankle disk for 10 to 15 minutes during practice sessions over a 10-month season had significantly fewer ankle injuries and fewer traumatic lower extremity injuries overall than control subjects.[72] In contrast, no difference was found in the occurrence of traumatic lower extremity injuries between female soccer players who participated in a program of 10 to 15 minutes of training on a balance board during the season and those who did not.[66] Differences in the instruction to subjects and the progression of the exercises may explain the conflicting results of these studies. Osborne and associates[53] found that control subjects and subjects with ankle sprains who partici-

pated in 8 weeks of ankle disk training showed a decreased tibialis anterior onset in response to an inversion perturbation, suggesting that balance training on an unstable disk may be able to induce changes in neuromuscular response. More research is necessary, though, to identify the effect of this type of training on neuromuscular responses in other muscles and the relationship of the change to function.

Another type of balance training involves the application of a perturbation to the surface on which the patient stands. Subjects with ACL deficiency who participated in rehabilitation with perturbation training have been found to be more successful in returning to sports without knee instability[18] and have a faster hamstring reaction time to forward movement of an isokinetic dynamometer arm, post-training.[4,32] Coordination of muscle activity during walking is also altered after this type of training in ways that are consistent with improved dynamic knee stability.[9] These results demonstrate that training with support surface perturbations changes neuromuscular control in the ACL-deficient knee. However, to date, no study has been published on the effect of this type of training in injury prevention or postoperative rehabilitation or the differential effect of this training in males compared with females.

CLINICAL PEARL #13

Balance training may normalize afferent input after injury, which in turn can normalize postinjury sway and alter neuromuscular responses

Perturbation training, similar to the other rehabilitation interventions presented in this chapter, should follow a logical progression. Fitzgerald and co-workers[18] described the initial application of support surface perturbations with upper limb support provided and verbal cues given for the onset of the perturbation. When the patient demonstrated the ability to maintain balance without difficulty, then support and verbal cues were removed and the perturbations were progressed by randomizing the timing, direction, and force of application.[18] During perturbation training, if a patient demonstrates an inability to maintain balance, it is likely that the progression was too difficult, and this often occurs when many variables (magnitude of force, direction, and timing) are progressed simultaneously. At least one variable should be reduced in difficulty such that the patient is sufficiently challenged but is able to perform the task. Perturbation training should also be progressed to include sport-specific tasks to encourage carryover to functional activity.[18] An example of this would be adding chest passes with a basketball while perturbations are being applied.

SUMMARY

Gender Differences

■ Anatomically, females exhibit a wider pelvis, greater Q-angle, greater femoral anteversion, a more externally rotated position of the tibia and greater genu valgum compared to males.

■ During athletic movements, females exhibit less knee flexion, greater genu valgum, greater femoral anteversion and hip abduction, and greater tibial external rotation compared to males doing the same tasks.

■ Compared to males, females exhibit reduced lower extremity active muscle stiffness; females also demonstrate earlier recruitment of the quadriceps muscle and slower hamstring activity onset after an unexpected force applied to the knee.

■ Female reproductive hormones may potentially influence ligament laxity.

Rehabilitation Interventions

■ Core stability training improves dynamic lower extremity alignment, produces more efficient movements and maintains the center of gravity over the base of support.

■ Jump training improves dynamic lower extremity alignment, improves neuromuscular response time and decreases landing forces.

■ Balance training improves neuromuscular response time, improves muscular coordination and improves functional ability.

REFERENCES

1. Aglietti, P., Insall, J.N., and Cerulli, G. (1983): Patellar pain and incongruence. I: Measurements of incongruence. Clin. Orthop., 176:217-224.
2. Almeida, S.A., Trone, D.W., Leone, D.M., et al. (1995): Gender differences in musculoskeletal injury rates: A function of symptom reporting? Med. Sci. Sports Exerc., 31:1807-1812.
3. Arendt, E. and Dick, R. (1995): Knee injury patterns among men and women in collegiate basketball and soccer. NCAA data and review of literature. Am. J. Sports Med., 23:694-701.
4. Beard, D.J., Kyberd, P.J., Fergusson, C.M., et al. (1993): Proprioception after rupture of the anterior cruciate ligament. An objective indication of the need for surgery? J. Bone Joint Surg. Br., 75:311-315.
5. Bendjaballah, M.Z., Shirazi-Adl, A., and Zukor, D.J. (1997): Finite element analysis of human knee joint in varus-valgus. Clin. Biomech., 12:139-148.
6. Beynnon, B.D., and Johnson, R.J. (1996): Anterior cruciate ligament injury rehabilitation in athletes. Biomechanical considerations. Sports Med., 22:54-64.
7. Beynnon, B.D., Ryder, S.H., Konradsen, L., et al. (1999): The effect of anterior cruciate ligament trauma and bracing on knee proprioception. Am. J. Sports Med., 27:150-155.
8. Caraffa, A., Cerulli, G., Projetti, M., et al. (1996): Prevention of anterior cruciate ligament injuries in soccer. A prospective controlled study of proprioceptive training. Knee Surg. Sports Traumatol. Arthrosc., 4:19-21.
9. Chmielewski, T.L., Rudolph, K.S., and Snyder-Mackler, L. (2002): Development of dynamic knee stability after acute ACL injury. J. Electromyogr. Kinesiol., 12:267-274.
10. Chmielewski, T.L., Wilk, K.E., and Snyder-Mackler, L. (2002): Changes in weight-bearing following injury or surgical reconstruction of the ACL: Relationship to quadriceps strength and function. Gait Posture, 16: 87-95.
11. Clark, M.A., Fater, D., and Reuteman, P. (2000): Core (trunk) stabilization and its importance for closed kinetic chain rehabilitation. Orthop. Phys. Ther. Clin. North Am., 9:119-135.
12. Cowan, D.N., Jones, B.H., Frykman, P.N., et al. (1996): Lower limb morphology and risk of overuse injury among male infantry trainees. Med. Sci. Sports Exerc., 28:945-952.
13. Cowling, E.J., and Steele, J.R. (2001): Is lower limb muscle synchrony during landing affected by gender? Implications for variations in ACL injury rates. J. Electromyogr. Kinesiol., 11:263-268.
14. Cresswell, A.G., Grundstrom, H., and Thorstensson, A. (1992): Observations on intra-abdominal pressure and patterns of abdominal intra-muscular activity in man. Acta Physiol. Scand., 144:409-418.

15. DeHaven, K.E., and Lintner, D.M. (1986): Athletic injuries: Comparison by age, sport, and gender. Am. J. Sports Med., 14:218-224.

16. Dufek, J.S., and Bates, B.T. (1991): Biomechanical factors associated with injury during landing in jump sports. Sports Med., 12:326-337.

17. Ferretti, A., Papandrea, P., Conteduca, F., et al. (1992): Knee ligament injuries in volleyball players. Am. J. Sports Med., 20:203-207.

18. Fitzgerald, G.K., Axe, M.J., and Snyder-Mackler, L. (2000): The efficacy of perturbation training in nonoperative anterior cruciate ligament rehabilitation programs for physical active individuals. Phys. Ther., 80:128-140.

19. Friden, T., Roberts, D., Zatterstrom, R., et al. (1996): Proprioception in the nearly extended knee. Measurements of position and movement in healthy individuals and in symptomatic anterior cruciate ligament injured patients. Knee Surg. Sports Traumatol. Arthrosc., 4: 217-224.

20. Good, L., Odensten, M., and Gillquist, J. (1991): Intercondylar notch measurements with special reference to anterior cruciate ligament surgery. Clin. Orthop., 263:185-189.

21. Gray, J., Taunton, J.E., McKenzie, D.C., et al. (1985): A survey of injuries to the anterior cruciate ligament of the knee in female basketball players. Int. J. Sports Med., 6:314-316.

22. Granata, K.P., Wilson, S.E., and Padua, D.A. (2002): Gender differences in active musculoskeletal stiffness. Part I. Quantification in controlled measurements of knee joint dynamics. J. Electromyogr. Kinesiol., 12:119-126.

23. Granata, K.P., Wilson, S.E., and Padua, D.A. (2002): Gender differences in active musculoskeletal stiffness. Part I. Quantification in controlled measurements of knee joint dynamics. J. Electromyogr. Kinesiol., 12:119-126.

24. Heidt, R.S., Jr, Sweeterman, L.M., Carlonas, R.L., et al. (2000): Avoidance of soccer injuries with preseason conditioning. Am. J. Sports Med., 28:659-662.

25. Heitz, N.A. (1999): Hormonal changes throughout the menstrual cycle and increased anterior cruciate ligament laxity in females. J. Ath. Train., 34:144-149.

26. Hewett, T.E., Stroupe, A.L., Nance, T.A., and Noyes, F.R. (1996): Plyometric training in female athletes. Decreased impact forces and increased hamstring torques. Am. J. Sports Med., 24:765-773.

27. Horton, M.G., and Hall, T.L. (1989): Quadriceps femoris muscle angle: Normal values and relationships with gender and selected skeletal measures. Phys. Ther., 69:897-901.

28. Hsu, R.W., Himeno, S., Coventry, M.B., and Chao, E.Y. (1990): Normal axial alignment of the lower extremity and load-bearing distribution at the knee. Clin. Orthop., 255:215-227.

29. Huston, L.J., Vibert, B., Ashton-Miller, J.A., and Wojtys, E.M. (2001): Gender differences in knee angle when landing from a drop-jump. Am. J. Knee Surg., 14:215-220.

30. Huston, L.J., and Wojtys, E.M. (1996): Neuromuscular performance characteristics in elite female athletes. Am. J. Sports Med., 24:427-436.

31. Hutchinson, M.R., and Ireland, M.L. (1995): Knee injuries in female athletes. Sports Med., 19:288-302.

32. Ihara, H., and Nakayama, A. (1986): Dynamic joint control training for knee ligament injuries. Am. J. Sports Med., 14: 309-315.

33. Ireland, M.L., Ballantyne, B.T., Little, K., and McClay, I.S. (2001): A radiographic analysis of the relationship between the size and shape of the intercondylar notch and anterior cruciate ligament injury. Knee Surg. Sports Traumatol. Arthrosc., 9:200-205.

34. James, S.L., Bates, B.T., and Osternig, L.R. (1978): Injuries to runners. Am. J. Sports Med., 6:40-50.

35. Johnson, P.J. (2002): Training the trunk in the athlete. Strength Cond. J., 24:52-59.

36. Kersnic, B., Iglic, A., Kralj-Iglic, V., et al. (1996): Determination of the femoral and pelvic geometrical parameters that are important for the hip joint contact stress: Differences between female and male. Pflugers Arch., 431:207-208.

37. Knapik, J.J., Sharp, M.A., Canham-Chervak, M., et al. (2001): Risk factors for training-related injuries among men and women in basic combat training. Med. Sci. Sports Exerc., 33:946-954.

38. Leanderson, J., Wykman, A., and Eriksson, E. (1993): Ankle sprain and postural sway in basketball players. Knee Surg. Sports Traumatol. Arthrosc., 1:203-305.

39. Lentell, G., Baas, B., Lopez, D., et al. (1995): The contributions of proprioceptive deficits, muscle function, and anatomic laxity to functional instability of the ankle. J. Orthop. Sports Phys. Ther., 21:206-215.

40. Lephart, S.M., Ferris, C.M., Riemann, B.L., et al. (2002): Gender differences in strength and lower extremity kinematics during landing. Clin. Orthop., 401:162-169.

41. Lephart, S.M., Pincivero, D.M., Giraldo, J.L., and Fu, F.H. (1997): The role of proprioception in the management and rehabilitation of athletic injuries. Am. J. Sports Med., 25: 130-137.

42. Livingston, L.A. (1998): The quadriceps angle: A review of the literature. J. Orthop. Sports Phys. Ther., 28:105-109.

43. Liu, S.H. (1997): Estrogen affects the cellular metabolism of the anterior cruciate ligament: A potential explanation for female athletic injury. Am. Orthop. Soc. Sports Med., 25:704-709.

44. Lund-Hanssen, H., Gannon, J., Engebretsen, L., et al. (1994): Intercondylar notch width and the risk for anterior cruciate ligament rupture. A case-control study in 46 female handball players. Acta. Orthop. Scand., 65:529-532.

45. Lysholm, M., Ledin, T., Odkvist, L.M., and Good, L. (1998): Postural control—A comparison between patients with chronic anterior cruciate ligament insufficiency and healthy individuals. Scand. J. Med. Sci. Sports, 8: 432-438.

46. Malinzak, R.A., Colby, S.M., Kirkendall, D.T., et al. (2001): A comparison of knee joint motion patterns between men and women in selected athletic tasks. Clin. Biomech., 16:438-445.

47. McLean, S.G., Neal, R.J., Myers, P.T., and Walters, M.R. (1999): Knee joint kinematics during the sidestep cutting maneuver: Potential for injury in women. Med. Sci. Sports Exerc., 31:959-968.

48. McNair, P.J., Prapavessis, H., and Callender, K. (2000): Decreasing landing forces: Effect of instruction. Br. J. Sports Med., 34:293-296.

49. Messier, S.P., Davis, S.E., Curl, W.W., et al. (1991): Etiologic factors associated with patellofemoral pain in runners. Med. Sci. Sports Exerc., 23:1008-1015.

50. Mizrahi, J., and Susak, Z. (1982): Analysis of parameters affecting impact force attenuation during landing in human vertical free fall. Eng. Med., 11:141-147.

51. Mizuno, Y., Kumagai, M., Mattessich, S.M., et al. (2001): Q-angle influences tibiofemoral and patellofemoral kinematics. J. Orthop. Res., 19:834-840.

52. Myklebust, G., Maehlum, S., Holm, I., and Bahr, R. (1998): A prospective cohort study of anterior cruciate ligament injuries in elite Norwegian team handball. Scand. J. Med. Sci. Sports, 8:149-153.

53. Osborne, M.D., Chou, L.S., Laskowski, E.R., et al. (2001): The effect of ankle disk training on muscle reaction time in subjects with a history of ankle sprain. Am. J. Sports Med., 29: 627-635.

54. Pester, S., and Smith, P.C. (1992): Stress fractures in the lower extremities of soldiers in basic training. Orthop. Rev., 21:297-303.

55. Porterfield, J.A., and DeRosa, C. (1991): Mechanical Low Back Pain: Perspectives in Functional Anatomy. Philadelphia, W.B. Saunders.

56. Prapavessis, H., and McNair, P.J. (1999): Effects of instruction in jumping technique and experience jumping on ground reaction forces. J. Orthop. Sports Phys. Ther., 29:352-356.

57. Reinker, K.A., and Ozburne, S. (1979): A comparison of male and female orthopaedic pathology in basic training. Mil. Med., 144:532-536.

58. Renstrom, P., Arms, S.W., Stanwyck, T.S., et al. (1986): Strain within the anterior cruciate ligament during hamstring and quadriceps activity. Am. J. Sports Med., 14:83-87.

59. Roetert, P. (2001): 3-D balance and core stability. In: Foran, B. (ed.): High Performance Sports Conditioning. Champaign, IL, Human Kinetics, p. 126.

60. Roniger, L.R. (2002): Training improves ACL outcomes in female athletes. Biomechanics, January, pp. 51-57.

61. Shelbourne, K.D., Facibene, W.A., Hunt, J.J. (1997): Radiographic and intraoperative intercondylar notch width measurements in men and women with unilateral and bilateral anterior cruciate ligament tears. Knee Surg. Sports Traumatol. Arthrosc., 5:229-233.

62. Shiraishi, M., Mizuta, H., Kubota, K., et al. (1996): Stabilometric assessment in the anterior cruciate ligament-reconstructed knee. Clin. J. Sport Med., 6:32-39.

63. Shultz, S.J., Perrin, D.H., Adams, J.M., et al. (2000): Assessment of neuromuscular response characteristics at the knee following a functional perturbation. J. Electromyogr. Kinesiol., 10:159-170.

64. Simoneau, G.G., Hoenig, K.J., Lepley, J.E., and Papanek, P.E. (1998): Influence of hip position and gender on active hip internal and external rotation. J. Orthop. Sports Phys. Ther., 28:158-164.

65. Slauterback, J.R., Fuzie, S.F., Smith, M.P., et al. (2002): The menstrual cycle, sex hormones, and anterior cruciate ligament injury. J. Ath. Train., 37: 275-280.

66. Soderman, K., Werner, S., Pietila, T., et al. (2000): Balance board training: Prevention of traumatic injuries of the lower extremities in female soccer players? A prospective randomized intervention study. Knee Surg. Sports Traumatol. Arthrosc., 8:356-363.

67. Solomonow, M., Baratta, R., Zhou, B.H., et al. (1987): The synergistic action of the anterior cruciate ligament and thigh muscles in maintaining joint stability. Am. J. Sports Med., 15:207-213.

68. Swanson, S.C., and Caldwell, G.E. (2000): An integrated biomechanical analysis of high speed incline and level treadmill running. Med. Sci. Sports Exerc., 32:1146-1155.

69. Teitz, C.C., Hu, S.S., and Arendt, E.A. (1997): The female athlete: Evaluation and treatment of sports-related problems. J. Am. Acad. Orthop. Surg., 5:87-96.

70. Tiberio, D. (1987): The effect of excessive subtalar joint pronation on patellofemoral mechanics: A theoretical model. J. Orthop. Sports Phys. Ther., 9:160-165.

71. Toth, A.P., and Cordasco, F.A. (2001): Anterior cruciate ligament injuries in the female athlete. J. Gend. Specif. Med., 4 25-34.

72. Wedderkopp, N., Kaltoft, M., Lundgaard, B., et al. (1999): Prevention of injuries in young female players in European team handball. A prospective intervention study. Scand. J. Med. Sci. Sports, 9:41-47.

73. Wojtys, E.M,, Ashton-Miller, J.A., and Huston, L.J. (2002): A gender-related difference in the contribution of the knee musculature to sagittal-plane shear stiffness in subjects with similar knee laxity. J. Bone Joint Surg. Am., 84-A:10-16.

74. Wojtys, E.M., Huston, L.J., Lindenfeld, T.N., et al. (1998): Association between the menstrual cycle and anterior cruciate ligament injuries in female athletes. Am. J. Sports Med., 26:614-619.

75. Woodland, L.H., and Francis, R.S. (1992): Parameters and comparisons of the quadriceps angle of college-aged men and women in the supine and standing positions. Am. J. Sports Med., 20: 208-221.

76. Wooley, S.M., Rubin, A.M., and Kantner, R.M., et al. (1993): Differentiation of balance deficits through examination of selected components of static stabilometry. J. Otolaryngol., 22:368-375.

77. Yoshioka, Y., Siu, D.W., Scudamore, R.A., and Cooke, T.D. (1989): Tibial anatomy and functional axes. J. Orthop. Res., 7:132-137.

78. Yu, W.D. (2001): Combined effects of estrogen and progesterone on the anterior cruciate ligament. Clin. Orthop. Relat. Res., 383:268-281.

CHAPTER 14

LEG, ANKLE, AND FOOT REHABILITATION

Edward P. Mulligan, M.S., P.T., S.C.S., ATC

CHAPTER OBJECTIVES

At the end of this chapter the reader will be able to:

- Explain the arthrokinematic considerations that influence motion in the joints of the foot and ankle.
- Explain the concentric and eccentric action of muscles in the lower leg, ankle, and foot.
- Recognize structural abnormalities in the alignment of the lower leg, rearfoot, and forefoot.
- Describe normal gait patterns and recognize common pathologic variations.
- Describe common athletic pathologic conditions and the rehabilitative management of the lower leg, ankle, and foot injuries.
- Explain the biomechanical principles and clinical practice of orthotic therapy.

The lower leg, ankle, and foot consist of 26 bones, all working as one unit to propel the body. The foot has three components: rearfoot, midfoot, and forefoot. The rearfoot and midfoot are composed of the tarsal bones. The rearfoot contains the subtalar joint, with the talus resting on top of the calcaneus. The midfoot is composed of the navicular and cuboid as they articulate with the talus and calcaneus to form the transverse tarsal joint. The three cuneiform bones are located within the midfoot. Five tarsal and 14 phalangeal bones make up the forefoot structure. The shape of the joint, orientation of its axis, supporting ligaments, and subtle accessory motions at the joint surface are important determinants of normal biomechanical behavior. The treatment of pathologic hypomobility or hypermobility is predicated on a thorough understanding of these principles and their functional intimacy.

ARTHROKINEMATIC CONSIDERATIONS
Tibiofibular Joint

The tibiofibular joint provides accessory motion to allow greater freedom of movement in the ankle. Fusion or hypomobility of this joint can restrict or impair ankle function. During ankle plantar flexion, the fibula slides caudal at the superior and inferior tibiofibular joint, while the lateral malleolus rotates medial to cause an approximation of the two malleoli. With dorsiflexion, the opposite accessory motions provide a slight spread of the malleoli and accommodate the wider portion of the anterior talus. Accessory motion of the tibiofibular joint also occurs with supination (calcaneal inversion) and pronation (calcaneal eversion). The head of the fibula slides distally and posteriorly with supination and proximally and anteriorly during pronation.[25]

Talocrural Joint

The talocrural articulation is a synovial joint with a structurally strong mortice and supporting collateral ligaments. The concave surface of the mortice is made up of the distal tibial plafond and the tibial (medial) and fibular (lateral) malleoli. Within the mortice sits the convex surface of the talar dome. The joint derives ligamentous support from the deltoid ligament medially and the anterior talofibular, calcaneofibular, and posterior talofibular ligaments laterally.

The lateral malleolus is positioned distally and posteriorly relative to the medial malleolus, causing the axis of motion for the ankle joint to run from posterolateral inferior to anteromedial superior (Fig. 14-1). This oblique orientation allows triplanar motion. Sagittal plane plantar flexion and dorsiflexion make up the primary movements of the joint and are coupled with adduction and abduction, respectively. Because the axis is nearly parallel to the transverse plane, inversion and eversion are negligible components of motion. Available range of motion is typically defined as approximately 20° of dorsiflexion and 50° of plantar flexion.[1]

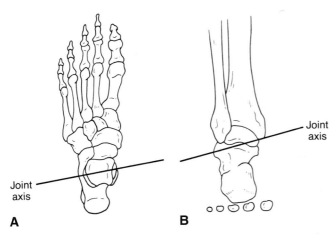

Figure 14-1. Joint axis for talocrural joint. *A*, Dorsal view. *B*, Posterior view. Axis of orientation runs from posterolateral inferior to anteromedial superior.

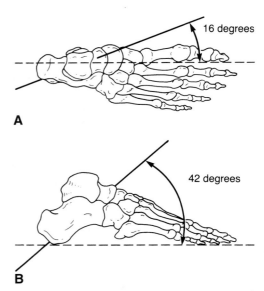

Figure 14-2. Subtalar joint axis lies approximately 16° from the sagittal plane (*A*) and 42° from the transverse plane (*B*). (Reproduced by permission from Mann, R.A. [1982]: Biomechanics of running. *In:* American Academy of Orthopaedic Surgeons: Symposium on the Foot and Leg in Running Sports. St. Louis, 1982, C.V. Mosby.)

A small amount of talocrural physiologic accessory motion also accompanies plantar flexion and dorsiflexion.[27] As the foot plantar flexes, the body of the talus slides anteriorly. Conversely, as the foot dorsiflexes, the direction of talar slide is posterior. Maximal stability to angular and torsional stresses occurs in the close-packed position of maximal dorsiflexion, in which the talus slides posteriorly and wedges within the mortice. The resting position of the ankle joint is 10° of plantar flexion (Table 14-1).

Subtalar Joint

The talocalcaneal articulation provides the triplanar motions of pronation and supination. The medial and lateral collateral, interosseous talocalcaneal, and posterior and lateral talocalcaneal ligaments support the joint.

The joint axis runs from dorsal, medial, and distal to plantar, lateral, and proximal. It is oriented approximately 16° from the sagittal plane and 42° from the transverse plane (Fig. 14-2). Because of this axis of orientation, the joint provides the triplanar motions of pronation and supination. The pronation components of motion in an open kinetic chain are calcaneal dorsiflexion, abduction, and eversion. Conversely, open kinetic chain supination consists of calcaneal plantar flexion, adduction, and inversion. Functionally, however, the subtalar joint operates like a closed kinetic chain. Closed kinetic chain motion occurs when the distal segment is fixed and the proximal segment becomes mobile, such as when the foot is in contact with the ground. The distal or terminal joints meet with considerable resistance, which prohibits or restrains free motion. During the weight-bearing portion of the stance phase of gait, friction and ground reaction forces prevent the abduction-adduction and plantar flexion-dorsiflexion elements of open kinetic chain subtalar motion. To counteract these forces, the talus functions to maintain the transverse and sagittal plane motions of supination and pronation.[31] Thus, in closed kinetic chain motion, subtalar joint pronation consists of talar plantar flexion-adduction and calcaneal eversion, whereas subtalar joint supination consists of talar dorsiflexion-abduction and calcaneal inversion (Fig. 14-3).[48] Note that calcaneal direction of

Table 14-1			
Joint Positional Treatment Considerations			
Joint	**Close-Packed Position**	**Resting Position**	**Capsular Pattern**
Talocrural	Maximal dorsiflexion	10° plantar flexion	Plantar flexion restricted greater than dorsiflexion
Subtalar	Maximal supination	Neutral	Increasing loss of varus until fixed in valgus
Midtarsal	Maximal supination	STJ neutral	Limitations in adduction and inversion
First MTP	Maximal dorsiflexion	Slight plantar flexion	Gross limitation of extension; slight limitation of flexion

MTP, Metatarsophalangeal; STJ, subtalar joint.

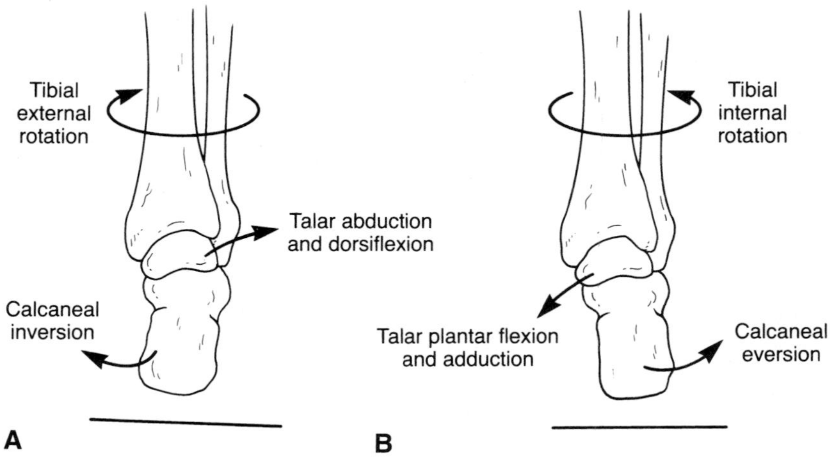

Figure 14-3. Closed-chain subtalar motion. *A*, Supination. *B*, Pronation.

movement is unaffected by the open-chain versus the closed-chain type of motion (Table 14-2).

The subtalar joint couples the function of the foot with the rest of the proximal kinetic chain. The prime function of the subtalar joint is to permit rotation of the leg in the transverse plane during gait. The rotation of the talus on the calcaneus allows the foot to become a directional transmitter and torque converter to the kinetic chain.[37] These characteristics allow the foot to be a loose adaptor to the terrain in midstance and a rigid lever for propulsion.

Because the subtalar joint is angulated approximately 45° from the transverse plane, there is 1° of inversion or eversion for every 1° of tibial internal or external rotation. This relationship can be observed in gait. As the subtalar joint pronates, the tibial tuberosity is seen to be rotating internally (Fig. 14-4). High angles of inclination (greater than 45°) of the subtalar joint axis cause a relative decrease in calcaneal inversion-eversion motion and an increased tibial rotation motion, leading to posture-related pathologic conditions due to poor absorption of ground reaction forces. Conversely, the athlete with a low angle of inclination (less than 45°) of the subtalar joint demonstrates a relative increase in calcaneal mobility, resulting in more foot-related overuse and fatigue problems due to the calcaneal hypermobility.[48]

The physiologic accessory motions of the subtalar joint occur in the frontal plane. The convex portion of the posterior calcaneus slides laterally during inversion (supination) and medially with eversion (pronation). The close-packed position of the subtalar joint is maximal supination, whereas the resting position is the subtalar neutral position. From its neutral position the subtalar joint can supinate approximately two times as much as it can pronate. This motion is measured in the frontal plane of calcaneal inversion and eversion. The normal subtalar range of motion is approximately 30°, with two thirds of that motion being represented as calcaneal inversion and one third as calcaneal eversion. Normal gait requires 8° to 12° of supination and 4° to 6° of pronation.[43]

Midtarsal Joint

The midtarsal joint consists of the talonavicular and calcaneocuboid articulations. They derive their ligamentous support from the calcaneonavicular (spring), deltoid, dorsal talonavicular, and calcaneocuboid (long and short plantar) ligaments.

The midtarsal joint has two separate axes. Functionally, these two axes work together to result in triplanar motion. The two axes of the midtarsal joint are the longitudinal and

Table 14-2		
Calcaneal and Talar Motion in Open and Closed		
Motion of Foot	**Open-Chain Component**	**Closed-Chain Component**
Pronation	Calcaneal eversion	Calcaneal eversion
	Calcaneal abduction	Talar adduction
	Calcaneal dorsiflexion	Talar plantar flexion
Supination	Calcaneal inversion	Calcaneal inversion
	Calcaneal adduction	Talar abduction
	Calcaneal plantar flexion	Talar dorsiflexion

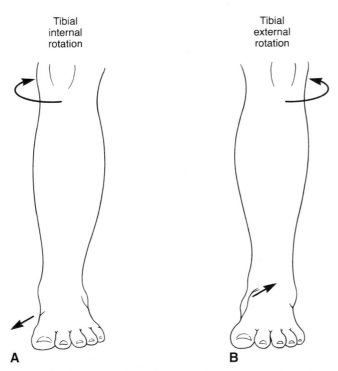

Figure 14-4. Relationship of the subtalar joint to the lower leg during gait. *A*, Subtalar pronation. *B*, Subtalar supination.

the oblique. The longitudinal axis is essentially parallel to the sagittal and transverse planes, allowing only frontal plane motions of inversion and eversion, whereas the oblique axis is parallel with the frontal plane, allowing motion in the sagittal (plantar flexion-dorsiflexion) and transverse (adduction-abduction) planes (Fig. 14-5). Because the oblique axis is angulated about equally for the sagittal and transverse planes, plantar flexion-adduction and dorsiflexion-abduction are coupled equally.

From a clinical standpoint, there is no reliable method of quantifying motion in the midtarsal joint. Midtarsal joint

motion is dictated by the position of the subtalar joint. When the subtalar joint is pronated, the axes of the talo-calcaneal and calcaneocuboid joints are parallel, allowing the midtarsal joint to unlock and become an adaptor with increased mobility. As the subtalar joint supinates, the midtarsal joint's motion decreases as the two axes diverge and "lock" the forefoot on the rearfoot in preparation for its rigid lever function during the propulsive phase of gait (Fig. 14-6).

The position of the midtarsal joint is dictated by ground reaction forces during the contact and midstance phases of gait and by muscular activity on the joint during the propulsive phase of gait.[39] The standard clinical index for determining midtarsal joint position is to compare the plantar plane position of the central three metatarsal heads to the plantar plane position of the neutral rearfoot when the midtarsal joint is maximally pronated about both its axes.

Physiologic accessory motions of the midtarsal joint that can be evaluated manually include dorsal and plantar glides of the navicular on the talus and of the cuboid on the calcaneus. Plantar glide accompanies supination, and dorsal glide accompanies pronation.

Tarsometatarsal, Metatarsophalangeal, and Interphalangeal Joints

The first ray represents a functional articulation consisting of the bones of the medial column. The joint axis runs from the distolateral to the proximomedial direction, almost parallel to the transverse plane. Motion occurs primarily in the sagittal (plantar flexion-dorsiflexion) and frontal (inversion-eversion) planes. The axis is angulated 45° from both these planes, so for every 1° of plantar flexion there is 1° of eversion (Fig. 14-7).

First-ray motion begins in the late-stance phase of gait and continues late into propulsion. As with the midtarsal joint, first-ray motion is influenced by the position of the

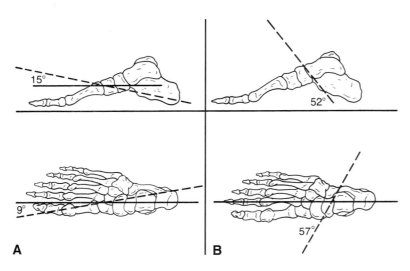

Figure 14-5. Axes of motion for the midtarsal joints. *A*, Longitudinal axis. *B*, Oblique axis.

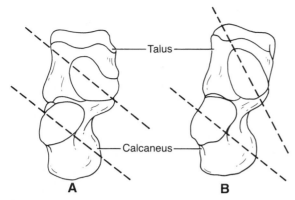

Figure 14-6. Axis of transverse tarsal joint. *A,* When calcaneus is in eversion, the conjoint axes between the talonavicular and calcaneocuboid joints are parallel to one another, so that increased motion occurs in the transverse tarsal joint. *B,* When the calcaneus is in inversion, the axes are no longer parallel, and there is decreased motion with increased stability of the transverse tarsal joint. (Reproduced by permission from Mann, R.A. [1982]: Biomechanics of running. *In:* American Academy of Orthopaedic Surgeons: Symposium on the Foot and Leg in Running Sports. St. Louis, 1982, C.V. Mosby.)

The fifth ray operates about an independent axis with the same directional orientation as the subtalar joint. The central three rays have an axis orientation parallel to the frontal and transverse planes. Consequently, there is only plantar flexion-dorsiflexion motion in the sagittal plane. The metatarsophalangeal (MTP) joints also have an additional vertical axis, which is parallel to the frontal and sagittal planes to allow abduction and adduction of the joints.

The first MTP joint represents the articulation between the first metatarsal and the proximal phalanx of the big toe. Minimal normal first MTP range of motion with the first ray stabilized is about 20° to 30° of hyperextension. Without stabilization, the first MTP joint should hyperextend to at least 60° to 70°.[30] The MTP joints also have an additional vertical axis, which is parallel to the frontal and sagittal planes to allow abduction and adduction of the joints.

Physiologic accessory motions of the MTP joints include plantar and dorsal glides. Plantar glide of the convex first metatarsal accompanies extension, whereas dorsal glide accompanies toe flexion.

subtalar joint. With the subtalar joint in pronation, the amount of first-ray motion is increased. As the subtalar joint supinates, the first-ray motion decreases. The normal extent of movement is 0.5 to 1 cm (a thumb's width) in the plantar and dorsal directions.[39]

The clinical standard for determining the neutral position of the first metatarsal head is to evaluate the position of the first ray relative to the three central metatarsal heads. It should lie in the same transverse plane, neither plantar flexed nor dorsiflexed.

MUSCULAR FUNCTION OF THE LOWER LEG, ANKLE, AND FOOT

The phasic action of the muscles of the lower leg and foot can be determined by examining the excursion of the musculotendinous unit from origin to insertion relative to the axis on which it acts (Fig. 14-8). Each muscle group has specific functions that control or provide the necessary forces to create movement. The muscles of the leg and foot can be divided into subgroups or compartments (Table 14-3 and Fig. 14-9).

Figure 14-7. First ray axis and motion. *A,* First ray axis of motion, dorsal view. *B,* First ray motion.

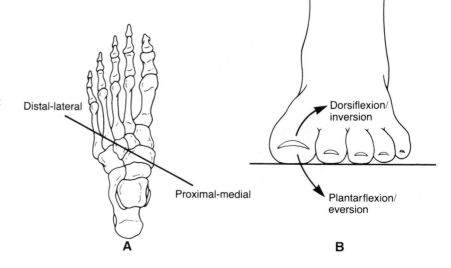

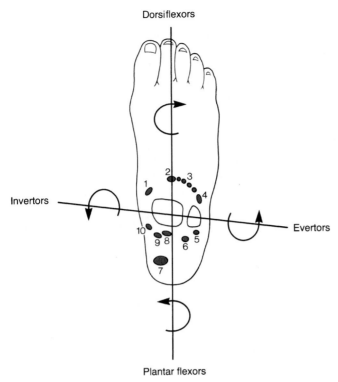

Dorsiflexors

Invertors

Evertors

Plantar flexors

Figure 14-8. Motion diagram of the ankle. Tibialis anterior (1), extensor hallucis longus (2), extensor digitorum longus (3), peroneus tertius (4), peroneus brevis (5), peroneus longus (6), Achilles tendon (7), flexor hallucis longus (8), flexor digitorum longus (9), and tibialis posterior (10). (From Magee, D.J. [1987]: Orthopedic Physical Assessment. Philadelphia, W.B. Saunders.)

CLINICAL PEARL #1

The action of a muscle can be determined by examining the musculotendinous unit's excursion from origin to insertion relative to the axis on which it acts.

Table 14-3	
Lower Leg Muscle Groups	
Group	**Muscles**
Posterior superficial	Gastrocnemius, soleus, plantaris
Lateral	Peroneal
Dorsal intrinsics	Extensor hallucis brevis, extensor digitorum brevis
Deep posterior	Posterior tibialis, flexor digitorum longus, flexor hallucis longus
Anterior pretibia	Anterior tibialis, extensor hallucis longus, extensor digitorum, peroneus tertius
Plantar intrinsic	Flexor digitorum brevis, flexor hallucis brevis, adductor and abductor hallucis, lumbricales

Posterior Superficial Muscle Group

The posterior superficial muscle group is composed of the gastrocnemius, soleus, and plantaris muscles. These muscles originate from above and below the knee joint and have a common insertion by way of the Achilles tendon on the posterior aspect of the calcaneus. In the open kinetic chain, the triceps surae provide flexion of the knee, plantar flexion of the ankle, and supination of the subtalar joint. With closed kinetic chain function, the gastrocnemius and soleus are active throughout the stance phase of gait. Initially, at heel strike, the gastrocnemius and soleus contract eccentrically to decelerate tibial internal rotation and forward progression of the tibia over the foot. Later, during midstance and heel-off, they provide subtalar joint supination (externally rotating the tibia) and ankle plantar flexion.

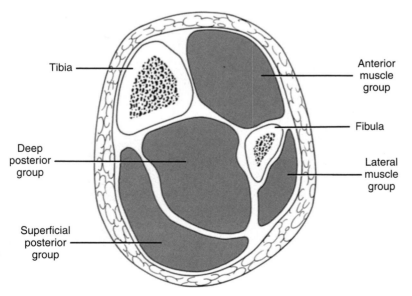

Tibia

Anterior muscle group

Fibula

Deep posterior group

Lateral muscle group

Superficial posterior group

Figure 14-9. Cross section of the lower leg muscle groups.

Posterior Deep Muscle Group

The posterior deep muscles of the lower leg include the posterior tibialis, flexor digitorum longus, and flexor hallucis longus. The posterior tibialis is a strong supinator and invertor of the subtalar joint and functions to control and reverse pronation during gait. It decelerates subtalar joint pronation and tibial internal rotation at heel strike and then reverses its function to accelerate subtalar joint supination and tibial external rotation during stance. The posterior tibialis also maintains the stability of the midtarsal joint in the direction of supination around its oblique axis during the stance phase of gait.

The flexor digitorum longus functions as a supinator of the subtalar joint and flexor of the second through fifth MTP joints in the open kinetic chain. When the foot is in contact with the ground and the digits are stable, the flexor digitorum longus actively stabilizes the foot as a weight-bearing platform for propulsion. If the flexor digitorum longus works unopposed by the action of the intrinsic muscles, clawing of the toes results.[21]

The flexor hallucis longus has a function similar to that of the flexor digitorum longus in that it flexes the first MTP joint in the open kinetic chain. Both of these long flexors help support the medial arch.

Lateral Muscle Group

The lateral muscle group includes the peroneus longus and brevis. The peroneus longus, because of its attachment to the first metatarsal and medial cuneiform on the plantar surface, functions to pronate the subtalar joint and to plantar flex and evert the first ray in the open kinetic chain. In the closed kinetic chain, the peroneus longus has many important functions. It provides support to the transverse and lateral longitudinal arches. During the latter portion of midstance and early heel-off, it actively stabilizes the first ray and everts the foot to transfer body weight from the lateral to the medial side of the foot.

The peroneus brevis is primarily an everter in open kinetic chain motion. During gait it functions in concert with the peroneus longus. Its primary role is to stabilize the calcaneocuboid joint, allowing the peroneus longus to work efficiently over the cuboid pulley.

Anterior Muscle Group

The pretibial muscles include the anterior tibialis, extensor digitorum longus, extensor hallucis longus, and peroneus tertius. As a group they are active during the swing phase and the heel-strike to foot-flat phases of gait.

The anterior tibialis is primarily a dorsiflexor of the talocrural joint in open kinetic chain function. In gait, the anterior tibialis basically operates concentrically in the swing phase and eccentrically in the stance phase. At the end of toe-off, the anterior tibialis begins to contract con-centrically to initiate dorsiflexion of the ankle and first ray, to assist in ground clearance at midswing, and then to supinate the foot slightly during late swing in preparation for heel strike. When the foot hits the ground, the anterior tibialis reverses its role to decelerate or control plantar flexion to foot-flat, prevent excessive pronation, and supinate the longitudinal axis of the midtarsal joint. A weak anterior tibialis can lead to "foot-slap," or uncontrolled pronation in gait.

In non–weight-bearing function, the long extensors (extensor digitorum and hallucis longus) provide dorsiflexion of the ankle and extension of the toes. Because, unlike the anterior tibialis, these tendons pass laterally to the subtalar joint axis, they provide a pronatory force at the joint. In fact, a prime responsibility of the long extensors is to hold the oblique axis of the midtarsal joint in a pronated position at heel strike and then to assist the controlled deceleration of plantar flexion to foot-flat.

Intrinsic Muscle Group

Generally, the intrinsic muscles of the foot act together during most of the stance phase of gait. Their function is to stabilize the midtarsal joint and digits while keeping the toes flat on the ground until lift-off. An unstable, pronated midtarsal joint during midstance necessitates that the intrinsic muscles work harder and longer. This phenomenon explains the common complaint of foot fatigue in the athlete with a hypermobile foot.

CLINICAL EXAMINATION

Anthropometric measurements of the leg, foot, and ankle provide objective evidence of effusion. Many techniques can be reliable. Volumetric displacement methods with submersion of the foot into a calibrated tank are highly reliable and easily performed. Other methods include girth assessments at selected sites or use of heel-lock and figure-eight tape measurement techniques (Fig. 14-10). Tatro-Adams[45] demonstrated excellent intratester and intertester reliability with the figure-eight method of measurement. Comparison with the uninvolved side is always appropriate.

Determination of Subtalar Joint Neutral Position

To assess inversion-eversion motion of the ankle, the clinician should first identify the subtalar neutral position. This can be found through palpation of the head of the talus as it articulates with the navicular. When the subtalar joint is pronated or supinated, the head of the talus is palpable medially or laterally. After the fourth and fifth metatarsal heads are loaded to pronate the forefoot to tissue resistance, the calcaneus is inverted and everted. When the subtalar joint is supinated, the medial side of the talus

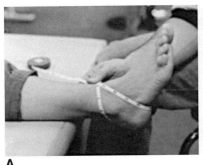

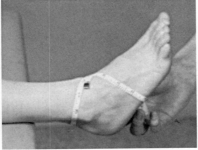

A   **B**

Figure 14-10. Ankle girth assessment. *A*, Heel-lock method. *B*, Figure-eight method.

disappears, and the lateral aspect of the talus becomes prominent. The reverse is true when the subtalar joint is pronated. The neutral position is defined as that point at which there is talonavicular congruency and neither the medial or lateral aspects of the talus are palpable or their protrusion is symmetric. This technique can be used in a closed-chain or open-chain assessment (Fig. 14-11). In a weight-bearing position, an easy visual assessment is to observe for equal concavities above and below the lateral malleolus.[39] A shallow curve superiorly and an accentuated curve inferiorly would suggest a pronated subtalar joint (Fig. 14-12).

Subtalar Range of Motion

Once the neutral position of the subtalar joint has been established, assessment of calcaneal inversion-eversion range of motion can take place. Initially, the neutral position of the subtalar joint is objectively quantified through goniometric measurement. Normal is considered to be 2° to 3° of inversion (calcaneal varus). The arms of the goniometer are

aligned with the longitudinal midline of the posterior calcaneus and the posterior bisection of the tibia (Fig. 14-13). Care must be taken to disregard the alignment of the Achilles tendon or the shape of the calcaneal fat pads, because they may produce unreliable measurements. Readings are recorded after maximal passive calcaneal inversion and eversion (Fig. 14-14). Inversion and eversion amounts of motion are then determined based on the initial neutral position. Differences may be noted, depending on whether this assessment was performed in a weight-bearing or non–weight-bearing posture. Lattanza and colleagues[29] found an average increase of 37% in subtalar eversion as a component of pronation when measured in the closed-chain weight-bearing posture rather than in the traditional non–weight-bearing position. The intratester and intertester reliabilities of these measurement techniques have been investigated by a number of authors.[18,35,40,42] Generally, the intratester reliability is considered to be fair and the intertester reliability poor. Measurement repeatability may be enhanced with experienced examiners using inclinometers in a weight-bearing assessment.

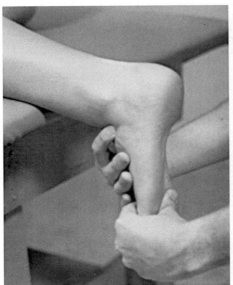

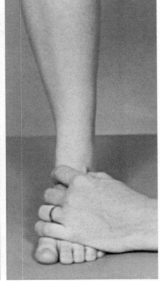

A   **B**

Figure 14-11. Subtalar neutral position. *A*, Non–weight-bearing palpation. *B*, Closed-chain palpation.

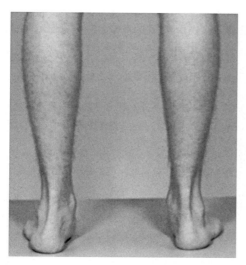

Figure 14-12. Pronated subtalar position with accentuated inferior curve.

Plantar Flexion-Dorsiflexion Range of Motion

Ankle dorsiflexion range of motion must be assessed while the subtalar joint is maintained in a neutral position. If the subtalar joint is not monitored, pronator substitution may provide an inaccurate portrayal of gastrocnemius-soleus flexibility. When the subtalar joint is pronated, midtarsal mobility is increased, and dorsiflexion of the foot can occur around the oblique axis of the midtarsal joint.

A minimum of 10° dorsiflexion is needed at heel-off to allow for normal ambulation.[4] Because the knee joint is fully extended at this point in the gait cycle, the two-joint gastrocnemius muscle is fully stretched over both joints. Consequently, the knee should be placed in full extension when the range of dorsiflexion excursion available in gait is evaluated. To differentiate soleus extensibility, dorsiflexion range of motion is assessed in a knee-flexed posture so that the gastrocnemius is slack. An increase of 10° dorsiflexion to a total of 20° is anticipated.

To measure ankle dorsiflexion range of motion, the athlete is placed prone with the ankle extended off the end of the table. The clinician then palpates and establishes the subtalar neutral position. The distal arm of the goniometer is placed parallel to the lateral aspect of the calcaneus and the fifth metatarsal head, and the proximal arm is aligned with the bisection of the lateral aspect of the lower leg and the head of the fibula. The clinician then passively forces dorsiflexion while the athlete actively assists (Fig. 14-15). This active assistance provides reciprocal inhibition of the passive tension stored in the triceps surae group. Pronator substitution tendencies are manifested by calcaneal eversion. Calcaneal stabilization may have to be provided manually. This procedure should be performed with the knee extended and flexed. If the dorsiflexion range is equal in the flexed and extended postures, ankle equinus (bony block caused by osseous lipping in the anterior ankle joint) or soleus equinus should be suspected.[4]

Plantar flexion range of motion is expected to be 50° to 60° and is assessed with similar goniometric placement techniques.

Subtalar Joint Position

Subtalar joint position is determined by comparing the orientation of the calcaneus relative to the distal third of the leg when the calcaneus is in its neutral position. Rearfoot varus is defined as an inverted calcaneus compared with the posterior bisection of the tibia in the non–weight-bearing position (Fig. 14-16A). Rearfoot valgus is the opposite situation, in which the calcaneus is everted relative to the tibia (Fig. 14-16B). *Calcaneal varus* and *calcaneal valgus* are terms used to describe calcaneal position relative to the supporting surface. This position may represent a compensated position dependent upon the range of motion available at the subtalar joint.

In identifying an athlete's foot type it is important to evaluate the feet in their position of function. The neutral and resting calcaneal stance positions are accurate

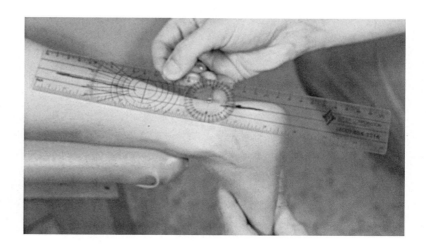

Figure 14-13. Measurement of subtalar neutral position.

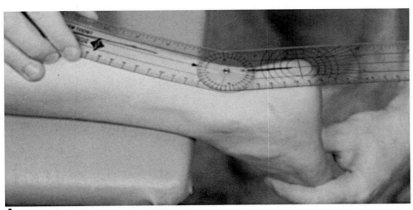

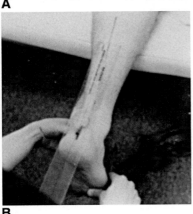

Figure 14-14. Measurement of subtalar range of motion. *A,* Inversion. *B,* Eversion.

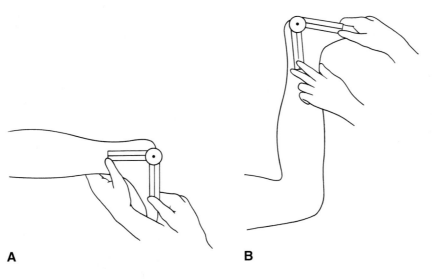

Figure 14-15. Goniometric assessment of ankle dorsiflexion range of motion. *A,* Knee extended. *B,* Knee flexed.

reflections of the way the kinetic chain of the lower extremity interacts with the supporting surfaces. The neutral calcaneal stance position is the angular relationship of the calcaneus and the ground with the subtalar joint in the neutral position. As described previously, this may be called a rearfoot varus or valgus posture. Resting calcaneal stance position is this same angular relationship in natural stance, in which compensation for deviations is allowed.

Subtalar joint position is assessed by placing the athlete in his or her angle and base of gait and measuring this relationship by placing one arm of a goniometer parallel to the ground and the other aligned with the posterior calcaneal bisection. Measurements are made in subtalar neutral and natural relaxed stances. Ideally, these values should be the same. The diagnostic hallmark of a rearfoot varus is an inverted neutral calcaneal stance position.[39] Compensation

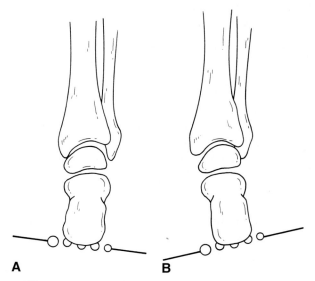

Figure 14-16. *A*, Rearfoot varus. *B*, Rearfoot valgus.

for these deformities depends on the availability of the subtalar range of motion. Rearfoot varus is considered fully compensated if the subtalar joint allows enough calcaneal eversion to reach a perpendicular position to the floor, where forces across the heel and forefoot are equilibrated (Fig. 14-17). Uncompensated rearfoot varus is indicated by having an inverted calcaneus in the neutral calcaneal stance position and less inversion in the resting or relaxed calcaneal stance position.

Midtarsal Joint Position

Midtarsal structure and foot type are determined by comparison of the forefoot position relative to the rearfoot.

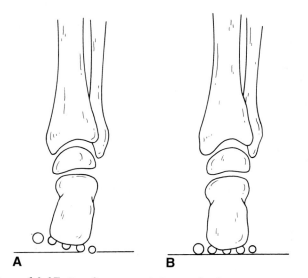

Figure 14-17. Rearfoot varus. *A*, Inverted calcaneus. *B*, Compensation accomplished by calcaneal eversion in relaxed stance position.

Forefoot varus is a structural abnormality in which the plantar plane of the forefoot is inverted relative to the plantar plane of the rearfoot, with the subtalar joint in its neutral position and the forefoot maximally pronated around both its midtarsal joint axes (Fig. 14-18*A*). Forefoot valgus is the opposite of forefoot varus in that the forefoot is everted relative to the rearfoot (Fig. 14-18*B*). An additional requirement for defining forefoot valgus is that the foot has a first ray, which has normal range of motion. This differentiates forefoot valgus from a plantar-flexed first ray. Often, a plantar-flexed first ray gives the appearance of a forefoot valgus but can be differentiated by the decreased range of motion associated with this deformity. A plantar-flexed first ray shows more plantar flexion than dorsiflexion range of motion (Fig. 14-18*C*).

Forefoot supinatus is a relatively fixed acquired soft tissue deformity that typically occurs in athletes whose

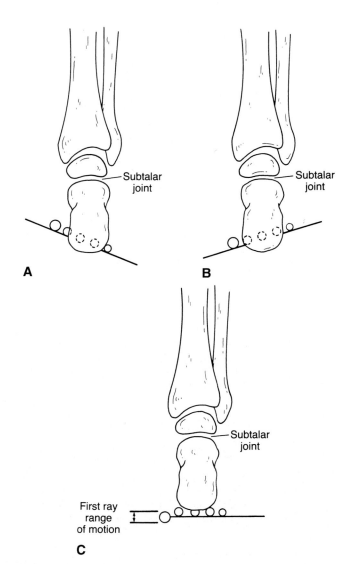

Figure 14-18. *A*, Forefoot varus, inverted forefoot. *B*, Forefoot valgus, everted forefoot. *C*, Plantar-flexed first ray.

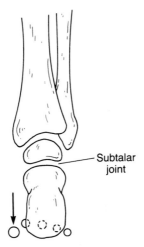

Figure 14-19. Forefoot supinatus: supinated forefoot with plantar-flexed first ray.

calcaneus is maintained in an everted position. The forefoot is supinated in relation to the rearfoot because of soft tissue adaptation, and the total midtarsal range of motion is reduced. The compensatory mechanism is the plantar-flexed attitude of the first ray to bring the medial forefoot in contact with the ground (Fig. 14-19).

When midtarsal foot type is assessed, it is important to assess the quality and quantity of midtarsal motion subjectively. Passive manual assessment techniques can identify the relative amounts of plantar flexion-dorsiflexion and abduction-adduction around the oblique axis and inversion-eversion of the longitudinal axis. Motion should be maximal with the subtalar joint held in pronation and should decrease as the subtalar joint is placed in a supinated position.

Proximal Considerations

Tibial Varum

Tibial varum is a structural deformity in which the distal tibia is closer to the midline than the proximal tibia. Its determination quantifies the amount of frontal plane deviation of the tibia. Tibial varum is assessed with the athlete bearing weight on the measured extremity in its angle and base of gait. The goniometer is placed with one arm parallel to the ground and the other parallel to the posterior bisection of the distal tibia (Fig. 14-20). The presence of tibial varum contributes to the total varus attitude of the lower extremity.

Tibial Torsion

To evaluate for tibial torsion, the clinician aligns the patient's legs straight so that the femoral condyles are in the frontal plane and the patellae face is straight up. The clinician then assesses the amount of torsion by measuring the angle of the malleoli relative to the shaft of the tibia. The normal value is considered to be approximately 13° to 18° of external tibial torsion (Fig. 14-21).

FUNCTIONAL RELATIONSHIPS

The entire kinetic chain is intimately linked with every movement in sport. Each segment of the body depends on the role and function of adjoining and distant structures. A prime example of this interdependence is displayed in over ground ambulation. The following is a description of "normal" gait. Normal gait is a difficult entity to quantify, but this description can serve as a basis by which to evaluate a potentially pathologic type of movement.

Normal Gait

At heel strike, the ankle is in a neutral position and then plantar flexes to foot-flat under the eccentric control of the

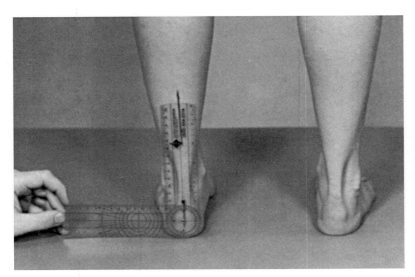

Figure 14-20. Measurement of tibial varum.

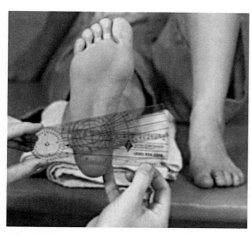

Figure 14-21. Measurement of tibial torsion.

pretibial muscles. The subtalar and midtarsal joints are supinated at heel contact and begin the process of pronation to unlock the midtarsal joint, which allows foot adaptation to the terrain. At the knee joint, the tibia follows the directional input of the subtalar joint by internally rotating and flexing. Normal subtalar pronation during this phase of gait is a passive activity in the closed kinetic chain that directs movement and attenuates ground reaction forces.[15]

During midstance, from foot-flat to heel-off, the subtalar joint undergoes supination as the body weight shifts anterior to the weight-bearing extremity. The ankle joint is moving toward its extreme of dorsiflexion. The supination movement of the subtalar joint dictates that the tibia rotate externally and allow the knee to reach full extension at the end of midstance. The posterior calf muscles eccentrically control the early pronation and concentrically shorten as the foot moves into supination. During this phase the foot reverses function, from that of a mobile adaptor to that of a rigid lever.

Propulsion from heel-off to toe-off shows the ankle joint plantar flexing while the midtarsal joint is locking on the supinating subtalar joint. This process prepares the foot for its role as a stable platform from which to push off. The MTP joints extend while the knee joint flexes in preparation for the swing phase of gait.

Swing-phase motion requires flexion of the knee and dorsiflexion of the ankle to provide ground clearance. The subtalar joint initially pronates in early swing to shorten the limb and assist in ground clearance. It then supinates in terminal swing to prepare for heel contact on the next step (Table 14-4 and Fig. 14-22).

Dynamic Gait Assessment

Whereas assessment of lower quarter injuries with the athlete in a static posture is the benchmark for evaluation, dynamic assessment of movement patterns offers the most valid means for determining the athlete's functional ability.

Assessment of gait should be incorporated into all evaluations of the lower extremity. This can be performed in any setting, but a treadmill greatly enhances the convenience of analysis.

Brandel and Williams[3] demonstrated a statistically insignificant difference in stride length, velocity, and cadence with treadmill analysis of gait versus normal walking at 2.5 to 3.2 miles per hour. A treadmill also allows easy control of gait speeds and inclination. With videotape-recording technology, an objective documentation of function is obtained, and the tape can be slowed down for careful analysis. A simple clinical setup requires only single positioning of the camera to allow anterior, posterior, and lateral views to be videotaped with the assistance of postural mirrors (Fig. 14-23).

General observations of gait should include head placement, shoulder height and position, arm swing and carry, cadence, step-stride length, weight acceptance, and single-limb stance stability. With knowledge of normal gait mechanics, joint position and motion in the different phases of the gait cycle can be compared with expected norms. Hypotheses on the source of deviations are then generated and correlated with static evaluation findings. Some subtle weaknesses, inflexibilities, and postural asymmetries can be detected with this method of evaluation. Points of observation for recognizing subtalar joint position during videotape analysis of gait are presented in Table 14-5.

CLINICAL PEARL #2

A hallmark of normal gait is that the calcaneus is vertical to the floor just before heel-off in the gait cycle. The subtalar joint should be supinating toward a closed-pack position during this time to lock the midtarsal axes and stiffen the foot in preparation for propulsion.

When gait is evaluated, it is important to recognize some of the general trends that differentiate walking, jogging, and running. As movement speed increases, the total range of motion that each joint undergoes must increase. This increased range of motion takes place during a shorter period of time because the gait cycle is occurring at a more rapid pace. As a result, velocity of joint motion must be increased. During the stance phase of gait, these higher velocities of motion cause high eccentric tensile contractions that must be dissipated and tolerated by the musculoskeletal system. Table 14-6 shows the parameters that define and differentiate walking, jogging, and running.

Pathologic Gait

Common Pronatory Disorders

By having the foot function as a rigid lever during propulsion, the weight of the body is propelled off that limb with

Table 14-4

Normal Gait Cycle

	STANCE PHASE			SWING PHASE		
	HEEL CONTACT	**FOOT-FLAT**	**HEEL-OFF**	**TOE-OFF**		
Joint	Forefoot Loading	Midstance	Propulsion	Early Swing	Midswing	Terminal Swing
Tibiofemoral position	Extended ——→ Mildly flexed ——→ Extended				Maximally flexed	
Motion	Flexion, tibial internal rotation	Extension, tibial external rotation	Flexion		Extension	
Talocrural position	Neutral ——→ Maximally plantar flexed ——→ Maximally dorsiflexed			Plantar flexed ——→ Neutral ——→ Dorsiflexed		
Motion	Plantar flexion	Dorsiflexion	Very rapid plantar flexion	Dorsiflexion		
Subtalar position	Mildly supinated ——→ Fully pronated ——→ Mildly supinated ——→ Fully supinated					
Motion	Pronation	Supination		Pronation		Supination
Midtarsal position	Everted ——→ Inverted					
Motion	Unlocking to adapt	Locking as rigid lever				
	0%	15%	30%	45%	60%	100%

STANCE PHASE | SWING PHASE

| Contact | Mid-Stance | Push Off | Balance Assist | Early Swing | Late Swing |
| 0% 10% | 20% 30% | 40% 50% | 60% | 70% 80% | 90% 100% |

Gastrocnemius
Soleus
Posterior tibial
Flexor digitorum longus
Flexor hallucis longus
Peroneus brevis
Peroneus longus
Anterior tibial
Extensor hallucis longus
Extensor digitorum longus
Peroneus tertius
Extensor digitorum brevis
Extensor hallucis brevis
Abductor hallucis
Flexor digitorum brevis
Quadratus plantae
Lumbricales
Flexor hallucis brevis
Transverse pedis
Adductor hallucis

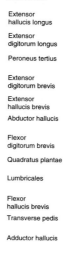

Figure 14-22. Muscular function in normal gait. (From McGlamry, E.D. [1987]: Fundamentals of Foot Surgery. Baltimore, Williams & Wilkins.)

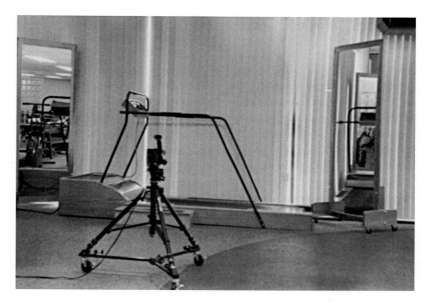

Figure 14-23. Video setup for gait analysis.

Table 14-5

Recognition of Subtalar Joint Position

View	Pronation	Supination
Posterior	Calcaneal inversion; calcaneal indentation concave to midline	Calcaneal eversion; calcaneal indentation convex to midline
Anterior	Internal rotation of tibia	External rotation of tibia
Lateral	Talar head adducts and plantar flexes; talar head bulges and medial arch flattens	Medial longitudinal arch heightens

Table 14-6

Contrast of Walking, Jogging, and Running

Parameter	Walking	Jogging	Running
Speed	2-4 mph	5-10 mph	10+ mph
Stance time duration	0.6 second	0.3 second	0.2 second
Stance:swing time ratio	3:2	3:4	1:2
Vertical forces	Body weight	2-3 × body weight	2-3 × body weight
Support phase	Double-limb support	Single-limb support	Single-limb support
Base of gait	2-3 cm	1 cm	None or crossover

maximum efficiency. If the subtalar joint cannot reach the neutral position, heading toward a supinated position just before heel-off, an unstable base of support is used for propulsion. If a condition does not allow the forefoot to lock on the rearfoot, a situation exists that is analogous to walking in sand, in which the base of support gives way under push-off forces. It takes significantly more muscle energy to push off such unstable platforms, resulting in foot and leg fatigue secondary to overuse.

Pronation is a normal and necessary component of gait. Only when the amount, timing, or sequence of the pronation-supination cycle is altered is pronation considered abnormal.[22] An athlete with rearfoot varus demonstrates this during midstance and, as a result, can have abnormal hypermobility and shearing forces within the foot. As can be seen in Figure 14-24, the athlete with rearfoot varus does obtain some supination in propulsion, but the subtalar joint is still in a pronated posture at the initiation of heel-off.

Forefoot varus is another condition that is compensated for by abnormal pronation of the subtalar joint. The subtalar joint remains pronated throughout the stance phase of gait to allow ground contact on the medial forefoot and creates an inefficient method of ambulation (Fig. 14-25).

Abnormal pronation can also be caused by soft tissue limitations or extrinsic factors proximal to the foot. Flexibility deficiencies, postural deviations, and muscular weaknesses can alter the normal pronation-supination sequence extrinsically.[49] Equinus deformities caused by a

tight gastrocnemius or soleus tend to cause a massive subtalar joint pronation just before propulsion begins.[39] A tight Achilles complex causes either early heel-off or prolonged subtalar joint pronation to compensate for the lack of adequate talocrural dorsiflexion range of motion. In both cases the subtalar joint has not supinated to neutral before heel-off.

Proximal inflexibilities, such as tight medial hamstrings, which shorten stride length or affect lower extremity external rotation during swing phase, are other examples of extrinsically induced abnormal pronation.[49] These inflexibilities do not allow enough time for full resupination of the subtalar joint during the late swing phase in its preparation for heel strike.

Postural deviations such as leg length discrepancies are a final example of abnormal pronation brought on by external causes. Subtalar pronation is a method by which leg length can be shortened in the closed kinetic chain.[28] Although this chapter deals with lower leg and foot pathologic conditions, it is important to note that dysfunction may originate proximal to the structure in which it is manifested.

Supinatory Disorders

Abnormal supination in gait is a less common occurrence than abnormal pronation but is seen in athletes who compensate for a forefoot valgus or a rigid, plantar-flexed first ray. Supinatory compensation is found first at the longitudinal axis of the midtarsal joint and then at the subtalar joint.[39] Rapid supination in midstance to bring the lateral

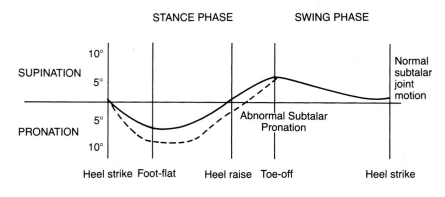

Figure 14-24. Graphic representation of subtalar joint motion in rearfoot varus.

STANCE PHASE   SWING PHASE

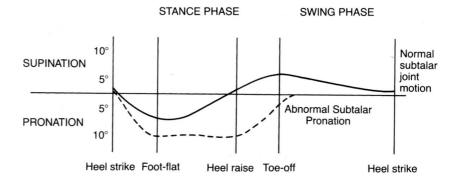

Figure 14-25. Graphic representation of subtalar joint motion in forefoot varus.

side of the foot to the floor creates lateral instability of the ankle, making the athlete prone to inversion injuries. As can be seen in Figure 14-26, rapid supination alters the timing sequence of normal subtalar motion, and the joint pronates late in propulsion.

LOWER LEG, ANKLE, AND FOOT INJURIES AND THEIR MANAGEMENT
Lower Leg Injuries

Tibiofibular Synostosis

Tibiofibular synostosis is a condition in which there is ossification of the interosseous membrane between the tibia and fibula at the inferior tibiofibular syndesmosis. The injury can occur because of a single inversion-internal rotation trauma or from recurrent, less severe episodes in which the anterior and posterior inferior tibiofibular ligaments and the interosseous membrane are damaged. Resultant spreading of the tibia and fibula allows bone formation from the periosteal insertions in the form of a flat exostosis or a synostosis that occurs proximally along the interosseous membrane.[20]

The athlete's chief complaint is difficulty in performing movements that require pivoting or cutting, and there is a sense of spasm and instability at the ankle joint. This injury should be suspected whenever an athlete cannot recover from an "ankle sprain" and remains symptomatic longer than usual.

Conservative management includes treatment of the initial injury with ice, compression, and rest.

Rehabilitation is focused on restoring normal joint stability. If there are continued complaints of pain and instability, a surgical synovectomy is indicated, when the bone is mature, to reduce risk of recurrence.

Achilles Tendon Rupture

The Achilles tendon complex is prone to injury if there is a sudden and powerful eccentric contraction of the gastrocnemius-soleus muscles (considered together as the triceps surae). This mechanism is best demonstrated during jumping and landing activities, in which the knee is extending while the ankle is dorsiflexing eccentrically. The tendon usually ruptures at a point just proximal to the calcaneus (Fig. 14-27). Vascular impairment, nonspecific degeneration leading to tissue necrosis, and use of injectable corticosteroids may weaken this area and predispose it to injury.

The athlete reports an audible snap and the sensation of being kicked in the leg. Immediate plantar flexion weakness and pain, swelling, and a palpable defect are usually present. The diagnosis is confirmed with a positive Thompson test, in which the athlete is prone, with the knee flexed and the foot relaxed. A firm squeeze to the calf should produce calcaneal plantar flexion. The test is positive when there is no movement of the foot.

Acute care consists of ice application, with the ankle immobilized in slight plantar flexion. A non–weight-bearing crutch gait should be used until the severity of injury has been determined. Table 14-7 provides a treatment rationale for lesions of the triceps surae mechanism. Postsurgical or closed nonsurgical care of complete

STANCE PHASE   SWING PHASE

Figure 14-26. Graphic representation of subtalar joint motion in forefoot valgus or rigid plantar-flexed first ray.

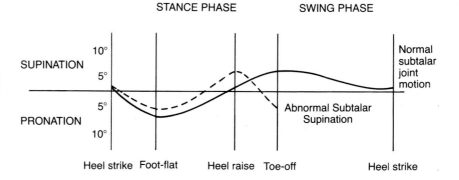

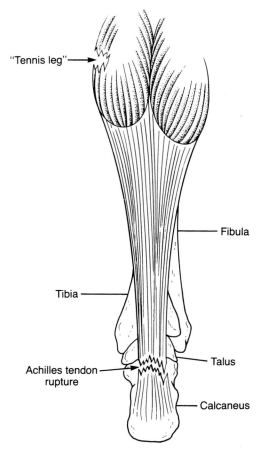

Figure 14-27. Tennis leg and Achilles tendon injury.

ruptures traditionally required 4 to 8 weeks of cast immobilization. However, recent trends have shown that protected (early and controlled) motion and functional orthoses are as safe and effective as less aggressive and more strict immobilization methods.[8] Protected-arc, active plantar flexion range-of-motion activities may be started as early as 2 to 4 weeks postinjury. This allows collagen fibers to be laid down along the line of stress. A 1-inch heel lift is used when weight bearing is allowed and the height of the lift is gradually decreased as the dorsiflexion range of motion improves. Surgical versus nonsurgical management decisions are based on the site and thickness of the tear in conjunction with the goals and ambitions of the patient. Results of both methods of management have been acceptable.[9]

Tennis Leg

Previously thought to be a tear of the plantaris muscle, "tennis leg" has now been proved through surgical exploration to be a musculotendinous lesion of the medial gastrocnemius head (see Fig. 14-27).[33] The usual mechanism of injury is sudden extension of the knee with the foot in a dorsiflexed position. This places a tremendous tensile stress on the two-joint expansion of the gastrocnemius. Middle-aged athletes or those with previous degenerative changes in this anatomic area may be predisposed to this type of trauma.

The athlete feels a sudden, sharp twinge in the upper medial calf and immediately has difficulty in full weight bearing. Typically, there is rapid swelling and ecchymosis,

Table 14-7

Gastrocnemius-Soleus Rehabilitation and Treatment

Parameter	Immediate (Acute Phase)	Intermediate (Subacute Phase)	Terminal (Chronic Phase)	Return to Activity (Functional Phase)
Goal	Rest Control inflammation and pain Promote healing Create "flexible" scar	Increase pain-free ROM Restore contractile capability	Increase musculotendinous tensile strength Modify, correct, or control abnormal biomechanics	Prepare and train for specific sport or activity
Modalities	Ice massage NSAIDs Gentle transverse friction massage to prevent adhesion formation HVGS in shortened position	Heat before rehabilitation Ice after rehabilitation Ultrasound (pulsed vs continuous) Myofascial–soft-tissue mobilization techniques	Heat before rehabilitation Ice after rehabilitation Iontophoresis/phonophoresis Deep transverse friction massage to improve gliding between tissue planes	Modality sequence: 1. Passive-active tissue and systemic warm-up 2. Static stretching 3. Activity or exercise 4. Stretch again—with mildly ballistic motion 5. Cool-down 6. Cryotherapy
ROM/flexibility	Immobilization or pain-free ROM dependent upon type and severity of pathologic condition	Temperature-assisted, prolonged-duration, low-intensity, static stretching Non–weight-bearing knee bent and straight towel stretches	Low-intensity, static stretching of involved musculotendinous unit Weight-bearing knee bent or straight wall leans Slant board stretching	Assess capability, tolerance, and response to ballistic motion of involved tissue

Table 14-7

Gastrocnemius-Soleus Rehabilitation and Treatment—cont'd

Parameter	Immediate (Acute Phase)	Intermediate (Subacute Phase)	Terminal (Chronic Phase)	Return to Activity (Functional Phase)
Exercise rationale	Isometrics progressing from submaximal to maximal intensity in protected ROM (knee flexed or ankle in plantar flexion); these exercises may have to be delayed 2-6 weeks in athletes with surgically repaired ruptures	Non–weight-bearing submaximal to maximal effort isokinetics in progressively larger arcs of motion; concentric contractions at highest attainable speeds in a velocity spectrum to minimize tensile stress in this subacute phase	Weight-bearing concentric and eccentric isotonic exercise at increasing speeds of contraction as dictated by tissue symptomatic response	Functional rehabilitation—activities such as tip-toe walking Plyometric progressions—hopping, bounding, depth jumps, and box drills Sport-specific training
Proprioceptive rehabilitation	BAPS board training in non–weight-bearing positions if not immobilized	BAPS board training in partial to full weight-bearing position with increasing levels of ROM difficulty	BAPS board training in full weight-bearing position with posterior peg overload	Unstable surface training
Alternative conditioning	UBE	Gravity-reduced running with assistance of unloading device or flotation device in water	Gravity-reduced running; stationary cycling	Stairclimbers Stationary cross-country skier
Complementary exercise	Hip-knee-trunk strengthening and conditioning activities	Dorsiflexion, inversion, and eversion strengthening Exercise of foot intrinsic musculature	Lower extremity stretching and continuation of activities from previous phase	Ensure normal plantar-to-dorsiflexion strength ratios and muscle balance 3-4:1 ratio at slow speeds of contraction
Activity education modification	Controlled immobilization and rest as needed Examine athletic shoes, training surface, and training regimens	Trial of low-amplitude rebounder running	Flat training surfaces only; avoid hilly and cambered terrain or muddy surfaces	Careful increases in training regimens; limit increase in program by more than 5%/week in intensity, duration, or frequency
Orthotic care	Crutches as necessary; weight-bearing status dictated by severity of pathologic condition	Viscoelastic heel lift inserts to reduce stress on Achilles tendon and decrease ground reaction forces	Custom orthotic insert to control excessive or abnormal compensatory subtalar joint motion	Orthotic or taping techniques

BAPS, Biomechanical Ankle Platform System; HVGS, high-voltage galvanic stimulation; NSAIDs, nonsteroidal anti–inflammatory drugs; ROM, range of motion; UBE, upper body ergometer.

with point tenderness or a palpable defect at the site of the lesion.

Acute care consists of immediate first-aid measures, including ice, compression, and elevation to the injured area. The ankle is placed in mild plantar flexion to alleviate stress on the area of injury. A non–weight-bearing crutch gait may be necessary, depending on the severity of the injury.

Gradual, gentle static stretching is initiated early in the subacute phase to align the healing scar tissue. Friction massage to the area also prevents random alignment of collagen fibers. As the athlete progresses to full weight bearing, heel lifts can be used in the shoe to protect against weight-bearing stresses. As Achilles tendon flexibility improves, the height of the lifts can be gradually reduced. Table 14-7 presents further details about the rehabilitation progression of Achilles tendon–related pathologic conditions.

Tendinopathies

Tendinous lesions of the muscles of the lower leg often occur in athletes involved in activities of a repetitious nature. Microtraumatic damage caused by overuse, fatigue, or biomechanical abnormalities may be manifested by an inflammatory reaction of these tendons.

Achilles Tendinitis

The Achilles tendon is the common tendon of the gastrocnemius and soleus muscles. It inserts into the posterosuperior aspect of the calcaneus and is a common site of pathologic changes in competitive and recreational athletes.[10,24] It is surrounded by the paratenon, which functions as an elastic sleeve that envelops the tendon and allows free movement against surrounding tissues. In areas in which the tendon passes over zones of potential pressure and friction, the paratenon is replaced by a synovial sheath or bursa.[11]

The major blood supply to the Achilles tendon is provided through the paratenon. An area of reduced vascularity is found 2 to 6 cm proximal to the insertion.[41] This region of relative avascularity may play an etiologic role in the frequent onset of symptoms at this level.[41]

Although an Achilles tendon overuse injury is a common problem, the nomenclature used to identify this injury is often confusing. Classification is based on whether the Achilles tendon itself or the peritendinous tissue that surrounds it is involved. Achilles tendinitis is defined as disruptive lesions within the substance of the tendon itself, whereas peritendinitis involves inflammation in the paratenon.[11] These conditions could occur simultaneously or in isolation.

The onset of Achilles tendinitis or peritendinitis is usually gradual and insidious, although some precipitating factor may be identified. The athlete complains of a dull, aching pain during or after activity. On physical examination, slight edema or tendon thickening may be present. Point tenderness is usually elicited 2 to 3 cm proximal to the calcaneal attachment. Because this is a contractile lesion, pain usually increases with passive dorsiflexion and resisted plantar flexion.[13] Crepitation may be noted in plantar flexion movements in the subacute and chronic stages.[26]

Table 14-8 presents a suggested rationale for the conservative management and treatment of tendinitis and peritendinitis. The four stages of injury define potential entry points into the treatment system. An athlete could initially be seen at any one of these stages. Progression from one

Table 14-8

Lower Leg Tendinopathy Rehabilitation and Treatment

Parameter	Immediate (Acute Phase)	Intermediate (Subacute Phase)	Terminal (Chronic Phase)	Return to Activity (Functional Phase)
Goal	Rest Control inflammation and pain Promote healing Create "flexible" scar	Rehabilitation of musculotendinous unit Increase ROM Increase muscle contractile capability	Increase musculotendinous tensile strength Modify, correct, or control abnormal biomechanics	Prepare and train for specific sport or activity
Modalities	Ice massage NSAIDs Gentle transverse friction massage to prevent adhesion formation	Heat before rehabilitation Ice after rehabilitation Ultrasound (pulsed vs. continuous) Myofascial–soft-tissue mobilization techniques	Heat before rehabilitation Ice after rehabilitation Iontophoresis/ phonophoresis Deep transverse friction massage to improve gliding between tissue planes	Modality sequence: 1. Passive-active tissue and systemic warm-up 2. Static stretching 3. Activity or exercise 4. Stretch again—with mildly ballistic motion 5. Cool-down 6. Cryotherapy
ROM/flexibility	Pain-free ROM exercises	Temperature-assisted, prolonged-duration, low-intensity, static stretching	Low-intensity, static stretching of involved musculotendinous unit	Assess capability, tolerance, and response to ballistic motion of involved tissue
Exercise rationale	Isometrics	Submaximal to maximal effort isokinetics in progressively larger arcs of motion; concentric contractions at highest attainable speeds in a velocity spectrum to minimize tensile stress in this subacute phase	Eccentric exercise at increasing speeds of contraction as dictated by tissue symptomatic response	Functional rehabilitation activities and plyometric progressions Sport-specific training

Table 14-8

Lower Leg Tendinopathy Rehabilitation and Treatment—cont'd

Parameter	Immediate (Acute Phase)	Intermediate (Subacute Phase)	Terminal (Chronic Phase)	Return to Activity (Functional Phase)
Proprioceptive rehabilitation	BAPS board training in non–weight-bearing positions	BAPS board training in partial to full weight-bearing position with increasing levels of ROM difficulty	BAPS board training in full weight-bearing position with resistance overload to appropriate muscle groups	Balance board training
Alternative conditioning	UBE	Gravity-reduced running with assistance of unloading device or flotation device in water	Gravity-reduced running; stationary cycling	Stairclimbers; Stationary cross-country skier
Complementary exercise	Hip-knee-trunk strengthening and conditioning activities	Exercise of foot intrinsic musculature	Lower extremity stretching and continuance of activities from previous phase	Ensure normal agonist-to-antagonist strength ratios and muscle balance
Activity education modification	Controlled immobilization and rest as needed. Examine athletic shoes, training surface, and training regimens	Trial of low-amplitude rebounder running	Flat training surfaces only; avoid hilly and cambered terrain or muddy surfaces	Careful increases in training regimens; limit increase in program by more than 5%/week in intensity, duration, or frequency
Orthotic care	Heel lift if appropriate	Viscoelastic inserts to decrease ground reaction forces (especially in rigid cavus feet)	Custom orthotic insert to control excessive or abnormal compensatory subtalar joint motion	Orthotic or taping techniques

BAPS, Biomechanical Ankle Platform System; NSAIDs, nonsteroidal anti-inflammatory drugs; ROM, range of motion; UBE, upper body ergometer.

stage to the next is variable and is dictated by time, symptoms, and individual response (Boxes 14-1 and 14-2).

As is usually true, the best treatment for microtraumatic injuries such as Achilles tendinitis is prevention of onset. The frequency or severity of inflammatory Achilles injuries may be reduced if some suggested guidelines are followed:

1. Select appropriate footwear. The athletic shoe should have a firm, notched heel counter to decrease tendon irritation and control rearfoot motion. The midsole should have a moderate heel flare, provide adequate wedging, and allow flexibility in the forefoot. It is also important to maintain a relatively consistent heel height in all shoes worn during the day.
2. Avoid training errors. Achilles tendon microtrauma can be magnified by errors in training. Steady, gradual increases of no more than 5% to 10% per week in training mileage and speed on appropriate terrain should be emphasized. Use of cross-training principles may also reduce cumulative stresses on the Achilles tendon.
3. Ensure gastrocnemius-soleus flexibility. The talocrural joint should have 10° of dorsiflexion with the knee joint extended and 20° with the knee flexed. Normal gait requires 10° of dorsiflexion just before heel-off, during which the subtalar joint is in neutral position and the knee is extending in stance phase.[4]
4. Control pronation forces. Abnormal compensatory pronation forces can cause a whipping or bowstring effect on the medial edge of the Achilles tendon. Orthotic correction may be indicated if this abnormal pronation is of structural origin.[11]
5. Ensure adequate strength. The triceps surae musculotendinous unit must have adequate concentric and eccentric contractile capabilities. This includes dynamic symmetry in bilateral comparisons and appropriate balance with its ipsilateral antagonist. A plantar flexion-to-dorsiflexion ratio of 3:1 or 4:1 has been suggested for slow isokinetic speeds (60°/sec) of contraction.[16]

Box 14-1

Management of Achilles Tendinitis

- Unload stress on tendon with heel lift and/or tape support
- Control abnormal subtalar joint motion
- Ensure adequate dorsiflexion range of motion
- Reduce eccentric loads during acute and subacute phases
- Restore normal plantar to dorsiflexion strength ratios and muscle balance
- Introduce plyometric progression gradually
- Carefully increase training regimens by not more than 5% to 10% per week in intensity, duration, or frequency

6. Perform postural screening for biomechanical malalignments. This may detect any abnormalities that could adversely affect the kinetic chain and increase stress on the Achilles tendon. Such conditions include leg length discrepancies, cavus foot resulting from metatarsal forefoot equinus, ankle equinus, tibial varum, and rotational influences of the femur or tibia.[4]

Anterior Tibialis Tendinitis

An inflammatory response of the anterior tibialis tendon occurs when it cannot absorb deceleration forces during the heel-strike phase to the foot-flat phase of gait. Uncontrolled or excessive pronation after heel strike stretches the anterior tibialis as it attempts to control the speed of forefoot loading.

Conditions that predispose the anterior tibialis to overuse usually include training errors and physical abnormalities. Often the combination of excessive extrinsic forces placed on intrinsic abnormalities produces stresses that cannot be dissipated or tolerated by the athlete. Extrinsic factors include dramatic increases in mileage, overstriding, and excessive hill running, all of which can cause fatigue and injury. The athlete with a tight Achilles complex requires increased muscular output of the anterior tibialis to overcome the inherent posterior tautness. This condition is then magnified with uphill running, which necessitates full dorsiflexion range of motion. In downhill running, increased eccentric forces are necessary to control forefoot loading over an increased range of motion. If the anterior tibialis has undergone adaptive shortening in response to chronic hyperpronation, the musculotendinous unit cannot provide the necessary range of motion and absorption of tensile forces needed during the early stance phase.

This injury is characterized by pain and swelling over the dorsum of the foot. There may be crepitation along the tendon or at its point of insertion onto the navicular. Examination reveals pain with stretching into the extremes of plantar flexion and pronation and pain-inhibited weakness with manual muscle testing of anterior tibialis function.

In Table 14-8 the treatment rationale for lower leg tendinopathies is summarized. Prime consideration should be given to correcting soft tissue imbalances, improving eccentric muscular capabilities, and selecting appropriate footwear. Selection of shoes should focus on midsole materials that attenuate shock and accommodate orthotic additions. A heel lift may be used for the athlete with structural equinus, or varus posting may be indicated if a forefoot varus or supinatus is prolonging the pronation process.

Peroneal Tendinitis

Inflammatory lesions of the peroneal muscle tendons or of their protective sheaths are common in athletes who, for compensatory reasons, overuse this musculature. The pathologic condition is due to chronic lateral ankle sprains or in athletes with hypermobile first rays. In both situations, the peroneal muscle tendons are worked excessively in an attempt to provide stability. Any mechanical stress caused by abnormal forefoot structures that force the foot into a valgus position can also amplify this inflammatory response.

Pain and swelling typically occur in the area just posterior to the lateral malleolus. Occasionally, symptoms are manifested at the musculotendinous junction.[13] Tendon crepitus may be present in more chronic conditions. Pain and weakness are evident with passive overstretching of these contractile structures and when resistance is provided to plantar flexion and eversion of the first ray. Compared with peroneal longus tendinitis, peroneal brevis tendinitis is more affected by resistance to calcaneal eversion and ankle plantar flexion. The differential diagnosis must be made among peroneal subluxation, inversion ankle sprain, sural nerve entrapment, and subacute lateral compartmental syndrome, because subsequent management differs for each of these conditions.

Rehabilitation is focused on providing symptomatic relief and identifying the causative factors. Muscular imbalances between the anterior or posterior tibialis and peroneal muscles should be explored. A metatarsal pad with a first ray cutout can provide orthotic relief of structural abnormalities. Transverse friction massage can be used to reduce symptoms and promote healing.[13] Table 14-8 presents further treatment considerations.

Posterior Tibialis Tendinitis

Posteromedial shin pain due to athletic overuse can indicate inflammatory microtrauma to the tendon of the posterior tibialis. Periosteal irritation and tibial stress reactions may also be suspected.

Medial tibial stress, whether tendinitis or periostitis, is generally the result of abnormal hyperpronation biomechanics (Fig. 14-28). The muscles in the superficial posterior compartment contract in a stretched position and are overworked in an attempt to stabilize the foot during propulsion. Common predisposing factors include

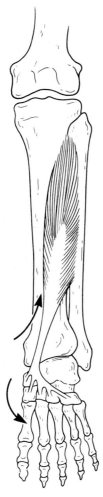

Figure 14-28. Etiology of posterior tibialis tendinitis: excessive traction stress placed on the posterior tibialis tendon with hyperpronation.

Box 14-2

Functional Exercises to Improve Control of Pronation

- BAPS board training with anteromedial and/or posteromedial overload
- Marble pick-ups with toes and lateral towel sweeps with foot
- Supro Dance—arch lift and drop
- Unilateral balancing activities progressing from stable to unstable surfaces
- Unilateral stance with opposite lower extremity frontal plane motion
- Bilateral progressing to unilateral stance trunk rotation with appropriate resistance and speed of motion

improper training on crowned or banked surfaces, inappropriate footwear, and any structural condition that increases the varus attitude of the lower extremity.

Pain and swelling are present over the posteromedial crest of the tibia along the origin of the posterior tibialis. Tenderness and crepitation may be found anywhere along the course of the tendon as it passes behind the medial malleolus and inserts distally on the navicular and first cuneiform. Manual resistance to plantar flexion and inversion localizes the complaint. In subacute phases, repeated unilateral heel raises, which require plantar flexion and supination of the calcaneus, can be a source of symptom aggravation.

Differential diagnosis is important to rule out a tibial stress reaction, in which there is pain at the junction of the lower and middle thirds of the posteromedial tibia. Tibial stress fractures can occur in this area if the bony osteoblastic activity cannot keep pace with the osteoclastic stress placed on it. At approximately 2 weeks after awareness of symptoms, a fracture through the tibial cortex may become evident on radiographs. Before this finding, a bone scan reveals increased calcium uptake in the area of injury. Clinical differentiation is accomplished by detection of tenderness in areas devoid of muscle on the tibial shaft or with percussion and tuning fork vibration techniques.

Treatment is focused on alleviating abnormal pronation using a semirigid orthosis with a medial heel wedge. Attention should also be given to the training regimen and to finding shoes with a stable, firm, and snug heel counter.

Flexor Hallucis Longus Tendinitis

The athlete who must perform repetitive push-off maneuvers is especially prone to developing tendinitis in the long flexor of the great toe. Hyperpronation during propulsion also places excessive stress on the tendon as it contracts from a lengthened position. This condition is similar to posterior tibial tendinitis and can be differentiated through selected manual muscle testing. Pain with passive extension of the first MTP joint while the ankle is dorsiflexed confirms the diagnosis. The condition is managed with appropriate varus posting and tape restriction for excessive dorsiflexion of the first MTP joint.

Flexor Digitorum Longus Tendinitis

The flexor digitorum longus is another musculotendinous unit in the superficial posterior compartment that is susceptible to overuse microtrauma. Pain is usually present in the posteromedial third of the leg as a result of overuse from forced, resistive dorsiflexion of the toes during propulsion.[21] The resultant cramping sensation in the forefoot and toes can be relieved with a viscoelastic metatarsal pad, which dorsally displaces the metatarsal heads and reduces the extension angle of the lesser four MTP joints. A more rigid sole in the athletic shoe may also help prevent excessive forced hyperextension of the digits in propulsion. Exercise rehabilitation focuses on correcting any intrinsic muscular imbalances that allow toe-clawing deformities and that require the flexor digitorum longus to work harder.[21] The intrinsic muscles of the foot can be isolated for emphasis during toe-curling exercises. This is accomplished by contracting the extensor hallucis longus to inhibit the ability of the long toe flexor to contract (Fig. 14-29).

Compartmental Compression Syndromes

There are four osseofascial compartments in the lower leg—the anterior, lateral, superficial posterior, and deep posterior. The anterior compartment is the most common site for compression ischemia. It is bordered by the interosseous membrane posteriorly, the tibia and fibula medially and laterally, and a tough, nonexpansive fascial covering anteriorly. If pressure increases within the compartment, there is no space for expansion or accommodation. With increasing pressure, circulation and tissue function can be quickly compromised. There are two types of anterior compartmental compression syndrome: acute and recurrent.

Acute Anterior Compartmental Compression Syndrome

This condition is usually traumatic in onset. Contusions, crush injuries, fractures, or severe overexertion can cause a rapid increase in compartmental volume from bleeding or muscular swelling. Increased intercompartmental pressure leads to venous collapse and increased resistance to arterial circulation. These physiologic changes produce an ischemic pain and, ultimately, tissue necrosis if the process is left uninterrupted.

The athlete's chief complaint is intense pain that is disproportionate to the injury and not relieved by rest. Palpation reveals a "woody tension" over the muscles of the anterior compartment, and passive plantar flexion evokes pain. In the advanced stages, neurologic changes may be evident, and the dorsalis pedis and anterior tibial pulses may be diminished. Table 14-9 presents the neurologic changes manifested in the later stages of lower leg compartmental syndrome.

This condition is considered an orthopedic emergency, because early muscle damage occurs in the first 4 to 6 hours, and irreversible tissue damage occurs within 18 hours after

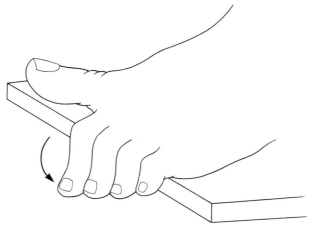

Figure 14-29. Isolation of intrinsic toe flexors to inhibit long toe flexor contribution.

Table 14-9

Late Neurologic Changes in Compression Syndromes

Compartment	Area of Paresthesia	Area of Weakness
Anterior	First dorsal web space	Dorsiflexion (drop foot)
Lateral	Anterior lateral leg	Eversion (peroneals)
Deep posterior	Medial arch	Inversion
Superficial posterior	Sural nerve distribution	Plantar flexion

injury. Acute care consists of ice application without compression and monitoring of the neurovascular status. If pain and swelling do not respond to conservative treatment, an emergency surgical fasciotomy must be performed.

Recurrent Compartmental Syndrome

Chronic, exertional compartmental syndrome has the same pathophysiologic characteristics as acute compartmental syndrome, but its presentation and care are different (Table 14-10). The athlete complains of lower leg pain and tightness that occur at a constant interval after the initiation of physical activity. The symptoms subside with rest but return on resumption of the activity. Most athletes have bilateral involvement with mild edema, tenderness, and occasional paresthesia. The diagnosis is confirmed with wick catheter measurement of intercompartmental pressure at rest and during activity.

Conservative management includes ice application before and after exercise, lower leg stretching, and balancing plantar flexion-dorsiflexion strength. Any alterations in the training program that decrease muscular workloads, including reduction in body weight may also be helpful. Bevel-heeled shoes, softer training surfaces, and energy-absorbing orthoses may accomplish this goal. If conservative measures fail, a surgical fasciotomy is indicated. Postoperative rehabilitation consists of gentle stretching and stationary cycling beginning 7 to 10 days post-surgery, with expected return to activity after 2 to 3 months.

Table 14-10

Symptom Presentation of Acute versus Recurrent Compartmental Syndromes

	Recurrent	Acute
Pathologic change	Reversible changes	Irreversible tissue damage possible
Effect of rest	Symptoms decrease	No change in symptoms
Nature of complaint	Cramping, aching	Intense pain
Involvement	Often bilateral	Usually unilateral

Ankle Injuries

Pathologic trauma to the ligamentous structures of the ankle is a common athletic injury. The majority of these injuries occur to the lateral side of the joint with an inversion mechanism of injury. In the neutral position of 0° dorsiflexion, the calcaneofibular ligament is taut, but as the foot plantar flexes, the anterior talofibular ligament tightens as its fibers become parallel to the axis. Eighty percent to 90% of ankle sprains occur as the result of this plantar flexion-inversion mechanism. Initial damage is to the anterior talofibular ligament because of the direction of force, and further stress affects the calcaneofibular and posterior talofibular ligaments. The posterior talofibular ligament is not involved or injured until the other two ligaments have ruptured and some degree of lower extremity rotation has occurred. Injuries to the medial side of the joint and the deltoid ligament are less common and typically involve a hyperpronation force, such as when an athlete plants the foot and then cuts in the opposite direction. Table 14-11 shows the common mechanisms of injury for bony and ligamentous structures of the ankle.

Inversion Sprains

The signs and symptoms of ankle ligamentous injuries vary according to the severity of injury, the tissues involved, and the extent of their involvement. Varying degrees of pain, swelling, point tenderness, and functional disability are usually evident. After inversion trauma, radiographic studies of the joint and bone structure are of paramount importance. Bony lesions must be ruled out before decisions about appropriate management of the injury can be made. Unstable bimalleolar fractures, proximal fibular fractures, and avulsion-type fractures all are possible and may require surgical fixation or longer periods of immobilization.

Table 14-12 presents some criteria for assessing the severity of injury in lateral ankle sprains. This grading process provides a basis for logically estimating the rate and intensity at which the athlete can progress through the phases of treatment and rehabilitation, as well as for estimating the length of time before the athlete can return to full participation.

Treatment and Rehabilitation

The functional or chronic disability associated with ankle sprains can be the result of various abnormalities. These include anterior, posterior, or varus instability of the talus in the ankle mortice, instability of or adhesion formation in the subtalar joint, inferior tibiofibular diastasis, peroneal muscle weakness, and motor incoordination due to articular deafferentation.[5,16,19,22,27,36]

Each potential problem must be addressed in the treatment and rehabilitation program. The damaged ligaments must be allowed to heal as a "flexible" restraint, the contractile elements must regain dynamic stabilization capabilities, and the proprioceptive system must be completely restored. Table 14-13 provides a suggested treatment plan for the conservative management of inversion ankle sprains. Each athlete's injury is unique, and progression through the various stages of rehabilitation may have

Table 14-11

Mechanism of Ankle Injuries

Mechanism of Injury	Comments	Ligamentous Injury (Progression of Increasing Severity of Pathology)	Potential Bony Lesions
Plantar flexion-inversion	Typical ankle sprain	ATF→ATF and CF→ATF, CF, and PTF	Transverse fracture of lateral malleolus Avulsion fracture of base of fifth metatarsal Medial malleolus fracture
Supinated position-adduction force			
Plantar flexion-inversion and rotation	Crossover cut on a plantar flexed and inverted foot	ATF and tibfib→ATF, tibfib, and CF	
Supinated position-eversion force			Spiral fracture of lateral malleolus or fracture of neck of fibula
Pure inversion	Rare; landing on another's foot	CF→CF and ATF→CF, ATF, and PTF	
Pronation: abduction-eversion-dorsiflexion	Open cut	Deltoid→deltoid, tibfib, and interosseus membrane	Avulsion fracture of medial malleolus
Pronated position-eversion force			Fibular fracture above the mortice line

ATF, Anterior talofibular ligament; CF, calcaneofibular ligament; PTF, posterior talofibular ligament; tibfib, anterior and posterior tibiofibular ligaments.

Table 14-12

Signs and Symptoms of Lateral Ankle Sprains

Grade	Severity	Involvement	Functional Status	Swelling	Pain/Tenderness	Ligament Laxity
I	Mild	Usually only ATF	Maintenance of joint integrity produces minimal functional disability	Variable, but usually slight	Mild, localized pain over ATF	Negative anterior drawer and talar tilt
II	Moderate	ATF and CF	Moderate disability, with difficulty in heel and toe walking	Variable, but more than in grade I and resultant ecchymosis	Moderate pain and tenderness over involved ligaments	Laxity evident but distinct end points to stress
III	Severe	ATF and CF; possibly PTF	Functional disability, with loss of ROM and complete inability to bear weight	Anterolateral and spreading diffusely around the joint	Marked tenderness to palpation	Positive anterior drawer or talar tilt

ATF, Anterior talofibular ligament; CF, calcaneofibular ligament; PTF, posterior talofibular ligament; ROM, range of motion.

Table 14-13

Conservative Management of Ankle Sprains

Phase	Immediate (Acute)	Intermediate (Subacute) (Postimmobilization)	Terminal (Chronic)	Return to Activity (Functional)
Goals	Protect joint integrity Control inflammatory response Control pain, edema, and spasm	Optimal stimulation for tissue regeneration	Functional progression Proprioceptive retraining Correct/control biomechanics	Preparation for return to sport or activity
Weight-bearing status	Non– to touch-down weight-bearing	Partial weight bearing progressing toward full weight bearing	Full weight bearing	Full weight bearing
Modalities	Ice Intermittent/constant compression Elevation TENS or HVGS Effleurage in elevated position	Cryotherapy (ice-ROM-ice) Contrast baths Friction massage at site of lesion	Cryokinetics (ice-exercise, activities-ice)	Ice after-participation
External support	Neutral orthotic Gibney open basket-weave taping Posterior splint to maintain neutral dorsiflexion	Stirrup splint with heel-lock support	Stirrup splint with heel-lock support	Taping or bracing
ROM/flexibility		Grade I or II joint mobilizations	Achilles stretching in sitting and standing positions	Achilles stretching in supinated positions
Open kinetic chain exercise	Isometrics	Alphabet ROM Toe curls and marble pickups Four-plane surgical tubing exercises Submaximal isokinetics in short arcs	Full-arc isokinetics	
Closed kinetic chain exercise		Standing trunk twists and squats Shuttle squats/heel raises/toe raises Soleus pumps Tubing lunge steps, TKEs, SKFI	Heel-raise progression Shuttle hops and bounds	Marching, running, sidesteps, backpedaling, cariocas, etc. Plyometric drills
Proprioception/agility/balance drills		BAPS in non– or partial weight-bearing position Stork stands Single plane tilt boards	BAPS in full weight bearing ProFitter or slide board Multiaxial tilt or balance boards Tubing walkaways/runaways Tubing contrakicks	Jump rope/jump platform Four-square hopping drills Functional running patterns Running in place tubing drills
Complementary alternative exercises	Gluteus medius strengthening	Pool therapy Stationary cycling	Rebounder minitrampoline drills Treadmill Stairmaster	Stationary cross-country skiing Lateral step-ups

BAPS, Biomechanical Ankle Platform System; CKC, closed kinetic chain; HVGS, high-voltage galvanic stimulation; ROM, range of motion; SKFI, single knee flexion initiation; TENS, transcutaneous electrical nerve stimulation; TKE, terminal knee extension.

to be altered, depending on the severity of tissue trauma, history, and goals of rehabilitation. Figures 14-30 to 14-42 illustrate some of the rehabilitation procedures used in the restoration of normal ankle joint function after ligamentous injury.

The goal of management is to provide dynamic stability to a potentially unstable joint (Box 14-3). During the acute immobilization phase, emphasis is placed on controlling symptoms and on maintaining general conditioning and neuromuscular continuity. Various modalities are used to minimize effusion and decrease pain. Edema within the ankle joint distorts the capsule's normal configuration and adversely affects articular mechanoreceptor function. Ice, focal compression around the periphery of

Box 14-3

Management of Inversion Ankle Sprains

- Aggressive management of acute swelling
- Normalization of gait pattern as soon as possible
- Maintenance of closed-pack position of neutral dorsiflexion during acute and subacute healing phases
- Addressing of structural abnormalities that would cause compensatory supination in gait
- Compensated forefoot valgus
- Uncompensated rearfoot varus
- >10° tibial varum without adequate compensatory calcaneal eversion range of motion
- Reestablishment of proprioceptive and kinesthetic skills and awareness
- Enhancement of gluteus medius and peroneal frontal plane muscle control and stabilization ability

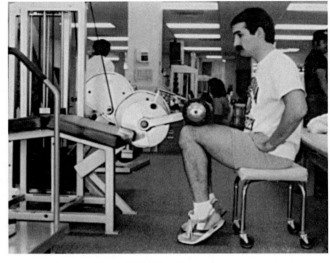

Figure 14-31. Soleus pumps.

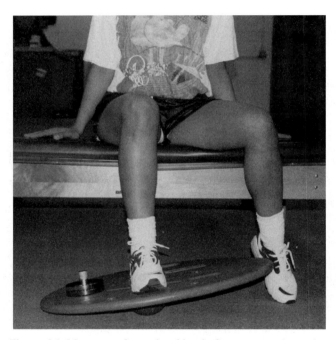

Figure 14-30. Biomechanical Ankle Platform System (BAPS): BAPS board with posterolateral overload.

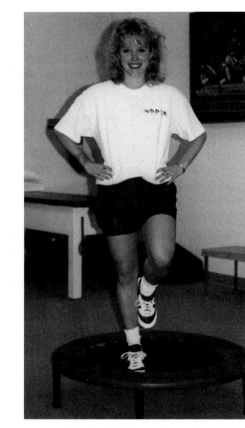

Figure 14-32. Stork stands.

the fibular malleolus, electrotherapy, and gentle effleurage with the ankle elevated all facilitate anesthesia and reduction of edema and reverse the neural inhibition of the dynamic stabilizers surrounding the joint. Support to the injured ligaments is provided by a neutral orthosis, Gibney's strapping (open basket-weave taping with a horseshoe pad to compress extracellular fluids back into circulation), and a posterior splint to maintain Achilles tendon flexibility. Because strict immobilization is no longer recommended, cautious and gentle motion in protected

arcs can be initiated through Biomechanical Ankle Platform System* board activity (see Fig. 14-30).

Early mobilization allows earlier return to function without increases in pain, residual symptoms, or rate of

---

*Available from Camp International, Jackson, Michigan.

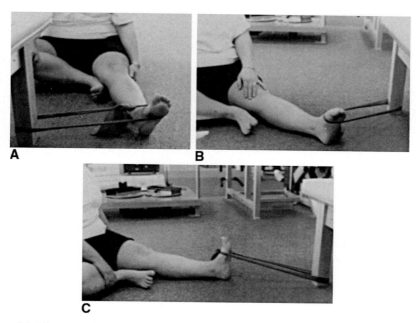

Figure 14-33. Surgical tubing resisted exercises. *A*, Eversion. *B*, Inversion. *C*, Dorsiflexion.

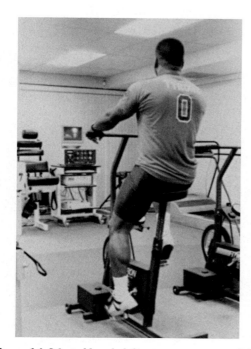

Figure 14-34. Ankle rehabilitation on stationary bike.

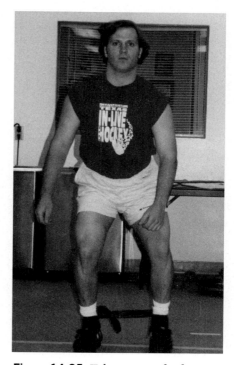

Figure 14-35. Tubing-resisted side steps.

reinjury.[17] Isometric exercises are also started during this phase to minimize or retard atrophy.

The weight-bearing status of the athlete is allowed to progress as symptoms and healing allow. Emphasis should be placed on maintaining a normal heel-to-toe gait and on keeping weight-bearing forces to below the pain symptom level. Early, pain-free weight bearing will maintain pro-

prioceptive input, prevent stiffness, and provide a means for an active muscle pump to mobilize effusion.

In the intermediate or postimmobilization phase, attention is focused on the healing ligaments. Subpathologic stress through joint mobilization is placed on the injured ligaments to stimulate organized collagen formation along the direction of normal fibers. Care must be

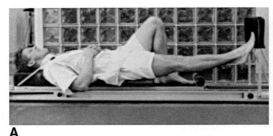

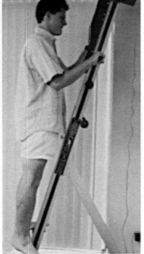

A

B

Figure 14-36. Closed-chain plantar flexion strengthening. *A*, Supine position with gravity eliminated on Shuttle 2000.* *B*, Standing on Versa-Climber.†

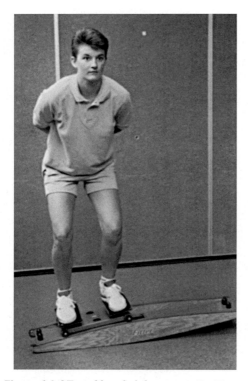

Figure 14-37. Ankle rehabilitation on ProFitter.

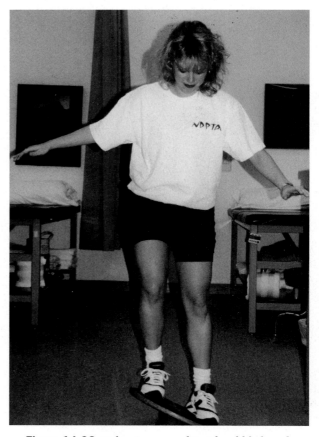

Figure 14-38. Balancing on multiaxial wobble board.

taken not to place traction forces on the joint with ankle-weight resistance on the foot. Closed-chain rehabilitation in a weight-bearing position is preferred because it can provide compressive forces that facilitate co-contraction and augment stability.

Weight bearing should progress in this stage to full weight bearing without ambulation assistance. The use of stirrup-type splints with heel-lock protection to limit excessive calcaneal inversion is indicated. Exercise

*Available from Versa Climber USA, Heart Rate, Inc., Costa Mesa, California.
†Available from Contemporary Design Company, Glacier, Washington.

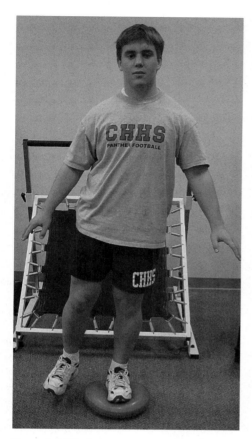

Figure 14-39. Balance training on Dyna-Disc.

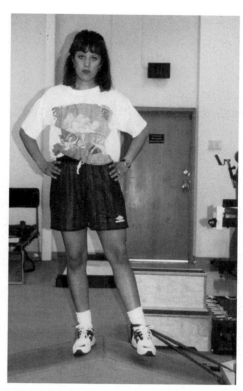

Figure 14-41. Proprioceptive training on inclined surface.

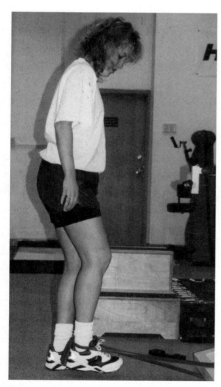

Figure 14-40. Contralateral kicks to simulate closed-chain pronation-supination.

rehabilitation may include Achilles tendon stretching; open-chain, cryotherapy-assisted active range of motion progressing toward submaximal effort isokinetics in limited arcs; and closed-chain functional activities such as soleus pumps, stork stands, stationary cycling, and body-weight transfers over stable or unstable surfaces (see Figs. 14-31 to 14-34).

In the terminal phase of rehabilitation, progressive closed-chain activities with emphasis on restoring kinesthetic awareness and proximal hip strength are given priority. Bullock-Saxton[6] showed that hip muscle function is compromised with severe ankle sprains. Gluteus maximus muscle recruitment may be delayed during hip extension in gait, and gluteus medius weakness may increase frontal plane inversion stress on the ankle due to a Trendelenburg gait. Tubing-resisted sidesteps is an excellent exercise to redevelop this strength deficit (see Fig. 14-35). Physical agents at this point are used only as needed, but after rehabilitation, ice is usually necessary. Exercise rehabilitation becomes aggressive and includes slant board Achilles tendon stretching without allowing subtalar joint substitution, full-arc isokinetics, and heel-raise progression (see Fig. 14-36). Balance and motor coordination are enhanced by the use of a ProFitter,° balance board, and DynaDisc† (see Figs. 14-37 to 14-39).

°Available from ProFitter, Calgary, Alberta, Canada.
†Available from Exertools, Novato, California.

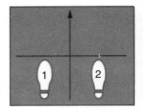

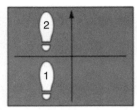

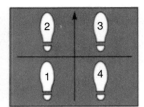

Side to side: Hop laterally between two quadrants.

Front to back: Hop forward and backward between two quadrants.

Four square: Hop from square to square in a circular pattern. Sets are performed clockwise and counterclockwise.

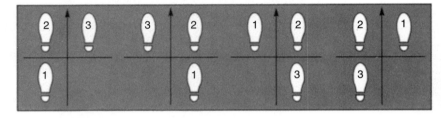

Triangles: Hop within three different quadrants. There are four triangles, each requiring a different diagonal hop.

Figure 14-42. Four-square hopping ankle rehabilitation. The eight basic hopping patterns in the four-square ankle rehabilitation program are arranged in order of increasing difficulty. The *arrows* denote the direction the athlete is facing. Number 1 is the starting point. (From Toomey, S.J. [1986]: Four-square ankle rehabilitation exercises. Physician Sportsmed., 14:281.)

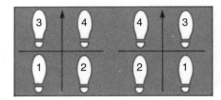

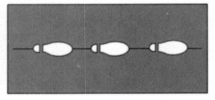

Crisscross: Hop in an X pattern.

Straight-line hop: Hop forward and then backward along a 15- to 20-ft. line.

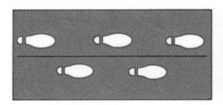

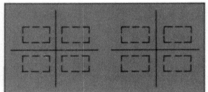

Line zigzag: Hop from side to side across a 15- to 20-ft. line while moving forward and then backward.

Disconnected squares: While performing the first five patterns, hop into squares marked in the quadrants.

As the athlete prepares to return to high-level activities, a functional progression should be used to simulate the stresses, forces, and motions inherent to the activity that caused the original injury. Elastic tubing resistance to weight-bearing activities improves ankle strength and coordination and stimulates proprioception for the entire lower extremity (see Fig. 14-40). Progression from resistance in marching to running to motion on inclines can be used (see Fig. 14-41). Tubing resistance can come from all directions, and progression is based on pain-free exercise without effusion or the tendency for the ankle to roll over.[36] Tape or external support should not be used during

these controlled activities to allow the full rehabilitative benefit. Clinical plyometrics on the Shuttle 2000 or with four-square hopping also represents an excellent means of recreating athletic activity (see Fig. 14-42). Finally, a functional movement progression that includes backpedaling, sidestepping, cariocas, pivoting, and cutting should be used in assessing the athlete's readiness for return to athletic activities.

Orthotic and external support should be used to prevent recurrence of trauma. Athletes with an uncompensated rearfoot varus, compensated forefoot valgus, or rigidly plantar-flexed first ray alter their gait pattern with prolonged or excessive supination in midstance and are extremely susceptible to reinjury. Because it takes at least 20 weeks for a ligament to regain its normal histologic characteristics, ankle taping or ankle support should be provided for at least 5 to 6 months after injury during participation in athletics.

Syndesmotic Ankle Sprains

The syndesmotic ankle sprain is often referred to as a "high" ankle sprain because of the anatomic location of the injury. Commonly, the athlete has tenderness and mild swelling over the anterior inferior tibiofibular ligament. The mechanism of injury is usually a combination of foot external rotation with lower leg internal rotation as pictured in Figure 14-43. External rotation stress to the foot and ankle with the knee held in 90° of flexion will reproduce pain over the ligament and syndesmosis. This type of injury is very slow to respond to conservative care. Boytin and colleagues[7] showed that players with syndesmotic ankle sprains missed significantly more games and required more treatment than did players who sustained lateral ankle sprains.

Postsurgical Management of Lateral Ankle Reconstructions

Sometimes surgical repair or reconstruction after lateral ligamentous injury is necessary to provide joint stability. Table 14-14 presents common reconstructive or reparative surgical procedures used in the management of chronic lateral ankle instability. Recent research has indicated that direct anatomic repair procedures that reproduce anterior talofibular and calcaneofibular orientation are mechanical restraints that are superior to anterior talar displacement and tilt without compromising subtalar joint range of motion. The postoperative therapeutic management of these procedures involves principles similar to those used in the conservative care of grade III ankle injuries. Typically, a short-leg cast or brace is applied for 6 weeks with the ankle in 0° dorsiflexion and mild eversion. During the first 2 weeks the athlete uses a non–weight-bearing crutch gait. In the final 4 weeks of immobilization partial

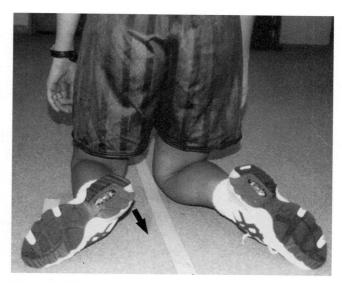

Figure 14-43. Mechanism of injury for syndesmotic ankle sprain.

weight bearing on crutches is allowed. Strict immobilization is discontinued at 6 weeks, and active-assisted range-of-motion exercises in the sagittal plane are begun. At 8 weeks, active range-of-motion exercises for calcaneal inversion and eversion are begun, along with resistive exercises for the plantar flexors and dorsiflexors. When the athlete can walk without a detectable limp, functional rehabilitation progression may commence. Return to activity is expected after 4 to 6 months.

Rehabilitation of Postimmobilization Fractures

Rehabilitation following cast removal after ankle fractures is focused on restoring joint mobility. The immobilization time necessary for ensuring union of fractures causes capsular restrictions, muscular atrophy, and proprioceptive deficits. Emphasis is then placed on joint mobilization and on appropriate exercises to strengthen and mobilize the soft tissues. The mechanics of the fracture and its surgical fixation must be understood and appreciated to avoid excessive force or stress on the initial injury. Figures 14-44 to 14-53 demonstrate joint mobilization techniques that

Table 14-14

Surgical Procedures for Lateral Ankle Instability

Nonanatomic reconstructions

Watson-Jones procedure	Peroneus brevis tendon used to reconstruct the anterior talofibular ligament
Evans procedure	Peroneus brevis tendon rerouted to limit inversion at the ankle and subtalar joints
Chrisman-Snook procedure	Anterior talofibular and calcaneofibular ligaments reconstructed using half of the peroneus tendon

Anatomic repairs

Modified Brostrom procedure	Direct repair of the anterior talofibular and calcaneofibular ligaments with reinforcement of the extensor retinaculum and lateral talocalcaneal ligament

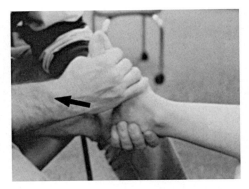

Figure 14-44. Talocrural joint traction to increase general mobility of ankle.

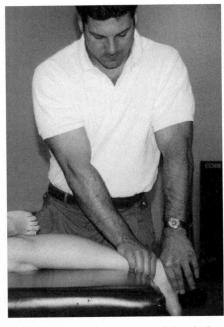

Figure 14-47. Talocrural joint: anterior glide of talus to increase plantar flexion range of motion.

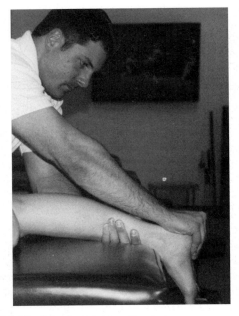

Figure 14-45. Subtalar joint traction to increase general mobility of subtalar joint.

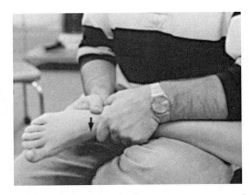

Figure 14-48. Medial glide of calcaneus to increase calcaneal eversion (pronation).

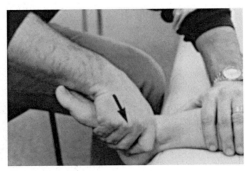

Figure 14-46. Talocrural joint: posterior glide of the talus to increase dorsiflexion range of motion.

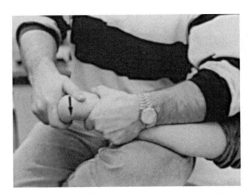

Figure 14-49. Lateral glide of calcaneus to increase calcaneal inversion (supination).

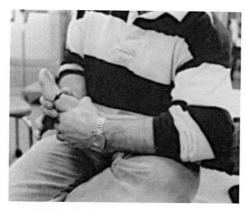

Figure 14-50. Plantar glide of midtarsal joint.

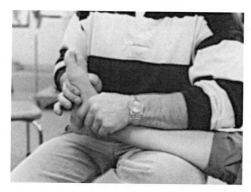

Figure 14-51. Dorsal glide of midtarsal joint.

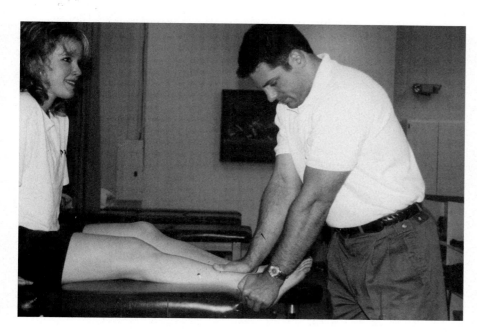

Figure 14-52. Tibiofibular joint: posterior glide of tibia.

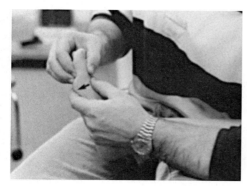

Figure 14-53. Plantar glide of first metatarsal at first metatarsophalangeal joint.

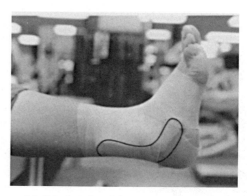

Figure 14-54. J-pad stabilization of peroneal tendons.

may be used carefully and rationally to restore accessory joint motion and normal joint arthrokinematics.

Peroneal Tendon Subluxation

The peroneal tendons lie in a deep groove posterior to the lateral malleolus. They are subject to subluxation out of this groove if sudden and violent dorsiflexion and eversion forces rupture the peroneal retinaculum. This is commonly seen when a novice skier falls forward while loading the inner edge of the skis.

This injury is commonly confused with inversion ankle sprains because of the similarity in symptoms. The athlete relates a feeling of tenderness, instability, and swelling in an area around the lateral malleolus. The correct diagnosis can be determined if there is complaint of intense retromalleolar pain with resistive dorsiflexion and eversion or, in patients with a chronic condition, marked instability and audible snapping of the tendon in and out of its groove.

Conservative management involves reducing the inflammatory response with ice, compression, and elevation. Peroneal stabilization can be attempted with taping techniques that limit excessive motion and that incorporate a J-shaped pad that compresses the tendons as they pass around the lateral malleolus (Fig. 14-54). If conservative management fails to control the symptoms, surgical intervention may be chosen. With surgery an attempt is made to reconstruct or reinforce the damaged peroneal retinaculum or use bony procedures to deepen the groove behind the lateral malleolus.

Calcaneal Injuries

Heel Bruises

Contusion injuries to the heel and calcaneal fat pad are among the most disabling in sports. Athletic activities that require frequent jumping or changes of direction seem to be especially likely to produce this type of injury. Runners with leg length discrepancy who overstride on the side of the short leg and who, as a result, have increased impact forces at the heel-strike area are also especially vulnerable to this type of trauma. Contusion injuries that cause subperiosteal bleeding and tender scar formation are sensitive to tissue compression monitored by pressure nerve endings in the area.

The athlete will complain of severe pain on the plantar aspect of the calcaneus, which is greatly aggravated by weight bearing. Treatment must include some element of rest to minimize continued, repetitive trauma. As the athlete returns to play, the heel should be taped and placed in a heel cup. It is also helpful if a shoe with a firm, well-fitting heel counter is selected for sports participation. The tape and heel cup strengthen and support the columnar septa and lobules, which provide the calcaneal fat pad with its impact-absorbing qualities.

Os Trigonum Injury

Injury to the os trigonum is common in athletes who function on their toes (e.g., ballet dancers) or who encounter resistance to dorsiflexion while in the extreme of plantar flexion (e.g., soccer players who have a kick blocked). Accessory bone fracture or soft tissue pinching produces severe local pain in the posterolateral portion of the ankle. Conservative treatment involves taping techniques to limit end-range plantar flexion. If this motion is necessary for performance, surgical excision may be necessary.

Calcaneal Apophysitis

Traction epiphyseal injuries in active adolescents are common when they wear shoes with cleats or when they rapidly alter the heel height of their athletic shoes. The tight Achilles tendon pulls on the calcaneal epiphyseal attachment, producing a disruption of circulation and possible fragmentation (also known as Sever's disease). The young athlete complains of pain on the posterior heel at the insertion point of the Achilles tendon, which is aggravated by activity and relieved by rest. This condition ends at skeletal maturity, when the epiphysis closes. Until then, judicious rest and insertion of bilateral heel lifts can help alleviate injurious stresses.

Retrocalcaneal Bursitis

Long-distance running and repetitive jumping can create a bursal inflammation between the Achilles tendon and calcaneus. This condition is aggravated by excessive compensatory pronation, which results in cumulative trauma and pressure to the posterolateral aspect of the heel. A structural predisposition to bursal inflammation may exist in the cavus foot if there is spurring on the posterosuperior aspect of the calcaneus.

This condition is characterized by pain, swelling, and discoloration on the posterolateral and posterosuperior aspects of the heel. Tenderness is elicited anterior to the Achilles tendon but posterior to the talus.

Ice, anti-inflammatory drugs, and orthotic control of the hypermobile calcaneus are used in treatment. If the subcutaneous bursa is involved, heel counter collar modification should also be used (Fig. 14-55). In selection of shoes a high priority should be placed on a stable heel counter. Structural predisposition may be alleviated by a heel lift; surgical excision of bony spurs in chronic conditions that do not respond to conservative management may be necessary.

Plantar Fasciitis

The plantar fascia is a dense band of fibrous connective tissue that originates from the calcaneal tuberosity and runs forward to insert on the metatarsal heads. As a tension band, it supports the medial longitudinal arch and assists in the push-off power of running and jumping.[44] Biomechanical abuse of this tissue results in microtrauma

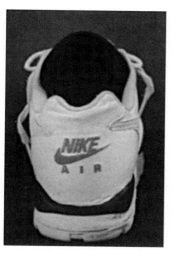

Figure 14-55. Notched heel collar on athletic shoe.

and inflammation. Chronic overuse and irritation can lead to bone formation in response to the traction forces of the plantar fascia and the muscles attaching to the calcaneal tuberosity.

This condition is most often seen in the running athlete who hyperpronates or has a rigid cavus foot and tight Achilles tendon. In both instances, excessive traction is placed on the fascia, which can be magnified with uphill or hard-surface training terrain. Creighton and Olson[12] have noted that decreased active and passive ranges of motion at the first MTP joint correlate with the onset of plantar fasciitis. Inadequate or inappropriate MTP motion can alter the windlass effect of the plantar fascia and decrease the inherent stability of the foot as the heel comes off the ground.

There is a gradual, insidious onset of pain, which can radiate along the path of the fascia, along the plantar aspect of the foot. Tenderness to palpation can be found at the medial aspect of the calcaneal tuberosity, in the medial arch, and occasionally at the distal insertion of the fascia on the metatarsal heads. The most consistent finding is exquisite pain with weight-bearing forces of the first few steps in the morning. The phenomenon of "physiologic creep," in which the tissues contract during the non–weight-bearing period at night and then are forcefully stretched with initial morning weight bearing, may explain this common complaint. Because the fascia is a noncontractile structure, active or passive dorsiflexion at the ankle and first MTP usually elicit the symptoms. These signs and symptoms can mimic those of other pathologic conditions but should be differentiated from medial plantar nerve irritation, tarsal tunnel syndrome, and infracalcaneal bursitis.

Treatment should initially be focused on controlling the inflammatory response and then on alleviating or reducing the excessive tension being placed on the plantar fascia and its associated structures, which have their origin at the calcaneal tuberosity. During the acute state, ice massage, anti-inflammatory medications, dexamethasone iontophoresis, and rest from aggravating activities are prescribed. A cold soda bottle with ridges can be used like a rolling pin under the arch of the foot to provide gentle stretch and cryomassage to the plantar fascia. Sponge-rubber heel lifts with a doughnut-shaped cutout may provide weight-bearing relief on the injured structures. In the subacute stage, pulsed phonophoresis, cross-fiber friction massage, and heel cord stretching are used to manage symptoms. A night splint will hold the ankle joint in dorsiflexion, the subtalar joint in neutral, and the first MTP in extension to reduce plantar fascia contracture. Correction of abnormal stresses can be provided through Low-Dye taping for the hyperpronator (Fig. 14-56), shock-absorbing inserts for the rigid cavus foot, and joint mobilization for the hypomobile first MTP joint (Fig. 14-57). Therapeutic exercise emphasis for the planus and cavus foot is detailed in boxes 14-4 and 14-5.

Box 14-4

Management of Plantar Fasciitis in the Rigid Cavus Foot—Stretching Emphasis

- Avoid or minimize the intensity, duration, and frequency of irritating activities
- Improve rearfoot and forefoot mobility
- Restore first metatarsophalangeal joint mobility through stretching and mobilization
- Use Gastroc-Soleus Stretching with control of hyperpronation tendencies
- Use massage and mobilization to tight plantar fascia soft tissue
- Use an accommodative orthosis to redirect plantar contact pressures to more tolerant areas of the foot

---

Box 14-5

Management of Plantar Fasciitis in the Flexible Planus Foot—Strengthening Emphasis

- Avoid or minimize the intensity, duration, and frequency of irritating activities
- Strengthen the muscles that control and reverse pronation
- Strengthen the intrinsic muscles of the foot
- Wear appropriate shoes that provide rearfoot stability and forefoot mobility
- Use taping to reduce strain on plantar fascia
- Use a semirigid to rigid biomechanical orthotic device to control compensatory pronation tendencies

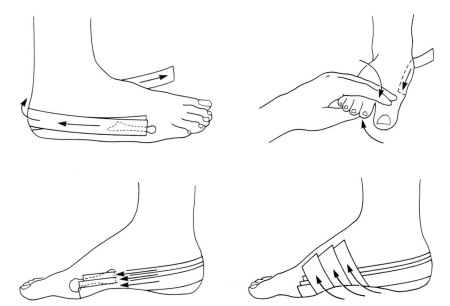

Figure 14-56. Modified Low-Dye taping technique to decrease traction stress on plantar fascia. (From Roy, S., and Irwin, R. [1983]: Sports Medicine: Prevention, Evaluation, Management, and Rehabilitation. Engelwood Cliffs, NJ, Prentice-Hall, p. 58.)

Foot Injuries

Tarsometatarsal Injuries

The tarsometatarsal joint is an articulation (Lisfranc's joint) that consists of the three cuneiform bones and the cuboid as they articulate with the five metatarsal bones. Transverse ligamentous supports span the base of the metatarsals with the exception of the first and second metatarsals. Midfoot sprains, dislocations, and fracture-dislocations, although not common, can occur in athletic competition. The joint can be injured through direct and indirect mechanisms. The direct crushing type of injury is less common and predictable in its pathologic course. Indirect injuries usually occur with an axial load to the heel with the foot in plantar flexion causing a hyperextension stress on the joint (Fig. 14-58).

Midfoot sprains have subtle examination findings that make diagnosis difficult. Swelling is usually mild. Pain with passive pronation-supination and tenderness on palpation are reliable indicators of this injury. The athlete will have pain or inability to perform unilateral heel raises, jumps, or cutting maneuvers. After the acute injury, initial evaluation should also include a circulatory assessment of the dorsalis pedis pulse and a neurologic screen for abnormal toe sensation.

After open or closed reduction, the foot is immobilized for a period of time, depending on the severity of the injury. Rehabilitation and weight-bearing progression can commence after immobilization with a gradual progression of functional activities on the toes. Recovery from medial midfoot sprains tends to progress at a slower rate and a longer time for return to full activity is seen.[32]

Tarsal Tunnel Syndrome

Tarsal tunnel syndrome is an entrapment neuropathy of the posterior tibial nerve as it passes through the osseofibrous tunnel between the flexor retinaculum and medial malleolus (Fig. 14-59). The typical mechanism of injury in athletes is excessive pronation, which causes a tightening of the flexor retinaculum. Hyperpronation of the forefoot can also cause the calcaneonavicular ligament to compress the medial plantar branch of the posterior tibial nerve. Direct trauma or chronic inflammation in this area produces a space-occupying lesion that can alter neurologic function.

The athlete reports intermittent burning, pain, tingling, and numbness in the medial foot, which are aggravated by weight bearing. A positive Tinel's sign may be elicited with tapping or compression over the affected nerve to reproduce the symptoms. In advanced stages, weakness in toe flexion and atrophy of the abductor hallucis may be evident.

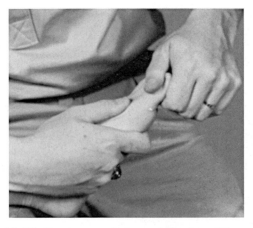

Figure 14-57. Traction-translation mobilization of first metatarsophalangeal joint to increase mobility.

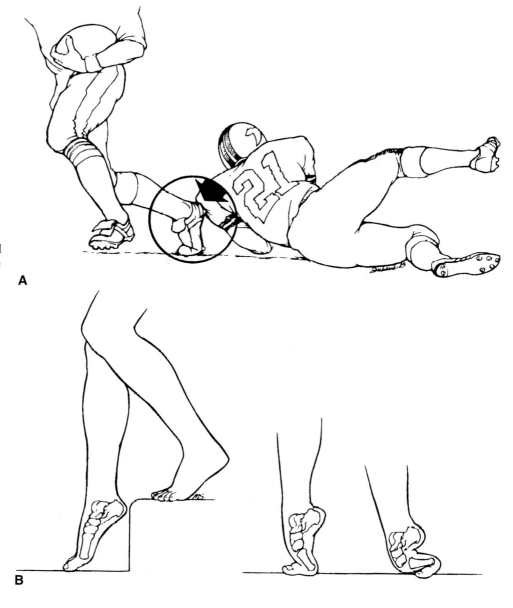

Figure 14-58. Mechanism of Lisfranc's fracture-dislocation. *A,* Axial load applied to heel with foot fixed in equinus. *B,* Axial load applied by body weight with ankle in extreme equinus. (From Heckman, J.D. [1991]: Fractures and dislocations of the foot. *In:* Rockwood, C.A. Jr., Green, D.P., and Bucholz, R.W. [eds.]: Rockwood and Green's Fractures in Adults, 3rd ed. Philadelphia, J.B. Lippincott, p. 2143.)

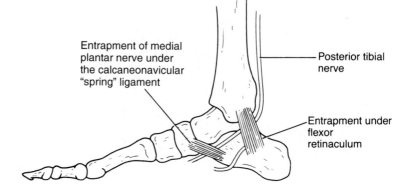

Figure 14-59. Tarsal tunnel syndrome (medial view).

The limb should be placed in a neutral-position orthosis to control pronation, and the athlete should be instructed in activity modifications. Therapeutic modalities such as ultrasound phonophoresis and ice massage may be tried to reduce edema and fibrosis in the area of entrapment. Resistant cases may require surgical release of the tissue that is causing compression.

Cuboid Syndrome

Cuboid syndrome describes a partial displacement of the cuboid bone by the pull of the peroneus longus. The onset can be gradual or traumatic. Acute pain and hypomobility can be induced with trauma or with a powerful contraction, with the foot in a plantar-flexed and inverted position. Gradual onset is more typical in the hyperpronated foot. Under these circumstances the peroneus longus is at a mechanical disadvantage, and it pulls the lateral portion of the cuboid dorsally and the medial portion in a plantar direction.[51]

The signs and symptoms of this injury include decreased or abnormal accessory motion of the calcaneocuboid joint and tenderness along the cuboid, peroneus longus, and lateral metatarsal heads. Treatment is focused on restoring normal arthrokinematics and protecting against further trauma or aggravation. After ice massage or a cold whirlpool bath, the athlete is prepared for bony manipulation. With the athlete prone and the knee mildly flexed to protect against excessive traction of the superficial peroneal nerve, a downward thrust of the thumbs is used to relocate the cuboid into its appropriate position (Fig. 14-60). After restoration of bony anatomy, a segmental balance pad may be used to unload stress on the fourth metatarsal and its cuboid articulation.[51] In athletes with chronic hyperpronation, Low-Dye taping or medial heel wedges can be used to counteract the damaging pull of the peroneus longus.

Metatarsal Stress Fractures

Metatarsal stress fractures occur when osteoclastic activity is greater than osteoblastic activity. Stress overload caused by prolonged pronation and excessive hypermobility of the first ray can begin a cycle of injury (Fig. 14-61). Hughes[23]

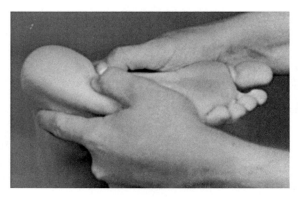

Figure 14-60. Cuboid mobilization.

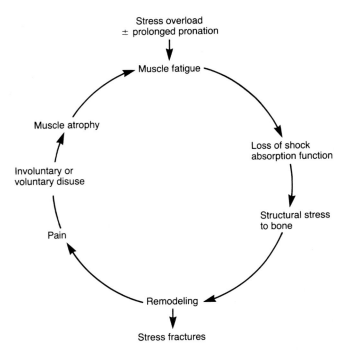

Figure 14-61. Stress fracture injury cycle. (From Taunton, J.E., Clement, D.B., and Webber, D. [1981]: Lower extremity stress fractures in athletes. Physician Sportsmed., 9:85.)

noted that predisposition to stress fractures is greatest in the presence of forefoot varus and decreased ankle dorsiflexion range of motion. Both of these conditions result in pronation during the propulsive phase of gait, placing considerable stress on the central three metatarsal bones, especially the second. Metatarsal stress fractures are most likely to occur at the beginning of the season in the deconditioned athlete or with sudden changes in training surfaces or athletic footwear.

There is localized pain and swelling over the metatarsal, which increase with activity and decrease with rest. Percussion and active flexion-extension of the toes also exacerbate the complaint.

Treatment is straightforward. The athlete must rest from weight-bearing or aggravating activities and find alternative methods of conditioning. In those in whom pain is present with ambulation or who may be suspected of not reducing activity levels, a short-leg walking cast may be appropriate. On return to activity, orthoses, tape, or a felt cutout to float the affected metatarsal should be used to relieve osteoclastic stresses.

During the subacute phase it is important for the athlete to correct the muscular, flexibility, and conditioning deficits that may have led to the initial injury.

Proximal Diaphysis Fracture of the Fifth Metatarsal Bone

Weight-bearing forces are great on the fifth metatarsal bone because of its many soft tissue attachments. Tension on the bone from the peroneus brevis, cubometatarsal ligament, lateral band of the plantar fascia, and peroneus tertius can lead to stress reactions, which can become a complete fracture with inversion trauma or a nonunion stress fracture with repetitive forces.[14] These lesions normally occur just distal to the base of the fifth metatarsal and are notoriously unpredictable in healing (Fig. 14-62).[50] Nonunion and reinjury are common. Management is therefore controversial and must be customized to the athlete. Some clinicians recommend early, aggressive surgical intervention with the use of percutaneous intermedullary screw fixation across the fracture site, whereas others simply use non–weight-bearing immobilization. The screw-fixation method has shown predictable healing and return to full athletic competition in an average of 8 weeks.[34] Conservative management allows 4 to 6 weeks of healing; the cast is then removed to determine whether the athlete can function with a nonfibrous union. Full athletic participation is contraindicated until there is full consolidation of the fracture site. When healing is complete, orthotic therapy should be considered to redistribute injurious forces.

Interdigital Neuroma

Compression and shearing forces at the bifurcation of the neurovascular bundle between the metatarsal heads can result in the formation of a benign tumor of fibrous tissue, called Morton's neuroma (Fig. 14-63). Pinching and squeezing of the neurovascular bundle between the

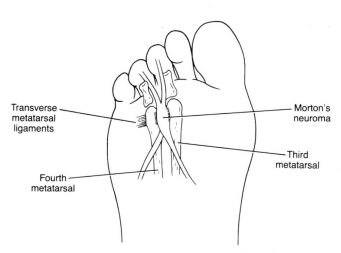

Figure 14-63. Plantar view of interdigital neuroma.

metatarsal heads and transverse metatarsal ligament occur in the hypermobile foot during midstance and propulsion.

The chief complaint is a burning or electric shock sensation in the forefoot that radiates into the toes. The lesion is usually located between the third and fourth metatarsal heads and is often mistaken for a stone in the shoe by the athlete. Pain can be relieved by removal of shoes and is aggravated by manual metatarsal head compression. A clicking or reproduction of symptoms can be elicited with simultaneous compression of the metatarsal heads in the transverse plane and plantar flexion of the affected MTP joints (Fig. 14-64).

Some success has been achieved with a metatarsal pad placed just proximal to the metatarsal heads, which increases their spatial spread and increases toe flexion. In selection of shoes a wide toe box should be considered, and orthotic inserts may be used to control hypermobility. Corticosteroid and anesthetic injections or oral

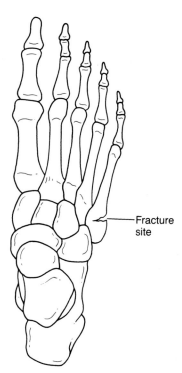

Figure 14-62. Proximal diaphysis fracture of fifth metatarsal (dorsal view).

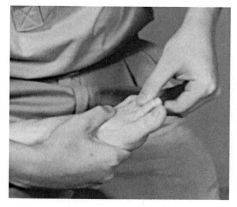

Figure 14-64. Metatarsal head compression in combination with plantar-dorsal glide to elicit pain from an interdigital neuroma.

anti-inflammatory medications can also be tried. Surgical excision of the neuroma is indicated when conservative measures fail.

Stairclimber's Transient Paresthesia

With the increase in popularity of stationary stair-climbing devices, a relatively new injury has become more common. In a study by Vereschagin and colleagues,[46] 39% of the individuals using these exercise machines experienced mild to moderate numbness or paresthesia in their feet during stair-climbing exercises. The symptoms are a result of persistent and prolonged weight-bearing compression of the interdigital nerve. It has been postulated that these transient paresthesia symptoms are magnified because there is no swing phase during the exercise movement to unload compressive forces under the foot. The following suggestions are offered to minimize neurologic irritation: (1) avoid repetitive MTP dorsiflexion by reducing step height and maintaining a flat-foot position on the pedals; (2) ensure wearing of proper footwear with ample toe-box depth, looser shoe lacing, and shock-absorbing insoles; and (3) limit the duration of the stair-climbing exercise according to the severity of the symptoms.

Turf Toe

Acute hyperdorsiflexion injuries to the first MTP joint occur as the toes are pressed down into an unyielding surface just before toe-off. This force causes hyperextension of the MTP joint as the phalanx is jammed into the metatarsal head.[47] Repetitive trauma of this nature results in plantar capsule tears, articular cartilage damage, and possible fracture of the medial sesamoid bone. Chronic trauma can lead to metatarsalgia, with ligamentous calcification and hallux rigidus.[38]

Sudden acceleration under high loads against unyielding AstroTurf is the usual mechanism of injury. Athletes who wear shoes that are extremely flexible and offer minimal support are especially prone to this injury. Also, athletes who wear a longer shoe to achieve greater width effectively lengthen the lever arm forces acting on the joint and subject the feet to repetitive trauma.

The athlete presents with a tender, red, and swollen first MTP joint that has increased pain with passive toe extension. Initial management calls for rest, ice, compression, elevation, and support to the injured joint. Tape immobilization can be used to limit excessive extension and valgus stresses that irritate the joint (Fig. 14-65). Rehabilitation procedures may include whirlpool range-of-motion exercises, ultrasound to mobilize scar tissue, and active range-of-motion exercises with the first ray stabilized. Figure 14-66 demonstrates an exercise to increase active range of motion for the hypomobile first MTP joint.

In the subacute stage, gentle plantar-dorsal glides of the first phalanx may be indicated to improve arthrokinematic mobility. On return to activity, the athlete should possess at least 90° of painless passive toe extension and have been screened for appropriate shoe selection.[38] A steel spring plate in the toe box or rigid taping into plantar flexion should be used initially when the athlete resumes full participation.

Sesamoiditis

The two small sesamoid bones of the foot are present on the plantar surface of the first metatarsal head, embedded within the tendon of the flexor hallucis brevis. The sesamoid bones enhance the windlass mechanism and help distribute and disperse weight-bearing forces during propulsion. The medial or tibial sesamoid bone is often

Step 1:   Prepare the plantar surface of the foot and toe with tape adherent. Encircle the first phalanx and midfoot with anchor strips. Do not extend the anchor strip to the IP joint as this will cause the MTP joint to extend during the taping technique.

Step 2:   Using precut moleskin or 1″ white tape, run a checkrein on the plantar-medial surface of the foot to limit dorsiflexion and adduction of the first MTP joint. Enclose the checkrein with elastic tape.

Step 3:   Modify the athletic shoe. Ensure proper length to decrease the lever arm effect on the joint. Place a spring steel, polyethylene, or orthoplast insert in the shoe to increase the rigidity of the distal forefoot.

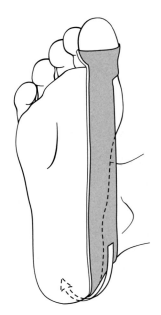

Figure 14-65. Turf toe taping technique to prevent excessive hyperextension of the first metatarsophalangeal (MTP) joint. IP, interphalangeal.

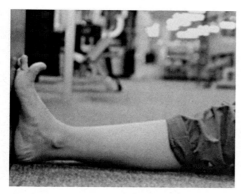

Figure 14-66. Active range of motion of first metatarsophalangeal joint, with first metatarsal head stabilized.

bipartite, and its appearance can be confused with a fracture.[48] Sesamoiditis describes an inflammatory condition of the tissues surrounding the sesamoid bones.

The athlete most prone to medial sesamoid pathologic conditions has a rigid cavus foot, tight Achilles tendon, and plantar-flexed first ray.[2] Sesamoid pain also occurs in athletes with normal foot structure but whose activities require maximal dorsiflexion of the first MTP joint, which allows excessive impact loading stresses on the sesamoids.

The athlete usually presents with tenderness and swelling of the first metatarsal head and pain with passive dorsiflexion. Pressure from improperly placed cleats on the athletic shoe may be a source of further aggravation.

Initial treatment in the acute stage involves ice massage, anti-inflammatory medications or cortisone injections, and rest. Pulsed phonophoresis and iontophoresis are alternative methods of combating the inflammatory response, which may be of value in reducing symptoms. Definitive treatment must include relief of weight-bearing stresses on the affected area. A semirigid orthosis with the first ray cut out or a Morton's extension can provide this relief.

ORTHOTIC THERAPY

The intent of orthotic therapy is to allow the subtalar joint to function near and around its neutral position. This is accomplished by balancing the forefoot to the rearfoot and by balancing the rearfoot with its supporting surface. There are a number of indications for the use of biomechanical orthoses:

1. Support and correction of intrinsic rearfoot and forefoot deformities
2. Support or restriction of range of motion
3. Treatment of postural problems
4. Dissipation of excessive ground reaction forces
5. Decrease of shear forces or tender spots on the plantar surface of the foot by redistributing weight bearing to more tolerant areas
6. Control of abnormal transverse rotation of the lower extremity

Contraindications to the use of orthotic therapy in the management of lower extremity injuries include the following:

1. Lack of intrinsic structural foot abnormality
2. Correction of soft tissue–induced equinus
3. Incomplete lower quarter biomechanical examination

The orthosis consists of the module (shell) and the post (Fig. 14-67). The module is the body of the orthosis, which conforms to the foot's plantar contours. The post is the "shim"; this is placed on the front or rear of the module and brings the ground up to the foot and places the subtalar joint in its neutral position.

Two main types of orthoses are used. The biomechanical orthosis is constructed of rigid materials such as high-density plastic or of semirigid materials called thermoplastics (Fig. 14-68). Biomechanical orthoses control and resist abnormal foot forces. Accommodative orthoses are constructed of soft materials, such as Plastazote.* These orthoses allow the foot to compensate, and the materials used in construction yield to abnormal foot forces. Posting on accommodative orthoses is referred to as bias. Table 14-15 offers the rationale and considerations for selecting the specific type of orthotic device that would be most appropriate for a particular athlete.

The post is the corrective portion of the orthosis and is analogous to the corrective lens of an eyeglass. Posts can be located in the rearfoot or forefoot and can be constructed intrinsically or extrinsically to provide a varus (medial) or valgus (lateral) angulation. For the biomechanical orthosis to be effective and for the athlete to comply in its use, it must meet the following requirements:

1. It must conform precisely to all contours of the foot, especially the heel seat and calcaneal and forefoot inclinations.
2. It must be rigid enough to maintain the shape, contour, and imposed angular relationships of the foot.
3. It must control abnormal motion, allow normal motion, and provide proper sequencing and timing of motion.
4. It must be able to withstand stress and wear.
5. It must be comfortable and ensure wearer compliance.
6. It must be adjustable.
7. It must end proximal to the weight-bearing surfaces of the metatarsal heads.
8. It must be narrow enough to fit on the shoe last and allow the first and fifth rays to function independently.

If an athlete is using orthoses, shoe selection should be appropriate. Criteria for shoe selection include a

---

*Available from AliMed, Dedham, Massachusetts.

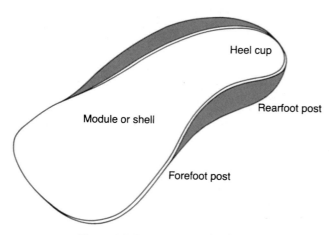

Figure 14-67. Anatomy of orthosis.

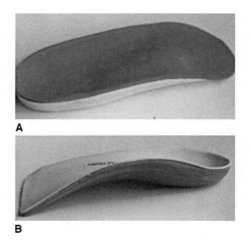

Figure 14-68. Orthoses. *A*, Semirigid. *B*, Rigid.

straight-last shoe with a snug, deep, and stable heel counter. The shoe should have minimal heel height and adequate shoe depth. For the narrow-shank shoe, the insoles and arch cookies may have to be removed and replaced with a "cobra pad" orthosis,[31] in which the entire insert consists of posting (Fig. 14-69). Feet that are high-arched or have an equinus attitude are difficult to fit with orthotic inserts.

When the orthosis has been fabricated, it should be placed in the athlete's shoe for a 5- to 10-minute running trial. Areas of irritation may have to be ground down, and correction of gait deviations will have to be assessed. The athlete should be instructed about gradually breaking in the orthosis, with the wear time not to exceed one additional hour of wear for each day the orthosis has been worn.

RETURN TO COMPETITION

The final component of lower leg rehabilitation is the functional progression and testing program, which must precede return to athletic competition. The concept of functional progression mandates a logical and ordered sequence of rehabilitative activities leading back to previous performance. Athletes must be educated to recognize that they cannot simply resume the activities that led to the initial injury when pain and swelling have subsided. Even the return of normal strength, flexibility, and endurance does not automatically ensure safe resumption of activity. Rehabilitative exercise programs cannot duplicate the speeds, forces, and stresses that normal high-speed athletic activities demand.

For these reasons, the athlete must be guided gradually back to activity by breaking down the component movements of the sport and addressing them in inverse order of difficulty. An example of this progression for an athlete with a lower extremity injury might be the following:

Non–weight-bearing exercise
Partial weight-bearing exercise
Full weight-bearing exercise
Stable surface balance training
Walking
Biomechanical Ankle Platform System or balance board activities

Table 14-15

Primary Considerations for Selecting an Orthosis

Physiologic age	Not chronologic age; the older the foot, the softer the orthosis
Foot type	The more mobile the foot, the more rigid the orthosis
Primary activity	Straight-ahead movements vs. pivoting or cutting
Chief complaint/diagnosis	Dictates need for specific accommodations (clips, extensions, metatarsal pads, etc.)
Subtalar motion	Control with more rigid device vs. bias with softer orthotic device
Shock absorbency	Softer orthosis to protect against proximal injuries up the chain or to improve dissipation of ground reaction forces
Weight of patient	Lower durometer for rigidity and firmness or for larger athlete

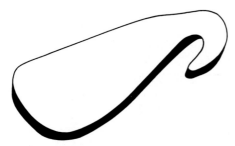

Figure 14-69. "Cobra pad" orthosis.

Rebounder running
Jogging
Running
Jumping and hopping
Backpedaling
Figure-eight running
Cutting and twisting
Zigzag running
Plyometrics

The program is structured according to the specific demands of the athlete's sport. Modifications are appropriate, depending on the goals and aspirations of the athlete. Specific criteria that dictate graduation from one functional level to the next must be defined precisely. It is the responsibility of the rehabilitation professional to provide the framework and specifics by which the athlete will function and progress.

After the athlete has completed the functional progression program and is psychologically prepared to return to competition, an objective evaluation of physical readiness should be performed. Criteria for return to activity should include absence or control of pain, swelling, and spasm; isokinetic symmetry in peak torque, total work, and average power; and functional normality with appropriate control, carriage, and confidence. Figure 14-70 is a sample functional evaluation form for lower leg injuries. It contains testing maneuvers and activities that can be used to judge an athlete's readiness to perform with symmetric functional normality.

SUMMARY

- Motion about a joint occurs in a direction that is perfectly perpendicular to the orientation of its axis.
- The resting position of a joint is the position in which to initiate treatment as the intracapsular space is large, the ligamentous support is lax, and arthrokinematic spin, glide, and roll are maximized.
- The closed pack position of a joint is a position that is dynamically stable as the joint surfaces are maximally congruent and the ligamentous support is taut.

- Physiologic accessory motions are necessary for full, pain-free range of motion.
- The position of the subtalar joint influences the mobility of the midtarsal joint and first ray while coupling the transverse plane rotation of the proximal kinetic chain.
- The muscles of the foot and leg work eccentrically early in the early stance phase of gait to control pronation and then reverse their function in late stance to concentrically accelerate propulsion.
- Normal gastrocnemius flexibility allows for 10 degrees of dorsiflexion with the knee extended and the subtalar joint in a neutral position. Normal soleus flexibility would allow for an additional 10 degrees of dorsiflexion motion when the knee is unlocked to put the gastrocnemius on slack.
- Ideal biomechanical structure requires that the posterior calcaneal bisection be parallel to the bisection of the distal third of the leg, the plantar plane of the rearfoot be parallel to the plantar plane of the central three metatarsal heads, and that the 1st and 5th metatarsal head be parallel to the central three met heads when the subtalar joint is in a neutral position.
- Observational gait analysis is a powerful examination tool that can be used in conjunction with static examination techniques to detect the source of pathology, impairments, or functional limitations.
- Prolonged or excessive subtalar hyperpronation during the stance phase of gait can be caused by a variety of skeletal or soft tissue abnormalities, asymmetries, and/or deviations.
- Tendinopathies are typically the result of abnormal anatomical structure, poor biomechanics, and improper training techniques or progressions.
- The rehabilitation of inversion sprains should focus on dynamic frontal plane muscular control, protection and support to the lateral ligaments, and restoration of proprioceptive abilities.
- Restoration of motion following prolonged immobilization may require manual intervention including specific, graded soft tissue and joint mobilization techniques.
- The cavus foot with plantar fasciitis typically responds more slowly to conservative intervention and emphasis should be placed on restoring joint mobility and soft tissue flexibility at the talocrual and 1st metatarsophalangeal joints.
- The planus foot with plantar fasciitis responds best with dynamic strengthening of the muscles that control subtalar pronation and orthotic correction or tape support along the medial longitudinal arch.
- Orthotic therapy is an important adjunct to the physical rehabilitation of injuries to the foot and ankle.

FOOT and ANKLE FUNCTIONAL TESTING

Name _____   Involved Extremity _____

HOP TESTS

TEST	PARAMETER	UNINVOLVED	INVOLVED	% DEFICIT
Unilateral Standing Long Jump Unilateral Standing Triple Jump	Distance in Inches	Trial 1 _____ Trial 2 _____ Trial 3 _____ Mean = _____	Trial 1 _____ Trial 2 _____ Trial 3 _____ Mean = _____	
Single Leg 20' Hop	Time in seconds	Trial 1 _____ Trial 2 _____ Trial 3 _____ Mean = _____	Trial 1 _____ Trial 2 _____ Trial 3 _____ Mean = _____	
Single Leg 20' Crossover Hop	Time in seconds	Trial 1 _____ Trial 2 _____ Trial 3 _____ Mean = _____	Trial 1 _____ Trial 2 _____ Trial 3 _____ Mean = _____	
4 Square Hop	# of Hops in _____ seconds	Trial 1 _____	Trial 1 _____	
Single Leg Vertical Jump	Distance in Inches	Trial 1 _____ Trial 2 _____ Trial 3 _____ Mean = _____	Trial 1 _____ Trial 2 _____ Trial 3 _____ Mean = _____	

STRENGTH TESTS

TEST	PARAMETER	UNINVOLVED	INVOLVED	% DEFICIT
Single Leg Squats @ _____% BW	# of repetitions Level _____	_____ reps	_____ reps	
Unilateral Heel Raises	# of repetitions Level _____	_____ reps	_____ reps	
Unilateral Toe Raises	# of repetitions Level _____	_____ reps	_____ reps	

FUNCTIONAL TESTS:

TEST	PARAMETER	UNINVOLVED	INVOLVED	% DEFICIT
Single Leg Knee Flexion	Knee Flexion Depth Ankle Dorsiflexion Range	_____ degrees _____ degrees	_____ degrees _____ degrees	
Frontal Plane Excursion Transverse Plane Excursion	Knee Valgus Hip Adduction Trunk Rotation	_____ cm _____ cm _____ degrees	_____ cm _____ cm _____ degrees	
Stork Stand (time)	Vision: Eyes Open vs. Closed Vestibular Influence – Neck rotation	_____ sec	_____ sec	
Stance Reach	Direction and Distance	_____ cm	_____ cm	
Lunge Step	Direction and Distance	_____ cm	_____ cm	
BAPS Board	Surface – Level - Overload			
Shuttle Run	Time	_____ sec	_____ sec	
_____ yard dash	Time	_____ sec	_____ sec	

SUMMARY:

RECOMMENDATIONS:

FUNCTIONAL SCORE = _____%   _____ Full Participation   _____ Participation with Restrictions   _____ No Participation

Clinician Signature _____   _____

Figure 14-70. Sample form for functional evaluation of lower leg injuries.

REFERENCES

1. American Academy of Orthopaedic Surgeons. (1965): Joint Motion: Methods of Measuring and Recording. Chicago, American Academy of Orthopaedic Surgeons.
2. Axe, M., and Ray, R. (1988): Orthotic treatment of sesamoid pain. Am. J. Sports Med., 16:411-416.
3. Brandel, B.K., and Williams, K. (1974): An analysis of cinematographic and electromyographic recordings of human gait. In: Nelson, R., and Morehouse, C. (eds.): Biomechanics, Vol. IV. Baltimore, University Park Press.
4. Bouche, R.T., and Kuwanda, K.T. (1984): Equinus deformity in the athlete. Physician Sportsmed., 12:81-91.
5. Bosien, W.R. (1955): Residual disability following acute ankle sprains. J. Bone Joint Surg. Am., 37:1237-1243.
6. Bullock-Saxton, J.E. (1994): Local sensation and altered hip muscle function following severe ankle sprain. Phys Ther., 74:17-31.
7. Boytin, M.J., Fischer, D.A., and Neuman, L. (1991): Syndesmotic ankle sprains. Am. J. Sports Med., 19:294-298.
8. Carter, T.R., Fowler, P.J., and Blokker, C. (1992): Functional postoperative treatment of Achilles tendon repair. Am. J. Sports Med., 20:459-462.
9. Cetti, R., Christensen, S., Ejsted, R., et al. (1993): Operative versus nonoperative treatment of Achilles tendon rupture. Am. J. Sports Med., 21:791-799.
10. Clancy, W.G., Neidhart, D., and Brand, D.L. (1976): Achilles tendinitis in runners. A report of five cases. Am. J. Sports Med., 4:46-57.
11. Clement, D.B., Taunton, J.E., and Smart, G.E. (1984): Achilles tendinitis and peritendinitis: Etiology and treatment. Am. J. Sports Med., 12:179-184.
12. Creighton, D., and Olson, V. (1987): Evaluation of range of motion of first metatarsophalangeal joint in runners with plantar fasciitis. J. Orthop. Sports Phys. Ther., 8:357-361.
13. Cyriax, J. (1978): Textbook of Orthopedic Medicine, 7th ed. London, Bailliere Tindall.
14. Dameron, T.B. (1975): Fractures and anatomical variations of the proximal portion of the fifth metatarsal. J. Bone Joint Surg. Am., 57:788-792.
15. Donatelli, R. (1985): Normal biomechanics of the foot and ankle. J. Orthop. Sports Phys. Ther., 7:91-95.
16. Davies, G. (1984): A Compendium of Isokinetics in Clinical Usage. La Crosse, WI, S & S.
17. Eiff, M.P., Smith, A.T., and Smith, G.E. (1994): Early mobilization versus immobilization in the treatment of lateral ankle sprains. Am. J. Sports Med., 22:83-87.
18. Elveru, R.A., Rothstein, J.M., and Lamb, R.L. (1988): Goniometric reliability in a clinical setting: subtalar and ankle joint measurements. Phys. Ther., 68:672-677.
19. Freeman, M.A.R., Dean, M.R.E., and Hanham, I.W.F. (1965): The etiology and prevention of functional instability of the foot. J. Bone Joint Surg. Br., 47:678-685.
20. Friedman, M. (1986): Injuries to the leg in athletes. In: Nicholas, J., and Hershman, E. (eds.): The Lower Extremity and Spine in Sports Medicine. St. Louis, C.V. Mosby.
21. Garth, W., and Miller, S. (1989): Evaluation of toe claw deformity, weakness of foot intrinsics, and posteromedial shin pain. Am. J. Sports Med., 17:821-827.
22. Gray, G. (1984): When the Foot Hits the Ground Everything Changes. Toledo, OH, American Physical Rehabilitation Network.
23. Hughes, L.Y. (1985): Biomechanical analysis of the foot and ankle to developing stress fractures. J. Orthop. Sports Phys. Ther., 7:96-101.
24. James, S.L., and Brubaker, C.E. (1973): Biomechanics of running. Orthop. Clin. North Am., 4:605-615.
25. Kapandji, I.A. (1970): The Physiology of Joints, Vol. II. Edinburgh, Churchill Livingstone.
26. Keene, S. (1985): Ligament and muscle-tendon unit injuries. In: Gould, J., and Davies, G. (eds.): Orthopedic and Sports Physical Therapy. St. Louis, C.V. Mosby, pp. 135-165.
27. Kisner, C., and Colby, L.A. (1985): Ankle and foot. In: Therapeutic Exercise: Foundation and Techniques. Philadelphia, F.A. Davis.
28. Klein, K. (1990): Biomechanics of running. Presented at Metroplex Trainer's Meeting, Fort Worth, TX, January 1990.
29. Lattanza, L., Gray, G., and Katner, R. (1988): Closed vs. open kinematic chain measurements of subtalar joint eversion: Implications for clinical practice. J. Orthop. Sports Phys. Ther., 9:310-314.
30. Magee, D.J. (1987): Orthopedic Physical Assessment. Philadelphia, W.B. Saunders.
31. McPoil, T., and Brocato, R. (1985): The foot and ankle: Biomechanical evaluation and treatment. In: Gould, J., and Davis, G. (eds.): Orthopedic and Sports Physical Therapy. St. Louis, C.V. Mosby, pp. 313-341.
32. Meyer, E.A., Callaghan, J.J., Albright, J.P., et al. (1994): Midfoot sprains in collegiate football players. Am. J. Sports Med., 22:392-400.
33. Miller, W.A. (1977): Rupture of musculotendinous junction of medial head of gastrocnemius. Am. J. Sports Med., 5:191-193.
34. Mindrebo, N., Shelbourne, K.D., Van Meter, C.D., and Rettig, A.C. (1993): Outpatient percutaneous screw fixation of the acute Jones fracture. Am. J. Sports Med., 21:720-723.
35. Picciano, A.M., Rowlands, M.S., and Worrell, T. (1993): Reliability of open and closed kinetic chain subtalar joint neutral positions and navicular drop test. J. Orthop. Sports Phys. Ther., 18:553-558.
36. Rebman, L. (1986): Suggestions from the clinic: Ankle injuries: Clinical observations. J. Orthop. Sports Phys. Ther., 8:153-156.
37. Root, W.L., Orient, W.P., and Weed, J.N. (1977): Clinical Biomechanics, Vol. II: Normal and Abnormal Function of the Foot. Los Angeles, Clinical Biomechanics.
38. Sammarco, G.J. (1988): How I manage turf toe. Physician Sportsmed., 16:113-199.
39. Seibel, M.O. (1988): Foot Function. Baltimore, Williams & Wilkins.
40. Sell, K.E., Verity, T.M., Worrell, T.W., et al. (1994): Two measurement techniques for assessing subtalar joint position: A reliability study. J. Orthop. Sports Phys. Ther., 19:162-167.
41. Smart, G.W., Tauton, J.E., and Clement, D.B. (1980): Achilles tendinitis and peritendinitis. Med. Sci. Sports Exerc., 17:731-743.
42. Smith-Oricchio, K., and Harris, B.A. (1990): Intertester reliability of subtalar neutral, calcaneal inversion, and eversion. J. Orthop. Sports Phys. Ther., 12:10-16.
43. Subotnick, S. (1989): Sports Medicine of the Lower Extremity. New York, Churchill-Livingstone.

44. Tanner, S., and Harvey, J. (1988): How we manage plantar fasciitis. Physician Sportsmed., 16:39-48.

45. Tatro-Adams, D., McGann, S.F., and Carbone, W. (1995): Reliability of the figure-of-eight method of ankle measurement. J. Orthop. Sports Phys., 22:161-163.

46. Vereschagin, K.S., Firtch, W.L., Caputo, L.J., and Hoffman, M.A. (1993): Stairclimber's transient paraesthesia. Physician Sportsmed., 21:63-69.

47. Visnick, A. (1987): A playing orthosis for turf toe. Athl. Train., 22:215.

48. Vogelbach, D. (1989): The foot and ankle. Presented at HEALTHSOUTH Continuing Education Program. Birmingham, AL.

49. Wallace, L. (1986): Lower quarter pain: Mechanical evaluation and treatment. Presented at Seventh Annual Conference of the Sports Physical Therapy Section, Williamsburg, VA.

50. Whittle, H.P. (1994): Fractures of the foot in athletes. Op. Tech. Sports Med., 2:43-57.

51. Woods, A., and Smith, W. (1983): Case report: Cuboid syndrome and the techniques for treatment. Athl. Train., 18:64-65.

CHAPTER 15

KNEE REHABILITATION

Mark D. Weber, Ph.D., ATC, P.T., S.C.S.
William R. Woodall, M.Ed., ATC, P.T., S.C.S

CHAPTER OBJECTIVES

At the end of this chapter the reader will be able to:

- Identify activities that may cause detrimental stresses to a healing/reconstructed anterior cruciate ligament, posterior cruciate ligament, medial collateral ligament, or lateral collateral ligament.
- Identify activities that may cause detrimental stresses to the patellofemoral joint.
- Develop appropriate rehabilitation programs for athletes with a variety of knee injuries.
- Determine when to progress an athlete's rehabilitation program using specific measurable criteria.
- Discuss the reliability, sensitivity, and specificity of arthrometry, lower extremity functional tests, and isokinetics.
- Interpret information obtained from an arthrometer, lower extremity functional tests, and isokinetics.

The knee joint is one of the most frequently injured joints in the body, especially in those engaging in athletic activity. In the functional anatomy section of this chapter some of the key information used in developing safe and effective rehabilitation programs is presented. The rehabilitation programs are goal oriented, modified by time instead of being driven by it. Also emphasized are knee rehabilitation of the entire kinetic chain, early controlled motion, a return to participation along a functional progression, and restoration of lower extremity muscular strength, power, endurance, and neuromuscular control.

FUNCTIONAL ANATOMY

To make appropriate clinical decisions for rehabilitation of knee injuries the clinician must have a thorough understanding of lower extremity anatomy and biomechanics. In the following sections some of the more important biomechanical factors related to rehabilitation of knee injuries are presented.

Ligaments

The knee is inherently unstable because of its location between the two longest bones in the body. Knee stability is maintained through static restraints (e.g., ligaments) and dynamic restraints (e.g., muscles). The role of the ligamentous restraints in controlling forces applied to the knee joint has been studied extensively. Loads produced on the knee by rehabilitation activities have been the subject of a number of investigations. The data gained from these studies provides the clinician with the information necessary to develop safe and effective rehabilitation programs.

Anterior Cruciate Ligament

The anterior cruciate ligament (ACL) is the primary restraint to anterior tibial translation on the femur. Grood and colleagues[74] reported that the ACL provides 85% of the ligamentous restraining force to anterior drawer at 30° and 90° of flexion. In addition to controlling anterior tibial translation, the ACL has several other functions that include the screw-home mechanism,[68] assisting in the control of varus and valgus stresses,[169] control of hyperextension stresses,[58,101,130] and a guiding function during tibiofemoral flexion-extension.[68,116] Because of its position in the femoral intercondylar notch, if there is a valgus stress on a flexed knee, the ACL becomes a restraint to external tibial rotation.[130] The ACL also assists the medial collateral ligament (MCL) in controlling tibial internal rotation.[65]

The stresses of rehabilitation exercises on the ACL have been studied in a number of investigations. Henning and associates[82] implanted a strain gauge in two patients with grade II ACL sprains. The patients then performed various rehabilitation activities and the strain was recorded. The strain on the ACL was reported as a percentage of the strain of an 80-pound Lachman test (Table 15-1). Although conclusions should be drawn with care from a study with only two subjects, it still provides some useful information about the relative rank of strain on the ACL with particular rehabilitation activities.

Beynnon and colleagues[20] implanted a Hall effect transducer in the knees of 11 subjects with normal ACLs

Table 15-1

Strain on the Anterior Cruciate Ligament

Activity	Relative ACL Strain*
Running downhill at 5 mph	125%
Isometric quad contraction at 22° of flexion against a 20-lb weight	62-121%
Isometric quad contraction at 0° of flexion against a 20-lb weight	87-107%
Jog on floor	89%
Leg lift with 22° of knee flexion	12-79%
Jog 5 mph on treadmill	62-64%
Isometric quad contraction at 45° of flexion against a 20-lb weight	50%
Walk without assistive device	36%
Half-squat, one leg	21%
Quad set	18%
Walk with crutches, weight bearing at 50 lb	7%
Stationary cycle	7%
Isometric hamstring contraction	−7%

Data compiled from Henning, C.E., Lynch, M.A., and Glick, K.R. (1985): An in vivo strain gauge study of elongation of the anterior cruciate ligament. Am. J. Sports Med., 13:22–26.
*Single recording indicates that the activity was reported for one subject only, whereas range indicates recording reported for both subjects.

and then determined the strain on the ACL during open-chain knee flexion and extension as well as during isometric contractions. They concluded that the following open-chain exercises produced either low or no strain on the ACL: isometric contractions of the hamstrings at 15°, 30°, 60°, and 90°; isometric quadriceps contractions at 60° and 90°; co-contractions of the quadriceps and hamstrings at 30°, 60°, and 90°; active knee flexion and extension between 35° and 90°; and knee flexion and extension with a 45-N (10-pound) weight between 45° and 90°. Exercises that proved to significantly increase the strain on the ACL included the following: knee extension exercise with a 45-N weight (particularly at 10° and 20° of knee flexion); isometric quadriceps contractions (at 15° and 30°); and iso-

metric co-contractions of the quadriceps and hamstrings at 15°. During knee extension exercise the transition from the unstrained ACL to the strained ACL shifted from 35° of flexion during active unweighted knee extension to 45° under the weighted knee extension condition.

Beynnon and associates[21] also compared closed-chain to open-chain exercises for peak strain on the ACL. They reported the following peak ACL strains: open-chain active knee flexion-extension with no load (2.8%), squatting (3.6%), open-chain knee flexion-extension with 45-N load (3.8%), squatting with Sport cord (4.0%), and 30 Nm isometric quadriceps contractions at 15° (4.4%). To put these ACL strain values into clinical perspective these authors reported the peak ACL strain to be 3.7% for a 150-N Lachman test and 1.7% for stationary bicycling.[19] The results of this study on the influence of open-chain quadriceps activities on ACL strain are predictable based on results of other studies.[56,106,182,183] The strain results during the closed-chain activities are somewhat surprising given that Escamilla and associates[56] reported no tensile load on the ACL during loaded squats or leg press.

Kvist and Gillquist[106] measured anterior tibial translation during knee extension exercises and several types of squats. During active knee extension, as loads increased so did the tibial translation with the ACL-deficient knee demonstrating a greater anterior translation than the uninjured knee. Anterior translation was greater during the eccentric phase compared with the concentric phase of the exercise. The greatest anterior translation occurred between 15° and 20° of knee flexion. This matches the range in which Escamilla and associates[56] reported the greatest tensile load on the ACL during weighted open-chain knee extension. Kvist and Gillquist also reported that there was less anterior translation under all squat conditions than with loaded open-chain knee extension exercise for the knees with deficient ACLs. Similar results were reported in two different studies by Yack and associates.[182,183]

In most studies investigating anterior shear during rehabilitation activities the results have been reported as strain on the ACL or anterior translation. A few researchers have calculated their results relative to body weight (BW). Table 15-2 contains such data.

Table 15-2

Anterior Shear Forces Across the Tibiofemoral Joint During Various Activities

Reference	Activity	Knee Position at Peak Anterior Shear	Calculated Force Times Body Weight
Ericson and Nisell[54]	Cycling, 60 RPM, 120 W workload	60-70°	0.05
Kaufman et al.[98]	Isokinetic knee extension at 60°/sec	25°	0.3
	Isokinetic knee extension at 180°/sec	25°	0.2
Nisell et at.[129]	Isokinetic knee extension at 30°/sec	45°	1.3
	Isokinetic knee extension at 180°/sec	40°	0.5

RPM, Rotations per minute; W, watts.

Posterior Cruciate Ligament

The primary function of the posterior cruciate ligament (PCL) is to limit posterior translations of the tibia on the femur.[71,75] It also assists in controlling varus, valgus, and hyperextension stresses to the knee.[62,74] The role of the PCL in controlling rotational forces appears to be minimal.[71,75] The importance of the PCL in normal knee arthrokinematics is indicated by the increased compression forces that are observed in the patellofemoral joint and medial compartment in cadaveric specimens when the PCL is sectioned.[154] This correlates with the common complaints of anterior knee pain and medial compartment arthrosis in patients with a PCL-deficient knee.[4,154,177] Rehabilitation activities that cause large posterior shear forces include isometric hamstring contractions, jogging, lunges, ascending and descending stairs, and squats greater than 60° of knee flexion (especially as hip flexion is increased).[4,30,137,167,177] In addition, during early PCL rehabilitation, the clinician may want to avoid activities that require high forces from the gastrocnemius, because there is evidence that these activities may produce significant strain on the PCL.[46] Isokinetic testing of the hamstrings also produces significant posterior shears of the tibiofemoral joint.[98] Table 15-3 contains calculated posterior shear data for several rehabilitation exercises. Box 15-1 contains a summary of exercises that may cause excessive stress during the early healing phase of an ACL or PCL reconstruction.

Collateral Ligaments

The medial collateral ligament (MCL) provides the primary restraint against valgus stresses to the knee.[74] The MCL provides some assistance in the control of internal rotation torsional forces through the knee, but this role decreases as the knee is flexed.[119] The MCL also assists in controlling excessive external rotation.[130] The MCL is taut in extension and external rotation.[159] Because of this, as flexion is initiated, tension within the ligament assists in reversal of the screw-home mechanism.[68] Rehabilitation activities that stress the MCL would include any adductor strengthening exercises in which the resistance is placed distal to the knee. In addition, care must be taken during closed kinetic chain activities if the athlete lacks hip control, because the hip has a tendency under these conditions to adduct and internally rotate, which creates a valgus stress to the knee.

The lateral collateral ligament (LCL) is the primary restraint to varus stresses at the knee.[74] The tendon of the biceps femoris overlaps the LCL[158] and may act as an active mechanism to bias the tension of the LCL.[74] The LCL, along with the posterolateral capsule, appears to play a large role in the control of external tibial rotation.[71,119] Rehabilitation activities that stress the LCL would include any abductor strengthening exercises in which the resistance is placed distal to the knee.

Capsular Restraints

The posterior medial and lateral "corners" of the knee joint capsule play an important role in the control of torsional forces through the knee. The posteromedial capsule is supported by the semimembranosus muscle and the oblique popliteal ligament, which is an expansion of the tendon of the semimembranosus.[158] The posterior medial corner provides some restraint to valgus stresses when the knee is in extension,[74] but it is primarily involved in the control of internal torsional stresses.[119]

The posterolateral capsule is reinforced by the arcuate ligament and popliteus tendon.[75] The posterior lateral corner, with the LCL, is primarily involved in the control of external rotation stresses; however, in the ACL-deficient knee, it also plays a role in controlling internal rotation of the knee.[71,75] The posterolateral corner plays a minor role in the control of varus stress to the knee when the knee is extended.[75] The posterior capsule is less prone to injury when the knee is in the flexed position because the structure is relatively slack.[74]

In vitro isolated sectioning of the ACL or PCL is generally not associated with rotational instabilities,[71,74,75,107,119] but when coupled with sectioning of either

Table 15-3

Posterior Shear Forces across the Tibiofemoral Joint during Various Activities

Reference	Activity	Knee Position at Peak Posterior Shear	Calculated Force Times Body Weight
Ericson and Nisell[54]	Cycling, 60 RPM, 120 W workload	105°	0.05
Kaufman et al.[98]	Isokinetic knee flexion at 60°/sec	75°	1.7
	Isokinetic knee flexion at 180°/sec	75°	1.4
Ohkoshi et al.[137]	Squat	15°	<0.25
		30°	<0.3
		60°	0.25-0.5
		90°	1.0-1.25

RPM, Rotations per minute; W, watts.

Box 15-1

Exercises to Avoid during Early Anterior Cruciate Ligament (ACL) or Posterior Cruciate Ligament (PCL) Rehabilitation

ACL
Loaded open-chain knee extensions from 50° to 5°
PCL
Open-chain hamstring exercises in any part of the range of motion
Loaded open-chain knee extensions from 90° to 50°
Closed-chain activities with the knee in greater than 50° of flexion

of the posterior corners, rotational instabilities become apparent. Clinically, this would suggest that an athlete with an acute rotational instability probably does not have an isolated cruciate injury.[107]

The Menisci

The meniscus serves a number of important functions including increasing of the stability and congruence of the knee joint,[6,13] load distribution and transmission,[6,13,66,122] shock absorption,[6,13] joint proprioception,[6] and aiding in joint lubrication and nutrition.[6,13] Its shape, attachments, and collagen arrangement allow the meniscus to effectively transmit compressive forces across the tibiofemoral joint. Removal of the meniscus reduces the contact area between the femur and tibia. This substantially increases the force per unit area between the two articular surfaces.[66] It is likely that the increase in force per unit area leads to the degenerative changes that often occur after removal of the meniscus.[57,122] The structure and attachments of the menisci also allow for early controlled weight bearing after longitudinal meniscal repairs because the sutured edges are approximated by weight-bearing stress.[122]

The peripheral 10% to 30% of the meniscus has a vascular supply from the perimeniscal capillary plexus.[6] The rest of the meniscus, 70% or more, receives nutrition by passive diffusion and mechanical pumping (intermittent compression during joint loading and unloading).[6] Because of the important role the meniscus plays in the health of the knee joint, meniscal tears in the vascular zone are usually repaired surgically.[6] By extrapolation from animal studies, the tensile strength of the meniscus 12 weeks after repair is approximately 80%.[99]

The menisci move or distort during tibiofemoral motion,[130] distorting posteriorly during flexion and anteriorly during extension. This distortion is caused by a shear from the oblique reaction force between the femur and the meniscus.[130] During active flexion, the contraction of the semimembranosus and popliteus muscles also assist in pulling the menisci posteriorly.[118] This is why open-chain

hamstring strengthening is usually avoided in the early rehabilitation phases after meniscal repairs. During internal and external rotation of the knee, the menisci distort in opposite directions. With internal rotation of the femur on the tibia, the medial meniscus distorts posteriorly, whereas the lateral meniscus distorts anteriorly.[130] The opposite occurs during external rotation of the femur on the tibia. In summary, during flexion and extension of the knee, the direction of meniscal distortion follows the direction of tibial plateau movement and during rotation the distortion follows the direction of femoral condyle movement. This means that during combined flexion-extension and internal-external rotation movements, the distortions for the anterior and posterior portions of one meniscus are in opposite directions, whereas in the other meniscus the distortion is primarily in one direction. This is why the frequent mechanism of isolated meniscal injury is combined knee flexion and rotation.[5]

PATELLOFEMORAL BIOMECHANICS

It is important to understand patellofemoral biomechanics when one prescribes knee exercises, regardless of the diagnosis. The connection between the tibiofemoral and patellofemoral joints must not be overlooked, nor should these joints be treated independently. Ignoring important aspects of the biomechanics of the patellofemoral joint during rehabilitation of a tibiofemoral joint problem often creates patellofemoral joint problems and unnecessarily extends the rehabilitation process.

The stability of the patellofemoral joint is based on the interplay among bony geometry, ligamentous-retinacular restraints, and muscles.[89] To function optimally, the patellofemoral joint must be able to control sagittal and frontal plane forces. Additionally, the hip and the foot must control transverse plane forces through the patellofemoral joint. Three factors play an important role in the sagittal plane mechanics of the patellofemoral joint: the quadriceps force of contraction, the sagittal plane angle of the knee, and the contact area between the patella and the femur. The interaction between the force of the quadriceps contraction and the knee angle determines the amount of compressive force that occurs between the patella and femur. The compression force is known as the patellofemoral joint reaction force (PFJR).[89,144,166] Increasing the quadriceps force of contraction and/or increasing the knee angle increases the PFJR[89,144] (Fig. 15-1). It is important to note that at knee angles of less than 25° to 30°, even large quadriceps forces do not produce tremendous compression forces because the magnitude of the posteriorly directed resultant force vector is sufficiently reduced.[89,144] During most rehabilitation activities, gravity has a profound influence on the force of the quadriceps contraction. As the torque of gravity increases during an exercise, the force of the quadriceps must

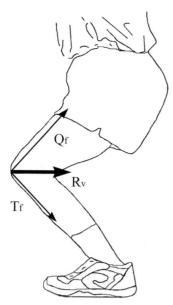

Figure 15-1. Resolution of quadriceps force (Qf) and patellar tendon force (Tf) produces a posteriorly directed resultant force (Rv).

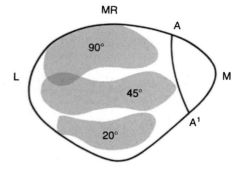

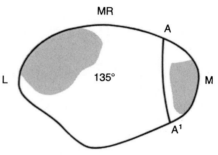

Figure 15-2. Patellofemoral contact pattern during knee flexion. L, lateral; M, medial; MR, median ridge; A-A[1], ridge separating medial and odd facets. (From Goodfellow, J., Hungerford, D.S., and Zindel, M. [1976]: Patellofemoral joint mechanics and pathology: 1. Functional anatomy of the patellofemoral joint. J. Bone Joint Surg. Br., 58:287-290.)

increase. For typical open-chain quadriceps exercises, as the knee moves toward extension, the torque of gravity increases and, therefore, the force of the quadriceps must increase. The opposite is true for common closed-chain activities in which the torque of gravity decreases as the knee moves toward extension and, thus, the force of the quadriceps decreases as well.

The third factor to consider in sagittal plane forces is the contact area between the patella and the femur. The contact area depends on the contact points between the patella and the femur, which change based on tibiofemoral joint flexion angle (Fig. 15-2).[67,72,88,89,166] In general, the contact area between the articular surfaces of the patella and femur increase as knee flexion progresses toward 90°.[88,89,166] Because the patellofemoral contact area varies it is important to account for it when the influence of the PFJR is examined. This relationship, PFJR applied per unit area of contact, is known as *patellofemoral contact stress*.

During typical open-chain quadriceps exercises, as the knee extends the patellofemoral joint contact stress increases significantly because of the increasing PFJR and decreasing contact area.[89,144,166] Experimentally, it appears that during open-chain quadriceps exercises, maximal contact stress peaks at approximately 35° to 40°. It then declines as extension continues, because of the reduced sagittal plane angle of the knee.[89,144] During typical closed-chain exercises, as the knee extends the patellofemoral joint contact stress decreases despite the decreasing contact area. This occurs because the PFJR is decreasing rapidly owing to the decreasing torque of gravity and decreasing sagittal plane angle of the knee. The

patellofemoral contact stress is also influenced by patellar position in the frontal and transverse planes. Inappropriate alignment in these planes can produce nonuniform pressure distribution with higher peak stresses in some areas and relative unloading in others.[88]

Fig. 15-3 is a graphic representation of data from several studies of patellofemoral contact stress versus knee flexion angle for both open- and closed-chain activities.[89,144,166] The lines for open- and closed-chain contact stress cross at approximately 50°. These data suggest that for the athlete with an extensor mechanism problem, open-chain strengthening activities for the quadriceps are safest from 90° to 50° and from 10° to 0°, whereas closed-chain activities are safest from 50° to 0°. These "safe" and "unsafe" ranges should be used only as a guide, with the truly detrimental ranges and loads being determined by the signs and symptoms of the athlete. Initially, athletes with extensor mechanism problems will often experience an increase in pain and symptoms if exercises are performed in the suggested unsafe ranges. However, as the athlete's condition improves, he or she will typically tolerate loads through greater ranges without symptoms, including the suggested unsafe ranges. The decision of

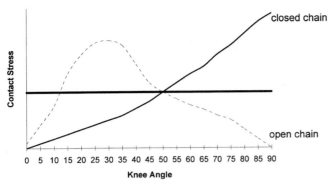

Figure 15-3. Patellofemoral contact stresses during open- and closed-chain activities. Area below horizontal line indicates relatively low contact stresses, a potentially "safe" zone. The area above the horizontal line indicates relatively high contact stresses and therefore is potentially an "unsafe" zone. (Graph developed from data reported by Hungerford, D.S., and Barry, M. [1979]: Biomechanics of the patellofemoral joint. Clin. Orthop., 144:9-15; Reilly, D.T., and Martens, M. [1972]: Experimental analysis of the quadriceps muscle force and patellofemoral joint reaction force for various activities. Acta Orthop. Scand., 43:126-137; and Steinkamp, L.A., Dillingham, M.F., Markel, M.D., et al. [1993]: Biomechanical considerations in patellofemoral joint rehabilitation. Am. J. Sports Med., 21:438-444.)

when and how to progress the exercise program should be based on the signs and symptoms of the athlete. Most athletic endeavors will require the athlete to tolerate loads through a wide range of motion (ROM) under a wide vari-

ety of situations. Therefore, in the late stages of the rehabilitation process, it is often necessary for the athlete to perform activities in the unsafe ranges if he or she is to tolerate these activities upon return to competition.

Table 15-4 contains calculated PFJR data for a variety of rehabilitation activities. Care must be taken in interpreting the data in this table, because these data do not account for the contact area through which the PFJR is being applied. Direct comparison should be made only between activities with peak compression forces at similar angles of knee flexion and, therefore, similar contact areas. For example, a comparison between knee extension with a 9-kg weight boot and cycling appear to have similar PFJR values (1.4 and 1.3, respectively) would be misleading. Because the patellofemoral contact area is greater at 83° than at 36°, the patellofemoral joint contact stress will be much greater for the knee extension exercise. Box 15-2 provides a summary of activities with high and low patellofemoral contact pressures.

The frontal plane forces that must be balanced by the extensor mechanism also originate from forces developed by the quadriceps. As with the sagittal plane forces, the contraction of the vastus lateralis (VL), vastus intermedius, rectus femoris, and vastus medialis longus (VML) produces a superiorly directed force that is resisted by an inferiorly directed force from the patellar tendon. In the frontal plane these two opposing forces do not form a straight line but instead form an angle similar to the physiologic valgus angulation between the femur and the tibia (Fig. 15-4).[67] Resolving these two forces provides a result-

Table 15-4

Patellofemoral Compressive Forces during Various Activities*

Reference	Activity	Knee Position at Peak Patellofemoral Compressive Force	Calculated Force Times Body Weight
Dahlkvist et al.[36]	Squat, slow ascent	45°	4.73
	Squat, slow descent		7.41
	Squat, fast ascent	55-60°	5.99
	Squat, fast descent	60°	7.62
Ericson and Nisell[55]	Cycling, 60 RPM, 120 W workload	83°	1.3
Flynn and Soutas-Little[61]	Forward running	35% of stance phase	5.6
	Backward running	52% of stance phase	3.0
Huberti and Hayes[88]	Squat	90°	6.5
Kaufman et al.[98]	Isokinetic knee extension 60°/sec	70°	5.1
	Isokinetic knee extension 180°/sec	80°	4.9
Reilly and Martens[144]	Walking	8°	0.5
	Straight leg raise	0°	0.5
	Knee extension with 9-kg weight boot	36°	1.4
	Ascending and descending stairs	40-60°	3.3
	Deep squat	135°	7.6
Scott and Winter[151]	Running	Midstance	7.0-11.1

*Because of the change in patellofemoral contact area at different points in the range of motion, it is appropriate to compare activities that occur only in similar ranges of motion.

Box 15-2

Contact Pressure and the Patellofemoral Joint

High contact pressure activities
Loaded open-chain knee extensions from 50° to 20°
Closed-chain activities with the knee in greater than 50° of
  flexion
Low contact pressure activities
Loaded open-chain knee extensions from 90° to 50° and
  from 20° to 0°
Closed-chain activities with the knee in less than 50° of
  flexion

ant force that is directed laterally. This resultant force is referred to as a valgus vector.[67] Thus, when the quadriceps contract, the patella has a tendency to shift laterally.[67,70,110] This tendency toward lateralization is dynamically balanced by the vastus medialis obliquus (VMO)[67,70,110] with assistance from the static restraints of the medial portion of the extensor retinaculum. Once the patella is seated in the femoral sulcus, the lateral wall of the sulcus will also assist in resisting the laterally directed resultant force vector.[67,145]

Several factors have been suggested to influence the magnitude of this valgus vector, including hip position, extensibility of lateral retinacular structures, competence of medial retinacular structures, femoral and tibial alignment, foot alignment, and ineffective firing or weakness of the VMO. Excessive hip internal rotation during the loading response in walking or running causes a functional increase in the physiologic valgus of the femur and

tibia.[17,85] This leads to a greater valgus vector, which can decrease the efficiency of the extensor mechanism. Several factors can contribute to excessive hip internal rotation during gait, including weakness of the gluteus medius, tightness of the tensor fasciae latae, weakness of the hip lateral rotators, and excessive foot pronation.[17,85] Tightness in the lateral retinaculum is associated with lateral compression syndrome of the patellofemoral joint.[17,67] Loss of static restraint from the medial retinacular structures can also allow for an increased tendency of the patella to track laterally.[67]

Lower extremity bony malalignment can contribute to an increased valgus vector. Such malalignments include genu valgus, anteversion of the femoral neck, and external tibial torsion.[17,85,90] Hughston and associates[90] referred to the combined femoral neck anteversion and external tibial torsion as the "treacherous extensor mechanism malalignment." Varus deformity of the foot that leads to excessive pronation during gait is another lower extremity alignment problem that contributes to an increased valgus vector.[17,50] Eng and Pierrynowski[50] reported that the use of a soft foot orthosis with medial posting was effective in reducing the pain in patients with symptomatic patellofemoral pain syndrome with varus foot deformities.

There is some evidence in the literature suggesting that closed-chain exercise may positively influence the tracking of the patellofemoral joint.[44,45,91] Ingersoll and Knight[91] compared the patellar tracking angles in a group of normal subjects trained in biofeedback and in a program using both open- and closed-chain activities with a group of normal individuals performing a program of entirely open-chain progressive resistance exercises. The group performing the combination open- and closed-chain exercises with biofeedback had improved tracking measures, whereas the open-chain only group actually had an increase in lateral glide. Doucette and Child[44] investigated the patellar congruency angle, using computed tomography, during an open-chain and a closed-chain activity in patients with lateral compression syndrome. In the closed-chain activity, the patellar congruence angle was improved compared with the open-chain activity at knee angles of 0°, 10°, and 20°. Their results also suggested that patellar tracking during open-chain activities improves with greater amounts of flexion. They concluded that open-chain exercise appeared to be more appropriate at angles greater than 30° of flexion, which corresponds to the safe ranges of patellofemoral joint contact stresses for open-chain activities.[44,89,166]

MUSCLE FUNCTION

The quadriceps femoris is the primary dynamic stabilizer of the knee and is responsible for knee extension. Functionally, it plays an important role in decelerating knee flexion and absorbing shock when one lands on the lower

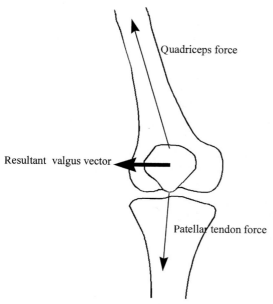

Figure 15-4. Frontal plane valgus vector created by the resolution of the quadriceps and patellar tendon forces.

Quadriceps force

Resultant valgus vector

Patellar tendon force

extremity.[27] As one would predict based on the influence of gravity, open-chain knee extension exercises with a 12 repetition maximum (RM) load produce greater quadriceps activity than squats or leg press with a 12 RM load as the knee extends from approximately 45° of flexion to 0°. Squats and leg presses produce more quadriceps activity from about 60° to 95° of knee flexion compared to a 12 RM open-chain knee extension load in the same ROM.[56]

The straight leg raise, isometric quadriceps contraction (quad set), and knee extension exercise are typical therapeutic exercises prescribed after knee injury or surgery. Total quadriceps activity is greater during a quad set than during a straight leg raise or unweighted knee extension exercise.[73,140] Soderberg and Cook[160] reported electromyographic (EMG) data for the rectus femoris and vastus medialis during a straight leg raise and quad sets. They noted an increase in rectus femoris activity with a straight leg raise and an increase in vastus medialis activity when a quad set was performed. These results were supported by the study of Karst and Jewett[96] of EMG activity from the VMO, VML, vastus lateralis, and rectus femoris. These authors also tested whether or not a straight leg raise performed with the hip in external rotation or while resisting an abduction force would preferentially recruit the VMO. They found no difference in VMO recruitment under these conditions. Karst and Jewett[96] concluded was that if the goal was to address the vasti group, the quad set was a better exercise than the straight leg raise.

There is currently no way to test the strength of the VMO in isolation from the rest of the quadriceps musculature, so it is impossible to directly measure isolated weakness in the VMO. Because of this, researchers have used electromyography to quantify the firing patterns and behaviors of the heads of the quadriceps. In particular, attention has centered around the firing patterns of the VMO and VL and the VMO-to-VL ratios.[31,44,45,78,80,96,97,150,175,181] Results of these studies have not been conclusive. It has been reported that in persons without patellofemoral pain syndrome, the VMO fires significantly faster than the VL, whereas in persons with patellofemoral pain, the VL fires first.[175] These results have not been supported by a more recent study.[97] The VMO-to-VL ratio for both symptomatic and asymptomatic individuals engaged in a variety of open- and closed-chain activities has been reported to be approximately 1:1 in two studies[31,150] and 2:1 in another.[181] The discrepancy between these results is, in part, due to the large individual variability in the VMO-to-VL ratio even within the normal asymptomatic population.[181] In normal individuals, Worrell and co-workers[181] reported a range of VMO-to-VL ratios from 0.35 to 17.21. Additionally, the reliability of the measurement is also problematic with reported intraclass correlation coefficients as low as 0.40.[181]

Probably the most comprehensive investigation of quadriceps activity during different rehabilitation exercises was performed by Cerny.[31] In this study EMG activity was measured from the VMO, VL, and adductor magnus during more than 20 exercises in both normal individuals and patients with patellofemoral pain. The exercises with the greatest quadriceps EMG activity in this study appeared to be quad sets and step-downs. Cerny concluded that none of the exercises studied selectively recruited the VMO in either normal individuals or patients with patellofemoral pain syndrome. In all of the studies discussed it should be noted that the VMO never functioned independently of any other head of the quadriceps during any of the exercises studied. Thus, the clinical results from these exercises would, in all likelihood, be a generalized quadriceps strengthening effect.[141]

There has been much debate about the different roles of the quadriceps musculature, especially the VMO, in the various ranges of motion. Historically, it was accepted that the VMO was responsible for terminal knee extension. Some of this interpretation was based on the fact that the atrophy of the vastus medialis is more visible because of the normal prominence of the muscle and the thinness of its fascial covering compared with that over the VL.[110] This visibility misled clinicians into the belief that there was specific, rather than general, quadriceps atrophy. At the same time clinicians noted that patients had difficulty performing terminal knee extension and that an extensor lag was often present.[161] A classic study by Lieb and Perry[111] defined the role of the VMO as a dynamic stabilizer against lateral displacement of the patella. Their study determined that the VMO in isolation could not produce any extension of the knee. Each of the other parts of the quadriceps, in isolation, could produce knee extension. Interestingly, this study was performed in 1968, and confusion still lingers over the role of the VMO. Some of this confusion can be related to the subtlety of the function of the VMO in relation to the other quadriceps muscles. Box 15-3 summarizes the function of the VMO using clinically relevant questions.

The hamstrings produce knee flexion, tibial rotation, and hip extension. Functionally, the hamstrings act more as hip extensors than knee flexors, because under most closed-chain conditions gravity produces the necessary knee flexion. For the knee joint, providing stability is a more important hamstring role than creating knee flexion. Hamstring contractions reduce loads on the ACL by creating a posterior shear of the tibia. Co-contraction with the quadriceps also stiffens the knee joint, making it more stable.[114] The semitendinosus has been found to contract against valgus loads on the knee whereas the biceps femoris contracts against varus loads.[28] The biceps femoris rotates the tibia externally, and the semimembranosus and semitendinosus rotate the tibia internally. In the presence of anterolateral rotatory instability or anteromedial rotatory instability, facilitation of enhanced neuromuscular control of the biceps femoris (anterolateral rotatory insta-

Box 15-3

Vastus Medialis Obliquus (VMO) Function

Is the VMO active during terminal knee extension? Yes, but so are the other parts of the quadriceps. In fact, the VMO is active through any range of knee extension when the other parts of the quadriceps are active.

Does the VMO become more active during open-chain terminal knee extension than during open-chain knee extension from 90° to 60°? Yes, but so do the other parts of the quadriceps. It is estimated that the terminal ranges of knee extension require twice as much quadriceps force to accomplish the last 15° of extension.[76,163] This is because of the lessening of the quadriceps mechanical advantage and an improvement in the mechanical advantage of gravity.[130]

Is the VMO strengthened with terminal knee extension exercises? Yes, but so are the other parts of the quadriceps.[141] It gets stronger through training, not because it is extending the knee, but because it is contracting against the patellar lateralizing force of the other parts of the quadriceps.

If the VMO is weak in isolation, can that weakness reduce the knee extension torque? Yes, because without the function of the VMO to stabilize the patella, the extension torque created by the other parts of the quadriceps is not being applied through an efficient patellofemoral mechanism.

Box 15-4

General Principles for Developing and Implementing Any Knee Rehabilitation Program

Awareness of the process of inflammation at the joint
Level of muscle control or strength
Amount of ROM available
Establishment of a weight-bearing status
Present functional status and desired outcomes

NOTE: The rehabilitation specialist should always be mindful of these principles when working within the time constraints placed on the rehabilitation program by any particular protocol.

bility) and of the semimembranosus and semitendinosus (anteromedial rotatory instability), respectively, may help deter abnormal tibial excursion.

AN OVERVIEW OF KNEE REHABILITATION PRINCIPLES

Before rehabilitation guidelines and protocols for specific knee pathologic conditions and surgical procedures can be addressed, an overview of general knee rehabilitation principles should be offered. Recently significant changes have occurred in the area of knee rehabilitation, with the greatest change being the speed at which patients are progressed through the rehabilitation process. Although the process has become much more rapid, the rehabilitation specialist should not simply focus on time frames to progress a patient's rehabilitation program but should always keep in mind certain basic rehabilitation principles when evaluating the patient's condition and appropriateness of the rehabilitation program (Box 15-4).

After trauma to the knee, whether from surgery or injury, the acute inflammatory process must be addressed. Specifically, joint effusion should be evaluated and treated and pain management techniques should be initiated. Appropriate, early treatment focused on controlling acute inflammation can significantly affect the rehabilitation program, both immediately and at the final outcome. This early anti-inflammatory treatment can help minimize both strength and ROM losses. Ice, compression, and elevation, applied in conjunction with safe, pain-free condition-appropriate exercise, can aid in progressing the patient through the acute stage of inflammation as rapidly as possible. Care should be taken by the rehabilitation specialist to not further irritate an acutely inflamed joint. Being too aggressive with exercises, weight-bearing status, or functional activities can keep the knee acutely inflamed and significantly lengthen the time of rehabilitation or even lead to permanent damage within the joint.

At the knee, achieving adequate quadriceps recruitment early in the rehabilitation process is extremely important. Quadriceps recruitment can be inhibited by the effects of acute inflammation. Kennedy and colleagues[100] determined that as little as 60 ml of saline injected into the knee decreased quadriceps recruitment by 30% to 50%. In the patient with true acute inflammation the presence of pain could further diminish his or her ability to recruit the quadriceps. Biofeedback units may be used to aid the patient in developing a strong voluntary quadriceps contraction. If any voluntary contraction is difficult, electrical muscle stimulation can be used to aid the patient in developing a contraction. Because Spencer and coorkers[162] related that as little as 20 ml of knee joint effusion may selectively inhibit contraction of the vastus medialis, this head of the quadriceps should be targeted when biofeedback or electrical stimulation is used.

Early knee motion after surgery or injury is critical to help prevent joint fibrosis, provide nutrition to the articular cartilage,[116] and initiate controlled stress. This stress will help align collagen fibers, providing for a flexible, strong scar and promoting the return of normal joint mechanics.[81] Active ROM at the knee, within case-appropriate range limitations, can be initiated as soon as pain allows. Supine heel slides can be used to aid in regaining knee flexion. However, these can be painful at the knee due to the contraction of the rectus femoris during flexion at the hip. Active knee flexion can also be done in either the seated or side-lying position. Active-assisted ROM can be very effective in regaining ROM. Techniques such as using a towel to pull the knee into more flexion or having the clinician aid the athlete in taking the knee into more flexion often allow for greater ROM gains to be achieved as long as the patient's complaints of pain are not increased significantly. Slow pedaling on the stationary bike is another excellent way to increase knee ROM as long as care is taken not to irritate the tibiofemoral or patellofemoral joints. The knee requires approximately 105° to 110° of flexion to complete a revolution on a properly fitted bike when no substitution is allowed.

Joint mobilization should be initiated at the patellofemoral joint during the early motion phase to help restore its normal arthrokinematics.[143] Without normal patellofemoral arthrokinematics, it is very difficult for the patient to regain normal, pain-free knee flexion and extension. The patella should be mobilized superiorly, inferiorly, medially, and laterally. A decrease in superior and inferior patellar glide can decrease knee extension and flexion ROM, respectively. Stretching of the lateral patellar retinaculum, as described by McConnell,[120] can possibly help decrease the incidence of patellofemoral pain by aiding in the restoration of normal patellofemoral arthrokinematics.

As progress out of the acute stage of knee inflammation is made, more aggressive rehabilitation techniques can be used. However, it is imperative that the rehabilitation specialist accurately determine the status of the joint. Signs such as increased temperature, effusion, and levels of pain should be used to classify the stage of inflammation. For example, when the clinician feels soft tissue resistance to passive ROM before the athlete complains of any joint pain, more aggressive passive ROM techniques may be used (Table 15-5). Knee extension is often the most difficult ROM to regain, but normal extension ROM is required before a normal gait pattern can be achieved. Regaining extension, both passive and, when appropriate, active should be set as a very high priority in any knee rehabilitation program. Various techniques can be used. One method involves placing the athlete prone with the

thigh resting on edge of the table, just proximal to the patella. As the athlete relaxes, the knee is pulled into extension. Weight can be added to the ankle to increase the force of the stretch. This method provides a low-load, long-duration stretch that can lead to plastic deformation of the tissues limiting extension (Fig. 15-5). There are spring-loaded splints available commercially, such as Dynasplint,* that can be used to deliver a low-load, long-duration stretch to tissues that surround the patient's knee.

Numerous techniques are available to use in the attempt to regain flexion at the athlete's knee. For example, supine wall slides can be used to regain early amounts of flexion. However, when the athlete achieves approximately 110° of flexion, wall slides may no longer be effective unless an additional outside force is applied, such as the athlete's other leg (Fig. 15-6). The final ranges of flexion can also be achieved by the athlete doing towel pulls while in a seated position. Passive flexion can also be achieved by the athlete using his or her body weight while sliding forward from a seated position (Fig. 15-7). Isokinetic machines can be used to gain flexion by manually pushing the athlete's leg back as far as pain will allow and then locking the machine in the isometric mode. This will allow for a prolonged, sustained stretch. One final method to increase flexion is by using a Total Gym† set-up as pictured in Fig. 15-8. The stress that is applied to the knee is controlled by the angle of the slide of the board and/or the range-limiting protection strap. Joint mobilization can be an extremely important adjunct treatment that can be used to aid in regaining flexion. Both inferior glides of the patella and posterior glides of the tibiofemoral joint can be used to aid in increasing the athlete's flexion.

Strengthening exercises should be initiated in a controlled fashion to ensure the athlete's proper execution of various strengthening exercises. These exercises should be progressed in a manner that both provides protection to healing structures and prevents abnormal muscle recruit-

---

*Available from Dynasplint Systems, Severna Park, Maryland.
†Available from Engineering Fitness International, San Diego, California.

Table 15-5

Pain Resistance Sequence

Reaction to Movement*	Joint Status	Treatment Action
Pain before resistance	Acute	Red light—No attempt should be made to gain ROM.
Pain with resistance	Subacute	Yellow light—Gentle attempt can be made to regain ROM, but should be done cautiously. (Vigorous attempts may cause reversion to acute state.)
Resistance before pain	Chronic	Green light—Vigorous intervention may be necessary to restore ROM.

From Wallace, L.A., Mangine, R.E., and Malone, T. (1985): The knee. *In:* Gould, J.A. III, and Davies, G.J. (eds.): Orthopaedic and Sports Physical Therapy. St. Louis, C.V. Mosby.
*Refers to passive movement through physiologic range.
ROM, range of motion.

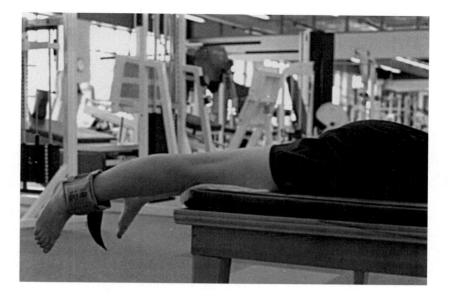

Figure 15-5. Prone passive knee extension with weight.

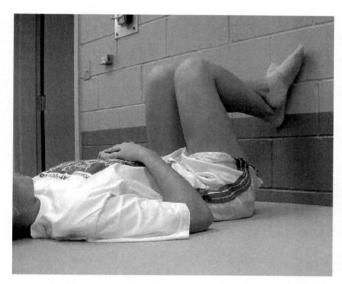

Figure 15-6. Supine wall slides with assist from uninvolved lower extremity.

ment patterns or habits to develop. For example, additional resistance should not be added to straight leg raises or terminal knee extension exercises until the athlete can go through the full, case-appropriate ROM. If additional resistance is added too soon, the athlete might not be able to exercise throughout the full ROM and weakness in certain areas of the range might develop. For example, if too much resistance is added to an athlete's terminal knee extension exercises and full extension ROM is not achieved during the exercise, an extensor lag could develop. This extensor lag could then manifest itself in a patient's functional activities as a deviation during gait.

Initially, simple exercises such as four-quadrant straight leg raises, multiple angle isometrics, and both supine and prone terminal knee extension exercises can be started.

These initial exercises are open-chain exercises that allow for muscle isolation. These simple, one-plane exercises allow the rehabilitation specialist to concentrate on single muscle groups or physiologic movements that can be considered components of larger functional movements or skills. For example, four-quadrant straight leg raises can be used to strengthen thigh and hip musculature in preparation for the athlete beginning more advanced functional activities such as single-leg squats.

CLINICAL PEARL #1

Use verbal, physical, and visual cues to assist the athlete in maintaining the correct lower extremity alignment during weight-bearing activities, examples include:
1. Verbal cues, remind the athlete to keep their knee directly over their foot during closed chain activities.
2. Physical cues, rubber tubing (or Thera-band) can be used to apply a valgus directed load on the knee. The athlete is then instructed to resist the pull of the tubing (keep the knee over the foot) as they perform squats, leg press, etc...
3. Visual cues, have the athlete perform the exercises in front of a full length mirror so they can see when the lower extremity alignment is inappropriate.

When weight bearing is allowed, the athlete can begin performing appropriate closed-chain exercises. This type of exercise uses muscles that cross joints both proximally and distally to assist with motion at the desired joint. These exercises allow the athlete to strengthen muscles throughout the ROM but do not provide for isolated strengthening of a particular muscle, which is why both open-chain and closed-chain exercises should be part of the rehabilitation program. Close attention must be paid to the proper performance of these exercises. During closed-chain

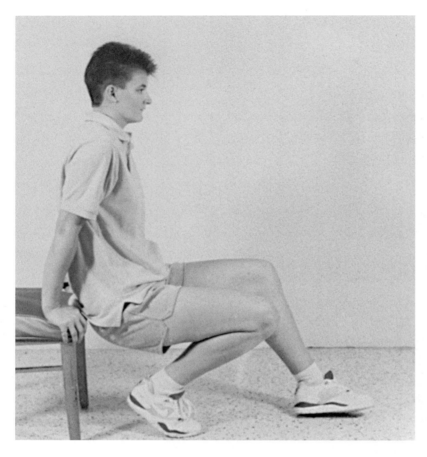

Figure 15-7. Passive knee flexion using body weight.

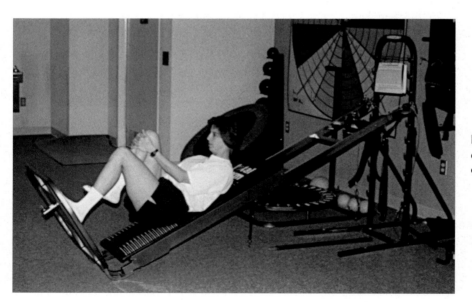

Figure 15-8. Total Gym. Passive flexion is controlled by the angle of the slide board or by the range-limiting protection strap.

exercises, each joint depends on other joints both proximally and distally to assist in proper body alignment. If closed-chain exercises are begun too early and/or an athlete's rehabilitation program is limited to just these types of exercise, weak muscles can be substituted for and abnormal habit patterns might develop. For example, if the hip musculature is not strong enough to control adduction and internal rotation of the thigh, the knee will assume a valgus alignment, and the foot will be pronated. This alignment increases the Q angle at the knee and predisposes the athlete to develop patellofemoral pain during the rehabilitation program. This can be seen occurring in a lateral step-up or leg press exercise (Figs. 15-9 and 15-10). If this pattern of movement then becomes ingrained into the athlete's movements during sporting activity, he or she can become more susceptible to both overuse and traumatic injuries.

As strength and ROM levels in the lower extremity improve, proprioception exercises can be added to the rehabilitation program. Proprioception, as defined by Sherrington, refers to all neural input from joints, muscles, tendons, and associated deep tissues.[148] Proprioception, also referred to as joint position sense, seems to be primarily determined by muscle spindle receptors. These muscle receptors are assisted to a lesser degree by the cutaneous and joint receptors, thereby providing the neuromuscular control required for a joint to perform efficiently. Proprioception can initially be addressed in the

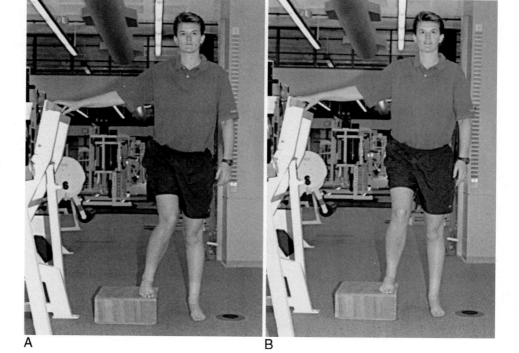

Figure 15-9. Lateral step-up. *A,* Performed incorrectly, allowing the hip to adduct and rotate internally. *B,* Performed correctly.

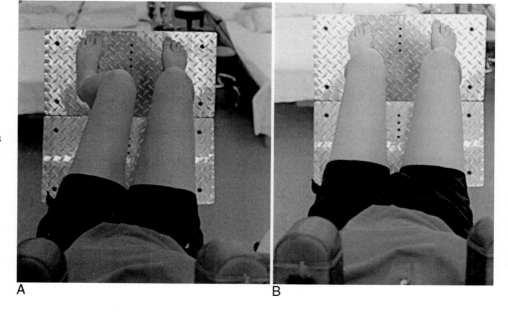

Figure 15-10. Leg press. *A,* Performed incorrectly. The hip is adducted and internally rotated. *B,* Performed correctly.

rehabilitation program even before the patient progresses to full weight bearing. Patients can perform partial weight-bearing activities on the Biomechanical Ankle Platform System (BAPS)* or Total Gym to begin stimulating the proprioceptive system. As the patient progresses to full weight-bearing activities the proprioceptive exercises can be progressed in difficulty in a variety of ways. A sequenced minisquat program (Table 15-6) is often a good method to begin this progression. To assist in the transition to single-leg full weight-bearing activities a sled-style leg press or Total Gym is useful. For example, the athlete can hop from spot to spot while on the leg press machine (Fig. 15-11). Progression of this exercise is accomplished by increasing load, increasing performance time, and changing the hop sequence.

As the athlete successfully progresses through a minisquat program he or she can be further challenged with a lunge program (Table 15-7 and Figs. 15-12 and 15-13) and finally can begin a hop/plyometric program (Table 15-8 and Fig. 15-14). Single-leg balance activities can also be performed using a Medi-Ball Rebounder (Fig. 15-15).† This type of activity can be progressed by

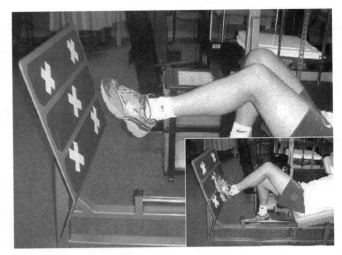

Figure 15-11. Leg press bounding. *Inset,* starting position.

Table 15-6

Example of Closed-Chain Progression of the Minisquat

Weight shifts with support
↓
Weight shifts without support
↓
Bilateral minisquats with support
↓
Bilateral minisquats without support
↓
Bilateral minisquats against wall
↓
Bilateral minisquats against wall with weights in hands
↓
One-legged minisquats with support
↓
One-legged minisquats without support
↓
One-legged minisquats against wall
↓
One-legged minisquats against wall with weight in hands
↓
Bilateral minisquats with tubing
↓
One-legged minisquats with tubing
↓
Gradually increase tubing strength and speed of movement

Table 15-7

Lunge Progression*

Balance and reach forward
Balance and reach backward
Balance and reach laterally
Forward lunge
Backward lunge
Lateral lunge
Diagonal lunge
Cross-over lunge
Cross-over diagonal lunge

*Lunges can be further progressed by having athlete carry dumbbells, toss medicine balls, or work against rubber tubing resistance.

changing from a stable weight-bearing surface to an unstable one, such as a wobble board. If a Rebounder is not available, Thera-Band‡ can be used to increase the difficulty of proprioception exercises. The athlete stands on the involved leg with the Thera-Band attached to the uninvolved leg (Fig. 15-16). He or she can then perform various activities with the Thera-Band, such as flutter kicks, hip abduction/adduction, or hip flexion with knee flexion and again the weight-bearing surface can be changed from stable to unstable as the exercises progress.

Other proprioception activities include use of devices such as the BAPS and the Slide Board§ (Fig. 15-17). Chapter 8 contains examples of lower extremity proprioceptive exercises. Care should be taken when one adds proprioception exercises to make sure the athlete has the strength and coordination to safely perform the exercises. All of the proprioception activities described force the

---

*Available from Camp International, Jackson, Michigan.
†Available from Engineering Fitness International, San Diego, California.

‡Available from The Hygenic Corporation, Akron, Ohio.
§Available from Don Courson, Don Courson Enterprises, Birmingham, Alabama.

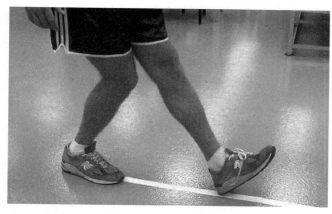

Figure 15-12. Forward balance and reach exercise, a low-level lunge activity.

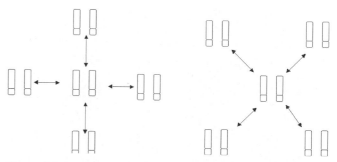

Figure 15-14. Dot drills are advanced hopping drills that can be progressed from two-leg hops to single-leg hops.

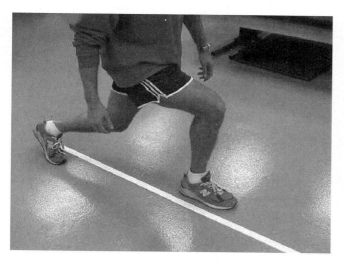

Figure 15-13. Crossover lunge, an advanced lunge activity.

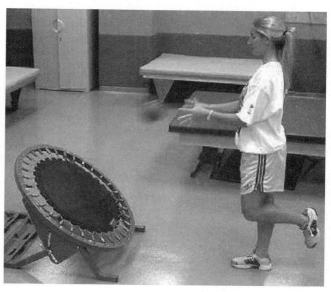

Figure 15-15. Medi-Ball Rebounder balance activity. Athlete stands on the involved leg.

Table 15-8	
Hop Functional Progression*	
Double Leg	**Single Leg**
Hop in place	Forward hop
Forward hop	Triple hop
Backward hop	Backward hop
Triple hop	Side-to-side
Side-to-side	Cross-over
Cross-over	Dot drills
Scissors hop	Lateral bounds
Dot drills	
180° hops	

*Athlete should land as quietly as possible with good knee flexion to dissipate forces. Difficulty is increased by increasing speed, distance, and time and adding cones to jump over and/or adding external loads. Lateral bounds are performed by taking-off and landing on different lower extremities.

involved leg to make numerous high-speed adjustments for the athlete to maintain his or her balance.

As ROM, strength, and proprioception improve, cardiovascular and muscular endurance must be addressed in preparation for the athlete to return to full functional levels. Biking can be used to increase endurance when knee ROM is adequate. Pool exercises, including swimming, kick board usage, or water running, can be used to increase endurance (see Chapter 12). Running can be used as an endurance activity, but care must be taken to not irritate the knee by progressing the program too aggressively. Table 15-9 contains an example of a running progression program. Threlkeld and colleagues[171] determined that backward running avoids the rapid initial loading of the knee that occurs with forward running because of the absence of heel strike. This may benefit an athlete who is unable to perform forward running because of pain.

Isokinetic equipment may be useful in the development of muscular power and endurance near the end of

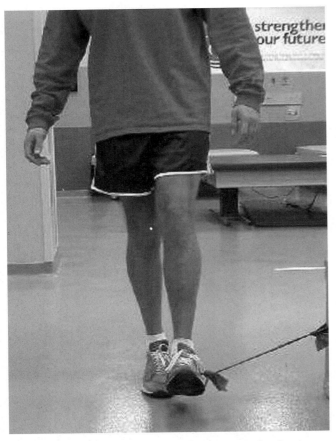

Figure 15-16. Proprioceptive exercise with use of a Thera-Band. The athlete stands on the involved leg and attaches the Thera-Band to the uninvolved ankle. The Thera-Band is pulled in each direction with the uninvolved leg while the involved leg attempts to maintain balance.

the rehabilitation process. Because anterior knee pain is often a complication of knee rehabilitation programs, caution must be used with these types of open-chain exercises. This is true both because of the potential for high patellofemoral joint compression values and the possibility

of excessive tibial translatory effects. For these reasons, one may have to limit the ROM the athlete exercises through on this equipment.

The final stage of any knee rehabilitation program should be a return to normal activities through the implementation of an appropriate progression of functional exercises. No patient should be released back to his or her sport simply on the basis of scores from various strength and ROM measurements. Functional activities should begin with exercises as simple as jogging in a straight line and progress from there. Both the speed and difficulty of the exercises should be increased until athletes are able to perform activities similar to those that they will be expected to perform when they return to their sport. Specific functional progressions will be discussed later in the chapter. Functional testing is covered later in the chapter as well.

In rehabilitation of the knee, every possible option should be offered to help the athlete return to the preinjury level. Each athlete should be constantly reevaluated throughout rehabilitation so that his or her program can be adjusted appropriately to address specific conditions and requirements. No two injuries are identical because every athlete's physical, mental, and healing capabilities are different. Therefore, there are no specific "cookbook" approaches, and each rehabilitation program should be designed to maximize the athlete's potential as quickly and as safely as possible.

REHABILITATION FOR SPECIFIC KNEE INJURIES
Patellofemoral Dysfunction

Patellofemoral joint dysfunction with pain is one of the most prevalent knee pathologic conditions seen in athletes.[97] This problem can either be the primary diagnosis or it can be a secondary complication found with other knee injuries or surgical procedures. Even if the patellofemoral joint is not the primary site of injury or dys-

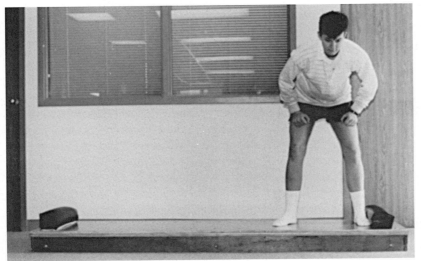

Figure 15-17. Slide board. This can be used to develop muscular strength, proprioception, eccentric firing of the hamstring muscles, and cardiovascular conditioning.

Table 15-9

Running Functional Progression

Jogging in place	Jogging figure-eights (large to small)
Jumping rope	Jog-sprint-jog (changing speeds)
Jogging	Sprinting/reversing/cutting on specified spot
Jogging forward/ reversing on command	Sprinting/reversing/cutting on command
Side-to-side sliding	Sport-specific drills

function, care must be taken not to irritate or damage the joint during other lower extremity rehabilitation programs.

Many conditions fall under the broad heading of patellofemoral dysfunction. Anterior knee pain is often the phrase used to describe any condition that leads to pain in the extensor mechanism at the knee. Because the diagnosis is often one of a very general nature, rehabilitation can be viewed as general in nature as well. As with other overuse injuries, rehabilitation is often done to correct or improve the biomechanics of the entire lower extremity in an attempt to decrease the patient's complaints of pain and dysfunction.

The need for a comprehensive lower extremity evaluation is paramount in athletes complaining of anterior knee pain. The functioning of the patella depends on a fine balance between ligaments and muscles because of the lack of inherent bony stability at the patellofemoral joint. When this balance is disrupted because of weakness, tightness, or other biomechanical problems, improper tracking of the patella can occur.[31] Lateral tracking of the patella is the most common tracking abnormality seen at the patellofemoral joint. Common causes of lateral tracking can include VMO dysfunction, tight lateral soft tissues, and various biomechanical problems that increase the tendency of the patella to track laterally. VMO dysfunction can be a weakness of the VMO due to disuse or effusion-induced neuromuscular shutdown. If the VMO is not pulling with enough force, it cannot offer the medially directed dynamic stability that is required to counteract the other heads of the quadriceps and keep the patella tracking appropriately. Tight lateral soft tissues around the knee can also increase the lateral tracking of the patella. If structures such as the patellar retinaculum, iliotibial band, gluteus medius, and tensor fascia lata are tight, they can cause the patella to track more laterally and possibly lead to pain in the area. Biomechanical problems anywhere along the lower extremity that affect the alignment of the femur on the tibia can affect the tracking of the patella. Many of these malalignment problems can be bony in nature, and it is not possible for the rehabilitation special-

ist to change them. For example, a wide pelvis that leads to an increased genu valgum angle at the knee cannot be "corrected" by rehabilitation. However, there are some malalignment problems that are able to be treated. For example, excessive pronation of the subtalar joint can lead to an increased Q angle at the knee and possibly increased lateral tracking at the patellofemoral joint. The rehabilitation specialist can treat this excessive pronation as described later in this chapter.

Rehabilitation of patellofemoral dysfunction, after a comprehensive evaluation, should concentrate on recruiting the VMO, normalizing patellar mobility, increasing general flexibility and muscular control of the entire lower extremity, and addressing any other biomechanical problems that can be altered by treatment (Box 15-5). The most important concept to keep in mind when the patellofemoral joint is rehabilitated is that no exercise should cause pain at the joint. Both the patient and the rehabilitation specialist should always proceed with this guiding factor in mind.

Although various exercises have been touted to isolate the VMO, there are no specific exercises that have been proven to isolate the VMO. Therefore, when the rehabilitation specialist is attempting to recruit and strengthen the VMO, no specific exercise should be considered superior to all others. Any knee extension exercise that elicits a contraction of the VMO and does not cause pain at the patellofemoral joint is appropriate. Use of a biofeedback unit to monitor VMO contraction is one method that is extremely helpful in ensuring that exercises are having an impact on the VMO. A biofeedback unit can be used in conjunction with a variety of open- and closed-chain exercises. Electrical stimulation units may also be used to obtain a strong contraction in the VMO.

CLINICAL PEARL #2

Lower extremity biomechanical problems frequently lead to or potentiate patello-femoral dysfunction. Key areas to evaluate and address during rehabilitation include hip abductor strength, foot alignment and the flexibility of the rectus femoris, hamstrings, gastroc-soleus, and tensor fascia latae.

Box 15-5

Patellofemoral Rehabilitation

After a comprehensive lower extremity evaluation:
- Facilitate recruitment of VMO
- Normalize patellar mobility
- Increase lower extremity flexibility
- Address any alterable lower extremity biomechanical problems
- Be sure that ALL activities are pain-free at the patellofemoral joint

Several techniques have been reported to be helpful in normalizing patellar mobility in patients who exhibit a laterally tracking patella due to tight lateral structures. The three most commonly reported techniques are manual patellar mobilization, patellar taping as described by McConnell, and iliotibial band/tensor fascia lata stretching. Kramer[104] reported success with manual lateral retinaculum stretching, when it was used as part of a comprehensive patellofemoral rehabilitation program. He described two manual maneuvers: (1) medial patellar glide held for 1 minute with the knee extended to stretch the lateral retinaculum; and (2) patellar compression with tracking. This second technique is performed with the athlete sitting and the knee flexed to 90°. The patella is compressed against the patellofemoral articular surface and tracked medially by the clinician as the athlete extends the knee (Fig. 15-18). Neither of these techniques should cause any pain in the athlete's patellofemoral joint. Another method of stretching the lateral structures involves flexing the knee to approximately 30° to 60° of flexion and then applying a posterolateral force against the medial border of the patella. This pushes the medial border of the patella down and lifts the lateral border, thereby stretching the lateral structures.

Patellar taping as described by McConnell[120] is presently one of the most controversial topics in patellofemoral rehabilitation. Although McConnell and others have reported a very high success rate in managing patellofemoral pain with these taping techniques, other researchers[26,103] have been unable to replicate these excellent results. McConnell described the taping techniques as a method to correct various malaligned patellar positions. At this time no radiologic studies have been performed to support this claim. However, because of the excellent results of McConnell and other researchers, the taping

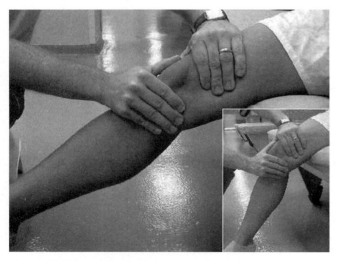

Figure 15-18. Patellar compression with tracking to stretch the lateral retinaculum performed as the knee is actively extended. *Inset*, starting position.

techniques should not be discounted just because of a lack of corroboration of McConnell's suggested hypothesis as to why the techniques work. If McConnell's taping techniques allow the athlete to exercise with no complaints of anterior knee pain, the taping techniques should be used.

McConnell based the application of tape on various evaluative measurements. She looked at several components of patellar orientation. These components are (1) the medial/lateral glide component, (2) the medial/lateral tilt component, (3) the rotation component, and (4) the anterior/posterior tilt component. It has been reported that these measurements are not able to be obtained reliably, either between testers or even by the same tester at different times.[176] However, there are other methods of determining which taping techniques should be used. It is rather simple to quickly ascertain whether or not the taping techniques will benefit a particular patient. One activity that reliably replicates a patient's complaints of patellofemoral pain must be found before the taping techniques can be used. This activity is referred to as the *asterisk sign*. Usually a lateral step-up or minisquat is found to be an asterisk sign for these patients. As individual pieces of tape are placed on the patient's knee the asterisk sign is reevaluated to determine if the tape has decreased the patient's complaints of pain. McConnell described four main types of tape application as follows: (1) correcting a lateral glide, (2) correcting a lateral tilt, (3) correcting an external rotation, and (4) correcting an anterior-posterior tilt, in which the inferior pole of the patella is tilted posterior (Fig. 15-19). Although whether or not these pieces of tape correct the position McConnell described is still being questioned, the tape still can be of clinical use. If after an individual piece of tape is applied, pain with the patient's asterisk sign is decreased or alleviated, that piece of tape is left on. If the tape does not have an impact on pain with the asterisk sign, that piece of tape is removed. This simple procedure is used for all four of the taping techniques that are described. Although attempting to answer why these techniques might work is very difficult, one may quite simply determine whether the tape is a reasonable adjunct to the treatment regimen. The authors have anecdotally found taping techniques to be a reasonable addition that can help many patients progress through a patellofemoral rehabilitation program, if they are used appropriately.

Finally, in the area of normalizing patellar mobility, specific attention should be paid to the iliotibial band and tensor fascia lata. If during the evaluation these structures are found to be tight in the patient, stretching should be instituted. It is important that stretches of these structures be performed correctly (Fig. 15-20). Ultrasound applied to these structures in conjunction with stretching may aid in flexibility gains.

The next area that should be addressed in patellofemoral rehabilitation is increasing general flexibility and muscular control of the entire lower extremity. It is espe-

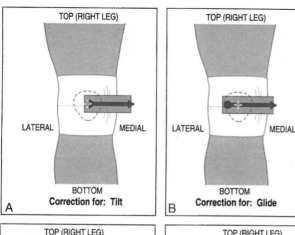

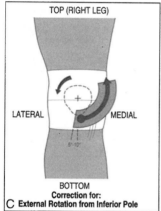

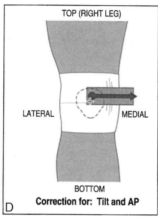

Figure 15-19. Tape correction. *A*, For lateral patellar tilt. *B*, For lateral patellar shift. *C*, For external rotation of the patella. *D*, For anteroposterior (AP) tilt of the patella. (Illustration courtesy of Smith & Nephew DonJoy Inc., Carlsbad, California.)

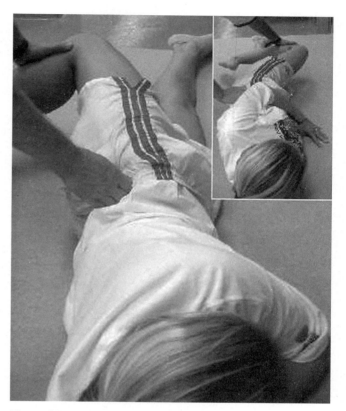

Figure 15-20. Method for stretching the tensor fascia lata. The correct position maintains hip extension and external rotation as the thigh is adducted. *Inset*, incorrect position allowing the hip to flexion during the adduction.

cially important that the athlete have normal levels of flexibility in their rectus femoris, iliopsoas, and hamstring muscles. A tight rectus femoris can cause increased patellofemoral joint pressures. Tight iliopsoas and hamstrings can lead to abnormal gait patterns that increase muscular activity at the knee and increase patellofemoral joint pressure. As flexibility and strength of the lower extremity increase, the athlete must be able to show good muscle control and coordination for the entire lower extremity. This idea of appropriate control at various speeds of activity was discussed earlier in this chapter.

One final topic to be discussed is that of correctable biomechanical problems that affect lower extremity alignment. The most common problem in this area is excessive pronation at the subtalar joint that can lead to an increased Q angle at the patellofemoral joint. This excessive pronation is often a compensation for a forefoot varus malalignment. Arch taping techniques, such as the Low-Dye (see Fig. 14-56) or Herzog technique, can be used to determine whether controlling pronation will affect the patient's patellofemoral pain. If taping does lessen the symptoms, orthotics can be used. For a patient with a forefoot varus,

the orthotic would be constructed with a medial forefoot post to control the forefoot motion. Appropriate shoe selection and replacement of worn shoes can also aid in control of excessive pronation.

If conservative treatment fails, surgery may be indicated. One of the most common procedures is a lateral retinaculum release in which the lateral retinaculum is cut, thus freeing the patella medially. Additionally, advancement of the VMO can be done in patients who have a VMO with a line of pull more vertical than normal. This is a type of proximal realignment. Table 15-10 shows a lateral release rehabilitation protocol for patients who have not undergone some sort of proximal realignment involving the VMO. The goals in this postoperative rehabilitation program are very similar to the goals of the conservative rehabilitation program for patellofemoral dysfunction. Emphasis should be placed on regaining patellar mobility and VMO/quadriceps control. Although this surgical procedure was quite popular in the past, it is presently performed less often and only after a course of conservative therapy has failed.

Other more involved surgical procedures, such as distal realignment, can be used if conservative therapy fails. In a distal realignment the tibial tubercle and patellar tendon are transferred to decrease the patient's Q angle. The main concern with this procedure is progressing knee flexion

Table 15-10

Rehabilitation Protocol for Lateral Release

	Week 1	Weeks 2-4	Weeks 4-6	Week 6
Functional progression Criteria	Begin WB and four-quadrant lifts As pain allows	Begin WB without crutches SLR with no extensor lag Full extension in gait No limp No increase in pain No increase in edema/ effusion	Begin strengthening Absence of pain No increase in edema/ effusion Full ROM	Return to athletics No effusion Functional testing >85% Quadriceps strength >85%
Evaluation	Pain Incision Effusion/edema Active flexion Quadriceps recruitment Passive extension Patellar mobility Hamstring flexibility Iliotibial band flexibility	Pain Gait Incision/scar Effusion/edema ROM/patellar mobility Quadriceps recruitment	ROM Quadriceps recruitment Patellar mobility Standing balance Self-report functional status	Functional testing Strength testing Self-report functional status
Treatment	Pain management Effusion/edema control Active flexion exercise Quadriceps recruitment exercises Passive extension Patellar mobilization Hamstring stretching IT band stretching	Pain management Effusion/edema control Scar massage Active ROM exercise Patellar mobilization Quadriceps recruitment General strengthening Flexibility exercise Minisquat progression	Strengthening Endurance exercise Proprioception exercise Hop and lunge progression Jogging progression	Strengthening Endurance exercise Sport-specific drills
Goals	75% WB Increase patellar mobility Full passive extension SLR without extensor lag	WB without crutches AROM 0-110° Normal patellar mobility Good flexibility	Full AROM Strengthening without pain	Return to athletics

AROM, active range of motion; IT, iliotibial; ROM, range of motion; WB, weight bearing; SLR, straight leg raise.

ROM and weight-bearing status in a fashion that does not excessively stress the tissues involved in surgery. The speed of the rehabilitation program is controlled by the quality of the fixation of the realigned bone. Overaggressive flexion ROM work or weight bearing can place too much stress on the fixation sight and lead to complications.

Anterior Cruciate Ligament Injuries

Rehabilitation after an injury to the ACL varies widely. Because of differences noted throughout the literature, we will present an overview using the most commonly accepted guidelines. The time frames discussed in the protocols can be adapted to fit various situations, but there are certain criteria that should be met before an athlete is progressed through any protocol.

After an injury to the ACL, immediate attention must be given to the hemarthrosis in the knee and the gen-eral inflammatory process. The athlete should be given crutches and instructed in a pain-free partial weight-bearing gait, and the traditional anti-inflammatory program of ice, compression, and elevation (I.C.E.) should be started. A brace is not required unless there are other associated injuries such as an MCL sprain. Motion exercises should be started immediately, concentrating on passive extension to help prevent rapid scarring in the intercondylar notch. Full extension also allows for greater ease in quadriceps recruitment, which is extremely important after ACL injury. Friden and associates[64] stated that there is a decrease in quadriceps strength after injury because of defects in afferent inflow from the ACL-deficient knee.[64] It is also thought that the lack of voluntary contraction of the quadriceps after ACL injury may be due to reflex inhibition or arthrogenous muscle inhibition.[157] Weight bearing should be increased as pain decreases, joint effusion decreases, quadriceps control increases, and full active knee extension is achieved. The athlete should not be progressed to full weight bearing until these goals have been accomplished.

Rehabilitation should progress with emphasis being placed on quadriceps strengthening as well as neuromuscular control of the hamstrings. Traditionally emphasis has been placed on strengthening of the hamstrings because of their role as the primary dynamic restraint in controlling anterior tibial translation.[77] Recently, however, the emphasis has changed to increasing general muscle control around the knee. A study by Friden and associates,[64] in which 26 patients with ACL-deficient knees were tested before and after rehabilitation, revealed that there was a minimal loss of strength of the hamstrings, and the best outcomes were obtained when both general muscular strength and coordination were addressed. The importance of the hamstrings in the ACL-deficient knee might lie more in hamstring control and proprioception. Studies indicate that athletes with complete tears of the ACL experience a decrease in proprioception at the knee.[116] The loss in proprioception may be due to the "ACL-mechanoreceptor reflex arc" to the hamstrings. Beard and colleagues found that the latency of reflex hamstring contraction in the ACL-deficient knee was twice that of the contralateral, uninjured knee.[63] It has been suggested that improving recruitment time of the hamstrings may place less stress on the ACL during functional activities.[116] Also it has been reported that using active hamstring control to reduce the pivot shift found with an ACL injury might be the key to successfully avoiding reconstructive surgery. Based on all of this information, the rehabilitation specialist should concentrate on facilitating control of the hamstrings, as opposed to simple strengthening in the sagittal plane. Engle and Canner[51-53] reported success in achieving this type of hamstring control in ACL-deficient knees with a program that uses proprioceptive neuromuscular facilitation (PNF) exercises for the hamstrings (Figs. 15-21 and 15-22). More advanced exercises, using devices such as the BAPS board, Slide Board, and Medi-Ball Rebounder, facilitate

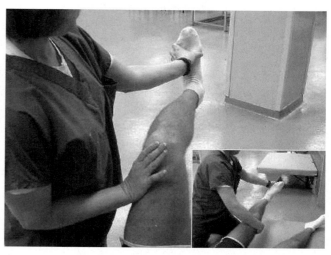

Figure 15-22. PNF pattern, D2 Flexion. *Inset,* starting position D2, Extension.

hamstring control and proprioception in functional positions and at higher speeds to control anterior tibial translation during more aggressive functional activities. PNF patterns and seated Thera-Band exercises can also be used to help incorporate the tibial rotation component of the function of the hamstrings. Recent studies have shown that patellofemoral arthrokinematics are altered in ACL-deficient knees. This should be kept in mind during rehabilitation of the ACL-deficient knee, and care should be taken to not irritate or damage the patellofemoral joint.[86,165]

Although surgery is usually the most common treatment option after injury to the ACL, the decision should be delayed until the acute inflammatory process has run its course at the knee. There is great concern that performing surgery on an acutely inflamed joint will lead to more complications during rehabilitation. When the period of acute inflammation has passed, the athlete, using information provided by the sports medicine team, must decide if a reconstructive procedure is the most appropriate treatment to choose. Whether to reconstruct the ACL or treat it with just a rehabilitation program continues to be a subject of debate. Many factors should be considered when this decision is made, the most important being the ultimate level of function the patient wishes to achieve. Noyes[131] has recommended that to have the best results, competitive or recreational athletes need surgical intervention, whereas light recreational athletes and nonathletes, both of whom can limit their activities, may be able to avoid surgery. Clinically, it appears that generally the competitive athlete does not perform well with an ACL-deficient knee. We are just beginning to understand the combinations of examination measures that may identify the few athletes who might function well without surgery.[49] Noyes and colleagues[136] used subjective and objective measurements to clinically evaluate 84 individuals with ACL-deficient knees. Their conclusion was that an ACL tear leads to functional disability for the majority of the patients. They found that one

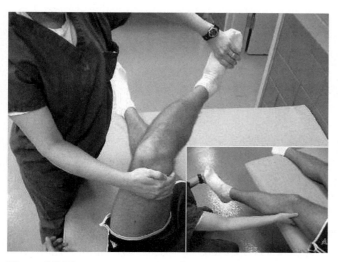

Figure 15-21. PNF pattern, D1 Flexion. *Inset,* starting position, D1 Extension.

third of the population compensated for the deficiency, knew their limits, and did well; one third of the population compensated for the deficiency, but found the instability aggravating; and one third of the population became worse and needed surgery to correct their instability. For the majority of patients who did not undergo surgical reconstructions, knee "giving way" episodes became a common problem.[135] These giving way episodes increase the possibility of occurrence of a meniscal tear or chondral injury. It is well documented that ACL-deficient knees demonstrate abnormal joint kinematics during gait and functional activities, both of which increase the possibility of developing early degenerative changes.[112,131,133]

When surgery is the chosen treatment, the ACL must be reconstructed because of the lack of success with direct repair of the ligament. The one exception to this rule might be for repair of a bony avulsion. If an adolescent has an avulsion fracture without significant ligament failure, primary repair can be a viable option. Concerns that must be addressed when surgery is the treatment of choice include timing of the procedure, graft selection, and surgical technique. The timing of surgery in relation to the inflammatory condition of the joint can greatly affect rehabilitation and ultimate outcomes. It has been shown that reconstructions performed on an acutely inflamed joint are more prone to postoperative complications such as ROM loss and functional deficits.[63,124] Allowing the patient to go through rehabilitation before surgery helps decrease the number and severity of postoperative complications.

Surgical technique is an area that includes both procedures that are chosen as well as how well these procedures are ultimately performed. Procedures relate mainly to intra-versus extra-articular reconstructions. Extra-articular procedures, such as the Ellison or Losee, have been shown to reduce the pivot shift but do not reliably limit the anterior translation of the tibia or restore the normal arthrokinematics through the axis of a normal ACL. Long-term control of knee instability with these extra-articular procedures is poor due to a gradual stretching that occurs in the soft tissues used in the surgical procedure. The one use for extra-articular procedures is with skeletally immature patients. Procedures that require drilling through an open physis are often avoided by surgeons because of the possibility of bone growth complications. Although the reports are inconsistent, studies have shown that complications, including leg length discrepancy and physis arrest with concomitant development of bony deformity, have occurred.[102,123] For these reasons, it is suggested that skeletally immature patients, especially those who are prepubescent, be treated with physis-sparing surgical procedures, if surgery is the treatment of choice.

Intra-articular procedures are by far the most commonly used in reconstruction of the ACL. Both graft fixation and graft placement are extremely important surgical variables that will affect the patient's outcome. After years of refinement the choice of fixation device is now less of a concern than the material that the surgeon is attempting to fixate. In other words, it is easier to obtain early stable fixation when the graft has a bony end as opposed to just tendon. Also it is imperative that an isometric graft placement be achieved at the time of surgery. If the graft placement sites are not appropriate, ROM deficits or abnormal ligament tension might be the result.

The most important decision before an intra-articular procedure is performed is to select the graft. The most important factors to take into consideration when deciding on graft material are graft strength, fixation required, and comorbid conditions that might be present (including factors such as donor site complications and the possibility of disease transmission). Many types of tissues have been used for intra-articular repairs of the ACL, including autografts (tissue transferred from one part of a person's body to another), allografts (human donor tissue), and prosthetics (synthetic materials). The most commonly used tissues for both autografts and allografts are the bone-tendon-bone graft taken from the central third of the patellar tendon (BTB) and the semitendinosus tendon from the hamstrings (HS). Other materials can be used as an allograft, including fascia lata and Achilles tendon. The strength characteristics of various types of materials used is listed in Table 15-11. Advantages of using the autograft BTB include high graft strength, good fixation due to bone-to-bone healing, and ease of obtaining graft material. Disadvantages are complications with the extensor mechanism, such as patellar fractures, patellar tendonitis, patellar tendon rupture, and anterior knee pain. Advantages in using the autograft HS include fewer complications with the extensor mechanism and results comparable to those with a BTB graft. Disadvantages with the HS graft include complications with fixation of the graft, possible hamstring weakness, and the technical difficulty of the procedure. Advantages in using an allograft include no complications with donor sites and increased availability of material. The disadvantages include higher cost, possible disease transmission, and possible recipient rejection (Table 15-12). At

Table 15-11

Strength of Anterior Cruciate Ligament (ACL) Substitutes

Graft	Percentage of ACL Strength
Patellar tendon	168
ACL	100
Semitendinosus	70
Gracilis	49
Iliotibial band	44
Fascia lata	36
Retinaculum	21

Compiled from data in Noyes, F.R., Butler, D.L., and Grood, E.S., et al. (1984): Biomechanical analysis of human ligament repairs and reconstruction. J. Bone Joint Surg. Am., 66:344.

Table 15-12

Anterior Cruciate Ligament Graft Advantages and Disadvantages

	Advantages	Disadvantages
Autograft patellar BTB	High graft strength Good fixation due to bone-to-bone healing Ease of obtaining graft material	Complications with the extensor mechanism, such as patellar fractures, patellar tendonitis, patellar tendon rupture, and anterior knee pain
Autograft hamstring tendon	Fewer complications with the extensor mechanism Comparable results to BTB	Complications with fixation of graft Possible hamstring weakness Technically it is a more complicated procedure
Allograft	No complications with donor sites Increased availability of material	Higher cost Possible disease transmission Possible recipient rejection

BTB, bone-tendon-bone graft.

this point in time the autograft BTB is still considered the "gold standard" in ACL reconstruction, and all other methods are compared to it. However, more studies are reporting equal, and in some cases, better long-term results with HS reconstructions.[9,16,153]

There has been much debate about the times and percentages of graft strength and revascularization. Noyes and colleagues[134] reported that at the time of harvesting, 14-mm-wide patellar tendon grafts exhibited 168% of the strength of a normal ACL. Cooper and colleagues[35] tested the strength of 10-mm-wide grafts. They chose 10-mm-wide grafts because they believed that most surgeons used this size of graft to minimize the possibility of graft impingement in the femoral intercondylar notch. They reported that at the time of harvest the 10-mm-wide graft exhibited 174% of the strength of a normal ACL. Others have reported 10-mm-wide BTB autograft strength to be less (107%) but still above normal values for the ACL. Unfortunately, due to the graft's loss of a vascular supply at the time of its harvest, its strength decreases significantly from the time of implantation, and it never regains its initial strength levels. The avascular necrosis that occurs after implantation causes the graft to be its weakest somewhere in the 4- to 8-week postoperative period. On the basis of data from animal models, it is generally accepted that the BTB autografts undergo a "ligamentization" process that results in a graft whose vascular and histologic appearance at 1 year postoperatively resembles that of a normal ACL.[3,7,33] Using the medial one third of the patellar tendon in rhesus monkeys, Clancy and colleagues[33] reported transplanted patellar tendon graft strength to be 53% of normal ACL strength at 3 months, 52% of normal at 6 months, 81% of normal at 9 months, and 81% of normal at 12 months. Although these values are below normal strength levels and far below the strength values at the time of harvesting and implantation, Noyes and colleagues[134] suggested that in most strenuous activities, the ACL is seldom exposed to more than 50% of its maximal load. Allografts appear to go through the same process of avascular necrosis followed by revascularization and cellular proliferation.[8] However, it is believed that patellar tendon allografts are generally weaker throughout the rehabilitation process, which accounts for the slight differences that are often seen in rehabilitation protocols.

Rehabilitation time frames and guidelines after BTB autograft ACL reconstruction vary widely. Although numerous protocols have been developed, the majority of the most commonly used protocols have certain common themes. Most protocols now emphasize early motion, developing quadriceps control early, obtaining full passive extension, controlled weight bearing, and initiation of closed-chain exercises. Even though the exact time frames vary from protocol to protocol, it has been found that achieving the early goals of full passive extension, good quadriceps control, and minimal joint effusion/inflammation leads to better ultimate outcomes for the patient (Box 15-6). Tables 15-13 and 15-14 show rehabilitation protocols for BTB autograft ACL reconstruction. These protocols emphasize quadriceps strengthening either with a closed-chain method or with the knee in full extension. Early in the rehabilitation protocol open-chain quadriceps strengthening is still blocked in extension. The amount of extension that is blocked varies from 30° to 60°, depending on the protocol. Full range, open-chain quadriceps strengthening is allowed any time from 2.5 to 3.5 months after surgery, depending on the specific protocol being followed. Because the speed of protocols for rehabilitation after ACL reconstruction has increased so much in recent

Box 15-6

Goals for Early Rehabilitation after ACL Reconstruction

Decrease knee joint effusion
Achieve full passive knee extension
Develop good quadriceps control, especially in extension
Develop/maintain patellar mobility

Table 15-13

Rehabilitation Protocol after Anterior Cruciate Ligament Reconstruction Using Bone–Patellar Tendon–Bone Autograft

	Week 1	Weeks 2-4	Weeks 5-8	3 Months	4-6 Months
Functional progression	PWB with 2 crutches	WB with 1 crutch or FWB exercises	Advance strengthening	Begin jogging	Return to sport
Criteria	As postoperative pain allows	Full knee extension during gait SLR with no extensor lag No increase in effusion	No increase in effusion AROM 0-125° Normal patellar mobility KT-1000 <2 mm increase	No increase in effusion No pain Full AROM Eccentric control with one-leg minisquat Leg press strength >70% KT-1000 unchanged	No increase in effusion Functional tests >85% Isokinetic tests >85% Pain free KT-1000 unchanged Self-report functional measures
Evaluation	Pain Effusion Patellar mobility AROM Passive extension Quadriceps recruitment Incision/portals	Pain Gait AROM/PROM Effusion Patellar mobility Quadriceps recruitment Incision/portals	Pain Gait AROM/PROM Effusion Patellar mobility Flexibility Standing balance KT-1000	Pain AROM Effusion KT-1000 Leg press strength test One-leg minisquat Lateral step-ups Self-report functional measures	Pain Effusion Functional tests Isokinetic tests KT-1000 Self-report functional measures Proprioception tests
Treatment	Pain management Control effusion Patellar mobilization Passive extension and flexion Active flexion Quadriceps NMES or biofeedback	Pain management Control effusion Patellar mobilization AROM/PROM Quadriceps NMES or biofeedback Closed-chain exercises Gait training General strengthening (hamstrings, hip, etc.) Scar mobility AROM 0-100° 75%-100% WB	Flexibility exercises Proprioception exercises Endurance exercises General strengthening (hamstrings, hip, etc.) Open-chain quadriceps strengthening from 60° to 90° Increase loads with closed-chain exercises	Increase isotonic exercise Aerobic conditioning Open-chain quadriceps strengthening full ROM Begin jogging progression Begin hop progression Proprioception exercises	Increase isotonic exercise Aerobic conditioning Running progression Hop activities Sport-specific activities Proprioception exercises
Goals	PROM 0-90° 50% WB SLR without extensor lag		Full AROM Normal gait Increase strength and endurance No increase in effusion with 20-30 minutes biking or ambulating	No pain or increase in effusion with increased resistance through full ROM 85% with functional and strength tests	Return to sport

Adapted from Mangine, R.E., Noyes, F.R. and DeMaio, M. (1992): Minimal protection program: Advanced weight bearing and range of motion after ACL reconstruction: Weeks 1 to 5 Orthopedics, 15:504-515, and DeMaio, M., Mangine, R.E., and Noyes, F.R. (1992): Advanced muscle training after ACL reconstruction: Weeks 6 to 52. Orthopedics, 15:757-767. AROM, active range of motion; FWB, full weight bearing; NMES, neuromuscular electrical stimulation; PROM, passive range of motion; PWB, partial weight bearing; ROM, range of motion; SLR, straight leg raise; WB, weight bearing.

Table 15-14

Accelerated Rehabilitation after Anterior Cruciate Ligament-Patellar Tendon Graft Reconstruction

Preoperative Phase

Goals
- Diminish inflammation, swelling, and pain
- Restore normal range of motion (especially knee extension)
- Restore voluntary muscle activation
- Provide patient education to prepare patient for surgery

Brace—Elastic wrap or knee sleeve to reduce swelling
Weight Bearing—As tolerated with or without crutches
Exercises
- Ankle pumps
- Passive knee extension to 0°
- Passive knee flexion to tolerance
- Straight leg raises (three-way, flexion, abduction, adduction)
- Quadriceps setting
- Closed kinetic chain exercises: minisquats, lunges, step-ups

Muscle Stimulation—Electrical muscle stimulation to quadriceps during voluntary quadriceps exercises (4 to 6 hours per day)
Neuromuscular/Proprioception Training
- Eliminate quad avoidance gait
- Retro stepping drills
- Joint repositioning on Sports RAC
  - Passive/active reposition at 90, 60, and 30°
  - Closed kinetic chain squat/lunge repositioning on screen

Cryotherapy/Elevation—Apply ice 20 minutes of every hour, elevate leg with knee in full extension (knee must be above heart)
Patient Education
- *Review postoperative rehabilitation program*
- Review instructional video (optional)
- Select appropriate surgical date

I. Immediate Postoperative Phase (Day 1 to Day 7)

Goals
- Restore full passive knee extension
- Diminish joint swelling and pain
- Restore patellar mobility
- Gradually improve knee flexion
- Reestablish quadriceps control
- Restore independent ambulation

Postoperative Day 1

Brace—EZ Wrap brace/immobilizer applied to knee, locked in full extension during ambulation of Protonics
Weight Bearing—Two crutches, weight bearing as tolerated
Exercises
- Ankle pumps
- Overpressure into full, passive knee extension
- Active and passive knee flexion (90° by day 5)
- Straight leg raises (flexion, abduction, adduction)
- Quadriceps isometric setting
- Hamstring stretches
- Closed kinetic chain exercises: minisquats, weight shifts

Muscle Stimulation—Use muscle stimulation during active muscle exercises (4 to 6 hours/day)
Continuous Passive Motion—As needed, 0 to 45/50° (as tolerated and as directed by physician)
Ice and Evaluation—Ice 20 minutes out of every hour and elevate with knee in full extension

Postoperative Days 2 to 3

Brace—EZ Wrap brace/Immobilizer, locked at 0° extension for ambulation and unlocked for sitting, etc.
Weight Bearing—Two crutches, weight bearing as tolerated
Range of Motion—Remove brace, perform range of motion exercises 4 to 6 times a day
Exercises
- Multiangle isometrics at 90 and 60° (knee extension)
- Knee extension 90-40°

(Continued)

Table 15-14

Accelerated Rehabilitation after Anterior Cruciate Ligament-Patellar Tendon Graft Reconstruction—cont'd

Postoperative Days 2 to 3—cont'd

- Overpressure into extension (knee extension should be at least 0° to slight hyperextension)
- Patellar mobilization
- Ankle pumps
- Straight leg raises (three directions)
- Minisquats and weight shifts
- Quadriceps isometric setting

Muscle Stimulation—Electrical muscle stimulation to quads (6 hours/day)

Continuous Passive Motion—0 to 90°, as needed

Ice and Evaluation—Ice 20 minutes out of every hour and elevate leg with knee in full extension

Postoperative Days 4 to 7

Brace—EZ Wrap brace/immobilizer, locked at 0° extension for ambulation and unlocked for sitting, etc.

Weight Bearing—Two crutches weight bearing as tolerated

Range of Motion—Remove brace to perform range of motion exercises 4 to 6 times per day, knee flexion 90° by day 5, approximately 100° by day 7

Exercises

- Multiangle isometrics at 90 and 60° (knee extension)
- Knee extension 90 to 40°
- Overpressure into extension (attain complete extension)
- Patellar mobilization (5 to 8 times daily)
- Ankle pumps
- Straight leg raises (three directions)
- Minisquats and weight shifts
- Standing hamstring curls
- Quadriceps isometric setting
- Proprioception and balance activities

Neuromuscular training/proprioception—Open kinetic chain passive/active joint repositioning at 90 and 60°; closed kinetic chain squats/weight shifts with repositioning on sports RAC

Muscle Stimulation—Electrical muscle stimulation (continue 6 hours daily)

Continue Passive Motion—0 to 90°, as needed

Ice and Elevation—Ice 20 minutes of every hour and elevate leg with knee full extension

II. Early Rehabilitation Phase (Weeks 2 to 4)

Criteria to Progress to Phase II

1. Quad control (ability to perform good quad set and straight leg raising)
2. Full passive knee extension
3. Passive range-of-motion 0 to 90°
4. Good patellar mobility
5. Minimal joint effusion
6. Independent ambulation

Goals

- Maintain full passive knee extension (maintain complete extension)
- Gradually increase knee flexion
- Diminish swelling and pain
- Muscle control and activation
- Restore proprioception/neuromuscular control
- Normalize patellar mobility

Week Two

Brace—Continue locked brace for ambulation

Weight Bearing—As tolerated (goal is to discontinue crutches 10 to 14 days postoperatively)

Passive Range of Motion—Self range-of-motion stretching (4 to 5 times daily), emphasis on maintaining full, passive range of motion

KT 2000 Test—(15-lb anterior-posterior test only)

Exercises

- Muscle stimulation to quadriceps exercises
- Isometric quadriceps sets
- Straight leg raises (four planes)
- Leg press (0 to 60°)

Table 15-14

Accelerated Rehabilitation after Anterior Cruciate Ligament-Patellar Tendon Graft Reconstruction—cont'd

- Knee extension 90 to 40°
- Half squats (0 to 40°)
- Weight shifts
- Front and side lunges
- Hamstring curls standing (active range of motion)
- Bicycle (if range of motion allows)
- Proprioception training
- Overpressure into extension
- Passive range of motion from 0 to 100°
- Patellar mobilization
- Well leg exercises
- Progressive resistance extension program—start with 1 lb, progress 1 lb per week

Proprioception/Neuromuscular Training

- Open kinetic chain passive/active joint repositioning at 90, 60, and 30°
- Closed kinetic chain joint repositioning during squats/lunges
- Initiate squats on tilt board; use sports RAC with repositioning

Swelling control—Ice, compression, elevation

Week Three

Brace—Discontinue locked brace (some patients use range-of-motion brace for ambulation)

Passive Range of Motion—Continue range-of-motion stretching and overpressure into extension (range of motion should be 0 to 100/105°)

Exercises

- Continue all exercises as in week 2
- Passive range of motion 0 to 105°
- Bicycle for range-of-motion stimulus and endurance
- Pool walking program (if incision is closed)
- Eccentric quadriceps program 40 to 100° (isotonic only)
- Lateral lunges (straight plane)
- Front step-downs
- Lateral step-overs (cones)
- Stair-stepper machine
- Progress proprioception drills, neuromuscular control drills
- Continue passive/active reposition drills on sports RAC (closed and open kinetic chain)

III. Progressive Strengthening/Neuromuscular Control Phase (Weeks 4 to 10)

Criteria to Enter Phase III

1. Active range of motion 0 to 115°
2. Quadriceps strength 60% > contralateral side (isometric test at 60° knee flexion)
3. Unchanged KT 2000 test bilateral values (+1 or less)
4. Minimal to no joint effusion
5. No joint line or patellofemoral pain

Goals

- Restore full knee range of motion (0 to 125°)
- Improve lower extremity strength
- Enhance proprioception, balance, and neuromuscular control
- Improve muscular endurance
- Restore limb confidence and function

Brace—No immobilizer or brace, may use knee sleeve to control swelling/support

Range of Motion

- Self range-of-motion (4 to 5 times daily using the other leg to provide range of motion), emphasis on maintaining 0° passive extension
- Passive range of motion 0 to 125° at 4 weeks

KT 2000 Test—Week 4, 20 lb anterior and posterior test

Week 4

Exercises

- Progress isometric strengthening program

(Continued)

Table 15-14

Accelerated Rehabilitation after Anterior Cruciate Ligament-Patellar Tendon Graft Reconstruction—cont'd

Week 4—cont'd

- Leg press (0 to 100°)
- Knee extension 90 to 40°
- Hamstring curls (isotonics)
- Hip abduction and adduction
- Hip flexion and extension
- Lateral step-overs
- Lateral lunges (straight plane and multiplane drills)
- Lateral step-ups
- Front step-downs
- Wall squats
- Vertical squats
- Standing toe calf raises
- Seated toe calf raises
- Biodex stability system (balance, squats, etc.)
- Proprioception drills
- Bicycle
- Stair-stepper machine
- Pool program (backward running, hip and leg exercises)

Proprioception/Neuromuscular Drills

- Tilt board squats (perturbation)
- Passive/active reposition open kinetic chain
- Closed kinetic chain repositioning on tilt board with sports RAC
- Closed kinetic chain lunges with sports RAC

Week 6

KT 2000 Test—20- and 30-lb anterior and posterior test
Exercises

- Continue all exercises
- Pool running (forward) and agility drills
- Balance on tilt boards
- Progress to balance and ball throws
- Wall slides/squats

Week 8

KT 2000 Test—20- and 30-lb anterior and posterior test
Exercises

- Continue all exercises listed in weeks 4 to 6
- Leg press sets (single leg) 0 to 100° and 40 to 100°
- Plyometric leg press
- Perturbation training
- Isokinetic exercises (90 to 40°) (120 to 240°/sec)
- Walking program
- Bicycle for endurance
- Stair-stepper machine for endurance
- Biodex stability system
- Sports RAC neuromuscular training on tilt board and Biodex stability

Week 10

KT 2000 Test—20 and 30 lb and manual maximum test
Isokinetic Test—Concentric knee extension/flexion at 180 and 300°/sec
Exercises

- Continue all exercises listed in weeks 6, 8 and 10
- Plyometric training drills
- Continue stretching drills
- Progress strengthening exercises and neuromuscular training

IV. Advanced Activity Phase (Weeks 10 to 16)

Criteria to Enter Phase IV

- Active range of motion 0 to 125° or greater
- Quad strength 75% of contralateral side, knee extension flexor:extensor ratio 70% to 75%

Table 15-14

Accelerated Rehabilitation after Anterior Cruciate Ligament-Patellar Tendon Graft Reconstruction—cont'd

- No change in KT 2000 values (comparable with contralateral side, within 2 mm)
- No pain or effusion
- Satisfactory clinical examination
- Satisfactory isokinetic test (values at 180°)
  - Quadriceps bilateral comparison 75%
  - Hamstrings equal bilateral
  - Quadriceps peak torque/body weight 65% at 180°/sec (males) 55% at 180°/sec (females)
  - Hamstrings/quadriceps ratio 66% to 75%
  - Hop test (80% of contralateral leg)
  - Subjective knee scoring (modified Noyes system), 80 points or better

Goals
- Normalize lower extremity strength
- Enhance muscular power and endurance
- Improve neuromuscular control
- Perform selected sport-specific drills

Exercises
- May initiate running program (weeks 10 to 12)
- May initiate light sport program (golf)
- Continue all strengthening drills
  - Leg press
  - Wall squats
  - Hip abduction/adduction
  - Hip flexion/extension
  - Knee extension 90 to 40°
  - Hamstring curls
  - Standing toe calf
  - Step-down
  - Lateral step-ups
  - Lateral lunges
- Neuromuscular training
- Lateral step-overs (cones)
- Lateral lunges
- Tilt board drills
- Sports RAC repositioning on tilt board

Weeks 14-16
- Progress program
- Continue all drills above
- May initiate lateral agility drills
- Backward running

V. Return to Activity Phase (Weeks 16 to 22)

Criteria to Enter Phase V
1. Full range of motion
2. Unchanged KT 2000 test (within 2.5 mm of opposite side)
3. Isokinetic test that fulfills criteria
4. Quadriceps bilateral comparison (80% or greater)
5. Hamstring bilateral comparison (110% or greater)
6. Quadriceps torque/body weight ratio (55% or greater)
7. Hamstrings/quadriceps ratio (70% or greater)
8. Proprioceptive test (100% of contralateral leg)
9. Functional test (85% or greater of contralateral side)
10. Satisfactory clinical exam
11. Subjective knee scoring (modified Noyes system) (90 points or better)

Goals
- Gradual return to full-unrestricted sports
- Achieve maximal strength and endurance
- Normalize neuromuscular control

Table 15-14

Accelerated Rehabilitation after Anterior Cruciate Ligament-Patellar Tendon Graft Reconstruction—cont'd

Goals—cont'd
- Progress skill training

Tests—KT 2000, Isokinetic, and Functional Tests before return

Exercises
- Continue strengthening exercises
- Continue neuromuscular control drills
- Continue plyometrics drills
- Progress running and agility program
- Progress sport specific training
  - Running/cutting/agility drills
  - Gradual return to sports drills

6-Month Follow-up
- Isokinetic test
- KT 2000 test
- Functional test

12-Month Follow-up
- Isokinetic test
- KT 2000 test
- Functional test

From HealthSouth Sports Medicine and Rehabilitation Center, Birmingham, Alabama.

years, it is imperative that the exercises chosen produce a safe amount of stress on the revascularizing ACL. These were presented earlier in this chapter in the section on functional anatomy of the ACL. An understanding of the exercises that place high loads on the ACL is necessary to determine safe exercises at different time frames in the rehabilitation program.

The time frames found within protocols vary widely; however, progression through a protocol should be based more on the athlete's achieving certain goals rather than simply reaching a certain date postoperatively. As mentioned earlier, the most important goals to strive for early in the rehabilitation period are decreasing joint effusion/inflammation, achieving full passive knee extension, developing good quadriceps control (especially in extension), and promoting patellar mobility. When the patellar tendon is used as the graft material, it is important to obtain normal patellar mobility so that scarring around the harvest site does not occur and lead to infrapatellar contracture syndrome.[124] If the patella loses mobility due to scarring, ROM and strength can be significantly decreased. Early in the rehabilitation process, the patellar area might be too tender, because of the incision from the graft harvest site, to allow for productive mobilization. Facilitation of early quadriceps recruitment will help in obtaining patellar movement.[117] Electrical stimulation can be extremely valuable in facilitating a quadriceps contraction great enough to result in superior mobilization of the patella. Keep in mind that when electrical stimulation is being used for quadriceps strengthening instead of merely facilitation, the knee should be placed in approximately 60° or more of flexion.[156]

Attempting maximal voluntary contractions with electrical stimulation while the knee is in full extension can be uncomfortable for the patient. Developing quadriceps control at full knee extension is extremely important for several reasons. Quadriceps contractions increase patellar mobility, these quadriceps contractions help maintain full extension ROM, and good quadriceps contractions at full extension are required before a patient can fully bear weight with a normal gait. When passive knee extension ROM is obtained during rehabilitation, it can be very difficult to maintain unless the patient has enough quadriceps strength to actively go into full extension.

Maintaining full passive extension often becomes increasingly difficult during the first two weeks postoperatively. In the initial period of rehabilitation, emphasis should be placed on gaining and maintaining extension, because flexion will increase as pain and effusion decrease. If the surgeon is confident about graft fixation, active terminal knee extension exercises can be initiated as soon as the postoperative pain has decreased. These exercises should be done with no more resistance than simply the weight of the leg. Traditionally any open-chain knee extension exercise in the 45° to 0° range has been avoided because of the stress placed on the graft. However, because the graft is strong when it is initially placed in the knee and only loses strength as it necroses and goes through its revascularization process, active terminal knee extension exercises with no added resistance can be used early in rehabilitation to aid in facilitating quadriceps recruitment. If the athlete has difficulty performing supine terminal knee extension exercises, they can be performed in the prone position where the hip extensors can aid in achieving full knee extension (Fig. 15-23).

When the patient can actively recruit the quadriceps, using biofeedback units to increase the level of recruitment can be extremely helpful. Biofeedback requires complete patient involvement because it only monitors what the patient is doing and offers no stimulation to the muscle. For patients who tolerate electrical stimulation, Snyder-Mackler and colleagues[156] found that it helped patients regain quadriceps strength at a faster rate. In a study of 110 patients, they found that high-intensity electrical stimulation performed at 65° of flexion in a closed-chain position resulted in a 70% recovery of quadriceps strength by 6 weeks postoperatively. This compared favorably to the 57% recovery of quadriceps strength in a group that only performed closed-chain strengthening exercises. Also the group that received electrical stimulation showed better knee control at midstance than the group that exercised without electrical stimulation.

Weight-bearing status varies between protocols, but most commonly at least partial weight bearing is initiated within days of surgery. It is extremely important to have patients walk with as normal a gait as possible while they are on crutches. Poor habits during gait can be developed in this early stage of rehabilitation and once a poor gait pattern becomes ingrained it can be very difficult to break the habit. The most common gait deviation is the patient ambulating with the knee in flexion and never going into full extension.[156] This lack of full extension in gait may be due to a lack of strength and/or ROM, a habit pattern developed before surgery due to instability at the knee, or a habit pattern developed after surgery. Some protocols require the patient to wear a brace at 0° immediately after surgery so ambulating with the knee in flexion is not as common a complication.

When gait has normalized, use of crutches can be discontinued, and strengthening should be progressed in a closed-chain fashion. Closed-chain exercises allow for strengthening of the lower extremity without creating stresses that are harmful to the graft. The decreased stress that is afforded by the use of closed-chain exercises is due to the compression forces at the tibiofemoral joint and the co-contraction of other muscles to help control motion at the hip, knee, and ankle. An excellent initial closed-chain exercise is terminal knee extension in the standing position using Thera-Band (Fig. 15-24).

Hip strength should be addressed to decrease excessive frontal plane motion that might occur as the resistance is increased during closed-chain exercises (see Figs. 15-9 and 15-10). Lack of control at the hip can contribute to lower extremity malalignment and lead to overuse problems such as patellofemoral pain. Hip-strengthening exercises can include both open- and closed-chain activities. Both the speed and the difficulty of these exercises can be increased as the patient works through the rehabilitation program.

As the athlete gains lower extremity strength and coordination, he or she can start the functional progression of the rehabilitation program (see Tables 15-6 and 15-7). The time postoperatively at which these various activities begin varies widely with different protocols. However, it is extremely important that the rehabilitation specialist remember that reaching specific postoperative dates is only one criterion for allowing an athlete to progress through the rehabilitation protocol. It is just as important that the athlete have the appropriate strength (concentric and eccentric), ROM, coordination, and stability in the lower extremity to progress the difficulty of their rehabilitation program. If the athlete's condition warrants it, running and more aggressive hopping progressions (see

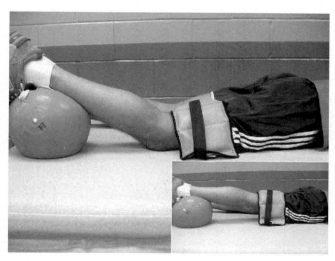

Figure 15-23. Prone terminal knee extension. The quadriceps are assisted in performing knee extension by the hip extensors. *Inset,* ending position.

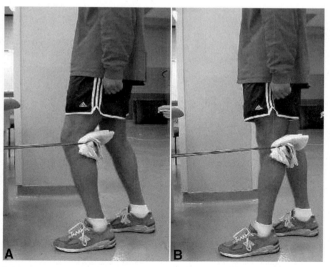

Figure 15-24. Closed-chain terminal knee extension. *A,* Starting position. *B,* Ending position.

Tables 15-8 and 15-9) are most often allowed at 3 to 4 months postoperatively, with a return to athletics commonly at 6 months postoperatively.

The type of graft that is used will dictate rehabilitation after an allograft. Generally, rehabilitation progression after reconstruction with an allograft is slightly slower than that with an autograft (Box 15-7). Weight bearing is often delayed, commonly from 4 to 6 weeks postoperatively. When weight bearing is allowed, the order and timing of rehabilitation progression for an allograft are similar to those for an autograft. It should be stressed that, regardless of the graft material used, objective criteria should be used to determine whether an athlete is ready to progress to the next stage of their rehabilitation program. Box 15-7 contains the key differences between the rehabilitation programs for a BTB autograft versus an allograft or hamstring autograft.

Functional Knee Braces

Functional braces, whether custom-made or off-the-shelf, are not able to control shear stresses through the knee under physiologic loads.[22,174] Even without the ability to control these stresses, some athletes report feeling more stable when they wear functional braces. Subjective improvements while an athlete wears a brace have been attributed to changes in proprioception.[25,34,125] There is evidence that braces alter timing and recruitment of thigh and calf musculature[128,180] and that patients with greater than 20% quadriceps deficit perform cutting maneuvers better while braced.[34] It has also been reported that 3 weeks after ACL reconstruction, patients ambulated with a more erect gait pattern including greater knee extension when they wore a functional brace.[43] When braced, the patients adopted a strategy that increased the use of the hip and ankle joint to control forces through the lower extremity while forces controlled by the knee were reduced. Risberg and associates[146] reported better Cincinnati Knee scores at 3 months after ACL reconstruction for patients randomly assigned to wear a functional brace. Despite this potential early benefit, there was no difference between the braced and nonbraced groups at 1 and 2 year follow-up on KT-1000° scores, Cincinnati Knee scores, functional hop test scores, pain scores, and patient satisfaction scores.

Based on the evidence presented above, the use of functional bracing after ACL reconstruction should probably be reserved for those athletes that are having difficulty returning to sport because of a lack of confidence in the reconstructed knee. Keeping in mind that the benefit to the brace is probably only improved proprioceptive function and not control of physiologic loads, the clinician and athlete must decide whether a custom-made brace is worth the extra cost to the athlete given the off-the-shelf alternatives. Additional consideration has to be given to the evidence that bracing increases energy expenditure, decreases maximal torque output from the quadriceps, and increases the rate of fatigue.[168]

Anterior Cruciate Ligament Injury Prevention Programs

A substantial number of ACL injuries occur in noncontact situations,[83] especially for female athletes. A number of factors have been proposed as potential causes of noncontact ACL injuries. These include the lack of control of abduction/adduction forces across the knee,[84] hamstring weakness,[84,114] electromechanical delay in hamstring activation,[178] reduced co-contraction of quadriceps and hamstring,[114] muscle fatigue,[32,178] reduced gastrocnemius

---

°Available from Medmetric, San Diego, California.

Box 15-7

Differences in Anterior Cruciate Ligament Rehabilitation Programs between Patellar Tendon Autograft and Allograft or Hamstring Autograft	
Patellar Bone-Tendon-Bone Autograft	**Allograft or Hamstring Autograft**
WBAT (with crutches) immediately	NWB for 4 weeks
	25% WB from 4 to 5 weeks
	50% WB from 5 to 6 weeks
	100% WB at 6 weeks
	OR
	PWB (with crutches) in brace locked in full extension for 1 week
	WBAT (with crutches) in brace locked in full extension from 1 to 2 weeks
	WBAT in brace locked in full extension from 2 to 6 weeks
Full ROM unloaded knee extension can begin as early as 2 weeks postoperatively	Full ROM unloaded knee extension can begin about 6 weeks postoperatively
Bilateral hopping can begin around 10 weeks	Bilateral hopping can begin around 12 weeks
Single-leg hopping can begin around 12 weeks	Single-leg hopping can begin around 14 weeks

WBAT, weight bearing as tolerated; NWB, non–weight-bearing; PWB, partial weight bearing; ROM, range of motion.

recruitment,[178] and insufficient ankle and hip balance and control.[32,178]

Several types of programs have been proposed to address these factors. These include plyometric programs,[83,84] wobble board training,[32,114] and perturbation training.[59] The results of studies using plyometric[83] or wobble board[32] training programs indicate that athletes participating in these training regimens have a reduced incidence of ACL injuries. A perturbation training study[59] has demonstrated that the ACL-deficient athlete was more successful in returning to sport if his or her rehabilitation included perturbation training. Wobble board and perturbation training programs progressively challenge the athlete's balance and thereby train the athlete to develop strategies that maintain control of the ankle, knee, and hip. Plyometric training improves the athlete's ability to control abduction/adduction forces especially when landing from a jump.[84] Plyometric training also improves hamstring strength[84] and hamstring activation time.[114] It is important to note that all three types of training are performed functionally with weight bearing through the lower extremity and are controlled "high"-speed activities rather than traditional strength training exercises. Because of the benefits, these activities should not only be used for ACL prevention programs, but they should also be incorporated into the functional progression, as appropriate, after ACL injuries or reconstruction.

Posterior Cruciate Ligament Injuries

Injury to the PCL is still relatively uncommon in the athletic population. An athlete is much more likely to injure his or her ACL or MCL. Literature on rehabilitation after PCL injury or surgery is, therefore, limited.[4]

A PCL-deficient knee can develop tibiofemoral and patellofemoral articular cartilage damage that can lead to very debilitating pain and dysfunction.[4] Although these degenerative changes do not occur in all PCL-deficient knees, it is a complication that must be considered when one is trying to decide whether surgery is the best option for the athlete.[149] Retropatellar pain can develop and become quite disabling in this patient population. This pain may be a result of excessive quadriceps activity that occurs in an attempt to control the posterior tibial translation found after the PCL is damaged. There is still much discussion on the topic of whether or not to reconstruct the PCL in patients with an isolated tear. If quadriceps strengthening programs do not control the laxity in athletes with a PCL-deficient knee, surgery becomes the best option.

When surgical reconstruction of the PCL is performed, a variety of tissues can be used. Autografts of bone-patellar tendon-bone, semitendinosus, or medial head of the gastrocnemius can be used. Also allografts of patellar tendon or Achilles tendon can be used. However, the surgical techniques for reconstruction are quite varied,

and no particular technique is presently viewed as the "gold standard." In fact, Anderson and Noyes[4] stated that there are incomplete data to date demonstrating the ability of any operative procedure to restore posterior stability at all angles of knee flexion.

The greatest concern after PCL reconstruction surgery is protection of the graft in the early stages of rehabilitation, which can be more difficult than after ACL reconstruction rehabilitation. In general, all of the time frames for progression of the rehabilitation program are slightly slower in PCL reconstruction rehabilitation compared with ACL reconstruction. The initial goals for the first 3 to 4 weeks in the postoperative rehabilitation program are to control inflammation/effusion, develop quadriceps control, maintain patellar mobility, and minimize stress to the graft. Most protocols call for bracing of the knee and limit weight bearing for 4 to 6 weeks. Isolated hamstring exercise is strictly controlled for 8 to 12 weeks to limit the amount of posterior tibial translation stress that is applied to the reconstructed PCL. Athletes are usually progressed to full weight bearing in the 6 to 10-week range as long as they have good quadriceps control and adequate ROM (especially extension), and the knee joint is not acutely inflamed.

CLINICAL PEARL #3

Following reconstruction of the ACL or PCL deficient knee, patello-femoral dysfunctions are one of the most common complications. Therefore, in planning and monitoring the rehabilitation program for athletes with these surgeries, care should be taken to avoid potentiating this complication. A simple rule-of-thumb is that all athletes with ligament reconstructions are patello-femoral problems waiting to happen.

As the rehabilitation program is advanced, closed-chain activities are emphasized so that co-contractions of lower extremity musculature aid in preventing posterior tibial translation. An example of a rehabilitation protocol after a two-tunnel autograft reconstruction is shown in Table 15-15. Rehabilitation for single-tunnel reconstructions are similar, but the progression of weight bearing and the ROM are often more conservative. Time of return to full activity and sports is extremely variable and is based on each individual athlete. Variables that affect this decision include the type of surgery, other structures involved in surgery, age and condition of the athlete, type of activities the athlete wishes to return to, and other complications that might have occurred during rehabilitation. Return to full function can vary from 6 to 12 months, depending on the athlete.

Medial Collateral Ligament Injuries

MCL injuries receive less attention today because of their nonoperative management and because of their frequent involvement with ACL injuries, which receive more

Table 15-15

Rehabilitation Protocol after Posterior Cruciate Ligament Two-Tunnel Autograft Reconstruction

	Week 1	Weeks 2-6	Weeks 6-12	3-5 Months	6-7 Months
Functional Progression Criteria	PWB with 2 crutches and brace locked at 0° As postoperative pain allows	PWB (single crutch) to FWB with brace locked at 0° No increase in effusion Pain controlled Good quadriceps recruitment	FWB with no brace No increase in effusion PROM 0-120° Normal patellar mobility SLR without extensor lag Isometric quadriceps strength 70% of contralateral side	Begin jogging progressing to running No increase in effusion No pain Full AROM Eccentric control with one-leg minisquat Leg press strength >70% Before initiating running functional tests >70% and no KT-1000 change	Return to sport No increase in effusion Functional tests >85% Isokinetic tests >85% Pain-free KT-1000 unchanged Self-report functional measures
Evaluation	Pain Effusion Patellar mobility PROM Passive extension Quadriceps recruitment Incision/portals	Pain Gait AROM extension PROM flexion Effusion Patellar mobility Quadriceps recruitment Balance Incision/portals	Pain Gait AROM extension Quad isometric strength PROM flexion Effusion Flexibility Balance KT-1000	Pain AROM Effusion KT-1000 Leg press strength test One-leg minisquat Self-report functional measures	Pain Effusion Functional tests Isokinetic tests KT-1000 Self-report functional measures Proprioception tests
Treatment	Pain management Inflammation management Patellar mobilization Passive extension to 0° Passive flexion to 60° Quadriceps sets with NMES or biofeedback Active knee extension 60-0° SLR Hamstring and calf stretching	Continue previous treatment PROM 0-90° progressing to 120° Knee extension PRE 50-0° Leg press 0-60° Total gym squats to 0-60° Gait training (weight shifts) Progress to minisquats 0-45° Scar mobility	Continue previous activities Proprioception exercises Stationary bike for endurance Single-leg balance activities Lateral step-ups 0-60° Wall squats 0-60° Initiate lunge progression 0-45° Begin active knee flexion against gravity ≈9 weeks	Continue previous activities with emphasis on quadriceps strengthening Jogging progression Initiate hamstring curls Begin light agility drills Double-leg hop drills Begin running ≈4 months	Emphasize quadriceps strengthening Aerobic conditioning Running progression Single-leg hop drills Plyometric training Cutting drills Sport-specific activities
Goals	PROM 0-60° 50% WB Control effusion/inflammation Good quadriceps recruitment Maintain patellar mobility	AROM 0-120° FWB SLR without extensor lag Isometric quadriceps strength 70% of contralateral side	Full AROM Normal gait No increase in effusion with 20-30 minutes of biking or ambulating	No pain or increase in effusion with increased exercise load 85% with functional and strength tests	Return to sport

Adapted from Wilk, K.E., Andrews, J.R., Clancy, W.G., et al. (1999): Rehabilitation programs for the PCL-injured and reconstructed knee. J Sport Rehabil, 8:333-361.
AROM, active range of motion; FWB, full weight bearing; NMES, neuromuscular electrical stimulation; PROM, passive range of motion; PWB, partial weight bearing; ROM, range of motion; SLR, straight leg raise.

attention. Isolated grade I and II MCL injuries are always managed nonoperatively, and general symptom-driven guidelines for knee rehabilitation are followed. Bracing is often used initially to control valgus stresses to the knee. Depending on the severity of the injury, the brace might be set to limit knee ROM. Brace settings vary from allowing full extension to blocking 15° of extension. Usually up to 90° of flexion is allowed. The patient is allowed to bear partial weight immediately if it is pain free. Weight bearing is progressed as tolerated and full weight bearing is allowed by 3 to 6 weeks for most grade II injuries. For grade I injuries, full activity is usually permitted in 3 to 4 weeks and for grade II injuries in 6 to 8 weeks. To return to activity the athlete should have (1) full, painless knee ROM, (2) no joint pain or functional instability, (3) normal muscle strength, and (4) normal levels of functional abilities.

Grade III MCL injuries can be managed either operatively or nonoperatively. Traditionally, grade III MCL injuries have been managed with 2 to 4 weeks of non–weight bearing and bracing with ROM limitations. Immediately after the injury the brace might even be locked at approximately 45°. The brace is then opened to

allow 0° to 90° of motion for the rest of the bracing period (4 to 6 weeks). Gentle ROM and strengthening exercises can be performed while the athlete is wearing the brace. Several studies report excellent results in isolated grade III MCL injuries that are managed nonoperatively and in which early motion activities are emphasized. After the initial 4 to 6 weeks of rehabilitation, the athlete with the grade III MCL injury can begin to progress through a more complete program of rehabilitation. Care should be taken to minimize valgus stress on the knee. It is not unusual for athletes with grade III MCL injuries to continue to exhibit some residual valgus laxity; however, this laxity does not appear to cause any functional limitations. These athletes can return to sports in 3 to 6 months, depending on their response to rehabilitation. An example of a rehabilitation protocol after an MCL injury is shown in Table 15-16.

Meniscal Injuries

Meniscal lesions have been treated by total meniscectomy, partial meniscectomy, and most recently, meniscal repair. Total meniscectomy by arthrotomy quickly alleviates the

Table 15-16

Rehabilitation Protocol for Isolated Medial Collateral Ligament Sprains Grades I, II, and III

	Week 1	Weeks 2-3	Weeks 4-8
Functional progression	Begin WB without crutches, grades I and II	Progress strengthening exercises	Return to athletics, grades I and II
Criteria	Full knee extension present during gait	No pain with exercises	No tenderness
	No limp	No increased effusion/edema	Functional testing >85%
	No pain at MCL	Patellar mobility normal	Quadriceps strength >85%
	No increased effusion	Full AROM	
	Full active extension ROM		
Evaluation	Pain	Pain	Functional testing
	Effusion/edema	Effusion/edema	Isokinetic testing
	Quadriceps recruitment	Patellar mobility	Self-report functional measure
	ROM	Quadriceps recruitment	
	Patellar mobility	Active ROM	
		Standing balance, grades I and II	
Treatment	Pain management	Pain management	Strengthening exercises
	Control of effusion/edema	Control of effusion/edema	Endurance exercises
	Quadriceps recruitment/biofeedback	Mobilization of patella	Sport-specific drills
	ROM exercises	Quadriceps strengthening	
	Flexibility exercises	AROM exercises	
	NWB, grade III only	Proprioception exercises	
	Rehabilitation brace, grades II and III	Endurance exercises	
Goals	Maximize ROM	Full ROM	Discontinue brace, grade II
	Good quadriceps recruitment	Absence of pain	Begin WB, grade III and progress through criteria beginning week 1
	Control valgus stress	FWB, grades I and II	
	75%-100% WB, grades I and II	Normal patellar mobility	Return to sports, grades I and II

AROM, active range of motion; FWB, full weight bearing; MCL, medial collateral ligament; NWB, non-weight bearing; ROM, range of motion; WB, weight bearing.

mechanical symptoms, and short-term results have usually been good.[41] However, long-term outcomes have been disappointing because of the degenerative articular changes that occur in knees after a total meniscectomy.[105,121] For this reason total meniscectomy is rarely indicated.

Meniscal lesions are now treated by partial meniscectomy or repair. Meniscal transplant, using either an allograft or a synthetic material, is also a possible option. At this time, this procedure has not been performed enough to determine long-term outcomes and efficacy. As this surgical procedure is progressed and refined, it may develop into a reasonable treatment option.

Partial meniscectomy is performed by removing as little of the meniscus as is possible. Maintaining as much of the meniscus as possible is felt to aid in minimizing long-term degenerative changes at the knee. Rehabilitation after a partial meniscectomy is symptom driven. The guidelines discussed in the section on the overview of knee rehabilitation principles show the rehabilitation process for the athlete who has undergone a partial meniscectomy. Usually athletes are able to return to sports rapidly, often within 2 to 3 weeks, after an uncomplicated partial meniscectomy. An example of a rehabilitation protocol after a partial meniscectomy is shown in Table 15-17.

Repair of the meniscus has become a viable surgical option in recent years. A greater understanding of the overall function of the meniscus has led surgeons to prefer to repair, rather than remove, parts of the meniscus whenever possible. Repairs are most often performed on the peripheral third of the meniscus because this area has a blood supply to allow for healing of the repair site. Repairs can be performed arthroscopically or through a small incision at the knee. The technique on the meniscus itself can be performed in a variety of ways.

Rehabilitation after a meniscal repair is much more guarded than that after a simple partial meniscectomy to protect the repair site. Table 15-18 shows an example of a rehabilitation protocol after a meniscal repair. In the first 4 weeks after surgery the athlete progresses from non–weight bearing to full weight bearing. Most often the knee is placed in a brace that is locked in full extension. Being in full extension produces an axial loading force on the meniscus that approximates the margins of the repair. Being locked in extension during gait in this early phase of rehabilitation also prevents knee flexion during weight bearing, which could lead to forces that could damage the repair. The brace can be removed and full ROM attempted while the athlete is still non–weight bearing;

Table 15-17

Rehabilitation Protocol for Partial Meniscectomy

	Week 1	Weeks 2-3	Weeks 4-8
Functional progression	Begin FWB without crutches	Progress strengthening exercises	Return to athletics
Criteria	Full extension present during gait	Absence of pain	Full AROM
	No limp	No increased effusion/edema	No effusion
	No increased effusion/edema		Functional testing >85%
	No increased pain		Quadriceps strength >85%
	Quadriceps control		
	Full active extension ROM		
Evaluation	Pain	Pain	Functional testing
	Gait	Gait	Isokinetic testing
	Quadriceps recruitment	Effusion/edema	Self-report functional measure
	AROM	Surgical incisions/portals	
	Patellar mobility	Quadriceps recruitment	
	Surgical incisions/portals	AROM	
	Effusion/edema	Patellar mobility	
		Standing balance	
Treatment	Pain management	Effusion/edema reduction	Strengthening exercises
	Control of effusion/edema	Strengthening exercises	Endurance exercises
	Quadriceps recruitment	Endurance exercises	Sport-specific drills
	ROM exercises	Proprioception exercises	
	Flexibility exercises	Flexibility exercises	
Goals	Maximum ROM	FWB	Return to athletics
	Normal patellar mobility	Full ROM	
	SLR without extensor lag	No pain with strengthening exercises	
	Full passive extension		

AROM, active range of motion; FWB, full weight bearing; ROM, range of motion; SLR, straight leg raise.

Table 15-18

Rehabilitation Protocol for Meniscus Repair

	Weeks 0-3	Weeks 4-11	Weeks 12-15	Weeks 16-24
Functional progression	Begin partial to full WB with brace locked in full extension	Begin full WB without brace	Begin jogging	Begin cutting and jumping activities
Criteria	As postoperative pain allows No increased effusion	SLR with no extensor lag Effusion continues to decrease Full extension during gait	Absence of effusion Absence of patellofemoral pain No gait deviations	No increased effusion with running No pain Isokinetic testing >85% Functional testing >85%
Evaluation	Pain Effusion Patellar mobility Quadriceps recruitment AROM/PROM Passive extension Incision/portals	Pain Effusion Patellar mobility Quadriceps recruitment AROM/PROM Standing balance	Gait Isokinetic testing Functional testing Effusion Self-report functional status	Gait Isokinetic testing Functional testing Effusion Self-report functional status
Treatment	Pain control Control of effusion/edema Patellar mobility AROM Quadriceps recruitment with biofeedback/electrical stimulation Passive extension FWB in brace locked at 0°	AROM/PROM Quadriceps recruitment/strengthening General strengthening Progress closed-chain exercises (no flexion greater than 60°) Endurance exercise Proprioception exercises	Strengthening exercises Endurance exercises Proprioception exercises	Strengthening exercises Endurance exercises Sport-specific drills
Goals	AROM 0-90° Full passive extension FWB in brace SLR with no extensor lag	Full AROM No gait deviations	Absence of effusion No pain	Return to athletics

Adapted from McLaughlin, J., DeMaio, M., Noyes, F.R., et al. (1994): Rehabilitation after meniscus repair. Orthopedics, 17:463-471.
AROM, active range of motion; FWB, full weight bearing; PROM, passive range of motion; WB, weight bearing; SLR, straight leg raise.

however, aggressive flexion is still not performed. As effusion decreases, active flexion should continue to progress, but if flexion measurements plateau, more aggressive passive flexion can be initiated at 4 weeks. The brace is usually removed in the 4- to 6-week range, and the athlete is permitted to be full weight bearing if there is minimal joint effusion, active ROM of between 0° and 10° of extension, 90° of flexion, and good quadriceps control.

At 4 to 6 weeks postoperatively, if the athlete's repair is progressing with no complications the rehabilitation program can be increased to include more aggressive strengthening and ROM exercises. This phase lasts 1 to 2 months and should aid the athlete in achieving full ROM, close to full strength, and full functional abilities in walking and activities of daily living, but not sports. At the end of this phase the athlete is progressed to an actual return to his or her sports program.

The final phase of return to sports activities will last 4 to 6 weeks and allow the athlete to return to full competition by 4 to 6 months postoperatively. This final phase should incorporate all aspects of the athlete's specific sport.

Rehabilitation after Combined Injuries of the Knee

When more than one structure is involved in a knee injury, rehabilitation of this type of combined injury is controlled by first analyzing which structures are involved. With combined injuries at the knee the rehabilitation program guidelines are controlled by the more serious of the injuries (Box 15-8). One of the most important initial steps the rehabilitation specialist can take is to determine which injury/surgical procedure is the one that will control the speed of the rehabilitation process. Fortunately, combined injuries at the knee that cause serious damage to multiple

structures are not common. However, when this type of situation does occur the rehabilitation specialist must determine which exercises are safe for an individual patient. The specialist must always remember that some exercises might be indicated for one part of the multiple structure injury and contraindicated for another part of the multiple structure injury.

The general guidelines on the inflammatory process and tissue healing times should be kept in mind with any rehabilitation program. With multiple structure injuries the inflammatory process and its common complications, such as ROM loss and excessive scar formation, can be more significant due to greater trauma at the joint. The initial goals of rehabilitation in patients with multiple structure injuries are still decreasing inflammation, regaining patellar mobility, and regaining quadriceps control (not necessarily strength). The ROM exercises in these patients should be limited based on the structures that are involved, but often at least limited-range ROM exercises are instituted.

One of the more common multiple structure injuries is damage to the ACL and MCL. When the ACL is damaged in combination with an MCL injury, the MCL is often left to heal on its own. The exception to this practice is when there is still significant joint laxity after the ACL graft is put in place. This laxity is seen if there is also a posterior oblique ligament injury at the knee. In this type of situation the surgeon may choose to reconstruct or repair the MCL as well. When injuries to both structures have occurred, rehabilitation follows the ACL rehabilitation protocol, with no significant valgus load being placed on the knee. Often times with this type of combined injury a rehabilitation brace is used for a longer time to aid in controlling valgus stresses at the knee. Because the longer time in a brace and the increased trauma to the knee from the combination injury, ROM work must be emphasized to limit the complication of ROM loss.

If both the ACL and PCL are injured, rehabilitation generally follows the PCL rehabilitation protocol. Often very significant trauma to the knee is required to rupture both the ACL and PCL so postoperative complications, such as ROM losses, can be a problem. Open-chain exercises involving the knee are often limited to low weight reeducation type exercises to minimize the anterior and posterior tibial translation at the knee. Strengthening is accomplished through closed-chain exercises. These closed-chain exercises are emphasized as the patient's weight-bearing status allows. Correctly performing exercises in a closed-chain fashion minimizes the anterior and posterior tibial translations due to the compression of weight bearing and co-contractions of the hip, thigh, and leg musculature. In doing a closed-chain activity such as a minisquat, the athlete needs to keep the knee between 0° and 60° of flexion, while keeping the trunk upright. This minimizes increasing hip flexion angles, which if not controlled can increase the muscular activity of the ham-

---

Box 15-8

Rehabilitation of Combined Injuries

Surgery	Dominant Rehabilitation Protocol
ACL and partial meniscectomy	ACL
ACL and meniscal repair	ACL first 3 months, meniscus in later rehabilitation stages
ACL and MCL	ACL with bracing
ACL and PCL	PCL
ACL and articular cartilage	Articular cartilage
ACL and posterolateral corner	ACL modified to protect posterior corner
PCL and articular cartilage	Articular cartilage with motion restrictions for PCL
PCL and posterolateral corner	PCL modified to protect posterior corner

strings. If a closed-chain exercise is performed incorrectly, excessive hamstring activity might increase the posterior translation of the tibia.

The posterolateral corner of the knee joint can be injured in conjunction with other ligament injuries at the knee. If this posterolateral corner is surgically reconstructed, care must be taken to avoid stress to the reconstruction. This includes avoiding hyperextension at the knee, guarding against excessive varus stresses to the knee, and controlling posterior tibial translation stresses early in the rehabilitation period.[92] When one works on regaining a patient's extension, support should be given to the tibia so that stress to the posterolateral corner is minimized. Some of the more traditional methods of increasing extension might have to be altered or avoided if the posterolateral corner is involved. If the posterolateral corner and the ACL are both reconstructed, the ACL rehabilitation protocol times guide the rehabilitation, but resistive hamstring exercises might be delayed by several weeks. Additionally,

deep flexion closed-chain exercises and strong open-chain quadriceps contractions between 60° and 130° should be delayed for several weeks compared with a traditional ACL rehabilitation protocol. Some surgeons might also delay full weight bearing by 2 to 3 weeks.

If the posterolateral corner and the PCL are both reconstructed, flexion ROM might be limited early in the rehabilitation program. In an athlete with any combined ligament injury that involves the posterolateral corner, a return to full athletic activities might be delayed from several weeks to several months. This delay varies based on the particular surgeon and the surgical procedure used, but it is common for a posterolateral reconstruction to slightly prolong the rehabilitation period (Table 15-19).

With ACL reconstruction and associated meniscal repairs, the ACL rehabilitation protocol is followed in an attempt to limit morbidity. However, care must be taken when closed-chain activities are performed early in rehabilitation. This type of loaded knee flexion can put

Table 15-19

Combined Reconstructive Surgery Rehabilitation Protocol: Posterior Cruciate Ligament and Posterolateral Reconstruction (Biceps Tenodesis)

Preoperative Instructions
- Gait training—Weight bearing as tolerated with crutches
- Instruction in immediate postoperative activities/hospital course
- Brace stays on for all exercises; can open brace to put muscle stimulator on and to do patella mobilizations

I. Immediate Postoperative Phase

Postoperative Days 1 to 4

Brace—EZY Wrap locked at 0° or full extension

Weight Bearing—Two crutches and progress to full weight bearing as tolerated

Exercises
- Ankle pumps
- Patella mobilization and passive extension to 0°
- Quad sets, adductor sets with quad sets, glut sets
- Leg raises in supine and on unaffected side

Ice and Elevation—Ice 20 minutes out of every hour and elevate with knee in extension.

II. Maximum Protection Phase (Postoperative Day 5 to Week 8)

Postoperative Day 5 to Week 2

Brace—Still locked in full extension

Weight Bearing—Progress to full weight bearing without crutches

Exercises
- Continue prior exercises and begin progressive-resistance exercise with leg raises

Postoperative Week 6

Brace—Discharge brace

Exercises
- Work toward regaining full active flexion seated—not against gravity
- Start exercise bike and swimming, emphasizing range of motion
- Start progressive-resistance exercise for quadriceps only

III. Minimal Protection Phase (Weeks 8 to 12)

Postoperative Week 10

Exercises
- Begin hamstring work against gravity and then start progressive-resistance exercises
- Continue all strengthening exercises

Postoperative Week 12

KT 2000 Test—Performed

Table 15-19

Combined Reconstructive Surgery Rehabilitation Protocol: Posterior Cruciate Ligament and Posterolateral Reconstruction (Biceps Tenodesis)—cont'd

Exercises
- Continue minisquats
- Initiate lateral step ups
- Initiate pool running (forward only)
- Hamstring curls (0 to 60°, low weight)
- Bicycle for endurance (30 minutes)
- Begin walking program

IV. Light Activity Phase (3 to 4 months)

Goals
- Development of strength, power, and endurance
- Begin to prepare for return to functional activities

Exercises
- Begin light running program
- Initiate isokinetics (high speed, full range of motion)
- Continue eccentric quadriceps program
- Continue minisquats/lateral step-ups
- Continue closed kinetic chain rehabilitation
- Continue endurance exercises

Tests
- Isokinetic test (15th week)
- KT 2000 test (before running program)
- Functional test (before running program)

Criteria for Running
- Isokinetic test interpretation satisfactory
- KT 2000 test unchanged
- Functional test 70% of contralateral leg

V. Return to Activity Phase (5 to 6 months)

Advance rehabilitation to competitive sports

Goals: Achieve maximal strength and further enhance neuromuscular coordination and endurance

Exercises
- Closed kinetic chain rehabilitation
- High-speed isokinetics
- Running program
- Agility drills
- Balance drills
- Plyometrics initiated
- Gradual return to sport activities

Criteria to return to sport activities
- Isokinetic quad torque to body weight ratio
- Isokinetic test 85% > contralateral side
- No change in laxity
- No pain/tenderness or swelling
- Satisfactory clinical exam

6-Month Follow-up
- Isokinetic test
- KT 2000 test
- Functional test

12-Month Follow-up
- Isokinetic test
- KT 2000 test
- Functional test

From HealthSouth Sports Medicine and Rehabilitation Center, Birmingham, Alabama.

the meniscal repair in danger of being damaged. For this reason, the weight-bearing guidelines in the traditional ACL rehabilitation protocol are slightly altered to protect the repair.

Articular Cartilage Injuries

Symptomatic articular cartilage lesions and osteochondral injuries of the knee pose a significant challenge to physicians and rehabilitation specialists. The true incidence of these injuries is unknown.[29] The mechanisms of injury for trauma-related lesions include impaction, shearing, or avulsion. Although the clinical significance of bone bruises (occult subchondral trabecular microfractures) is not fully understood, these lesions have been reported in 80% of patients with acute ACL tears.[95] Treatment options for symptomatic osteochondral lesions include nonsurgical treatments, arthroscopic lavage and debridement, abrasion arthroplasty, microfracture, MosaicPlasty (articular cartilage autographs), autologous chondrocyte transplantation, and allografts.[2]

Conservative management of symptomatic individuals has limited indications, and the relief from arthroscopic lavage and debridement appears to be short-lived.[69] Abrasion arthroplasty and microfracture, while differing in technique, are both methods used to introduce bleeding from the subchondral bone into the lesion. The clot that forms over the region reorganizes into a predominantly fibrocartilaginous tissue.[2] In mosaicplasty the lesion is filled with osteochondral plugs taken from low load/contact areas of the joint. Autologous chondrocyte transplantation is a two-step surgical procedure. During the initial arthroscopic inspection of the lesion a chondral biopsy is obtained. This sample sent to a laboratory* where the chondrocytes are placed in a culture that allows them to multiply until there are approximately 12 million cells.[69] During the second surgical procedure, a periosteal flap is placed over the defect, and the cell culture is injected into the defect to fill the space between the flap and subchondral bone. Because of a lack of long-term studies with sufficient numbers of patients, there is no clear consensus as to which procedure—microfracture, mosaicplasty, or autologous chondrocyte transplantation—is superior.[2] Regardless of surgical procedure used, the rehabilitation program must be designed so that the healing lesion receives enough stress to enhance healing while excessive stress, especially shear forces, during the initial postoperative period is avoided (Box 15-9). This is accomplished primarily by unloaded joint ROM. Joint motion enhances articular cartilage healing and the use of a continuous passive motion machine for 6 to 8 hours/day during the first 4 to 8 weeks after surgery is advocated.[155]

---

*Available from Genzyme Tissue Repair, Cambridge, Massachusetts.

Box 15-9

Early Rehabilitation of Articular Cartilage Lesions

Unloaded range of motion is critical to enhance the healing of the cartilage repair

Emphasize active and active-assisted range of motion when not in continuous passive motion

Rehabilitation guidelines are currently evolving as our understanding of articular cartilage healing and surgical techniques improve. In general, during the first 2 weeks after surgery the athlete will be non–weight bearing.[69,93,155] Depending on the location and size of the lesion, as well as the procedure performed, toe-touch weight bearing may begin between the second and fourth week. Weight bearing may be progressed to partial weight bearing between the sixth and eighth week and to full weight bearing with crutches around 8 weeks after surgery. Some protocols require the use of a brace locked at 0° during this weight-bearing progression.[69] Large or multiple lesions in weight-bearing regions of the femur or tibia may require a non–weight-bearing status for 8 weeks.[155] When full weight bearing is allowed, athletes may discontinue the use of crutches if they have at least 0° to 100° of motion, effusion, if present, is minimal and stable, they are able to perform a straight leg raise without extensor lag, and they do not experience an increase in symptoms.[93]

During the protective rehabilitation phase (0 to 8 weeks) controlled ROM activities are critical.[69,93,155] These can include passive, active-assistive, and unloaded active ROM. As stated earlier the use of a continuous passive motion machine is highly recommended for at least 4 weeks. If the athlete does not have access to a continuous passive motion machine, it is recommended that they perform 500 repetitions of appropriate motion activities three times a day.[155] Isometric exercises for the quadriceps and hamstrings can be performed at joint angles that do not load the region of the lesion. Biofeedback and electrical stimulation may be useful in activating the quadriceps during these multi-angle isometrics. If the chondral defect was located on the patella and or femoral sulcus, isometrics may need to be limited to 0°.[155] Ice, compression, and elevation should be used to reduce joint effusion. In many cases a stationary bike with minimal or no resistance can be used for ROM exercise when the athlete has gained enough knee motion to allow for normal pedaling.[69,155] Pool ROM activities can be initiated when the incisions are healed[155]; however, the athlete must be careful to maintain their appropriate weight-bearing status especially when entering and exiting the pool.

During the transition rehabilitation phase, the athlete is allowed to progress from partial to full weight-bearing status. Low-load leg presses, Total Gym activities at lower angles of inclination, and treadmills with unloading devices may be useful in assisting the athlete in the transition from partial- to full-weight acceptance on the involved lower extremity.[93,155] Progression of weight-bearing activities in the pool is also useful. When the athlete can discontinue the use of crutches (see earlier guidelines), the focus of the rehabilitation program can shift toward controlled strength training, proprioceptive, and balance activities. The athlete can begin a minisquat program, leg press (0° to 60°), and Total Gym strengthening exercises.[69,155] Open-chain knee extension exercises should be avoided for most athletes with patellar lesions during this phase of rehabilitation (and quite possibly throughout the entire rehabilitation process).[155] Athletes with tibial or femoral lesions may be allowed to begin open-chain knee extension exercises in this phase.[69] If allowed, these exercises should be progressed very slowly in terms of load and the ROM may need to be limited. Because of relatively high tibiofemoral compression forces, lunges,[167] and hopping drills should be avoided during this stage,[155] but it may be possible to begin lateral step-ups.[69] Stationary bicycling and treadmill walking can be used to begin aerobic conditioning.[69] The transition phase will commonly last until about 12 to 16 weeks after surgery. Any increase in effusion or symptoms will necessitate a reduction in rehabilitation intensity.

From 4 to about 6 months postoperatively the rehabilitation program should focus on continued progressive strengthening and endurance exercises. The intensity of the activities begun in the transitional rehabilitation phase can be increased, and a lunge program can be initiated. A jogging progression may be initiated between the fifth and sixth month.[69] After the sixth month, the athlete may be allowed to begin sport-specific drills as long as he or she has full ROM, quadriceps and hamstring strength within 10% of the uninvolved leg, and no pain or effusion. At this time a hop program tailored to the sport requirements can be initiated; as before any evidence of pain or effusion suggests the need to reduce the impact and load intensity of the program. After surgery, it is generally possible for the athlete to return to low-impact sports at approximately 6 months, whereas a return to high-impact sports will usually require about 1 year.[69]

INSTRUMENTED AND FUNCTIONAL TESTING
Arthrometry

Arthrometers provide the clinician with a quantifiable method of testing ligamentous laxity of the anterior and posterior cruciate ligaments. Introduced in 1983 by Daniel and co-workers[39] the KT-1000 was one of the first commercially produced arthrometers used clinically for measuring anterior-posterior laxity (Fig. 15-25).[79] A number of other devices have been developed, but the KT1000 (and KT2000, a KT1000 with an X-Y plotter) remains one of the most commonly cited and clinically used arthrometers.

A number of investigations have been undertaken to evaluate the validity and reliability of arthrometry.[11,38,40,79,113] When one interprets, compares, and applies these results, several factors that must be considered are the displacement force used, the displacement difference considered diagnostic, and study design issues (single testers, multiple testers, etc.).

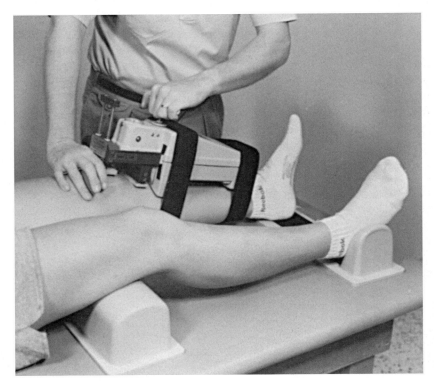

Figure 15-25. KT-1000 arthrometer.

Reliability of arthrometry can be estimated by a statistical technique called intraclass correlation coefficients (ICCs). Depending on the formula used, this test provides either a measure of reproducibility of individual evaluators or the reproducibility of a measure between evaluators. ICCs can range from 0 (totally unreliable) to 1 (perfect reliability). Reported ICCs for ACL testing using a KT-1000 or a KT-2000 range from 0.65 to 0.99.[12,18,27,126,142] In general, results from testers experienced in arthrometry are more reliable than those from novices, and serial measures between testers are less reliable than serial measures from the same tester. The active quadriceps tests are generally less reliable than any of the passive displacement force tests. The reliability results of the common passive displacement forces (67 N, 89 N, 134 N, maximum manual) are mixed, with no one particular displacement force being consistently more reliable than the others.

PCL arthrometry appears to be somewhat less reliable than ACL arthrometry. Huber and associates[87] reported ICCs ranging from 0.59 to 0.84 for PCL testing using a KT-1000. Similar to ACL testing, results from novice testers were generally less reliable than those from experienced testers and reliability of results between different testers was less than for serial measures from the same tester.

Sensitivity and specificity are statistical methods that can be used as measures of validity for arthrometric testing. Sensitivity refers to the ability of the arthrometer to detect ligamentous deficiency when a ligament deficiency truly exists. The more sensitive an arthrometer test is, the less likely that someone with a ligament deficiency will be missed, in other words the less likely that there will be a false-negative result from the test. Specificity refers to the ability of the arthrometer to classify a result as negative when there is no ligamentous deficiency. An arthrometer with high specificity is less likely to produce false-positive findings (classify someone as ligamentous deficient when they are truly not). Both sensitivity and specificity scores range from 0% to 100%, with 100% being perfect (no false-negative or false-positive results, respectively).

The reported sensitivity for the KT-1000 in differentiating ACL tears ranges from 49% to 97% and the reported specificity for ACL tears ranges from 64% to 95%, depending on the displacement force applied and the side-to-side difference considered diagnostic.[11,113] The sensitivity is better with the manual maximum test, whereas specificity is better with the 89-N (20-pound) force test. The sensitivity and specificity of the instrument is also influenced by the difference in displacement between involved and uninvolved knees used as the diagnostic criterion. Sensitivity is better if a 2-mm side-to-side difference is used whereas specificity is better if a 3-mm difference is considered diagnostic. Based on their results of 97% sensitivity for a manual maximum test and 95% sensitivity for a Lachman test, Liu and colleagues[113] suggested that these examinations were more accurate in predicting acute ACL tears than a magnetic resonance imaging scan (reported sensitivity of 82%).

The sensitivity and specificity of arthrometric PCL testing have been reported for the Knee Ligament Testing arthrometer.[48] Using a side-to-side difference of 3 mm as diagnostic for a PCL injury and a posterior displacement force of 178 N (40 lb), Eakin and Cannon[48] reported a sensitivity of 90% and a specificity of 100%.

Regardless of the accuracy and reliability reported in the literature, the clinician performing the arthrometry must be meticulous in their measurement technique. Daniel[37] suggested that the two greatest sources of error in KT-1000 measures are inappropriate patellar pad stabilization and lack of muscle relaxation. Other key points suggested by Daniel to reduce measurement error include proper lower extremities are alignment, accurate placement of the arthrometer, and consistent speed and direction of force application.[37]

The arthrometer may also be valuable for monitoring the graft laxity during the rehabilitation process. Queale and colleagues[142] suggested that an increase in anterior translation of greater than 2 mm (89-N displacement force) between successive measures indicates increasing laxity. DeMaio and associates[42] recommended a decrease in exercise intensity, modification of the rehabilitation program, or possible continuance of or regression back to crutch ambulation if there is an increase of greater than 2 mm during the first 5 weeks after ACL reconstruction. Another modification that has been suggested[94] for patients with increasing anterior laxity postoperatively is the use of a functional brace during all weight-bearing activities. Arthrometric monitoring may be especially important for athletes with a reconstruction for chronic ACL deficiency.[15] There is evidence to suggest that patients with chronic ACL deficiency are at greater risk for graft stretching during the first 24 weeks after reconstruction. If used wisely, the arthrometer can provide quantitative information about the surgical and rehabilitation techniques being used. Also, by detecting increased tibial translation early, the arthrometer may help head off early graft and knee problems that may not be detected by physical examination.

The prognostic value of arthrometry after ACL reconstruction for functional outcome has yet to be established. Sgaglione and colleagues[152] reported that side-to-side differences (89-N anterior displacement force) of greater than 3 mm were significantly correlated with positive pivot shifts, lower scores using the Hospital for Special Surgery knee scoring system, and greater patient dissatisfaction with the reconstructive surgery. In contrast, in another study[127] no association was reported between KT-1000 measures (89 N) and single-leg hop tests, timed hop tests, Lysholom scores, Sports Activity Rating System scores, or Factor Occupational Rating System Scales. Tyler and colleagues[173] and Bach and associates[10] also reported the lack of association between arthrometry and functional tests or knee scoring systems. The results from these studies suggest that relying solely on arthrometric scores to define reconstruction failure may not be the most appropriate criteria. Tyler and colleagues[173] hypothesized that the reestablishment of a firm end point was more important to dynamic function of the knee than the amount of passive anterior displacement.

Isokinetic Tests

The knee has been studied isokinetically more than has any other joint.[47] Isokinetic testing can provide the clinician with valuable information about the isolated strength of muscles groups, either those damaged by injury or those that provide support to injured joints. Isokinetic testing of the knee has been shown to be extremely reliable, with ICCs as high as 0.99[109] for concentric contraction in asymptomatic subjects. Most of the studies reviewed by Perrin[138] had ICCs between 0.80 and 0.99. For eccentric contraction measures, isokinetic testing is still reliable but not to the same extent that concentric testing is, especially in subjects with knee injuries.[164] With eccentric testing, Steiner and colleagues[164] reported ICCs ranging from 0.58 to 0.96 for average peak torque, with the symptomatic subjects scoring lower. To ensure high retest reliability the clinician should make sure that the dynamometer axis is closely matched to the knee joint axis and that the athlete is positioned identically each time the test is performed.[138] This includes the accurate replacement of the resistance pad of the dynamometer on the leg. The joint should be tested only through pain-free motion. Allowing the athlete to warm up and perform practice repetitions at the testing speed also improves the reliability of the test.[138]

Isokinetic testing generally provides information on torque (peak or average), total work, and power. When test results of the quadriceps are compared to those of the hamstrings (agonist-to-antagonist comparisons), it is important to apply a gravity correction factor.[138] The often-quoted normal concentric peak torque hamstring-to-quadriceps ratio is 60%. This ratio for gravity-corrected measures is fairly accurate for slower testing velocities (60° per second), but as testing velocities increase, the ratio is usually greater than 60%. This occurs because the decrease in hamstring torque with increasing velocities is usually less than that of the quadriceps.[47,138] Dvir[47] has suggested that the hamstring-to-quadriceps ratio is generally not as important as the ratio developed by dividing the involved side measure by the uninvolved side measure. To illustrate this point, if an athlete produces 100 Nm of torque with the right quadriceps and 60 Nm of torque with the right hamstrings, the hamstring-to-quadriceps ratio is 60%. If an athlete produces a left quadriceps torque of 200 Nm and left hamstring torque of 120 Nm, then the left

side hamstring-to-quadriceps ratio is also 60%. A side-to-side comparison between the hamstring-to-quadriceps ratios would suggest that the legs were equal, but there is certainly a large deficit for the right thigh musculature torque production. Therefore, in most instances, it is recommended that injured-side muscle group test results be compared to results from the same muscle group on the uninjured-side. Another form of the hamstring-to-quadriceps ratio called the functional hamstring quadriceps ratio has been proposed.[1] The ratio for knee extension is determined by dividing the eccentric hamstring torque by concentric quadriceps torque. The ratio for knee flexion is determined by dividing the concentric hamstring torque by the eccentric quadriceps torque. Proponents of these ratios suggest that they are more in line with how the thigh muscles function during activities; however these ratios are not immune to the same problems illustrated above for the conventional hamstring-to-quadriceps ratio.

In making side-to-side comparisons it is important to consider the following testing principles. The placement of the dynamometer resistance pad must be the same on both legs, and both knees should be tested through the same ROM. Isokinetic total work measure is determined by the area under the torque curve. The y-axis for this measure is torque, and the x-axis is ROM. Thus, if the uninjured side is tested through a greater ROM, the total work for that side could be higher merely because it was performed through a greater ROM and not because it produced a higher torque curve.[138]

Using isokinetic testing with injured athletes does have to be done with caution and with an understanding of the joint forces produced during testing. Kaufman and associates[98] studied the joint forces during dynamic isokinetic testing and found significant compression forces for both the patellofemoral and the tibiofemoral joint. Patellofemoral joint compression forces were calculated to reach approximately 5.1 times BW at a knee angle of 70° to 75° during concentric testing at 60° per second. During concentric testing at 180° per second, the compression force was almost as high at 4.9 times BW. This suggests that the common premise that tests at higher speeds produce less joint compression is false. Fortunately at angles less than 20°, the patellofemoral compression forces dropped to less than BW. In this study tibiofemoral compression forces during knee extension peaked at approximately 55° of knee flexion during the 60° per second test and produced a force four times BW. The 180° per second test produced a force of 3.8 times BW. During knee extension, anterior shear of the tibiofemoral joint was greatest at about 25° of flexion and was calculated to be 0.3 times BW for testing at 60° per second and 0.2 times BW for the 180° per second test. Posterior shear force of the tibiofemoral joint during knee flexion peaked at approximately 75° of flexion force measured 1.7 times BW for the 60° per second test and 1.4 times BW for the 180° per second test.

Again, it is important to note that testing at 180° per second did very little to reduce the anterior and posterior shear forces compared with those that occurred at 60° per second.

It must be stressed that although isokinetic testing provides accurate measures of muscle torque, work, and power, this is not the only information that should be used to determine the readiness of an athlete to return to play. Results are mixed in studies examining the relationship between function and isokinetic tests. For example, Lephart and co-workers[108] reported very low, nonsignificant correlations between isokinetic tests and functional tests in ACL-deficient athletes. This study was designed to explore the differences between athletes who were able to return to sports with an ACL-deficient knee and those who were not. The scores on the functional tests in this study were significantly higher for those who returned to sports versus those unable to return.[108] On the other hand, Wilk and colleagues[179] reported correlation coefficients of 0.71 and 0.67 for the relationship between subjective knee scores and isokinetic scores in 50 patients with ACL reconstruction. They also reported significant correlations as high as 0.69 for the relationship between isokinetic performance and functional tests. Differences in methodology probably account for at least some of the discrepancies between studies. In general, there appears to be low to modest correlations between isokinetic test results and many of the functional hop and jump tests, especially when the subject sample was patients after a reconstruction of the ACL.[139,147] A possible reason for low to moderate correlations is that most of the studies used statistical analyses designed for testing the presence of a linear relationship between isokinetic test results and other measures of function. It is more likely that a curvilinear relationship exists, in that when the quadriceps and/or hamstrings are very weak there is a more profound impact on function, compared with minimal to moderate weakness. This effect would reduce the strength of relationships tested by statistics that assume a consistent linear relationship between variables.

Functional Tests

Functional testing of the lower extremity aids in determining the functional capabilities of the knee joint during sports activities. Functional tests can be used to determine limitations, which cannot be determined through muscle testing or arthrometry. This is evidenced by a report from Tibone and colleagues,[172] who examined functional abilities in ACL-deficient individuals. They reported isokinetic peak torque data for quadriceps and hamstrings of 86% and 96%, respectively, but this was not sufficient to eliminate the subjective need for ACL reconstruction.

Several functional tests have been used to assess functional performance objectively after ACL injury. Tegner and associates[170] have used one-legged hopping, figure-eight running, running up and down a spiral staircase, and running up and down a slope to evaluate functional knee integrity. They reported that athletes with ACL injuries performed significantly worse on these tests than uninjured athletes.

Barber and coworkers[14] evaluated the effectiveness of hopping and shuttle runs in determining lower extremity functional limitations in athletes with ACL-deficient knees. The hop tests included in this study were the one-legged hop for distance, the one-legged vertical jump, and the one-legged timed hop test. The scores on these tests were indexed and were considered abnormal if the performance of the involved lower extremity performance was less than 85% of that of the noninvolved lower extremity. The vertical jump test did not consistently detect functional limitations. By using results from either the one single-leg hop for distance or time test, 50% of patients with ACL-deficiency were identified; however, all patients with an ACL deficiency reported giving-way episodes, indicating a lack of sensitivity of these tests in defining functional limitations. If the results from both single-leg hop tests were combined, then 60% of the athletes with ACL-deficient knees performed abnormally (index less than 85%) on at least one of the two tests. Based on these findings, the authors[14] recommended that clinicians use two one-legged hop tests as a screening procedure to determine lower limb function, in addition to subjective complaints of giving-way.

A follow-up study from the same group[132] supported their previous results and further elucidated the clinical significance of hop test results on function. Four tests for appraising functional stability (Fig. 15-26): (1) one-legged hop for distance; (2) one-legged hop for time; (3) one-legged triple hop for distance; and (4) one-legged crossover hop for distance were examined. Using a side-to-side comparison of less than 85% to indicate an abnormal test result, they reported the sensitivity of the single-leg hop test to be 52% and the specificity to be 97%. The sensitivity of the timed single-leg hop test was 49% and the specificity was 94%. They only reported the sensitivity results for the cross-over hop and triple hop tests, which were 58% and 50%, respectively. Once again combining the test results from any two tests (which two did not matter) improved the overall sensitivity to 62%. From a clinical perspective these results indicate that in an athlete who has an abnormal hop test (index of less than 85%), functional status is compromised and he or she is probably not ready to return to sport. A normal hop test result, on the other hand, does not by itself indicate that the athlete is functionally ready to return to competition. The clinician needs to also consider the results from other assessments e.g., (arthrometry, isokinetics, and self-report functional status measures) in making the decision about the athlete's readiness to return to sport. This approach is supported by results from the study of Eastlack and associates[49] on pre-

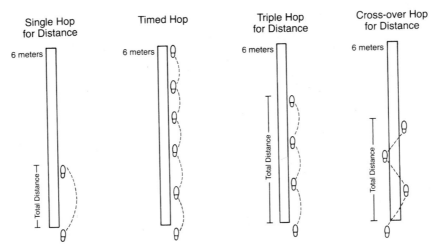

Figure 15-26. Four tests for appraising functional stability. (From Noyes, F.R., Barber, S.D., and Mangine, R.E. [1991]: Abnormal lower limb symmetry determined by function hop tests after anterior cruciate ligament rupture. Am. J. Sports Med., 19:513-518.)

dicting copers, those persons who can return to all preinjury activities without limitation after ACL injury. The subjects in this study performed a battery of functional tests, clinical tests, and self-report functional status measures. Combining the results from four of the study measures (global rating score, Knee Outcome Survey Sports portion, quadriceps strength, and crossover single-leg hop test), the authors reported a sensitivity of 97% and specificity of 92% in being able to separate copers from noncopers in their sample.

CLINICAL PEARL #4

When can the athlete return to play? The answer should be based at least in part on isolated muscle strength, self-report functional measures, a minimum of two functional tests, and arthrometry. With strength and functional side-to-side comparison tests, if an athlete scores less than 85% on any single test, they will probably have difficulty returning to sport. However, just because they score higher than 85% on any one or all tests does not necessarily mean they will not experience any difficulty returning to sport. It is always easier to determine who is not ready to return to sport than it is to determine who is ready.

The reliability of several functional hop tests has been established. The one-legged hop for distance appears to be one of the most reliable, with an ICC reported as high as 0.99.[24] The single-legged 6-m hop for time has a reported ICC of 0.77.[24] The ICC for a 30-m single-legged agility hop has been reported to be 0.09.[24] However, Booher and associates[24] still contend that the agility hop is a stable measure for clinical use because in their study the mean difference between trials was less than 0.5 second. Based on their 95% confidence intervals for the agility hop, a clinical difference of greater than ±2 seconds is probably

significant. The single-leg triple hop,[23] 6-m single-leg crossover hop,[23] and single-leg vertical jump[27] have reported ICC of 0.95, 0.97, and 0.96, respectively.

Most of the research efforts related to functional tests of the knee have been primarily concerned with the use of these tests for examining the function of the knee after a ligamentous injury. A number of functional tests have been described for the examination of athletes with patellofemoral dysfunction, but until recently the reliability of such tests has not been studied. Loudon and colleagues[115] reported the intrarater reliability of the following tests: crossover lunge (ICC = 0.82), 8 inch-step-down (ICC = 0.94), single-leg press (ICC = 0.82), bilateral squat (ICC = 0.79), and balance and reach (ICC = 0.83). The number of correctly performed repetitions the subject completed in 30 seconds served as the measure for all of these tests. In the unilateral tests, subjects with patellofemoral dysfunction performed significantly fewer repetitions with the involved lower extremity compared with the uninvolved side. Limb symmetry indexes (involved knee score/uninvolved knee score) for subjects with patellofemoral problems ranged from 80% to 90%, whereas indexes for those without patellofemoral problems ranged from 95% to 100%.

In their literature review of the use of hop tests to predict dynamic knee stability, Fitzgerald and associates[60] noted weak to no correlation between hop tests and arthrometry or self-report functional status measures and weak to moderate correlations between hop tests and isokinetic measures. By examining the results presented in their review it becomes apparent that each of these tests provides the clinician with a different measure of the injured athlete's status. In isolation, these measures do not sufficiently represent the athlete's ability to return to practice or competition. However, combining the data from arthrometry, functional tests, strength tests, and self-report measures of functional status, the clinician can reasonably extrapolate how an athlete will perform on the field and thus reduce the risk of reinjury.

SUMMARY

▓ Rehabilitation of the lower extremity should incorporate the appropriate balance of closed- and open-chain exercises along an increasing continuum of difficulty.

▓ In choosing exercises, one must understand the effect the exercises will have on both the tibiofemoral and the patellofemoral joint.

▓ Controlled motion, muscle recruitment, restoration of joint arthrokinematics, and control of inflammation should be the focus of any early phase rehabilitation program regardless of injury.

▓ The transition and advanced phases of rehabilitation should focus on developing muscle strength, power, endurance, and balance.

▓ Progression through all phases of rehabilitation should be guided by the athlete's ability to meet specific criteria and not simply by time alone.

▓ Functional testing and other measurements, such as arthrometry, self reported functional status, and isokinetic testing, should be used to assist in the determination of when an athlete can return to competition.

REFERENCES

1. Aagaard, P., Simonsen, E.B., Magnusson, S.P., et al. (1998): A new concept for isokinetic hamstring:quadriceps muscle strength ratio. Am. J. Sports Med., 26:231-237.

2. Alleyne, K.R., and Galloway, M.T. (2001): Management of osteochondral injuries of the knee. Clin. Sports Med., 10:343-364.

3. Amiel, D., Kleiner, J.B., and Akeson, W.H. (1986): The natural history of the anterior cruciate ligament autograft of patellar tendon origin. Am. J. Sports Med., 14:449-462.

4. Anderson, J.K., and Noyes, F.R. (1995): Principles of posterior cruciate ligament rehabilitation. Orthopedics, 18:493-500.

5. Arnheim, D.D. (1989): The knee and related structures. In: Modern Principles of Athletic Training, 7th ed. St. Louis, Times Mirror/Mosby College Publishing.

6. Arnoczky, S.P. (1994): Meniscus. In: Fu, F.H., Harner, C.D., and Vince, K.G. (eds.): Knee Surgery, Vol 1. Baltimore, Williams & Wilkins, pp. 131-140.

7. Arnoczky, S.P., Tarvin, G.B., and Marshall, J.L. (1982): Anterior cruciate ligament replacement using patellar tendon. J. Bone Joint Surg. Am., 64:217-224.

8. Arnoczky S.P., Warren R.F., and Ashlock MA. (1986): Replacement of the anterior cruciate ligament using a patellar tendon allograft. J. Bone Joint Surg. Am., 68: 376-385.

9. Aune, A.K., Holm, I., Risberg, M.A., et al. (2001): Four-strand hamstring tendon autograft compared with patellar tendon-bone autograft for anterior cruciate ligament reconstruction. Am. J. Sports Med., 29:722-728.

10. Bach, B.R., Jones, G.T., Hager, C.A., et al. (1995): Arthrometric results of arthroscopically assisted anterior cruciate ligament reconstruction using autograft patellar tendon substitution. Am. J. Sports Med., 23:179-185.

11. Bach, B.R., Warren, R.F., Flynn, W.M., et al. (1990): Arthrometric evaluation of knees that have a torn anterior cruciate ligament. J. Bone Joint Surg. Am., 12-A:1299-1306.

12. Ballantyne, B.T., French, A.K., Heimsoth, S.L., et al. (1995): Influence of examiner experience and gender on interrater reliability of KT-1000 arthrometer measurements. Phys. Ther., 75:898-906.

13. Barber, F.A. (1994): Accelerated rehabilitation for meniscus repairs. Arthroscopy, 10:206-210.

14. Barber, S.D., Noyes, F.R., Mangine, R.B., et al. (1990): Quantitative assessment of functional limitations in normal and anterior cruciate ligament-deficient knee. Clin. Orthop., 255:204-214.

15. Barber-Westin, S.D., Noyes, F.R., Heckmann, T.P., et al. (1999): The effect of exercise and rehabilitation on anterior-posterior knee displacements after anterior cruciate ligament autograft reconstruction. Am. J. Sports Med., 27:84-93.

16. Beard, D.J., Anderson, J.L., Davies, S., et al. (2001): Hamstrings vs. patella tendon for anterior cruciate ligament reconstruction: A randomised controlled trial. Knee, 8:45-50.

17. Beckman, M., Craig, R., and Lehman, R.C. (1989): Rehabilitation of patellofemoral dysfunction in the athlete. Clin. Sports Med., 8:841-861.

18. Berry, J., Kramer, K., Binkley, J., et al. (1999): Error estimates in novice and expert raters for the KT-1000 arthrometer. J. Orthop. Sports Phys. Ther., 29:49-55.

19. Beynnon, B.D., and Fleming, B.C. (1998): Anterior cruciate ligament strain in-vivo: A review of previous work. J. Biomech., 31:519-525.

20. Beynnon, B.D., Fleming, B.C., Johnson, R.J., et al. (1995): Anterior cruciate ligament strain behavior during rehabilitation exercises in vivo. Am. J. Sports Med., 23:24-34.

21. Beynnon, B.D., Johnson, R.J., Fleming, B.C., et al. (1997): The strain behavior of the anterior cruciate ligament during squatting and active flexion-extension: A comparison of an open and closed kinetic chain exercise. Am. J. Sports Med., 25:823-829.

22. Beynnon, B.D., Pope, M.H., Wertheimer, C.M., et al. (1992): The effect of functional knee-braces on strain on anterior cruciate ligament in vivo. J. Bone Joint Surg. Am., 74:1298-1312.

23. Bolgla, L.A., and Keskula, D.R. (1997): Reliability of lower extremity functional performance tests. J. Orthop. Sports Phys. Ther., 26:138-142.

24. Booher, L.D., Hench, K.M., and Worrell, T.W. (1993): Reliability of three single-leg hop tests. J. Sports Rehabil., 2:165-170.

25. Branch, T., Hunter, R., and Reynolds, P. (1988): Controlling anterior tibial displacement under static load: A comparison of two braces. Orthopedics, 11:1249-1252.

26. Brockroth, K., Wooden, C., Worrell, T., et al. (1993): The effects of patellar taping on patellar position and perceived pain. Med. Sci. Sports Exerc., 25:989-992.

27. Brosky, J.A., Nitz, A.J., Malone, T.R., et al. (1999): Intrarater reliability of selected clinical outcome measures following anterior cruciate ligament reconstruction. J. Orthop. Sports Phys. Ther., 19:39-48.

28. Buchanan, T.S., Kim, A.W., and Lloyd, D.G. (1996): Selective muscle activation following rapid varus/valgus perturbations at the knee. Med. Sci. Sports Exerc., 28:870-876.

29. Buckwalter, J.A. (1998): Articular cartilage: Injuries and potential for healing. J. Orthop. Sports Phys. Ther., 18:192-202.

30. Castle, T.H., Noyes, F.R., and Grood, E.S. (1992): Posterior tibial subluxation of the posterior cruciate-deficient knee. Clin. Orthop., 284:193-202.

31. Cerny, K. (1995): Vastus medialis oblique/vastus lateralis muscle activity ratios for selected exercises in person with and without patellofemoral pain syndrome. Phys. Ther., 75: 672-683.

32. Cerulli, G., Benoit, D.L., Caraffa, A., et al. (2001): Proprioceptive training and prevention of anterior cruciate ligament injuries in soccer. J. Orthop. Sports Phys. Ther., 31:655-660.

33. Clancy, W.G., Narechania, R.G., Rosenberg, T.D., et al. (1981): Anterior and posterior cruciate ligament reconstruction in rhesus monkeys. J. Bone Joint Surg. Am., 63:1270-1284.

34. Cook, F.F., Tibone, J.E., and Redfern, F.C. (1989): A dynamic analysis of a functional brace for anterior cruciate ligament insufficiency. Am. J. Sports Med., 17:519-524.

35. Cooper, D.E., Deng, X.H., Burstein, A.L., and Warren, R.F. (1993): The strength of the central third patellar tendon graft: A biomechanical study. Am. J. Sports Med., 21: 818-824.

36. Dahlkvist, N.J., Mayo, P., and Seedhom, B.B. (1982): Forces during squatting and rising from a deep squat. Eng. Med., 11: 69-76.

37. Daniel, D.M. (1990): The accuracy and reproducibility of the KT-1000 knee ligament arthrometer. http://medmetric.com/acc.htm, accessed 7/24/2002.

38. Daniel, D.M., Malcom, L.L., and Losse, G., et al. (1985): Instrumented measurement of anterior laxity of the knee. J. Bone Joint Surg. Am., 67:720-726.

39. Daniel, D.M., Stone, M.L., and Malcom, L., et al. (1983): Instrumented measurement of ACL disruption. Orthop. Res. Soc., 8:12-17.

40. Daniel, D.M., Stone, M.L., Sachs, R., et al. (1985): Instrumented measurement of anterior knee laxity in patients with acute anterior cruciate ligament disruption. Am. J. Sports Med., 13:401-407.

41. DeHaven, K.E. (1985): Rationale for meniscus repair or excision. Clin. Sports Med., 4:267-273.

42. DeMaio, M., Mangine, R.E., and Noyes, F.R. (1992): Advanced muscle training after ACL reconstruction: Weeks 6 to 52. Orthopedics, 15:757-767.

43. DeVita, P., Lassiter, T., Hortobagyi, T., et al. (1998): Functional knee brace effects during walking in patients with anterior cruciate ligament reconstruction. Am. J. Sports Med., 26:778-784.

44. Doucette, S.A., and Child, D.D. (1996): The effect of open and closed chain exercise and knee joint position on patellar tracking in lateral patellar compression syndrome. J. Orthop. Sports Phys. Ther., 23:104-110.

45. Doucette, S.A., and Goble, E.M. (1992): The effect of exercise on patellar tracking in lateral patellar compression syndrome. Am. J. Sports Med., 20:434-440.

46. Durselen, L., Claes, L., and Kiefer, H. (1995): The influence of muscle forces and external loads on cruciate ligament strain. Am. J. Sports Med., 23:129-136.

47. Dvir, Z. (1995): Isokinetics: Muscle Testing Interpretation and Clinical Applications. Edinburgh, Churchill Livingstone.

48. Eakin, C.L., and Cannon, W.D. (1998): Arthrometric evaluation of posterior cruciate ligament injuries. Am. J. Sports Med., 26:96-102.

49. Eastlack, M.E., Axe, M.J., and Snyder-Mackler, L. (1999): Laxity, instability, and functional outcome after ACL injury: Copers versus noncopers. Med. Sci. Sports Exerc., 31:210-215.

50. Eng, J.J., and Pierrynowski, M.R. (1993): Evaluation of soft foot orthotics in the treatment of patellofemoral pain syndrome. Phys. Ther., 73:62-68.

51. Engle, R.P. (1988): Hamstring facilitation in anterior instability of the knee. Athl. Train., 23:226-228, 285.

52. Engle, R.P., and Canner, G.G. (1989): Proprioceptive neuromuscular facilitation (PNF) and modified procedures for anterior cruciate ligament (ACL) instability. J. Orthop. Sports Phys. Ther., 11:230-236.

53. Engle, R.P., and Canner, G.C. (1989): Rehabilitation of symptomatic anterolateral knee instability. J. Orthop. Sports Phys. Ther., 11:237-244.

54. Ericson, M.O., and Nisell, R. (1986): Tibiofemoral joint forces during ergometer cycling. Am. J. Sports Med., 14:285-290.

55. Ericson, M.O., and Nisell, R. (1987): Patellofemoral joint forces during ergometer cycling. Phys. Ther., 67:1365-1369.

56. Escamilla, R.F., Fleisig, G.S., Zheng, N., et al. (1998): Biomechanics of the knee during closed kinetic chain and open kinetic chain exercises. Med. Sci. Sports Exerc., 30:556-569.

57. Fairbank, T.J. (1948): Knee joint changes after meniscectomy. J. Bone Joint Surg. Br., 30:664-670.

58. Fiebert, I., Gresly, J., Hoffman, S., et al. (1994). Comparative measurements of anterior tibial translation using a KT-1000 knee arthrometer with the leg in neutral, internal rotation, and external rotation. J. Orthop. Sports Phys. Ther., 19:331-334.

59. Fitzgerald, G.K., Axe, M.J., Snyder-Mackler, L., et al. (2000): The efficacy of perturbation training in nonoperative anterior cruciate ligament rehabilitation programs for physically active individuals. Phys. Ther., 80:128-140.

60. Fitzgerald, G.K., Lephart, S.M., Hwang, J.H., et al. (2001): Hop tests as predictors of dynamic knee stability. J. Orthop. Sports Phys. Ther., 31:588-597.

61. Flynn, T.W., and Soutas-Little, R.W. (1995): Patellofemoral joint compressive forces in forward and backward running. J. Orthop. Sports Phys. Ther., 21:277-282.

62. Fowler, P.J., and Lubliner, J. (1995): Functional anatomy and biomechanics of the knee joint. In: Griffin, L.Y. (ed.): Rehabilitation of the Injured Knee. St. Louis, C.V. Mosby.

63. Fowler, P.S. (1994): The ACL injury. In: 1994 Advances on the Knee and Shoulder. Cincinnati, Cincinnati Sports Medicine and Deaconess Hospital.

64. Friden, T., Zatterstrom, R., Anders, L., et al. (1991): Anterior cruciate-insufficient knees treated with physiotherapy. Clin. Orthop., 263:190-199.

65. Fu, F.H., Harner, C.D., Johnson, D.L., et al. (1993): Biomechanics of knee ligaments—Basic concepts and clinical application. J. Bone Joint Surg., 75A:1716-1727.

66. Fukubayashi, T., and Kurosawa, H. (1980): The contact area and pressure distribution pattern of the knee. Acta Orthop. Scand., 51:871-879.

67. Fulkerson, J.P., and Hungerford, D.S. (1990). Biomechanics of the patellofemoral joint. Disorders of the Patellofemoral Joint, 2nd ed. Baltimore, Williams & Wilkins, pp. 25-39.

68. Fuss, F.K. (1992): Principles and mechanisms of automatic rotation during terminal extension in the human knee joint. J. Anat., 180: 297-304.

69. Gillogly, S.D., Voight, M., and Blackburn, T. (1998): Treatment of articular cartilage defects of the knee with autologous chondrocyte implantation. J. Orthop. Sports Phys. Ther., 18:241-251.

70. Goh, J.C., Lee, PY.C., and Bose, K. (1995): A cadaver study of the function of the oblique part of vastus medialis. J. Bone Joint Surg. Br., 77: 225-231.

71. Gollehon, D.L., Torzilli, P.A., and Warren, R.F. (1987): The role of the posterolateral and cruciate ligaments in the stability of the human knee. J. Bone Joint Surg. Am., 69:233-242.

72. Goodfellow, J., Hungerford, D.S., and Zindel, M. (1976): Patellofemoral joint mechanics and pathology: 1. Functional anatomy of the patellofemoral joint. J. Bone Joint Surg. Br., 58:287-290.

73. Gough, J.V., and Ladley, G. (1971): An investigation into the effectiveness of various forms of quadriceps exercises. Physiotherapy, 57:356-361.

74. Grood, E.S., Noyes, F.R., Butler, D.L., et al. (1981): Ligamentous and capsular restraints preventing straight medial and lateral laxity in intact human cadaver knees. J. Bone Joint Surg. Am., 63:1257-1269.

75. Grood, E.S., Stowers, S.F., and Noyes, F.R. (1988): Limits of movement in the human knee. J. Bone Joint Surg. Am., 70: 88-97.

76. Grood, E.S., Suntay, W.J., Noyes, F.R., et al. (1984): Biomechanics of the knee-extension exercise. J. Bone Joint Surg. Am., 66:725-733.

77. Gross, M.T., Tyson, A.D., and Burns, C.B.B. (1993): Effect of knee angle and ligament insufficiency on anterior tibial translation during quadriceps muscle contraction: A preliminary report. J. Orthop. Sports Phys. Ther., 17:133-143.

78. Gryzlo, S.M., Patek, R.M., Pink, M., et al. (1994): Electromyographic analysis of knee rehabilitation exercises. J. Orthop. Sports Phys. Ther., 20:36-43.

79. Hanten, W.P., and Pace, M.B. (1987): Reliability of measuring anterior laxity of the knee joint using a knee ligament arthrometer. Phys. Ther., 67:357-359.

80. Hanten, W.P., and Schulthies, S.S. (1990): Exercise effect on electromyographic activity of the vastus medialis oblique and vastus lateralis muscles. Phys. Ther., 70:561-565.

81. Hardy, M.A. (1989): The biology of scar formation. Phys. Ther., 69:1014-1024.

82. Henning, C.E., Lynch, M.A., and Glick, K.R. (1985): An in vivo strain gauge study of elongation of the anterior cruciate ligament. Am. J. Sports Med., 13:22-26.

83. Hewett, T.E., Lindenfeld, T.N., Riccobene, J.V., et al. (1999): The effect of neuromuscular training on the incidence of knee injury in female athletes: A prospective study. Am. J. Sports Med., 27:699-706.

84. Hewett, T.E., Stroupe, A.L., Nance, T.A., et al. (1996): Plyometric training in female athletes: Decreased impact forces and increased hamstring torques. Am. J. Sports Med., 24: 765-773.

85. Host, J.V., Craig, R., and Lehman, R.C. (1995): Patellofemoral dysfunction in tennis players. Clin. Sports Med., 14:177-203.

86. Hsieh, Y.F., Draganich, L.F., Ho, S.H., et al. (2002): The effects of removal and reconstruction of the anterior cruciate ligament on the contact characteristics of the patellofemoral joint. Am. J. Sports Med., 30:121-127.

87. Huber, F.E., Irrgang, J.J., Harner, C., et al. (1997): Intratester and intertester reliability of the KT-1000 arthrometer in the assessment of posterior laxity of the knee. Am. J. Sports Med., 25:479-485.

88. Huberti, H.H., and Hayes, W.C. (1984): Patellofemoral contact pressure. J. Bone Joint Surg. Am., 55:715-724.

89. Hungerford, D.S., and Barry, M. (1979): Biomechanics of the patellofemoral joint. Clin. Orthop., 144:9-15.

90. Hughston, J.C., Walsh, W.M., and Puddu, G. (1984). Patellar Subluxation and Dislocation. Philadelphia, W.B. Saunders, pp. 1-20.

91. Ingersoll, C.D., and Knight, K.L. (1991): Patellar location changes following EMG biofeedback or progressive resistive exercises. Med. Sci. Sports Exerc., 23:1122-1127.

92. Irrgang, J.J., and Fitzgerald, G.K. (2000): Rehabilitation of the multiple-ligament-injured knee. Clin. Sports Med., 19:545-569.

93. Irrgang, J.J., and Pezzullo, D. (1998): Rehabilitation following surgical procedures to address articular cartilage lesions in the knee. J. Orthop. Sports Phys. Ther., 28:232-240.

94. Jenkins, W.L., Munns, S.W., and Loudon, J. (1998): Knee joint accessory motion following anterior cruciate ligament allograft reconstruction: A preliminary report. J. Orthop. Sports Phys. Ther., 28:32-39.

95. Johnson, D.L., Urban, W.P., Caborn, D.N.M., et al. (1998): Articular cartilage changes seen with magnetic resonance imaging, detected bone bruises associated with acute anterior cruciate ligament rupture. Am. J. Sports Med., 16:409-414.

96. Karst, G.M., and Jewett, P.D. (1993): Electromyographic analysis of exercises proposed for differential activation of medial and lateral quadriceps femoris muscle components. Phys. Ther., 73:286-295.

97. Karst, G.M, and Willett, G.M. (1995): Onset timing of electromyographic activity in the vastus medialis oblique and vastus lateralis muscle in subjects with and without patellofemoral pain syndrome. Phys. Ther., 75:813-823.

98. Kaufman, K.R., An, K., Litchy, W.J., et al. (1991): Dynamic joint forces during knee isokinetic exercise. Am. J. Sports Med., 19:305-316.

99. Kawai, Y., Fukubayashi, T., and Nishino, J. (1989): Meniscal suture: An experimental study in the dog. Clin. Orthop., 243:286-293.

100. Kennedy, J.C., Alexander, I.J., and Hayes, K.C. (1982): Nerve supply of the human knee and its functional importance. Am. J. Sports Med., 10:329-335.

101. King, S., Butterwick, D.J., and Cuerrier, J.P. (1986): The anterior cruciate ligament: A review of recent concepts. J. Orthop. Sports Phys. Ther., 8:110-122.

102. Kocher, M.S., Saxon, H.S., Hovis, W.D., et al. (2002): Management and complications of anterior cruciate ligament injuries in skeletally immature patients: Survey of the Herodicus Society and the ACL Study Group. J. Pediatr. Orthop., 22:452-457.

103. Kowall, M.G., Kolk, G., Nuber, G.W., et al. (1996): Patellar taping in the treatment of patellofemoral pain. A prospective radiographic study. Am. J. Sports Med., 24: 61-66.

104. Kramer, P.G. (1986): Patella malalignment syndrome: Rationale to reduce excessive lateral pressure. J. Orthop. Sports Phys. Ther., 8:301-309.

105. Krause, W.R., Pope, M.H., Johnson, R.J., et al. (1976): Mechanical changes in the knee after meniscectomy. J. Bone Joint Surg. Am., 58:599-604.

106. Kvist, J., and Gillquist, J. (2001): Sagittal plane knee translation and electromyographic activity during closed and open kinetic

chain exercises in anterior cruciate ligament-deficient patients and control subjects. Am. J. Sports Med., 29:72-82.

107. Lane, J.G., Irby, S.E., Kaufman, K., et al. (1994): The anterior cruciate ligament in controlling axial rotation. Am. J. Sports Med., 22:289-293.

108. Lephart, S.M., Perrin, D.H., Fu, F.H., et al. (1992): Relationship between selected physical characteristics and functional capacity in the anterior cruciate ligament-insufficient athlete. J. Orthop. Sports Phys. Ther., 16:174-181.

109. Levene, J.A., Hart, B.A., Seeds, R.H., et al. (1991): Reliability of reciprocal isokinetic testing of the knee extensors and flexors. J. Orthop. Sports Phys. Ther., 14:1221-1227.

110. Lieb, F.J., and Perry, J. (1968): Quadriceps function: An anatomical and mechanical study using amputated limbs. J. Bone Joint Surg. Am., 50:1535-1548.

111. Lieb, F.J., and Perry, J. (1971): Quadriceps function: An electromyographic study under isometric conditions. J. Bone Joint Surg. Am., 53:749-758.

112. Limbird, T.J., Shiavi, R., Frazer, M., et al. (1988): EMG profiles of knee joint musculature during walking: Changes induced by anterior cruciate ligament deficiency. J. Orthop. Res., 6:630-638.

113. Liu, S.H., Ost, L., Henry, M., et al. (1995): The diagnosis of acute complete tears of the anterior cruciate ligament: Comparison of MRI, arthrometry, and clinical examination. J Bone Joint Surg Br., 77-B:586-588.

114. Lloyd, D.G. (2001): Rationale for training programs to reduce anterior cruciate ligament injuries in Australian football. J. Orthop. Sports Phys. Ther., 31:645-654.

115. Loudon, J.K., Wiesner, D., Goist-Foley, H.L., et al. (2002): Intrarater reliability of functional performance tests for subjects with patellofemoral pain syndrome. J. Athl. Train., 37:256-261.

116. Lutz, G.E., Stuart, M.J., and Sim, F.H. (1990): Rehabilitative techniques for athletes after reconstruction of the anterior cruciate ligament. Mayo Clin. Proc., 65:1322-1329.

117. Mangine, R.E., Noyes, F.R., and DeMaio, M. (1992): Minimal protection program: Advanced weight bearing and range of motion after ACL reconstruction—Weeks 1 to 5. Orthopedics, 15:504-515.

118. Markolf, K.L., Bargar, W.L., Shoemaker, S.C., et al. (1981): The role of joint load in knee stability. J. Bone Joint Surg. Am., 63:570-585.

119. Markolf, K.L., Mensch, J.S., and Amstutz, H.C. (1976): Stiffness and laxity of the knee—The contributions of the supporting structures. J. Bone Joint Surg. Am., 58, 583.

120. McConnell, J. (1986): The management of chondromalacia patellae: A long-term solution. Aust. J. Physiother., 32:215-223.

121. McGinty, J.B., Guess, L.F., and Marvin, R.A. (1977): Partial or total meniscectomy: A comparative analysis. J. Bone Joint Surg. Am., 59:763-766.

122. McLaughlin, J., DeMaio, M., Noyes, F.R., et al. (1994): Rehabilitation after meniscus repair. Orthopedics, 17:463-471.

123. Micheli, L.J., Rask, B., and Gerberg, L. (1999): Anterior cruciate ligament reconstruction in patients who are prepubescent. Clin. Orthop., 364:40-47.

124. Millett, P.J., Wickiewicz, T.L., and Warren, R.F. (2001): Motion loss after ligament injuries to the knee. Am. J. Sports Med., 29:664-675.

125. Mishra, D.V., Daniel, D.M., and Stone, M.L. (1989): The use of functional knee braces in the control of pathologic anterior knee laxity. Clin. Orthop., 241:213-220.

126. Myrer, J.W., Schulthies, S.S., and Fellingham, G.W. (1996): Relative and absolute reliability of the KT-2000 arthrometer for uninjured knees. Am. J. Sports Med., 24:104-108.

127. Neeb, T.B., Aufdemkampe, G., Wagener, J.H.D., et al. (1997): Assessing anterior cruciate ligament injuries: The association and differential value of questionnaires, clinical tests, and functional tests. J. Orthop. Sports Phys. Ther., 26:324-331.

128. Nemeth, G., Lamontagne, M., Tho, K.S., et al. (1997): Electromyographic activity in expert downhill skiers using functional knee braces after anterior cruciate ligament injuries. Am. J. Sports Med., 25:635-641.

129. Nisell, R., Ericson, M.O., Nemeth, G., et al. (1989): Tibiofemoral joint forces during isokinetic knee extension. Am. J. Sports Med., 17:49-54.

130. Norkin, C.C., and Levange, P.K. (1992): The knee complex. In: Joint Structure and Function: A Comprehensive Analysis, 2nd ed. Philadelphia, F.A. Davis, pp. 337-377.

131. Noyes, F.R. (1989): Rules for surgical indications in ACL surgery. In: 1989 Advances on the Knee and Shoulder. Cincinnati, Cincinnati Sports Medicine and Deaconess Hospital.

132. Noyes, F.R., Barber, S.D., and Mangine, R.E. (1991): Abnormal lower limb symmetry determined by function hop test after anterior cruciate ligament rupture. Am. J. Sports Med., 19:513-518.

133. Noyes, F.R., Barber-Westin, S., and Roberts, C. (1994): Use of allografts after failed treatment of rupture of the anterior cruciate ligament. J. Bone Joint Surg. Am., 76:1019-1031.

134. Noyes, F.R., Butler, D.L., Grood, E.S., et al. (1984): Biomechanical analysis of human ligament grafts used in knee-ligament repairs and reconstructions. J. Bone Joint Surg. Am., 66:344-352.

135. Noyes, F.R., Matthews, D.S., Mooar, P.A., et al. (1983): The symptomatic anterior cruciate-deficient knee. Part I: The long-term functional disability in athletically active individuals. J. Bone Joint Surg. Am., 65:163-174.

136. Noyes, F.R., Matthews, D.S., Mooar, P.A., et al. (1983): The symptomatic anterior cruciate-deficient knee. Part II: The results of rehabilitation, activity modification, and counseling on functional disability. J. Bone Joint Surg. Am., 65:154-162.

137. Ohkoshi, Y., Yasuda, K., Kaneda, K., et al. (1991): Biomechanical analysis of rehabilitation in the standing position. Am. J. Sports Med., 19:605-611.

138. Perrin, D.H. (1993): Isokinetic Exercise and Assessment. Champaign, IL, Human Kinetics.

139. Petschnig, R., Baron, R., and Albrecht, M. (1998): The relationship between isokinetic quadriceps strength test and hop tests for distance and one-legged vertical jump test following anterior cruciate ligament reconstruction. J. Orthop. Sports Phys. Ther., 28:23-31.

140. Pocock, G.S. (1963): Electromyographic study of the quadriceps during resistive exercise. J. Am. Phys. Ther. Assoc., 43:427-434.

141. Powers, C.M. (1998): Rehabilitation of patellofemoral joint disorders: A critical review. J. Orthop. Sports Phys. Ther., 28:345-354.

142. Queale, W.S., Snyder-Mackler, L., Handling, K.A., et al. (1994): Instrumented examination of knee laxity in patients with ante-

rior cruciate deficiency: A comparison of the KT-2000, Knee Signature System, and Genucom. J. Orthop. Sports Phys. Ther., 19:345-351.

143. Quillen, W.S., and Gieck, J.H. (1988): Manual therapy: Mobilization of the motion restricted knee. Athl. Train., 23: 123-130.

144. Reilly, D.T., and Martens, M. (1972): Experimental analysis of the quadriceps muscle force and patellofemoral joint reaction force for various activities. Acta Orthop. Scand., 43:126-137.

145. Reynolds, L., Levin, T.A., Medeiros, J.M., et al. (1983): EMG activity of the vastus medialis oblique and the vastus lateralis in their role in patellar alignment. Am. J. Phys. Med., 62:61-70.

146. Risberg, M.A., Holm, I., Steen H., et al. (1999): The effect of knee bracing after anterior cruciate ligament reconstruction: A prospective, randomized study with two years' follow-up. Am. J. Sports Med., 27:76-83.

147. Risberg, M.A., Holm, I., Tjomsland, O., et al. (1999): Prospective study of changes in impairments and disabilities after anterior cruciate ligament reconstruction. J. Orthop. Sports Phys. Ther., 29:400-412.

148. Rowinski, M.J. (1985): Afferent neurobiology of the joint. In: Gould, J.A., and Davies, G.J. (eds.): Orthopedic and Sports Physical Therapy. St. Louis, C.V. Mosby.

149. Rubenstein, R.A., and Shelbourne, K.D. (1993): Diagnosis of posterior cruciate ligament injuries and indications for nonoperative and operative treatment. Operative Tech. Sports Med., 1:118-127.

150. Schaub, P.A., and Worrell, T.W. (1995): EMG activity of six muscles and VMO:VL ratio determination during a maximal squat exercise. J. Sports Rehabil., 4:195-202.

151. Scott, S.H, and Winter, D.A. (1990): Internal forces at chronic running injury sites. Med. Sci. Sports Exerc., 22: 357-369.

152. Sgaglione, N.A., Warren, R.F., Wickiewicz, T.L., et al. (1990): Primary repair with semitendinosus tendon augmentation of acute anterior cruciate ligament injuries. Am. J. Sports Med., 18:64-73.

153. Shaieb, M.D., Kan, D.M., Chang, S.K., et al. (2002): A prospective randomized comparison of patellar tendon versus semitendinosus and gracilis tendon autografts for anterior cruciate ligament reconstruction. Am. J. Sports Med., 30: 214-220.

154. Skyhar, M.J., Warren, R.F., Ortiz, G.J., et al. (1993): The effects of sectioning the posterior cruciate ligament and posterolateral complex on the articular pressures within the knee. J. Bone Joint Surg. Am., 75:694-699.

155. Sledge, S.L. (2001): Microfracture techniques in the treatment of osteochondral injuries. Clin. Sports Med., 20:365-377.

156. Snyder-Mackler, L., DeLitto, A., Bailey, S.I., et al. (1995): Strength of the quadriceps femoris muscle and functional recovery after reconstruction of the anterior cruciate ligament. J. Bone Joint Surg. Am., 77:1166-1173.

157. Snyder-Mackler, L., DeLuca, P.F., Williams, P.R., et al. (1994): Reflex inhibition of the quadriceps femoris muscle after injury or reconstruction of the anterior cruciate ligament. J. Bone Joint Surg. Am., 76:555-560.

158. Soames, R.W. (1995): Skeletal system. In: Gray's Anatomy, 38th ed. New York, Churchill Livingstone.

159. Soderberg, G.L. (1986): Kinesiology: Application to Pathological Motion. Baltimore, Williams & Wilkins.

160. Soderberg, G.L., and Cook, T.M. (1983): An electromyographic analysis of quadriceps femoris muscle setting and straight leg raising. Phys. Ther., 63:1434-1438.

161. Speakman, H.G.B., and Weisberg, J. (1977): The vastus medialis controversy. Physiotherapy, 63:249-254.

162. Spencer, J.D., Hayes, K.C., and Alexander, I.J. (1984): Knee joint effusion and quadriceps reflex inhibition in man. Arch. Phys. Med. Rehabil., 65:171-177.

163. Sprague, R.B. (1982): Factors related to extension lag at the knee joint. J. Orthop. Sports Phys. Ther., 3:178-181.

164. Steiner, L.A., Harris, B.A., and Krebs, D.E. (1993): Reliability of eccentric isokinetic knee flexion and extension measurements. Arch. Phys. Med. Rehabil., 74:1327-1335.

165. Steiner, M.E., Koskinen, S.K., Winalski, C.S., et al. (2001): Dynamic lateral patellar tilt in the anterior cruciate ligament-deficient knee. Am. J. Sports Med., 29:593-599.

166. Steinkamp, L.A., Dillingham, M.F., Markel, M.D., et al. (1993): Biomechanical considerations in patellofemoral joint rehabilitation. Am. J. Sports Med., 21:438-444.

167. Stuart, M.J., Meglan, D.A., Lutz, E.S., et al. (1996): Comparison of intersegmental tibiofemoral joint forces and muscle activity during various closed chain exercises. Am. J. Sports Med., 14:792-799.

168. Styf, J. (1999): The effects of functional bracing on muscle function and performance. Sports Med., 28:77-81.

169. Takeda, Y., Xerogeanes, J.W., Livesay, G.A., et al. (1994): Biomechanical function of the human anterior cruciate ligament. Arthroscopy, 10:140-147.

170. Tegner, Y., Lysholm, J., Lysholm, M., et al. (1986): A performance test to monitor rehabilitation and evaluate anterior cruciate ligament injuries. Am. J. Sports Med., 14:156-159.

171. Threlkeld, A.J., Horn, T.S., Wojtowicz, G.M., et al. (1989): Kinematics, ground reaction force, and muscle balance produced by backward running. Orthop. Sports Phys. Ther., 11:56-63.

172. Tibone, J.E., and Antich, T.J. (1988): A biomechanical analysis of anterior cruciate ligament reconstruction with the patellar tendon. Am. J. Sports Med., 16:332-333.

173. Tyler, T.F., McHugh, M.P., Gleim, G.W., et al. (1999): Association of KT-1000 measurements with clinical tests of knee stability 1 year following anterior cruciate ligament reconstruction. J. Orthop. Sports Phys. Ther., 29:540-545.

174. Vailas, J.C., and Pink, M. (1993): Biomechanical effects of functional knee bracing. Sports Med., 15:210-218.

175. Voight, M.L., and Wieder, D.L. (1991): Comparative reflex response times of vastus medialis obliquus and vastus lateralis in normal subjects and subjects with extensor mechanism dysfunction. Am. J. Sports Med., 19:131-137.

176. Watson, C.J., Propps, M., Galt, W., et al. (1999): Reliability of McConnell's classification of patellar orientation in symptomatic and asymptomatic subjects. J. Orthop. Sports Phys. Ther., 19:378-385.

177. Wilk, K.E. (1994): Rehabilitation of isolated and combined posterior cruciate ligament injuries. Clin. Sports Med., 13:649-677.

178. Wilk, K.E., Arrigo, C., Andrews, A.R., et al. (1999): Rehabilitation after anterior cruciate ligament reconstruction in the female athlete. J. Athl. Train., 34:177-193.

179. Wilk, K.E., Romaniello, W.T., Soscia, S.M., et al. (1994): The relationship between subjective knee scores, isokinetic testing, and functional testing in the ACL-reconstructed knee. J. Orthop. Sports Phys Ther., 20:60-73.

180. Wojtys, E.M., Kothari S.U., and Huston, L.J. (1996): Anterior cruciate ligament functional brace use in sports. Am. J. Sports Med., 24:539-546.

181. Worrell, T.W., Connelly, S., and Hilvert, J. (1995): VMO:VL ratios and torque comparisons at four angles of knee flexion. J. Sports Rehabil., 4:264-272.

182. Yack, H.J., Collins, C.E., and Whieldon, T.J. (1993): Comparison of closed and open kinetic chain exercise in the anterior cruciate ligament-deficient knee. Am. J. Sports Med., 21:49-54.

183. Yack, H.J., Riley, L.M., and Whieldon, T.R. (1994): Anterior tibial translation during progressive loading of the ACL-deficient knee during weight-bearing and nonweight-bearing isometric exercise. J. Orthop. Sports Phys. Ther., 20:247-253.

CHAPTER 16

HAMSTRING, QUADRICEPS, AND GROIN REHABILITATION

Greg Gardner, Ed.D., ATC
James B. Gallaspy, M.Ed., ATC

CHAPTER OBJECTIVES

At the end of this chapter the reader will be able to:

- Identify common muscular injuries to the quadriceps, hamstring, and groin areas.
- Explain the application of cryostretching in the rehabilitation of muscular injuries to the quadriceps, hamstring, and groin muscle groups.
- Recognize appropriate activities to increase muscular strength and endurance for the hamstring, quadriceps, and groin muscle groups.
- Identify appropriate functional activities for rehabilitation of quadriceps, hamstring, and groin injuries.

The quadriceps, hamstrings, adductor group, sartorius, and tensor fasciae latae constitute the thigh muscles and are subject to extreme forces as they propel the body under various degrees of resistance.[7] Muscle strains are the most common injury to the hamstrings and adductors, whereas contusions rank as the primary injury to the quadriceps.[3] Strains involving the quadriceps occur less often than do hamstring strains because of the great strength and size of the quadriceps muscle.[10] Strains involve injury to the muscle, tendon, musculotendinous junction, or tendon-bone attachment. They can result from muscle imbalance, poor flexibility, overstretching, violent muscle contraction against heavy resistance, idiosyncrasy of nerve innervation, or leg length discrepancy.[2,3,5,10,13,17]

Strains are graded by their degree of severity. Each is determined by the amount of muscle or tendon damage and is labeled as mild, moderate, or severe (or first, second, or third degree). Athletes suffering a muscle strain present with the signs and symptoms shown in Table 16-1. The use of magnetic resonance imaging in the evaluation of muscle injuries offers definitive evidence of the severity of the injury.[4] This information can also act as a valuable guide in predicting the length of the rehabilitation process.[19]

The goals in treating muscle strains are to reduce pain, restore muscle function, and reduce the likelihood of reinjury. Restoration of muscle length is important in reinjury prevention, because a shortened muscle is more susceptible to strains.[1,5,18]

Initial treatment of strains and contusions consists of ice, compression, elevation, and rest, along with the use of nonsteroidal anti-inflammatory drugs to decrease inflammation.[3,9,10] Additional modalities such as pulsed ultrasound to decrease hematoma formation, without the adverse effects of increasing tissue temperature (as with continuous ultrasound in the early stages of healing), and electrical stimulation to decrease pain and inflammation can be beneficial.[22] The use of deep-water pool exercises is excellent during the early phases of the rehabilitation program (see Chapter 12). An elastic wrap (e.g., SurgiGrip*) or other supporting orthosis should be used in the early stages of treatment to provide compression, and use should be continued throughout the rehabilitation program to support the thigh.

The restoration of muscle length precedes muscle strengthening unless the length of the injured muscle is equal to or greater than that of the uninjured muscle.[6] The passive stretching process used in restoration of muscle length, when appropriate, actually aids in increasing the tensile strength of the replacement scar tissue.[14] The decision on when to begin restoring muscle length is critical and depends on the athlete's response to stretching. If intense or moderate pain develops in the injured muscle before the athlete perceives a stretch, the injured muscle is not ready for stretching.[6] When the athlete can feel the muscle stretch before or with pain, stretching may begin.

---

*Available from Western Medical Ltd., Tenatly, New Jersey.

Table 16-1

Signs and Symptoms of Muscle Strains

Severity	Symptoms	Signs
Mild (first degree)	Local pain, mild pain on passive stretch and active contraction of the involved muscle; minor disability	Mild spasm, swelling, ecchymosis; local tenderness; minor loss of function and strength
Moderate (second degree)	Local pain; moderate pain on passive stretch and active contraction of the involved muscle; moderate disability	Moderate spasm, swelling, ecchymosis, local tenderness; impaired muscle function and strength
Severe (third degree)	Severe pain; disability	Severe spasm; swelling, ecchymosis, hematoma; tenderness, loss of muscle function; palpable defect may be present

In mild to moderate strains, stretching can begin within 2 to 7 days of injury. Muscle strengthening can begin when the muscle can tolerate strengthening with light resistance that is pain-free. The rehabilitation program should include active and passive stretching, proprioceptive neuromuscular facilitation (PNF) stretching and strengthening techniques, and isometric, isotonic, and isokinetic strengthening exercises.

CLINICAL PEARL #1

Restoration of muscle length must precede the initiation of muscular strengthening activities.

If low-grade muscle spasm is present, the use of cryostretching, as described by Knight,[15] may be beneficial. This technique consists of cold applications and the PNF technique of hold-relax[15] (Box 16-1). Although it is similar to cryokinetics in that exercise is performed while the body part is numbed, cryostretching differs with regard to the number of exercise sets and the exercise itself.[15] During cryostretch the affected muscle is alternately stretched statically and contracted isometrically.[15]

Knight[15] has also proposed a neuromuscular training session before the first initial exercise session; this may be done before or immediately after ice application but before the first exercise bout. The purpose of this session is to help the athlete "get the feel" of contracting the proper muscle group. Sometimes, without this session, the athlete contracts both the agonist and the antagonist muscle group when asked to contract the muscle in spasm. During the neuromuscular training session the clinician moves the appropriate body part in a direction that elongates the muscle in spasm. The athlete is then asked to return the body part to the anatomic position, which requires contracting the affected muscle. This is repeated three to four times, always within a comfortable range of motion.

The stretchings consist of 65-second exercise bouts, with a static stretch interspersed with three isometric contractions of about 5 seconds each, as outlined in Box 16-1. The exercise is begun by stretching the affected muscle until pain or tightness is incurred; the athlete backs off just a little until the pain disappears and holds the limb in that position for 20 seconds. The athlete then begins a slow contraction of the muscle with the spasm, building up to a maximal muscle contraction. A second stretch is held for 10 seconds, followed by a second isometric contraction of about 5 seconds. The athlete moves forward again so that tightness or slight pain is felt in the traumatized area, and a 10-second stretch is repeated. Finally, the body part is rested in the anatomic position for 20 seconds, and the 65-second exercise bout is repeated as outlined above.

Box 16-1

Cryostretching Procedure

1. Numb with ice (20 minutes maximum)
2. Exercise
   A. First exercise bout (65 seconds total)
      (1) Static stretch (20 seconds)
      (2) Isometric contraction (5 seconds)
      (3) Static stretch (10 seconds)
      (4) Isometric contraction (5 seconds)
      (5) Static stretch (10 seconds)
      (6) Isometric contraction (5 seconds)
      (7) Static stretch (10 seconds)
   B. Rest (20 seconds)
   C. Second exercise bout (65 seconds total; same as first exercise bout)
3. Renumb with ice (3 to 5 minutes)
4. Exercise—two bouts and rest as in step 2
5. Renumb with ice (3 to 5 minutes)
6. Exercise—two bouts and rest as in step 2

Data from Knight, K.L. (1995): Cryotherapy in Sports Injury Management. Champaign, IL, Human Kinetics, pp. 233-239.

Box 16-2

Procedure for Combination of Cryostretching and Cryokinetics

1. Numb with ice for 15 to 20 minutes
2. Perform cryostretch exercise
3. Renumb
4. Perform cryokinetic exercise
5. Renumb
6. Perform cryokinetic exercise
7. Renumb
8. Perform cryokinetic exercise
9. Renumb
10. Perform cryostretch exercise

Data from Knight, K.L. (1995): Cryotherapy in Sports Injury Management. Champaign, IL, Human Kinetics, pp. 233-239.

Second and third renumbing sequences are also carried out.

Once muscle spasm begins to abate (often within 2 or 3 days) a combination of cryostretching and cryokinetics can be implemented[15] (Box 16-2).

Cryokinetic exercise should begin with manual, resisted muscle contractions through a full range of motion and progress to isotonic, isokinetic, and functional drills. The use of cryostretch and cryokinetic techniques should not be overlooked in the early phases of rehabilitation as methods to return muscular strength and endurance to their preinjury level sooner. Progressive-resistance exercise can begin when tolerated, with an emphasis on eccentric exercises.[3,9,10]

CLINICAL PEARL #2

Therapeutic objectives for the initial phase of hamstring, quadriceps, and groin injuries focus on controlling and/or reducing symptoms of the injury.

HAMSTRING REHABILITATION

Hamstring strain is one of the most common and frustrating injuries that an athlete can incur; it can also recur often.[10,12,13,16,23] The biceps femoris, laterally, and the semitendinosus and semimembranosus, medially, compose the hamstring muscle group. These muscles function in knee flexion, hip extension, and internal and external rotation of the tibia and antagonistically resist knee extension.[1,2,8] The semimembranosus also dynamically reinforces the posterior and medial knee capsular structures, retracts the medial meniscus posteriorly, and supports the anterior cruciate ligament to prevent anterior tibial translation.[25] The tendons of insertion of the semitendinosus, sartorius, and gracilis form the pes anserinus, which inserts on the proximomedial aspect of the tibia.[25] Cumulatively, the hamstrings support the anterior cruciate ligament to help prevent anterior excursion of the tibia on the femur and to assist the medial capsule and medial collateral ligament.[8] The hamstrings perform an important role in walking and assume an extensor action with heel strike.[12,25] During running, the hamstrings are active longer during the swing and early stance phases of gait.[12]

Hamstring injuries usually occur during sprinting or high-speed exercises (e.g., in a sprinter leaving the block, in the lead leg of a hurdler, or in a jumper's takeoff leg).[12,17] Hamstring strains can have various causes: (1) a sudden change from a stabilizing flexor to an active extensor, combined with muscle imbalance between the quadriceps and hamstrings; (2) poor flexibility; (3) faulty posture; and (4) leg length discrepancy. All are potential mechanisms for hamstring injuries.[2,3,10,13,17] The short head of the biceps femoris is most often injured; it is believed to contract simultaneously with the quadriceps muscle as a result of an idiosyncrasy in nerve innervation, thus contributing to the high injury rate of this hamstring muscle.[3,8,13,18] It has been suggested that hamstring strength should be 60% to 70% that of the antagonist quadriceps to help prevent hamstring injuries.[1,3,17]

The clinician should perform active, passive, and resisted knee flexion and hip extension tests to determine injury severity. Usually, the amount of knee extension the athlete can achieve while prone indicates injury severity. Once severity has been ascertained, treatment can proceed as outlined in Table 16-2.

In the acute stage, emphasis is on reducing inflammation, pain, and spasm through the use of appropriate modalities. Depending on injury severity, at about day 2 to 4 postinjury, athletes can begin a stretching program within their pain-free range. Initially, the injured extremity can be stretched in the prone position using the uninvolved extremity to control the amount of hamstring stretch achieved (Fig. 16-1). As pain decreases and elasticity increases, a more aggressive stretching program can be implemented (Fig. 16-2). The exercise session should be terminated with cryotherapy, and a traction weight is used above the knee to facilitate lengthening of the hamstring muscle with the spasm (Fig. 16-3).

Later in the rehabilitation process, isokinetic equipment can be used at higher speeds because of the high percentage of type II or fast-twitch muscle fibers located in the hamstrings.[12,25] The hamstrings can be isolated isokinetically to a greater degree by having the athlete lie prone or by having the athlete lean forward while in the traditional seated position. Isokinetic equipment can also be used to obtain data that can aid in determining when the athlete has reached the optimal hamstring-to-quadriceps ratio for deterring injury.

The athlete can also use surgical tubing (Fig. 16-4) for high-speed resistance exercise to fatigue in hip flexion, extension, abduction, and adduction and in knee flexion

Table 16-2

Progression for Hamstring Rehabilitation

I. Initial Phase
    A. R.I.C.E. (rest, ice, compression, elevation)
    B. Tubi-Grip for effusion
    C. Modalities
        1. Pulsed ultrasound
        2. Electrical stimulation
        3. Ice postexercise
    D. Cryostretching and cryokinetics with the following exercises:
        1. Hamstring setting
        2. Co-contractions
        3. Heel slides (seated and supine)
        4. Active hamstring curls
        5. Active hip extensions
        6. Single-leg hamstring stretches to tolerance
    E. Aquatic therapy
    F. Active range of motion, as tolerated

II. Intermediate Phase
    A. Stationary bike, StairMaster
    B. Modalities
        1. Continuous ultrasound
        2. Moist heat
    C. Hamstring stretching
        1. Single-leg hamstring stretches
        2. Straddle groin and hamstring stretches
        3. Side straddle and hamstring stretches
        4. Supine assisted hamstring stretches
    D. Progressive-resistance exercise
        1. Hamstring curl
        2. Hip extensions
        3. Hip adduction and abduction
        4. Straight leg raises
    E. Proprioceptive exercise
    F. Prophylactic cryotherapy
    G. Increased pool program
    H. Proprioceptive neuromuscular facilitation patterns
    I. Beginning of functional activity progression
        1. Forward and backward walking or jogging (use neoprene sleeve for support)

III. Advanced Phase
    A. High-speed isokinetic exercise (seated and prone)
    B. Eccentric hamstring curls
    C. Functional drills
        1. Jogging or running (forward and backward)
        2. Jogging or running (uphill, backward)
        3. Slide Board, if available
        4. Lateral drills
    D. High-speed surgical tubing exercises in hip flexion, extension, abduction, and adduction and in knee flexion and minisquats
    E. Protective wrapping

(hamstring curls) or can use the Inertia machine*, if available, in the above planes.

The athlete may return to unlimited participation, wearing a neoprene sleeve for support and proprioception, when the following criteria are met:

---

*Available from E.M.A., Newnan, Georgia.

1. Hamstring flexibility is equal bilaterally.
2. Muscular strength, power, endurance, and time to peak torque, as measured by an isokinetic dynamometer, are 85% to 90% of those of the contralateral limb.
3. Hamstring strength is 60% to 70% that of the quadriceps.
4. No symptoms are noted with functional activities.

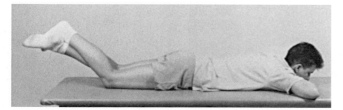

Figure 16-1. Use of the prone position and the uninvolved leg to promote hamstring elasticity. This can be used in conjunction with cryotherapy techniques.

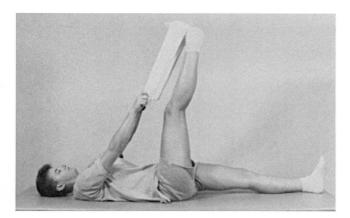

Figure 16-2. Single-leg hamstring stretch with towel. The uninvolved leg is kept flat on the table.

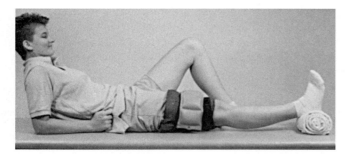

Figure 16-3. Use of a traction weight with cryotherapy postexercise to facilitate the return of hamstring length.

QUADRICEPS REHABILITATION

Quadriceps injuries are a common occurrence in sports. The quadriceps muscle is subject to both strains and contusions, with the latter having a higher incidence.[2,3] The quadriceps musculature is composed of the rectus femoris, vastus medialis, vastus lateralis, and vastus intermedius muscles. Its static role is to prevent knee buckling while standing, and its dynamic function is to extend the knee forcefully, as in running or jumping exercises. The rectus

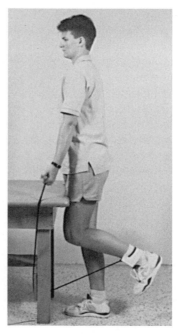

Figure 16-4. Hamstring curls with surgical tubing can be performed at varying rates to fatigue to help increase muscle endurance.

femoris is a biarticular muscle, functioning in knee extension and hip flexion. The tensor fasciae latae and the sartorius are also considered part of the anterior thigh.

Contusions

The quadriceps is constantly exposed to direct contact in various vigorous sports such as football, soccer, and basketball.[2,3] A quadriceps contusion can vary from a mild bruise to a large, deep hematoma that may take months to resolve.[2] The mechanism of injury is usually a direct blow to the thigh, compressing the muscle against the femur. The anterior or anterolateral aspect of the quadriceps is most often involved, because the medial aspect is protected by the athlete's contralateral leg.[17,19,23] A quadriceps contusion displays the standard signs and symptoms as seen with other muscle injuries, but the symptoms are less localized than those in a more subcutaneous area.[19] The athlete may exhibit local pain, stiffness, pain on passive stretching, disability that varies with the site and extent of injury, tenderness, ecchymosis, hematoma formation, and loss of active extension.[2,3,5,17,20,23] Injury severity can usually be determined by the degree of limitation of active knee flexion.

Moderate to severe quadriceps contusions should be treated nonaggressively to prevent the development of myositis ossificans, and exercise is progressed according to the athlete's tolerance. Some authors[3,10] have advocated the use of cryotherapy with simultaneous prolonged knee flexion at 20-minute intervals to help prevent the transitory loss of knee flexion that usually accompanies a quadriceps contusion. The degree of active knee flexion is determined by the athlete's pain tolerance. Modalities such as massage, heat, and forced stretching of the muscle during the acute phase are contraindicated.[2,20,23,24] Quadriceps setting can be performed and electrical muscle stimulation can be used to help diminish muscle atrophy and to promote quadriceps reeducation if these treatments cause no pain.[1,3,11] Also, passive range-of-motion devices can be useful in the early stages of injury. Figures 16-5 to 16-12 depict stretching exercises that can be used at various stages of the healing process to increase the elasticity of the quadriceps muscle. Table 16-3 presents an outline of a rehabilitation program progression after quadriceps injury.

In contusions, if the hematoma is not readily resolved, the clinician should suspect the development of myositis ossificans. Third-degree injuries need protective rest, cryotherapy, isometric exercise, and gentle active range of motion, as tolerated, before aggressive rehabilitation can begin. With severe thigh contusions, the use of massage, heat, and forced stretching or running is contraindicated in the early phases of healing.

The athlete may return to unlimited participation when the following criteria are met:

1. Quadriceps flexibility is equal bilaterally.
2. Muscular strength, power, endurance, and time to peak torque, as measured by an isokinetic dynamometer, are 85% to 90% of those of the contralateral limb.
3. Minimal or no tenderness is present in the quadriceps.
4. No symptoms are noted with functional activities at full speed.

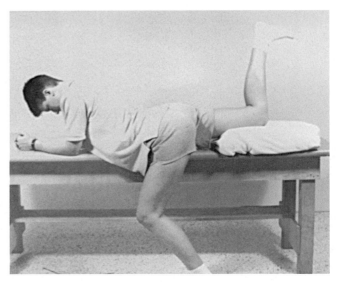

Figure 16-6. Passive hip flexor stretch. The amount of passive stretch can be modified by the amount of hip extension, which is based on the athlete's tolerance to stretch. It can be used in conjunction with cryotherapy techniques.

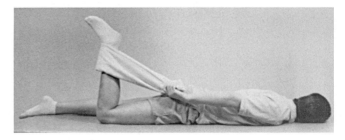

Figure 16-7. Single-leg quadriceps stretch. A towel is used to stretch the quadriceps muscle gradually. In the later stages of rehabilitation the proprioceptive neuromuscular facilitation contract-relax technique can be used to facilitate the range of motion.

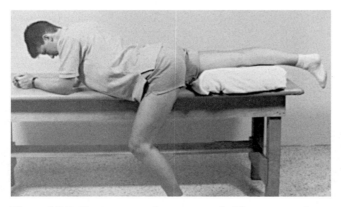

Figure 16-5. Passive rectus femoris stretch. The amount of passive stretch can be modified by the amount of hip extension, which is based on the athlete's tolerance to stretch. It can be used in conjunction with cryotherapy techniques.

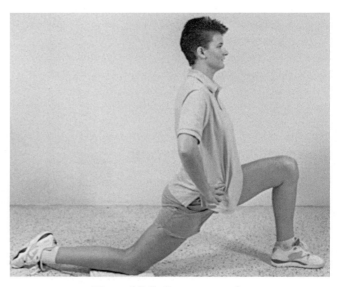

Figure 16-8. Iliopsoas stretch.

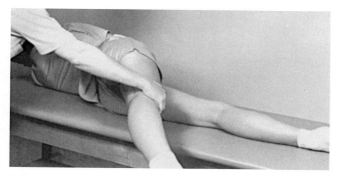

Figure 16-9. Manual iliopsoas stretch. This can later be adapted into the proprioceptive neuromuscular facilitation contract-relax technique or into other proprioceptive neuromuscular facilitation patterns.

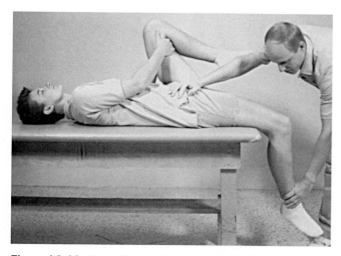

Figure 16-10. Manual rectus femoris stretch. This can be used to stretch the rectus femoris muscle and can also be used as a test to determine its length.

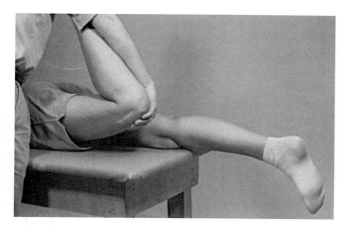

Figure 16-11. Manual hip flexor stretch. This can be adapted into the proprioceptive neuromuscular facilitation contract-relax technique to increase the range of motion.

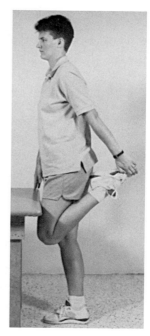

Figure 16-12. Single-leg standing quadriceps stretch. The athlete can also pull the hip into extension to accentuate the stretch.

5. The traumatized area is protected. Use of a pad made of Orthoplast*, with a raised section over the injured area, is recommended.

Strains

Quadriceps strains usually involve the rectus femoris muscle.[10,23] Strains to this area occur less often than do hamstring strains because of the great strength, size, and flexibility of the quadriceps muscle group.[10] The injury is usually a result of insufficient warm-up, poor stretching, tight quadriceps, bilateral quadriceps imbalance, or a short leg.[20] Signs and symptoms vary with injury severity but are characterized by pain down the entire length of the rectus femoris and tenderness in the area of the strain. The athlete exhibits pain on active quadriceps contraction and passive stretching. If the muscle is ruptured, swelling may initially mask a muscle defect, but a permanent bulge in the thigh is present as the swelling subsides.[1,10,11]

Rehabilitation for a quadriceps strain is similar to that for strains of other muscles. The severity of injury determines when active rehabilitation may begin, and all exercises should be performed within a pain-free range of motion. Static stretching is begun as tolerated (see Figs. 16-5 to 16-7) along with passive range-of-motion exercises. Progression should be made to active range-of-motion and resistive exercises with emphasis on knee extension and hip flexion.

*Available from Johnson & Johnson, New Brunswick, New Jersey.

Table 16-3

Progression for Quadriceps Rehabilitation

I. Initial Phase
 A. R.I.C.E. (rest, ice, compression, elevation)
 B. Modalities
  1. Pulsed ultrasound
  2. Electrical muscle stimulation
  3. Ice postexercise
 C. Tubi-Grip for effusion
 D. Active range of motion, as tolerated
 E. Cryostretch and cryokinetics with the following exercises:
  1. Active straight leg raises
  2. Active terminal knee extensions
  3. Active hip flexion
  4. Heel slides (seated and supine)
  5. Quadriceps sets
  6. Co-contractions
 F. Aquatic therapy
II. Intermediate Phase
 A. Stationary cycling
 B. Modalities
  1. Continuous ultrasound
  2. Moist heat
 C. Increase in aquatic program
 D. Quadriceps stretching
 E. Concentric 90° to 45° knee extensions
 F. Proprioceptive neuromuscular facilitation patterns
 G. Proprioception exercises
 H. Progressive-resistance exercise with exercises initiated in initial phase
 I. Active-assisted flexion
 J. Closed-chain exercises
  1. Terminal knee extensions with Thera-Band
  2. Lateral step-ups
III. Advanced Phase
 A. High-speed isokinetic exercises (seated and supine)
 B. Functional drills
 C. Eccentric 90° to 0° knee extensions
 D. High-speed surgical tubing exercises in hip flexion, extension, abduction, and adduction and in minisquats
 E. Protective wrapping

In the late phases of rehabilitation, isokinetic equipment can be used, at higher speeds, with the athlete in the supine position to accentuate the quadriceps muscle or in the traditional seated position.

Additionally, surgical tubing can be used for exercising in the planes of hip flexion, extension, adduction, abduction, and knee extension at high contractile speeds to fatigue for endurance (Fig. 16-13). The quadriceps rehabilitation progression in Table 16-3 can be used as a guideline for quadriceps strains. Although designed for quadriceps contusions, the program can be accelerated to accommodate quadriceps strains, because this injury can usually be rehabilitated more quickly than a quadriceps contusion.

The athlete may return to unlimited participation, wearing a neoprene sleeve for support and proprioception, when the following criteria are met:

1. Muscular strength, power, endurance, and time to peak torque, as measured by an isokinetic dynamometer, are 85% to 90% of those of the contralateral limb.
2. Quadriceps flexibility is equal bilaterally.
3. No symptoms are noted with functional activities at full speed.

GROIN REHABILITATION

The groin is the depressed region that lies between the thigh and abdominal area. The muscles of this region

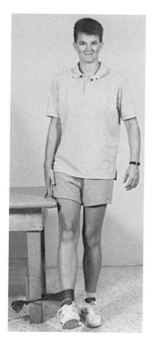

Figure 16-13. Hip flexion and extension using a Thera-Band° at varying speeds. The knee is straight, and the athlete flexes and extends the hip at varying speeds. In the final stages of rehabilitation, the athlete performs this exercise as fast as possible to fatigue, but not at the expense of good mechanics.

include the adductor group, rectus femoris, and iliopsoas. The adductor group is composed of the adductor longus, adductor brevis, adductor magnus, pectineus, and gracilis. These muscles adduct the thigh and flex and externally and internally rotate the hip.[25] The adductors function dynamically to adduct the thigh and serve as hip flexors and extensors, depending on their anterior or posterior relationship to the flexion-extension axis of the hips. During walking and running, contraction of the adductors contributes to the forward and backward swing motion of the leg. The static effect of these muscles is to stabilize the trunk by constantly adjusting the position of the pelvis. Twisting of the pelvis is prevented by the adducting and the internal-external rotating components of the adductor group.[25]

Groin strains can result from any forced adduction, overextension, twisting, running, or jumping with external rotation.[2,3,10,20,21] This stretching usually occurs when the muscular unit is overloaded during the eccentric phase of muscular contraction.[11,16,26] The athlete complains of a sudden, sharp pain located along the ischiopubic ramus, the lesser trochanter, or the adductor's musculotendinous junction.[1,8,9] The athlete complains of pain on passive

abduction and resisted adduction. The pain may begin at the origin of the traumatized muscle and radiate along the medial aspect of the thigh into the rectus abdominis area.[24]

The injury should be assessed by administering active, passive, and resisted tests in hip flexion, extension, adduction, abduction, and internal and external rotation and in knee extension.[3] The use of a hip spica with the hip internally rotated may help to alleviate some of the pain and discomfort experienced with activities of daily living and during the rehabilitation program (Fig. 16-14). Lateral movements and abduction with external rotation should be avoided until symptoms subside. Table 16-4 presents an outline of a rehabilitation program progression for groin strains.

The athlete may return to unlimited participation when the following criteria are met:

1. Muscular strength is equal bilaterally, as determined by manual muscle testing.
2. Full, pain-free hip range of motion is present.
3. The athlete can perform the sport-specific functional activities required, asymptomatically, at full speed.

Most injuries to the thigh region usually result in trauma to the soft tissue, particularly muscle. Although fractures can occur to this area, they are not as prevalent as muscle strains and contusions. Strains are most often produced indirectly though poor muscle flexibility, abnormal agonist-to-strength or antagonist-to-strength ratios, or eccentric muscle contraction. Contusions are generally incurred more in contact sports and result from a direct blow to the soft tissue.

Soft tissue injuries of the thigh are treated initially with emphasis on decreasing pain, spasm, and inflammation of the traumatized region. Early range-of-motion and stretching exercises can be instituted as tolerated, except for quadriceps contusions, in which the potential for myositis ossificans exists. Early aggressive motion, stretching, heat, and massage to quadriceps contusions are contraindicated.

As muscle elasticity is restored and inflammation subsides, the athlete can begin active progressive-resistance exercise, as tolerated. Later stages of rehabilitation should concentrate on high functional speed and eccentric exercise. Isokinetic machines can be used at higher speeds, and surgical tubing can be used for exercises at varying speeds to aid in reconditioning the type II muscle fibers. The athlete should also perform sport-specific functional activities at 50%, 75%, and then full speed. This allows the clinician to judge how the athlete performs in the sport. The athlete should be able to perform these functional activities asymptomatically before returning to participation. Once the athlete returns to competition, the area should be supported or protected with an appropriate orthosis. Most muscular strains to this region can be prevented through an adequate stretching and warm-up program before participation.

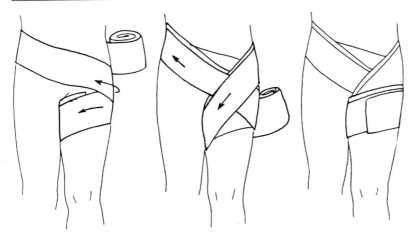

Figure 16-14. Hip spica. With the leg internally rotated to relax the adductor muscles, a 6-inch extralong elastic bandage is used to help support the groin area. (From Arnheim, D. [1989]: Modern Principles of Athletic Training, 7th ed. St. Louis, C.V. Mosby, p. 341.)

Table 16-4

Progression for Groin Rehabilitation

I. Initial Phase
 A. R.I.C.E. (rest, ice, compression, elevation)
 B. Modalities
  1. Pulsed ultrasound
  2. Electrical stimulation
  3. Ice postexercise
 C. Cryostretch and cryokinetics with the following exercises:
  1. Active hip abduction
  2. Active straight leg raises
  3. Active hip flexion
  4. Isometric hip adduction
 D. Hip active range of motion
 E. Aquatic therapy
 F. Stationary cycling

II. Intermediate Phase
 A. Modalities
  1. Continuous ultrasound
  2. Moist heat
 B. Proprioceptive exercises
 C. Progressive-resistance exercise with active exercises initiated in initial phase
 D. Active adduction
 E. Groin stretching
  1. Straddle groin and hamstring stretches
  2. Side straddle groin and hamstring stretches
  3. Groin stretches
  4. Wall groin stretches
 F. Increase of aquatic program
 G. Prophylactic cryotherapy
 H. Proprioceptive neuromuscular facilitation patterns
 I. Stationary cycling

III. Advanced Phase
 A. Concentric and eccentric hip abduction and adduction
 B. High-speed surgical tubing exercises in hip abduction, adduction, flexion, and extension
 C. Functional drills
  1. Running
  2. Cariocas
  3. Cutting
  4. Lateral movements
  5. Slide Board, if available
 D. Protective wrapping—hip spica

APPLICATION TECHNIQUES

Hamstring and Groin Exercises

Hamstring Stretch. The athlete lies supine on a table, and an object is placed under the foot to apply a gentle stretch of the hamstring. The quadriceps should be relaxed.

Straddle Groin and Hamstring Stretch. The athlete sits on the floor with the legs spread and the back straight (Fig. 16-15). The athlete then leans forward until a stretch is felt, holds for 10 seconds, relaxes, and repeats the exercise.

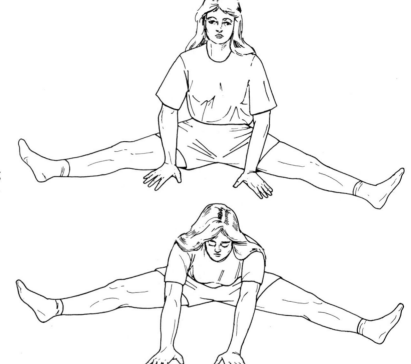

Figure 16-15. Straddle groin and hamstring stretch.

Side Straddle Groin and Hamstring Stretch. The athlete sits on the floor with the legs spread and the back straight (Fig. 16-16). The athlete leans to the left and tries to grasp as far down the leg as possible, holds 10 seconds, relaxes, and repeats on the opposite side.

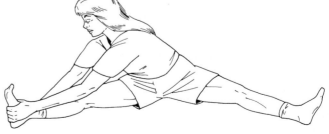

Figure 16-16. Side straddle groin and hamstring stretch.

Continued

A P P L I C A T I O N   T E C H N I Q U E S — c o n t ' d

Hamstring and Groin Exercises—cont'd

Supine Assisted Hamstring Stretch. With the help of a partner or towel, the athlete raises the leg until a stretch is felt in the hamstring, holds for 10 seconds, relaxes, and then repeats the exercise (see Fig. 16-2). PNF contract-relax can also be performed easily in this position.

Single Hamstring Stretch. The athlete straightens the supported leg with the other leg off to the side (Fig. 16-17) and slowly leans forward until a stretch is felt in the back of the hamstring. This is held for 10 seconds, and then the athlete relaxes and repeats the exercise. The stretch is performed with the chin up and the back straight and without bouncing.

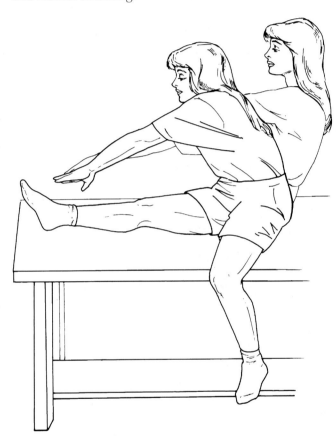

Figure 16-17. Single hamstring stretch.

Groin Stretch. In the sitting position, with the back straight, the athlete bends the knees, places the feet together, and pulls the feet toward the groin (Fig. 16-18). The elbows are placed on the knees and pressed down. This position is held for 10 seconds, followed by the athlete's relaxing and repeating the exercise.

Wall Groin Stretch. The athlete lies on the back with the buttocks and legs against the wall. The legs are spread enough so that a stretch is felt in the groin region (Fig. 16-19). A small amount of weight can be used around the ankles to increase the stretch and allow it to be more passive. This is held for 10 seconds. The athlete then relaxes and repeats the exercise.

Quadriceps Exercise

Standing Quadriceps Stretch. The athlete holds on with one arm for balance, grasps the foot of the injured extremity with the hand, and brings the heel to the buttocks (Fig. 16-20). While standing up straight, the athlete slowly extends the leg, maintaining the hold on the foot, and holds for 10 seconds. A stretch should be felt in the quadriceps. The athlete then relaxes and repeats the exercise.

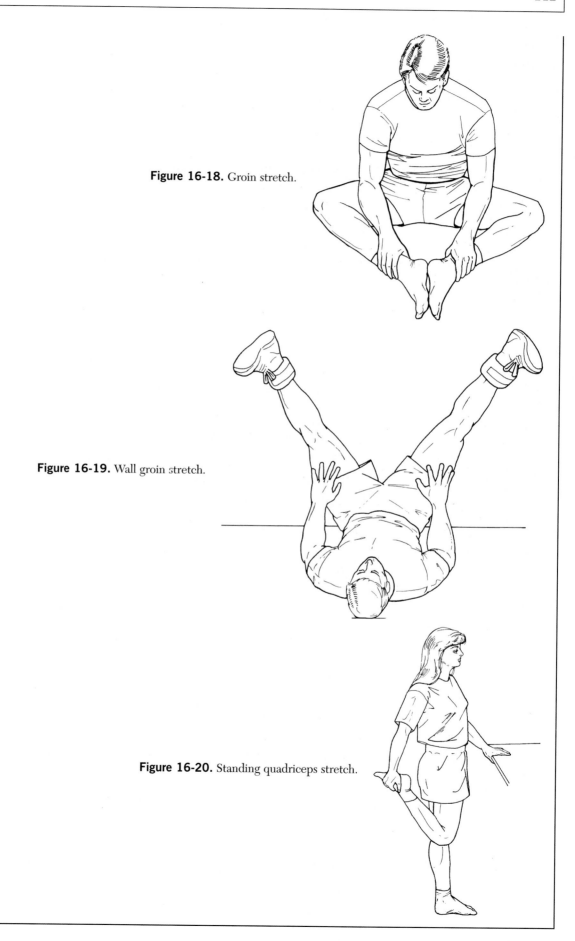

Figure 16-18. Groin stretch.

Figure 16-19. Wall groin stretch.

Figure 16-20. Standing quadriceps stretch.

SUMMARY

Introduction

■ Muscle strains are the most common injury to the hamstrings and adductors, whereas contusions rank as the primary injury to the quadriceps.

■ The use of magnetic resonance imaging in the evaluation of muscle injuries offers definitive evidence of the severity of the injury. This information can also provide a valuable guide in predicting the length of the rehabilitation process.

■ The goals in treating muscle strains are to reduce pain, restore muscle function, and reduce the likelihood of reinjury. Restoration of muscle length is important in reinjury prevention, because a shortened muscle is more susceptible to strains.

■ If low-grade muscle spasm is present, the use of cryostretching may be beneficial.

Hamstring Rehabilitation

■ Hamstring strain is one of the most common and frustrating injuries that an athlete can incur; it can also recur often.

■ Hamstring injuries usually occur during sprinting or high-speed exercises or activities.

■ Hamstring strains can have various causes: (1) a sudden change from a stabilizing flexor to an active extensor, combined with muscle imbalance between the quadriceps and hamstrings; (2) poor flexibility; (3) faulty posture; and (4) leg length discrepancy.

■ There is some evidence to suggest that hamstring strength should be 60% to 70% that of the antagonist quadriceps to help prevent hamstring injuries.

Quadriceps Rehabilitation

Contusions

■ Moderate to severe quadriceps contusions should be treated nonaggressively to prevent the development of myositis ossificans, and exercise is progressed according to the athlete's tolerance.

■ It is advocated by some that the use of cryotherapy with simultaneous prolonged knee flexion at 20-minute intervals helps to prevent the transitory loss of knee flexion that usually accompanies a quadriceps contusion.

■ With severe thigh contusions, the use of massage, heat, and forced stretching or running is contraindicated in the early phases of healing.

Strains

■ The injury is usually a result of insufficient warm-up, poor stretching, tight quadriceps, bilateral quadriceps imbalance, or a short leg.

■ Rehabilitation for a quadriceps strain is similar to that for strains of other muscles. The severity of injury determines when active rehabilitation may begin, and all exercises should be performed within a pain-free range of motion.

Groin Rehabilitation

■ Groin strains can result from any forced adduction, overextension, twisting, running, or jumping with external rotation.

■ Strains usually occur when the muscular unit is overloaded during the eccentric phase of muscular contraction.

■ The use of a hip spica with the hip internally rotated may help to alleviate some of the pain and discomfort experienced with activities of daily living and during the rehabilitation program.

■ Lateral movements and abduction with external rotation should be avoided until symptoms subside.

REFERENCES

1. Agre, J.C. (1985): Hamstring injuries: Proposed etiological factors, prevention, and treatment. Sports Med., 2:21-33.
2. American Academy of Orthopaedic Surgeons (1984): Athletic Training and Sports Medicine. Chicago, American Academy of Orthopaedic Surgeons.
3. Arnheim, D.H., and Prentice, W.E. (2000): Modern Principles of Athletic Training, 10th ed. St. Louis, C.V. Mosby, pp. 565-598.
4. Askling, C., Tengvar M., Saartok, T., and Thorstensson, A. (2000): Sports related hamstring strains—Two cases with different etiologies and injury sites. Scand. J. Med. Sci. Sports, 10:304-307.
5. Booher, J.M., and Thibodeau, G.A. (2000): Athletic Injury Assessment, 4th ed. St. Louis, McGraw-Hill.
6. Cibulka, M.T. (1989): Rehabilitation of the pelvis, hip, and thigh. Clin. Sports Med., 8:777-803.
7. Colby, S., Francisco, A., Yu, B., et al. (2000): Electromyograph and kinetic analysis of cutting maneuvers: Implications for anterior cruciate ligament injury. Am. J. Sports. Med. 28: 234-240.
8. Distefano, V. (1978): Functional anatomy and biomechanics of the knee. Athl. Train., 13:113-118.
9. Estwanik, J.J., Sloane, B., and Rosenberg, M.A. (1990): Groin strain and other possible causes of groin pain. Physician Sportsmed., 18:54-65.
10. Fahey, T.D. (1986): Athletic Training: Principles and Practice. Palo Alto, CA, Mayfield, pp. 77, 340-343.
11. Gardner, L. (1977): Hip abductors and adductors in rehabilitation. Physician Sportsmed., 5:103-104.
12. Garrett, W.E., Califf, J.C., and Gassett, F.H. (1984): Histochemical correlates of hamstring injuries. Am. J. Sports Med., 12:98-103.
13. Heiser, T.M., Weber, J., Sullivan, G., et al. (1984): Prophylaxis and management of hamstring muscle injuries in intercollegiate football. Am. J. Sports Med., 12:368-370.
14. Kaariainen, M., Jarvinen, T., Jarvinen, M., et al. (2000). Relation between myofibers and connective tissue during muscle injury repair. Scand. J. Med. Sci. Sports, 10:332-337.

15. Knight, K.L. (1995): Cryotherapy in Sports Injury Management. Champaign, IL, Human Kinetics, pp. 233-239.
16. Knight, K.L. (1985): Strengthening hip abductors and adductors. Physician Sportsmed., 13:161-163.
17. Kulund, D.N. (1982): The Injured Athlete. Philadelphia, J.B. Lippincott, pp. 356-358.
18. Liemohn, W. (1978): Factors related to hamstring strains. J. Sports Med. Phys. Fitness, 18:71-75.
19. Mintz, D.N. (2000): Imaging of sports injuries. Phys. Med. Rehabil. Clin. North Am., 11:435-469.
20. O'Donoghue, D.H. (1984): Treatment of Injuries to Athletes, 4th ed. Philadelphia, W.B. Saunders, pp. 433-442.
21. Peterson, L., and Renstrom, P. (1986): Sports Injuries. Chicago, Year Book Medical, pp. 440-443.
22. Prentice, W.E. (1994): Therapeutic Modalities in Sports Medicine. St. Louis, C.V. Mosby, pp. 7, 268-269.
23. Roy, S., and Irvin, R. (1983): Sports Medicine: Prevention, Evaluation, Management, and Rehabilitation. Englewood Cliffs, NJ, Prentice-Hall, pp. 299-305.
24. Torg, J.S., Vegso, J.J., and Torg, E. (1987): Rehabilitation of Athletic Injuries. Chicago, Year Book Medical, pp. 97-101, 110-115.
25. Weineck, J. (1986): Functional Anatomy in Sports. Chicago, Year Book Medical, pp. 102-115.
26. Zarins, B., and Ciullo, J.V. (1983): Acute muscle and tendon injuries in athletes. Clin. Sports Med., 2:167-182.

CHAPTER 17

LOW BACK REHABILITATION

Julie Fritz, Ph.D., P.T., ATC

CHAPTER OBJECTIVES

At the end of this chapter the reader will be able to:

- Explain the need for classification methods designed to direct the treatment of patients with low back pain.
- Recognize red flags indicating the potential for a serious underlying condition.
- Explain the importance of yellow flags to the management of patients with low back pain.
- Determine the stage of a patient with low back pain.
- Identify key signs and symptoms and determine the classification of the patient and the treatments associated with a patient classified to be in stage I.
- Identify key impairments and the treatments designed to eliminate these impairments for those patients determined to be in a stage II classification.

Low back pain (LBP) is a nearly universal experience among the adult population. Studies have documented the lifetime prevalence rate of LBP to be as high as 80%.[88] Although most cases are self-limiting and recover with little intervention, those who recover are prone to recurrences at a rate of up to 60%.[114] The past few decades have witnessed numerous advances in the medical community's understanding of the lumbar spine. The functional anatomy of the lumbar spine has been investigated in detail, the biomechanics of the lumbar motion segments have been studied, and new technology has allowed for more precise diagnostic imaging of the spine. Despite these advances, the prevalence of LBP and the associated costs have been growing at an alarming rate in recent decades, leading to the characterization of back pain as an epidemic.[126]

LBP is also a prevalent and problematic condition in athletes. Up to 20% of all sports-related injuries are reported to involve the spine.[18] Athletes in certain sports appear to be particularly prone to LBP. For example, high rates of LBP in athletes participating in the following sports have been reported: gymnastics, swimming, tennis, volleyball, football, and others.[43,53,90,103,112] The rehabilitation of individuals with LBP, including athletes, remains largely enigmatic. Numerous approaches to rehabilitation have been advocated, yet for any given individual with LBP, the selection of a treatment method from among the many competing approaches has been said to take on the characteristics of a lottery,[106] often leaving the rehabilitation specialist uncertain of the best course of action to undertake with any particular patient. This chapter presents a classification-based approach to the evaluation and treatment of patients with LBP. This approach seeks to classify patients with LBP on the basis of clusters of signs and symptoms. The patient's classification is then matched to a treatment strategy believed to be most effective for that individual patient.

EVALUATION AND TREATMENT: THE IMPORTANCE OF CLASSIFICATION

Identifying the anatomic structure responsible for LBP is often difficult, and up to 90% of patients cannot be given a precise diagnosis on the basis of pathology.[116] This large group of patients is typically given a nominal diagnosis, such as "lumbar strain" or "back pain," and has been considered as a homogenous entity. Although it is generally agreed that most of these patients should be treated conservatively, the search for effective conservative treatment measures has been elusive. It has been suggested that undiagnosed LBP is not actually a homogeneous entity, but instead consists of subtypes or classifications of patients who can be identified on the basis of specific signs and symptoms noted during the examination.[22] The classification in turn directs the clinician to a specific treatment intervention. An effective classification system for LBP should improve the clinician's decision-making and may be necessary before the therapeutic benefit of specific conservative treatment interventions can be documented in research studies.

Delitto and colleagues[22,38] have proposed a treatment-based classification system for use in the evaluation and treatment of individuals with LBP. This system uses information gathered from the physical examination and from patient self-reports to guide patient management. Three basic levels of decision-making or classification are required: (1) the athlete must be screened for red flags and yellow flags to ascertain his or her suitability for rehabilitation, (2) the acuity (or stage) of the low back condition must be determined, and finally (3) a treatment approach is selected.

Assessing for Red and Yellow Flags: First Level Classification

Red Flags

Even though a specific pathoanatomic source cannot be identified for most individuals with LBP, the cause for most cases can be attributed to mechanical factors. In a much smaller percentage of patients, the cause may be something more serious such as a fracture, cauda equina syndrome, neoplastic condition, or inflammatory disease.[54] Red flags are signs or symptoms that suggest a more serious underlying pathology and may necessitate a referral for medical or surgical interventions.

Several findings from the patient's history should alert the clinician to the potential of a serious underlying pathology. Spinal fractures can occur as a result of major trauma or falls. Compression fractures most commonly occur in postmenopausal women or in individuals with other bone-weakening conditions such as chronic corticosteroid use. Stress fractures are also not uncommon in athletes with persistent LBP. Stress fractures of the sacrum have been reported as a cause of LBP in athletes.[104] The pars interarticularis of the vertebral arch is the most common site of stress fractures in the spine, particularly among athletes involved in sports activities that involve repeated extension and rotation movements. The term spondylolysis describes a bony defect in the pars interarticularis region.[133] Rates of spondylolysis are particularly high in gymnasts, weightlifters, throwing athletes in track and field, divers, and rowers.[108,109] Spondylolysis may progress to spondylolisthesis, a forward slippage of one vertebra in relation to the vertebra below (Fig. 17-1).[33] Red flags that may indicate the presence of spondylolysis or spondylolisthesis include teenage athletes with LBP, participation in sports involving repetitive hyperextension of the spine, and pain with extension activities. If a spondylolytic lesion is suspected, a referral for further diagnostic imaging should be considered. Early identification of these conditions may prevent a nonunion fracture or progression of the slippage.[85] Treatment may involve bracing and activity limitation. Rehabilitation typically focuses on stabilization exercises.

LBP caused by a spinal neoplasm is rare, occurring in less than 1% of cases of LBP.[23] A missed or delayed diagnosis is possible if an awareness of red flags for the condition is lacking. Deyo and Diehl[23] identified several red flags that should raise a suspicion of spinal tumors includ-

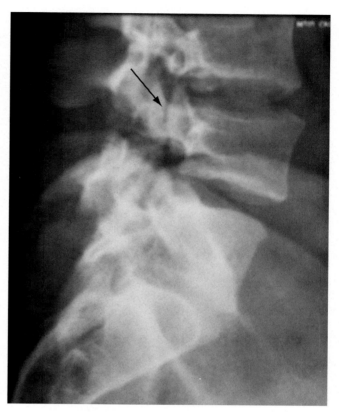

Figure 17-1. Grade 1 spondylolisthesis of L4 vertebra in a 17 year-old football offensive lineman with low back pain.

ing: age older than 50, unexplained weight loss, and no relief with bed rest. The most significant red flag is a prior history of cancer. The most common cancers that may result in metastases to the spine are the breast, lung, and prostate.[118] LBP caused by infectious conditions such as osteomyelitis or septic discitis are also rare; red flags include fever, chills, a recent history of an infectious condition such as a urinary tract infection, or intravenous drug use.[127] The medical history may also provide the first clues for detecting ankylosing spondylitis, a rheumatic inflammatory disorder more common in male individuals, and characterized by fibrosus and ossification of ligaments and joint capsules. Most affected individuals are younger than 35 years old when they first experience symptoms and will describe morning stiffness. The findings of relief with exercise and the need to get out of bed at night are also important in raising suspicion of ankylosing spondylitis.[11,44]

Cauda equina syndrome occurs when a large, midline disc herniation causes compression of the cauda equina nerve roots. The condition is rare, estimated to occur in less than 0.01% of patients with LBP,[54] but when present it represents a surgical emergency that requires immediate referral. Red flags for cauda equina syndrome are sensory deficits in the perineal (i.e., "saddle") region, urinary retention, or loss of sphincter control.[24] Table 17-1 pro-

Table 17-1

Red Flags for Potentially Serious Conditions Causing Low Back Pain

Fractures	Cauda Equina Syndrome	Neoplastic Conditions	Ankylosing Spondylitis	Spinal Infection
Spinal Fractures: Major trauma, such as motor vehicle accident, a fall from a height, or a direct blow to the lumbar spine	Saddle anesthesia Recent onset of bladder dysfunction, such as urinary retention, increased frequency, or overflow incontinence	Age older than 50 years Prior history of cancer Unexplained weight loss No relief with bed rest	Get out of bed at night Morning stiffness Male gender Age at onset younger than 35 years	Recent fever and chills Recent bacterial infection, intravenous drug abuse, or immune suppression (from steroids, transplant, or HIV)
Compression Fracture: Minor trauma or strenuous lifting in older or potentially osteoporotic individuals; prolonged corticosteroid use	Serious or progressive neurologic deficit in the lower extremity		No relief when lying down Relief with exercise and activity	
Pars Interarticularis Stress Fracture: Persistent back pain in younger individuals involved in repetitive hyperextension activities				

Data from References 5 and 23.

vides a contrasting view of red flags that could potentially be a serious condition causing LBP.

Yellow Flags

LBP is a common experience, and most affected individuals are able to recover and resume normal activities within a few weeks.[111] Research has shown that psychosocial variables are far more important than physical examination findings for predicting which patients are at risk for not making a rapid recovery.[39,71] Yellow flags are findings that indicate an increased risk for prolonged pain and disability because of psychosocial factors.[97] Research suggests that fear-avoidance beliefs may be the most important psychosocial yellow flag indicating an increased risk for prolonged LBP.[40,124]

The Fear-Avoidance Model was developed to help explain why some individuals with acute painful conditions progress to chronic pain whereas others are able to recover.[67] The model proposes that pain perceptions have both a sensory component and an emotional reaction component. During normal conditions these two components have a proportional relationship. In some instances, however, the relationship between the sensory component and the emotional reaction component can become dissociated, resulting in pain experience or behavior, or both, that

is out of proportion to demonstrable pathology.[107] The most important determinant of the relationship between the sensory and emotional components of pain perceptions is proposed to be an individual's fear of pain and subsequent avoidance behaviors.[67,107]

The response of an individual to a painful experience may fall somewhere along a continuum between two extremes: avoidance and confrontation.[96] Confrontation is seen as an adaptive response in which the individual resumes activities in a graded manner, eventually returning to a normal level of activity. Conversely, avoidance is viewed as a maladaptive response in which activities anticipated to cause pain are avoided. Avoidance may result in decreased activity levels, continued disability, and adverse psychological consequences.

CLINICAL PEARL #1

Fear-avoidance beliefs may be the most important psychosocial factor that increases the risk for prolonged disability caused by LBP. Patients with high levels of fear-avoidance beliefs need to be managed with an active rehabilitation approach with ample positive reinforcement when functional goals are achieved.

The presence of an avoidance response to LBP has been associated with an increased risk for prolonged disability and work loss.[17,39,62,124] Yellow flags indicating an increased risk for prolonged disability caused by heightened fear avoidance beliefs can be assessed through the clinical assessment or by using a questionnaire. Several attitudes and behaviors may represent yellow flags.[58] Waddell and colleagues[124] developed the Fear-Avoidance Beliefs Questionnaire (FABQ) to quantify fear-avoidance beliefs in patients with LBP (Fig. 17-2). The questionnaire is designed to assess the impact of fear-avoidance beliefs on two aspects of function: physical activity and work.

Once yellow flags are identified, the rehabilitation approach used with the patient may need to be modified. An emphasis on active rehabilitation and positive reinforcement of functional accomplishments is recommended for patients with increased fear-avoidance beliefs.[86] Graded exercise programs that direct attention toward attaining certain functional goals and away from the symptom of pain also have been recommended.[68] Finally, graduated exposure to specific activities that a patient fears as potentially painful or difficult to perform may be helpful.[122] Table 17-2 summarizes the attitudes and behaviors that may be associated with yellow flags.

Staging the Patient: Second Level Classification

Determining the acuity of the patient's LBP is an important consideration for rehabilitation. Acuity is not strictly based on the duration of symptoms, but also on the nature of the patient's examination and the goals for rehabilitation. Patients who have difficulty performing basic daily activities such as sitting, standing, or walking are considered to be in stage I (i.e., acute). Patients in stage I tend to have increased levels of pain and disability, and the goals for rehabilitation are directed toward reducing the patient's symptoms and permitting him or her to move on to stage II of treatment. Patients who are able to perform basic daily activities, but experience difficulties with more demanding activities such as running, lifting, sporting activities, and so on, are considered to be in stage II. Patients in stage II generally will have less severe symptoms, but they tend to have had symptoms for a longer duration of time, possibly limiting their ability to work or engage in sports activities. The goals of rehabilitation for patients in stage II focus on reducing impairments of strength, flexibility, endurance and neuromuscular control, and returning to full participation in work or sports activities.

Fear-Avoidance Beliefs Questionnaire

Here are some of the things other patients have told us about their pain. For each statement please mark the number from 0 to 6 to indicate how much physical activities such as bending, lifting, walking or driving affect or would affect your back pain.

	Completely Disagree			Unsure			Completely Agree
1. My pain was caused by physical activity	0	1	2	3	4	5	6
2. Physical activity makes my pain worse	0	1	2	3	4	5	6
3. Physical activity might harm my back	0	1	2	3	4	5	6
4. I should not do physical activities which (might) make my pain worse	0	1	2	3	4	5	6
5. I cannot do physical activities which (might) make my pain worse	0	1	2	3	4	5	6

The following statements are about how your normal work affects or would affect your back pain.

	Completely Disagree			Unsure			Completely Agree
6. My pain was caused by my work or by an accident at work	0	1	2	3	4	5	6
7. My work aggravated my pain	0	1	2	3	4	5	6
8. I have a claim for compensation for my pain	0	1	2	3	4	5	6
9. My work is too heavy for me	0	1	2	3	4	5	6
10. My work makes or would make my pain worse	0	1	2	3	4	5	6
11. My work might harm by back	0	1	2	3	4	5	6
12. I should not do my regular work with my present pain	0	1	2	3	4	5	6
13. I cannot do my normal work with my present pain	0	1	2	3	4	5	6
14. I cannot do my normal work until my pain is treated	0	1	2	3	4	5	6
15. I do not think that I will be back to my normal work within 3 months	0	1	2	3	4	5	6
16. I do not think that I will ever be able to go back to that work	0	1	2	3	4	5	6

Figure 17-2. The Fear-Avoidance Beliefs Questionnaire.[126] The physical activity subscale is computed as the sum of questions 2 through 5. The work subscale is computed as the sum of questions 6, 7, 9-12, and 15. (From Waddell, G., Newton, M., Henderson, I., et al. (1993): A Fear-Avoidance Beliefs Questionnaire (FABQ) and the role of fear-avoidance beliefs in chronic low back pain and disability. Pain, 52:157-168.

Table 17-2

Attitudes and Behaviors That May Represent Yellow Flags

Attitudes and Beliefs	Behaviors
Belief that pain is harmful or disabling resulting in guarding and fear of movement	Use of extended rest
Belief that all pain must be abolished before returning to activity	Reduced activity level with significant withdrawal from daily activities
Expectation of increased pain with activity or work, lack of ability to predict capabilities	Avoidance of normal activity and progressive substitution of lifestyle away from productive activity
Catastrophe focused, expecting the worst	Reports of extremely high pain intensity
Belief that pain is uncontrollable	Excessive reliance on aids (braces, crutches, and so on)
Passive attitude to rehabilitation	Sleep quality reduced after the onset of back pain
	High intake of alcohol or other substances with an increase since the onset of back pain
	Smoking

Determining the Best Treatment Approach: Third Level Classification

Once the patient has been screened for red and yellow flags and the stage of the condition has been judged, the next decision is determining which treatment approach is most likely to benefit the patient. Instead of focusing on a pathoanatomic diagnosis, the clinician should seek to classify the patient's condition on the basis of clusters of signs and symptoms. The classification assignment should in turn assist in the determination of the most appropriate treatment approach. The treatment-based classification system used in this chapter was originally described by Delitto and colleagues in 1995,[22] and has been updated and modified based on research developments since that time.[31,34,36-38] The system uses information gathered from the patient's medical history and physical examination to place the patient into a classification, which in turn guides the treatment of the patient. Four basic classifications are used for patients in stage I: manipulation/mobilization, specific exercise (flexion, extension, and lateral shift patterns), stabilization, and traction. Each of these classifications is associated with several key examination findings and a unique treatment approach. The examination components are assessed through patient self-report measures, the neurologic assessment, and the patient's medical history and physical examination. Table 17-3 summarizes the key examination findings and treatments for stage I classification.

Self-Report Measures

Several self-report measures provide useful information for the classification process and may also serve as useful indicators of the effectiveness of treatment. Three self-report measures are recommended: a pain diagram and pain rating scale, the FABQ, and a disability measure.

Pain Diagram and Rating

A pain body diagram is used to determine the nature and distribution of the patient's symptoms. The patient is asked to indicate the location and nature (i.e., aching, burning, numbness, and others) of symptoms on the body diagram. If symptoms are noted to extend distal to the knee, a classification of manipulation/mobilization becomes less likely.[31] The presence of symptoms distal to the knee, or symptoms of numbness and tingling, increase the likelihood of a specific exercise or traction classification. A pain diagram may also serve as an additional yellow flag screening tool. Nondermatomal or widespread distributions of symptoms may indicate psychosocial factors are impacting the patient's pain perceptions.[13] A pain rating scale asks the patient to rate his or her level of pain on a 0 to 10 scale, with 0 indicating no pain, and 10 the worst imaginable pain. Ratings of pain may serve as a useful outcome measure to document treatment success or failure.

Fear-Avoidance Beliefs Questionnaire

The FABQ is a helpful screening tool for yellow flags. The FABQ has both a work and physical activity subscale (see Fig. 17-2). The work subscale of the FABQ may be particularly helpful for classifying the patient. The work subscale contains seven items, each scored 0 to 6, with higher numbers indicating greater levels of fear-avoidance beliefs. Research has found that total scores greater than 34 should raise concerns about prolonged disability.[40] Total scores greater than 18 have been associated with a reduced likelihood of success with a manipulation treatment approach,[31] and these patients may need a more active rehabilitation program.

Modified Oswestry Disability Questionnaire

The two most commonly used self-report disability scales are the Modified Oswestry and Roland Morris Questionnaires.[7] We have used the Oswestry for the purposes of staging the patient and assessing the outcomes of treatment. The Oswestry has 10 sections: 1 section for pain severity and the other 9 representing various functional activities (Fig. 17-3). The patient indicates his or her

Table 17-3

Key Examination Findings and Treatments for Stage I Classifications

Classification	Key Examination Findings	Treatments
Stabilization	Frequent prior episodes of low back pain Increasing frequency of episodes of low back pain "Instability catch" or painful arcs during lumbar flexion/extension ROM Hypermobility of the lumbar spine Positive prone segmental instability test	Trunk strengthening stabilization exercises
Manipulation/ Mobilization	No symptoms distal to the knee Recent onset of symptoms Low levels of fear-avoidance beliefs Hypomobility of the lumbar spine Increased hip internal rotation (>35°) or discrepancy in hip internal rotation ROM between the right and left hip	Manipulation or mobilization techniques targeted to the sacroiliac or lumbar region. ROM exercises.
Specific Exercise		
Extension Pattern	Symptoms distal to the knee Signs and symptoms of nerve root compression Symptoms centralize with lumbar extension Symptoms peripheralize with lumbar flexion	Extension exercises Mobilization to promote extension
Flexion Pattern	Older age (>55 years) Symptoms distal to the knee Signs and symptoms of nerve root compression and/or neurogenic claudication Symptoms peripheralize with lumbar extension Symptoms centralize with lumbar flexion	Avoidance of flexion activities Flexion exercises Mobilization to promote flexion Deweighted ambulation Avoidance of extension activities
Lateral Shift Pattern	Visible frontal plane deviation of the shoulders relative to the pelvis Asymmetrical side-bending active ROM Painful and restricted extension active ROM	Pelvic translocation exercises Autotraction
Traction	Signs and symptoms of nerve root compression No movements centralize symptoms	Mechanical or autotraction

ROM, range of motion.

Modified Oswestry Low Back Pain Disability Questionnaire

This questionnaire has been designed to give your therapist information as to how your back pain has affected your ability to manage in every day life. Please answer every question by placing a mark in the **one** box that best describes your condition today. We realize you may feel that two of the statements may describe your condition, but **please mark only the box which most closely describes your current condition.**

Pain Intensity
- ☐ I can tolerate the pain I have without having to use pain medication.
- ☐ The pain is bad but I can manage without having to take pain medication.
- ☐ Pain medication provides me complete relief from pain.
- ☐ Pain medication provides me with moderate relief from pain.
- ☐ Pain medication provides me with little relief from pain.
- ☐ Pain medication has no effect on my pain.

Personal Care (Washing, Dressing, etc.)
- ☐ I can take care of myself normally without causing increased pain.
- ☐ I can take care of myself normally but it increases my pain.
- ☐ It is painful to take care of myself and I am slow and careful.
- ☐ I need help but I am able to manage most of my personal care.
- ☐ I need help every day in most aspects of my care.
- ☐ I do not get dressed, wash with difficulty and stay in bed.

Lifting
- ☐ I can lift heavy weights without increased pain.
- ☐ I can lift heavy weights but it causes increased pain.
- ☐ Pain prevents me from lifting heavy weights off the floor, but I can manage if weights are conveniently positioned (ex. On a table).
- ☐ Pain prevents me from lifting heavy weights, but I can manage light to medium weights if they are conveniently positioned.
- ☐ I can lift only very light weights.
- ☐ I cannot lift or carry anything at all.

Walking
- ☐ Pain does not prevent me from walking any distance.
- ☐ Pain prevents me from walking more than 1 mile.
- ☐ Pain prevents me from walking more than ½ mile.
- ☐ Pain prevents me from walking more than ¼ mile.
- ☐ I can only walk with crutches or a cane.
- ☐ I am in bed most of the time and have to crawl to the toilet.

Sitting
- ☐ I can sit in any chair as long as I like.
- ☐ I can only sit in my favorite chair as long as I like.
- ☐ Pain prevents me from sitting for more than 1 hour.
- ☐ Pain prevents me from sitting for more than ½ hour.
- ☐ Pain prevents me from sitting for more than 10 minutes.
- ☐ Pain prevents me from sitting at all.

Standing
- ☐ I can stand as long as I want without increased pain.
- ☐ I can stand as long as I want but increases my pain.
- ☐ Pain prevents me from standing more than 1 hour.
- ☐ Pain prevents me from standing more than ½ hour.
- ☐ Pain prevents me from standing more than 10 minutes.
- ☐ Pain prevents me from standing at all.

Sleeping
- ☐ Pain does not prevent me from sleeping well.
- ☐ I can sleep well only by using pain medication.
- ☐ Even when I take pain medication, I sleep less than 6 hours.
- ☐ Even when I take pain medication, I sleep less than 4 hours.
- ☐ Even when I take pain medication, I sleep less than 2 hours.
- ☐ Pain prevents me from sleeping at all.

Social Life
- ☐ My social life is normal and does not increase my pain.
- ☐ My social life is normal, but it increases my level of pain.
- ☐ Pain prevents me from participating in more energetic activities (ex. sports, dancing, etc.)
- ☐ Pain prevents me from going out very often.
- ☐ Pain has restricted my social life to my home.
- ☐ I have hardly any social life because of my pain.

Traveling
- ☐ I can travel anywhere without increased pain.
- ☐ I can travel anywhere but it increases my pain.
- ☐ Pain restricts travel over 2 hours.
- ☐ Pain restricts my travel over 1 hour.
- ☐ Pain restricts my travel to short necessary journeys under ½ hour.
- ☐ Pain prevents all travel except for visits to the doctor/therapist or hospital.

Employment/Homemaking
- ☐ My normal homemaking/job activities do not cause pain.
- ☐ My normal homemaking/job activities increase my pain, but I can still perform all that is required of me.
- ☐ I can perform most of my homemaking/job duties, but pain prevents me from performing more physically stressful activities (ex. lifting, vacuuming).
- ☐ Pain prevents me from doing anything but light duties.
- ☐ Pain prevents me from doing even light duties.
- ☐ Pain prevents me from performing any job/homemaking chores.

Figure 17-3. The Modified Oswestry Disability Questionnaire. (Reprinted with permission from Fritz, J.M., and Irrgang, J.J. [2001]: A comparison of a Modified Owestry Low Back Pain Disability Questionaire and the Quebec Back Pain Disability Scale. Phys. Ther., 81:776-788.)

degree of limitation in that activity because of LBP. Each section contains six responses, scored from 0 to 5. Each section score is summed to obtain the final score. The final score is then multiplied by two, and the degree of disability is expressed as a percentage. Higher scores on the Oswestry indicate greater levels of perceived disability.[41] The Oswestry score can assist with staging the patient.

Generally, patients in stage I will have Oswestry scores at or greater than 30%, and patients in stage II will have scores less than 30%.

Neurologic Assessment

A neurologic assessment is required for any patient who has symptoms that extend below the buttock. The neurologic examination consists of four components: (1) strength of key muscles for each lumbar and sacral myotomes, (2) sensation within dermatomes of the lower quarter, (3) deep tendon reflexes of the lower quarter, and (4) signs of neural tension. The results of the neurologic examination will determine if signs of nerve root compression are present and need to be monitored throughout treatment. Results of the neurologic assessment may also provide prognostic information. Individuals with positive findings on the neurologic examination may be more likely to experience long-term pain and disability.[2]

Strength Assessment

Evaluation of key muscles to each lumbar and sacral myotome is performed. Myotomal weakness may be indicative of lower motor neuron lesions, most commonly a nerve root compression caused by intervertebral disc herniation. More generalized weakness may indicate more serious pathology or simply generalized disuse atrophy of the lower limb. The key muscles to be tested and corresponding myotomes are listed in Table 17-4.

Sensory Assessment

Evaluation for sensory loss is performed by lightly brushing the hand over key dermatomal areas. Any region of diminished or absent sensation should be tested further with the use of a pin to clearly map out the area of sensory deficit. Box 17-1 contains the key areas used to assess specific dermatomes. Considerable overlap and individual variations in dermatomal patterns are known to exist. The results of sensory testing should be collaborated with the results of other components of the neurologic assessment to determine the presence and extent of nerve root compression.

Deep Tendon Reflex Assessment

Diminished deep tendon reflexes may represent nerve root compression. Hyperactive reflexes can represent another area of concern related to upper motor neuron disturbances (e.g., myelopathy). At the same time, hyperactive reflexes can be a normal variant. If encountered, the clinician should at least *suspect* a myelopathic process or an upper motor neuron pathology. Confirming evidence for these conditions would be clonus or the presence of a Babinski response. If these findings exist, referral for further diagnostic work-up is likely required. Table 17-5 describes two lower extremity reflexes that are assessed.

Neural Tension Tests

These tests are procedures designed to place tension on neural structures to assist in the diagnosis of nerve root compression that is typically caused by lumbar intervertebral disc herniation. Two different neural tension tests are used (Fig. 17-4A and B).

Straight Leg Raise (see Fig. 17-4A)

Straight leg raise is used to place tension on the sciatic nerve to aid in the diagnosis of the presence of nerve root compression of the lower lumbar nerve roots (L4-S1). The patient is prone and the lower extremity is raised by the clinician to the maximum tolerable level of hip flexion range of motion (ROM). The test must be performed passively and the patient's knee is maintained in full extension and the hip in a neutral rotation. The opposite leg is kept in extension. For each test, the clinician notes any symptoms produced during the test and also the degree of hip flexion at which the symptoms are produced. A positive

---

Table 17-4

Key Muscles to Be Tested and Corresponding Myotomes

Muscles	How to Test
Hip flexion (L1-L2)	The hip is flexed to near end range and pressure is applied to the anterior thigh into hip extension.
Knee extension (L3-L4)	The knee is placed in a position slightly less than full extension. One hand stabilizes the patient's thigh, the other applies pressure on the anterior tibia into knee flexion.
Dorsiflexion (L4-L5)	Dorsiflexion is best tested by having the patient walk on the heels. Nonweight-bearing assessment of dorsiflexion strength can be performed, but may be less sensitive to subtle strength deficits. For nonweight-bearing assessment, the foot is placed in full dorsiflexion with some inversion. One hand stabilizes the distal tibia, the other hand applies pressure on the dorsum of the foot into plantarflexion with some eversion.
Great toe extension (L5)	With the shoes off, the great toe is placed in extension. One hand stabilizes the foot, the other hand applies pressure on the dorsum of the distal phalanx of the great toe into flexion.
Ankle plantarflexion (S1-S2)	Plantarflexion is best tested by having the patient walk on the toes. Nonweight-bearing assessment of plantarflexion strength can be performed, but may be less sensitive to subtle deficits. For nonweight-bearing assessment, the foot is placed in full plantarflexion. One hand stabilizes the distal tibia, the other applies pressure on the plantar aspect of the foot into plantarflexion. (With the knee flexed the soleus muscle is the primary plantarflexor.)

Box 17-1

Key Areas Used to Assess Specific Dermatomes

- Inguinal area (L1)
- Anterior mid-thigh (L2)
- Distal anterior thigh and medial knee (L3)
- Medial lower leg and foot (L4)
- Lateral lower leg and foot (L5)
- Posterior calf (S1)

test requires the reproduction of the patient's familiar leg symptoms between 30° and 70° of hip flexion. It is important to distinguish between the reproduction of familiar symptoms and hamstring tightness.

Both the symptomatic and contralateral lower extremities are examined. A positive contralateral straight leg raise test occurs when the straight leg raise of the asymptomatic lower extremity reproduces the symptoms in the symptomatic extremity. A positive contralateral straight leg raise test is highly specific for a lower lumbar disc herniation.[110]

Femoral Nerve Stretch (see Fig. 17-4B)

Femoral nerve stretch is a neural tension test used to place tension on the femoral nerve to diagnose nerve root compression of the mid-lumbar nerve roots (L2-L4). The femoral nerve stretch is performed with the patient prone. The clinician first passively extends the patient's hip, and then passively flexes the knee. If the patient's familiar anterior thigh symptoms are reproduced or intensified with these maneuvers, the test is considered positive. It is important to distinguish between reproduction of the patient's familiar symptoms caused by tension on the femoral nerve and stretching of the rectus femoris muscle.

STAGE I MANAGEMENT
Manipulation/Mobilization Classification

Spinal manipulation is an intervention for which there is at least some supporting evidence of its effectiveness. Several randomized trials have found spinal manipulation to be more effective than placebo or other interventions for patients with LBP.[5,21,28,63] Manipulation/mobilization techniques may be directed at either the sacroiliac (SI) region or the lumbar spine. Many theoretic approaches to identifying patients likely to benefit from spinal manipulation have been proposed; however, there is little to no evidence to support their use and reliability. These approaches are frequently based on pathoanatomic and biomechanical theories that use various examination procedures to identify a pathologic motion segment, or a biomechanical dysfunction toward which a manipulative intervention is then directed.

An alternative to the traditional tests used to classify patients is the development of a clinical prediction rule. A clinical prediction rule is a tool designed to assist in the classification process and improve decision-making for clinicians.[65] Flynn and colleagues[31] developed a clinical prediction rule consisting of multiple factors from the medical history and physical examination to predict *a priori* which patients will most likely benefit from spinal manipulation. The results of this study identified a set of five criteria that accurately identified patients who would benefit from the manipulative intervention. The five criteria are listed in Box 17-2. The presence of at least four of five of these findings was strongly predictive of a dramatic response to the manipulative intervention, and the presence of three findings was moderately predictive of success.[31] Therefore, a classification of manipulation/mobilization should be strongly considered when at least three of these findings are present.

Table 17-5

Lower Extremity Reflex Tests

Reflex	Test Integrity of Nerve Roots	Technique
Patellar tendon reflex	L3-L4 nerve roots	The patient is seated with the knee flexed to approximately 90°. The patellar tendon is struck with the reflex hammer and reflexive knee extension is observed.
Achilles tendon reflex	S1-S2 nerve roots	The patient is seated, the ankle is supported at approximately neutral dorsiflexion. The ankle dorsiflexor muscles must be relaxed. The Achilles tendon is struck with the reflex hammer and reflexive plantarflexion is observed and felt with the supporting hand.

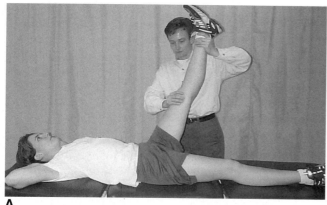

Straight Leg Raise — The hip is passively flexed with the knee maintained in extension. The test is positive if the patient's familiar leg symptoms are reproduced between 30°-70° of hip flexion.

A

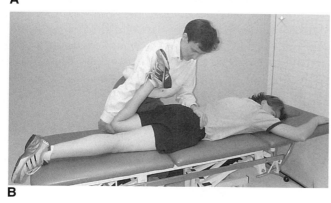

Femoral Nerve Stretch — The knee and hip are passively flexed. The test is positive if the patient's familiar anterior thigh symptoms are reproduced or intensified with these maneuvers.

B

Figure 17-4. *A*, Straight leg raise: The hip is passively flexed with the knee maintained in extension. The test is positive if the patient's familiar leg symptoms are reproduced between 30° and 70° of hip flexion. *B*, Femoral nerve stretch: The knee and hip are passively flexed. The test is positive if the patient's familiar anterior thigh symptoms are reproduced or intensified with these maneuvers.

Box 17-2

Key Examination Findings Leading to a Classification of Manipulation/Mobilization[31]

- Low Fear Avoidance Beliefs Questionnaire (FABQ)—work subscale score (<19 points)
- Short duration of current symptoms (<16 days)
- No symptoms extending distal to the knee
- At least one hypomobile lumbar spine segment (judged from lumbar spring testing)
- At least one hip with more than 35° of internal rotation ROM

No increasing frequency of low back pain episodes noted by the patient

No signs of nerve root compression

No peripheralization during lumbar active movement testing

The five findings that make up the clinical prediction rule.

Examination for the Manipulation/Mobilization Classification

Patients who are most likely to respond to a manipulation/mobilization intervention are generally those with a more recent onset of symptoms, with symptoms localized to the low back, buttock, and possibly into the thigh.

Patients with signs of nerve root compression (i.e., positive straight leg raise and strength, reflex, or sensory deficits) are likely to respond more favorably to an alternative treatment approach. Traditionally, classifying a patient for a manipulation/mobilization intervention has relied predominately on mobility assessments and special tests. Many of these diagnostic tests have been found to have poor reliability and questionable validity,[27,31,102] and therefore clinicians should be cautious about making classification decisions on the basis of any one of these findings in isolation. Confirmatory findings from the physical examination are outlined later in this chapter.

Further Examination of the Sacroiliac (SI) Region
Tests of Bony Landmark Symmetry

The clinician assesses the symmetry of the pelvic landmarks including the posterior superior iliac spine (PSIS), anterior superior iliac spines (ASIS), and the iliac crests with the patient standing. The iliac crests are evaluated from the posterior aspect of the patient using the clinician's hands or a pelvic level. The clinician judges the symmetry of the heights of the iliac crests. A difference between right and left sides can indicate a leg length discrepancy, an iliac rotation, or both. Asymmetry of the iliac crests must be correlated with the positional findings of the PSIS and ASIS. The PSIS levels are determined by placing the tips of the index fingers directly beneath the inferior aspect of the PSIS on each side and visually comparing the height. The same procedure is used in comparing the ASIS heights.

After each of the landmarks has been palpated, the results are compiled to arrive at one of three possible determinations:

- long leg: symmetrically increased height of the ASIS, PSIS, and iliac crests on one side
- innominate rotation: asymmetrical heights of ASIS, PSIS, and iliac crests (e.g., low PSIS on right, high iliac crest on right, and high ASIS on right)
- normal: even pelvic landmarks in standing

The PSIS levels are palpated in a similar manner with the patient sitting. Palpation of the ASIS is difficult with the patient seated and is not performed. Interpretation of the

position of the PSIS with the patient sitting is correlated with the results of palpation in the standing position. Asymmetry that was present in standing and remains in sitting may indicate SI region dysfunction. If the asymmetry is eliminated in sitting, a leg length discrepancy should be suspected.

The Standing and Seated Flexion Tests

The clinician places the tips of their index fingers directly beneath the PSIS on both sides. The fingers are directed against the inferior margin of the PSIS with maintenance of upward pressure. The patient is instructed to bend forward as far as possible while the clinician continues to monitor the position of the PSIS and observes for symmetry of cranial movement of these bony landmarks (Fig. 17-5A). Normally, the superior movement of each PSIS should be equal. A positive finding occurs when the cranial

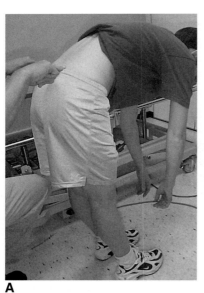

Standing Flexion Test— The clinician palpates the PSIS while the patient flexes forward. The test is positive if one PSIS moves further in a cranial direction.

A

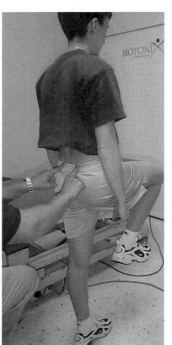

B

Gillet Test— The clinician palpates the PSIS while the patient flexes the hip and knee. The test is postitive if the PSIS does not move in a caudal direction.

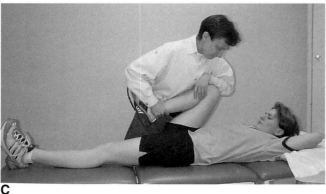

C

Gaenslen's Test— The clinician flexes the knee and hip, then applies overpressure. The test is positive if the patient's familiar symptoms are reproduced.

Figure 17-5. *A*, Standing flexion test: The clinician palpates the posterior superior iliac spine (PSIS) while the patient flexes forward. The test is positive if one PSIS moves further in a cranial direction. *B*, Gillet test: The clinician palpates the PSIS while the patient flexes the hip and knee. The test is positive if the PSIS does not move in a caudal direction. *C*, Gaenslen's test: The clinician flexes the knee and hip and then applies overpressure. The test is positive if the patient's familiar symptoms are reproduced.

excursion of one PSIS is judged to be greater than the other. The side that moves further in a cranial direction is presumed to be the hypomobile side that requires manipulation/mobilization.

The seated flexion test is performed and interpreted in an identical manner, except the patient is seated. The clinician palpates the PSIS on both sides and the patient is then asked to flex forward while the clinician continues to monitor the position of the PSIS. If one PSIS is found to move further in a cranial direction than the other, the test is considered to be positive. The side that moves further in a cranial direction is presumed to be the hypomobile side.

The Gillet Test

With the patient standing, the clinician places one thumb under the PSIS on the side being tested. The other thumb is placed in the midline over the S2 spinous process. The patient is instructed to stand on one leg, and flex the hip and knee on the side being testing, bringing the leg toward the chest. The clinician continues to palpate the PSIS on the tested side. The test is considered to be positive if the PSIS fails to move posterior and inferior with respect to the S2 spinous process (see Fig. 17-5B).

Gaenslen's Test

Gaenslen's test is a provocation test for SI region dysfunction. The patient is supine with both legs extended. The leg being tested is passively brought into full hip flexion and knee flexion, while the opposite hip is maintained in an extended position. Overpressure is applied by the clinician to the flexed extremity (see Fig. 17-5C). A positive test occurs when the patient's familiar symptoms are reproduced in either SI region with application of the overpressure.

Further Examination of the Lumbar Region
Lumbar Active Motion Assessment: The Movement Diagram

Active ROM is performed with the patient standing. In performing these procedures, the clinician needs to determine the ROM present in each direction, as well as the behavior of the patient's symptoms during and immediately after the movement in question. The patient is asked to perform the following movements:

- side-bending to the right and left
- extension
- forward bending

Reliable methods of measurement have been described for quantification of forward bending and extension using a single inclinometer.[125] For ease of recording the ROM present and the location of symptoms, we have developed a movement diagram and a shorthand system to denote the effect of movements on the patient's symptoms and to record the pattern of motion restriction present (Fig. 17-6).

For the classification of manipulation/mobilization, the focus of active movement testing is on the identification of a noncapsular pattern of movement restriction that may indicate the need for manipulation or mobilization of the lumbar spine. Noncapsular patterns in the lumbar region were characterized by Cyriax[19] as occurring when a gross limitation of side-bending is present in only one direction. Noncapsular patterns may be further distinguished as either opening or closing restrictions.[22] A closing restriction theoretically occurs when side-bending is limited toward the side of pain, and extension is also limited. The movement diagram of a left closing restriction is shown in Figure 17-7. An opening restriction is proposed to occur when the restricted motions are side-bending away from the painful side and flexion. The movement diagram of a left opening restriction is shown in Figure 17-8.

Passive Segmental Motion Testing

Passive segmental motion tests are both provocation and tests of mobility of the lumbar motion segments. The patient lies prone and the clinician places the hypothenar eminence over the spinous process of the vertebra to be tested. The contact point of the hand is just distal to the pisiform. Once the clinician's hand is positioned appropriately, the wrist and elbow are extended and a gentle but firm anteriorly directed pressure is applied to the spinous process. The force is applied not by pushing with the arms but by allowing the body weight to be lowered. The patient is instructed to report any change in symptoms during the performance of the test. The clinician also judges the mobility as normal, hypomobile, or hypermobile. The presence of hypomobile lumbar motion segments is an indication for a manipulation/mobilization classification.

Treatment for the Manipulation/Mobilization Classification

Although it has not been studied extensively, a few studies have found greater benefit from manipulation techniques versus mobilization of the lumbosacral region.[46,84] Patients with diagnoses of spondylolisthesis, lumbar instability, osteoporosis, or any concerns of a stress fracture should be approached with caution, and manipulation techniques are generally contraindicated in these individuals. Many different manipulation and mobilization techniques have been described, but there is currently no evidence for the superiority of one approach over another. The correct identification of the patient who actually needs manipulation/mobilization interventions is likely more important than the particular technique chosen by the clinician. Several manipulation/mobilization techniques are described

Treatment for the Lumbar Region

For lumbar region techniques, the lumbar motion segment to be manipulated or mobilized is determined from the accessory motion testing. The segment that seems to be the most hypomobile or painful should be treated first. After performing the manipulation or mobilization technique, active movement and passive motion should be reassessed. If impairments remain, other lumbar segments may need to be treated. Three treatment techniques for the lumbar region will be described: a lumbar manipulation technique and mobilization procedures for opening and closing restrictions (see Fig. 17-9A-C).

Lumbar Manipulation

The patient is placed in side-lying with the side to be manipulated up. The clinician should palpate this motion segment for movement as the patient's top leg is flexed. For example, if the clinician is attempting to manipulate the L4-L5 motion segment on the right, the patient should be in left side-lying and the clinician should palpate in the L4-L5 interspace. The patient's right leg should be flexed until motion is felt at the L4-L5 interspace. Rotation of the trunk is induced through the patient's left arm until motion is felt at the L4-L5 interspace. The clinician then uses the arm on the patient's pelvis to induce a thrust in the anterior direction (see Fig. 17-9A)

Lumbar Opening Mobilization

The patient is side-lying with the side to be mobilized up. If possible, the table is positioned to side-bend the patient away from the painful side. For example, if the patient has a left opening restriction at L4-L5, he or she would be in right side-lying with the table positioned in right side-bending. The clinician should palpate the L4-L5 interspace while flexing the patient's hips and knees until motion is felt at that segment. The patient's upper leg is flexed further to allow the foot to rest behind the opposite knee. The clinician next palpates the L4-L5 interspace with inducing flexion and rotation of the trunk to that level by pulling the patient's right arm parallel to the table. The clinician places one arm against the patient's trunk and the other arm over the pelvis. The fingertips of both hands are placed at the segment with pressure directed against the lower side of the spinous processes. Mobilization is performed by lifting the spinous processes with the fingertips while a downward force is created by the forearms (see Fig. 17-9B).

Lumbar Closing Mobilization

The patient is side-lying with the side to be mobilized up. The table is positioned to place the patient into side-bending toward the top side. For example, for a right closing restriction at L4-L5, the patient would be in left side-lying with the

table positioned into right side-bending. The clinician palpates the L4-L5 interspace and extends the patient's lower hip until motion is felt at the interspace. The clinician next palpates the interspace while producing trunk rotation and extension by pulling the patient's lower arm toward the ceiling. The clinician places the right arm against the patient's trunk. The hand is positioned with the thumb on the superior side of the spinous process of L4. The opposite arm blocks the patient's pelvis. The fingertips are placed on the inferior side of the lower vertebra in the motion segment. The mobilization is achieved through a force against the superior spinous process in a caudal and downward direction (see Fig. 17-9C). The force can be accentuated by the superior arm pushing into further extension and side-bending.

Treatment for the Sacroiliac Region

Many manipulation and mobilization techniques have been described for the SI region.[8,45] The manipulation technique described below has been demonstrated to be effective in several studies for many patients with SI region findings.[21,28]

Sacroiliac Region Manipulation

The patient is supine. The clinician stands on the side opposite of that to be manipulated. The patient is passively moved into side-bending toward the side to be manipulated. The patient interlocks the fingers behind the head. The therapist passively rotates the patient, then delivers a quick thrust to the ASIS in a posterior and inferior direction (see Fig. 17-9D). For example, if the patient's left side is to be manipulated, the patient is moved into left side-bending, followed by right rotation. The side to be manipulated may be determined from the results of the SI region special tests. Although the manipulation is directed toward one side, Cibulka and colleagues[15] found changes in innominate tilt on both sides of the pelvis after the performance of this manipulation, and therefore the choice of side to manipulate may not be that important to the outcome of the technique.

> ## CLINICAL PEARL #2
>
> Although the SI manipulation technique is described as targeting the SI region, it is often helpful for patients with pain and hypomobility of the lumbar spine as well.

Stabilization Classification

Strengthening the muscles of the lumbar spine is often the focus of exercise programs for patients with LBP. Although a link between LBP and lumbar muscle weakness may appear intuitive, research has produced some conflicting results. Some researchers report strength differences between asymptomatic subjects and those with back pain,[79] whereas others report little association.[92]

More recent investigations focus on aspects of muscle performance other than maximal force output. These studies indicate that the properties of muscular endurance,[52] muscle balance,[66] and neuromuscular control[70] may be more important than maximum muscle strength in preventing and rehabilitating LBP.

The lumbar spine devoid of any muscle activity is highly unstable, even under very low loads.[93] Muscle activity is therefore important for maintaining spinal stability. Stability during lifting and rotational movements has been studied most extensively. The erector spinae muscles provide most of the extensor force needed for lifting.[6] Rotation is mostly produced by the oblique abdominal muscles.[75] The oblique abdominals and the majority of the lumbar erector spinae muscle fibers lack direct attachment to the lumbar spinal motion segments, and therefore are unable to stabilize individual motion segments. The multifidus muscle is better suited for the purpose of segmental stabilization. The multifidus originates from the spinous processes of the lumbar vertebrae and forms a series of repeating fascicles attaching to the inferior lumbar transverse processes, the ilium, and sacrum. The multifidus is proposed to function as a stabilizer during lifting and rotational movements of the lumbar spine.[73] The quadratus lumborum has been proposed to be the primary stabilizer for side-bending movements.[80]

The oblique abdominals and transversus abdominus also contribute to spinal stabilization. These muscles have a more horizontal orientation and have been proposed to contribute to spinal stability by creating a rigid cylinder and increasing the stiffness of the lumbar spine.[42,50] This hypothesis is supported by studies demonstrating continuous activity of the transversus abdominus muscle throughout flexion and extension movements of the lumbar spine.[16]

Examination for the Stabilization Classification

Many of the findings leading to a stabilization classification come from the patient's medical history, including frequent recurrent episodes of LBP precipitated by minimal perturbations, deformity (e.g., lateral shift) with prior episodes, short-term relief from manipulation, a history of trauma, use of oral contraceptives, or an improvement of symptoms with the use of a brace.[22] Other authors recommend palpatory techniques for the presence of a "step-off" between the spinous processes of adjacent vertebrae, or hypermobility with passive intervertebral motion testing.[77,94] The reliability of these techniques, however, has been questioned, and their validity has not been demonstrated.[76] Others emphasize aberrant motions such as the "instability catch" occurring during active ROM testing of the motion.[61,94] The instability catch has been described by numerous authors as a sign of segmental instability[61,87,92]; however, its presence has never been related to symptoms or abnormal movements on diagnostic imaging studies.

Hicks[47] investigated a clinical prediction rule for predicting which patients with LBP are likely to benefit from a stabilization treatment approach. The most important factors were numerous pervious episodes of LBP, particularly if the patient reports that episode frequency is increasing (Box 17-3). From the physical examination, the most important factors were aberrant motions during active ROM, hypermobility detected during passive accessory motion testing, and a positive prone segmental instability test. These examination findings are detailed in the following sections.

Aberrant Motions

While standing, the patient is asked to perform flexion and extension ROM. Several different aberrations may occur that are considered to be signs of a stabilization classification. Most aberrations will occur during flexion, or on return from a forward flexed position. An "instability catch" is a sudden movement that occurs out of the plane of the intended motion.[93] For example, the patient may suddenly rotate, or side-bend, or both, while performing flexion. "Thigh climbing" occurs when the patient is attempting to return from a flexed position, and he or she uses an external support to assist in extending the spine.[22] Often the patient will be observed to assist spinal extension by pushing on the thighs. A "painful arc" is defined as symptoms occurring during the midrange of a motion that are not present at the beginning or end of the motion.[19] A painful arc may occur in flexion or return from flexion. Any of these aberrations (instability catch, thigh climbing, or a painful arc) are considered signs of a stabilization classification.

Passive Accessory Motion Testing

Passive accessory motion testing was described previously. For the stabilization classification, the clinician is looking for hypermobility at any level of the lumbar spine. The presence of hypermobility is an indication for a classification of stabilization.

Box 17-3

Key Examination Findings Leading to a Classification of Stabilization[47]

Increasing frequency of episodes of low back pain
Greater than three previous episodes of low back pain
At least one hypermobile lumbar spine segment (judged from lumbar spring testing)
Aberrant movements during lumbar flexion/extension active range of motion
Positive prone segmental instability test

Prone Instability Test

The patient lies prone with the trunk on the examining table and legs over the edge with feet resting on the floor (Fig. 17-10*A* and *B*). While the patient rests in this position, the clinician performs passive accessory motion testing on each level of the lumbar spine. The patient is asked to report any provocation of pain during the motion testing. Next, the patient is asked to lift his or her legs off the floor (hand-holding to the table may be used to maintain this position). With the patient holding this position, the motion testing is repeated. The test is positive if a lumbar segment was painful in the resting position, but is not painful or the pain is markedly reduced in the leg lifting position. Lifting the legs causes the spinal extensor muscles to activate, which assists in spinal stabilization. If the prone instability test is positive, a stabilization classification is indicated.[47]

Treatment for the Stabilization Classification

The treatment of patients in the stabilization classification begins with patient education. Education should focus on avoiding end-range movements of the lumbar spine to avoid positions that may overload the passive stabilizing structures of the spine. Lifting even light loads from a position of near end-range spinal flexion should be avoided because of the potentially damaging forces created in the ligaments and intervertebral discs of the spine by such movements.[81] Although important for anyone with LBP, patients in the stabilization classification need to be educated regarding the importance of maintaining trunk strength and overall endurance. Fatigue can adversely impact the ability of the spinal musculature to respond to imposed loads, which may further compromise the stabilizing structures.[131]

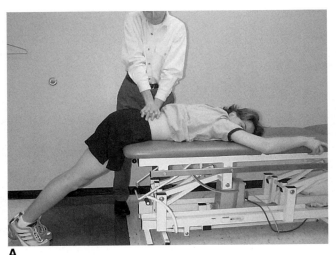

A

Step 1 — With the patient's feet on the floor, the clinician identifies any lumbar segments that are painful with passive motion testing.

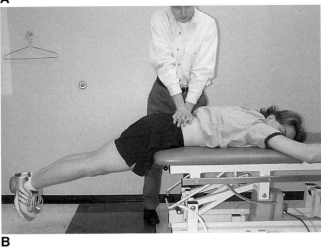

B

Step 2 — The patient lifts the legs off the floor and the clinician re-tests any lumber segments that were painful in step 1. A postive test occurs when the pain is substantially reduced or eliminated in step 2.

Figure 17-10. *A*, Step 1: With the patient's feet on the floor, the clinician identifies any lumbar segments that are painful with passive motion testing. *B*, Step 2: The patient lifts the legs off the floor and the clinician retests any lumbar segments that were painful in step 1. A positive test occurs when the pain is substantially reduced or eliminated in step 2.

Many exercise programs have been advocated for spinal stabilization. Although the literature supports the usefulness of active strengthening exercise programs, studies comparing different stabilization strengthening routines have generally not found any differences.[20,78] One approach is to identify exercises that optimally challenge important stabilizing muscles without imposing any potentially dangerous loads on the spine.[21,80] Important stabilizing muscles of the lumbar spine include the abdominal muscles, erector spinae and multifidus, and the quadratus lumborum. Basic exercises can be identified to address each of these muscle groups (Fig. 17-11A-E).

Abdominal Muscles and Transversus Abdominus

The muscles of the abdominal wall include the rectus abdominus, external and internal oblique, and the transverse abdominus. The primary function of these muscles is flexion and rotation of the trunk.[75] The oblique abdominals have a somewhat horizontal orientation, and contribute to spine stability by increasing the stiffness of the lumbar spine. The oblique abdominals have been shown to co-contract with the spinal extensors during side-bending or extension movements, increasing the stiffness and stability of the torso.[42] The rectus abdominus, because of its midline orientation, is primarily a trunk flexor and is not emphasized during the rehabilitation of patients with LBP. Transversus abdominus is a deep abdominal muscle with a horizontal orientation that helps to stabilize the spine by forming a rigid cylinder. Recent evidence demonstrates that a feedforward postural response occurs in regards to transversus abdominus contraction and limb movement.[50,51] In subjects without LBP, the transversus abdominus contracts before extremity movement, theoretically to stabilize the spine in preparation for movement. However, in patients with back pain, there is a delay in the onset of transversus abdominus contraction.[49] This has led to the hypothesis that the transversus abdominus plays an important role in spine stabilization.

Training the transversus abdominus may be initiated by teaching the patient the abdominal hollowing maneuver.[101] The patient is instructed to draw the navel up toward the head and in toward the spine so that the stomach flattens but the spine remains in its neutral position. Patients with LBP may have difficulty performing this seemingly simple maneuver. The key to the exercise is to isolate the deep abdominals and avoid substitution with the rectus abdominus. Palpation for muscle contraction by the patient just medial to the ASIS will often provide helpful feedback for proper performance of the exercise. The quadruped position is also useful for learning the hollowing maneuver because it may be more difficult to substitute with the rectus abdominus in this position.

Once the patient can perform the abdominal hollowing maneuver properly, more challenging activities can be added. From the supine position, leg movements (i.e., marching or leg raises) can be incorporated while maintaining the hollowing. Performing bridging exercises while maintaining the hollowing is also a challenge both to the transversus abdominus and gluteus maximus muscle (see Fig. 17-11A). It is recommended that hollowing should be combined with other aspects of the stabilization exercise program, and eventually should be incorporated into more functional positions and postures that would challenge each individual patient in his or her everyday activities. For example, if the patient complains of pain while sitting at work, the hollowing maneuver should be used in that position to control symptoms.

The oblique abdominal muscles can be exercised effectively with the horizontal side support exercise. This exercise produces high levels of activity in the oblique abdominals (50% maximal voluntary contraction [MVC]) with low compression forces.[1] To perform the horizontal side support, the patient is side-lying with the knees bent and upper body supported on the lower elbow. The patient then lifts the pelvis from the table (see Fig. 17-11B and C). The side support should be performed on both sides to achieve a balance of strength. If a patient has unilateral low back symptoms, it may be more difficult for the patient to perform the exercise on the symptomatic side. The patient should perform the side support exercise for progressively longer sustained periods of time and more repetitions. If asymmetry exists, it should be a goal to achieve equality in strength and endurance between the left and right sides. The side support exercise can also be progressed by extending the knees and using the ankles as the distal contact instead of the knees.

Performing curl-ups with a rotation of the torso has also been found to target the oblique abdominals while imposing relatively low compressive loads.[1] Performing curl-ups without any trunk rotation will target mostly the rectus abdominus muscle and therefore is less useful to the rehabilitation process. The position of the legs during the curl-up does not appear to affect muscle activity or compression on the spine.[1] A more challenging exercise for the oblique abdominals is a hanging straight leg raise. To perform this exercise the patient is hanging, supporting his or her body weight with the upper extremities. The legs are lifted to the horizontal position (90° of hip flexion). This exercise provides high levels of oblique abdominal activity (nearly 100% MVC), whereas producing low levels of compressive force on the spine.[1]

Erector Spinae and Multifidus

Strengthening of the erector spinae muscles may be important because they are the primary source of extension torque for lifting tasks.[6] The lumbar extensors can be divided into two groups: the multisegmental erector spinae muscles that attach to the thoracic spine and the pelvis, with most fibers spanning the lumbar region without any

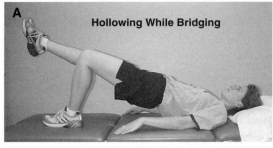

Hollowing While Bridging

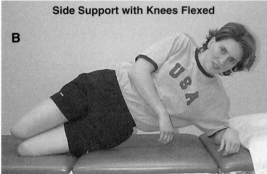

Side Support with Knees Flexed

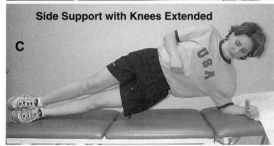

Side Support with Knees Extended

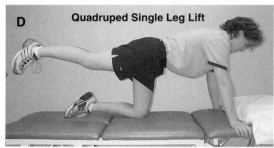

Quadruped Single Leg Lift

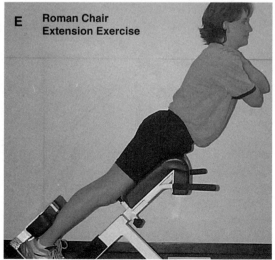

**Roman Chair
Extension Exercise**

Transversus Abdominus

Abdominal Hollowing

↓

Hollowing with leg movements, bridging, etc.

↓

Hollowing with functional activities

Oblique Abdominals

Horizontal Side Support

↓

Curl-ups with Trunk Rotation

↓

Hanging Leg Lifts

Quadratus Lumborum

Horizontal Side Support

Erector Spinae and Multifidus

Quadruped Single Arm or Leg Lifts

↓

Quadruped Opposite Arm and Leg Lifts

Prone Extension Exercises
Dynamic Extension Exercises
(e.g., Roman Chair)

Figure 17-11. Stabilization Exercise Treatment Program. *A*, Hollowing while bridging. *B*, Side support with knees flexed. *C*, Side support with knees extended. *D*, Quadruped single leg lift. *E*, Roman chair extension exercise.

attachment; and the segmental extensors, which attach to individual lumbar vertebrae.[60,74] The erector spinae muscles produce the extensor force needed for lifting, whereas the segmental extensors, primarily the multifidus muscle, provide stabilization of individual lumbar motion segments.[72,73] The multifidi originate from the spinous processes of the lumbar vertebrae and form a series of repeating fascicles attaching to the lumbar transverse processes below, as well as the ilium and sacrum. The multifidus is proposed to function as a segmental stabilizer during both lifting and rotational movements. Current evidence suggests that decreased endurance of multifidus and erector spinae muscles may be a risk factor for recurrence of LBP.[105] Research has also shown that the multifidi do not automatically recover full strength and endurance after the first episode of LBP, unless specific exercises are performed.[48] These findings emphasize the need for clinicians to focus attention on rehabilitation of the extensor musculature, with a particular focus on regaining endurance.

The erector spinae and multifidus muscles can be trained using extension exercises. Caution must be employed, however, because extension exercises also tend to produce high levels of compression on the lumbar spine, which may not be tolerated by all patients.[12] The safest position to begin an extension exercise program is quadruped. While in the quadruped position, the patient is asked to extend one leg or one arm to a horizontal position while maintaining the abdominal hollowing (see Fig. 17-11D). Raising the opposite arm and leg simultaneously offers more efficient training of multifidus and erector spinae with muscle activity levels in the realm of 30% of the MVC, while maintaining safe levels of lumbar compression.[82] Abdominal hollowing should be maintained while performing quadruped extension exercises to stabilize the spine in a neutral position, avoiding flexion or extension.

Extension exercises can be progressed to the prone position and performed dynamically instead of statically when a greater challenge to the extensor muscles is desired, which is often true for athletes. From a prone lying position, the patient is asked to raise the trunk and legs off of the table while keeping the pelvis in contact. Alternatively, the patient may perform active extension using a Roman chair to vary the angle of extension (see Fig. 17-11E).[120] For these exercises the patient's legs are fixed and the trunk is unsupported. The patient flexes the trunk forward and then extends against gravity to return to the starting position. These exercises produce high levels of activity in the erector spinae and multifidus muscles (40% to 60% MVC); however, the compressive loads on the lumbar spine increase over the quadruped position and may not be tolerated early in rehabilitation.[21] The use of prone extension exercises as described should be limited to patients who are hopeful of returning to athletic competi-

tion or demanding work activities, and who can tolerate the compression forces produced by such exercises. Quadruped exercises will be sufficient for the majority of patients, for whom the emphasis of retraining will be on endurance, and high levels of MVC are not required.

Quadratus Lumborum

The quadratus lumborum appears to play a key role in the stabilization of the spine during side-bending movements in the frontal plane or during compression of the spine. When compression is applied to the spine in an upright position, activity of the quadratus lumborum most closely correlates with the increased need for stability because of compressive loads.[80] The horizontal side support exercise described previously produces the greatest muscle activity in the quadratus lumborum (54% MVC) with low compressive loads. The horizontal side support exercise effectively targets both the oblique abdominals and quadratus lumborum, and is a key component of a stabilization exercise program.

CLINICAL PEARL #3

The horizontal side support exercise promotes high levels of activity in the oblique abdominal and quadratus lumborum muscles, whereas placing low compressive loads on the spine. This exercise is quite useful for patients in the stabilization classification and for patients who have progressed to stage II management.

Specific Exercise Classifications

The important clinical characteristic of patients in stage I likely to benefit from specific exercise routines is the presence of the centralization phenomenon. Centralization was originally described by McKenzie[83] as a phenomenon occurring during lumbar movement testing when the patient reports that the pain moves from an area more distal or lateral to a location more central or near midline position in the lumbar spine. Peripheralization occurs when the patient reports the movement of pain from an area more proximal in the lumbar spine to an area more distal or lateral. Movements that do not produce centralization or peripheralization are judged to be status quo.[34,83]

The centralization phenomenon is an important finding in patients with LBP. Patients with LBP, particularly when there is radiation into the buttock, thigh, or calf, who do not exhibit centralization are less likely to have a successful treatment outcome.[26,128] Long[69] studied patients with chronic LBP entering a work hardening program and found that the presence of centralization during the initial evaluation was associated with greater reductions in pain and greater percentages of return to work after completion of the program. Karas and colleagues[56] found that the inability to centralize symptoms during the initial evaluation decreased the likelihood of return to work within 6 months.

The presence of centralization has also been proposed to be an important finding for classifying patients into treatment-based subgroups.[22,83] When patients are found to centralize during the examination, the movements producing the centralization are then used as treatment techniques. Three different movements are typically found to centralize symptoms: extension, flexion, or pelvic translocations for a patient with a lateral shift. The three subgroups of patients in the specific exercise classification are defined by which movement is found to produce the centralization.

Other examination factors are also used to make a classification of specific exercise. Patients who centralize with extension and fit an extension classification often have signs and symptoms consistent with an intervertebral disc herniation. These patients will likely report that standing or walking is preferable to sitting, and sitting tolerance may be limited to less than a few minutes. These patients are also likely to report symptoms that extend into the buttock or lower extremity, or both, and may have signs of nerve root compression.

Patients fitting a flexion classification frequently report a clear preference for sitting versus standing or walking, and they may not have any symptoms at all when sitting.[35,57] Patients who centralize with flexion tend to be somewhat older and often have degenerative or stenotic spinal conditions.[38] Spinal stenosis causes a narrowing of the spinal canals. This narrowing is exacerbated with spinal extension and is relieved with spinal flexion.[95] Patients with spinal stenosis, therefore, often will be found to centralize with flexion movements and peripheralize with extension movements. Neurogenic claudication, defined as poorly localized pain, paraesthesias, and cramping of one or both lower extremities of a neurologic origin, which is brought on by walking and relieved when sitting,[99] frequently occurs with lumbar spinal stenosis.[114] Signs of nerve root compression may also be present on examination.

Patients fitting a lateral shift classification usually have a visible lateral shift deformity. A lateral shift deformity can be defined as a shifting of the patient's trunk and shoulders relative to the pelvis in the frontal plane.[59] Patients with a lateral shift will most often have symptoms into the lower extremity and signs of nerve root compression.[22] Lumbar intervertebral disc pathology is also common among patients fitting a lateral shift classification.[98]

On examination, patients fitting a lateral shift classification will typically have substantially asymmetric side-bending ROM, with a gross limitation of side-bending ROM in the direction opposite the lateral shift.[25]

Examination for the Specific Exercise Classifications

The portion of the physical examination most central to the specific exercise classifications is the active motion assessment. The focus of the active movement testing is not ROM, but rather the response of symptoms to movement (i.e., centralization or peripheralization). In addition, the neurologic assessment for signs of nerve root compression is often required for patients fitting specific exercise classifications because distal symptoms are common.

Lumbar Active Motion Assessment: Centralization/Peripheralization

The lumbar motion assessment begins with testing side-bending, flexion, and extension with the patient standing. For the purpose of detecting centralization/peripheralization, it is important to establish the baseline symptoms of the patient before any movements. The patient is asked to explain the symptoms experienced before the motion testing in terms of both location and intensity, and is then instructed to report any change in these factors that occurs with testing. The patient is then asked to side-bend to the left and right, to extend backward, and flex forward. After each movement the patient is asked about the effect of the movement on symptoms. If symptoms are abolished or move centrally, centralization has occurred. If symptoms fluctuate in intensity but do not centralize, the patient is judged to be status quo with that movement. If symptoms move peripherally, away from the spine, the patient is judged to have peripheralized with the movement. Any movement producing centralization is noted. This movement will be used as the basis for the patient's specific exercise program. Any movement causing peripheralization is also noted, and these movements are avoided in further motion assessment and treatment procedures.

For patients with a visible lateral shift deformity, pelvic translocation movements are also assessed with the patient standing. The clinician stands at the patient's side, on the same side toward which the patient has shifted. The clinician then stabilizes the patient's shoulders and trunk with his or her body and translates the pelvis in the frontal plane in the direction that corrects the shift. For example, if the patient had a right lateral shift deformity, the clinician would stand on the patient's right side and translate the patient's pelvis to the right (i.e., right pelvic translocation). The status of the patient's symptoms with this movement is judged as either centralized, peripheralized, or status quo.

If single movements produce centralization, these movements will form the basis for the patient's classification and treatment. If single movements cause peripheralization, these movements are avoided. However, many patients will remain status quo with single movement testing performed with the patient standing. If the patient's history suggests a specific exercise classification, but single movements in standing are judged to be status quo, further movement testing may be performed. The clinical decision-making scheme for movement test is pictured in Figure 17-12. Further movement testing may be accomplished by changing the patient's position, performing repeated movements, or sustaining the end-range movement position. Spinal flexion or extension, or both, may be assessed in the seated, supine, prone, or quadruped positions, as well as in the standing position. The quadruped position is particularly useful for evaluation because both flexion and extension can be assessed by having the patient rock back and forth, and the position decreases the weight-bearing stresses on the spine. The movement tests in any position can be repeated 5 to 10 times consecutively, or can be sustained for 20 to 30 seconds. After each test the patient is questioned regarding the impact on symptoms and the same judgments are made: centralization, peripheralization, or status quo. If centralization occurs with flexion, extension, or lateral shifts with any movement testing, the patient is assigned to the corresponding specific exercise classification. Box 17-4 summarizes the key examination findings leading to a classification of specific exercises.

Treatment for the Specific Exercise Classifications

The basic principle for treating patients in a specific exercise classification is to use the motions that were found to

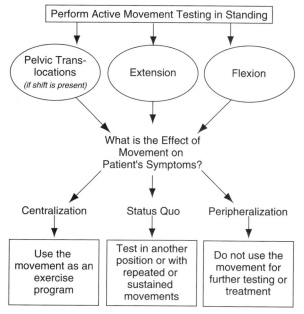

Figure 17-12. Decision-making with lumbar active movement testing.

Box 17-4

Key Examination Findings Leading to a Classification of Specific Exercise

Centralization during lumbar active movement assessment
Symptoms distal to the knee
Signs of nerve root compression
Clear preference for flexed or extended postures (sitting vs. standing/walking)
Visible lateral shift deformity

---

produce centralization on examination as interventions. The overall goal of interventions is to produce a lasting centralization of symptoms and permit the patient to progress on to later stages of treatment.

Treatment for Flexion Classification
Exercises to Promote Flexion

Flexion exercises are usually easiest to perform in the supine or quadruped positions. Patients fitting a flexion classification will frequently find the position of supine with the hips and knees flexed (i.e., the "hook-lying position") to be a comfortable position from which to exercise, and therefore a good place to begin a program. From this position, the patient may bring a single knee or both knees to the chest creating further flexion of the lumbar spine. The knee-to-chest position can be sustained for 20 to 30 seconds and repeated. Another simple flexion exercise to perform from this position is a posterior pelvic tilt. The patient is instructed to flatten his or her back against the support surface, reducing the lumbar lordosis and increasing lumbar flexion. The quadruped position is also a useful position for performing flexion exercises. From the quadruped position, the patient can move from the neutral position back onto the heels to promote lumbar flexion (Fig. 17-13A). This motion can be repeated as a gentle rocking movement from neutral into lumbar flexion.

Mobilizations to Promote Flexion

Joint mobilization can serve as a useful adjunct treatment for patients fitting a flexion classification. Because patients in this classification tend to be older, with degenerative changes, stiffness of the lumbar spine and hip joints is not uncommon. If stiffness is detected in the lumbar spine with passive accessory mobility testing, mobilizations may be performed. Several techniques may be used. Prone posterior-to-anterior mobilization is useful for many patients. The patient is prone and then positioned with the lumbar spine in flexion. This may be accomplished either by positioning the table into flexion or by using pillows under the patient's abdomen. The clinician contacts

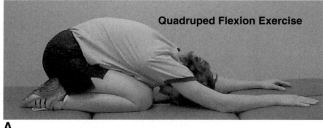

Quadruped Flexion Exercise

A

Hip Extension Mobilization

B

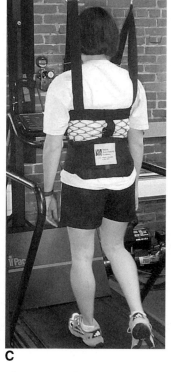

C

Exercises to Promote Lumbar Flexion

Supine flexion exercises

Quadruped flexion exercises

Mobilization to Promote Lumbar Flexion

Lumber mobilization in flexion

Hip extension mobilization

De-Weighted Ambulation

Aquatic ambulation

De-weighted treadmill ambulation

Figure 17-13. Treatment for flexion specific exercise classification. *A,* Quadruped flexion exercise. *B,* Hip extension mobilization. *C,* De-weighted ambulation.

the lumbar spinous process to be mobilized with the hypothenar eminence of the hand. An oscillatory mobilization force is produced through the clinician's trunk while the elbows are maintained in extension[130] (see Fig. 17-13B).

Mobilization or flexibility exercises, or both, for the hip joints are often indicated for patients fitting a flexion classification. If hip joint mobility is limited, particularly hip joint extension, an increased demand for extension ROM in the lumbar spine may be created. Patients fitting a flexion classification often cannot tolerate lumbar extension; therefore, improving mobility of the hip joints may help reduce stress on the lumbar spine. Stretching techniques for the hip joint flexor muscles (i.e., iliopsoas, rectus femoris, and tensor fascia latae) may be used. Mobilization of the hip joint to improve extension ROM is indicated when hypomobility of the joint is detected. Mobilization to improve hip joint extension is performed with the patient prone. A posterior-to-anterior mobilization force is directed to the proximal femur. The angle of hip extension can be increased to progress the mobilization technique (see Fig. 17-13B).

De-weighted Treadmill Ambulation

Patients fitting a flexion classification often have substantial limitations in walking tolerance[98]; therefore, addressing this functional limitation is an important goal of treatment. The limitation in walking with these patients is at least partly caused by the narrowing of the spinal canals that results from axial loading and extension that occur during walking.[132] De-weighted treadmill ambulation uses harness support to provide a vertical traction force, thereby reducing axial loading during walking (see Fig. 17-13C). Flynn and colleagues[32] found an average 24% reduction in vertical ground reaction forces during walking with 20% of body weight supported. Training with de-weighted treadmill ambulation is begun with sufficient

traction force to reduce or abolish the patient's lower extremity symptoms while walking. Usually a traction force equal to 20% to 40% of the patient's body weight is sufficient to accomplish this goal.[37] Over the course of treatment, the amount of walking time is gradually increased while the amount of traction force is gradually diminished.

Treatment for Extension Classification
Exercises to Promote Extension

Extension exercises can be performed in a variety of ways. Quadruped is usually a comfortable position for beginning an extension exercise program. Extension is achieved by having the patient rock forward over the arms then returning to the starting position (Fig. 17-14A). This gentle rocking motion is repeated 10 to 20 times. The patient should not rock back into flexion at this stage of treatment. Another basic activity that may be useful early in treatment is having the patient lie prone. Lying prone promotes extension of the lumbar spine. The prone position is sustained from 30 seconds up to a few minutes. With all exercises the response of the patient's symptoms is the key to determining their effectiveness. Exercises that help to centralize the patient's pain are continued; those that do not

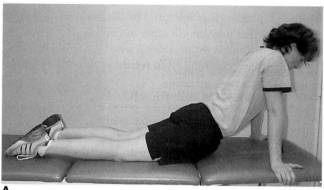

Exercises to Promote Lumbar Extension

Quadruped extension exercises

Prone lying

Prone on elbows

Prone press-ups

Mobilization to Promote Lumbar Extension

Lumber mobilization in prone lying

Lumber mobilization in prone on elbows

Lumber mobilization with prone press-up

Figure 17-14. Treatment for extension specific exercise classification. A, Prone press-up. B, Lumbar mobilization in prone lying.

to the patient because the table can be positioned. Mechanical traction may be performed with the patient either prone or supine. If the patient is supine, flexing the hips and knees will tend to place the lumbar spine into more flexion, and may be better tolerated by older patients with imaging findings suggesting lumbar spinal stenosis. The goal of treatment with mechanical traction is to centralize the patient's symptoms and to permit the patient to progress into another classification, such as specific exercise. Patients in the traction classification should be monitored closely. If reassessment shows that the patient is able to centralize symptoms with active movements, progression to a specific exercise classification would be indicated. If the patient's symptoms and signs of nerve root compression continue to worsen, referral for surgery, injections, or other treatment options is warranted.

Treatment with autotraction may be preferred to mechanical traction for patients in the traction classification. Autotraction is particularly indicated for patients with a lateral shift deformity who are unable to centralize symptoms, or who actually experience peripheralization of symptoms, with pelvic translocation. Autotraction uses a specially designed table that allows the patient to be positioned in a variety of ways. The patient is initially positioned in a manner that centralizes symptoms to the greatest extent possible. For patients with a lateral shift, this is most often accomplished by having the patient lie supine with lumbar flexion, or side-lying on the side opposite the direction of the shift. After positioning the patient, the table can be elevated, and the patient is asked to produce the traction force by pulling with the arms and pushing with one or both feet (Fig. 17-16). As the patient is producing the traction force, the table can be gradually

repositioned to move the patient away from the accommodated position into a more neutral posture.

STAGE II MANAGEMENT

The goal of stage I management, regardless of the classification, is to reduce pain and disability and progress the patient into stage II treatment. The goals for management of patients with LBP in stage II are more focused on improving functional abilities and addressing any impairments of strength or flexibility that can be identified. Another goal of stage II management is to reduce the likelihood of the patient experiencing a recurrence of LBP. Rates of recurrence are reported to be as high as 60% to 80%.[3,123] Stage II treatment approach has three basic components: specific trunk strengthening, general strength and flexibility exercises, and aerobic conditioning.

Specific Trunk Strengthening

Some evidence suggests that failure to regain strength of the important trunk stabilizing muscles may increase the risk for poor recovery from, or a recurrence of an episode of, LBP.[14,100] Hides and colleagues[48] have shown that a program of trunk strengthening and stabilization exercises can reduce the likelihood of recurrence after an episode of LBP. If patients did not receive specific trunk strengthening exercises as part of stage I treatment, those exercises should be initiated once the patient moves into stage II. Strengthening exercises for the abdominal muscles, erector spinae and multifidus, and quadratus lumborum should be used as were previously described (see Fig. 17-11A-E).

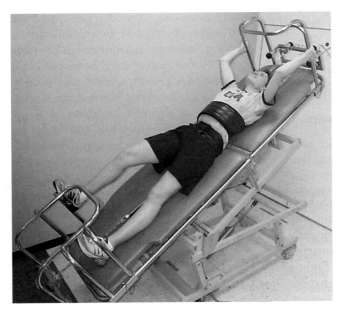

The patient produces the traction force by pulling with the arms and pushing with the legs.

Figure 17-16. Auto-Traction Treatment for Traction Classification. The patient produces the traction force by pulling with the arms and pushing with the legs.

CLINICAL PEARL #5

Adequate strength of the trunk stabilizing muscles may be an important factor in preventing the recurrence of LBP. Once a patient reaches stage II, specific stabilizing exercises should be initiated if not done already.

General Strength and Flexibility Exercises

In addition to training the stabilizing muscles of the trunk, the clinician may also need to focus a portion of the stage II rehabilitation program on some of the large muscle groups of the lower extremities. This is particularly important when a patient is having difficulty performing lifting tasks. Current theory suggests that the proper way to perform a lifting task is to lift from a squatted position, flexing the hips and knees while minimizing flexion of the lumbar spine.[82] When lumbar flexion predominates a lifting task, the risk for injury is increased. To lift from a squatted position, an individual must have adequate strength and endurance of the gluteus maximus and quadriceps muscle groups in particular. If the gluteus maximus and quadriceps are deconditioned, correct lifting may not be performed and the risk for recurrence of LBP may be increased. The gluteus maximus in particular is often weak in individuals with chronic LBP and has been found to be more fatigable than those of healthy individuals.[55] Strengthening of the gluteus maximus can be achieved with bridging exercises or quadruped single leg extension exercises with the knee flexed to reduce the contribution of the hamstring muscles. It has also been reported that the performance of balance exercises in the standing position may improve the strength and timing of gluteus maximus contractions.[9] The performance of squatting exercises will incorporate both the quadriceps and gluteus maximus muscles.[115]

Although a link between lower extremity flexibility and LBP is often assumed, research has not shown this to be the case.[89] A few studies have suggested a relationship between flexibility of the hamstring and hip flexor muscle and LBP, particularly in adolescents.[29,64] Stretching of these muscle groups may be important for some patients during stage II treatment. The flexibility of the hamstring muscles can be assessed with the straight leg raise test described earlier. Hip flexor flexibility is best evaluated using the Thomas test (see Reference 45, pp 462-464). Caution may need to be exercised when instructing a patient with LBP in proper stretching techniques. When stretching the hamstrings, the patient should be instructed to avoid excessive lumbar flexion. This may be accomplished by instructing the patient to maintain a neutral to slightly lordotic lumbar spine while stretching, or by using the supine position for stretching. The best position for stretching the hip flexors while avoiding undue stress on the lumbar spine is often a kneeling position. The patient kneels on the side to be stretched and is taught to perform a posterior tilt of the pelvis to stretch the hip flexors, particularly the iliopsoas (Fig. 17-17). Careful instruction may be required to ensure that the patient is able to achieve the stretch with a posterior tilt of the pelvis and not by extending the lumbar spine. Placing the hip into slight adduction will place greater emphasis on the iliotibial band.

Aerobic Exercises

Increased levels of aerobic fitness have been linked to a decreased incidence of low back injury, and may help to avoid recurrence.[10] There is also evidence that low stress aerobic exercise may be effective in the treatment of patients with acute or chronic LBP.[5,119] An aerobic exercise component should be incorporated into all stage II treatment programs. The particular aerobic activity used depends on the preferences and tolerance of the individual patient. Walking results in low levels of compression on the lumbar spine and is well tolerated by most patients in stage II. Because walking also requires constant, submaximal effort from the stabilizing muscles of the trunk while placing low compressive loads on the spine,[21] it is as an effective aerobic exercise for patient with LBP who have progressed to stage II treatment. Progressive walking programs can generally be initiated early in the rehabilitation process and can be progressed as the patient's activity tolerance increases.

Not all patients with LBP, even those in stage II treatment, will be able to tolerate walking as an aerobic activity. Walking places the lumbar spine into a more extended position and this position may not be tolerated for prolonged periods of time by all patients. These patients may be better suited to stationary cycling as an aerobic exercise. Another option for aerobic activity in patients who experience an increase in symptoms while walking is the use of aquatic exercise. Having the patient walk while in a pool permits the buoyancy of the water to reduce the compressive forces of gravity (see Chapter 12). This usually allows a patient to walk without any increase in symptoms. The depth of the water will correspond to the amount of reduction in compression. Exercise progression can therefore be achieved by having the patient walk in progressively more shallow water, until such time as the patient can tolerate walking outside of the water without any increase in symptoms.

De-weighted treadmill ambulation may also be an option for patients who do not tolerate regular walking because of increased symptoms. As described earlier, de-weighted treadmill walking uses a traction harness system to decrease the weight that the body must support during walking, thereby reducing the compressive forces on the lumbar spine, and likely reducing the symptoms experienced when walking. When beginning an aerobic exercise program using de-weighted treadmill ambulation, the clinician should use sufficient traction force to permit the

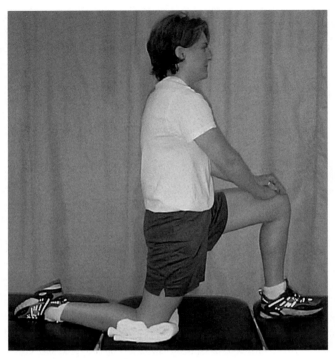

To stretch the right hip flexor, the patient is instructed to kneel on the right knee, then perform a posterior pelvic tilt to produce hip extension. Extension of the lumbar spine should be avoided.

Figure 17-17. Kneeling Hip Flexor Stretch for Stage II. To stretch the right hip flexor, the patient is instructed to kneel on the right knee, then perform a posterior pelvic tilt to produce hip extension. Extension of the lumbar spine should be avoided.

patient to walk without any increase in symptoms. The amount of traction force can then be gradually reduced over the course of treatment until the patient is able to walk without any external support or increase in symptoms.

Another popular and effective aerobic exercise is jogging or running. Running has not been associated with an increased risk for developing LBP, and running has actually been found to place participants at a lower risk for development of degenerative changes of the lumbar intervertebral discs than participants in other activities such as soccer or weightlifting.[121] Running has been found to create increased compressive loads on the lumbar spine,[130] and therefore may not be tolerated by some patients in stage II rehabilitation after an episode of LBP. If return to running is a goal of a patient, caution should be exercised and a gradual return emphasized. If a patient experiences difficulty in returning, the use of a de-weighting device to reduce compression along with running on a treadmill may be helpful.

SUMMARY

Background

- Low back pain is a common occurrence resulting in substantial pain and disability.
- It is frequently not possible to identify the underlying cause of low back pain.

- Classification systems seek to group patients on the basis of clusters on examination findings, instead of seeking to identify the underlying cause.
- Each classification category has a specific treatment approach associated with it that is believed to be most effective for patients in that category.

Screening for Red and Yellow Flags: First Level Classification

- Red flags are findings that may indicate a serious underlying pathology.
- Clinicians should be aware of red flags for conditions such as fracture, cancer, cauda equina syndrome, and other conditions that would warrant a referral to a physician.
- Yellow flags are findings that indicate the patient may be at risk for prolonged disability because of psychosocial factors.
- The most important psychosocial factor for patients with low back pain is fear-avoidance beliefs.
- Patients with high levels of fear-avoidance beliefs should be treated with active interventions, emphasizing functional ability rather than pain.

Staging the Patient: Second Level Classification

- Staging is not based strictly on acuity, but also on the presentation of the patient and the goals for rehabilitation.

- Patients in stage I have high levels of disability and difficulty performing basic daily activities. The goals for rehabilitation are to reduce symptoms and progress to stage II.
- Patients in stage II have lower levels of disability but difficulty performing more complex tasks. The goals for rehabilitation are to resume full functioning and to prevent recurrence.

Determining the Best Treatment: Third Level Classification

- Information from the medical history and physical examination is used to classify the patient.
- For patients in stage I, four classifications exist: manipulation/mobilization, specific exercise, stabilization, and traction.
- Patients in the manipulation/mobilization classification tend to have a more recent onset of symptoms, stiffness in the spine, and no symptoms distal to the knee. Interventions include manipulation and mobilization techniques and ROM exercises.
- Patients in the stabilization classification tend to have frequent previous episodes that are increasing in frequency, hypermobility in the spine, and a positive prone instability test. Interventions include strengthening exercises for trunk stabilizing muscles.
- Patients in the specific exercise classification are characterized by the presence of centralization during lumbar ROM testing. Interventions involve repeated end-range exercises in the direction that produces the centralization (flexion, extension, or lateral shift).
- Patients in the traction classification tend to have signs of nerve root compression and do not centralize with lumbar ROM testing. Interventions include mechanical or autotraction.
- Interventions for patients in stage II focus on eliminating impairments of trunk strength, lower extremity strength and flexibility, and aerobic conditioning.

REFERENCES

1. Axler, C.T., and McGill, S.M. (1997): Low back loads over a variety of abdominal exercises: Searching for the safest abdominal challenge. Med. Sci. Sports Exerc., 29:804-811.
2. Balagué, F., Nordin, M., Sheikhzadeh, A., et al. (1999): Recovery of severe sciatica. Spine, 24:2516-2524.
3. Bergquist-Ulman, M., and Larsson, U. (1970): Acute low back pain in industry: A controlled prospective study with special reference to therapy and confounding factors. Acta. Orthop. Scand., 170(suppl):S1-S117.
4. Beursken, A.J., de Vet, H.C., Köke, A.J., et al. (1997): Efficacy of traction for nonspecific low back pain. 12-week and 6-month results of a randomized clinical trial. Spine, 22:2756-2762.
5. Bigos S., Bowyer, O., Braen, G., et al. (1994): Acute low back problems in adults. AHCPR Publication 95-0642. Rockville, MD, Agency for Health Care Policy and Research, Public Health Service, US Department of Health and Human Services.
6. Bogduk, N., Macintosh, J.E., and Pearcy, M.J. (1992): A universal model of the lumbar back muscles in the upright position. Spine, 17:897-913.
7. Bombardier, C. (2000): Outcome assessment in the evaluation of treatment of spinal disorders: Summary and general recommendations. Spine, 25:3100-3103.
8. Boyling, J.D., Palastanga, N., and Grieve, G.P. (1994): Grieve's Modern Manual Therapy: The Vertebral Column, 2nd ed. St. Louis, MO, Churchill Livingstone.
9. Bullock-Saxton, J.E., Janda, V., Bullock, M.I. (1993): Reflex activation of gluteal muscles during walking. An approach to restoration of muscle function for patients with low-back pain. Spine, 18:704-709.
10. Cady, L.D., Bischoff, D.P., O'Connell, E.R. (1979): Strength and fitness and subsequent back injuries in firefighters. J. Occup. Med., 21:269-279.
11. Calin, A., Porta, J., Fries, J.F., and Schurman, D.J. (1977): Clinical history as a screening tool for ankylosing spondylitis. JAMA, 237:2613-2614.
12. Callaghan, J.P., Gunning, J.L., and McGill, S.M. (1998): The relationship between lumbar spine load and muscle activity during extensor exercises. Phys. Ther., 78:8-18.
13. Chan, C.W., Goldman, S., Ilstrup, D.M., Kunselman, A.R, and O'Neill, P.I. (1993): The pain drawing and Waddell's nonorganic physical signs in chronic low back pain. Spine, 18:1717-1722.
14. Cholewicki, J., and McGill, S.M. (1996): Mechanical stability of the in vivo lumbar spine: Implications for injury and low back pain. Clin. Biomech., 11:1-15.
15. Cibulka, M.T., Delitto, A., and Koldehoff, R.M. (1988): Changes in innominate tilt after manipulation of the sacroiliac joint in patients with low back pain. An experimental study. Phys. Ther., 68:1359-1363.
16. Cresswell, A.G., Grundstrom, H., and Thorstensson, A. (1992): Observations on intra-abdominal pressure and patterns of abdominal intra-muscular activity in man. Acta. Physiol. Scand., 144:409-418.
17. Crombez, G., Vlaeyen, J.W., Heuts, P.H., and Lysens, R. (1999): Pain-related fear is more disabling than pain itself: Evidence on the role of pain-related fear in chronic back pain disability. Pain, 80:329-339.
18. Cypress, B.K. (1983): Characteristics of physician visits for back symptoms: A national perspective. Am. J. Pub. Health., 73:389.
19. Cyriax, J. (1982): Textbook of Orthopaedic Medicine, Vol 1: Diagnosis of Soft Tissue Lesions, 6th ed. London, UK, Bailliere Tindall.
20. Danneels, L., Vanderstraeten, G., Cambier, D., et al. (2001): Effects of three different training modalities on cross-sectional area of the lumbar multifidus muscle in patients with chronic low back pain. Br. J. Sports Med., 35:186-192.
21. Delitto, A., Cibulka, M.T., Erhard, R.E., et al. (1993): Evidence for use of an extension-mobilization category in acute low back syndrome: a prescriptive validation pilot study. Phys. Ther., 73:216-222.
22. Delitto, A., Erhard, R.E., and Bowling, R.W. (1995): A treatment-based classification approach to low back syndrome: Identifying and staging patients for conservative treatment. Phys. Ther., 75:470-489.
23. Deyo, R.A., and Diehl, A.K. (1988): Cancer as a cause of back pain: Frequency, clinical presentation, and diagnostic strategies. J. Gen. Intern. Med., 3:230-238.

24. Deyo, R.A., Rainville, J., and Kent, D.L. (1992): What can the history and physical examination tell us about low back pain? JAMA, 268:760-765.

25. Donahue, M.S., Riddle, D.L., and Sullivan, M.S. (1996): Intertester reliability of a modified version of McKenzie's lateral shift assessments obtained on patients with low back pain. Phys. Ther., 76:706-716.

26. Donelson, R., Silva, G., and Murphy, K. (1990): Centralization phenomenon: Its usefulness in evaluating and treating referred pain. Spine, 15:211-213.

27. Dreyfuss, P., Michaelsen, M., Pauza, K., et al. (1996): The value of medical history and physical examination in diagnosing sacroiliac joint pain. Spine, 21:2594-2602.

28. Erhard, R.E., Delitto, A., Cibulka, M.T. (1994): Relative effectiveness of an extension program and a combined program of manipulation and flexion and extension exercises in patients with acute low back syndrome. Phys. Ther., 74:1093-1100.

29. Feldman, D.E., Shrier, I., Rossignol, M., and Abenhaim, L. (2001): Risk factors for the development of low back pain in adolescence. Am. J. Epidemiol., 154:30-36.

30. Fiebert, I., and Keller, C.D. (1994): Are "passive" extension exercises really passive? J. Orthop. Sports Phys. Ther., 19: 111-117.

31. Flynn, T., Fritz, J., Whitman, J., et al. (2002): A clinical prediction rule for classifying patients with low back pain who demonstrate short-term improvement with spinal manipulation. Spine, 27:2835-2843.

32. Flynn, T.W., Canavan, P.K., Cavanagh, P.R., et al. (1997): Plantar pressure reduction in an incremental weight-bearing system. Phys Ther., 77:410-419.

33. Fredrickson, B.E., Baker, D., McHolick, et al. (1984): The natural history of spondylolysis and spondylolisthesis. J. Bone Joint Surg., 66-A:699-707.

34. Fritz, J.M., Delitto, A., Vignovic, M., and Busse, R.G. (2000): Inter-rater reliability of judgments of the centralization phenomenon and status change during movement testing in patients with low back pain. Arch. Phys. Med. Rehabil., 81:57-61.

35. Fritz, J.M., Erhard, R.E., Delitto, A., et al. (1997): Preliminary results of the use of a two-stage treadmill test as a clinical diagnostic tool in the differential diagnosis of lumbar spinal stenosis. J. Spinal Dis., 10:410-416.

36. Fritz, J.M., Erhard, R.E., and Hagen, B.F. (1998): Update: Segmental instability of the lumbar spine. Phys. Ther., 78:889-896.

37. Fritz, J.M., Erhard, R.E., and Vignovic, M. (1997): A nonsurgical treatment approach for patients with lumbar spinal stenosis. A case report. Phys. Ther., 77:962-973.

38. Fritz, J.M., and George, S. (2000): The use of a classification approach to identify subgroups of patients with acute low back pain: Inter-rater reliability and short-term treatment outcomes. Spine, 25:106-114.

39. Fritz, J.M., George, S.Z., and Delitto, A. (2001): The role of fear avoidance beliefs in acute low back pain: Relationships with current and future disability and work status. Pain, 94:7-15.

40. Fritz, J.M., and George, S.Z. (2002): Identifying specific psychosocial factors in patients with acute, work-related low back pain: The importance of fear-avoidance beliefs. Phys. Ther., 82:973-983.

41. Fritz, J.M., and Irrgang, J.J. (2001): A comparison of a Modified Oswestry Disability Questionnaire and the Quebec Back Pain Disability Scale. Phys. Ther., 81:776-788.

42. Gardner-Morse, M.G., and Stokes, I.A.F. (1998): The effects of abdominal muscle coactivation on lumbar spine stability. Spine, 23:86-92.

43. Goldstein, J.D., Berger, P.E., Windler, G.E., and Jackson, J.W. (1991): Spine injuries in gymnasts and swimmers. An epidemiologic investigation. Am. J. Sports Med., 19:463-468.

44. Gran, J.T. (1985): An epidemiological survey of the signs and symptoms of ankylosing spondylitis. Clin. Rheumatol., 4: 161-169.

45. Greenman, P.E. (1996): Principles of Manual Medicine, 2nd ed. Philadelphia, PA, Lippincott Williams & Wilkins.

46. Hadler, N.M., Curtis, P., Gillings, D.B., and Stinnett, S. (1987): A benefit of spinal manipulation as an adjunctive therapy for acute low-back pain: A stratified controlled study. Spine, 12: 703-705.

47. Hicks, G.E. (2002): Predictive validity of clinical variables used in the determination of patient prognosis following a lumbar stabilization program. Doctoral Dissertation, University of Pittsburgh.

48. Hides, J.A, Jull, G.A., and Richardson, C.A. (2001): Long-term effects of specific stabilizing exercises for first-episode low back pain. Spine, 26:E243-E248.

49. Hodges, P.W., and Richardson, C.A. (1997): Contraction of the abdominal muscles associated with movement of the lower limb. Phys. Ther., 77:132-141.

50. Hodges, P.W., and Richardson, C.A. (1996): Inefficient muscular stabilization of the lumbar spine associated with low back pain. Spine, 21:2640-2649.

51. Hodges, P.W., and Richardson, C.A. (1998): Delayed postural contraction of transversus abdominis in low back pain associated with movement of the lower limb. J. Spinal Dis., 11:46-52.

52. Hultman, G., Nordin, M., Saraste, H., et al. (1993): Body composition, endurance, strength, cross-sectional area, and density of erector spinae in men with and without low back pain. J. Spinal Dis., 6:114-120.

53. Hutchinson, M.R., Laprade, R.F., Burnett, Q.M., et al. (1995): Injury surveillance at the USTA Boys' Tennis Championships: A 6-yr study. Med. Sci. Sports Exerc., 27:826-830.

54. Jarvik, J.G., and Deyo, R.A. (2002): Diagnostic evaluation of low back pain with emphasis on imaging. Ann. Intern. Med., 137:586-597.

55. Kankaanpaa, M., Taimela, S., Laaksonen, D., et al. (1998): Back and hip extensor muscle fatigability in chronic low back pain patients and controls. Arch. Phys. Med. Rehabil., 79:412-418.

56. Karas, R., McIntosh, G., Hall, H., et al. (1997): The relationship between nonorganic signs and centralization of symptoms in the prediction of return to work for patients with low back pain. Phys. Ther., 77:354-360.

57. Katz, J.N., Dalgas, M., Stucki, G., and Lipson, S.G. (1995): Degenerative lumbar spinal stenosis. Diagnostic value of the history and physical examination. Arthritis Rheum., 38: 1236-1241.

58. Kendall, N.A., Linton, S.J., and Main, C.J. (1997): Guide to assessing psychosocial yellow flags in acute low back pain: Risk factors for long-term disability and work loss. Wellington, New Zealand, Accident Rehabilitation & Compensation Insurance Corporation of New Zealand and the National Health Committee.

59. Kilpikoski, S., Airaksinen, O., Kankaanpaa, M., et al. (2002): Interexaminer reliability of low back pain assessment using the McKenzie method. Spine, 27:E207-E214.

60. Kippers, V., and Parker, A.W. (1984): Posture related to myoelectric silence of erectores spinae during trunk flexion. Spine, 7:740-745.

61. Kirkaldy-Willis, W.H., and Farfan, H.F. (1982): Instability of the lumbar spine. Clin. Orthop., 165:110-123.

62. Klenerman, L., Plade, P.D., Stanley, M., et al. (1995): The prediction of chronicity in patients with an acute attack of low back pain in a general practice setting. Spine, 20:478-484.

63. Koes, B.W., Bouter, L.M., van Mameren, H., et al. (1992): The effectiveness of manual therapy, physiotherapy, and treatment by the general practitioner for nonspecific back and neck complaints. A randomized clinical trial. Spine, 17:28-35.

64. Kujala, U.M., Salminen, J.J., Taimela, S., et al. (1992): Subject characteristics and low back pain in young athletes and nonathletes. Med. Sci. Sports Exer., 24:627-632.

65. Laupacis, A., Sekar, N., and Stiell, I.G. (1997): Clinical prediction rules. A review and suggested modifications of methodological standards. JAMA, 277:488-494.

66. Lee, J.H., Hoshino, Y., Nakamura, K., et al. (1999): Trunk muscle weakness as a risk factor for low back pain: A 5-year prospective study. Spine, 24:54-61.

67. Lethem, J., Slade, P.D., Troup, J.D.G., and Bentley, G. (1983): Outline of a fear avoidance model of exaggerated pain perception-I. Behav. Res. Ther., 21:401-408.

68. Linton, S.J., and Andersson, T. (2000): Can chronic disability be prevented? A randomized trial of a cognitive-behavioral intervention for spinal pain patients. Spine, 25:2585-2591.

69. Long, A.L. (1995): The centralization phenomenon: Its usefulness as a predictor of outcome in conservative treatment of low back pain (a pilot study). Spine, 20:2513-2521.

70. Luoto, S., Taimela, S., Hurri, H., et al. (1996): Psychomotor speed and postural control in chronic low back pain patients: A controlled follow-up study. Spine, 21:2621-2629.

71. Macfarlane, G.J., Thomas, E., Croft, P.R., et al. (1999): Predictors of early improvement in low back pain amongst consulters to general practice: The influence of pre-morbid and episode-related factors. Pain, 80:113-119.

72. MacIntosh, J.E., and Bogduk, N. (1996): The anatomy and function of the lumbar back muscles. In: Boyling, J.D., Palastanga, N. (eds.), Grieve's Modern Manual Therapy. The Vertebral Column, 2nd ed. New York, Churchill Livingstone, pp. 189-209.

73. Macintosh, J.E., and Bogduk, N. (1986): The biomechanics of the lumbar multifidus. Clin Biomech., 1:205-213.

74. MacIntosh, J.E., and Bogduk, N. (1987): The morphology of the lumbar erector spinae. Spine, 12:658-668.

75. MacIntosh, J.E., Pearcy, M.J., and Bogduk, N. (1993): The axial torque of the lumbar back muscles: Torsion strength of the back muscles. Aust. NZ J. Surg., 63:205-212.

76. Maher, C., and Adams, R. (1994): Reliability of pain and stiffness assessments in clinical manual lumbar spine examination. Phys. Ther., 74:801-811.

77. Maitland, G.D. (1986): Vertebral Manipulation, 5th ed. Oxford, Butterworth Heinemann, pp. 74-76.

78. Mannion, A., Taimela, S., Montener, M., and Dvorak, J. (2001): Active therapy for chronic low back pain. Part 1. Effects on back muscle activation, fatigability, and strength. Spine, 26:897-908.

79. Mayer, T.G., Smith, S.S., Keeley, J., et al. (1985): Quantification of lumbar function. Part 2. Sagittal plane trunk strength in chronic low back pain patients. Spine, 10:765-770.

80. McGill, S.M. (1997): Distribution of tissue loads in the low back during a variety of daily and rehabilitation tasks. J. Rehabil. Res. Dev., 34:448-458.

81. McGill, S.M. (1988): Estimation of force and extensor moment contributions of the disc and ligaments at L4-L5. Spine, 13:1395-1402.

82. McGill, S.M. (1998): Low back exercises: Evidence for improving exercise regimens. Phys. Ther., 78:754-766.

83. McKenzie, R.A. (1989): The lumbar spine: Mechanical diagnosis and therapy. Waikanae, New Zealand: Spinal Publications Limited.

84. Meade, T.W., Dyer, S., Browne, W., et al. (1990): Low back pain of mechanical origin: Randomised comparison of chiropractic and hospital outpatient treatment. BMJ, 300:1431-1437.

85. Micheli, L.J., and Wood, R. (1995): Back pain in young athletes: Significant differences from adults in causes and patterns. Arch. Pediatr. Adolesc. Med., 149:15-18.

86. Moore, J.E., Von Korff, M., Cherkin, D., et al. (2000): A randomized trial of a cognitive-behavioral program for enhancing back pain self-care in primary care setting. Pain, 88:145-153.

87. Nachemson, A. (1985): Lumbar spine instability: A critical update and symposium summary. Spine, 10:290-291.

88. Nachemson, A.L. (1985): Advances in low back pain. Clin. Orthop., 200:266-278.

89. Nadler, S.F., Wu, K.D., Galski, T., and Feinberg, J.H. (1998): Low back pain in college athletes. A prospective study correlating lower extremity overuse or acquired ligamentous laxity with low back pain. Spine, 23:828-833.

90. NCAA. (1998): NCAA Injury Surveillance System (1997-1998): Overland Park, KS, National Collegiate Athletic Association.

91. Newton, M., Thow, M., Somerville, D., et al. (1993): Trunk strength testing with iso-machines. Part II: experimental evaluation of the Cybex II back testing system in normal subjects and patients with chronic low back pain. Spine, 18:812-820.

92. Ogon, M., Bender, B.R., Hooper, D.M., et al. (1997): A dynamic approach to spinal instability. Part II. Hesitation and giving-way during interspinal motion. Spine, 22:2859-2866.

93. Panjabi, M.M. (1992): The stabilizing system of the spine. Part II. Neutral zone and instability hypothesis. J. Spinal Disord., 5:390-398.

94. Paris, S.V. (1985): Physical signs of instability. Spine, 10:277-279.

95. Penning, L. (1992): Functional pathology of lumbar spinal stenosis. Clin. Biomech., 7:3-15.

96. Phillips, H.C. (1987): Avoidance behaviour and its role in sustaining chronic pain. Behav Res Ther., 25:273-279.

97. Pincus, T., Vlaeyen, J.W., Kendall, N.A, et al. (2002): Cognitive-behavioral therapy and psychosocial factors in low back pain. Spine, 27:E133-E138.

98. Porter, R.W., and Miller, C.G. (1986): Back pain and trunk list. Spine, 11:596-600.

99. Porter, R.W. (1996): Spinal stenosis and neurogenic claudication. Spine, 21:2046-2052.

100. Rantenen, J., Hurme, M., Ralck, B., et al. (1993): The lumbar multifidus muscle five years after surgery for a lumbar intervertebral disc herniation. Spine, 18:568-574.

101. Richardson, C.A., and Jull, G.A. (1995): Muscle control-pain control: What exercises would you prescribe? Manual Therapy, 1:2-11.

102. Riddle, D.L., and Freburger, J.K. (2002): Evaluation of the presence of sacroiliac joint region dysfunction using a combination of tests: A multicenter intertester reliability study. Phys. Ther., 82:772-781.

103. Sands, W.A., Shultz, B.B., and Newman, A.P. (1993): Women's gymnastics injuries. A 5-year study. Am. J. Sports Med., 21:271-276.

104. Shah, M.K., and Stewart, G.W. (2002): Sacral stress fractures: An unusual cause of low back pain in an athlete. Spine, 27:E104-E108.

105. Sihvonen, T., Lindgren, K.A., Airaksinen, O., et al. (1997): Movement disturbances of the lumbar spine and abnormal back muscle electromyographic findings in recurrent low back pain. Spine, 22:289-297.

106. Sikorski, J.M. (1985): A rationalized approach to physiotherapy for low back pain. Spine, 10:571-578.

107. Slade, P.D., Troup, J.D.G., Lethem, J., and Bentley, G. (1983): The fear-avoidance model of exaggerated pain perception-II. Behav. Res. Ther., 21:409-416.

108. Soler, T., and Calderon, C. (2000): The prevalence of spondylolysis in the Spanish elite athlete. Am. J. Sports Med., 28:57-62.

109. Standaert, C.J., and Herring, S.A. (2000): Spondylolysis: A critical review. Br. J. Sports Med., 34:415-422.

110. Supik, L.F., and Broom, M.J. (1994): Sciatic tension signs and lumbar disc herniation. Spine, 19:1066-1069.

111. Thomas, E., Silman, A.J., Croft, P.R., et al. (1999): Predicting who develops chronic low back pain in primary care: A prospective study. BMJ, 318:1662-1667.

112. Thompson, N., Halpern, B., Curl, W.W., et al. (1987): High school football injuries: Evaluation. Am. J. Sports Med., 15:117-124.

113. Troup, J.D.G., Martin, J.W., and Lloyd, D.C. (1981): Back pain in industry. A prospective survey. Spine, 6:61-67.

114. Turner, J.A., Ersek, M., Herron, L., and Deyo, R. (1992): Surgery for lumbar spinal stenosis. Attempted meta-analysis of the literature. Spine, 17:1-8.

115. Vakos, J.P., Nitz, A.J., Threlkeld, A.J., et al. (1994): Electromyographic activity of selected trunk and hip muscles during a squat lift. Effect of varying the lumbar posture. Spine, 19:687-694.

116. Valkenburg, H.A., and Haanen, H.C.M. (1982): The epidemiology of low back pain. In: White, A.A., Gordon, S. (eds.), American Academy of Orthopedic Surgeons Symposium on Low Back Pain. St. Louis, MO, CV Mosby, pp. 9-22.

117. van der Heijden, G.J., Beurskens, A.J., Dirx, M.J., et al. (1995): Efficacy of lumbar traction: A randomized clinical trial. Physiotherapy, 81:29-35.

118. van Tulder, M.W., Assendelft, W.J., Koes, B.W., and Bouter, L.M. (1997): Spinal radiographic findings and nonspecific low back pain. A systematic review of observational studies. Spine, 22:427-434.

119. van Tulder, M.W., Koes, B.W., and Bouter, L.M. (1997): Conservative treatment of acute and chronic nonspecific low back pain. A systematic review of randomized controlled trials of the most common interventions. Spine, 22:2128-2156.

120. Verna, J.L., Mayer, J.M., Mooney, V., et al. (2002): Back extension endurance and strength: The effect of variable-angle Roman chair exercise training. Spine, 27:1772-1777.

121. Videman, T., Sarna, S., and Battie, M.C. (1995): The long-term effects of physical loading and exercise lifestyles on back-related symptoms, disability and spinal pathology among men. Spine, 20:700-705.

122. Vlaeyen, J.W., de Jong, J., Geilen, M., et al. (2001): Graded exposure in vivo in the treatment of pain-related fear: A replicated single-case experimental design in four patients with chronic low back pain. Behav. Res. Ther., 39:151-166.

123. Von Korff, M., Deyo, R.A., Cherkin, D., et al. (1993): Back pain in primary care: Outcomes at one year. Spine, 18:855-862.

124. Waddell, G., Newton, M., Henderson, I., et al. (1993): A Fear-Avoidance Beliefs Questionnaire (FABQ) and the role of fear-avoidance beliefs in chronic low back pain and disability. Pain, 52:157-168.

125. Waddell, G., Somerville, D., Henderson, I., and Newton, M. (1992): Objective clinical evaluation of physical impairment in chronic low back pain. Spine, 17:617-628.

126. Waddell, G. (1987): A new clinical model for the treatment of low back pain. Spine, 12:632-639.

127. Waldvogel, F.A., and Papageorgiou, P.S. (1980): Osteomyelitis: The past decade. N Engl J Med., 303:360-370.

128. Werneke, M., and Hart, D.L. (2001): Centralization phenomenon as a prognostic factor for chronic low back pain and disability. Spine, 26:758-764.

129. White, T.L., and Malone, T.R. (1990): Effects of running on intervertebral disc height. J. Orthop. Sports Phys. Ther., 12:139-146.

130. Whitman, J.M., Flynn, T.W., and Fritz, J.M. (2003): Non-surgical management of patients with lumbar spinal stenosis: A literature review and a case series of three patients managed with physical therapy. Phys. Med. Clin. N. Am., 14:1-23.

131. Wilder, D.G., Aleksiev, A.R., Magnusson, M.L., et al. (1996): Muscular response to sudden load: A tool to evaluate fatigue and rehabilitation. Spine, 21:2628-2637.

132. Willen, J., Danielson, B., Gaulitz, A., et al. (1997): Dynamic effects on the lumbar spinal canal. Axially loaded CT-myelography and MRI in patients with sciatica and/or neurogenic claudication. Spine, 22:2968-2976.

133. Wiltse, L.L., Newman, P.H., and Macnab, I. (1976): Classification of spondylolysis and spondylolisthesis. Clin. Orthop., 117:23-29.

CHAPTER 18

CERVICAL SPINE REHABILITATION

Todd R. Hooks, P.T.

CHAPTER OBJECTIVES

At the end of this chapter the reader will be able to:

- Describe the orientation and function of the anatomic structures in the cervical spine.
- Explain the arthrokinematics and biomechanics of the cervical spine during active range of motion and joint mobilizations.
- Perform special tests for the cervical spine, including explaining the technique and differentiating positive and negative test findings.
- Appreciate the clinical thought process involved during the evaluation.
- Design and implement a therapeutic program on the basis of the clinical findings during the evaluation.
- Describe common pathologic conditions in the cervical spine and the therapeutic considerations needed to address the pathology.

The cervical spine is one of the most commonly injured areas in the human body, with pathologies ranging from chronic in nature because of poor postural habits, to those occurring from acute, traumatic injuries. Rehabilitation techniques have changed in recent years because of a more thorough understanding of this region. This has allowed rehabilitation to evolve from structured protocols, to programs that address the need for normalization for the tissues tolerance to functional loading (forces causing stretching or compression) that have relied solely on static, isometric exercises, to programs that institute dynamic, isotonic exercises that restore postural deficits and regain neuromuscular control, strength, and endurance. This chapter addresses the anatomic, arthrokinematic, and biomechanical considerations that are needed during the evaluation and treatment process. Differential assessment of the tissues related to the cervical spine and evaluating joint play and mobility will allow the clinician to determine

tissue lesions and whether a pathologic hypermobility or hypomobility is present, and to address this through manual techniques and the application of an exercise regimen to expedite the healing process. Various special tests are presented that allow the clinician to determine the specific cause of pain and loss of function. It is through performing a complete evaluation procedure that the sports rehabilitation specialist will develop a clearer understanding of the exact tissue that is in lesion and allow the clinician to provide the optimal stimulus to help facilitate healing for that tissue.

ANATOMY

It is imperative that the clinician is competent in locating the anatomic structures of the cervical spine and has a proficient understanding of their biomechanical function(s) to allow for a thorough evaluation and institute a proper rehabilitation program. Therefore, this section addresses the cervical vertebral column and its surrounding ligaments, muscles, and neurovasculature structures. Because various pathologic conditions can affect one or more of these systems, it is important that the rehabilitation specialist has a thorough functional understanding of these structures.

Bony Configuration

The cervical spine consists of seven vertebrae. The anatomic structure of the midcervical spine (C3-C6) is similar to that of the thoracic and lumbar spine in that they each have a vertebral body, pedicle, lamina, and spinous process. However, the midcervical spine has a number of anatomic structures that are unique to this region (Fig. 18-1). Each midcervical vertebra has an uncinate process, a foramen transversarium, and their spinous processes are bifid. The foramen transversarium accommodates the vertebral artery and vein and is found in all cervical vertebrae except C7, although variations do exist. The spinous processes are bifid to allow for greater range of motion (ROM) into extension and to provide a mechanical advantage for muscular attachments.

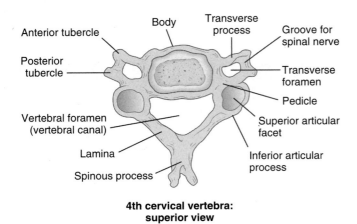

**4th cervical vertebra:
superior view**

Figure 18-1. Superior view of midcervical vertebrae.

The superior surfaces of the vertebral bodies in the midcervical spine are concave in the frontal plane and convex in the sagittal plane, and the opposite is true for the inferior surfaces. These cervical vertebrae have two superior and two inferior facets that are located on the pedicles. The superior facets are oriented in a posterior direction, and the inferior facets are oriented in an anterior direction. The biplanar orientation of these joints requires that rotation and lateral flexion are coupled movements. These facets articulate with the adjacent vertebrae to form facet joints (zygapophyseal joints). They have an approximate angle of 45° from the horizontal plane in the midcervical region (C3-C6) that decreases to approximately 30° in the lower cervical region (C7-T3) (Fig. 18-2). The facet joints are planar synovial joints with articular cartilage on the surfaces that is enclosed in a fibrosis joint capsule. Found within the joint capsule is a meniscoid, adipose tissue, and connective tissue.[5] The medial branch of the dorsal primary ramus innervates the facet joints.

The first cervical vertebrae (C1), the atlas, articulates with the occiput superiorly and the axis (C2) inferiorly. The atlas does not have a spinous process or a real vertebral body; however, the odontoid process (dens) of the axis functions as the body of C1 (see Fig. 18-4). The atlas consists of two lateral masses, which are connected by anterior and posterior arches, with transverse processes that provide for weight acceptance through the articular processes. The posterior surface of the anterior arch has a facet lined with hyaline cartilage that articulates with the odontoid process of C2 (Fig. 18-3). The superior articular processes are biconcave to articulate with the biconvex occipital condyles, and the inferior articular processes are biconvex and articulate with the biconvex superior facets of the axis.

The axis (C2) contains a superior projection, the odontoid process, which articulates with the posterior aspect of the anterior arch of the atlas. The axis, like the atlas, has small transverse processes and a posterior arch instead of pedicles (Fig. 18-4). In the upper cervical spine (C1-C2), the foramen transversarium is located more laterally than in the midcervical spine, therefore requiring the vertebral artery to ascend in a lateral direction in this region. Weight bearing is absorbed superiorly as the axis articulates with the inferior facets located on the lateral masses of the atlas and is transmitted inferiorly through inferior facet joints that are more posteriorly located on the axis, resembling those of the midcervical region.

Uncovertebral joints (joints of Luschka), first described by von Luschka, are believed to develop because of degenerative changes in the annulus fibrosus (Fig. 18-5). They are located on the lateral aspect of the midcervical vertebra and on the posterolateral aspect of C7-T1.[20] Uncovertebral joints function to deepen the articular surface and provide stability as they articulate with the adjacent vertebral body. However, because of their close proximity to the spinal nerves, osteophyte formation in this region can encroach on these structures. They also limit motion, especially lateral flexion, and serve to prevent lateral disc herniations.

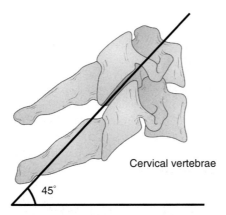

Figure 18-2. Lateral view of midcervical vertebrae depicting the plane of the facet joints. (From Temporomandibular joint and the cervical spine. Richardson, J.K., Iglarsh, Z.A., and Snyder-Mackler, L. [1994]: Clinical Orthopaedic Physical Therapy. Philadelphia, WB Saunders, p. 12.)

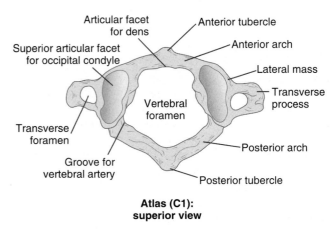

**Atlas (C1):
superior view**

Figure 18-3. Superior view of the atlas (C1).

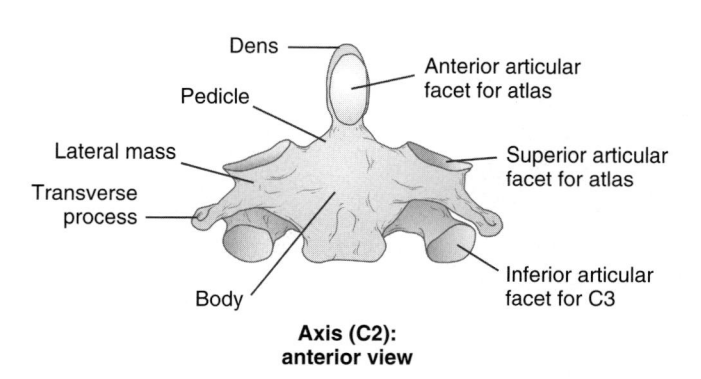

Figure 18-4. Anterior view of the axis (C2).

Intervertebral Disc

An intervertebral disc (IVD) is present between each cervical vertebra except the occiput and atlas (C0-C1) and the atlas and axis (C1-C2). The discs in the cervical spine are relatively thicker than those in the thoracic and lumbar spine, which allows for a greater ROM. The cervical discs are slightly higher anteriorly, thereby contributing to the lordotic curve in the cervical spine. The IVD is divided into a central region, the nucleus pulposus, and a peripheral ring, the annulus fibrosus. There is not a true demarcation between the nucleus and the annulus, but rather a gradual change in tissue structure from the inner layer to the outer ring. Because of the collagenous properties of the nucleus pulposus, containing primarily Type II collagen, it functions to resist axial compression and distrib-

utes these forces. The annulus fibrosis is composed of primarily type I collagen and functions to resist tensile forces within the disc. As a person ages, the amount of proteoglycan and therefore the amount of water begins to diminish.[10] The IVDs are avascular and depend on diffusion from the vertebral end-plates for their nutrition. The disc is innervated along the periphery of the annulus fibrosus through the sinuvertebral nerve.[19]

Nerve Roots

Although there are seven cervical vertebrae, there are eight pairs of nerve roots in the cervical spine. This occurs because the first nerve root (C1) exits between the occiput and the atlas, as do nerves 2 through 7 also exit above the vertebrae for which they are named. The transition of the nerve root exiting below the vertebrae for which it derives its name occurs at C8, and continues this throughout the thoracic and lumbar spine. As an example, because the C5 nerve root exists above C5 vertebra, a protrusion of the C4-C5 IVD would most likely affect this nerve. Nerve roots exit the vertebral column in the intervertebral foramen and divide into the anterior (ventral) and posterior (dorsal) primary rami. The posterior primary rami innervate the deep erector spinae muscles and the facet joints. The anterior primary rami of C5-T1 combine to form the brachial plexus supplying the upper arms.[28]

Ligamentous Support

Because the upper cervical spine has sacrificed osteokinematic stability to allow for greater arthrokinematic mobility, it is dependent on ligamentous support to allow for basic function and to avoid injuries. Because of the unique and complex articulations present in the upper cervical region, there are specialized ligaments to provide the needed stability. The dens are connected to the anterior rim of the foramen magnum by the apical ligament and the two obliquely oriented alar ligaments. The alar ligaments limit the amount of contralateral rotation that occurs at the atlantoaxial joint.[11] The cruciform (cruciate) ligament consists of three bands of fibers that are oriented in a superior, inferior, and transverse direction (Fig. 18-6). The transverse band is approximately 7 to 8 mm in thickness,[20] making it the largest and strongest of all atlantoaxial ligaments. The cruciform ligament functions to stabilize the dens against the posterior aspect of the anterior arch of the atlas and to prevent subluxation into the spinal canal. Posterior to the cruciform ligaments is the tectorial membrane. It originates at the basilar occipital bone and forms the continuation of the posterior longitudinal ligament (PLL). The PLL attaches to the IVD of adjacent vertebrae and their vertebral margins and functions to prevent cervical disc herniations and excessive flexion of the vertebral bodies.[3] In the cervical spine the PLL is broader and thicker

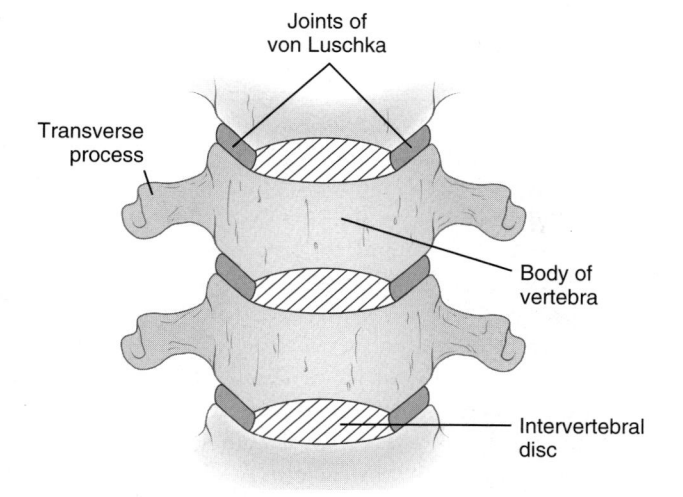

Figure 18-5. Anterior view of midcervical vertebrae displaying uncovertebral joints (Joints of von Luschka). (From Temporomandibular joint and the cervical spine. Richardson, J.K., Iglarsh, Z.A., and Snyder-Mackler, L. [1994]: Clinical Orthopaedic Physical Therapy. Philadelphia, WB Saunders, p. 12.)

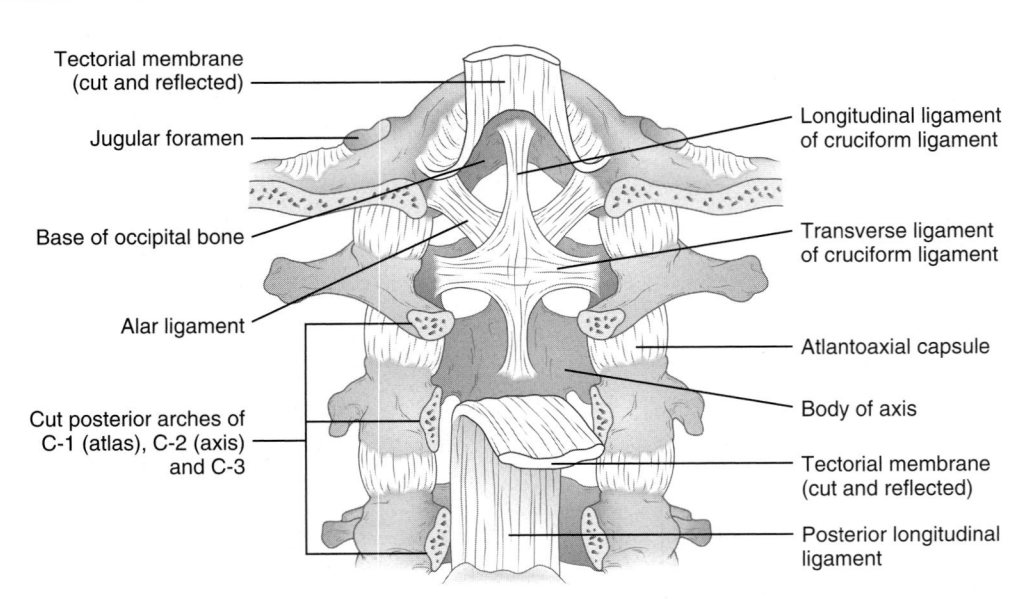

Figure 18-6. Posterior view of ligaments in the upper cervical spine. (From Temporomandibular joint and the cervical spine. Richardson, J.K., and Iglarsh, Z.A., Snyder-Mackler, L. [1994]: Clinical Orthopaedic Physical Therapy. Philadelphia, Saunders, p. 12, Fig. 1-11.)

compared with the lumbar spine. The anterior longitudinal ligament (ALL) originates from inferior surface of the basilar occiput bone and extends to the sacrum. It attaches to the vertebral bodies and IVD, but not to the bony rims.[16] This ligament functions in preventing hyperextension of the vertebral bodies.

The posterior vertebral elements have specialized ligaments to provide stability. The ligamentum flavum connects adjoining laminae and because of their attachment to the anterior aspect of the facet joint, they serve to prevent entrapment of the facet capsule and meniscus in the facet joints. The ligamentum nuchae is posterior to the ligamentum flavum and is a fibroelastic membrane that functions to limit cervical flexion. The posterior cervical ligament originates at the occiput and inserts into the spinous processes of the cervical spine before terminating at C7. It functions to resist excessive flexion and divides the posterior cervical muscles into right and left sides.

Muscular Arrangement

The cervical spine has numerous muscles that have influences on proprioceptive input and postural control and provide active movements for the occiput, cervical spine, and upper trunk. These muscles can be divided into anterior and posterior groups according to their attachment in relation to the transverse processes. Tables 18-1 and 18-2 list these muscles including the origin, insertion, action, and innervation of each muscle.

BIOMECHANICS

CLINICAL PEARL #1

The forces and stresses that are controlled and generated by the body ensure the proper histologic, biomechanical, and physiologic properties of each tissue.

"Structure governs function and function dictates structure."

—*Rob Tillman, P.T., M.O.M.T.*

The osteokinematic motion in the cervical spine is a result of the interaction of the cervical vertebrae, IVD, ligaments, joint capsule, and the orientation of the facet joints working together to control and dictate the movements that occur in this region. Active ROM is a result of the interaction of the entire cervical spine to produce a desired movement. However, because of the anatomic differences between the upper and midcervical spine, the upper cervical spine is able to perform motions independent of those of the midcervical region. This allows for the cervical spine to correctly position the head for optimal orientation of the visual, auditory, and olfactory nervous systems.

The arthrokinematic motions of the upper cervical spine are discussed in detail because of the complex articulations in this region. Notably, the desired motion occurs

Table 18-1

Origin, Insertion, Action, and Innervation of the Anterior Cervical Spine Musculature

| | | Anterior Musculature | | |
Muscle	Origin	Insertion	Action	Innervation
Sternocleidomastoid	Sternal head: anterior sternum	Mastoid process	Bilaterally: flexes head	C2
	Clavicular head: medial third of clavicle		Unilaterally: side-bends head toward and rotates head to opposite side	Spinal accessory nerve (Cranial nerve XI)
Scalene anterior	Anterior tubercles of transverse processes of C3-C6	Scalene tubercle of first rib	Elevates first rib Unilaterally: side-bends neck toward and rotates neck to opposite side Bilaterally: flexes neck	C5-C8
Scalene medius	Posterior tubercles of transverse processes C2-C7	Superior surface of first rib behind subclavian groove	Elevates first rib Unilaterally: side-bends neck toward and rotates neck to opposite side Bilaterally: flexes neck	C3-C4
Scalene posterior	Posterior tubercles of transverse processes C4-C6	Second rib posterior to serratus anterior attachment	Elevates second rib Unilaterally: side-bends neck toward and rotates neck to opposite side Bilaterally: flexes neck	C4-C8
Longus capitis	Anterior tubercles of transverse processes C3-C6	Basilar part of occipital bone	Flexes head and neck and assists with rotation	C1-C4
Longus colli	Vertebral bodies C5-T3 and anterior tubercles of transverse processes C3-C5	Vertebral bodies C2-C4 Anterior tubercle of atlas Anterior tubercles of transverse processes C5-C6	Flexes head and neck and assists with rotation Unilaterally: side-bends neck	C2-C8
Rectus capitis anterior	Lateral mass of the atlas	Basilar part of occipital bone	Bilaterally: flexes head Unilaterally: side-bends and rotates head ipsilaterally	C1-C2
Rectus capitis lateralis	Anterior tubercle of transverse process of the atlas	Jugular process of occiput	Bilaterally: flexes head Unilaterally: side-bends head	C1-C2

as a result of these actions occurring in unison. The following processes described are a teaching tool, which is meant to allow for a biomechanical understanding of what occurs, although functionally these movements are occurring together and in synchrony. Because normal variations occur in osseous and connective tissue properties and orientation, structural discrepancies can exist that produce altered arthrokinematic movements.

During flexion of the upper cervical spine (Fig. 18-7), the convex condyles of the occiput glide in a posterior direction on the concave facets of the atlas, which produces an anterior tilt of the occiput. The atlas is pushed in an anterior direction approximately 2 to 3 mm because of the force created in the facet joints. The translation creates approximation between the dens and the transverse ligament, which restricts further motion. The atlas tilts 15° to 20° anteriorly causing its anterior arch to move inferiorly 2 to 4 mm as the posterior arch is elevated. The superior tilt of the posterior arch increases the tension on the posterior ligamentous structures between C1 and C2. As

Table 18-2

Origin, Insertion, Action, and Innervation of the Posterior Cervical Spine Musculature

		Posterior Musculature		
Muscle	**Origin**	**Insertion**	**Action**	**Innervation**
Upper trapezius	Medial third of superior nuchal line, external occipital protuberance, and ligamentum nuchae	Lateral third of clavicle	Extends, side-bends, and rotates head to opposite side. Elevates scapula	Spinal accessory nerve (Cranial nerve XI) C3-C4
Levator scapulae	Transverse processes of the upper 3-4 cervical vertebrae	Medial border of scapula above spine	Extends, side-bends, and rotates neck to ipsilateral side. Elevates and downwardly rotates scapula	Dorsal scapular nerve (C5) C3-C4
Splenius capitis	Ligamentum nuchae, spinous processes of C7 and upper 4-5 thoracic vertebrae	Mastoid process and superior nuchal line	Extends, side-bends, and rotates head and neck to ipsilateral side	C4-C6
Splenius cervicis	Spinous processes of T3-T6	Posterior tubercles of transverse processes of upper 3-4 cervical vertebrae	Extends, side-bends, and rotates neck to ipsilateral side	C4-C6
Longissimus capitis	Transverse processes of upper 4-5 thoracic vertebrae	Mastoid process	Extends, side-bends, and rotates head to ipsilateral side	C6-C8
Longissimus cervicis	Transverse processes of upper 4-5 thoracic vertebrae	Posterior tubercles of transverse processes of C2-C6	Side-bends and rotates neck to ipsilateral side	C6-C8
Semispinalis capitis	Transverse processes C7 and upper 6-7 thoracic vertebrae, C4-C6 articular processes	Between superior and inferior nuchal lines	Extends, side-bends, and rotates head to ipsilateral side	C1-C8
Semispinalis cervicis	Transverse processes of upper 5-6 thoracic vertebrae	Spinous processes of C2-C5	Extends, side-bends, and rotates neck to ipsilateral side	C1-C8
Obliquus capitis inferior	Spinous process of the axis	Transverse process of atlas	Extends, side-bends, and rotates head to ipsilateral side. Side-bends and rotates neck to ipsilateral side	C1-C2
Obliquus capitis superior	Transverse process of the atlas	Above inferior nuchal line	Extends and side bends head	C1
Rectus capitis posterior major	Spinous process of the axis	Lateral aspect of inferior nuchal line	Extends, side-bends, and rotates head to ipsilateral side	C1
Rectus capitis posterior minor	Posterior tubercle of the atlas	Medial third of inferior nuchal line	Extends and side-bends head	C1

the tension increases, this causes movement between C2 and C3.[14]

Extension of the upper cervical spine occurs (Fig. 18-8) as a result of the convex occipital condyles gliding forward on the concave facet joints of the atlas, which produces a posterior tilt of the occiput. The compressive forces cause the atlas to translate posterior 2 to 3 mm, which is restrained by the anterior arch of the atlas approximating against the odontoid process. The atlas tilts posteriorly approximately 12°, which causes its anterior arch to

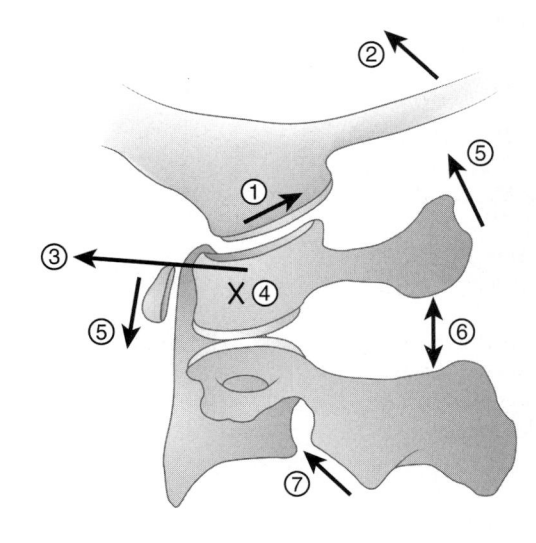

Upper Cs mechanics: flexion

Figure 18-7. Biomechanics of the upper cervical spine during flexion. (Cervical Biomechanics. Residency Course Notes; Systems Course [680]:33. ©1998 The Ola Grimsby Institute.)

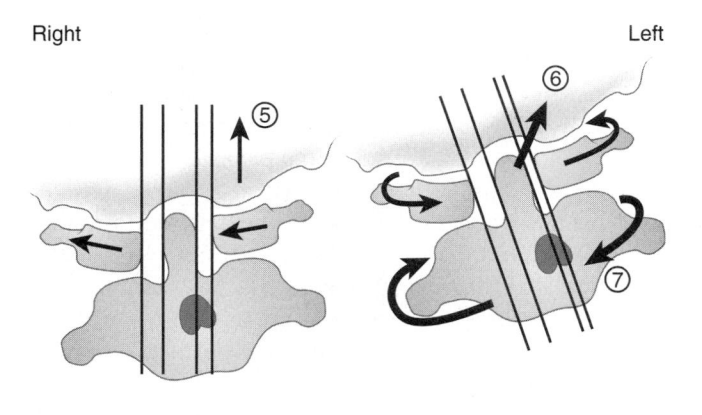

Upper Cs mechanics: rotation

Figure 18-9. Biomechanics of the upper cervical spine during lateral flexion. (Cervical Biomechanics. Residency Course Notes; Systems Course [680]:35-36. ©1998 The Ola Grimsby Institute.)

translate superiorly on the dens 2 to 4 mm as the posterior arch moves inferiorly. As the anterior ligamentous structures become taut, it causes the axis to glide posteriorly on C3.[14]

Right lateral flexion of the upper cervical spine (Fig. 18-9) is produced as the convex condyles of the occiput glide 3° to 5° to the left, which causes a relative right translation of the atlas. This translation is prevented as the dens approximates against the lateral mass of the atlas. Lateral flexion between C1 and C2 does not occur because

of the approximation between the odontoid process and the atlas and their biconvex articulating surfaces. Because of the lateral forces exerted by the occiput and atlas, the axis side-bends to the right 5° on C3 as a result of the inability of C1 to glide laterally on C2. The atlas will then rotate immediately on the axis to the left to maintain an anterior orientation of the face. The left occipital condyle elevates as a result of the wedge-shaped lateral masses of the atlas gliding to the right. This elevation causes tension in the left alar ligament, thus producing compression between C2 and C1 as the axis is elevated. The joint compression between the biconvex surfaces of both the atlas and the axis produces a right rotation of the axis. As lateral flexion is increased, the occiput and atlas will rotate to the left on the axis to allow anterior orientation of the face.[14]

Rotation of the upper cervical spine (Fig. 18-10) to the right begins with the occiput rotating on the atlas a minute

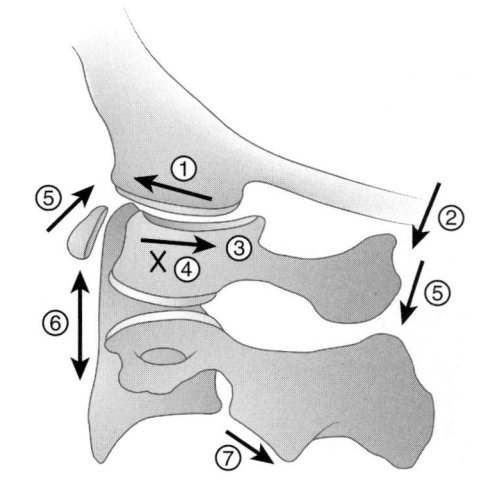

Upper Cs mechanics: extension

Figure 18-8. Biomechanics of the upper cervical spine during extension. (Cervical Biomechanics. Residency Course Notes; Systems Course [680]:34. ©1998 The Ola Grimsby Institute.)

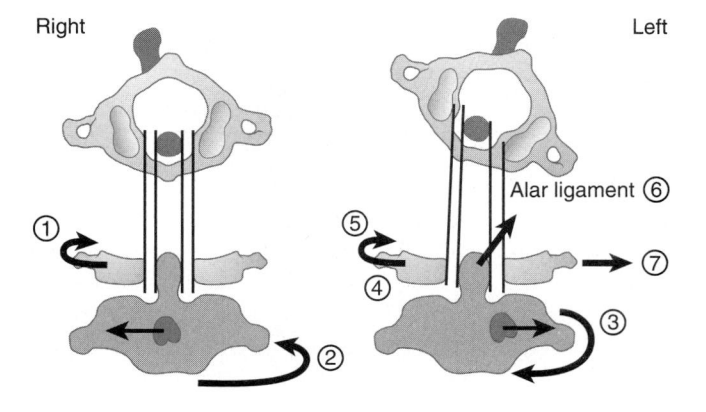

Upper Cs mechanics: rotation

Figure 18-10. Biomechanics of the upper cervical spine during rotation. (Cervical Biomechanics. Residency Course Notes; Systems Course [680]:37. ©1998 The Ola Grimsby Institute.)

amount (approximately 1°). As joint approximation occurs, the atlas is pulled into right rotation bringing the left lateral mass of C1 closer to the dens. The compressive forces that occur between the atlas and the axis produce 2° to 3° of left rotation of C2 caused by the biconvex surfaces. The occiput and atlas rotate to the right approximately 40° applying tension on the left alar ligament, which brings the axis into right rotation. The axis will continue to rotate and side-bend to the right approximately 10°, which allows the occiput and atlas to rotate to the available end ROM. The increased tension on the left alar ligament produces left side-bending of the occiput. The atlas is forced to glide to the left because of the compressive forces of the left occipital condyle. As the atlas side glides to the left, it produces an increase in the amount of left side-bending of the occiput as the wedge-shaped lateral masses of the atlas tilts the occiput.[14]

In the midcervical spine, the superior facets are oriented in a superior, posterior, and medial direction, whereas the inferior facets are oriented in an anterior, inferior, and lateral direction. As a result, during cervical rotation the contralateral inferior facet glides in a superior and medial direction, which produces lateral flexion in the same direction. Therefore, in the cervical region, rotation and lateral flexion always occur together in the same direction.

During flexion, the superior vertebral body slides and tilts anteriorly on the inferior vertebra, which causes separation of the facet joints. During extension, the superior vertebral body slides and tilts posteriorly. This motion is limited because of joint approximation and tension in the ALL. The facet joints are oriented to allow for an increase in the amount of flexion and extension.

EVALUATION

CLINICAL PEARL #2

"The least reliable way to diagnose in soft tissue lesions is to palpate immediately for tenderness in the area outlined by the patient."

—*James Cyriax, M.D.*

During the evaluation of the cervical spine, it is important to perform a screening examination of the thoracic spine, temporomandibular joint, and upper extremities to ensure that the pathology is cervical in nature. Table 18-3 outlines an examination flow. It is helpful to have a systemic approach to the evaluation process; this will ensure that the clinician does not overlook a step of the assessment and will allow for a smooth, systematic flow of the examination. By performing all of the listed aspects of the examination it will allow the sports rehabilitation specialist to determine which tissues(s) is in lesion as a result of the tissue's response to the test imposed. Each tissue is

---

Table 18-3

Examination Flow

Initial Observation
Patient Subjective History
Active Motion
Flexion
Extension
Lateral flexion
Rotation
Combined motions
Repetitive motions
Prolonged positions
Passive Motion
Flexion
Extension
Lateral flexion
Rotation
Prolonged positions
Overpressure
Resisted Motion
Each motion tested in three positions
Flexion
Extension
Lateral flexion
Rotation
Palpation
Note temperature variations, atrophy, swelling, tenderness, thickness, dryness, moisture, abnormalities, crepitus, and pain
Neurologic Tests
Sensation tests
Reflexes
Myotomes
Special Tests
Vascular tests
  DeKleyn's test
  Hautant's test
  Underburg's test
Neurologic tests
  Distraction
  Compression
  Shoulder abduction test
  Valsalva maneuver
Upper limb tension tests
  ULTT1
  ULTT2
  ULTT3
  ULTT4
Instability tests
  Odontoid fracture
  Transverse ligament integrity
  Alar ligament integrity
Thoracic outlet syndrome tests
  Roos test
  Adson test
  Allen test
  Costoclavicular compression maneuver
  Pectoralis minor test
  Wright's hyperabduction test

Table 18-3

Examination Flow—cont'd

Mobility Tests
Upper and Midcervical Spine
  Flexion
  Extension
  Lateral flexion
  Rotation
Diagnostic Tests
  X-rays, magnetic resonance imaging, computed tomography,
    myelogram, electromyograph, laboratory tests

suspected as a potential source of pain until that tissue has been cleared through careful examination. To clear a tissue, the clinician must perform tests that create stress or tension on that tissue. If a positive response does not occur, the tissue can be excluded as a source of pain.

Visual Observation

The examination process begins with the visual observation of the athlete. The clinician watches the athlete walk into the room and observes the athlete's positioning of their head, neck, and shoulder girdle. The sports rehabilitation specialist may be able to detect any defects or abnormalities that may exist and develop an understanding of how the patient's pain is affecting his or her functional ability. The clinician may be able to detect the athlete's ability, speed, and willingness to move his or her head and upper limbs, which can give an indication to the degree of injury present.

History

The athlete's subjective history is an important aspect of the evaluation process. By performing a complete history, the clinician can get clues to the patient's diagnosis. The rehabilitation specialist will develop a better understanding of the athlete's condition and will gain insight as to the direction and intensity of the examination and treatment.

It is important to allow the athlete to describe his or her current complaint and any previous related conditions. The athlete should be encouraged to describe the symptoms including the location and nature of their pain, as well as any conditions that increase or relieve these symptoms. A visual analogue pain-rating scale is commonly used to allow the athlete to indicate the severity of the pain. Although many different types of analogue scales are available for use, it is important to use the same scale to allow for consistency.[18] The clinician should be aware of what the athlete's goals are and his or her time frame for achieving these goals. This will ensure that both the clinician and the athlete clearly understand one another and will allow insight into the athlete's motivation.

Structural Inspection

The clinician begins an inspection of the athlete in a standing position after the patient has undressed. The visual inspection can include the patient as they are standing in a normal, habitual stance and in the anatomic position. The clinician should briefly perform a full examination of the entire patient in an anterior, lateral, and posterior view observing the body contours and looking for any structural abnormalities or postural faults that may be present. The clinician can observe the athlete's respiratory pattern to assess the rate and rhythm, and to determine if inspiration originates from the diaphragm or from the upper thoracic region. The clinician may also choose to perform an inspection while the patient is in both a habitual and upright sitting posture. Because postural abnormalities (i.e., forward head, rounded shoulders) are a profound amplifier for decreased ROM and function, the clinician should make note of their presence because of the potential contribution to tissue irritation.

Active Movements

The first motions performed by the athlete are active movements. This allows the clinician not only to observe the patient's available ROM, but also the quality of motion, pain elicited, and the speed and willingness to move. The athlete will begin by performing cardinal plane motions. As the patient performs the active movements, the clinician should observe for segmental areas that have either an abrupt or reduced angulation. This may indicate areas where segmental motion is altered compared with the rest of the cervical spine.

Those movements that are most painful should be performed last to ensure a carryover of pain does not occur during the remaining motions.[7] If an athlete complains of pain with repetitive movements, prolonged positions (i.e., cervical flexion, extension, sitting, standing, and so on), or a combined motion, the clinician should instruct the patient to perform these actions last. Therefore, it may be necessary to have the athlete repeat a movement (5 to 10 times), maintain a position (15 to 20 seconds), or perform combined movements attempting to reproduce the symptoms.

Passive Movements

The rehabilitation specialist performs passive ROM to assess the cervical spine for possible restrictions and to determine each motions endfeel. In the cervical spine, the normal endfeel for all cardinal plane movements is a tissue stretch. If the ROM is restricted in multiple directions, the clinician should determine if the limitation presents as a capsular or noncapsular pattern. The capsular pattern of the cervical spine is: side flexion and rotation equally limited, slight limitation into extension, and full flexion.[7] A noncapsular pattern will have ROM limitations, but does not resemble that of the capsular pattern. This noncapsular restriction may result from pain, adhesions, or an internal derangement.[7] During assessment of passive ROM, it is important to remember that a greater ROM will occur if the passive movements are assessed while the athlete is supine as opposed to when the patient is seated. This is a result of the increased muscular tone present in the seated position to maintain an erect head.

The clinician may choose to hold a movement for a sustained period, or apply overpressure at end range. The clinician may also opt to bias the amount of overpressure to the upper or lower cervical spine to evoke symptoms.[8] For example, overpressure into extension for the upper cervical spine (Fig. 18-11A) can be performed by passively flex-ing the midcervical and cervicothoracic spine followed by extending the upper cervical segments. Extension overpressure to the lower cervical spine (see Fig. 18-11B) can be created by flexing the upper cervical spine then introducing extension into the lower segments. The clinician must be careful not to generally overstress the system without the appropriate differential assessment, which may require radiologic testing.

Resisted Motion

During resisted motion testing, the athlete is asked to repeat the same movements as performed during the active and passive parts of the examination (flexion, extension, side-bending, and rotation) and will be instructed to maintain a static, isometric position during the test. Each movement is tested in three positions of the patient's available ROM. The athlete is first tested with the cervical

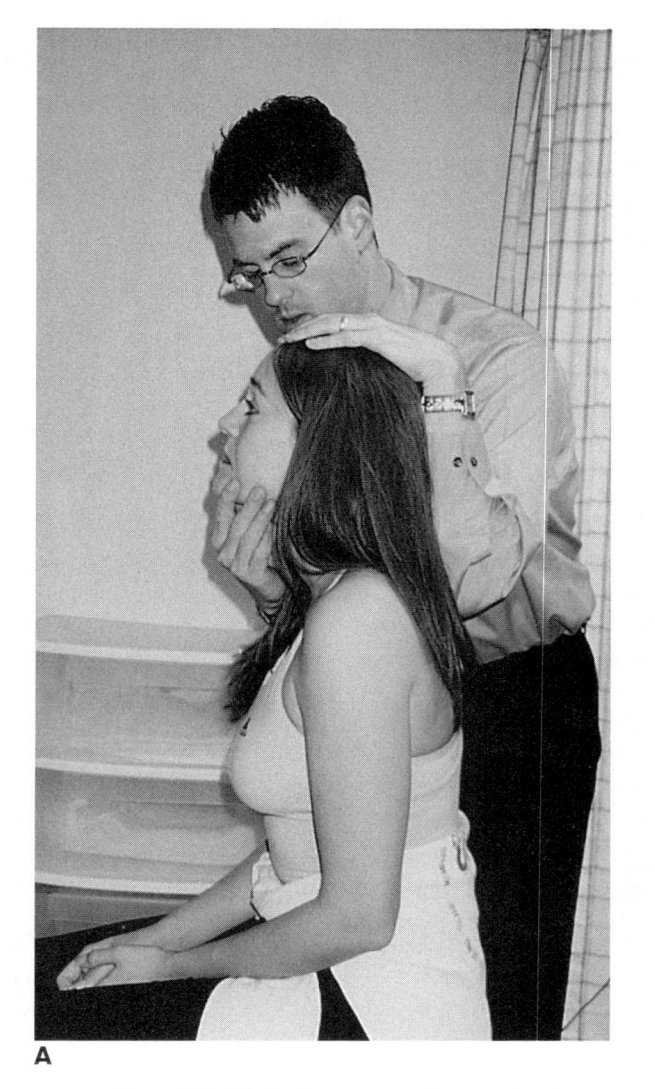

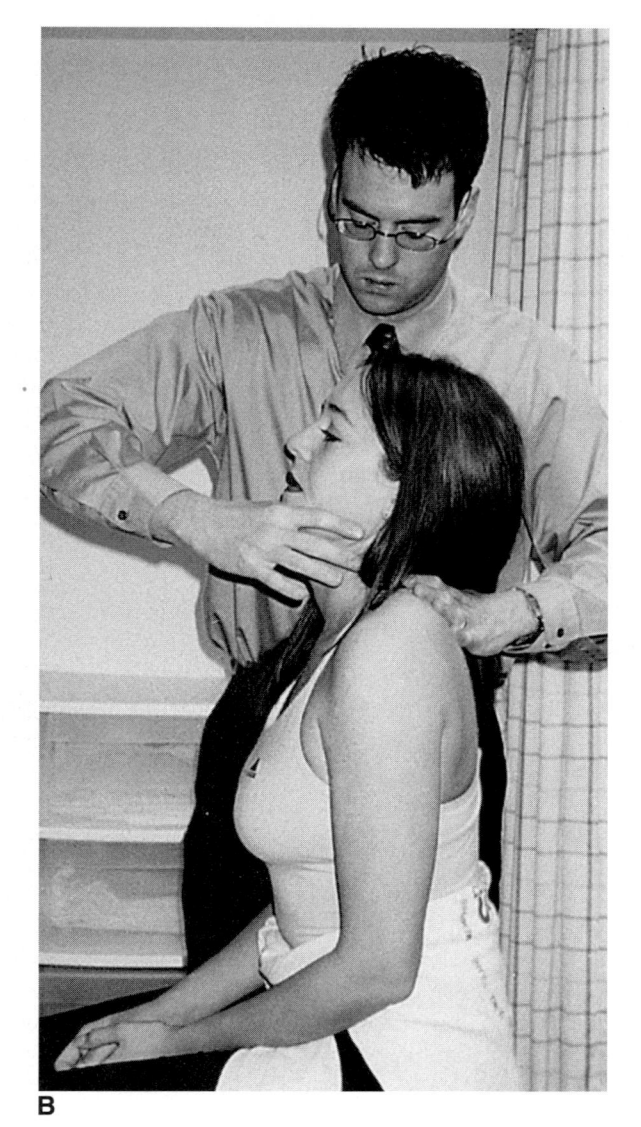

Figure 18-11. *A*, Overpressure bias to the upper cervical spine. *B*, Overpressure bias to the lower cervical spine.

spine in a midrange position, and then in the beginning of the available ROM, followed by the outer limits of the available ROM. Each movement is tested in similar fashion with the athlete's head positioned in three different positions. By testing each motion in three positions, various amounts of joint compressive forces and tensile forces are generated in the contractile and noncontractile tissues.

The purpose of this part of the examination is not to determine muscular strength, but to give the clinician insight as to the feedback of the affected tissues response when tensile forces and joint compression/decompression occur as a result of muscle activation. If, however, muscle weakness is noted, the clinician must determine if this is a result of pain inhibition, injury to the contractile tissues, or the presence of a neurologic pathology. It may be necessary to perform more muscle-specific manual muscle testing to allow for appropriate muscle differentiation.[12,17] In addition, a neurologic examination should be conducted to rule out any possible upper or lower motor neuron lesion.

CLINICAL PEARL #3

The clinician can determine whether the tissue in lesion is inert tissue or contractile tissue after performing the active, passive, and resisted motions. If active and passive motions are painful in the same direction and no pain is reported with resistive isometric movements, an inert tissue is suspected.[7] If active and passive motions are painful in the opposite direction, and pain presents with resisted isometrics in the same direction as active motion, this is indicative of a contractile tissue lesion.[7]

Palpation

Palpation allows the clinician to assess the status of the athlete's tissues. Although the clinician will make note of any tenderness occurring during palpation, because of the possibility of referred symptoms, the clinician must rely on his or her manual skills while palpating the athlete. Irritation of a spinal nerve or a structure innervated by that spinal nerve can cause referred pain in a dermatomal, myotomal, or sclerotomal pattern (Fig. 18-12).[7] Therefore, to rely solely on patient feedback to identify tissue lesions can be misleading.

Palpation begins superficially with the skin progressing to deeper underlying structures. The rehabilitation specialist can identify skin temperature variations that may be present in the cervical spine area using the back of his or her hand. A histamine reaction can be observed and compared bilaterally by performing a light scratch of the skin, in the cervical spine area, using the dorsum of the thumb. To assess the skin and subcutaneous tissues the clinician can roll the skin in multiple directions. Skin rolling is performed by grasping the dermis and superficial fascia between the fingers and thumb, the skin is then lifted and

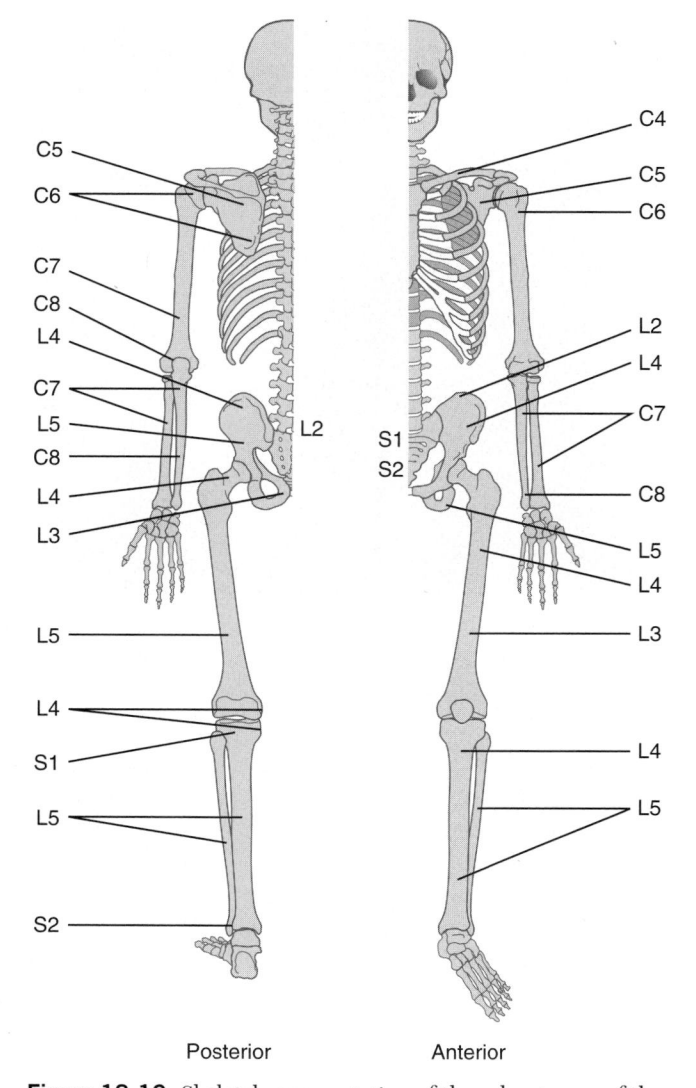

Figure 18-12. Skeletal representation of the sclerotomes of the body. (From Principles and concepts. Magee, D.J. [1997]: Orthopedic Physical Assessment, 3rd ed. Philadelphia, WB Saunders, p. 14.)

rolled (Fig. 18-14). The clinician may notice restrictions or abnormalities in the consistency of the tissues that may indicate fibrosis.

During palpation, the clinician should make note of tenderness, altered muscular tone, crepitus, bony abnormalities or defects, or any other indication of pathologic conditions. Table 18-4 contains a list of commonly palpated anterior and posterior structures. Proper orientation to bony landmarks and surrounding soft tissue is imperative during the evaluation process.[13]

Neurologic Tests

A neurologic evaluation should be performed on every athlete to assess the status of the neurologic system and to

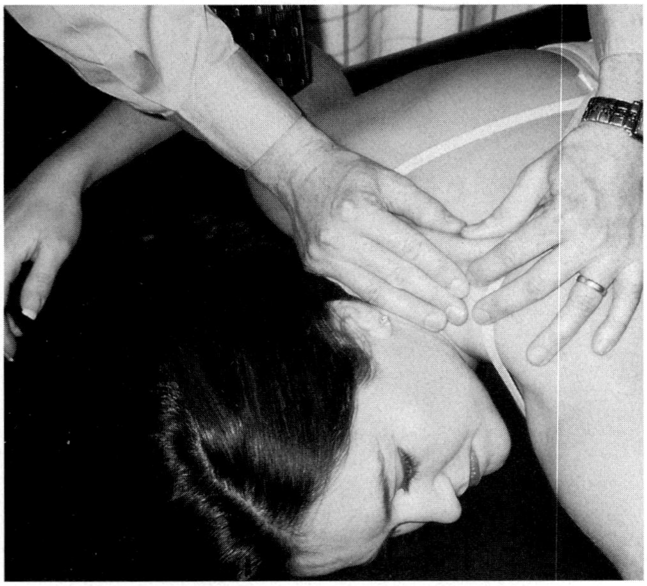

Figure 18-13. Skin rolling technique used during evaluation and treatment of the mobility of the skin and underlying fascia.

verify that the athlete does not have a previously undetected neurologic dysfunction. The clinician examines the reflexes and the sensory and motor functions of the athlete to determine if an upper or lower motor neuron lesion is present (Table 18-5).

To prevent any visual cues during sensation testing, the athlete closes his or her eyes as the clinician lightly runs his or her hands in a dermatomal pattern on the patient. The

Table 18-4

Commonly Palpated Structures in the Assessment of the Cervical Spine

Posteriorly	Anteriorly
External occipital protuberance	Sternum
	Clavicle
Superior nuchal line	Supraclavicular fossa
Mastoid process	First rib
Ligamentum nuchae	Sternocleidomastoid muscle
Upper trapezius	
Levator scapulae	Scalene muscles
Spinous processes	Hyoid bone
Transverse processes	Thyroid cartilage
Facet joints	Thyroid gland
	First cricoid ring
	Lymph nodes
	Carotid pulse
	Temporomandibular joints
	Mandible
	Parotid gland

Table 18-5

Comparison of an Upper and Lower Motor Neuron Lesion

Upper Motor Neuron Lesion	Lower Motor Neuron Lesion
Spasticity	Flaccidity
Hyperreflexia	Hyporeflexia
Hypertonicity	Hypotonicity
Muscle weakness distal to lesion	Weakness of innervated muscles
Pathologic reflexes positive bilaterally	Pathologic reflexes absent

clinician notes any areas of hyposensitivity or hypersensitivity. If a deficit is present, the rehabilitation specialist can perform more extensive testing of the patient's sensitivity to superficial pain, temperature, vibration, and two-point discrimination. The rehabilitation specialist determines if the altered sensation presents in a dermatomal pattern (Fig. 18-14) or follows the distribution of a peripheral nerve.

The deep tendon reflexes of the biceps (C5-C6), brachioradialis (C5-C6), triceps (C7-C8), and abductor digiti minimi (C8-T1) are tested and graded bilaterally. If the clinician is having difficulty obtaining a reflexive response, the athlete can be instructed to perform a Jendrassik maneuver[9] by pressing his or her legs together, thereby facilitating the nervous system. The deep tendon reflexes of the athlete are compared bilaterally to determine if any hyporeflexes or hyperreflexes are present.

Because reflexes can vary from person to person, the clinician should not be alarmed if the athlete has a weakened or heightened reflexive response bilaterally, although an altered unilaterally response should be noted. A hyporeflexive response indicates a lower motor neuron lesion, whereas a hyperreflexive response is indicative of an upper motor neuron lesion.

If signs of an upper motor neuron lesion are present, pathologic reflex testing is indicated. Babinski's sign (Fig. 18-15) for the lower extremity and Hoffmann's sign (Fig. 18-16) for the upper extremity are two examples of pathologic reflex tests that are commonly used. The pathologic reflexes should be examined bilaterally to note a difference in either side.

The rehabilitation specialist also assesses the athlete's motor responses of the cervical myotomes (Table 18-6) to determine if neurologic weakness is present. The athlete is instructed to maintain an isometric contraction while the joint being tested is held in a neutral position. Because most muscles receive innervation from more than one neurologic level, a lesion of a single nerve root may not result in complete paralysis of a muscle. This can result in only a mild muscle weakness in the early stages

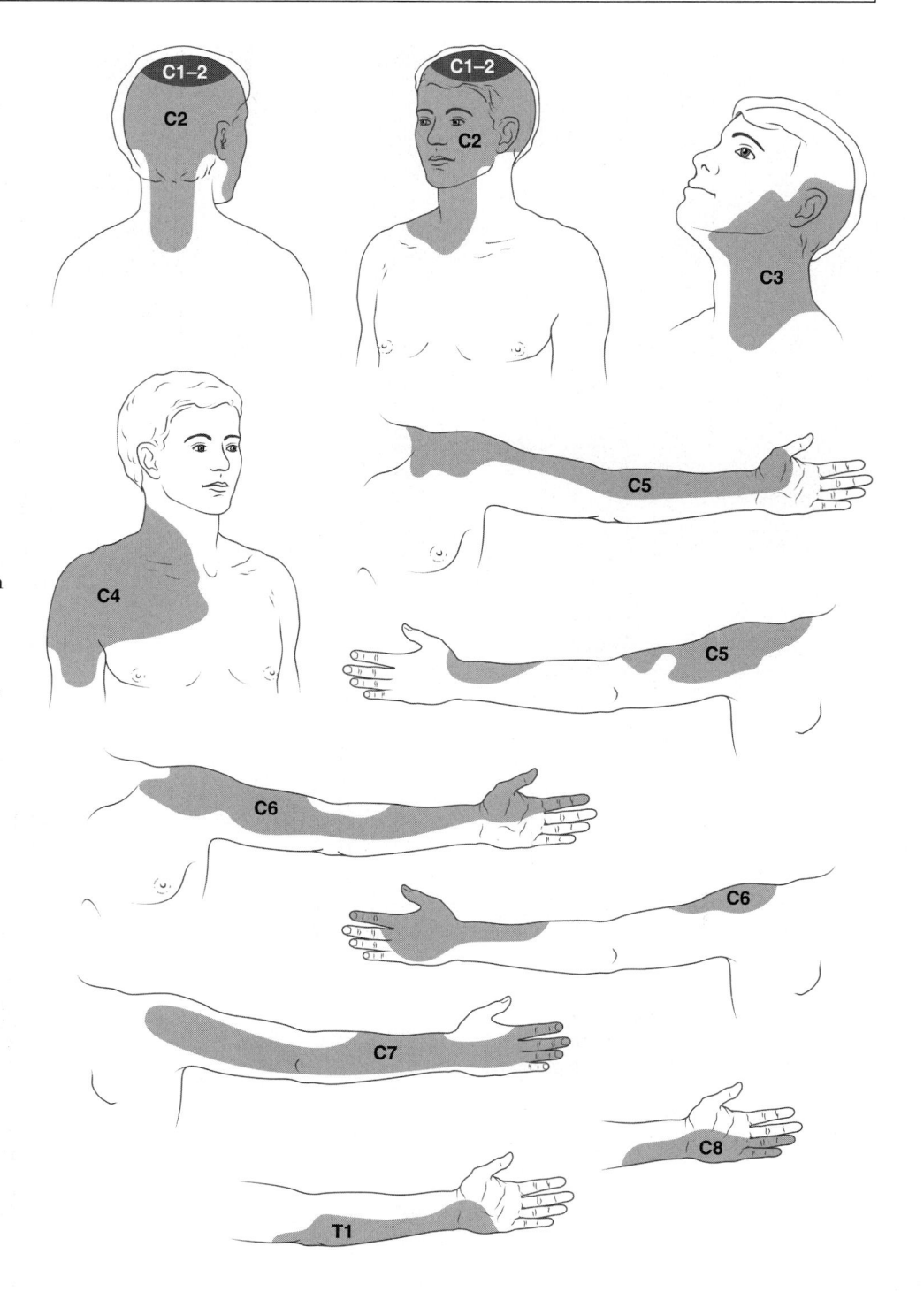

Figure 18-14. Dermatomal pattern of the upper extremity. (From Cervial spine. Magee, D.J. [1997]: Orthopedic Physical Assessment, 3rd ed. Philadelphia, WB Saunders, p. 135.)

of injury that can cause difficulty for the clinician to detect a difference. The clinician should therefore require the athlete to maintain an isometric contraction for a minimum of 5 seconds to allow for subtle weakness to manifest itself.

Although the pathologic cause of the patient's symptoms may not yet be determined, the clinician will at this point be able to conclude if the neurologic tests are indicative of an upper or lower motor neuron lesion. Table 18-7

provides the clinical findings to help differentiate a nerve root lesion from a peripheral nerve injury.

SPECIAL TESTS

A variety of special tests exist to assist the clinician in determining the status of the osseous, neurovascular, and ligamentous structures. Although many tests are available to evaluate the cervical spine, the rehabilitation

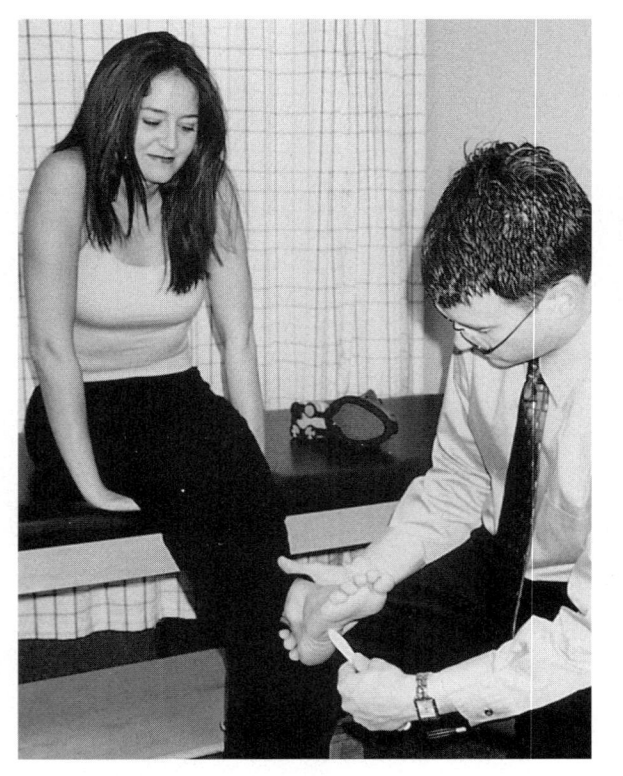

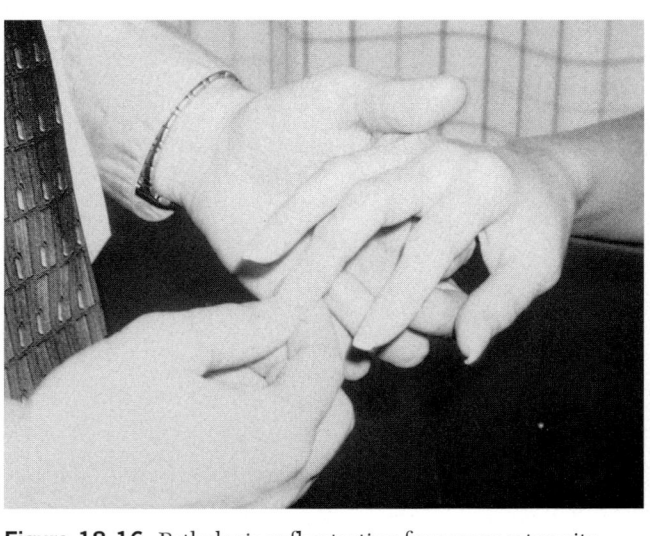

Figure 18-16. Pathologic reflex testing for upper extremity. Hoffmann's reflex is performed by flicking the terminal phalanx of the middle finger. Positive test: Reflexive flexion of distal phalanx of thumb and index finger.

Figure 18-15. Pathologic reflex testing for lower extremity. Babinski's reflex is performed by stroking the lateral sole of foot. Positive test: Dorsiflexion of great toe and fanning of other toes.

specialist must use his or her clinical judgment to determine which tests are clinically relevant to perform according to the athlete's subject history and objective findings. The rehabilitation specialist should also use the subjective history and objective information in determining whether to perform a test in a unilateral or bilateral manner. This will ensure a more efficient and stream-lined evaluation for the clinician. The special tests presented in this section include vascular, neurologic, and instability tests (see Figures 18-17 through 18-25 for descriptions).

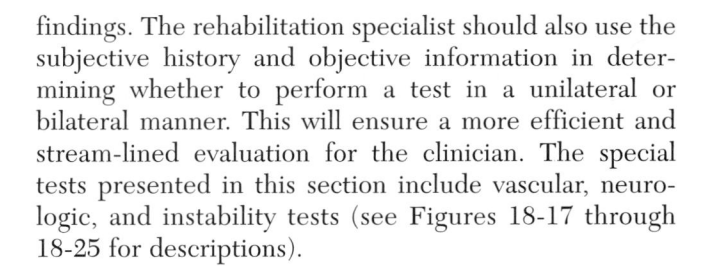

Table 18-6

Cervical Myotomes

Action	Nerve Root	Muscles
Chin tuck	C1-C2	Rectus capitis anterior
		Rectus capitis lateralis
Head side flexion	C3	Longus capitis
		Longus cervicis
		Scalene
Shoulder elevation	C4	Trapezius
		Levator scapulae
Shoulder abduction	C5	Deltoid
Elbow flexion	C6	Biceps
Wrist extension		Extensor carpi radialis brevis
		Extensor carpi radialis longus
Elbow extension	C7	Triceps
Wrist flexion		Flexor carpi radialis
		Flexor digitorum superficialis
Thumb extension	C8	Extensor pollicis longus
		Extensor pollicis brevis
Finger abduction/adduction	T1	Intrinsic muscles of the hand

Table 18-7

Differential Diagnosis Between a C6 Nerve Root Lesion and a Radial Nerve Lesion

	Altered Sensation	Muscle Deficits	Abnormal Reflexes
C6 nerve root	Lateral arm and forearm, radial side of wrist, thumb, and index finger	Biceps, brachioradialis, supinator, extensor carpi radialis longus	Biceps Brachioradialis
Radial nerve C5, 6, 7, 8, T1	Posterior lateral aspect of arm, posterior forearm, hand into thumb, index, middle, and radial side of ring fingers excluding finger tips	Triceps, anconeus, brachioradialis, extensor carpi radialis longus, supinator, extensor carpi radialis brevis, extensor carpi ulnaris, extensor digitorum, extensor digiti minimi, extensor indicis, abductor pollicis longus, extensor pollicis brevis	None

Vascular Tests

Procedure	Positive Test	Figure
DeKlyn's Test[9]*		
1. The athlete lies supine with his or her head over the edge of the table with the clinician supporting the head.	Considered positive for vertebral artery compromise if the athlete describes dizziness, nausea, tinnitus, or displays signs of nystagmus during testing.	Fig. 18-17
2. The clinician slowly rotates and extends the athlete's head while maintaining constant visual and verbal contact with the patient for approximately 30 seconds.		
Hautant's Test[9]		
1. Athlete is seated, with shoulders flexed to 90°, elbows extended and forearms supinated.	Considered positive for diminished blood supply to the brain if the athlete's arm drops while the head is placed in an extended and rotated position.	Fig. 18-18*A* Fig. 18-18*B*
2. The athlete is asked to maintain this position while closing his or her eyes.		
3. The test is repeated with the clinician extending and rotating the athlete's head to one side.	**Not** considered positive for vascular insufficiency if a change in arm position occurs with the head in a neutral position, this could occur because of vertigo.	
Underburg's Test[9]		
1. The athlete is standing, with shoulders flexed to 90°, elbows extended and the forearms supinated.	Considered positive for vascular insufficiency if the athlete has a loss of balance or is unable to maintain the arm position.	
2. The athlete is asked to close his or her eyes and march in place with his or her head held in an extended and rotated position to each side.		

*DeKlyn's test is used to determine if a vascular insufficiency is present. The vertebral artery can become compromised during cervical rotation in athletes with conditions such as cervical instability or arthritis.

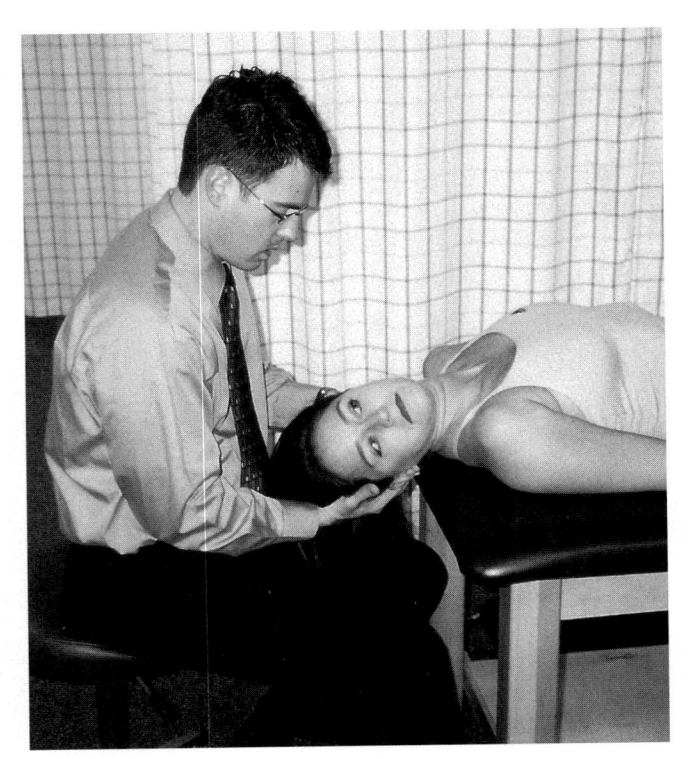

Figure 18-17. Vertebral artery test.

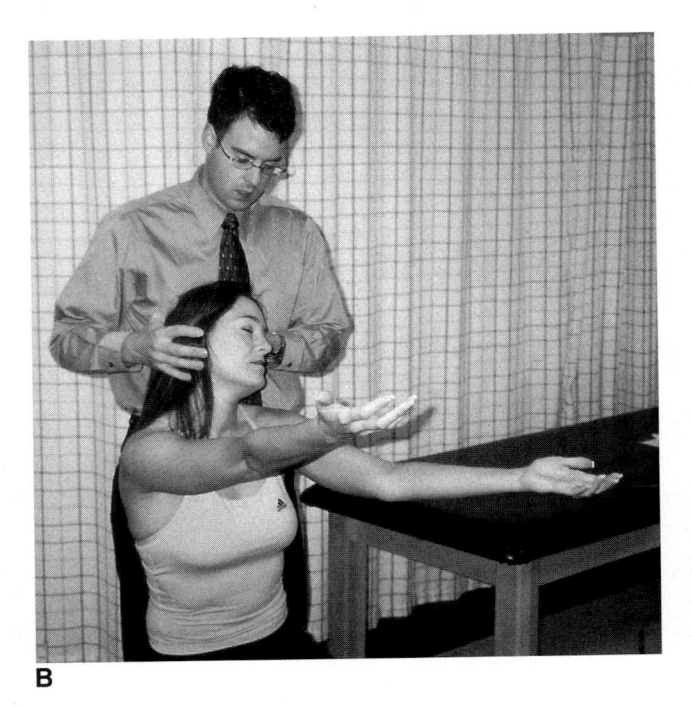

A

B

Figure 18-18. *A-B*, Hautant's test.

Neurologic Tests

Procedure	Positive Test	Figure
Distraction Test		
The clinician stands behind the athlete while bilaterally cupping the mastoid processes and gently applying a superiorly directed force.	Considered positive if the athlete reports a decrease in symptoms while the head is held in a distracted position. This occurs because of the relief of compressive forces on the weight-bearing structures of the cervical spine. **Note:** Occasionally a patient may report an increase of symptoms during distraction. This could result from increased tension applied to soft tissues such as the facet capsule, cervical ligaments, or muscle fibers.	Fig. 18-19
Compression Test[*†] **Spurling's test**[24]: 1. The clinician stands behind the seated patient. 2. The clinician carefully places the athlete's head in a rotated, side-bent, and extended position while applying a compressive force through the top of the head.	Considered positive for foraminal compression if the athlete reports pain radiating down the arm on the ipsilateral side to which the head is side-bent. Not considered positive if the patient only reports pain in the cervical region with no radiating symptoms. **Note:** The athlete may describe a pain or change in sensation in a dermatomal pattern, which can give the clinician clues as to the affected nerve root.	Fig. 18-20
Shoulder Abduction Test The athlete is seated and actively elevates his or her arm, placing it on top of his or her head.	By having the arm in an abducted position, decreased pressure will be placed on the nerves and nerve roots by shortening the nerve pathway. Therefore, if the athlete were to have compression on either a nerve or nerve root, he or she will express a relief of symptoms with the arm in an elevated position. **Note:** Occasionally an athlete may report an increase in pain with the arm in the abducted position, this can be caused by an increase in pressure in the interscalene triangle.	Fig. 18-21
Valsalva Maneuver 1. Performed with the athlete sitting in an upright position. 2. Ask the athlete to take a deep breath, hold it, and bear down as if trying to move their bowels.	Reproduction of symptoms is caused by an increase in intrathecal pressure and is indicative of a space-occupying lesion, such as a herniated disc, tumor, or osteophyte.	

Tension Testing

Introduction	Upper limb tension tests (ULTT), first described by Elvey.[8] Butler[4] adapted them into a series of four tests to place emphasis on specific peripheral nerves. By altering the position of the upper limb, the clinician can bias the particular nerve being tested by causing elongation of the neural pathway (Table 18-8).
Caution	Notably, stress testing is considered contraindicated if an athlete displays signs of an acute neurologic injury, worsening of symptoms, a lesion of the spinal cord, or diabetes or other pathologic condition involving the nervous system.[4]
Procedure	1. The athlete lies supine as the clinician applies and maintains a constant depressive force to the shoulder. 2. Depending on the nerve being tested, the upper limb is carried through various ranges of motion to provide for symptom provocation (Fig. 18-23*A-D*).

Continued

Neurologic Tests—cont'd

Procedure—cont'd	In the example of a radial nerve bias test (ULTT 3) the shoulder is depressed and brought into slight abduction, approximately 10°, and internally rotated, the elbow is extended, the forearm is pronated, and the wrist and fingers are flexed and ulnarly deviated (Fig. 18-23C). Each joint is taken through a full range of motion until symptoms appear. If the patient's symptoms do not appear, the cervical spine can be side-bent away from the side being tested to create a further increase in tension.
	3. Perform these tests bilaterally to allow a comparison of results.
Positive Test	Considered positive if the athlete reports neurologic symptoms such as a burning pain or numbness.
	Not considered a positive test due to the subjective description of the pain. The athlete may describe the pain or altered sensation in the distribution of a dermatome or a peripheral nerve, thus giving the clinician an indication of the affected nerve root level or peripheral nerve.
	Note: Because the tests create increased tension throughout the upper limb, the athlete may report a dull or aching pain, or a muscle stretch.

*Compression tests are commonly performed to assess the weight-bearing structures in the neck.
†Yoo[29] demonstrated that the diameter of the intervertebral foramina can be increased or decreased by flexing and extending the cervical spine. To bias the weight-bearing structures that are tested, the position of the athlete's head can be altered while applying a compressive force.[14] A compressive force applied with the head held in a flexed position will bias the intervertebral disc, an extended position examines the facet joints, and testing in a slightly flexed and sidebent position will bias the uncovertebral joints.

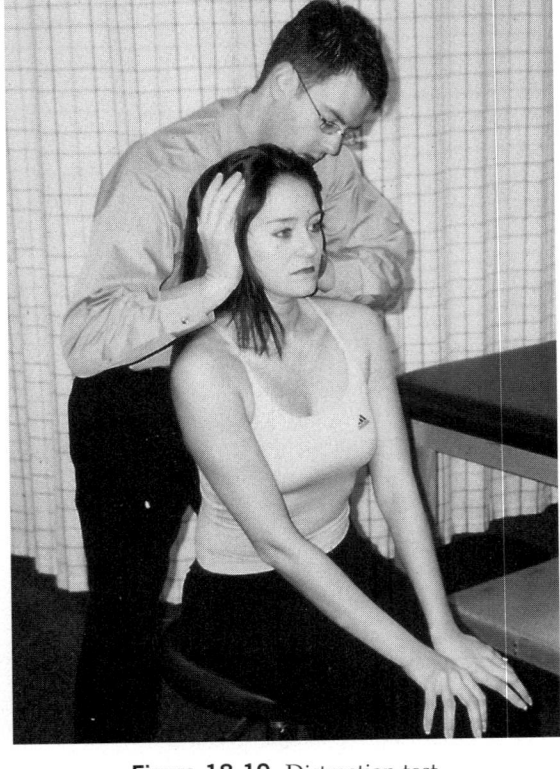

Figure 18-19. Distraction test.

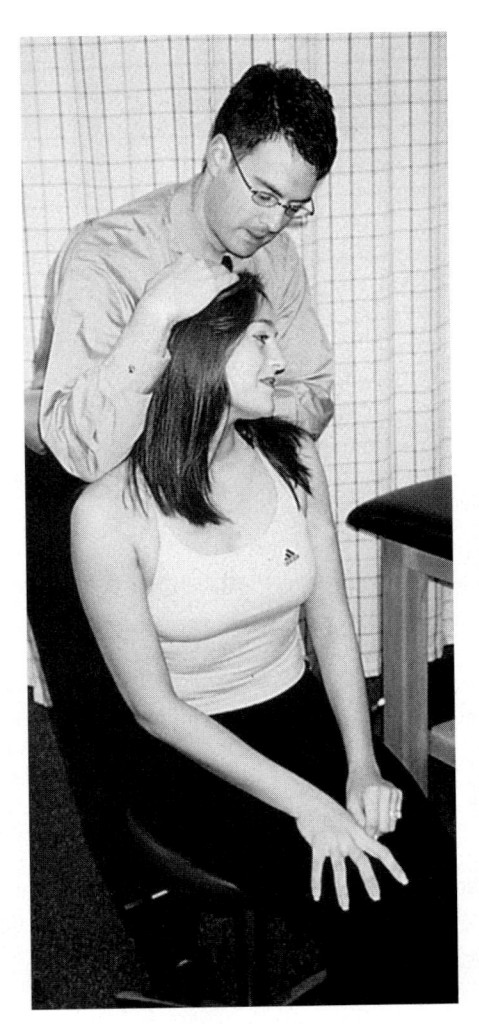

Figure 18-20. Spurling's test.

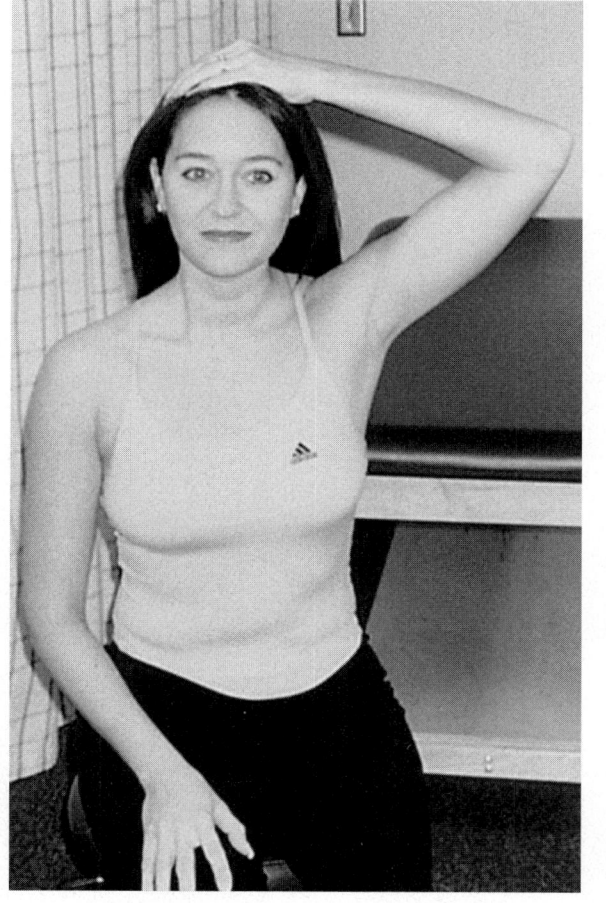

Figure 18-21. Shoulder abduction test.

Table 18-8

Cervical Spine and Extremity Positioning for Upper Limb Tension Testing

	Nerve Tested	Cervical Spine	Shoulder	Elbow	Forearm	Wrist	Fingers
ULTT1	Median nerve	Side-bent contralateral direction	Depressed and abducted to 110°	Extended	Supinated	Extended	Extended
ULTT2	Median nerve	Side-bent contralateral direction	Depressed and abducted to 110°	Extended	Supinated	Extended	Extended
ULTT3	Radial nerve	Side-bent contralateral direction	Depressed and abducted to 10°	Extended	Pronated	Flexed and ulnarly deviated	Flexed
ULTT4	Ulnar nerve	Side-bent contralateral direction	Depressed and abducted to 10°	Flexed	Supinated	Extended and radially deviated	Extended

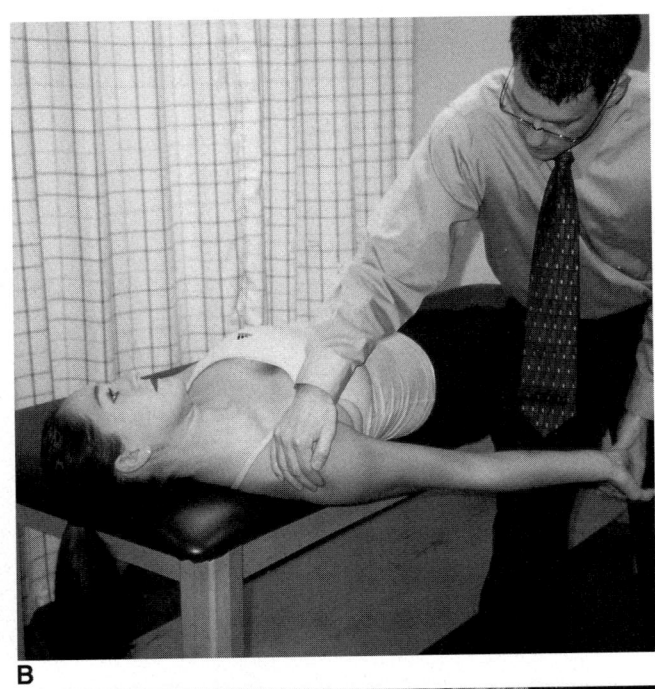

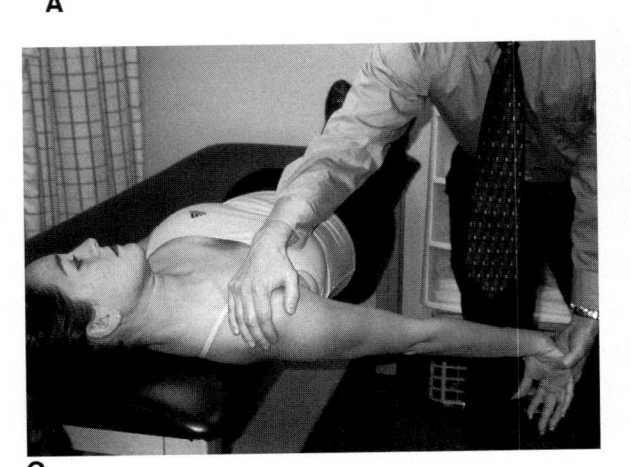

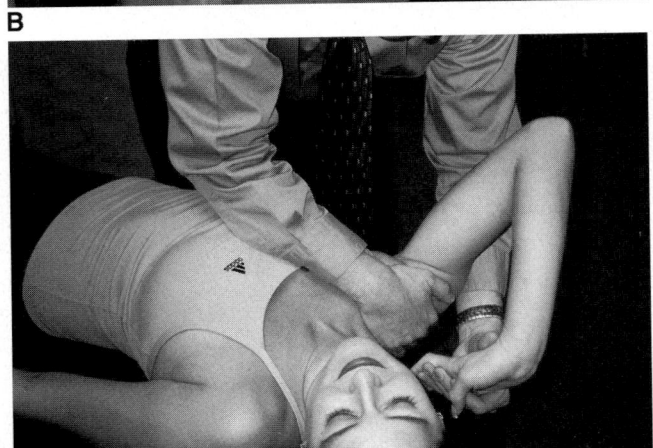

Figure 18-22. End position in upper limb tension tests. *A*, ULTT1. *B*, ULTT2. *C*, ULTT3. *D*, ULTT4.

Instability Testing

Procedure	Positive Test	Figure
Sharp-Purser Test* 1. Athlete is seated and the clinician places one hand on the athlete's forehead and the other hand stabilizes the spinous process of the axis with a pinch grip. 2. The clinician applies a posteriorly directed force to the forehead. **WARNING!** Perform this test with extreme caution.	Considered positive if the clinician feels the atlas translate on the axis. **Note:** Because of a restoration of normal joint alignment, the athlete may report alleviation of symptoms.	Fig. 18-23
Odontoid Fracture Test† 1. Athlete lies supine and the clinician uses his or her left hand to stabilize the athlete's head. 2. The clinician positions his or her right index finger and thumb along the sides of the spinous process of the axis. 3. The clinician applies an anterior directed force to the spinous process.	If the odontoid process is intact, the clinician will detect a hard endfeel with little to no movement occurring. A positive test will result in an increase in the amount of translation present with the athlete possibly complaining of pressure on the esophagus or neurologic symptoms, or both.[14]	Fig. 18-24

Continued

Instability Testing—cont'd

Procedure	Positive Test	Figure
Transverse Ligament Test[‡21]		
1. Athlete lies supine and the clinician supports his or her head in a neutral position.	If the transverse ligament is intact the clinician should note a firm, abrupt end point.	
2. The clinician places his or her index fingers over the posterior arches of the atlas.	If a rupture is present, the clinician may detect a soft end point, and signs of vertebral/basilar insufficiency.	
3. The head and the atlas are lifted in an anterior direction.		
Alar Ligament Test[§]		
1. Athlete lies supine.	If the alar ligament is intact, the clinician will detect the spinous process of C2 immediately pressing into the clinician's finger.	Fig. 18-25
2. The clinician supports the athlete's head using both hands and positions the middle finger of each hand along each side of the spinous process of the axis.		
3. The athlete's head is then flexed laterally away from the clinician's finger.	A positive test would result in a delay of movement occurring at the axis indicating a possible injury to the alar ligament.	

The clinician should perform instability testing of the upper cervical spine to determine if the athlete has had an injury to the odontoid process or surrounding ligaments. Signs and symptoms of vertebral instability and/or vertebral/basilar insufficiency can include oral/facial paresthesia, limb paresthesia, drop attacks, and nystagmus. These symptoms may be constant or induced by head movement.[21] Upper cervical instability testing should be performed on all athletes that have sustained a traumatic injury to the head and neck. These tests should be performed with extreme caution to avoid injury to any neurovascular structures.

*Used to determine if the atlas is subluxated on the axis.

†Assesses for possible odontoid fracture by creating an anterior shear of the axis on the atlas.

‡Assesses the integrity of the transverse ligament.

§Assesses the integrity of the alar ligament.

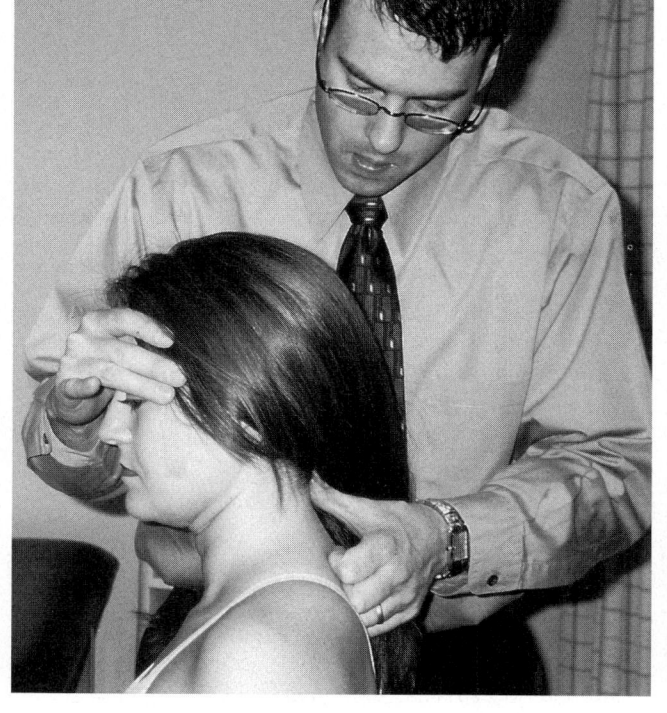

Figure 18-23. Sharp-Purser test.

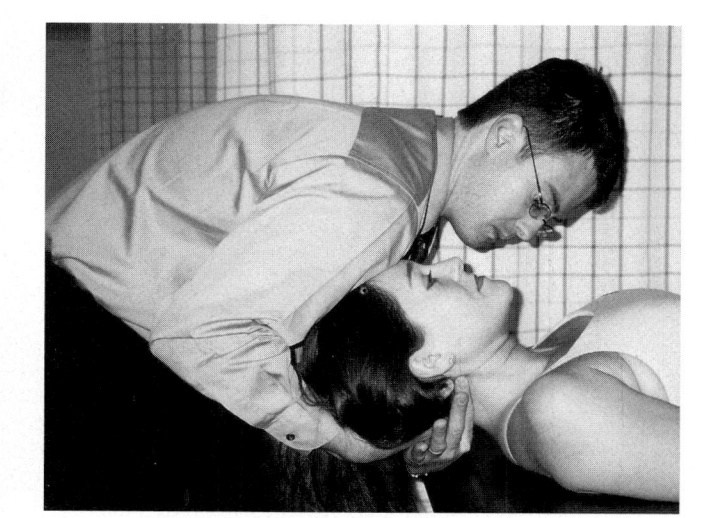

Figure 18-24. Odontoid fracture test.

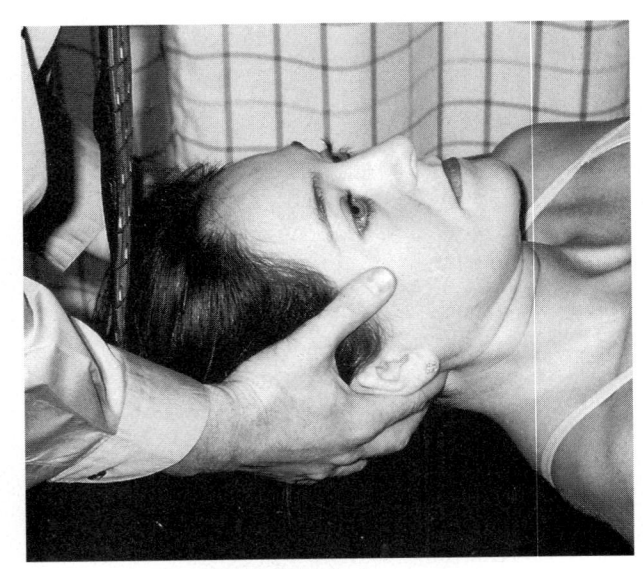

Figure 18-25. Alar ligament test.

THORACIC OUTLET SYNDROME

Thoracic outlet syndrome is the compromise of the brachial plexus and/or the subclavian artery or vein in the neck or upper extremity by the surrounding anatomic structures. In 95% of all cases the brachial plexus is involved, the arterial system is involved in 5%, and the venous system is involved in 2%.[6,23] Although the condition most often affects middle-aged women who have respiratory dysfunctions and a forward head posture, the condition should not be dismissed in individuals not meeting this stereotype. Thoracic outlet syndrome can result from congenital anomalies, postural faults, or environmental or traumatic stresses.

The athlete will have different symptoms depending on the structures that are compressed. Athletes with irritation to the nerves will describe radiating pain down the arm in a segmental distribution and hypersensitivity or hyposensitivity in these regions. Patients with obstruction of the vascular system will describe an ischemic pain in the whole hand. Common patient complaints include the following: pain, grip weakness, and numbness and tingling that is frequently present in the ulnar nerve distribution. The athlete may also report vascular symptoms that include temperature changes of the upper extremity and hand, feeling of heaviness, swelling, and fatiguing quickly that is relieved with rest.

The neurologic and vascular structures of the upper extremity pass through four possible anatomic spaces that serve as potential pathologic sites for thoracic outlet syndrome. These are the sternocostovertebral space, the scalene triangle, the costoclavicular space, and the pectoralis minor space.

Sternocostovertebral Space

The sternocostovertebral space is formed by the sternum anteriorly, the spine posteriorly, and the first rib laterally.

The subclavian artery and vein and the brachial plexus travel through this space. Although unusual, compression can occur in this region because of a tumor of the thyroid, lymph nodes, or a Pancoast tumor present at the lung.

Scalene Triangle

The scalene triangle is formed by the anterior scalene anteriorly, the middle scalene posteriorly, and the first rib inferiorly. Muscle tightness is commonly found in the scalenes in patients exhibiting a forward head postural dysfunction. Athletes with respiratory problems may recruit the scalenes to assist in inspiration. Conditions that cause muscle tightness or hyperactivity of the scalene muscles can produce neurovascular compression between the anterior and middle scalene muscles, or can elevate the first rib, which causes a reduction in the dimensions of the scalene triangle.

Costoclavicular Space

The costoclavicular space is formed by the medial one third of the clavicle anteriorly, the first rib posteriorly, and the scapula posterolaterally. The costoclavicular syndrome occurs as a result of depression of the shoulder girdle and fixation of the clavicle onto the first rib.[25,27] When the shoulder is in a depressed and retracted position, the clavicle is approximated on the neurovascular structures as traction is placed on these structures. The first rib may become elevated in someone with an abnormal breathing pattern that originates from the accessory respiratory muscles (scalenes) or because of muscle tightness in this muscle group. This elevation of the first rib can create a reduced volume in this space causing a compression of the neurovascular structures.

Pectoralis Minor Space

The pectoralis minor space is formed by the pectoralis minor tendon anteriorly, and the ribs posteriorly. Compression can occur in this region when the arm is taken into an abducted position causing the neurovascular structures to curve around the coracoid process as the pectoralis minor and subclavius muscles are placed on stretch, causing compression. Hyperactivity of the pectoralis minor muscle can also cause compression in this region; this can be seen in conditions that cause the muscle to be used as an accessory muscle for respiration. Other conditions that can create compression of the neurovascular structures in this region include postural kyphosis or trauma to the pectoralis minor or upper rib.

Thoracic Outlet Testing

There are several special tests that can be performed to aid in the determination of the presence of thoracic outlet syndrome. These tests are described in Figures 18-26 through 18-31.

Thoracic Outlet Syndrome Tests

Procedure	Positive Test	Figure
Roos Test[22]	Considered positive if the patient describes numbness or tingling, weakness, ischemic pain, or decreased speed and coordination of hand movements. **Not** considered positive if the patient reports only minor fatigue.	Fig. 18-26
1. Patient stands and is instructed to retract and depress his or her shoulder girdles, abduct the arms to 90°, laterally rotate the arms, and flex the elbows to 90°.		
2. Ask the patient to completely open and close both hands repeatedly for 3 minutes.		
Adson[1] and Allen[2] Tests* **Adson Test**	Considered positive if the pulse disappears and patient's symptoms reappear.	Fig. 18-27
1. Locate the radial pulse on the affected side.		
2. Rotate the athlete's head to the same side as being tested and extended backward.		
3. Clinician extends and laterally rotates the patient's shoulder.		
4. Ask the athlete to take a deep breath and hold it as the clinician continues to check the radial pulse.		
Allen Test Performed in a similar manner as the Adson test.	Considered positive if the radial pulse is diminished and patient's symptoms are reproduced.	Fig. 18-28
1. Extend the athlete's shoulder and laterally rotate with elbow extension.		
2. Clinician locates the radial pulse.		
3. Instruct the athlete to rotate their head away from the affected side.		
Costoclavicular Compression Maneuver	Considered positive if the radial pulse is diminished and patient's symptoms are reproduced.	Fig. 18-29
1. The athlete sits with his or her shoulders in a depressed and retracted position (military posture) and the chin tucked.[14]		
2. Clinician palpates the radial pulse.		
3. Ask the athlete to take a deep breath and hold it as the clinician applies a depressive force to the clavicles with his or her forearms.		
Pectoralis Minor Test†	Considered positive if the pulse is diminished or a reproduction of symptoms is produced.	Fig. 18-30
1. Clinician passively retracts the affected shoulder into a pain free position.		
2. Ask the athlete to actively protract the shoulder.		
Wright's Hyperabduction Test	Considered positive if the pulse is diminished or a reproduction of symptoms is produced.	Fig. 18-31
1. The clinician locates the radial pulse on the affected side.[14]		
2. Flex the athlete's shoulder and horizontally abducted to apply a stretch to the anterior capsule of the shoulder.		
3. Clinician may choose to have the patient hold a deep breath or rotate their head to create additional tension.		

*Assess for thoracic outlet syndrome that originates in the scalene triangle.
†Used to assess the neurovascular structures as they pass under the pectoralis minor.[14]

MOBILITY TESTING

The rehabilitation specialist can perform passive joint movements to the cervical vertebrae to examine the intervertebral mobility and assess for a possible hypomobility or hypermobility that may be present. Because normal joint mobility is relative from person to person, it is important for the clinician to examine the surrounding joints for comparison. It is possible for a joint to be hypomobile with certain movements and hypermobile during other movements. Because an athlete may have sufficient neuromuscular control of a joint's translational movements, it is important to remember that the presence of a hypomobility or hypermobility is not necessarily indicative of a pathologic condition.

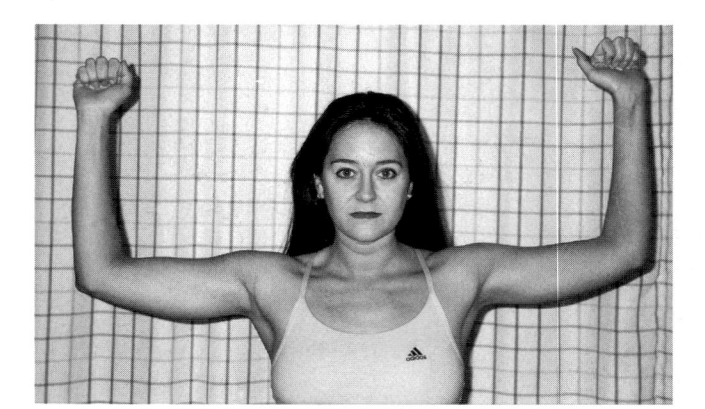

Figure 18-26. Roos test.

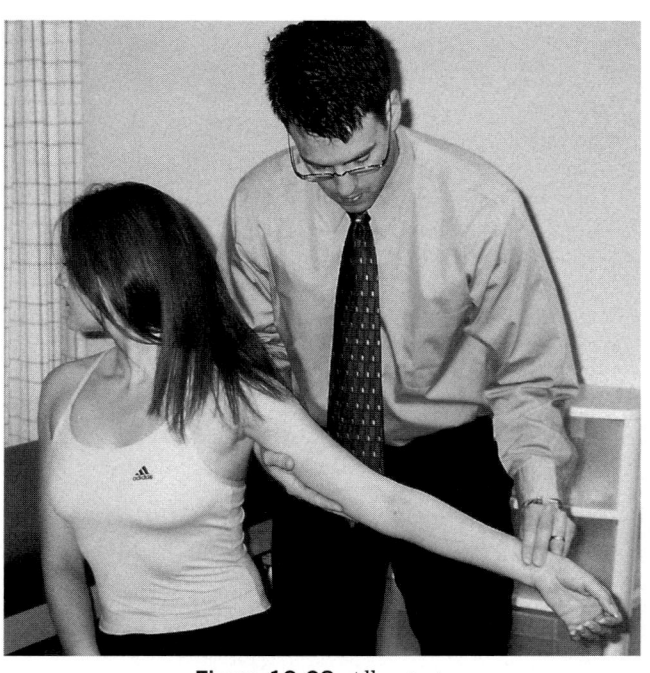

Figure 18-28. Allen test.

The clinician may inspect the mobility of the entire cervical spine or a particular joint or region. The passive intervertebral movement is examined for the same movements as during the active and passive ROM parts of the examination—that is, flexion, extension, rotation, and lateral flexion.

The upper cervical spine can be assessed with the athlete in the seated or supine position. Testing flexion of the occiput on C1 (Fig. 18-33) is performed by the clinician holding the athlete's head in a neutral position as the clinician places his or her index fingers on the lateral aspect of the patient's neck between the transverse processes of the atlas and the mastoid processes of the occiput.[14] The clinician introduces flexion into the upper cervical spine by passively nodding the athlete's head as the clinician detects

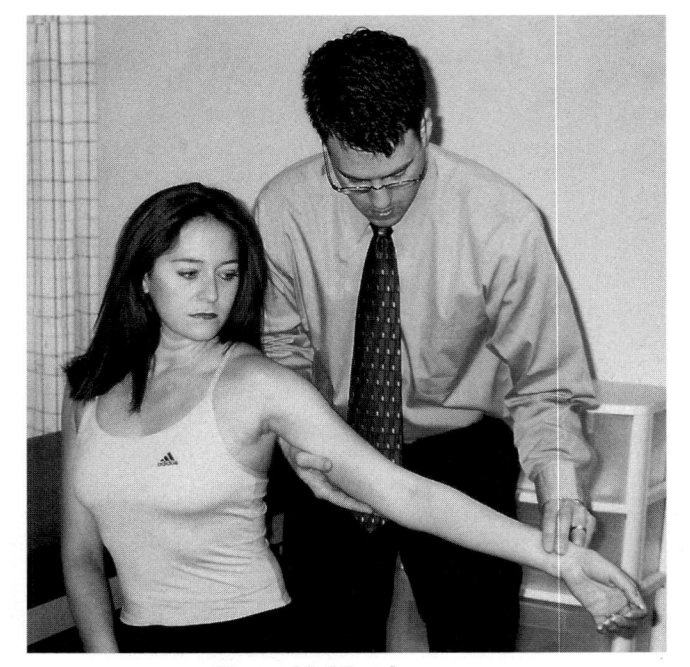

Figure 18-27. Adson test.

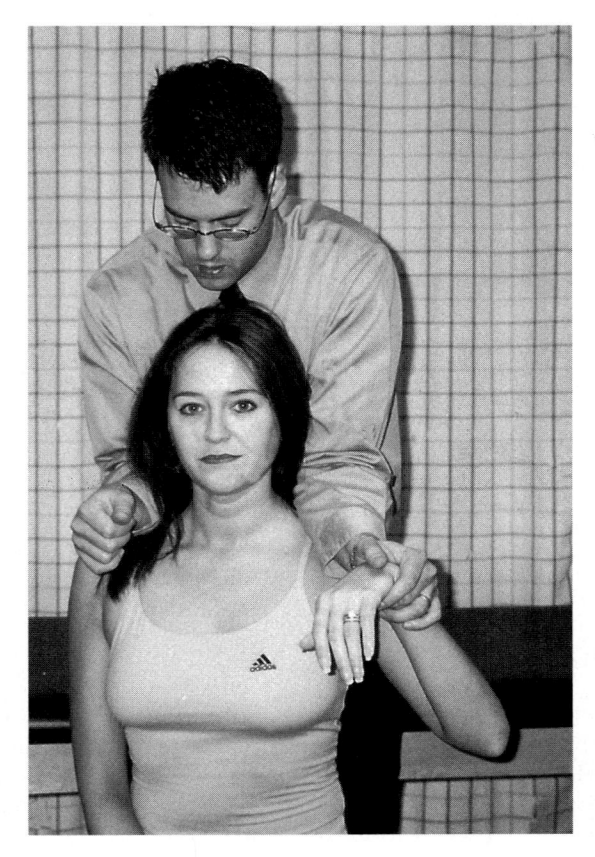

Figure 18-29. Costoclavicular compression maneuver.

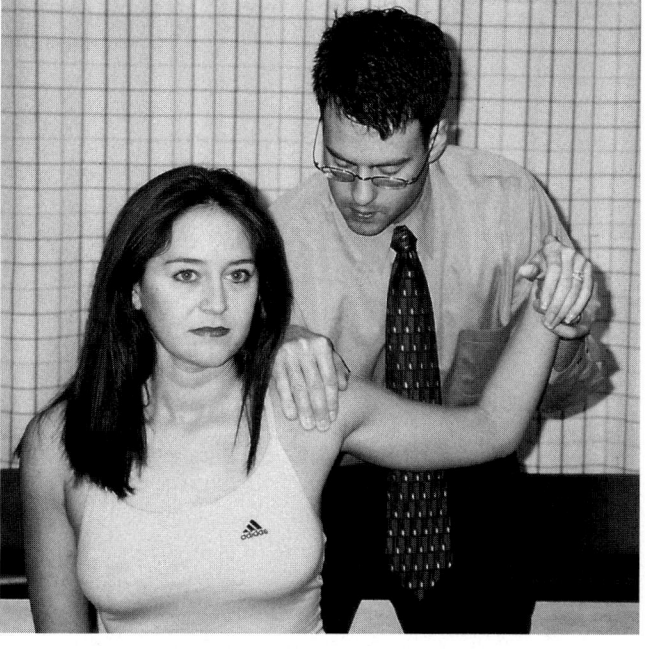

Figure 18-30. Pectoralis minor test.

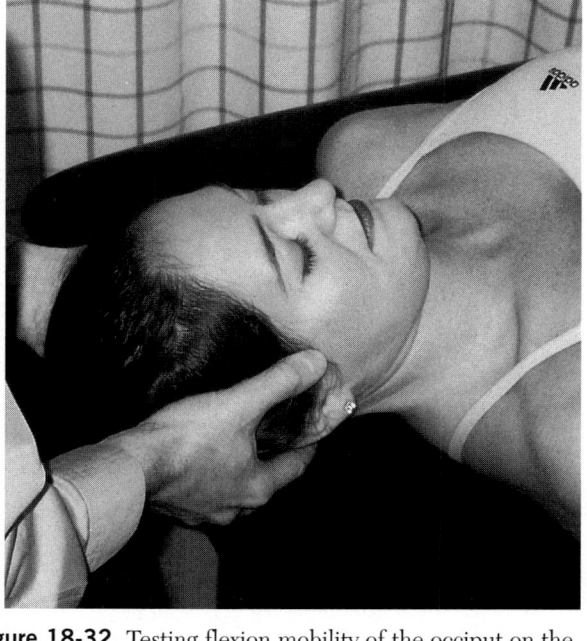

Figure 18-32. Testing flexion mobility of the occiput on the atlas. The clinician detects for the amount of motion occurring as the head is flexed.

the motion occurring as a separation between the mastoid processes and the transverse processes of the atlas. The clinician can assess extension, lateral flexion, and rotation of the occiput and atlas in a similar manner performed during flexion.

Rotation of the atlas on the axis is examined with the athlete in a seated position. The clinician's right hand is positioned on top of the athlete's head and the left hand is placed in the midline of the spine with the index finger

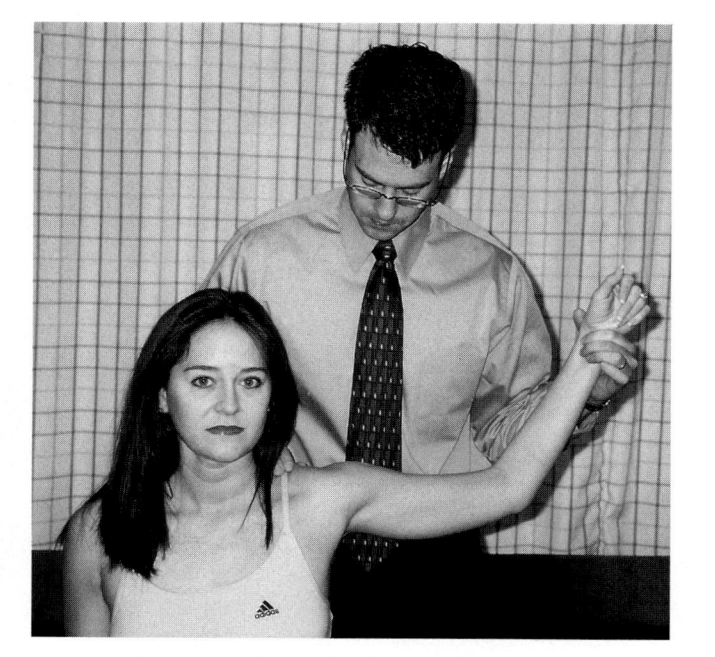

Figure 18-31. Wright's hyperabduction test.

over the spinous process of the axis. The clinician rotates the head to the right while palpating to detect the C2 spinous process rotating to the left. The axis will begin to rotate to the left as the C1-C2 joint is taken to end range, which occurs at approximately 40°. A comparison is made between right and left rotation to assess for a possible hypomobility or hypermobility. The sports rehabilitation specialist may also inspect lateral flexion of C1-C2 in a similar fashion to determine the available motion during this movement.

The clinician can examine flexion, extension, and rotation mobility of the midcervical spine with the athlete supine. To examine passive intervertebral right lateral flexion of C4-C5, the clinician places his or her fingers over these facet joints while supporting the patient's head (Fig. 18-33). The clinician laterally flexes the cervical spine while palpating the right inferior facet of C4 translating inferiorly and posteriorly onto the C5 right superior facet. This is repeated on the other side for bilateral comparison. This process can be repeated in the remaining vertebral segments in this region.

The mobility of the first rib is often included in the assessment of the cervical spine. The first rib serves as an attachment site for the anterior and middle scalenes. Tightness or neurologic facilitation of this musculature or other conditions could cause decreased mobility in this region. The athlete is examined in a supine position as the clinician uses their web space between the thumb and index finger to apply a force directed in an anterior

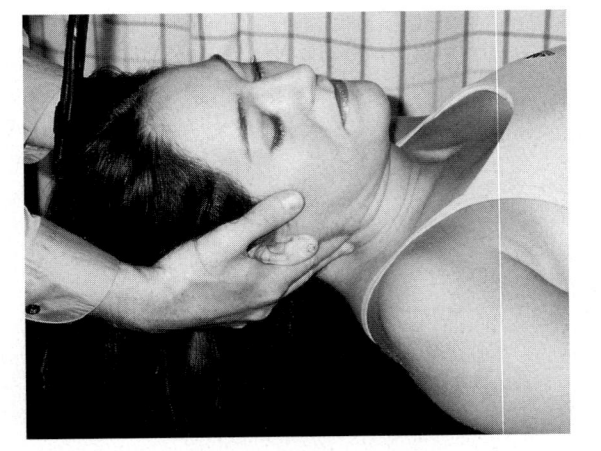

Figure 18-33. Right lateral flexion mobility testing of C4-C5. The athlete's head is laterally flexed while the clinician palpates C4 translating posteriorly and inferiorly onto C5 on the right side.

and caudal direction to the first rib (Fig. 18-34). The clinician will compare the available motion and endfeel of the first rib bilaterally.

DIAGNOSTIC TESTS

After the clinical examination of the athlete, the clinician should review any diagnostic testing that the athlete has undergone to verify the clinical findings of the evaluation. Plain film radiographs are commonly taken with musculoskeletal injuries. These allow for determination of possible vertebral fractures, dislocations, developmental vertebral abnormalities, metabolic bone diseases, and

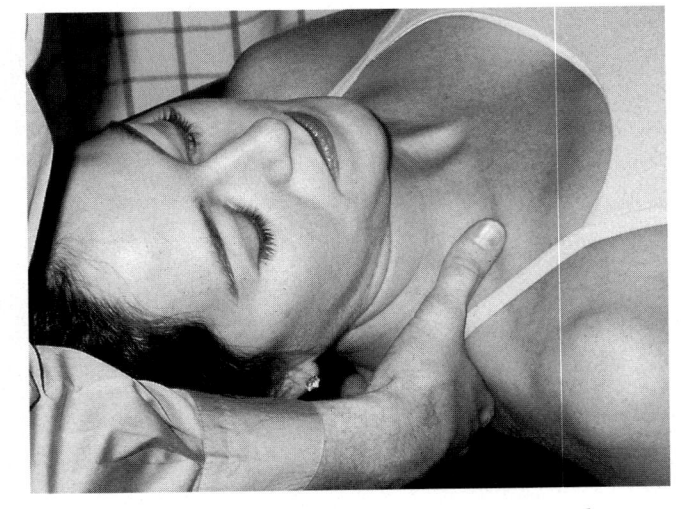

Figure 18-34. Mobility testing or joint mobilization technique of the first rib. The clinician uses the web space between the thumb and index finger and directs a force in an anterior and caudal direction.

tumors. Anteroposterior, lateral, and oblique views are routinely taken, which allows for a complete examination of the entire cervical spine.

In addition, the athlete may have had further studies performed, such as magnetic resonance imaging, computed tomography, or a myelogram. If a nerve injury is suspected, electromyographic studies can be used to determine the grade of nerve injury present. Laboratory tests can assist in determining if an infection or disease is present, such as osteoporosis, osteomalacia, rheumatoid arthritis, hyperthyroidism, and hypothyroidism.

REHABILITATION TECHNIQUES FOR THE CERVICAL SPINE

After completing a thorough evaluation, the sports rehabilitation specialist should be able to determine pathologic tissue(s) that are contributing to the athlete's condition. The athlete can have a wide variety of symptoms and limitations that will determine and dictate the treatment intensity and direction. The athlete's injury can be treated with various modalities, manual techniques, and therapeutic exercise programs. It is important that the rehabilitation program chosen addresses the athlete's individual injuries and deficiencies. This allows for a therapeutic program that is both patient- and tissue-specific. It is also important that the sports rehabilitation specialist continuously monitors the athlete's current conditions and symptoms. This will ensure an optimal therapeutic program at all times and will allow for adjustments as needed and dictated by the athlete's condition.

Modalities

During the acute phase of treatment, therapeutic modalities are commonly used to allow for pain reduction, reducing muscle tone and spasticity, decreasing stiffness, increasing blood flow and metabolic rate, and reduction of edema. The modality chosen should be determined by the target tissue and the desired therapeutic benefit. It is also important that the modality chosen is not contraindicated for the athlete's current condition (e.g., the application of ultrasound to a hypermobile joint).

Soft Tissue Mobilization

After a sports-induced cervical injury it is common for musculoskeletal dysfunctions to develop in the athlete. Sports rehabilitation specialists commonly perform various soft tissue mobilization techniques to decrease muscle soreness, stiffness, spasm, hypertonicities, and edema, and to prepare the tissues for therapeutic activities. The clinician should also be aware of conditions such as infections or a fracture, which may be a contraindication for soft tissue mobilization at that time.

Before the clinician begins implementing a soft tissue mobilization program, he or she must decide on the desired treatment goals and outcomes to determine which specific technique is used. Dysfunctions of the neuromusculoskeletal system often require an implementation of a multitechnique approach. Effleurage and kneading techniques are useful in increasing circulation and neuromodulating pain. Decreased mobility is often found in the muscle, fascia, and skin surrounding postural muscles after trauma and chronically habitual postures. Myofascial mobilization techniques such as skin rolling (see Fig. 18-14) and transverse massaging can be used to restore the decreased mobility and to reduce the associated pain. Transverse massage is performed by placing the target muscle on slack and beginning with light pressure, the clinician's finger pads (palmar surfaces of the interphalangeal bone) apply a rhythmic cross-fiber massage (Fig. 18-36.)

Flexibility Exercises

Stretching exercises can be performed in cases of muscle spasms, hypertonicity, and adaptive shortening. It is important for the rehabilitation specialist to determine before beginning a stretching program whether the muscle tightness or increase tone are present as a result of a cervical hypermobility or a facilitated segment (reactive innervated level) that is producing a protective muscle splint. Although a light-stretching program to relax the muscles can be implemented, a therapeutic program aimed at addressing the causative factor is needed to ensure and to provide long-term symptom relief.

The clinician can use various flexibility exercise programs. A vapor coolant spray, such as Fluorimethane (Gebauer Chemical Co., Cleveland, OH), can be used to stimulate the sensory receptors of the skin allowing for an increase in passive stretch without causing pain. The spray

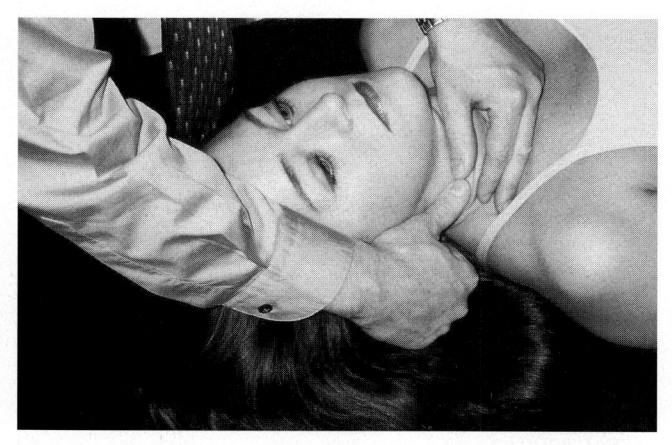

Figure 18-35. Transverse massage to the sternocleidomastoid. The muscle is initially placed on slack as the clinician performs a cross-fiber massage technique.

and stretch technique is performed with the patient sitting upright with the head supported allowing for relaxation of the cervical musculature. The Fluorimethane bottle is held approximately 18 inches and at an angle from the targeted muscle and is applied in a unidirectional motion parallel to the muscle fibers. The clinician simultaneously stretches the muscle while the Fluorimethane spray is being applied. The work by Travell and Simons[26] describes patient positioning and the direction for stretching and vapor coolant spray. (See Chapter 6 for additional information regarding the spray and stretch technique.)

Contract-relax or contract-relax contract-antagonist techniques can also be used to stretch tight musculature. A contract-relax stretch is performed by taking the muscle to a position of mild stretch and instructing the patient to match the applied resistance of the therapist by mildly contracting the target muscle. This contraction is maintained for 3 to 5 seconds followed by the clinician applying a further stretch for 5 to 10 seconds as the patient exhales and relaxes. This process is repeated throughout a full ROM. The contract-relax contract-antagonist stretch is performed in a similar manner, except that after the contraction of the agonist muscle there is a contraction of the antagonist muscle that provides a reciprocal inhibition as a stretch is applied (see Chapter 6).

Joint Mobilization

Joint mobilization techniques can be performed not only to restore motion, but also to provide a neurophysiologic effect thus reducing pain and muscle spasms. The sports rehabilitation specialist must evaluate the intervertebral mobility and the possible presence of pain originating from a cervical segment or surrounding tissue to determine the justification and application of joint mobilizations. It is important for the clinician to understand the role and application of joint mobilization techniques to allow for optimal use in a rehabilitation setting. When performing a joint mobilization technique, the practitioner should maintain a close approximation to the joint being mobilized and also use his or her legs and body to create weight transfer to provide the force needed for the mobilization. This technique allows the clinician to produce the needed movement while generating a minimum amount of force, and also allows for a greater palpatory sense. A few examples of mobilization techniques are described in Figures 18-36 through 18-41. The cervical spine can be mobilized in motions other than those described earlier by applying the arthrokinematic principles of the cervical joints. There are also other techniques that can be used depending on the joint mobilization school of thought adhered to by the rehabilitation specialist.

Joint mobilization techniques for the upper cervical spine can be applied with the athlete in a supine or seated position. A flexion mobilization of the occiput on the atlas

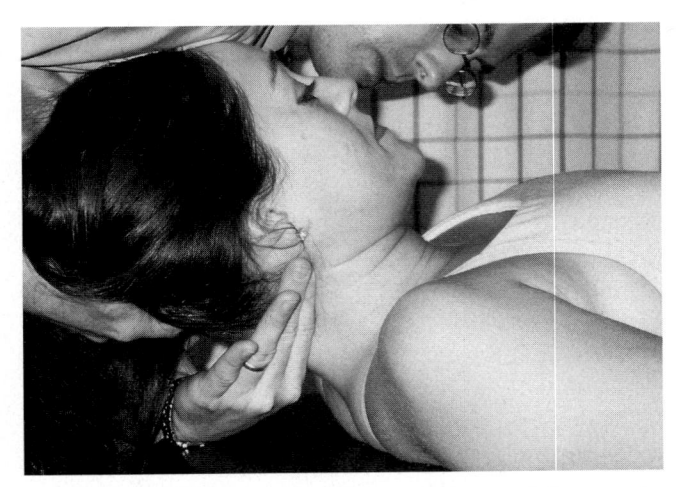

Figure 18-36. The clinician performs a flexion mobilization of the occiput on the atlas by stabilizing the atlas as the head is moved into a flexed position.

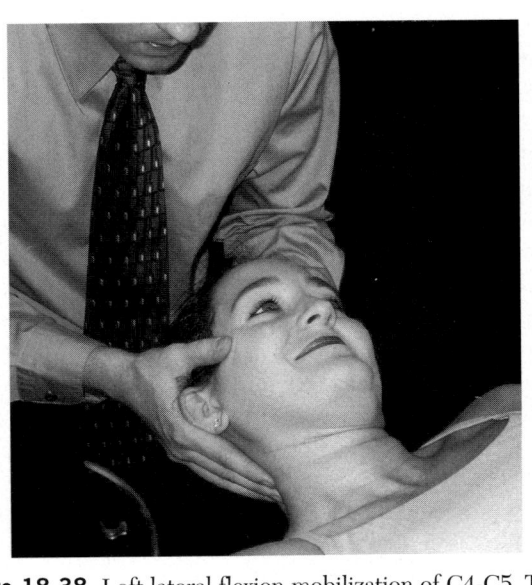

Figure 18-38. Left lateral flexion mobilization of C4-C5. The left transverse process of C5 is stabilized while mobilizing C4 into left side bending.

is performed with the athlete in a supine position as the head is placed in a neutral position. The clinician stabilizes the atlas by placing his or her thumb and index finger on its transverse processes (see Fig. 18-36). The athlete's head is supported between the clinician's opposing forearm and shoulder as the occiput is held in the hand. The occiput is moved into a flexed position while maintaining a fixated position of the atlas. The clinician can also mobilize into extension, side-bending, and rotation, as needed, using the same hand placements and altering the direction of mobilization.[14]

Mobilization of the atlas on the axis into left rotation in a supine position is illustrated in Figure 18-37. The athlete is supine with the head held in a neutral position. The rehabilitation specialist uses his or her left hand to stabilize

the axis by placing his thumb over the right transverse process. As the athlete's head is held between the clinician's right hand and chest, the clinician rotates his or her body to the left. Due to the motion of the axis being restricted, this will cause mobilization between the atlas and the axis. The rehabilitation specialist can mobilize C2-C3 using the same technique.[14]

Mobilization of the midcervical vertebrae is more efficiently performed with the patient in the supine position

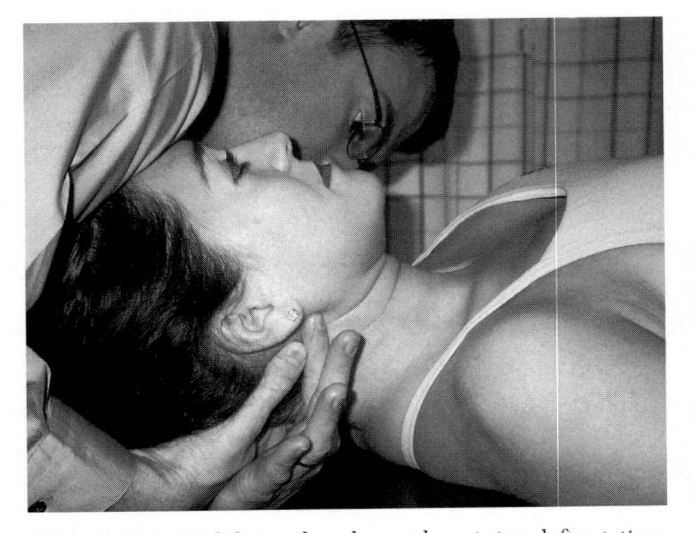

Figure 18-37. Mobilizing the atlas on the axis into left rotation. The left transverse process of the axis is stabilized as the therapist rotates the athlete's head into left rotation.

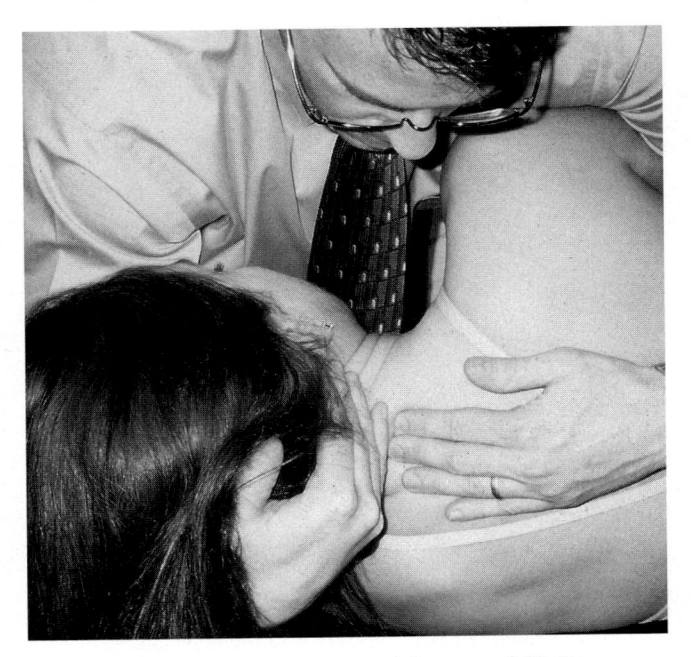

Figure 18-39. Extension mobilization of C3-C4.

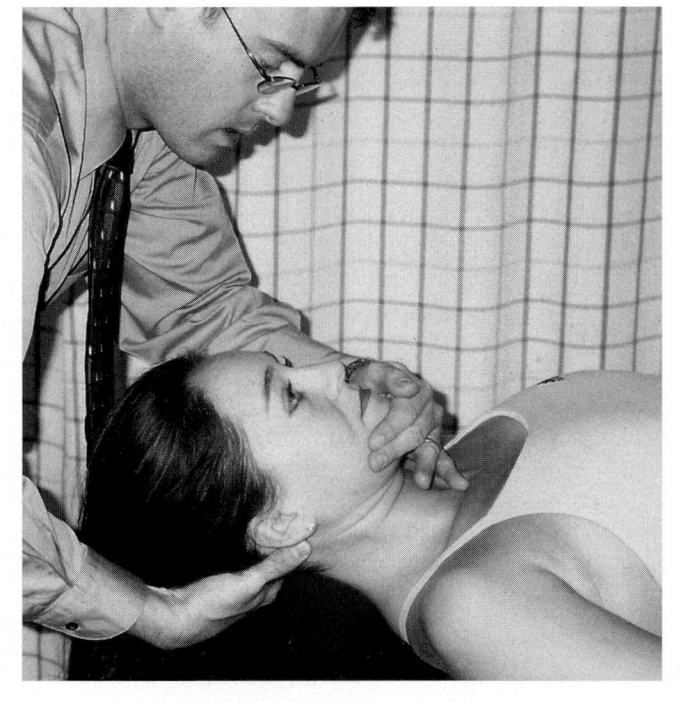

Figure 18-40. Manual cervical traction.

because of the otherwise longer arm movement occurring with the clinician generating motion through the occiput in a seated position. Mobilization of C4-C5 into left side-bending is illustrated in Figure 18-38. The clinician supports the athlete's head in a neutral position and positions his or her thumbs over the left transverse process of C5

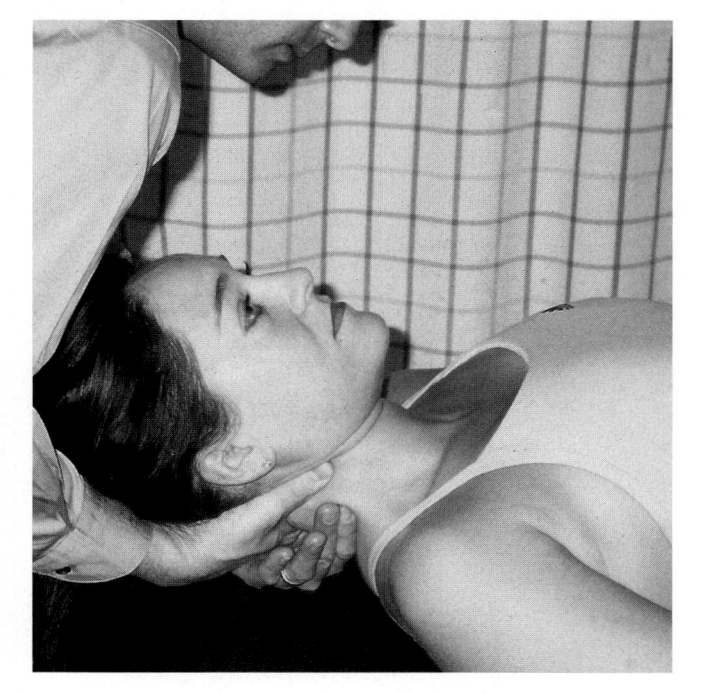

Figure 18-41. Joint-specific manual traction.

and right transverse process of C4. The clinician stabilizes C5 as C4 is side-bent to the left by using the right hand and forearm to induce motion of the head and upper segments of the cervical spine. The rehabilitation specialist can mobilize the midcervical spine into flexion, extension, and rotation by applying the same principles of stabilizing the inferior spinal segment and mobilizing the superior spinal segment.

An extension mobilization of C3-C4 can be performed with the athlete in a side-lying position (see Fig. 18-40). The athlete's head is supported and cradled between the clinician's hand and the anterior aspect of the arm as his or her left fingers are placed over C3. The clinician positions his or her right fingers over the spinous process of C4 to provide stabilization. The rehabilitation specialist introduces motion by shifting his or her weight.[14]

Cervical traction is often performed as a generalized technique when initiating joint mobilizations. The athlete is placed in a supine position and the clinician supports the athlete's head with one hand cupping the occiput. The other hand is placed under the athlete's chin to provide positioning, as no force is translated into the chin (see Fig. 18-40). A traction force is introduced as the clinician shifts his or her body weight back. This technique can also be modified to allow the traction forces to be specific to an intervertebral joint. The clinician would perform a joint-specific traction mobilization by stabilizing the spinous process of the inferior vertebrae with one hand as motion is introduced to that intervertebral level as the other hand applies a distractive force to the superior vertebrae (see Fig. 18-41). During both traction techniques, the clinician should mobilize the cervical spine in a superior and anterior direction to allow for motion to occur along the longitudinal axes.[14]

Fundamental Exercises

CLINICAL PEARL #4

To provide the optimal stimulus for tissue repair, regeneration, and growth, the clinician should provide adequate stresses and forces (resistance) to the athlete's rehabilitation program while avoiding stresses that can create deleterious effects in pathologic tissue. Therefore, to adequately prepare an athlete for a return to sports, the tissues must be able to tolerate functional loads.

"Challenge the tissue."
—*Rob Tillman, P.T., M.O.M.T.*

Various pathologic conditions can have extreme variability in symptoms and can affect the athlete's ability to voluntarily move and control movement in the cervical spine. Therefore, the rehabilitation specialist's therapeutic exercise program must be specific in nature to address the athlete's symptoms and causative pathology. Cervical isometrics or isotonics performed in a ROM near the midline can be performed to promote stabilization. The clinician can address postural concerns by having the patient perform exercises with high repetitions while in a corrected posture. The athlete's neuromuscular system can be challenged by adding a proprioceptive component into their rehabilitation. If the athlete reports pain and is unable to perform exercises in a seated (weight-bearing) position, the athlete is assessed for his or her ability to begin exercises in a nonweight-bearing (supine) position. The clinician therefore cannot only alter the rehabilitation program by changing the exercises that the athlete performs, but by adjusting the athlete's position, repetition, level of proprioceptive difficulty, and ROM of the exercises. This allows the athlete to be prescribed a program that addresses his or her individual needs.

If the athlete has pain originating from a weight-bearing structure (facet joints, disc), he or she may be unable to perform exercises in an upright posture during the early phases of rehabilitation because of an increase in pain. Therefore, it may be necessary to have the athlete perform ROM activities while in a supine, nonweight-bearing position. The athlete is encouraged to perform active movements within a pain-free ROM while in a gravity-eliminated position. The athlete may also be able to tolerate external resistance such as Theraband (Akron, OH) (Fig. 18-42), pulley system, or manual resistance sooner than in an upright position. This allows an earlier initiation of exercises to avoid the deleterious effects as a result of immobilization.

Cervical isometrics are commonly performed to allow for early initiation of the rehabilitation program by having the athlete resist a self-administered manual resistance. As the athlete's condition improves, the sports rehabilitation specialist can further challenge the athlete's ability to stabilize and control the cervical spine by adding external resistance to the exercise. This is typically performed with a pulley system (Fig. 18-43A-B) or Theraband. The plane of the resistance can be altered to allow the clinician to target different muscle groups (Fig. 18-44). The athlete may also be instructed to perform upper extremity resistance exercises while maintaining a static, isometric position of the cervical spine (Fig. 18-45).

Postural faults that may cause or attribute to the pathologic condition of the athlete must be addressed. A typical posture identified is a forward head, rounded-shoulder posture. This posture can elevate the inferior angle of the scapula and depress the acromion as the scapula fulcrums at its ventral midpoint on the resultant increased thoracic

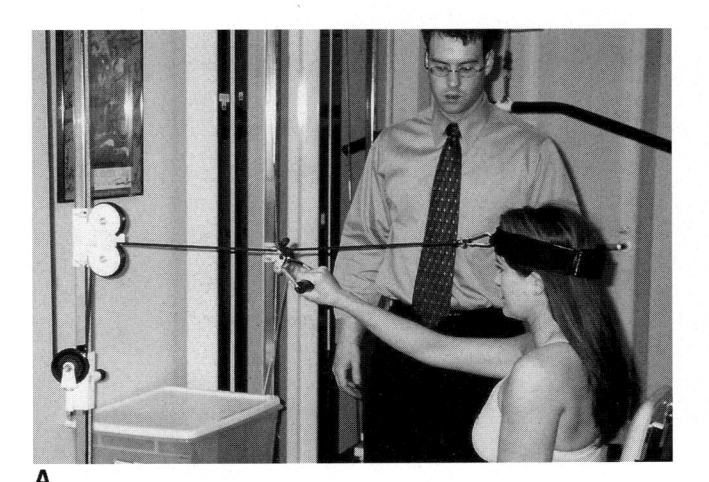

A

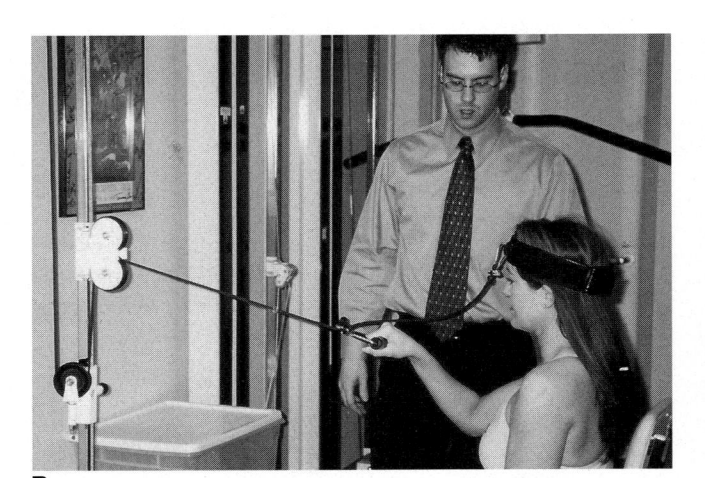

B

Figure 18-43. Seated cervical isometric extension using a pulley system. *A,* Contraction phase. *B,* Handle attached to allow for rest between repetitions.

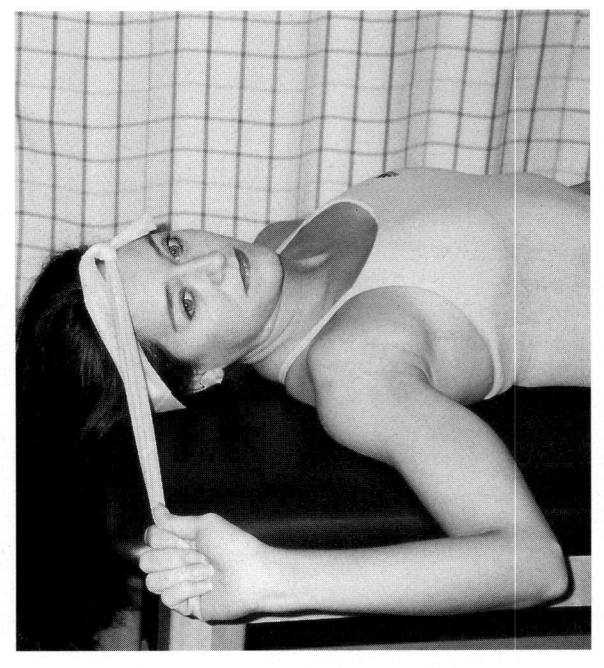

Figure 18-42. Using Theraband (Akron, OH) to increase resistance during supine cervical rotation.

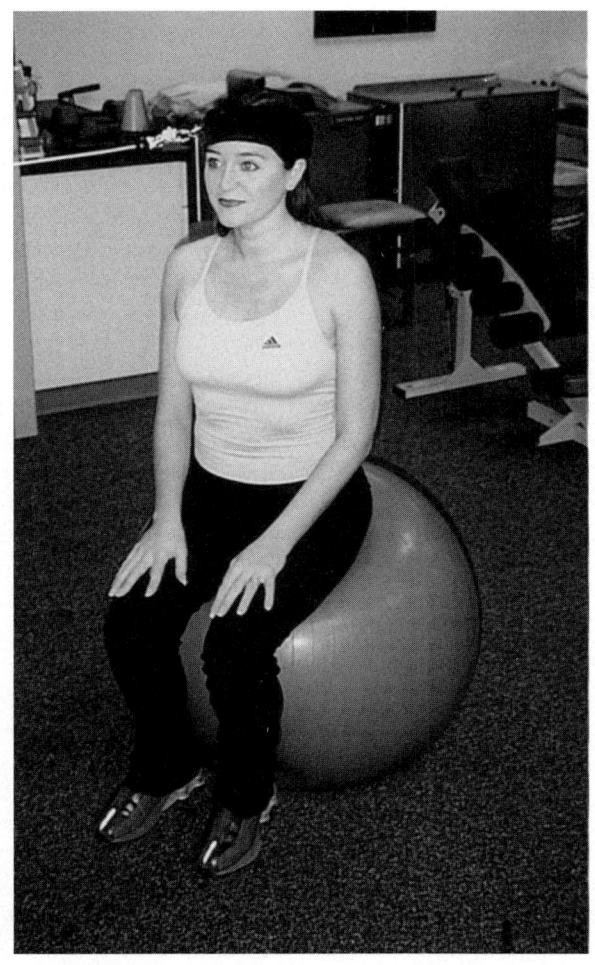

Figure 18-44. Seated cervical isometrics performed at an oblique angle.

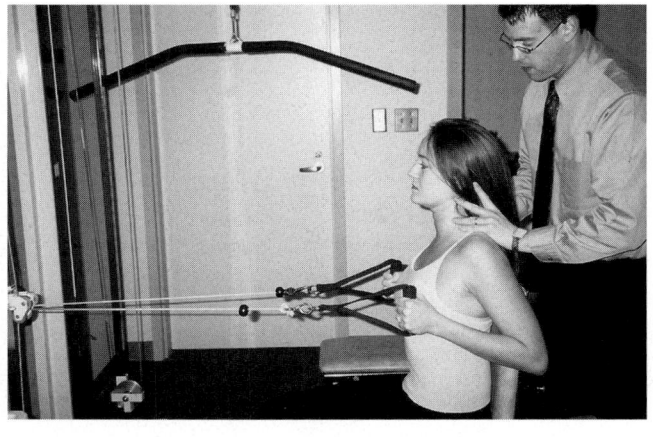

Figure 18-46. Seated rows. The athlete is instructed to retract the scapula and the cervical spine. The clinician can provide tactile cueing to ensure proper technique.

exercises for the anterior musculature and strengthening exercises for the posterior musculature. Seated rows can be performed to target the scapula retractors and the thoracic and cervical extensors. The athlete is instructed to retract the scapula as he or she extends the thoracic spine and retracts the cervical spine. The clinician may provide tactile cueing for the athlete to allow for proper form during the exercise (Fig. 18-46). In similar fashion, the athlete can perform prone dumbbell flies. A hinged bench can be used to allow the athlete to simultaneously extend the thoracic spine and retract the cervical spine and scapula (Fig. 18-47). The athlete can perform pectoralis stretches using a door frame or corner of a room (Fig. 18-48).

A proprioceptive component can be added to the exercise regimen. This is achieved by having the athlete lie, sit,

kyphosis.[15] This can result in adaptive shortening of the pectoralis minor and place the lower trapezius on stretch. This excessive stretching is referred to as *stretch weakness* because of the resultant weakness that occurs after prolonged elongation.[17] The athlete performs flexibility

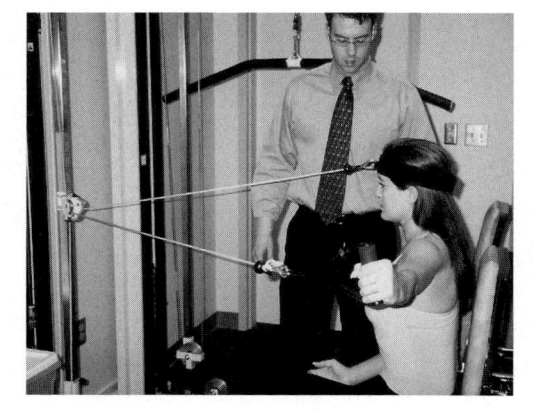

Figure 18-45. Seated cervical isometrics while performing isotonic shoulder horizontal abduction.

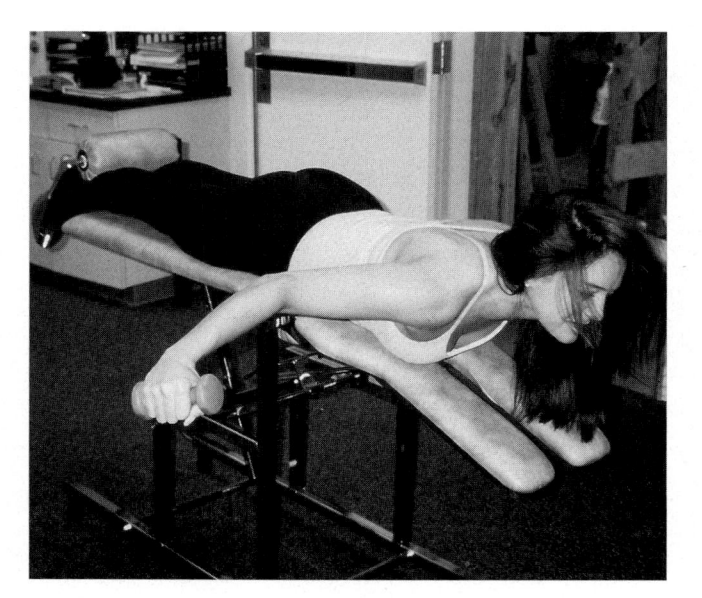

Figure 18-47. Prone dumbbell flies performed on a hinged bench to allow for a greater range of motion of the thoracic and cervical spine.

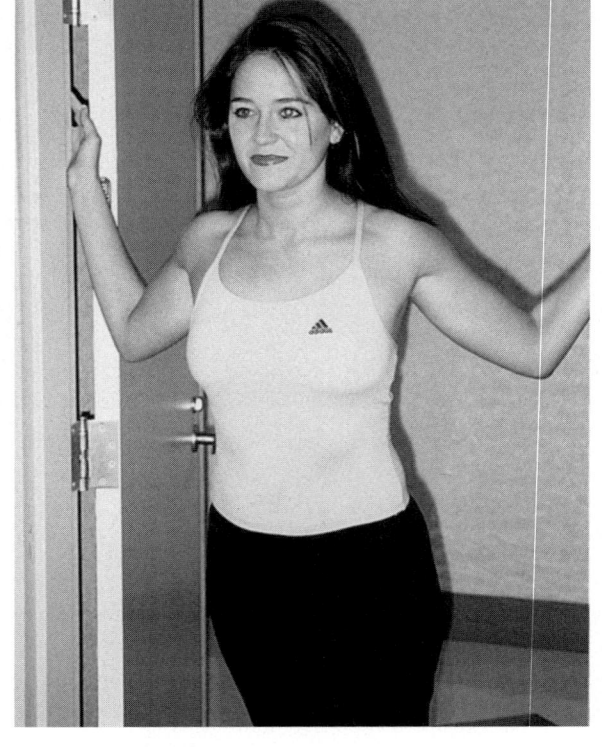

Figure 18-48. Door stretch for the pectoralis muscle.

or stand on an unstable surface. The athlete performs stabilization, postural re-education, and strengthening exercises in similar fashion to those performed with a stable base of support. Figure 18-49A-C illustrates some examples of incorporating proprioceptive training into a cervical rehabilitation program.

Because of the high physical demands associated with athletics, the rehabilitation program should also include exercises that strengthen the upper extremities, improve core stability, and increase the cardiovascular endurance of the athlete.

Pathologic Rehabilitation Considerations

Cervical Spondylosis

Cervical spondylosis can develop due to many different conditions and can have a wide array of presentations. Depending on its severity and location, the athlete may have a compromise of the neurovascular system. Spondylosis can be a result of numerous factors including the following: a genetically small diameter of the intervertebral foramen or spinal canal, or large nerve root caused by tumors, hematoma, or cyst. Osteophytes can develop at the facet or uncovertebral joint as a result of excessive tensile forces and joint motion. Ligaments, such as the PLL or the ligamentum flavum, can become thickened and calcified as a result of excessive traction forces or trauma. The clinician should be aware of the anatomic structure that is causing encroachment on the neurovascular system

and whether the athlete has any genetically, predisposing factors that possibly attributed to this condition.

Treatment of this athlete will consist of restoring the mobility in the hypomobile vertebral segments that occur as a result of spurring and calcifications through active and passive movements. Frequently, the athlete will also display hypermobility in adjacent segments to compensate for the lack of mobility. The athlete needs to perform stabilization exercises (i.e., cervical isometrics, midline ROM exercises, and others) to control this excessive motion. The surrounding cervical soft tissue commonly displays signs of tightness and spasm caused by neuromuscular facilitation. Therefore, the sports rehabilitation specialist will need to perform soft tissue mobilization techniques to restore mobility and decrease spasms. If the athlete has any associated postural adaptations, such as a forward head, round-shoulder posture, the clinician should address this with flexibility (see Fig. 18-48), strengthening (Figs. 18-50 and 18-51), and postural exercises.

Facet Joint Lock

Facet joint impingement occurs as a result of the facet joint capsule or a meniscoid body becoming entrapped between a facet joint in the cervical spine. This can occur as a result of a rapid approximation of the joint surfaces, such as extension, side-bending, and rotation, or holding the head in an awkward position for an extended period, such as sleeping in an uncomfortable position. The athlete will present with the head in a side-bent and rotated position, with complaints of a "locked" neck and unilateral neck pain. Assessment will reveal pain and decreased motion into contralateral side-bending and rotation. Tenderness will be elicited on palpation of the affected facet joint, and muscle guarding will be detected in the surrounding musculature.

Because of the presence of pain and muscle guarding, the clinician may provide inhibition through modalities or soft tissue mobilization techniques, or both. The rehabilitation specialist can administer manual traction while simultaneously passively side-bending and rotating the athlete's head. This is initially performed in the pain-free direction and is gradually progressed into the restricted direction. The clinician can also provide manual resistance into ipsilateral cervical rotation throughout a full available ROM while also providing manual traction to help reduce muscle guarding and neuromodulate the athlete's pain (Fig. 18-52).

Cervical Sprain

A cervical sprain is a common injury because of the strenuous nature of athletics. This can be a result of a traumatic injury such as fall or tackle that causes excessive motion or tension in the cervical spine. A cervical sprain can cause injury to muscular and ligamentous structures. Therefore, the sports rehabilitation specialist should determine the status of the cervical ligaments through palpation and provocation tests (see Figs. 18-23 through 18-25).

Initially after the injury, the athlete may require modalities to help control pain and inflammation. The clinician will initiate passive and active ROM exercises and soft tissue mobilization to help neuromodulate the athlete's pain and facilitate soft tissue repair and regeneration. If the athlete does not have gross ligamentous instability, light stretches can be performed to help reduce muscle spasms. As soon as the athlete can tolerate it, he or she should begin performing isometric exercises, progressing to an isotonic program to increase the strength and stabilization of the cervical spine.

Thoracic Outlet Syndrome

Treatment of thoracic outlet syndrome, along with any other pathologic condition, is dependent on the clinician's findings during the examination. Compression of the

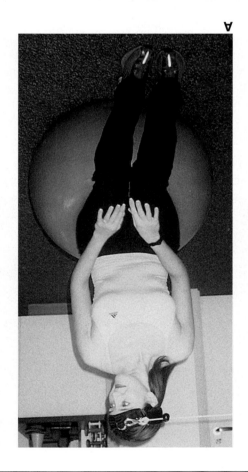
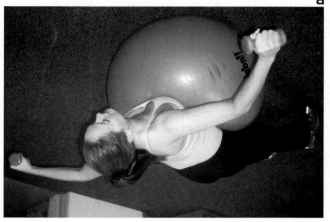
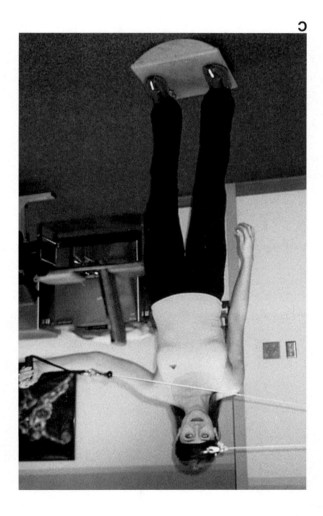

Figure 18-49. *A,* Cervical isotonic rotation sitting on Swiss ball. *B,* Prone horizontal abduction on Swiss ball. *C,* Cervical extension isometric with upper extremity movement standing on unstable surface.

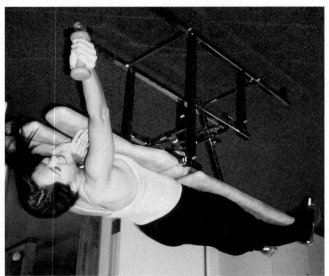

Figure 18-50. Prone horizontal abduction at 100° with full external rotation. Strengthening exercises for the lower trapezius and scapular retractors can help restore the normal positioning of the scapula.

neurovascular structures can result from altered kinematics related to posture or decreased mobility in the surrounding joints or soft tissue, or both. The athlete typically receives exercises that address postural concerns, through flexibility and strengthening exercises with special attention on the posterior rotator cuff, scapular retractors, and the cervical and thoracic extensors.

The athlete may display signs of decreased joint mobility in the cervical and thoracic regions because of an increase in cervical lordosis and thoracic kyphosis. Although

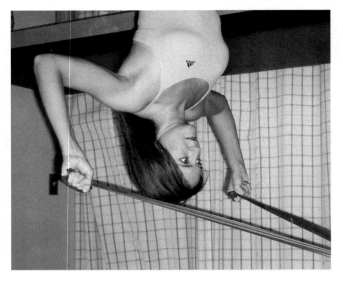

Figure 18-51. Bilateral scapular retraction with external rotation with exercise tubing.

thoracic function has not been addressed in this chapter, the clinician can perform soft tissue and joint mobilization techniques to correct both of these. Compression of the neurovascular structures can be caused by an elevated and hypomobile first rib. This can be caused by an overuse of the upper respiratory muscles, the sternocleidomastoid and scalenes, during inspiration. Normal mobility in this case will need to be restored through joint mobilizations to the first rib (see Fig. 18-34). If the athlete does not breathe from the diaphragm but rather from the upper thoracic region, the clinician should instruct the athlete in diaphragmatic breathing (Fig. 18-53). The clinician should

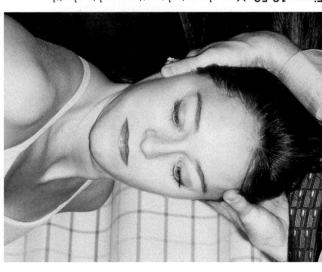

Figure 18-52. Manual cervical traction combined with isometric cervical rotation and passive range of motion can release an entrapped meniscoid and restore range of motion.

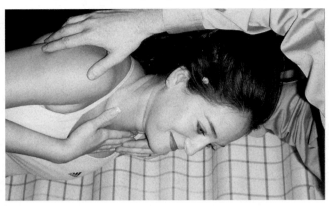

Figure 18-53. Diaphragmatic breathing technique. The clinician can assess the athlete's breathing pattern in this manner and instruct the athlete if needed. If treatment is warranted, the athlete is instructed to place one hand on the upper chest and one hand over the stomach and is given verbal and tactic cueing to breathe using the diaphragm.

also rule out any pathology involving the C3 vertebrae that could cause irritation of the phrenic nerve.[14] The athlete will also perform flexibility and strengthen exercises to restore normal mobility and to regain normal postural alignment.

SUMMARY

Principles

■ Because of the complexity of the cervical region, pain has many possibly origins.

■ The osseous and connective tissues in the cervical spine interact to allow for a balance between functional mobility and stability.

■ The facet joint planes, ligamentous tension, and muscle actions act together to provide the necessary arthrokinematic movements.

Evaluation

■ The clinician should be cautious not to assume the source of pain without performing a thorough evaluation to determine what tissue is in lesion.

■ The clinician does not have to perform all special tests, only those that are deemed clinically relevant.

■ In cases of traumatic injuries to the head and neck with resultant paresthesia or vertebral insufficiency, or both, upper cervical instability can be ruled out using radiologic and instability tests.

■ The clinician can determine whether hypermobilities or hypomobilities are present through mobility testing of the cervical region.

Rehabilitation

■ The clinician should base the treatment program on addressing the cause of pain and providing for a return to function.

■ Soft tissue mobilization techniques can be implemented to provide relaxation to allow for joint mobilizations and therapeutic exercises.

■ The clinician can perform joint mobilization techniques to neuromodulate pain and address hypomobilities.

■ The clinician can ensure that the athlete is given a customized rehabilitation program by altering the fundamental exercises through the use of isometrics, isotonics, adjusting the range of motion of the exercise, and adding a proprioceptive component.

REFERENCES

1. Adson, A.W., and Coffey, J.R. (1927): Cervical rib: A method of anterior approach for relief of symptoms by division of the scalenes anticus. Ann. Surg., 85:839-857.

2. Allen, E.V. (1929): Thromboangiitis obliterans: Methods of diagnosis of chronic occlusive arterial lesions distal to the wrist with illustrative cases. Am. J. Med. Sci., 178:237-244.

3. Bland, J.H. (1994): Disorders of the Cervical Spine. Philadelphia, WB Saunders.

4. Butler, D.S. (1991): Mobilisation of the Nervous System. Melbourne, Australia, Churchill Livingstone.

5. Calliet, R. (1996): Soft Tissue Pain and Disability. Philadelphia, FA Davis.

6. Cuetter, A.C., and Bartoszek, D.M. (1989): The thoracic outlet syndrome: Controversies, overdiagnosis, overtreatment and recommendations for management. Muscle Nerve, 12:410-419.

7. Cyriax, J.C. (1982): Textbook of Orthopaedic Medicine, Vol 1: Diagnosis of Soft Tissue Lesions, 8th ed. London, Bailliere Tindall.

8. Elvey, R.L. (1994): The investigation of arm pain. In: Boyling, J.D., and Palastanga, N. (eds.), Grieve's Modern Manual Therapy: The Vertebral Column. Edinburgh, UK, Churchill Livingstone.

9. Evans, R.C. (1994): Illustrated Essentials in Orthopedic Physical Assessment. St. Louis, MO, Mosby-Year Book.

10. Gower, W.E., and Pedrini, V. (1969): Age-related variations in protein polysaccharides from human nucleus pulposus, annulus fibrosus and costal cartilage. J. Bone Joint Surg., 51A:1154-1162.

11. Greenberg, A.D. (1968): Atlanto-axial dislocations. Brain, 91:655-684.

12. Hislop, H.J., and Montgomery, J. (2002): Daniels and Worthington's Muscle Testing: Techniques of Manual Examination, 7th ed. Philadelphia, WB Saunders.

13. Hoppenfeld, S. (1976): Physical Examination of the Spine and Extremities. New York, Appleton-Century-Crofts.

14. Institute, T.O.G. (1998): Cervical Biomechanics: Residency Course. In: Systems Course 680.

15. Kaltenborn, F.M. (1980): Mobilization of the Extremity Joints: Examination and Basic Treatment Techniques. Oslo, Norway, Olaf Norlis Bokhandel.

16. Kapandji, I.A. (1974): The Physiology of Joints, Vol 3: The Trunk and the Vertebral Column. New York, Churchill Livingstone.

17. Kendall, F.P., and McCreary, E.K. (1993): Muscles Testing and Function, 4th ed. Baltimore, MD, Lippincott Williams & Wilkins.

18. Magee, D.J. (1997): Orthopedic Physical Assessment, 3rd ed. Philadelphia, WB Saunders.

19. Mednel, T., Wink, C.S., and Zimny, M.L. (1992): Neural elements in human cervical intervertebral discs. Spine, 17:132-135.

20. Panjabi, M.M., and White, A.A. (1978): Clinical Biomechanics of the Spine. Philadelphia, JB Lippincott.

21. Pettman, E. (1994): Stress tests of the craniovertebral joints. In: Boyling, J.D., and Palastange, N. (eds.), Grieve's Modern Manual Therapy: The Vertebral Column. Edinburgh, UK, Churchill Livingstone.

22. Roos, D.B. (1976): Congenital anomalies associated with thoracic outlet syndrome. J. Surg., 132:771-778.

23. Roos, D.B., and Wilbourn, A.J. (1990): The thoracic outlet syndrome is underrated. Arch. Neurol., 47:327-328.

24. Spurling, R.G., and Scoville, W.B. (1944): Lateral rupture of the cervical intervertebral disc. Surg. Gynecol. Obstet., 78:350-358.

25. Stanton, P.E., Wo, N.M., Haley, T., et al. (1988): Thoracic outlet syndrome: A comprehensive evaluation. Am. Surg., 54:129-133.

26. Travell, J.G., and Simons, D.G. (1983): Myofascial Pain and Dysfunction: The Trigger Point Manual. Baltimore, Williams & Wilkins.

27. Turek, S. (1967): Orthopaedics: Principles and Their Applications. Philadelphia, WB Saunders.

28. Williams, P.L., and Warwick, R. (1983): Gray's Anatomy. 36th British ed. Baltimore, MD, Williams & Wilkins.

29. Yoo, J.U., Zou, D., Edwards, W.T., et al. (1992): Effect of cervical spine motion on the neuroforaminal dimensions of human cervical spine. Spine, 17:1131-1136.

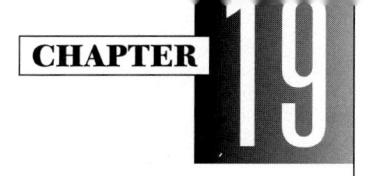

CHAPTER 19

SHOULDER REHABILITATION

Kevin E. Wilk, P.T.
Gary L. Harrelson, Ed.D., ATC
Christopher Arrigo, M.S., P.T., ATC

CHAPTER OBJECTIVES

At the end of this chapter the reader will be able to:

- Incorporate biomechanical principles of the shoulder as they relate to the prevention and postinjury or postsurgical rehabilitation for specific injuries.
- Associate anatomical structures of the shoulder to particular injuries based on the structures function during the pitching act.
- Explain the role of the rotator cuff in shoulder arthrokinematics and injury prevention.
- Develop a rehabilitation program for specific shoulder pathologic conditions that take into account the biomechanical function and healing parameters for the anatomical structures involved.
- Progress an athlete through phases of shoulder rehabilitation based on specific criteria for advancement.
- Incorporate rehabilitation limitations and concerns for specific postinjury and postsurgical shoulder pathologic conditions.

Most athletic shoulder injuries are due to one of two mechanisms: (1) repetitive overhead activity (microtrauma) or (2) a significant force (macrotrauma) to the shoulder complex. The violent act of throwing and other similar overhead movements result in the repeated application of high stresses to both the shoulder and elbow. Most of these injuries can be classified as microtraumatic and result from repetitive overuse mechanisms. Tullos and King[181] reported that at least 50% of all baseball players experience sufficient shoulder or elbow joint symptoms to keep them from throwing for varying periods of time during their careers. The synchronous kinematics of throwing can be influenced by a number of factors including glenohumeral and scapulothoracic motions, connective tissue flexibility, osseous structure, and dynamic muscle balance and symmetry. The glenohumeral joint complex is also susceptible to traumatic injuries such as dislocations, subluxations, acromioclavicular joint sprains, soft tissue injuries, and other types of injuries that commonly occur during collision and contact sports. The shoulder region is further predisposed to athletic injury because the tremendous mobility afforded by the joint is the result of inherently poor glenohumeral stability. In this chapter we will discuss the anatomy, biomechanics, common injuries and rehabilitation programs specific to the shoulder joint complex.

ANATOMY AND BIOMECHANICS

The shoulder complex is composed of three synovial joints and one physiologic articulation. The sternoclavicular, acromioclavicular, and glenohumeral components are true joints, whereas the physiologic articulation is usually referred to as the scapulothoracic joint. These four articulations, along with the ligaments (Fig. 19-1), rotator cuff complex, and the primary mover musculature of the upper quarter, work in unison to produce and control the various movements of the shoulder complex. Dysfunction in any one of these interdependent structures can result in limited performance of the entire shoulder complex.

Sternoclavicular Joint

Functionally, the sternoclavicular joint is the only bony articulation connecting the shoulder complex to the thorax. It is a modified saddle joint with a joint capsule, three major ligaments, and an intra-articular disc. The costoclavicular ligament is the primary stabilizer of the joint. It stabilizes the clavicle against the pull of the sternocleidomastoid muscle and controls motion about the joint that produces elevation-depression and protraction-retraction.[143] The costoclavicular ligament also functions to check elevation of the clavicle.[43] The sternoclavicular ligament stabilizes the joint anteriorly and posteriorly by controlling anterior and posterior movements of the clavicular head on the sternum. The proximal end of the clavicle is separated

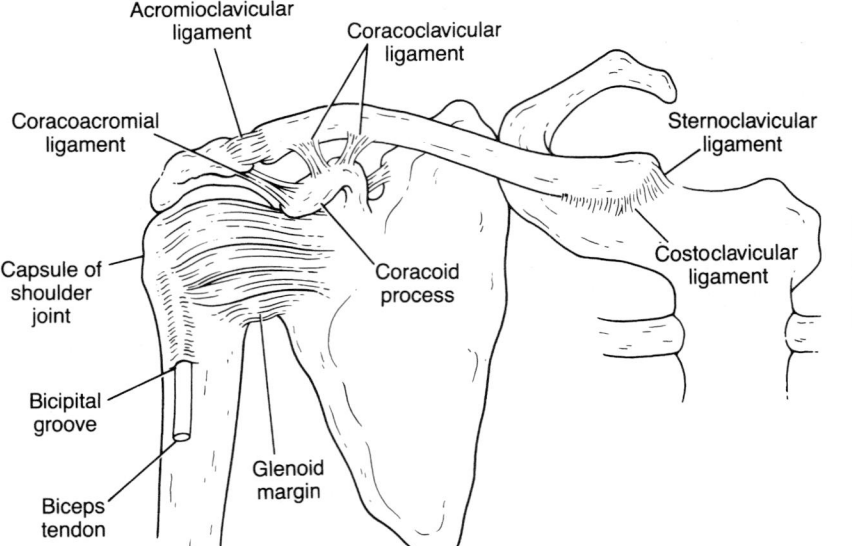

Figure 19-1. Ligamentous structures of the shoulder girdle. (From O'Donoghue, D.H. [1984]: Treatment of Injuries to Athletes, 4th ed. Philadelphia, W.B. Saunders, p. 119.)

from the sternal manubrium by an intra-articular disc or meniscus. This joint disc helps to absorb centrally directed forces that are transmitted along the clavicle and improves the incongruence of the articular surfaces, thus decreasing the tendency of the clavicle to dislocate medially on the manubrium.[132]

Acromioclavicular Joint

The acromioclavicular joint is a plane joint that consists of two major ligament complexes and an intra-articular meniscus. The two primary functions of the acromioclavicular joint are (1) to maintain the appropriate clavicle-scapula relationship during the early stages of upper limb elevation and (2) to allow the scapula additional range of rotation on the thorax in the later stages of limb elevation.[143]

The integrity of the articulation between the acromion and the distal clavicle is maintained by the surrounding ligaments rather than by the bony configuration of the joint. The coracoclavicular ligaments are the primary acromioclavicular joint stabilizers. The ligaments consist of a lateral portion, the trapezoid ligament, and a medial portion, the conoid ligament. It is these ligaments that are responsible for controlling the longitudinal rotation of the clavicle necessary for full unrestricted upper extremity elevation. The joint capsule is reinforced by the anterior, inferior, posterior, and superior acromioclavicular ligaments. The fibers of the deltoid and upper trapezius muscles, which attach to the superior aspect of the clavicle and acromion process, function to reinforce the acromioclavicular ligaments and further stabilize the joint.

A fall onto an outstretched arm tends to translate the scapula medially, and the small acromioclavicular joint alone cannot adequately control scapular motion, which frequently results in joint dislocation. As the scapula and its coracoid process attempt to move medially, the trapezoid ligament tightens, shifting the force to the clavicle and, ultimately, to the strong sternoclavicular joint.[143] Therefore, anterior-posterior stability of the acromioclavicular joint is maintained by the joint capsule whereas vertical stability is provided by the coracoclavicular ligaments.

Glenohumeral Joint

The glenohumeral joint is the most mobile and the least stable of all the joints in the human body.[203] It is also the most commonly dislocated major joint in the human body.[46,111] Even though the glenohumeral joint exhibits significant physiologic motion, only a few millimeters of humeral head displacement occur during any of these movements in normal individuals.[4,83,84,95,156,157,186] Conversely, on clinical examination, Matsen[128] demonstrated excessive passive displacement of 10 mm inferiorly and 8 mm anteriorly in normal asymptomatic shoulders. Therefore, stabilization of the humeral head within the glenoid is accomplished via the combined efforts of the static and dynamic glenohumeral stabilizers. These two categories of joint stabilizers can be classified into passive and active stabilizing mechanisms (Table 19-1).

The Static Stabilizers: Bony Geometry

The bony geometry of the glenohumeral joint sacrifices osseous stability to facilitate excessive joint mobility. The articular surface of the glenoid is pear-shaped with the inferior half being 20% larger than the superior half.[150] Additionally, the articular surface of the glenoid is much smaller than the articular surface of the humeral head, which is approximately three to four times that of the glenoid.[175] At any given time during normal motion, only

Table 19-1

The Passive and Active Mechanisms for Glenohumeral Joint Stability

Passive Mechanisms	Active Mechanisms
Bony	Joint compression
Glenoid labrum	Dynamic ligament
Intra-articular pressure	Tension
Joint cohesion	Neuromuscular control
Glenohumeral capsule	Scapulothoracic joint
Glenohumeral ligaments	

25% to 30% of the humeral head is actually in contact with the glenoid.[33,50,176] This lack of articular contact contributes to the inherent instability of the glenohumeral joint.[49]

The glenoid faces superiorly, anteriorly, and laterally. This superior tilt of the inferior glenoid limits inferior translation of the humeral head on the glenoid.[20] The glenoid articular surface is within 10° of being perpendicular to the blade of the scapula; thus, the glenoid fossa is retroverted approximately 6°.[167] Excessive retroversion of the glenoid is considered a primary etiology predisposing an individual to posterior glenohumeral instability and increased glenoid anteversion is found in individuals suffering from recurrent anterior dislocations.[39,167]

The areas of contact between the articular surfaces of the humeral head and the glenoid vary based on arm position with the greatest amount of articular contact occurring in mid-elevation between 60° and 120°.[175] With increasing arm elevation, contact points on the humeral head move from inferior to posterosuperior while the glenoid contact shifts from a central location posteriorly.

At the extremes of normal motion the glenohumeral joint does not function in a strict ball-and-socket fashion. In these extremes, rotation is coupled with humeral head translation on the glenoid.[81,94,156] Normally, external rotation produces posterior translation and vice versa, whereas subjects with known anterior instability demonstrate anterior humeral head translation in extreme external rotation.[34,81,95]

Bony defects on either the humeral head or the glenoid are commonly associated with glenohumeral instability.[169] With recurrent anterior instability an osseous defect is commonly noted on the posterolateral portion of the humeral head (Hill-Sachs lesion).[90] In contrast, an anteromedial lesion is often noted with recurrent posterior instability (reverse Hill-Sachs lesion). Bony defects of the anterior or posterior glenoid rim may also occur with recurrent glenohumeral instability.[152,161,164] Both of these lesions represent impaction fractures, occurring as the humeral head subluxates and then reduces repetitively over the glenoid rim.

The Glenoid Labrum

The glenoid labrum is a fibrous rim that serves to slightly deepen the glenoid fossa and allows for the attachment of the glenohumeral ligaments on the glenoid. The superior attachment of the labrum is loose and approximates the mobility of the meniscus within the knee joint, whereas the inferior attachment is firm and unyielding.[145] The labrum functions to deepen the glenoid anywhere from 2.5 to 5 mm.[94] The labrum may function in tandem with joint compression forces to stabilize the joint in the mid-range of glenohumeral motion where the ligamentous structures are lax.[123,155] The labrum also serves as a buttress that assists in controlling glenohumeral translation, similar to a chock-block, which would prevent a wheel from rolling downhill. Finally, Bowen and co-workers[34] noted that the labrum also contributes to glenohumeral joint stability by increasing the surface area and acting as a load-bearing structure for the humeral head. Also, the long head of the biceps brachii muscle inserts into the superior portion of the labrum.

Shoulder Capsule and Ligaments

The shoulder joint capsule is large, loose and redundant, which also allows for the large range of glenohumeral motion naturally available at the glenohumeral joint. The capsule is composed of multilayer collagen fiber bundles of differing strengths and orientation. The anteroinferior capsule is the thickest and strongest portion of the joint capsule.[77] The collagen fibers within this portion of the joint capsule have two distinct orientations, radial fibers that are linked to each other by circular fibers. In this manner, rotational forces create tension within the fibers producing compression of the joint surfaces while centering the articular surfaces.[77]

The glenohumeral joint capsule is reinforced with district capsular ligaments that contribute greatly to joint stability. There is a wide variation in the size, strength, and orientation of these capsular ligaments, which typically function when the joint is placed in extremes of motion to protect against instability.[62,139,146]

The anterior glenohumeral joint capsule consists of three distinct ligaments: the superior glenohumeral ligament, the middle glenohumeral ligament, and the inferior glenohumeral ligament complex.[62,146,182] The superior glenohumeral ligament arises from the anterosuperior labrum anterior to the biceps tendon and inserts superior into the lesser tuberosity of the humerus. The middle glenohumeral ligament originates adjacent to the superior glenohumeral ligament and extends laterally to attach on the lesser tuberosity with the subscapularis tendon. The inferior glenohumeral ligament complex is composed of three functional portions: an anterior band, a posterior band, and an axillary pouch. There is tremendous variation in these structures, with the middle glenohumeral ligament exhibiting the greatest degree of variation.[62,66] Posteriorly, the capsule is the thinnest and exhibits no distinct capsular ligaments except for the posterior band of the inferior glenohumeral ligament complex.

The anterior glenohumeral ligaments function as primary restrains to anterior translation of the humerus on the glenoid.[148,171] The superior and middle glenohumeral ligaments are the primary restraints to anterior translation with the arm completely abducted.[35] The middle glenohumeral ligament plays a significant role in limiting translation of the humeral head in the mid-range of shoulder abduction.[36,66,149] The inferior glenohumeral ligament complex, particularly the anterior band, is responsible for preventing translation of the humeral head with the arm abducted to 90° and beyond.[147,148,170]

The constraints to posterior translation are also based on arm position. The posteroinferior portion of the inferior glenohumeral ligament complex is the primary passive stabilizer against posterior instability with the arm in 90° of abduction. At less than 90° of abduction, the posterior capsule is the primary restraint against posterior forces.

During the combined motion of abduction and external rotation, the anterior band of the inferior glenohumeral ligament complex fans out and surrounds the anteroinferior aspect of the humeral head like a hammock restraining anterior displacement while the posterior band provides inferior support.[145] In abduction and internal rotation the anterior band of the inferior glenohumeral ligament complex moves inferiorly to resist inferior displacement and the posterior band shifts posterosuperiorly to prevent posterior translation.[145] Additionally, when the arm is positioned in 90° of abduction and 30° extension, the anterior band of the inferior glenohumeral ligament complex becomes the primary stabilizer to both anterior and posterior forces. Finally, as a general rule, the superior capsular structures play significant roles in glenohumeral joint stability when the arm is adducted whereas the inferior structures are the primary providers of joint stability between 90° of abduction and full elevation.

The forces required to dislocate the shoulder change with age. Less force is required in individuals younger than 20 and older than 40 years of age.[17,18,110] Bankart described the "essential lesion" responsible for shoulder instability as a detached labrum and capsule from the glenoid (referred to subsequently as a *Bankart lesion*). It is interesting to note that the Bankart lesion is not one specific anatomic defect, but rather a wide spectrum of pathologic conditions related to detachment of the capsulolabral complex of the glenohumeral joint. Baker and associates[16] identified three types of Bankart lesions present as a result of initial acute anterior glenohumeral dislocations (Box 19-1). It is also interesting to note that the degree of instability present during examination under anesthesia varies depending on the grade of the lesion present (Box 19-1).[16]

Box 19-1

Three Types of Bankart Lesions

Grade	Definition	Instability Present Under Anesthesia
I	Capsular tears without labral lesions	Stable
II	Capsular tears with partial labral detachments	Mildly unstable
III	Complete capsular-labral detachments	Grossly unstable

From Baker, C.L., Uribe, J.W., and Whitman, C. (1990): Arthroscopic evaluation of acute initial anterior shoulder dislocations. Am. J. Sports Med., 18:25-28.

Approximately 85% of patients with traumatic anterior glenohumeral dislocations exhibit detachment of the glenoid labrum from the anterior glenoid rim whereas the remaining individuals show interstitial stretch or rupture of the capsule without loosening or detachment of the labrum.[131]

Intra-Articular Pressure and Joint Cohesion

Normally, the capsule of the glenohumeral joint is sealed airtight and contains very little (less than 1 ml) fluid.[131] This limited fluid volume contributes to joint stability in a manner similar to syringe-type suction, which serves to hold the articular surfaces together with viscous and intermolecular forces.[131] The normal intra-articular pressure of the glenohumeral joint is negative, which creates a relative vacuum that also helps resist translation.[41,75,119] This is a relatively small force, only exerting approximately 20 to 30 pounds of stabilizing pressure, but when these properties are disrupted via a capsular puncture or tear, subluxation tends to occur.[75,119] In the unstable shoulder this vacuum effect of viscous and intermolecular forces is lost because the labrum is no longer able to function as a seal or gasket.[79]

The Dynamic Stabilizers: Neuromuscular Control

The primary active stabilizers of the glenohumeral joint and the secondary stabilizers are listed in Box 19-2. The most important function the primary glenohumeral stabilizers provide is the production of a combined muscular contraction that enhances humeral head stability during active arm movements. These muscles act together in an agonist/antagonist relationship to both effect movement of the arm and at the same time stabilizing the glenohumeral joint. The combined effect of the rotator cuff musculature is a synergistic action that creates humeral

Box 19-2

Dynamic Stabilizers of the Shoulder

Primary Stabilizers	Secondary Stabilizers
Rotator cuff muscles (supraspinatus, infraspinatus, teres minor, subscapularis)	Teres major
Deltoid	Latissimi dorsi
Long head of the biceps brachii	Pectoralis major

head compression within the glenoid and counterbalances the shearing forces generated by the deltoid.[153,205]

The second method of active glenohumeral joint stability is provided through the blending of the rotator cuff tendons into the shoulder capsule, producing tension with the capsular ligaments. This tension serves to actively tighten the glenohumeral ligamentous capsule, which accentuates centering of the humeral head within the glenoid fossa.

The third component that contributes to dynamic shoulder stability is *neuromuscular control*.[198,199] This refers to the continuous interplay of afferent input and efferent output in an individual's awareness of joint position (proprioception) and his or her ability to produce a voluntary muscular contraction to stabilize the joint and/or alter joint position that can prevent excessive humeral head translation. The authors refer to the ability to control the shoulder joint during active motions as *reactive neuromuscular control*. We feel that this factor is more important to normal shoulder function than joint position or repositioning abilities.[199] Reactive neuromuscular control is an individual's ability to integrate proprioceptive information and motor control to react to the information.

Scapulothoracic Joint

The scapulothoracic joint is not a true anatomic joint because it has none of the usual joint characteristics, such as a joint capsule. However, it is a free-floating physiologic joint without any ligamentous restraints, except where it pivots about the acromioclavicular joint.[29] According to Steindler[177] the primary force holding the scapula to the thorax is atmospheric pressure. The ultimate function of scapular motion is to orient the glenoid fossa for optimal contact with the maneuvering arm and to provide a stable base of support for the controlled rolling and gliding of the articular surface of the humeral head.[143] This relationship allows for optimal function of the upper extremity in space by continually adjusting the length-tension relationships of all vital musculature as the scapula constantly repositions itself on the thoracic wall. The muscles of the scapulothoracic joint play a significant role in maintaining optimal scapular position and posture. Five muscles directly control the scapula. These include the trapezius (upper,

middle, and lower), the rhomboids, the levator scapulae, the serratus anterior, and to a lesser extent, the pectoralis minor. These muscles act in a synchronous fashion, providing both mobility and stability to the scapulothoracic joint.

Coracoacromial Arch

The coracoacromial arch, or subacromial space, has also been considered a physiologic joint by some authors.[115] It provides protection against direct trauma to the subacromial structures and prevents the humeral head from dislocating superiorly. It is bordered by the acromion process and acromioclavicular joint superiorly, the coracoid process anteromedially, and the rotator cuff and greater tuberosity of the humeral head inferiorly. The coracoacromial ligament, which serves as a "roof" over the greater tubercle of the humerus, rotator cuff tendons, portions of the biceps tendon, and subdeltoid bursa, further decreases the available space with the arch. The space between the humeral head on the inferior aspect of the acromion depends on arm position and varies from approximately 30 ± 4.9 mm (when arm is at 0° of abduction) and 6 ± 2.4 mm (when arm is at 90° of abduction).[34] Additionally, this space can be decreased in the presence of inflamed or swollen soft tissues. Soft tissue structures, such as the supraspinatus and infraspinatus tendons, lying between the two unyielding joint borders, are at risk for impingement or compressive injuries in the presence of abnormal glenohumeral joint mechanics or trauma.

Rotator Cuff

The supraspinatus, infraspinatus, teres minor, and subscapularis muscles comprise the rotator cuff (Fig. 19-2). Collectively, each tendon blends with and reinforces the glenohumeral capsule, and all contribute significantly to the dynamic stability of the glenohumeral joint.[141] The rotator cuff muscles could be considered the fine tuners of the glenohumeral joint and shoulder girdle, whereas the latissimus dorsi, teres major, deltoid, and pectoralis muscles are the prime movers.[92] All the rotator cuff muscles contribute in some degree to glenohumeral abduction, with the supraspinatus and deltoid muscles functioning as the primary abductors. The rotator cuff muscles also function to compress the glenohumeral joint and act to reduce or control vertical shear imparted onto the humeral head.[58,162] The infraspinatus is considered the next most active rotator cuff muscle, after the supraspinatus.[97,104,106] Selective nerve blocks have shown that the supraspinatus and infraspinatus muscles are responsible for 90% of the external rotation strength of the shoulder.[19] The teres minor also contributes to external rotation of the glenohumeral joint. The subscapularis is the primary internal rotator, with abduction activity peaking around 90°.[19]

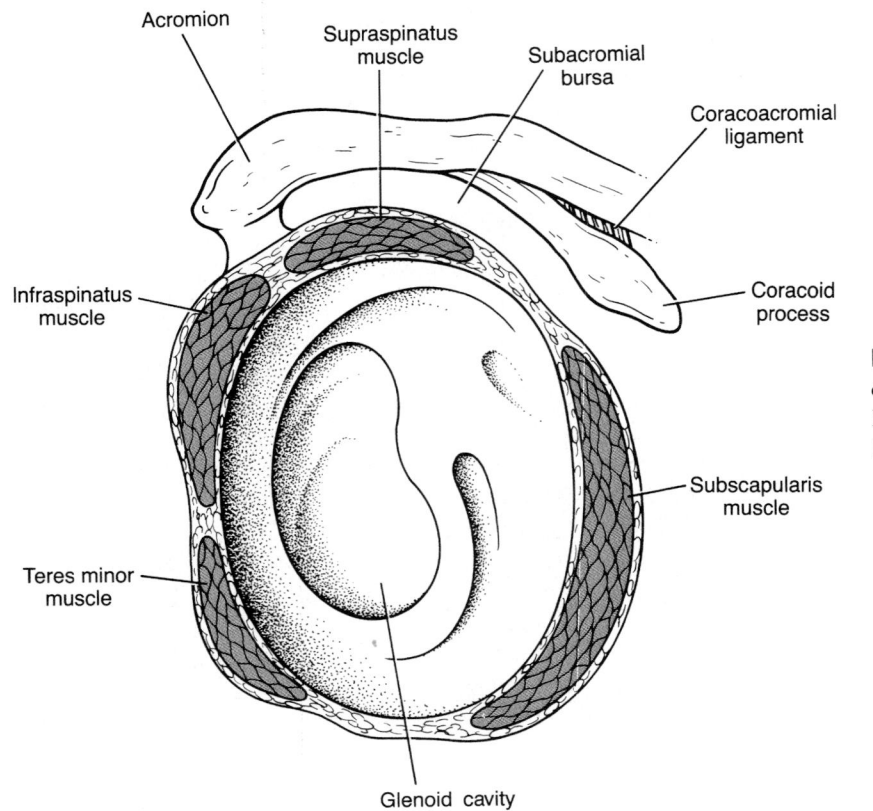

Acromion   Supraspinatus   Subacromial
                 muscle   bursa

                                              Coracoacromial
                                              ligament

Infraspinatus   Coracoid
muscle   process

                                                      Subscapularis
                                                      muscle

Teres minor
muscle

Glenoid cavity

Figure 19-2. Anatomic view of the glenoid cavity with its surrounding structures. (From Hill, J.A. [1988]: Rotator cuff injuries. Sports Med. Update, 3:5.)

SHOULDER ELEVATION

Most glenohumeral motion occurs around the plane of the scapula. This plane of motion is approximately 30° to 45° anterior to the frontal plane.[156] Codman[51] first reported that abduction of the humerus to 180° overhead requires that the clavicle, scapula, and humerus move through essentially their full range of motion in a specific pattern of interaction. When internally rotated, the humerus can abduct on the scapula to approximately 90° before the greater tubercle strikes up against the acromion. If the humerus is fully rotated externally, however, the greater tubercle and accompanying rotator cuff tendons clear the acromion, coracoacromial ligament, and superior edge of the glenoid fossa,[114,124,166] thereby allowing another 30° of abduction (Fig. 19-3). Thus, the glenohumeral joint contributes 90° to 120° of shoulder abduction, depending on the rotational position of the humeral head.[43,100,124] The remaining 60° is supplied by scapular elevation. This combined motion between the scapula and the humerus is known as scapulohumeral rhythm. During the first 30° of glenohumeral abduction, the contribution of scapular elevation is negligible and is not coordinated with the movement of the humerus.[100,124] This is referred to as the setting phase, during which the scapula is seeking a position of stability on the thoracic wall in relationship to the humerus.[100] The purpose of scapular

rotation is twofold[143]: (1) to achieve a ratio of motion for maintaining the glenoid fossa in an optimal position to receive the head of the humerus, thus increasing the range of motion and (2) to ensure that the accompanying motion of the scapula permits muscles acting on the humerus to maintain a satisfactory length-tension relationship. After the initial 30° of humeral elevation, scapular motion becomes better coordinated. Toward the end range of glenohumeral elevation, however, the scapula contributes more motion and the humerus less.[99,114] In gross terms, it is generally agreed that every 1° of scapular motion is accompanied by 2° of humeral elevation. Scapulohumeral rhythm therefore is considered to be a ratio of 1:2.[100] If scapular movement is prevented, only 120° of passive abduction and 90° of active motion are possible.[124]

Clavicular motion at both the acromioclavicular and sternoclavicular joints is essential for full shoulder elevation. Inman and Saunders[99] have demonstrated that for full abduction of the arm to occur, the clavicle must rotate 50° posteriorly. Surgical pinning of the clavicle to the coracoid process, which has been performed in some cases in which a complete tear of the coracoclavicular ligament is present, dramatically limits shoulder abduction.

Glenohumeral elevation in abduction is the primary function of the deltoid and supraspinatus muscles. The contribution of the deltoid and supraspinatus to shoulder abduction has been extensively investigated. It was

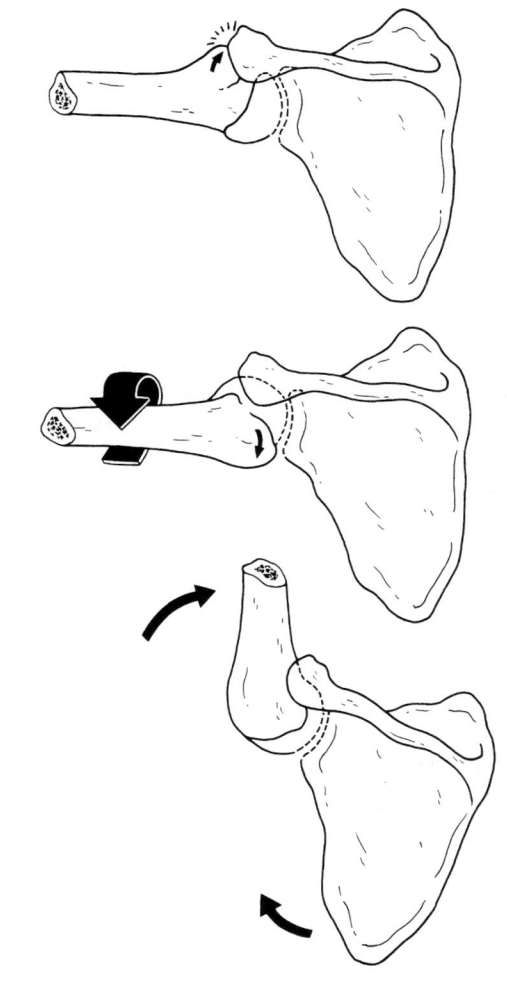

Figure 19-3. Clearing of the greater tuberosity from under the acromion to gain full abduction at the glenohumeral joint. (From Gould, J.A. [1990]: Orthopaedic and Sports Physical Therapy, 2nd ed. St. Louis, C.V. Mosby, p. 488.)

commonly assumed that abduction of the arm is initiated by the supraspinatus and is continued by the deltoid.[92] Studies in which selective nerve blocks were used to deactivate the deltoid and supraspinatus muscles have shown that complete abduction still occurs, although with a 50% loss in power, when one or the other muscle is deactivated.[52,53] Simultaneous nerve blocks of both these muscles result in the inability to raise the arm.[52] Thus, each muscle can elevate the arm independently, but there is a resultant loss of approximately 50% of the normal power generated in abduction.[22]

Additionally, the other three rotator cuff muscles—the teres minor, the infraspinatus, and the subscapularis—are active to some degree throughout the full abduction range of motion.[100] These three rotator cuff muscles work as a functional unit to compress the humeral head to counteract the superior shear of the deltoid during arm elevation.[100,114]

THROWING MECHANISM

Throwing is an integral part of many sports, but different techniques are required, depending on the endeavor. High-speed motion analysis has allowed investigators to slow down the pitching act and examine the kinetics and kinematics involved (Fig. 19-4). The throwing act, as performed by the baseball pitcher, is a series of complex and synchronized movements involving both the upper and the lower extremities. As described by several authors,[70,132] the throwing mechanism can be divided into five phases (Fig. 19-5): (1) wind-up, (2) cocking, (3) acceleration, (4) release and deceleration, and (5) follow-through. Injuries to the shoulder joint can occur during the cocking, acceleration, or deceleration phases. The overhead throw is the fastest human movement and takes approximately 0.5 second to complete (from wind-up to ball release).

Wind-Up

The purpose of the wind-up is to put the athlete in an advantageous starting position from which to throw. In addition, it can serve as a distraction to the hitter. The wind-up is a relatively slow maneuver that prepares the pitcher for correct body posture and balance while leading the body into the cocking phase (Fig. 19-5). It can last from 0.5 to 1.0 second[185] and is characterized by a shifting of the shoulder away from the direction of the pitch, with the opposite leg being cocked quite high and the baseball being removed from the glove.[132] It is also during this phase that the head of the humerus can wear and roughen from leverage on the posterior glenoid labrum.

Cocking

The cocking phase is most often divided into early and late cocking phases. During the cocking phase (Fig. 19-5), the shoulder is abducted to approximately 90°, externally rotated 90° or more, and horizontally abducted to approximately 30°.[70,132] This is primarily accomplished by the deltoid and stabilized by the rotator cuff muscles that pull the humeral head into the glenohumeral joint.[37] The anterior, middle, and posterior deltoids reach peak electromyographic (EMG) activity in the early cocking phase when the arm is abducted to 90°.[154] During late cocking, the activity of the deltoids decreases as the rotator cuff musculature becomes more dominant. Additionally, the pectoralis major, subscapularis, and latissimus dorsi act eccentrically to stabilize the humeral head during the late cocking phase. This position places the anterior joint capsule and internal rotators, which are used to accelerate the ball, in maximum tension. Also, the opposite leg is kicked forward and placed directly in front of the body. Kinetic energy begins to be transferred from the lower extremities

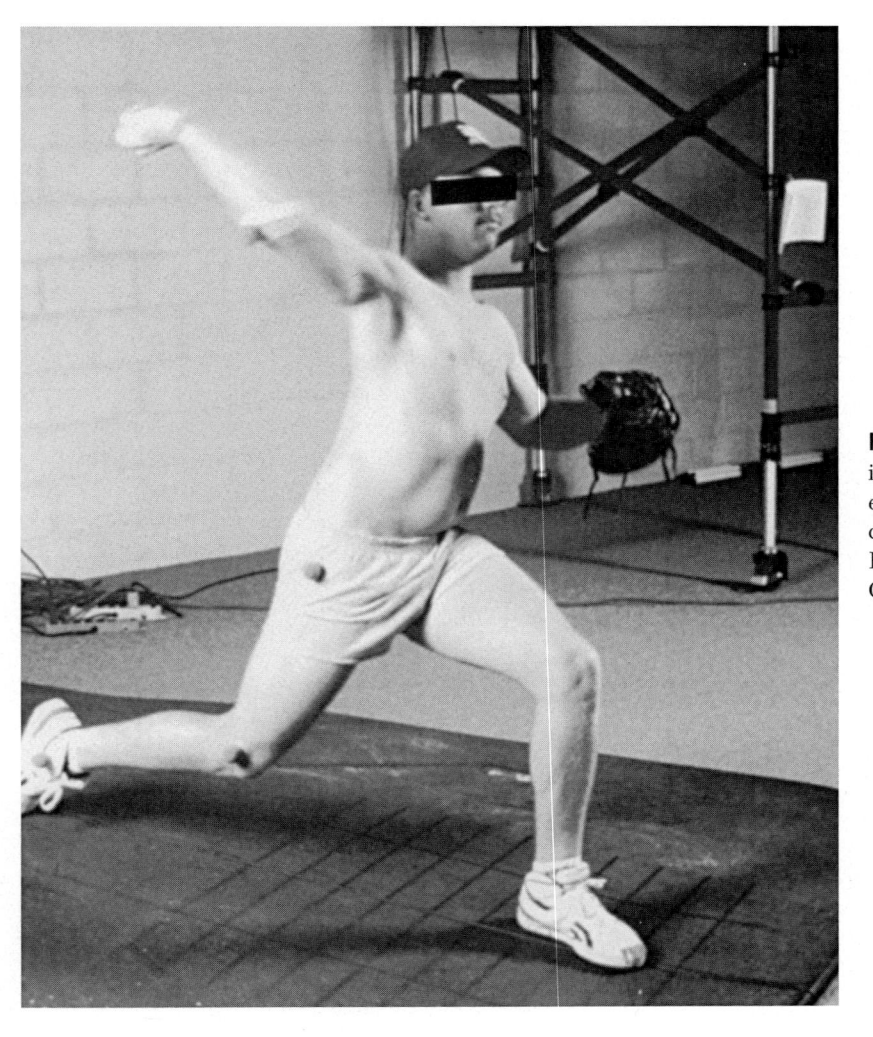

Figure 19-4. High-speed photography allows investigators to slow down the pitching act and examine the arthrokinematics involved. (Photo courtesy of Sports Medicine Update. Birmingham, AL. HealthSouth Rehabilitation Corporation.)

and trunk to the arm and hand in which the ball is held.[185] Because of the significant stresses placed on the anterior shoulder capsule, the capsule may "stretch out" with continuous throwing. If the anterior capsule is significantly stretched out, increased humeral head displacement during the late cocking phase can occur. This may present clinically as "internal impingement" and will be discussed in detail later. Furthermore, this extreme external rotation position (late cocking) may also lead to glenoid labrum lesions. This type of glenoid labrum lesion has been referred to as a *peel back lesion* and will also be discussed later.

Acceleration

The acceleration phase (Fig. 19-5) begins at the point of maximal external rotation and ends at ball release.[133] This phase lasts an average of 50 msec, approximately 2% of the duration of the pitching act.[70,151] Muscles that once were on a stretch in the cocking phase become the accelerators in a powerful concentric muscular contraction. The body is brought forward, with the arm following behind. The energy developed by the body's forward motion is transferred to the throwing arm to accelerate the humerus.[181] This energy is enhanced via contraction of the internal rotators (primarily the subscapularis) as the humerus is rotated internally from its previously externally rotated position, and the ball is accelerated to delivery speed.[132] During this phase, the maximum internal rotation angular velocity is approximately $7365 \pm 1503°$/sec.[70] During this phase there is also an anterior displacement force of approximately 50% of body weight. Rotatory torque at the shoulder can start at approximately 14,000 inch-pounds and builds up to approximately 27,000 inch-pounds of kinetic energy at ball release.[37]

During the acceleration phase, the pectoralis major and latissimus dorsi are the main muscles that actively generate velocity and arm speed.[63] The subscapularis muscle is active in steering the humeral head. At ball release, the throwing shoulder should be abducted about 90° to 100°, regardless of the type of pitch being thrown or the style of the thrower. The difference between an "overhead" and a "sidearm" baseball pitcher is not the degree of glenohumeral abduction, but rather the degree of lateral tilt at

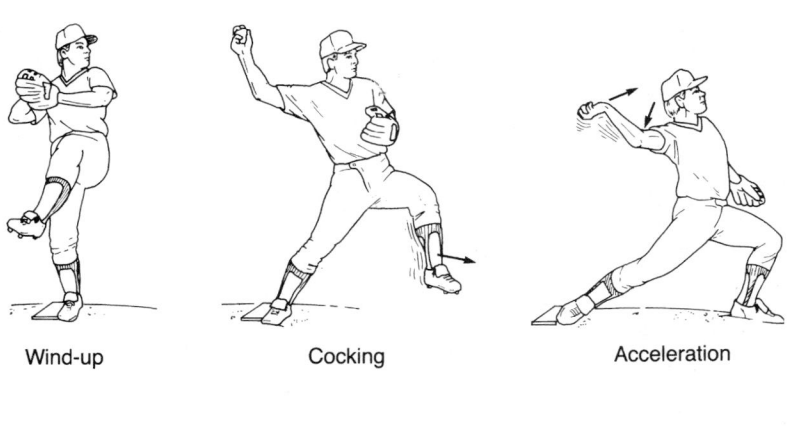

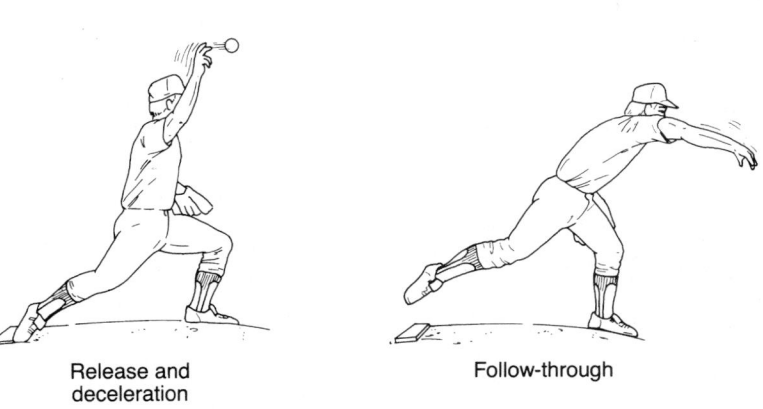

Wind-up   Cocking   Acceleration

Release and
deceleration   Follow-through

Figure 19-5. Dynamic phases of pitching. (From Walsh, D.A. [1989]: Shoulder evaluation of the throwing athlete. Sports Med. Update, 4:24.)

the trunk.[70] Because of the tremendous forces acting at the glenohumeral joint, numerous injuries can result during this phase of overhead throwing, such as instability, labral tears, overuse tendinitis, and tendon ruptures.[185]

Release and Deceleration

In the release and deceleration phases of throwing, the ball is released, and the shoulder and arm are decelerated (Fig. 19-5). Generally, deceleration forces are approximately twice as great as acceleration forces but act for a shorter period of time (approximately 40 msec).[132] Initially, in the deceleration phase, the humerus has a relatively high rate of internal rotation, and the elbow extends rapidly.[132] Great eccentric forces are applied to the posterior rotator cuff muscles to slow the internal rotation and horizontal adduction of the humerus and to stabilize the humeral head within the glenoid cavity. Jobe and colleagues[106,108] analyzed the throwing mechanism using electromyography and found that the muscles of the rotator cuff are extremely active during the deceleration phase. It has been reported that the posterior rotator cuff must resist as much as 200 pounds of distraction force that is attempting to pull the arm out of the glenohumeral joint in the direction the ball has been thrown.[28] Labral tears at the attachment of the long head of the biceps, subluxation of the long head of the biceps by tearing of the transverse

ligament, and various lesions of the rotator cuff, such as undersurface tearing or tensile overload, can be incurred during this phase of throwing.[185]

Follow-Through

During the follow-through phase (Fig. 19-5) the body moves forward with the arm, effectively reducing the distraction forces applied to the shoulder.[72] This results in relief of tension on the rotator cuff muscles.

Because of the repetitive action of throwing, the baseball pitcher's shoulder undergoes adaptive changes that should be recognized and distinguished from pathologic lesions. The throwing shoulder has significantly increased external rotation and decreased internal rotation compared with that of the nonthrowing side. This is considered a functional adaptation to throwing but may lead to specific pathologic conditions that will be discussed later. The various shoulder injuries that can occur in each phase of throwing are summarized in Box 19-3.

Glousman and associates[76] have compared the EMG activity of the shoulder girdle muscles in pitchers with isolated anterior glenohumeral instability and in normal subjects. In pitchers, the supraspinatus and serratus anterior exhibited increased activity throughout late cocking and acceleration, the infraspinatus muscle exhibited enhanced activity during early cocking and acceleration, and the

Box 19-3

Potential Shoulder Injuries Associated with Each Throwing Phase

Phase	Potential injuries
Wind-up	None that are common
Cocking	Anterior subluxation
	Internal impingement
	Glenoid labrum lesions
Acceleration	Shoulder instability
	Labral tears
	Overuse tendinitis
	Tendon ruptures
Release and deceleration	Labral tears at the attachment of the long head of the biceps
	Subluxation of the long head of the biceps by tearing of the transverse ligament
	Lesions to the rotator cuff, such as undersurface or tensile overload
Follow-through	Tear of the superior aspect of the glenoid labrum at the origin of the biceps tendon
	Tight posterior shoulder structures can cause abnormal glenohumeral kinematics by forcing the humeral head anteriorly and superiorly into the acromial arch during this phase

biceps brachii was noted to have an increase in activity during the acceleration phase. Additionally, the subscapularis, latissimus dorsi, and pectoralis major demonstrated less EMG activity in subjects with anterior instability during all phases of the throwing motion.

Wick and colleagues[188] noted numerous significant differences between throwing a baseball overhead and throwing a football. During the acceleration phase, the angular velocity for baseball throwing was 7365 ± 1503°/sec compared with 4586 ± 843°/sec for throwing a football. At ball release, the shoulder was externally rotated approximately 21° more for throwing a football. Also at ball release, shoulder abduction was calculated to be 99° during baseball throwing and 114° during football throwing. The duration of the football throw was also significantly longer (0.20 second) than a baseball throw (0.15 second).

OVERVIEW OF THE REHABILITATION PROGRAM

The shoulder rehabilitation program presented in this chapter is designed to restore shoulder range of motion and strength in a functional and progressive manner. The exercises may be implemented with specific limitations for certain motions, depending on the injury sustained or surgical procedure performed. Often, emphasis is placed on the rotator cuff musculature and the scapular stabilizers. Rehabilitation exercises that concentrate on the rotator cuff musculature are paramount after any shoulder injury. With shoulder rehabilitation the clinician should concentrate on increasing dynamic stability, particularly that of the rotator cuff, because of the relatively weak nature of the static restraints of the glenohumeral joint.

The entire upper kinematic chain should be evaluated when a shoulder rehabilitation program is designed in consideration of the importance of proximal stability for distal mobility. The synchronous interplay among each of the joints of the shoulder complex is vital to active, balanced joint stability and normal glenohumeral function. The scapular stabilizers (e.g., trapezius, latissimus dorsi, rhomboids, and serratus anterior) are often overlooked when shoulder injuries are addressed. The scapular stabilizers maintain the appropriate scapula-glenohumeral joint relationship, allowing for normal kinematics during functional activities. This is particularly true in the pitching motion in which these muscles play a large role during the deceleration phase of throwing.

Strengthening exercises for the shoulder musculature, especially the rotator cuff, have been critically analyzed by numerous investigators.[69] Jobe and Moynes[105] first examined the effect of specific exercises on the rotator cuff musculature. They reported that the supraspinatus can best be exercised apart from the other cuff muscles with the arm abducted to 90°, horizontally adducted to 30°, and fully internally rotated, which is referred to as the *empty can* position (Fig. 19-6). The infraspinatus and teres minor

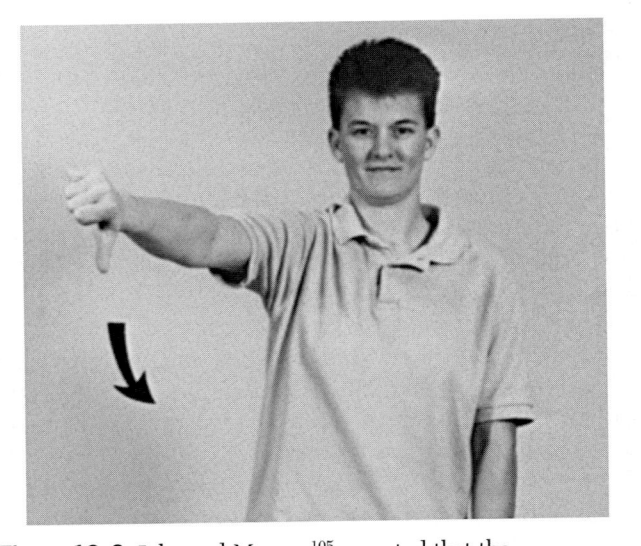

Figure 19-6. Jobe and Moynes[105] reported that the supraspinatus muscle is best exercised with the arm abducted to 90°, horizontally flexed to 30°, and internally rotated.

can be exercised in the side-lying position with the arm held close to the side and the elbow flexed to 90°. The subscapularis can be strengthened with the individual in the supine position, the affected arm held close to the side, and the elbow flexed to 90°.

Since the study of Jobe and Moynes,[105] Blackburn and co-workers[29] investigated rotator cuff activation, using intramuscular electromyography, while subjects performed specific rotator cuff exercises. Although Jobe and Moynes[105] reported that the supraspinatus is best isolated and exercised with the arm abducted to 90°, horizontally flexed 30°, and fully internally rotated (see Fig. 19-6), Blackburn and co-workers[29] noted that the supraspinatus is involved whenever the arm is elevated, whether the subject is standing or prone. Isolation of supraspinatus function appears to occur during pure abduction, with neutral rotation of the arm while standing. Also, Blackburn and co-workers[29] noted that a significant increase in supraspinatus function can be achieved in the prone position, with the arm in maximal external rotation and in 100° of horizontal abduction (Fig. 19-7). Recently, Malanga and associates[127] analyzed the EMG activity of the rotator cuff and deltoid muscles in the empty can and the prone positions advocated by Blackburn and co-workers.[29] The empty can position produced high levels of EMG activity of the supraspinatus (107% maximum voluntary isometric contraction), but the middle deltoid (104%) and anterior deltoid (96%) were also extremely active. Conversely, during prone horizontal abduction (at approximately 100°) with external rotation, the most active muscles were the middle deltoid (111%), the posterior deltoid (96%), and the supraspinatus (94%). The investigators concluded that neither position isolated the supraspinatus, but both positions could be used for exercising. In addition, Kelly and colleagues[112] have reported that the best test position to isolate the supraspinatus, with the least activation from the infraspinatus, is with the arm positioned at 90° of elevation in the scapular plane with 45° of humeral external rotation. This position is referred to as the *full can* position. We recommend this position for manual muscle testing of the supraspinatus (Fig. 19-8). Townsend and associates[179] studied seven glenohumeral muscles during 17 traditional shoulder exercises and reported that certain exercises were better for recruiting selected muscles. For instance, the best exercise noted in the study to recruit the teres minor muscle was side-lying external rotation followed by prone horizontal abduction with external rotation. Table 19-2 provides detailed information about specific exercises and muscular activity.

In a recent study performed at our center, Fleisig[69] reported the exercise movement, which produced the highest EMG activity of the posterior rotator cuff was side-lying external rotation, followed by prone external rotation, then standing external rotation at 90° abduction. Furthermore, the investigators noted that use of a towel roll between the humerus and body enhanced EMG activity of the infraspinatus and teres minor by 18% to 20%.

After injury or surgery, modalities may be used as needed. Cryotherapy both pre- and postexercise is recommended in the acute stages of healing to reduce the

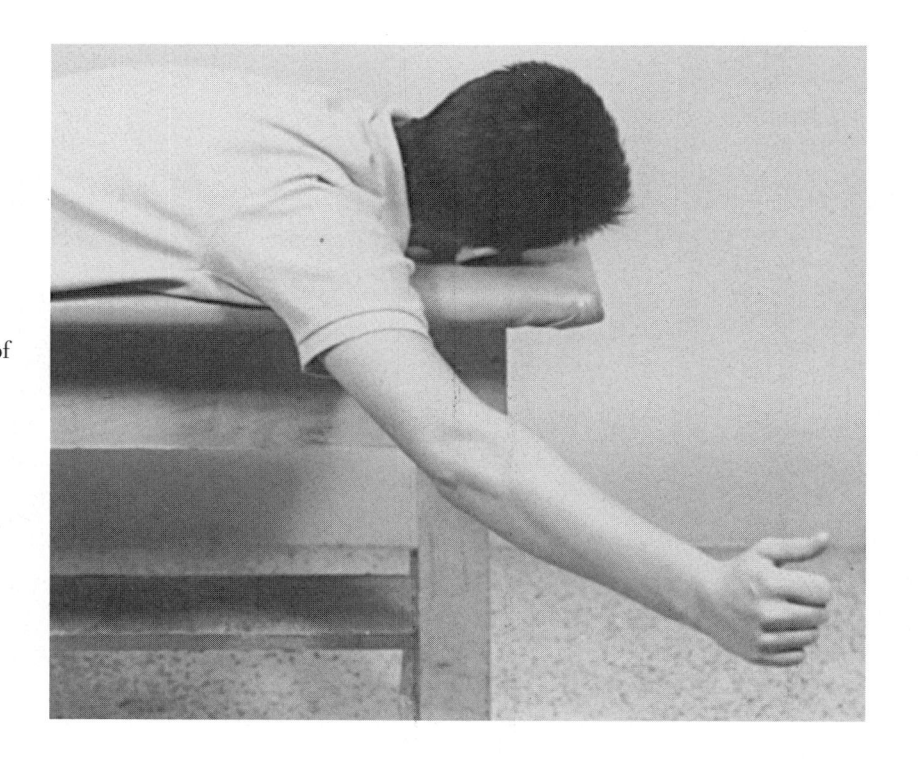

Figure 19-7. Blackburn and co-workers[15] reported significant electromyographic activity of the supraspinatus in the prone position. The subject is performing horizontal abduction at 100° of abduction, with full external rotation.

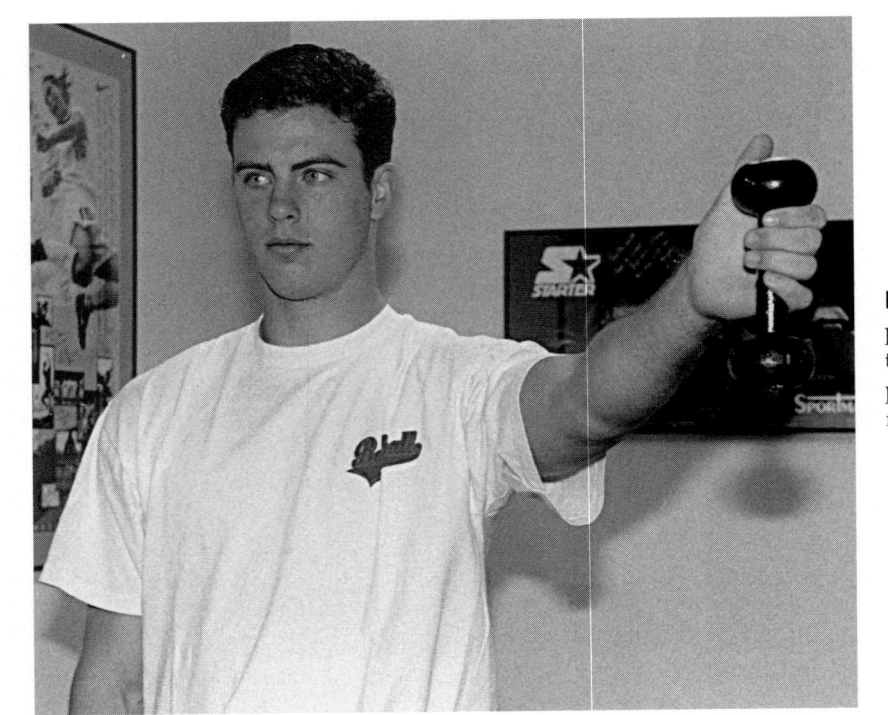

Figure 19-8. The "full can" position. This position has been suggested to be the best way to isolate the supraspinatus muscle while producing minimal activation of surrounding muscles.

Table 19-2

Electromyographic Activity of Specific Muscles during Selected Exercises

Muscle and Exercise	Electromyographic Activity (% MVIC ± SD)	Peak Arc Range (°)
Anterior deltoid		
Scaption internal rotation	72 ± 23	90-150
Scaption external rotation	71 ± 39	90-120
Flexion	69 ± 24	90-120
Middle deltoid		
Scaption internal rotation	83 ± 13	90-120
Horizontal abduction internal rotation	80 ± 23	90-120
Horizontal abduction external rotation	79 ± 20	90-120
Posterior deltoid		
Horizontal abduction interval rotation	93 ± 45	90-120
Horizontal abduction external rotation	92 ± 49	90-120
Rowing	88 ± 40	90-120
Supraspinatus		
Military press	80 ± 48	0-30
Scaption internal rotation	74 ± 33	90-120
Flexion	67 ± 14	90-120
Subscapularis		
Scaption internal rotation	62 ± 33	90-150
Military press	56 ± 48	60-90
Flexion	52 ± 42	120-150
Infraspinatus		
Horizontal abduction external rotation	88 ± 25	90-120
External rotation	85 ± 26	60-90
Horizontal abduction internal rotation	74 ± 32	90-120
Teres minor		
External rotation	80 ± 14	60-90
Horizontal abduction external rotation	74 ± 28	60-90
Horizontal abduction internal rotation	68 ± 36	90-120

Modified from Townsend, H., Jobe, F.W., Pink, M., et al. (1992): EMG analysis of the glenohumeral muscles during a baseball rehabilitation program. Am. J. Sports Med., 19:264-269.
MVIC, maximum voluntary isometric contraction.

inflammatory process. Cryotherapy may also be used prophylactically after the acute phase has subsided. Iontophoresis, moist heat, or ultrasound may be indicated for chronic overuse injuries of the shoulder.

Therapeutic exercises for the shoulder should address strength, endurance, and dynamic stability. A variety of machines and techniques can be used to accomplish specific goals. The upper body ergometer can be used in the early phases of rehabilitation for restoration of range of motion and in later phases for muscular endurance (Fig. 19-9). Exercises that result in an eccentric contraction are particularly important for athlete performing overhead movements, especially for the muscles involved in deceleration movements of the shoulder. Isokinetic equipment can be used at high speeds to help increase muscular power and endurance. Some isokinetic machines allow eccentric contraction of the posterior cuff muscles and concentric contraction of the anterior muscles, which can be used to strengthen the muscles functionally. In addition, most isokinetic machines can be set up in functional planes, such as with proprioceptive neuromuscular facilitation (PNF) patterns (Fig. 19-10). Care must be taken when using isokinetics eccentrically at the shoulder, because the learning curve for performing this type of exercise properly is significant, and delayed-onset muscle soreness often results. Manual resistance exercises, such as rhythmic stabilization exercises, can be used to promote co-contractions and facilitate muscle synergies (Fig. 19-11). Finally, surgical tubing is a versatile tool that can be used to strengthen in diagonal patterns or through simulation of the throwing act (Figs. 19-12 and 19-13). The use of each of these exercise types during the rehabilitation process depends on the goals of the particular phase.

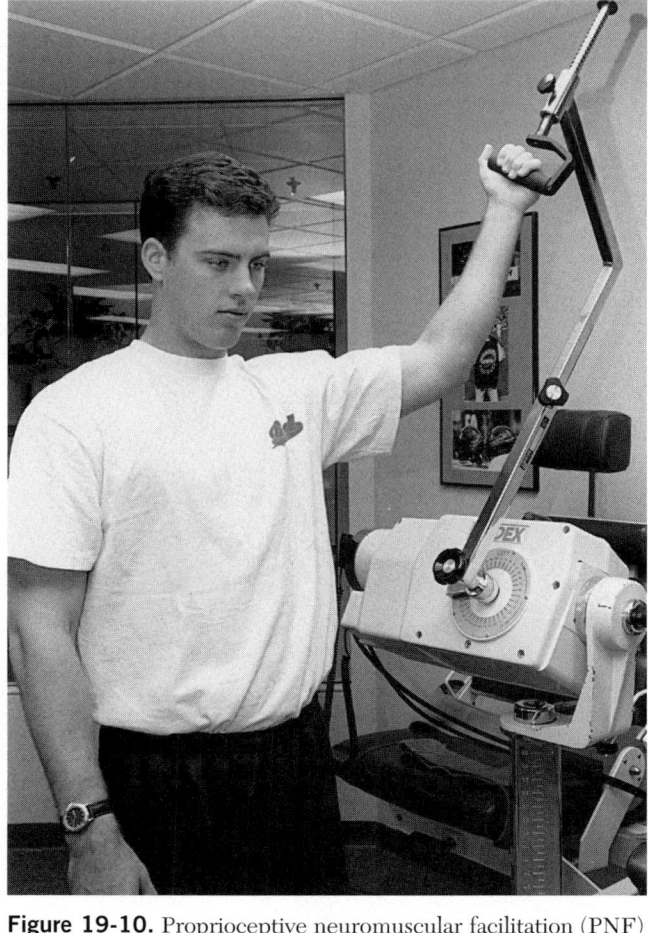

Figure 19-10. Proprioceptive neuromuscular facilitation (PNF) patterns can be used to simulate functional planes and enhance neuromuscular control of the shoulder girdle. This PNF pattern is being performed on the Biodex isokinetic device.

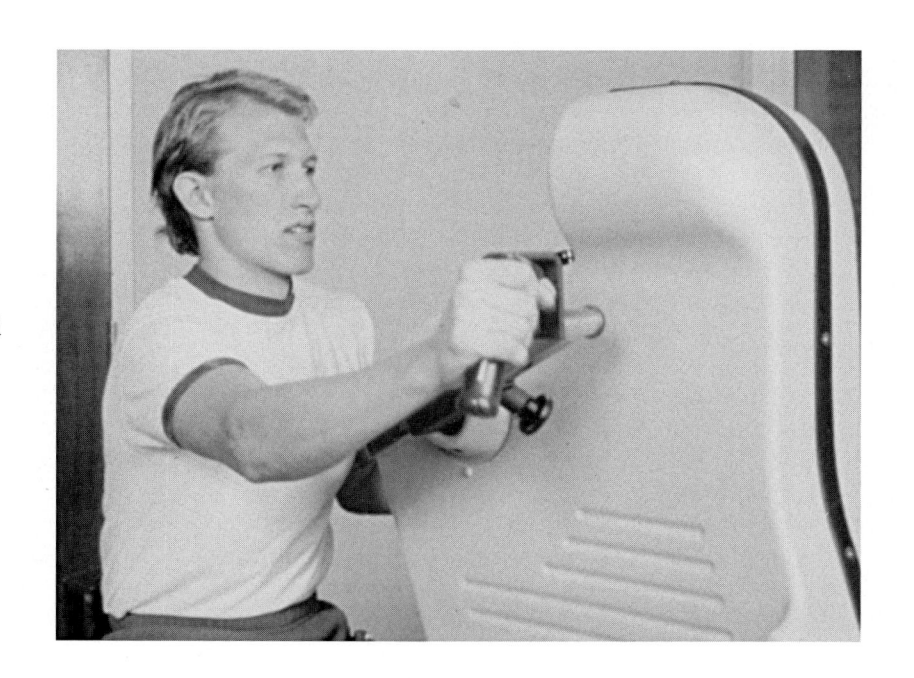

Figure 19-9. The upper body ergometer is used for range of motion and muscular endurance.

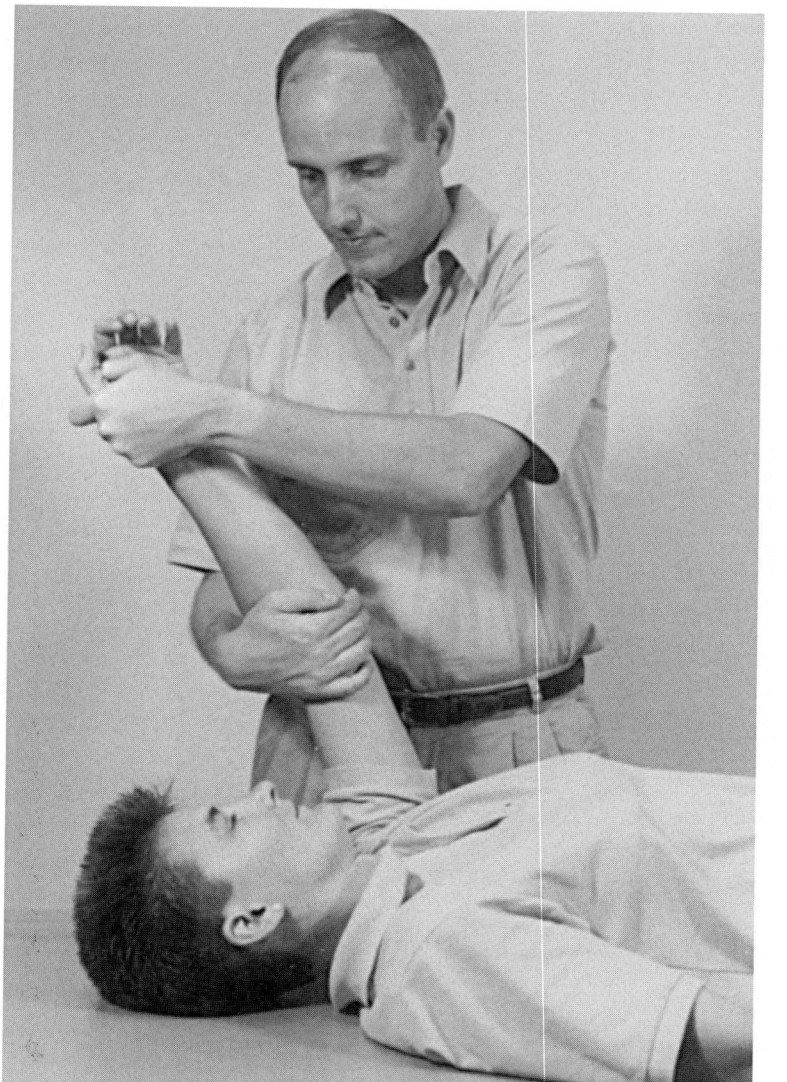

Figure 19-11. Proprioceptive neuromuscular facilitation patterns being performed against manual resistance.

Specific uses for each exercise will be explained throughout the treatment sections.

Glenohumeral mobilization techniques (see Chapter 6) are important for attaining accessory motion in the early stages of healing without subjecting the joint to the high forces of passive stretching. Grade I and/or II anterior-posterior, inferior-superior, and long arm distraction mobilizations can be used early in the rehabilitation program to neuromodulate the athlete's pain. Grade III or IV mobilizations can be added in later phases of rehabilitation to increase flexibility within the capsule. In older patients (aged 45 to 60) it is imperative to restore inferior capsular mobility early in the rehabilitation process (especially after rotator cuff repair).

Glenohumeral flexibility, particularly flexibility of the posterior shoulder structures, is paramount for athlete using overhead movements. This is particularly evident with inflexibility of the posterior capsule and musculature

that presents as decreased motion in horizontal adduction and internal rotation. Tightness in the posterior shoulder leads to increased stress on the posterior shoulder structures during the follow-through phase of pitching. Tight posterior shoulder structures can also cause abnormal glenohumeral kinematics by forcing the humeral head anteriorly and superiorly into the acromial arch.[82] The flexibility exercises illustrated at the end of this chapter (Figs. 19-30 through 19-41) should be undertaken not only after injury or surgery but also during the off-season to help prevent posterior glenohumeral restriction and injury.

Muscular strength and endurance of the scapular stabilizing musculature are important in maintaining correct joint arthrokinematics. The role of the scapulothoracic joint and surrounding musculature in maintaining a normally functioning shoulder is critical. Muscular spasm, weakness, and poor neuromuscular coordination of these stabilizing muscles directly affects glenohumeral motion.

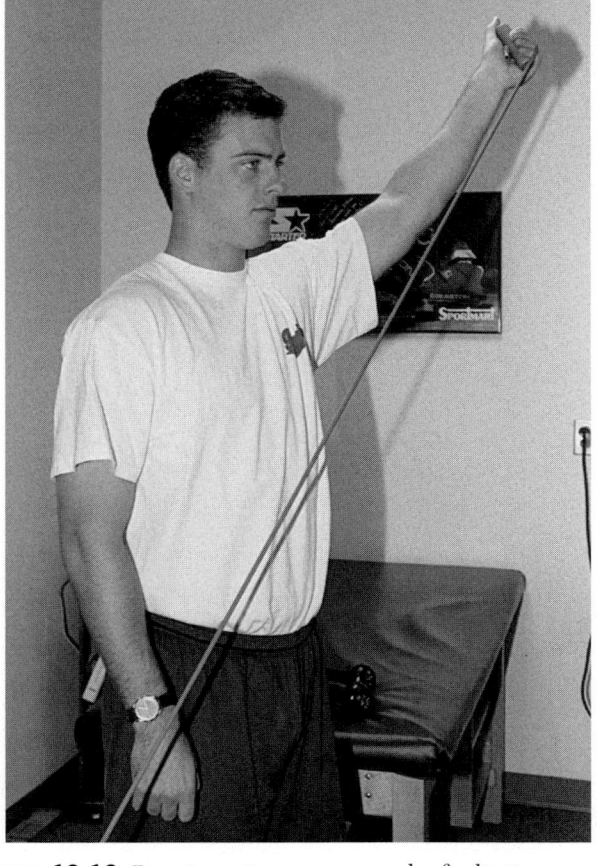

Figure 19-12. Proprioceptive neuromuscular facilitation pattern using surgical or exercise tubing.

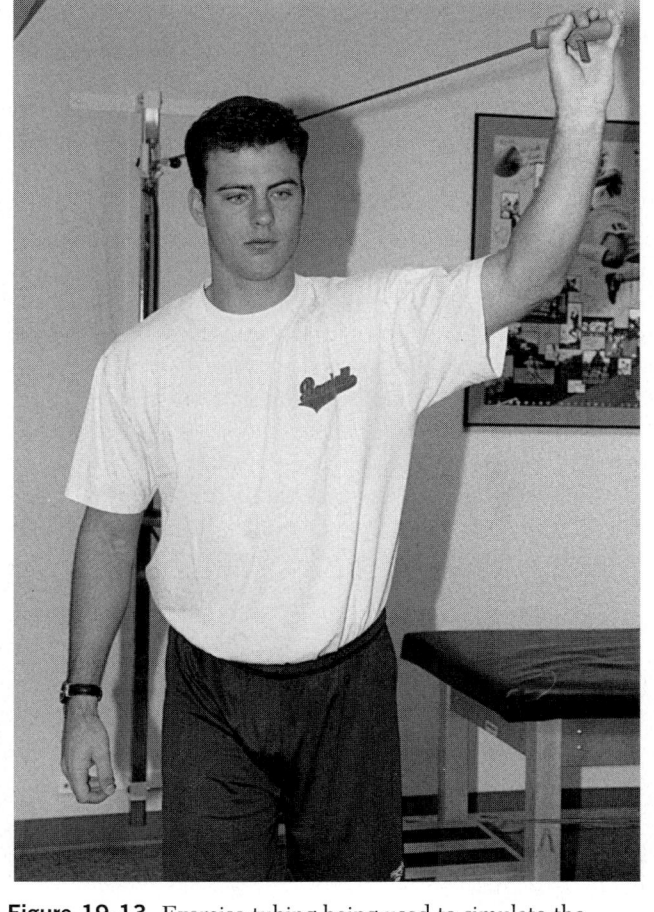

Figure 19-13. Exercise tubing being used to simulate the throwing motion.

If the scapula cannot rotate on the thoracic cage, maintain the correct length-tension muscular relationship, or properly orient the glenoid fossa with the humeral head, asynchronous motion at the shoulder complex will lead to injury. Scapula stabilizers can be strengthened by having the athlete perform push-ups, prone horizontal abduction, scapular retraction exercises, and neuromuscular control drills.

Because the rotator cuff muscles are mainly endurance-type muscles, the progressive resistance exercise (PRE) program is based on low weight and high repetition.[23] This not only increases muscular endurance but also decreases the potential for perpetuating the inflammatory process by performing the exercises with too much weight. A common view, held by numerous clinicians, is that the PRE program should be progressed by having the athlete work from 30 to 50 total repetitions and not add weight until 50 repetitions can be performed comfortably (see Chapter 7). The PRE program is begun with a gradual progression toward more dynamic exercises as healing progresses. This decreases the chance of rotator cuff inflammation and trauma while still producing muscle strength and endurance of the rotator cuff.

On the basis of numerous studies and their EMG results during specific movements, Wilk and associates[197] developed a core exercise program for athletes who use overhead movements called the Throwers' Ten Exercise Program (described in Appendix A). The program emphasizes the key muscles and muscle groups responsible for the throwing motion. The goal of this exercise program is to reestablish glenohumeral joint dynamic stability through rotator cuff musculature strength and neuromuscular control. Athletes should begin with a traditional PRE program and stretching exercises and gradually progress into eccentric and isokinetic exercises and then into a more dynamic program consisting of high-speed movements performed to muscular fatigue, proprioception exercises, use of inertia machines, and upper extremity plyometrics. The athlete should return to throwing gradually by progressing through an appropriate interval rehabilitation program, as outlined in Appendix B.

A plyometric exercise program can be extremely useful in the advanced phases of rehabilitation of an injured athlete. Plyometric exercise combines strength with speed of movement and has significant implications for the overhead thrower.[191,202] The drills apply a stretch-shortening cycle to the muscle, that is, an eccentric contraction followed by a concentric contraction. This stimulates the neurophysiologic components of the muscle to produce greater force. Box 19-4 presents the three phases of a plyometric drill. Successful plyometric training relies heavily on the rate of stretch rather than on the length of stretch. With plyometric exercise the neuromuscular system is trained by using the stretch reflex, proprioceptive stimulus, and muscular activation. Plyometrics should be performed only two or three times weekly because of the microtrauma that may occur with this type of aggressive exercise. Performing plyometrics daily can result in additional trauma to a healing shoulder in some athletes.

The upper extremity plyometric program is organized into four different exercise groupings: (1) warm-up drills, (2) throwing movements, (3) trunk drills, and (4) wall drills. Some of the plyometric drills are illustrated in Appendix C and others can be found in Chapter 11. For a complete description, the reader is encouraged to review several articles.[47,73,191,202]

The nonoperative rehabilitation program for the overhead thrower can be divided into four distinct phases. Each phase should represent specific goals and contain various exercises to accomplish these goals. Table 19-3 provides an overview of the program.

NONOPERATIVE REHABILITATION GUIDELINES
Range of Motion

Most throwers exhibit an obvious motion disparity whereby external rotation is excessive and internal rotation is limited in 90° of abduction.[25,40,109,200] Several investigators have documented the fact that pitchers exhibit greater external rotation than position players.[40,200] Brown and associates[40] reported that professional pitchers exhibited $141 \pm 15°$ of external rotation measured at 90° of abduction. This was approximately 9° more than the external rotation of the nonthrowing shoulder and approximately 9° more than that of the throwing shoulder of positional players measured in 90° of abduction. Bigliani and co-workers[25] examined range of motion of 148 professional

Table 19-3
Nonoperative Rehabilitation of the Overhead Thrower

I. Phase I: Acute Phase
Goals
- Diminish pain and inflammation
- Normalize or improve motion and flexibility
- Retard muscular atrophy
- Enhance dynamic stabilization

II. Phase II: Intermediate Phase
Goals
- Improve muscular strength and endurance
- Maintain or improve flexibility
- Promote concentric-eccentric muscular training
- Maintain dynamic stabilization

III. Phase III: Advanced Phase
Goals
- Initiate sport-specific training
- Enhance power and speed (plyometrics)
- Maintain rotator cuff strength program
- Improve muscular endurance

IV. Phase IV: Return to Activity
Goals
- Gradually return to sports activities
- Maintain strength, power, endurance, and flexibility gains

players. They reported that a pitcher's external rotation at 90° of abduction averaged 118° (range 95 to 145°) on the dominant shoulder, whereas the external rotation of a position player's dominant shoulder averaged 108° (range 80 to 105°). In an ongoing study of professional baseball players, Wilk and colleagues[201] assessed the range of motion of 372 professional baseball players. They noted that pitchers exhibit an average of $129.9 \pm 10°$ of external rotation and $62.6 \pm 9°$ of internal rotation when passively assessed at 90° of abduction. In pitchers, external rotation is approximately 7° greater on the throwing shoulder compared with that on the nonthrowing shoulder, whereas internal rotation is 7° greater on the nonthrowing shoulder. They also noted that pitchers exhibit the greatest total arc of motion, i.e., external and internal rotation at 90° abduction, followed closely by catchers, then outfielders, and finally infielders. Furthermore, when left-handed pitchers are compared with right-handed pitchers, the left-handed throwers exhibit approximately 7° more external rotation, and 12° more total motion than the right-handed throwers. These findings were statistically significant ($p < 0.01$).

Laxity

Most throwers exhibit significant laxity of the glenohumeral joint, which permits excessive range of motion. The

Box 19-4
Three Phases of a Plyometric Drill

Phase	Description
I	Stretch phase or the eccentric muscle loading that activates the muscle spindle
II	Amortization phase that represents the time between the eccentric and concentric phases
III	Shortening phase or the response or concentric phase

hypermobility of the thrower's shoulder has been referred to as thrower's laxity.[102] The laxity of the anterior and inferior glenohumeral joint capsule can be recognized by the clinician during the stability assessment of the overhead thrower's shoulder joint. Some clinicians have reported that the excessive laxity exhibited by the thrower is the result of repetitive throwing and have referred to this as *acquired laxity*[8] whereas others have documented that the overhead thrower exhibits *congenital laxity*.[25] Bigliani and co-workers[25] examined the laxity in 72 professional baseball pitchers and 76 position players. They noted a high degree of inferior glenohumeral joint laxity, with 61% of pitchers and 47% of position players exhibiting a positive sulcus sign on the throwing shoulder. Additionally, in the players who also exhibited a positive sulcus sign on the dominant shoulder, 89% of the pitchers and 100% of the position players exhibited a positive sulcus sign on the

nondominant shoulder. Thus, it would appear that some baseball players exhibit inherent congenital laxity, with superimposed acquired laxity as a result of adaptive changes from throwing.

Muscular Strength

Several investigators have examined muscular strength parameters in the overhead throwing athlete[3,21,55,91,195,196] with varying results and conclusions. Wilk and colleagues[195,196] performed isokinetic testing on professional baseball players as part of their physical examinations during spring training (Table 19-4). They demonstrated that external rotation strength of the pitcher's throwing shoulder is significantly weaker ($p > 0.05$) than that of the nonthrowing shoulder by 6%. Conversely, internal rotation strength of the throwing shoulder was significantly stronger

Table 19-4

Muscular Strength Values in Professional Baseball Players

A. Bilateral Comparisons—Glenohumeral Joint

	180°/s	300°/s	450°/s
ER	95-109%	85-95%	80-80%
IR	105-120%	100-115%	100-110%
Abd	100-110%	100-110%	—
Add	120-135%	115-130%	—

B. Unilateral Muscle Ratios—Glenohumeral Joint

180°/s	300°/s	450°/s
external/internal rotation| 63-70%	65-72%	62-70%
Abd/Add	82-87%	92-97%	—
ER/Abd	64-69%	66-71%	—

C. Isokinetic Torque/Body Weight Ratios—Glenohumeral Joint

	180°/s	300°/s
ER	18-23%	15-20%
IR	27-33%	25-30%
Abd	26-32%	20-26%
Add	32-36%	28-33%

D. Scapular Muscle

| | Protract | | Retract | | Elevation | | Depression | |
	D	ND	D	ND	D	ND	D	ND
Pitchers								
Catchers	71 ± 10	74 ± 13	62 ± 8	60 ± 7	83 ± 14	84 ± 5	22 ± 6	18 ± 5
Position players	68 ± 10	73 ± 10	63 ± 5	59 ± 7	88 ± 15	85 ± 8	21 ± 4	16 ± 5

E. Unilateral Muscle Ratios—Scapular

| | Protraction/Refraction | | Elevation/Depression | |
	D	ND	D	ND
Pitchers	87%	81%	27%	21%
Catchers	93%	81%	24%	19%
Position players	98%	94%	29%	27%

Data condensed from Wilk, K.E., Andrews, J.R., Arrigo, C.A., et al. (1993): The strength characteristics of internal and external rotator muscles in professional baseball pitchers. Am. J. Sports Med., 21:61-69, and Wilk, K.E., Andrews, J.R., Arrigo, C.A. (1995): The abductor and adductor strength characteristics of professional baseball pitchers. Am. J. Sports Med., 23:307-311.

Abd, abduction; Add, adduction; ER, external rotation; IR, internal rotation; D, dominant; ND, nondominant.

($p < 0.05$) by 3% compared with that of the nonthrowing shoulder. In addition, adduction strength of the throwing shoulder is also significantly stronger than that of the nonthrowing shoulder by approximately 9% to 10%. The authors believe that important isokinetic values are the unilateral muscle ratios, which describe the antagonist/agonist muscle strength relationship. A proper balance between agonist and antagonist muscle groups is thought to provide dynamic stabilization to the shoulder joint. To provide proper muscular balance, the external rotators should be at least 65% of the strength of the internal rotators.[195] Optimally, the external to internal rotator muscles strength ratio should be 66% to 75%.[195,196,200] This provides proper muscular balance. Magnusson and co-workers[126] measured isometric muscular strength values of professional pitchers using a hand-held dynamometer and compared them to those of a control group of nonthrowing, nonathletic individuals. In pitchers, the supraspinatus muscle was significantly weaker on the throwing side compared with the nonthrowing side when measured by an isometric manual muscle test (the empty can maneuver).[126] Additionally, shoulder abduction, external rotation, internal rotation, and the supraspinatus muscle were weaker in pitchers than in the control group of non–baseball players.

The scapular muscles play a vital role during the overhead throwing motion.[63] Proper scapular movement and stability are imperative to asymptomatic shoulder function.[116,117] These muscles work in a synchronized fashion and act as force couples about the scapula, providing both movement and stabilization. Wilk and colleagues[196] documented the isometric scapular muscular strength values of professional baseball players. Their results indicated that pitchers and catchers exhibited a significantly different strength increase of the scapular protractors and elevators than position players (Table 19-4). All players (except infielders) exhibited significantly stronger scapular depressors on the throwing side than on the nonthrowing shoulder. In addition, they believed that agonist/antagonist muscular ratios are important values for the scapular muscles in providing stability, mobility, and symptom-free shoulder function.

Proprioception

Proprioception is defined as the conscious or unconscious awareness of joint position, whereas neuromuscular control is the efferent motor response to afferent (sensory) information.[56] The thrower relies on enhanced proprioception to influence the neuromuscular system to dynamically stabilize the glenohumeral joint because of significant capsular laxity and excessive range of motion. Allegrucci and associates[7] tested shoulder proprioception in 20 healthy athletes participating in various overhead sports. Testing of joint proprioception was performed on a motorized system with the subject attempting to reproduce a specific joint

angle. These investigators noted that the dominant shoulder exhibited diminished proprioception compared with that of the nondominant shoulder. They also noted improved proprioception near the end range of motion compared with that at the starting point. Blasier and associates[30] reported that individuals who have clinically appreciable generalized joint laxity are significantly less sensitive during proprioceptive testing. Wilk, Reed, Creedhou, Reinold, and Andrews (unpublished data, 2000) studied the proprioception capability of 120 professional baseball players. They passively positioned the players at a documented point within the players' external rotation range of motion. The athletes were then instructed to actively reposition the shoulder in the same position. The researchers noted no significant difference between the throwing shoulder and nonthrowing shoulder. In addition, Wilk, Reed, Creedhou, Reinold, and Andrews (unpublished data, 2000) compared the proprioception ability in 60 professional baseball players with that of 60 non–overhead throwing athletes. They noted no significant differences between baseball players and non–overhead throwing athletes. However, baseball players exhibited slightly improved proprioception abilities at external rotation end range of motion compared with non–overhead throwing athletes, but these results were not significantly different.

Painful Arc

A painful arc or "catching point," particularly with shoulder abduction (but also possibly present in other planes), is characterized by specific points throughout a range of motion at which pain intensifies but dissipates once past that point. There may be as many as three or four catching points through an arc of motion. The most common range of motion in which patients demonstrate a painful arc is from 70 to 120° of arm elevation.[60] The athlete may attempt to exercise through these points of pain, which often dissipate within 5 to 7 days after initiation of treatment. Painful arcs in the young athlete can develop because of structural factors such as a hooked acromion, fracture malunion, or bursal swelling or may develop from a loss of dynamic humeral head stability, causing the humeral head to displace superiorly during arm elevation. If the clinician determines the latter to be the cause, exercises that enhance dynamic stability should be emphasized immediately.

Crepitus

Crepitus within the shoulder joint is a common occurrence and is usually asymptomatic. Generally, crepitus can be detected after shoulder surgery or rotator cuff tendinitis. If the crepitus remains asymptomatic, the athlete should attempt to exercise through it. Crepitus should also dissipate within 7 to 10 days after initiation of an appropriate rotator cuff exercise program.

Middle Deltoid and Elbow Pain

Middle deltoid and elbow pain can be referred from the shoulder, often from a tight shoulder capsule. It is usually exacerbated with external rotation in the supine position with 90° of abduction and 90° of elbow flexion (90/90 position). This pain is usually seen in individuals with chronic shoulder problems or in individuals who have undergone prolonged immobilization. Often, the elbow pain at the end range of shoulder external rotation may be greater than that of the actual shoulder pain. This condition usually responds well to moist heat and application of ultrasound to the shoulder capsule and to glenohumeral joint mobilization. A shoulder with a limitation of external rotation should not be stretched aggressively in the 90/90 position, because this will tend to exacerbate the elbow pain. Most patients can tolerate long arm distraction with imposed external rotation better than aggressive external rotation stretching in the 90/90 position. As treatment proceeds and normal synchronous glenohumeral motion is restored, the athlete should report a decrease in elbow and middle deltoid pain.

Pain beyond 90° of Elevation

If impingement or rotator cuff tendinitis is present, pain beyond 90° of elevation is a common occurrence. Athletes with this complaint should begin active-assisted range-of-motion (AAROM) exercises through a full range of motion, and joint mobilization techniques should be used as indicated. The pain is often propagated by a decrease in muscular strength and usually improves with a rotator cuff therapeutic exercise program. If symptoms are severe and the athlete has radiographic changes indicative of a grade III (or hooked acromion) type of injury, the prognosis is poor for nonoperative therapy.[27]

SHOULDER INJURIES
Scapulothoracic Joint Lesions

The scapulothoracic joint should also be assessed after any shoulder injury or surgery. Scapulothoracic pathologic conditions occur in chronic pain conditions in which glenohumeral motion has gradually decreased or in which the glenohumeral joint has been immobilized for a long period. In most instances the scapulothoracic joint becomes involved as a secondary problem. Increased shoulder pain can result in muscle spasm within the supraspinatus, trapezius, rhomboids, latissimus dorsi, and subscapularis. As mentioned earlier, for every 2° of glenohumeral abduction there must be approximately 1° of associated scapular motion to achieve 180° of arm elevation. If the scapulothoracic joint is not functioning properly, the athlete may be able to attain only 100 to 120° of passive abduction, and active abduction may be even more limited.

The scapulothoracic joint should be evaluated for spasm in the rhomboids, latissimus dorsi, upper and lower trapezius, subscapularis, teres minor, infraspinatus, and supraspinatus muscles. These areas should also be assessed for active trigger points, as discussed by Travell and Simons.[180] The activation of trigger points in these muscles may refer pain to the middle deltoid and elbow and, in severe spasm, down the arm. In addition, the clinician may find that the vertebral scapular border cannot be distracted off the thoracic cage, which results not only in increased pain for the athlete but also in an increase in localized muscle spasm.

Before decreased glenohumeral motion can be treated, scapulothoracic motion must be restored. This is usually accomplished by reducing the muscle spasm with moist heat, ultrasound, soft tissue mobilization, trigger point release, and scapular mobilization (Figs. 19-14 and 19-15). In severe spasm, the spray-and-stretch technique of Travell and Simons,[180] which uses Fluori-Methane spray* to desensitize the trigger points, may be indicated. Trigger point injection may also be considered.[180] As trigger points are diminished, the athlete should report a decrease in shoulder pain, neck stiffness, and referred pain, with an associated increase in glenohumeral abduction. A careful cervical and thoracic spine evaluation is necessary any time a patient describes scapular pain and muscle spasm.

ROTATOR CUFF LESIONS

The rotator cuff can become injured through a variety of mechanisms. Most commonly, the cuff can become frayed, which can progress to a full-thickness tear after repetitive wear, and it gradually degenerates. However, in young

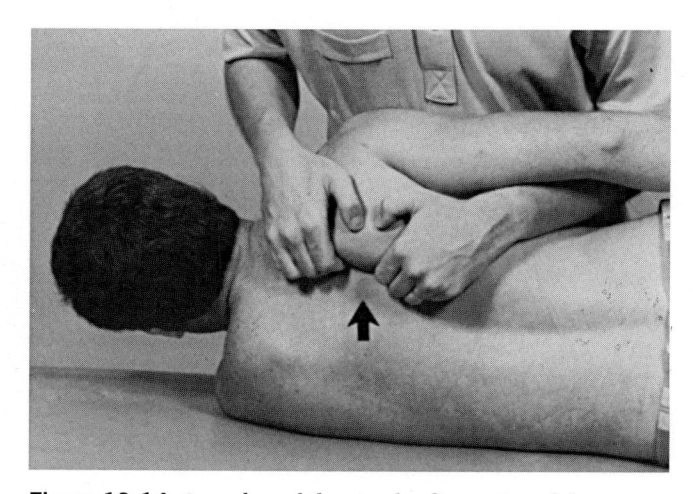

Figure 19-14. Scapula mobilization by distraction of the vertebral border of the scapula and lateral glide.

*Available from Gebauer Chemical Co., Cleveland Ohio.

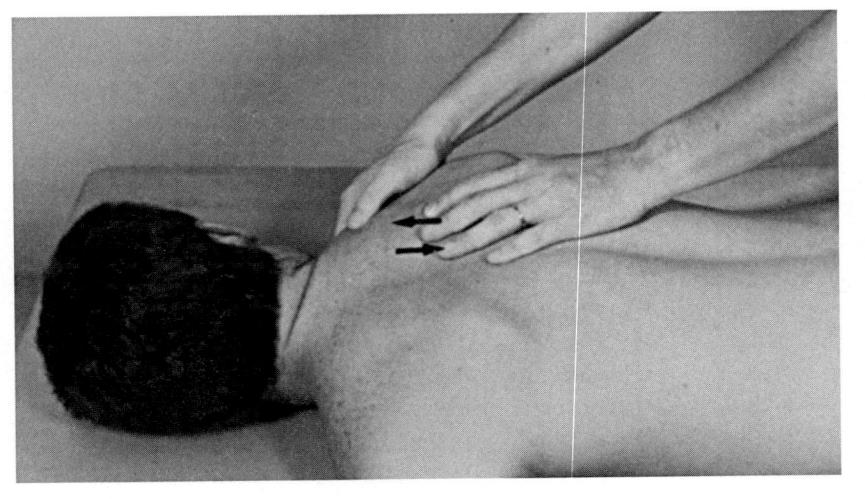

Figure 19-15. Scapula mobilization by superior and inferior scapula glides.

athletes, the cuff most commonly exhibits partial tearing or fraying, with symptoms of tendinitis. Andrews and Meister[12] classified rotator cuff lesions into categories based on the specific pathomechanics (Table 19-5). We will briefly discuss a few of these categories as they pertain to the athlete with a shoulder injury. First, the athlete involved in overhead sports (i.e., thrower or swimmer) is prone to capsular laxity, which contributes to the clinical syndrome referred to as *posterior impingementi*. In addition, such athletes are susceptible to undersurface rotator cuff tearing (tensile overload) and occasionally to compressive cuff disease. In contrast, athletes involved in collision sports such as football, lacrosse, or hockey are more likely to sustain a traumatic rotator cuff tear because of the athlete's arm being forcefully abducted or violently pulled away from the body. Full-thickness tears of the rotator cuff are unusual in young athletes.

Impingement Syndrome

The term *impingement syndrome* was popularized by Neer in 1972.[140] He emphasized that both the supraspinatus insertion to the greater tubercle and the bicipital groove lie anterior to the coracoacromial arch with the shoulder in the neutral position and that with forward flexion of the shoulder, these structures must pass

Table 19-5		
Classification of Rotator Cuff Disease		
Type	**Classification**	
I	Primary compressive disease	
II	Instability with secondary compressive disease	
III	Primary tensile overload failure	
IV	Tensile overload failure due to capsular instability	
V	Macrotraumatic failure	

beneath the coracoacromial arch, providing the opportunity for impingement.[130] He introduced the concept of a continuum in the impingement syndrome from chronic bursitis to partial or complete tears of the supraspinatus tendon, which may extend to involve ruptures of other parts of the rotator cuff.[130]

Impingement of the rotator cuff may occur in some athletes such as baseball players, quarterbacks, swimmers, and others whose activities involve repetitive use of the arm at or above 90° of shoulder abduction. Matsen and Arntz[130] defined impingement as the encroachment of the acromion, coracoacromial ligament, coracoid process, or acromioclavicular joint on the rotator cuff mechanism that passes beneath them as the glenohumeral joint is moved, particularly in flexion and internal rotation. Impingement usually involves the supraspinatus tendon. When the supraspinatus muscle assists in stabilizing the head of the humerus within the glenoid, the greater tubercle cannot butt against the coracoacromial arch (Fig. 19-16).[162] Whether impingement is the primary event causing rotator cuff tendinitis or whether rotator cuff impingement results from rotator cuff disease is undetermined.[162] In all likelihood both mechanisms of injury can occur.

There is approximately 5 to 10 mm of space between the humeral head and the undersurface of the acromial arch at 90° of shoulder abduction (depending on anatomy). Thus, whenever the arm is elevated, some degree of rotator cuff impingement may occur.[67,162] The shoulder is most vulnerable to impingement when the arm is at 90° of abduction and the scapula has not rotated sufficiently upward to free the rotator cuff of the overhanging acromion and coracoacromial ligament. Impingement of the glenohumeral joint can occur with horizontal adduction of the arm, which causes impingement against the coracoid process.[86] Forward flexion with internal rotation of the humerus also jams the greater tubercle under the acromion, the coracoacromial ligament, and, at times, the coracoid process.[90] If the arm is raised in external

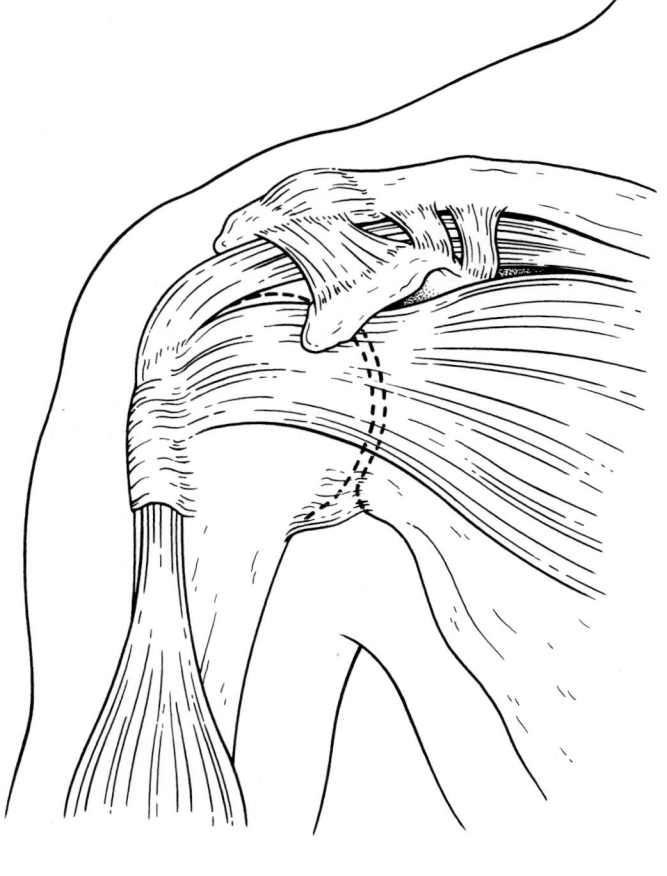

Figure 19-16. Anatomy relative to the impingement syndrome. The supraspinatus tendon is seen passing beneath the coracoacromial arch. (Redrawn from Matsen, F.A., III, and Arntz, C.T. [1990]: Subacromial impingement. *In:* Rockwood, C.A., Jr., and Matsen, F.A., III [eds.]: The Shoulder. Philadelphia, W.B. Saunders, p. 624.)

rotation, however, the greater tubercle is turned away from the acromial arch, and the arm can be elevated without impingement.

Impingement syndrome is perpetuated by the cumulative effect of many passages of the rotator cuff beneath the coracoacromial arch. This results in irritation of the supraspinatus and, possibly, the infraspinatus tendon, as well as in enlargement of the subacromial bursa, which can become fibrotic, thus further decreasing the already compromised subacromial space. Furthermore, with time and progression of wearing and attrition, microtears and partial-thickness rotator cuff tears may result. If these continue, secondary bony changes (osteophytes) can occur under the acromial arch, propagating full-thickness rotator cuff tears.

The etiology of the impingement syndrome is usually multifocal, and the supraspinatus tendon is the most likely structure to be involved. Several factors have been proposed as contributing to the development of impingement syndrome. Tendon avascularity has long been thought to contribute to impingement. Lindblom in 1939,[122] first reported avascularity of the rotator cuff at the supraspinatus attachment to the greater tubercle, describing this as the "critical zone"[50] in which many lesions occur. However, from their work, Moseley and Goldie[138] concluded that the critical zone is no more avascular than the rest of the rotator cuff. Finally, Iannotti and co-workers[98] using laser

Doppler technology, reported substantial blood flow in the critical zone of the rotator cuff.

Although it now appears that the rotator cuff is not a completely avascular structure, Rathbun and Macnab[159] and Sigholm and associates[173] proposed two mechanisms that may compromise supraspinatus blood flow. Rathbun and Macnab[159] noted that shoulder adduction places the supraspinatus under tension and "wrings out" its vessels, resulting in tissue necrosis. Sigholm and associates[173] demonstrated that active forward flexion increases subacromial pressure to a level sufficient to reduce tendon microcirculation substantially. However, in interpreting these findings, Matsen and Arntz[130] point out that "since the shoulder is frequently moved, it is unclear whether either of these mechanisms could produce ischemia of sufficient duration to cause tendon damage." Brewer[38] reported that the blood supply to the critical zone diminishes with age. The relationship among cuff vascularity, impingement, and rotator cuff lesions is still speculative, and more research is needed. However, it appears that the critical zone is an area of hypovascularity and is prone to impingement and thus to tendon damage. This is especially true in the aging patient with a shoulder injury.

The shape of the acromion has been studied in individuals with impingement syndrome.[27,140] Fig. 19-17 illustrates the three types of acromial shapes. It appears that rotator cuff lesions are more likely to occur if a hooked

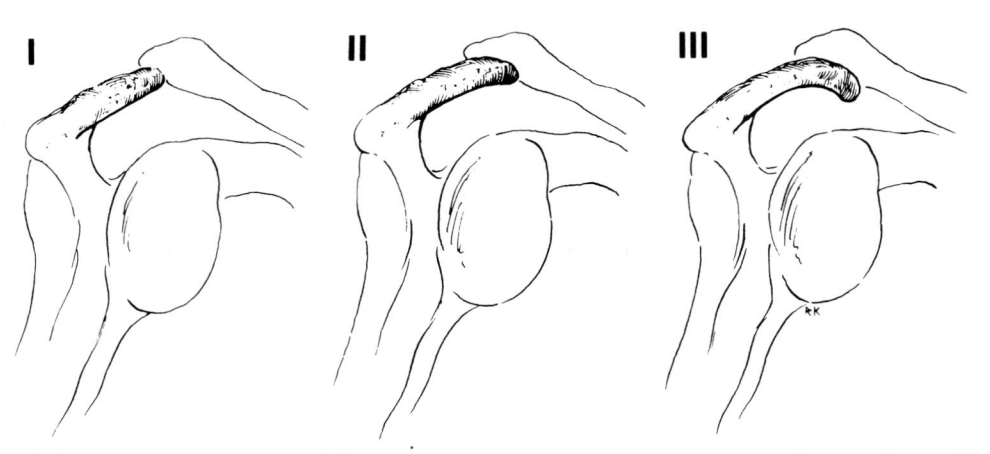

Figure 19-17. Biglianni and co-workers[27] identified three different shapes of the acromion: type I—smooth; type II—curved; and type III—hooked. (From Jobe, C.M. [1990]: Gross Anatomy of the Shoulder. *In:* Rockwood, C.A., Jr., and Matsen, F.A. [eds.], The Shoulder. Philadelphia, W.B. Saunders, p. 45.)

acromion is present,[27,140] but it cannot be determined whether the acromial shape is caused by or results from a cuff tear.[130,137]

Finally, a weakened rotator cuff mechanism can predispose an athlete to rotator cuff impingement. The rotator cuff functions to stabilize the shoulder against the actions of the deltoid and pectoralis major muscles. In the presence of a weakened cuff mechanism, contraction of the deltoid causes upward displacement of the humeral head, squeezing the remaining cuff against the coracoacromial arch (Fig. 19-18).[125] Other factors that

can result in rotator cuff impingement include degenerative spurs, chronic bursal thickening, rotator cuff thickening related to chronic calcium deposits, tightness of the posterior shoulder capsule, and capsular laxity.[130]

Neer[141] has described three progressive stages of impingement syndrome (Fig. 19-19). Stage I is a reversible lesion usually seen in individuals younger than 25 years of age. These patients present with an aching type of discomfort in the shoulder. This stage usually involves only inflammation of the supraspinatus tendon and long head of the biceps brachii. Stage II is generally seen in individuals

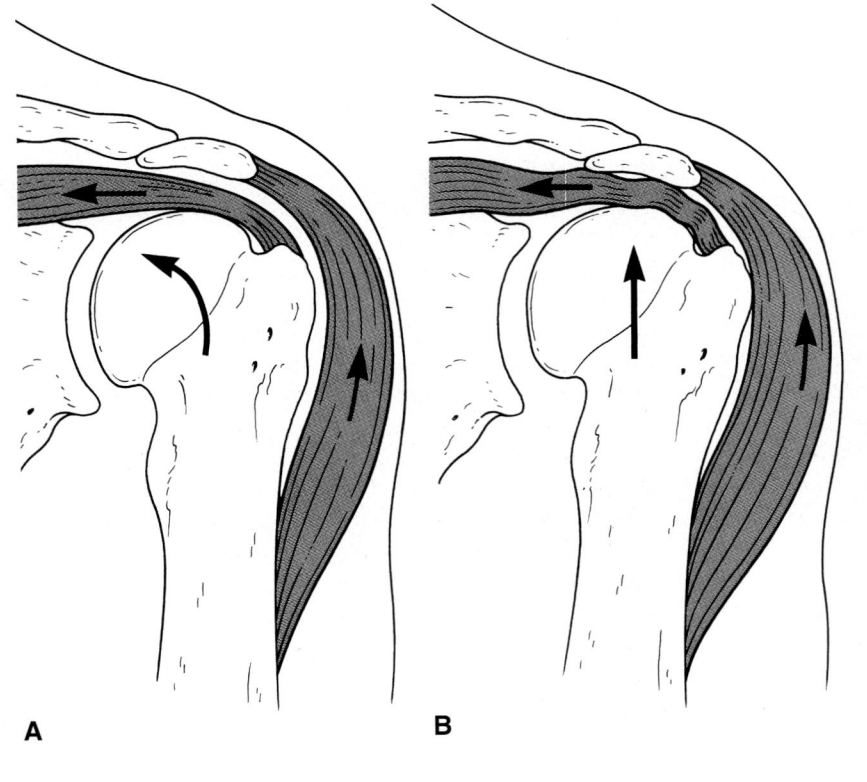

A   **B**

Figure 19-18. The supraspinatus helps stabilize the head of the humerus against the upward pull of the deltoid. *A,* Subacromial impingement is prevented by normal cuff function. *B,* Deep surface tearing of the supraspinatus weakens the ability of the cuff to hold the humeral head down, resulting in impingement of the tendon against the acromion. (Redrawn from Matsen, F.A., III, and Arntz, C.T. [1990]: Subacromial impingement. *In:* Rockwood, C.A., Jr., and Matsen, F.A., III [eds.]: The Shoulder. Philadelphia, W.B. Saunders, p. 624.)

Stage I: Edema and hemorrhage

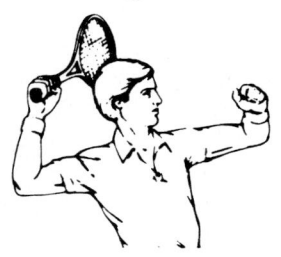

Typical age:	<25 years
Differential diagnosis:	Subluxation; A/C arthritis
Clinical course:	Reversible
Treatment:	Conservative

Stage II: Fibrosis and tendinitis

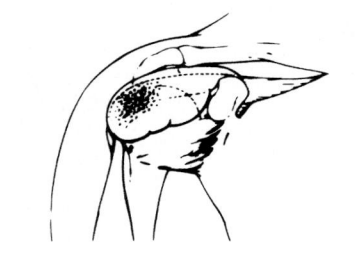

Typical age:	25-40 years
Differential diagnosis:	Frozen shoulder; calcium
Clinical course:	Recurrent pain with activity
Treatment:	Consider bursectomy; C/A ligament division

Stage III: Bone spurs and tendon rupture

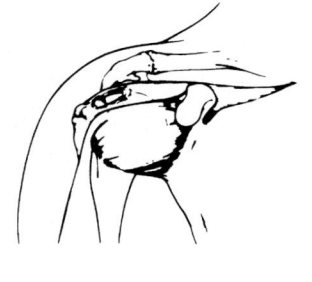

Typical age:	>40
Differential diagnosis:	Cervical radiculitis; Neoplasm
Clinical course:	Progressive disability
Treatment:	Anterior acromioplasty; rotator cuff repair

Figure 19-19. Neer's three-stage classification of impingement syndrome. A/C, acromioclavicular joint; C/A, coracoacromial. (Reprinted with permission from Neer, C.S. [1983]: Impingement lesions. Clin. Orthop., 173:70.)

24 to 40 years of age and involves fibrotic changes of the supraspinatus tendon and subacromial bursa. Again, an aching type of pain is present, which may increase at night, and there may be an inability to perform the movement that produces in the impingement syndrome. Injuries in this stage sometimes respond to conservative treatment, but it may require surgical intervention. Stage III seldom occurs in those younger than age 40. In this stage, the individual has had a long history of shoulder pain, and often there is osteophyte formation, a partial-thickness or eventually a full-thickness rotator cuff tear,[74] and an obvious wasting of the supraspinatus and infraspinatus muscles. Injuries in this stage usually do not respond well to conservative treatment.

Rotator cuff impingement is a self-perpetuating process. Matsen and Arntz[130] noted the following: (1) muscle or cuff tendon weakness causes impingement from a loss of the humeral head stabilizing function leading to tendon damage, disuse atrophy, and additional cuff weakness (Fig. 19-20); (2) bursal thickening causes

impingement from subacromial crowding, producing greater thickening of the bursa; and (3) posterior capsular tightness can lead to impingement, disuse, and stiffness, because the tight capsule forces the humeral head to rise up against the acromion. Numerous factors, both structural and functional, contribute to impingement,[185] especially in young athletes. Additionally, if the capsule is especially lax and if the dynamic stabilizers are not sufficient, the humeral head may displace anterosuperiorly, leading to complaints of impingement.

The goal in treating athletes with an impingement syndrome, either nonoperatively or surgically, is to reduce the compression and friction between the rotator cuff and subacromial space. Box 19-5 lists several factors[129,130] that are necessary to minimize the compression. The primary complication of impingement syndrome is a rotator cuff tear. If the impingement syndrome is diagnosed in its early stages, the prognosis is encouraging. In an acute impingement syndrome, time, rest from noxious stimuli, nonsteroidal anti-inflammatory drugs, local modalities such as

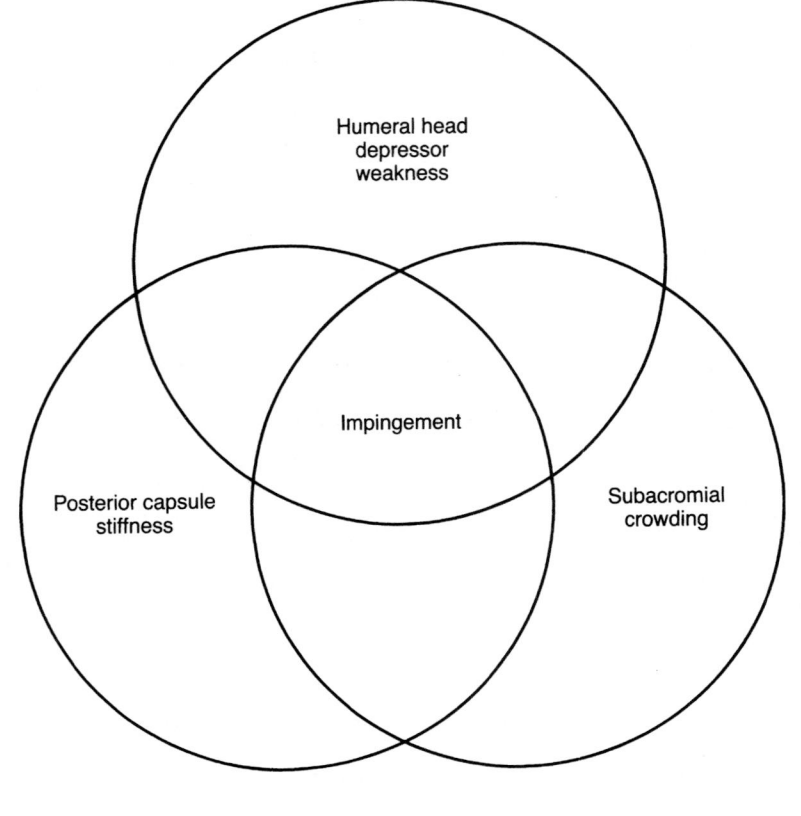

Figure 19-20. Normal shoulder tendon function depends on normal function of the humeral head depressors, normal capsular laxity, and adequate subacromial space. Some effects of impingement (e.g., weakness of the humeral head depressors, stiffness of the posterior capsule, and crowding of the subacromial space with thickened bursa) may further intensify impingement, producing a self-perpetuating process. (Modified from Matsen, F.A., III, and Arntz, C.T. [1990]: Subacromial impingement. *In:* Rockwood, C.A., Jr., and Matsen, F.A., III [eds.]: The Shoulder. Philadelphia, W.B. Saunders, p. 624.)

cold, heat, and electrical stimulation, and a general shoulder rehabilitation program of flexibility, and a PRE program (as outlined at the end of this chapter) are indicated.

On evaluation, active range of motion may be limited with an empty or muscular guarding endfeel as a result of pain. This may be caused by posterior capsule stiffness. In such instances, moist heat, ultrasound, joint mobilization, and a general shoulder flexibility program with emphasis

on supine internal and external rotation and horizontal adduction are appropriate. Most young throwers will exhibit a functional loss of internal rotation and, therefore, have a tight posterior capsule. It is important to stretch the posterior capsule (if tight) and inferior capsule and normalize the degree of internal rotation. Table 19-6 provides an outline of the protocol for nonoperative treatment of shoulder impingement syndrome.

Injection of the subacromial space with lidocaine in an athlete with impingement syndrome decreases pain. Steroid injections into the tendons of the rotator cuff and biceps tendon may produce tendon atrophy or reduce the ability of a damaged tendon to repair itself.[130] Kennedy and Willis[113] found a degenerative effect in the rabbit Achilles tendon after steroid injection. They concluded that physiologic doses of local steroids injected directly *into* a normal tendon weaken it significantly for up to 14 days postinjection. This weakness was attributed to cellular necrosis. When developing a rehabilitation program, the clinician must be aware of the potential effects of steroid injection.

Surgical intervention for patients with grade III impingement syndromes or for those that do not respond to nonoperative care consists of subacromial decompression, referred to as an *acromioplasty*. The goal of performing a subacromial decompression is to relieve the mechanical impingement and to prevent wear at the critical areas of the rotator cuff. Subacromial decompression consists of resection of the anteroinferior acromial

---

Box 19-5

Factors Necessary to Minimize Compression in the Subacromial Space

- Shape of the coracoacromial arch, which allows passage of the adjacent rotator cuff mechanism
- Normal undersurface of the acromioclavicular joint
- Normal bursa
- Normal function of the humeral head stabilizers (rotator cuff)
- Normal capsular laxity
- Smooth upper surface of the rotator cuff mechanism
- Normal function of the scapular stabilizers

Data from Matsen, F.A., III, and Arntz, C.T.: Rotator cuff tendon failure. *In:* Rockwood, C.A., Jr., and Matsen, F.A., III (eds.), The Shoulder, Vol. II. Philadelphia, W.B. Saunders, pp. 647-677, and Matsen, F.A., III and Arntz, C.T. (1990): Subacromial impingement. *In:* Rockwood, C.A., Jr., and Matsen, F.A., III (eds.), The Shoulder, Vol. II. Philadelphia, W.B. Saunders, pp. 623-646.

Table 19-6

Nonoperative Treatment of Subacromial Impingement Rehabilitation Protocol

Subacromial impingement is a chronic inflammatory process produced as one of the rotator cuff muscles and the subdeltoid bursa are "pinched" against the coracoacromial ligament and/or the anterior acromion when the arm is raised above the head. The supraspinatus portion of the rotator cuff is the most common area of impingement. This syndrome is commonly seen in individuals who use their arms repetitively in a position above the shoulder height. This condition also occurs in golfers, tennis players, and swimmers.

This four-phase program can be used for conservative management of impingement. The protocol is designed to attain maximal function in minimal time. This systematic approach allows specific goals and criteria to be met and ensures the safe progression of the rehabilitation process. Client compliance is critical.

Maximal Protection—Acute Phase

Goals
1. Relieve pain and inflammation
2. Normalize range of motion
3. Reestablish muscular balance
4. Educate patient and improve posture

Avoidance
- The elimination of any activity that causes an increase in symptoms

Range of Motion
- L-bar
  - Flexion
  - Elevation in scapular plane
  - External and internal rotation in scapular plane at 45° abduction
    - Progress to 90° abduction
- Horizontal abduction/adduction
- Pendulum exercises
- Active-assisted range of motion—Limited symptom-free available range of motion
  - Rope and pulley
    - Flexion

Joint Mobilizations
- Emphasize
- Inferior and posterior glides in scapular plane
- Goal is to establish balance in the glenohumeral joint capsular

Modalities
- Cryotherapy
- Iontophoresis

Strengthening Exercises
- Rhythmic stabilization exercises for external/internal rotation
- Rhythmic stabilization drills: flexion/extension
- External rotation strengthening
- Submaximal isometrics (external rotation, internal rotation, abduction)
- Scapular strengthening
- Retractors
- Depressors
- Protractors

Patient Education
- Activity level, activities
- Pathologic condition avoidance of overhead activity, reaching, and lifting activity
- Correct seating posture (consider lumbar roll)
- Seated posture with shoulder retraction

Guideline for Progression
1. Decreased pain and/or symptoms
2. Normal range of motion
3. Elimination of painful arc
4. Muscular balance

Intermediate Phase

Goals
1. Reestablish non-painful range of motion
2. Normalize athrokinematics of shoulder complex
3. Normalize muscular strength
4. Maintain reduced inflammation and pain

Range of Motion
- L-bar
- Flexion
  - External rotation at 90° of abduction
  - Internal rotation at 90° of abduction
  - Horizontal abduction/adduction at 90°
- Rope and pulley
  - Flexion
  - Abduction (symptom free motion)

Joint Mobilization
- Continue joint mobilization techniques to the tight aspect of the shoulder (especially inferior)
- Initiate self-capsular stretching
- Grade II/III/IV
- Inferior, anterior, and posterior glides
- Combined glides as required

Modalities (as needed)
- Cryotherapy
- Ultrasound/phonophoresis
- Iontophoresis

Strengthening Exercises
- Progress to complete shoulder exercise program
- Emphasize rotator cuff and scapular muscular training
  - External rotation tubing
  - Side-lying external rotation
  - Full can
  - Shoulder abduction
  - Prone horizontal abduction
  - Prone rowing
  - Prone horizontal abduction external rotation
  - Biceps/triceps
  - Standing lower trapezius muscular strengthening

Functional Activities
- Gradually allow an increase in functional activities
- No prolonged overhead activities
- No lifting activities overhead

Table 19-6

Nonoperative Treatment of Subacromial Impingement Rehabilitation Protocol—cont'd

Advanced Strengthening Phase

Goals
1. Improve muscular strength and endurance
2. Maintain flexibility and range of motion
3. Gradual increase in functional activity level

Flexibility and Stretching
- Continue all stretching and range of motion exercises
- L-bar external/internal rotation at 90° abduction
- Continue capsular stretch
- Maintain/increase posterior/inferior flexibility

Strengthening Exercises
- Start fundamental shoulder exercises
  - Tubing external/internal rotation
  - Lateral raises to 90° dumbbell
  - Full can dumbbell
  - Side-lying external rotation
  - Prone horizontal abduction
  - Prone extension
  - Push-ups
  - Biceps/triceps

Guideline for Progression
1. Full nonpainful range of motion
2. No pain or tenderness
3. Strength test fulfills criteria
4. Satisfactory clinical examination

Return to Activity Phase

Goals
1. Unrestricted symptom free activity

Initiate Interval Sport Program
- Throwing
- Tennis
- Golf

Maintenance Exercise Program
- Flexibility exercises
  - L-bar
    - Flexion
    - External rotation and internal rotation at 90° abduction
    - Self-capsular stretches
  - Isotonic exercises
    - Fundamental shoulder exercises
      - Perform 3 times a week

---

undersurface to increase the space between the undersurface of the acromion and the rotator cuff/humeral head. Often, partial or complete resection of the coracoacromial ligament is also performed to further increase the available space. An acromioplasty may be performed in conjunction with a rotator cuff débridement or repair.

The impingement syndrome can be corrected surgically by arthroscopy or arthrotomy. For open subacromial decompression, use of a technique that does not compromise the deltoid attachments is recommended, rather than a separation of the deltoid from its insertion during the surgical procedure. This approach results in less morbidity and allows for early postoperative motion, with almost no need for postoperative immobilization.[130] If the deltoid is detached from the acromion and distal clavicle, the rehabilitation program should proceed more slowly to allow for deltoid healing.[193,194]

Modalities can be used initially after surgery to help control pain and inflammation, with the concurrent initiation of early range-of-motion exercises. In the early stages the athlete may complain of joint crepitus and a painful arc or catching points; these should be worked through as tolerated. The crepitus and painful arc should subside in 7 to 10 days after the initiation of exercises. We expect full passive range of motion (PROM) or AAROM to be restored in 2 to 3 weeks after arthroscopic decompression. As active range of motion is restored, a PRE program can be initiated. Coracoacromial ligament resection has no effect on the course of the rehabilitation. If a rotator cuff repair is

performed in conjunction with the acromioplasty, a rotator cuff repair rehabilitation protocol should be followed.

Internal impingement has been described in the literature by Walch and associates.[184] Andrews and colleagues[10] originally identified the lesion in the overhead thrower. This cuff lesion develops when the arm is abducted and externally rotated, such as in the cocking phase of throwing. During this movement, the humeral head tends to glide anteriorly (especially when the anterior capsule is hypermobile). As this motion occurs, the supraspinatus and infraspinatus impinge (or produce friction) on the posterosuperior edge of the glenoid rim, resulting in an undersurface tearing of the rotator cuff and fraying of the posterosuperior glenoid labrum (Fig. 19-21). This lesion is extremely common in athletes using overhead movements.

Posterosuperior glenoid impingement, often referred to, as internal impingement is one of the most commonly observed injuries to the overhead throwing athlete.[9,10,11,101-103,184] We believe that one of the underlying causes of symptomatic internal impingement is excessive anterior shoulder laxity. One of the primary goals of the rehabilitation program is to enhance the athletics' dynamic stabilization capacity, thus, controlling anterior humeral head translation. In addition, another essential goal is to restore flexibility to the posterior rotator cuff muscles of the glenohumeral joint. We strongly caution against aggressive stretching of the anterior and inferior glenohumeral structures; this may result in increased anterior translation. Additionally, the program should emphasize

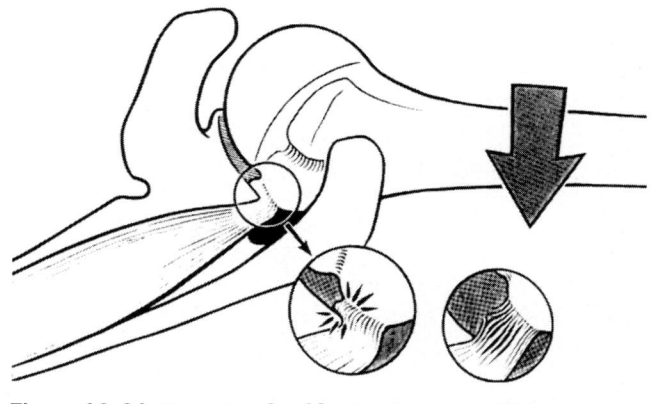

Figure 19-21. Posterior shoulder impingement. This occurs when the arm is abducted and externally rotated; the supraspinatus and infraspinatus muscles impinge (rub) on the posterosuperior rim of the glenoid cavity, leading to fraying of the cuff or labrum. (From Walch, G., Boileau, P., Noel, E., and Donell, T. [1992]: Impingement of the deep surface of the supraspinatus tendon on the glenoid rim. J. Shoulder Elbow Surg., 1:239-245.)

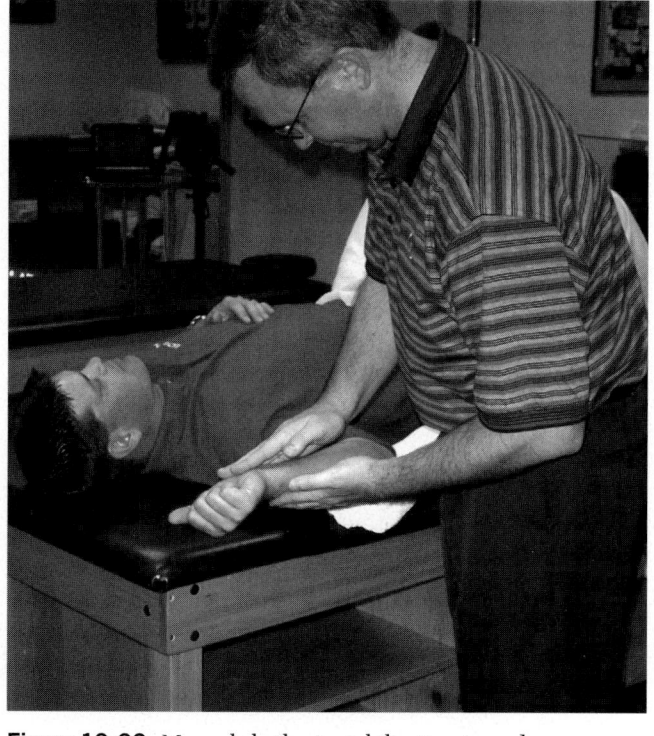

Figure 19-22. Manual rhythmic stabilization in end range glenohumeral external rotation.

muscular strengthening of the posterior rotator cuff to reestablish muscular balance and improve joint compression abilities. The scapular muscles must be an area of increased focus as well. Restoring dynamic stabilization is an essential goal to minimize the anterior translation of the humeral head during the late cocking and early acceleration phases of throwing. Exercise drills such as PNF patterns with rhythmic stabilization are incorporated.[199,200] Also, stabilization drills performed at the end range of external rotation are beneficial in enhancing dynamic stabilization (Fig. 19-22). Perturbation training to the shoulder joint is performed to enhance proprioception, dynamic stabilization, and neuromuscular control during this phase (see Chapter 8). It is the authors' opinion that this form of training has been extremely effective in treating the thrower with posterior/superior impingement.

After the clinician has restored posterior flexibility, normalized glenohumeral strength ratios, enhanced scapular muscular strength, and diminished the patient's symptoms, an interval throwing program may be initiated (Appendix B). Jobe[101] suggested abstinence from throwing for 2 to 12 weeks depending on the thrower's symptoms. Once the thrower begins their interval throwing program, the clinician or pitching coach should observe the athlete's throwing mechanics often. Occasionally, throwers who exhibit internal impingement will allow their arm to lag behind the scapula, thus, throwing with excessive horizontal abduction and not throwing with the humerus in the plane of the scapula. Jobe[101-103] referred to this as *hyperangulation of the arm*. This type of fault leads to excessive strain on the anterior capsule and internal impingement of the posterior rotator cuff.[101,102] Correction of throwing

pathomechanics is critical to returning the athlete to asymptomatic and effective throwing.

Rotator Cuff Tears

The primary function of the rotator cuff is to provide dynamic stabilization and steer the humeral head. It appears that the cuff is well designed to bear tension and resist upward displacement of the humerus.[48,49] The cuff balances the major forces applied by the prime mover muscles during motions such as flexion and abduction.

The role of the rotator cuff in shoulder movements has long been, and still remains, somewhat controversial. Poppen and Walker[156,157] reported that the pull of the supraspinatus is fairly constant throughout the range of motion and actually exceeds that of the deltoid until 60° of shoulder abduction has been reached. Norkin and Levangie[143] found that EMG activity of the deltoid in abduction shows a gradual increase in activity, peaking at 90° of humeral abduction and not plateauing until 180° has been reached. Colachis and associates[52,53] used selective nerve blocks and noted that the supraspinatus and infraspinatus provide 45% of abduction and 90% of external rotation strength. Additionally, Howell and co-workers[96] measured the torque produced by the supraspinatus and deltoid in the forward flexion and elevation planes. They found that the supraspinatus and deltoid muscles are equally responsible for producing torque about the shoulder joint in functional planes of motions. Currently, it appears that both the deltoid and the supraspinatus contribute to abduction throughout the full range of motion. Active abduction is possible with loss of the deltoid or supraspinatus, with a corresponding loss in power.[52,53]

The etiology of rotator cuff tears can be one or a combination of the following: repetitive microtrauma, disuse, overuse tendinitis, anatomic factors, and attrition. Neer[141] reported that acute cuff tears occurring as a result of trauma account for approximately 3% to 8% of all tears. It has been postulated that rotator cuff tears result after the commonly diagnosed "cuff tendinitis" and that rotator cuff tears may actually represent failure of the rotator cuff fibers. This may explain why individuals with this injury usually recover with time and conservative treatment.[129] Matsen and Arntz[129] suggested the following explanation for perpetuation of rotator cuff failure:

> The traumatic and degenerative theories of cuff tendon failure can be synthesized into a unified view of pathogenesis. Let us assume that the normal cuff starts out well vascularized and with a full complement of fibers. Through its life it is subjected to various adverse factors such as traction, contusion, impingement, inflammation, injections, and age-related degeneration. Each of these factors places fibers of the cuff tendons at risk. Even though laboratory studies show that normal tendon does not fail before failure of the musculotendinous junction or the tendon bone junction, in the clinical situation the rotator cuff tendon ruptures both at its insertion to bone and in its mid-substance. With the application of loads (whether repetitive or abrupt, compressive, or tensile), each fiber fails when the applied load exceeds its strength. Fibers may fail a few at a time or in mass. Because these fibers are under load even with the arm at rest, they retract after their rupture. Each instance of fiber failure has at least three adverse effects: (1) it increases the load on the neighboring fibers (fewer fibers to share the load); (2) it detaches muscle fibers from bone (diminishing the force that the cuff muscles can deliver); and (3) it risks the vascular elements in close proximity by distorting their anatomy (a particularly important factor owing to the fact that the rotator cuff tendons contain the anastomoses between the osseous and muscular vessels). Thus, the initially well-vascularized rotator cuff tendon becomes progressively less vascular with succeeding injuries. Although some tendons, such as the Achilles tendon, have a remarkable propensity to heal after rupture, cuff ruptures communicate with joint and bursal fluid, which removes any hematoma that could contribute to cuff healing. Even if the tendon could heal with scar, scar tissue lacks the normal resilience of tendon and is, therefore, under increased risk for failure with subsequent loading (minor or major). These events weaken the substance of the cuff, impair its function, and render the cuff weaker, more prone to additional failure with less load, and less able to heal.

Arthroscopy has allowed investigators to examine rotator cuff lesions and make observations regarding these lesions (Box 19-6).

Box 19-6

Arthroscopy Observations Regarding Rotator Cuff Lesions

- Failure of the musculotendinous cuff is almost always peripheral, near the attachment of the cuff to the greater tuberosity, and it nearly always begins in the supraspinatus part of the cuff near the biceps tendon.[130]
- Partial-thickness tears appear to be two to three times as common as full-thickness lesions.[141,206]
- Often partial tears occur on the joint side and not on the bursal side.[72,206]
- Rotator cuff tears often begin deep and extend outward, therefore challenging the concept of subacromial impingement as the primary cause of defects.[61,129,204]
- Full-thickness cuff tears appear to occur in tendons that are weakened by some combination of age, repeated small episodes of trauma, steroid injections, subacromial impingement, hypovascularity of the tendon, major injury, and previous partial tearing.[129]

Athletes presenting with rotator cuff tendinitis generally respond favorably to a well-designed rehabilitation program. The involved shoulder is usually stiff, especially in the posterior capsule, with appreciable glenohumeral crepitus. The stiffness limits one or a combination of the following motions: forward flexion, internal and external rotation, and horizontal adduction. The emphasis of the program is to correct any asymmetric capsular tightness. The athlete may also have difficulty reaching behind the back, because this movement elongates the musculotendinous unit and compresses it as it is pulled under the coracoacromial arch with internal rotation.[32] Modalities (such as moist heat, iontophoresis, and ultrasound), mobilization, and stretching exercises for the posterior capsule and muscles may be indicated. Rest from the noxious stimuli and use of nonsteroidal anti-inflammatory drugs are also appropriate. Initiation of a general shoulder flexibility program and a rotator cuff PRE program, as outlined at the end of this chapter, are necessary to prevent progressive cuff degradation. The PRE program should concentrate on the posterior rotator cuff muscles, because these muscles are responsible for humeral head depression and contract eccentrically to slow the arm down during the deceleration phase of throwing.

Return to throwing should not begin until the entire rehabilitation program has been completed. The patient must exhibit specific criteria before a throwing program is initiated. The criteria used by the authors include full non-painful range of motion, satisfactory muscular strength, satisfactory clinical examination, and appropriate progression through the rehabilitation program. Once these criteria have been satisfied, an interval throwing program (Appendix B) may be initiated. The athlete should continue with a program that includes strengthening and flexibility exercise after the throwing program has been initiated.

Anterior Instability

Shoulder instability is a common clinical problem, with anterior instability occurring most commonly. The anatomy of the glenohumeral joint predisposes the shoulder to instability. The glenoid cavity is relatively small and shallow, and the capsule tends to be loose in young, athletic individuals. These factors combine to make the shoulder susceptible to dislocations anteriorly.[43,100,158,162] Anterior glenohumeral instability can be divided into acute traumatic dislocation and recurrent dislocation or subluxation. Most acute anterior dislocations occur with the arm abducted to 90°, extended, and externally rotated such as when an athlete is attempting an arm tackle in football or when an abnormal force is applied to an arm that is executing a throw. The dislocated shoulder is characterized by a flattened deltoid contour, an inability to move the arm, and severe pain. With this injury the head of the humerus is forced out of its articulation, past the glenoid labrum and then upward, to rest under the coracoid process.[13]

The dislocated shoulder is usually readily detectable, but symptoms of a subluxating shoulder can be more subtle and may be overlooked. Anterior subluxation of the glenohumeral joint may develop without a history of trauma and is common in throwers. The subluxating shoulder is often referred to as the *dead arm syndrome*, because it is characterized by a loss in shoulder strength and power. Rowe and Zarins[161,162] reported that in 60 instances of dead arm syndrome, 26 patients were aware of shoulder subluxation, and 32 patients were not aware of its occurrence. Clinically, the athlete has soreness over the anterior aspect of the shoulder and reports a reproduction of the signs and symptoms in the cocking or acceleration phase of the throwing act. Athletes may also report a loss in shoulder strength and power and a feeling of clicking or sliding within the shoulder.

Several mechanisms of injury can explain the insidious onset of anterior instability. One of the most prevalent views is that in the cocking phase of throwing, extreme external rotation places repeated stress on the anterior capsule and results in capsule attenuation and, ultimately, in anterior instability.

Weakness of the scapula stabilizers is also believed to contribute to anterior instability.[57] The function of the scapula rotators (e.g., trapezius, rhomboids, and serratus anterior) is to place the glenoid in the optimal position for the activities being performed. The rotator cuff seeks to stabilize the humeral head, and the glenohumeral ligament, particularly the inferior aspect, provides a static restraint at the margins of the joint.[107] Damage to the static restraints (gradual attenuation) results in instability, causing asynchronous firing of the scapular rotators and

rotator cuff muscles. Greater stress is placed on the rotator cuff muscles in an attempt to stabilize the humeral head, producing rotator cuff damage and leading to rotator cuff impingement (described earlier). Thus, Jobe and associates[107] reported that impingement problems are due to the primary lesion, glenohumeral instability.

Shoulder instability can be associated with an anterior glenoid labrum tear as the humeral head slips past the anterior aspect of the labrum and then reduces itself. A small portion of the anterior labrum may be torn, especially with recurrent episodes of instability. Additionally, Hill-Sachs and Bankart lesions (Fig. 19-23) are common with anterior instability, and their presence can be used to confirm this diagnosis. Bankart lesions result from an avulsion of the capsule and labrum from the glenoid rim and occur as the result of a traumatic glenohumeral joint dislocation. Individuals who have had a subluxation generally do not have a Bankart lesion. A Hill-Sachs lesion is a bony injury involving the posterolateral aspect of the humeral head as it strikes the rim of the glenoid at the time of dislocation.[163] Therefore, greater forces are required to dislocate a shoulder than to subluxate it, and greater tissue damage results.

Whether the injury is a subluxation or a dislocation, nonoperative treatment is often attempted first. The success of nonoperative care varies.[14,15,74,93] Athletes who have dislocated their shoulders and thus have Bankart lesions are less likely to return to unrestricted sports participation than are individuals who do not have Bankart lesions. Rehabilitation should initially concentrate on decreasing the acute inflammation and pain and then gradually restoring full shoulder

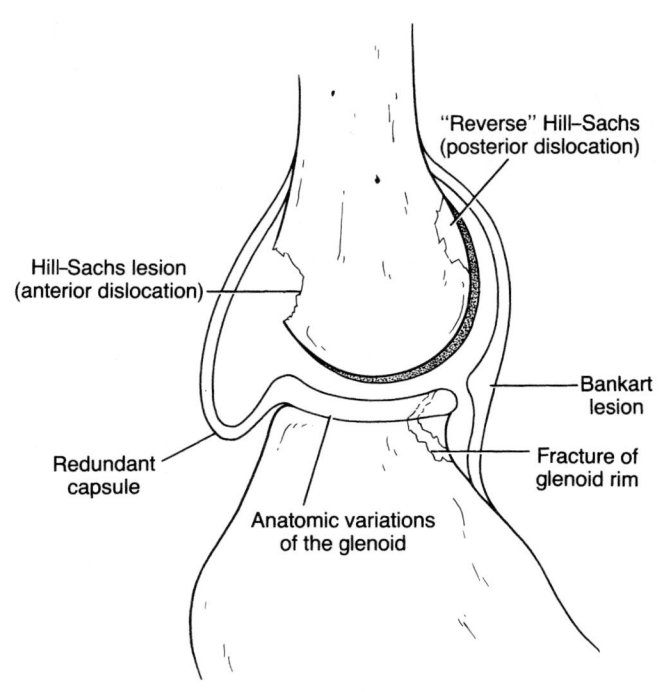

Figure 19-23. Anatomic lesions produced from shoulder instability. (From Rowe, C.R. [1988]: The Shoulder. New York, Churchill Livingstone, p. 177.)

motion. After normal motion is restored, an aggressive shoulder flexibility program is contraindicated because of the attenuation of the tissues. A strengthening program for the rotator cuff should be implemented, with a focus on the rotator cuff muscles and scapular stabilizers.[44] Historically, non-anatomic extra-articular surgical procedures such as the Bristow, Magnuson-Stack, and Putti-Plate have been performed with limited success to address glenohumeral listability.[2,5,31,36,54,118,121,134] By-in-large these have been replaced with the anatomic stabilization techniques detailed later in this chapter, which restore normal anatomy and facilitate early aggressive rehabilitation.

In some athletes who exhibit recurrent anterior instability and who are not required to abduct and externally rotate their arms above shoulder height, a shoulder brace may be used. Numerous devices are available, and these are designed to restrict combined abduction and external rotation. The Shoulder Subluxation Inhibitor* is custom fitted and is made of low- and high-density polyethylene. The SAWA shoulder orthosis† is an off-the-shelf brace made of cotton and rubber, with Velcro straps to limit motion. The Sully Brace‡ is another off-the-shelf brace made of neoprene. Use of these types of braces has proven to be beneficial in athletes such as interior linemen, hockey players, and soccer players, but their use has been completely unsuccessful for athletes who have to throw or catch a ball.

Posterior Instability

Posterior dislocation or subluxation is not as common as anterior instability, but it does occur. Usually, posterior subluxation results from traumatic forces that injure the posterior capsule. This can occur in football linemen who use their hands during blocking or rushing; with the elbow locked in extension and the shoulder flexed, the arm can be forcefully pushed posteriorly. Posterior dislocation may occur because of a fall onto an extended arm. The diagnosis is often missed because physical findings are not as dramatic as with an anterior dislocation.

Again, nonoperative treatment should be attempted first, using a balanced strengthening program for the anterior and posterior rotator cuff musculature. Strengthening of the posterior rotator cuff should be accomplished without placing the shoulder into a subluxated or apprehensive position.[144] An aggressive shoulder flexibility regimen is contraindicated because of the attenuated tissues. Engle and Canner[65] have reported success with a rehabilitation program that emphasizes PNF exercise techniques centered around development of the posterior cuff muscles. Success of the nonoperative program depends greatly on

the type of athlete and the sport. Athletes who use their arms in an extended position in front of their body are more susceptible to recurrent symptoms.

Surgical management of those athletes whose injuries do not respond to nonoperative care is controversial. The results after surgical reconstruction for posterior instability have been disappointing.[87,165] Surgical techniques include shifting of the posterior capsule (capsulorrhaphy), posterior Bankart repair, or posterior osteotomy to help prevent dislocation. The posterior capsule tends to be much thinner than the anterior capsule and is thus prone to stretch out, which may contribute to diminished surgical success.

Rehabilitation after posterior capsulorrhaphy advances more slowly compared with rehabilitation after anterior capsulorrhaphy. The most significant differences from the anterior capsulorrhaphy rehabilitation program include: (1) no forward flexion above 90° and no horizontal adduction for 4 weeks to avoid stress on the repaired capsule; (2) slower restoration of internal rotation-internal rotation in the 90/90 position should not begin until approximately 6 weeks after surgery; and (3) a slower return to functional or sports activities.

Multidirectional Instability

Athletes who exhibit atraumatic (congenital), multidirectional instability pose a difficult problem, not only to the clinician but also to the surgeon. These individuals typically have generalized ligamentous and capsular laxity.[207] Most commonly these athletes are swimmers, gymnasts, and occasionally overhead throwing athletes. The most common treatment plan for these individuals is a thorough nonoperative strengthening program. Although the program is usually successful, it is not uncommon for the athlete to experience intermittent symptoms.

Nonoperative treatment focuses on dynamic stabilization, proprioception, and neuromuscular control exercises. Rehabilitation techniques such as rhythmic stabilization, co-contractions, proprioceptive training, and motor control drills are the hallmark of a well-structured program. In the program the posterior and anterior musculature should be balanced in an attempt to control and stabilize the glenohumeral joint. In patients with atraumatic instability, it is critical that scapular muscle strength be improved through an aggressive rehabilitation program.

If nonsurgical treatment fails and the athlete is unable to participate in sports, surgical intervention may be indicated. Bigliani[24] suggested that a capsular shift may correct redundancy on all three sides: anterior, posterior, and inferior.

Glenoid Labrum Lesions

In recent years, increasing attention has been paid to the glenoid labrum. Glenoid labrum lesions are extremely common in athletes and can be classified as either

---

*Available from SSI, Physical Support Systems, Inc., Windham, New Hampshire.
†Available from Brace International, Scottsdale, Arizona.
‡Available from The Saunders Group, Chaska, Minnesota.

atraumatic or traumatic. Traumatic injuries to the glenoid capsulolabral complex are known to occur with glenohumeral dislocations or subluxations. With this mechanism of injury, a wide spectrum of glenoid labral injuries may occur, including a detachment of the labrum from the glenoid, a frank tear, or a combination of these lesions. Additionally, the labrum can be injured because of repetitive stresses during the throwing motion. Andrews and colleagues[9,10] described a tear of the superior aspect of the glenoid labrum at the origin of the biceps tendon. The authors theorized that this lesion may be due to repetitive forceful contraction of the biceps brachii during the follow-through phase of throwing.

Snyder and associates[174] described an anterosuperior labral complex lesion. This superior labrum, anterior, and posterior (SLAP) lesion begins posteriorly and extends anteriorly and involves the "anchor" of the long head of the biceps brachii to the labrum. Numerous mechanisms may produce this lesion. A labral tear may result from a fall onto an outstretched arm, from forceful muscular contraction of the biceps, or from repetitive strenuous overhead sport movements. Snyder and associates[174] classified SLAP lesions into four types (Fig. 19-24 and Box 19-7). Specific treatment recommendations are based on the type of labral lesion present (Box 19-7). The rehabilitation

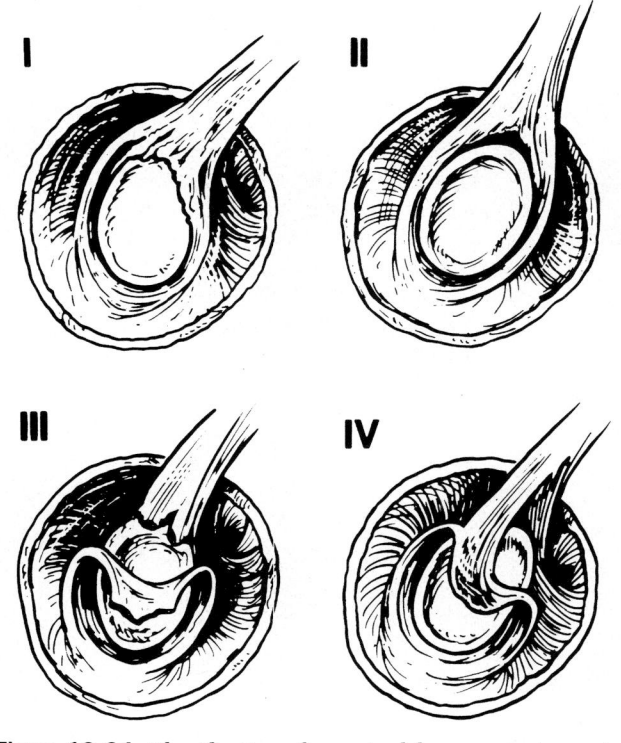

Figure 19-24. Classification of superior labrum, anterior, and posterior lesions according to Snyder and associates.[174] (From Zuckerman, J.D. [1993]: Glenoid labrum lesions. *In:* Andrews, J.R. and Wilk, K.E. [eds.], The Athlete's Shoulder. New York, Churchill Livingstone, p. 232.)

Box 19-7

Classification of Superior Labrum, Anterior, and Posterior (SLAP) Lesions

Type	Description	Treatment Recommendations
I	The superior labrum is markedly frayed, but the attachments of the labrum and biceps tendon remain intact.	The frayed labral tissue should be débrided back to the intact labrum.
II	Similar in appearance to the type I lesion, except that the attachment of the superior labrum is compromised, resulting in instability of the labrum-biceps complex.	Débridement and the superior glenoid labrum should be reattached to the superior glenoid with an absorbable tack or with a similar surgical technique.

Note: Within the type II SLAP lesion group there is a sub group referred to as a peel-back lesion.[42] A peel-back lesion most commonly occurs in the overhead athlete due to the extreme of external rotation.[42]

Type	Description	Treatment Recommendations
III	Lesion consists of a bucket-handle tear of the labrum, which can displace into the joint.	The bucket-handle tear is excised.
IV	Lesions are similar to type III lesions, except that the labral tear extends into the biceps tendon, allowing it to subluxate into the joint.	Tear is excised and biceps repair on tenodosis.

From Snyder, S.J., Karzel, R.P., DelPizzo, W., et al. (1990) SLAP lesions of the shoulder. Arthroscopy, 6:274-276.

program for these pathologic conditions will be discussed later in this chapter.

Acromioclavicular Separation

Injuries involving the acromioclavicular joint can occur insidiously from activities requiring repetitive overhead activity. Acute injuries occur either from direct trauma, in which the athlete falls on the tip of the shoulder and depresses the acromion process inferiorly, or from a fall on the outstretched arm, in which the forces are transmitted superiorly through the acromion process. The extent of acromioclavicular sprain or separation depends on whether the coracoclavicular ligaments are traumatized or the main stabilizing acromioclavicular ligaments are damaged. Rockwood and Young[160] identified six types of acromioclavicular joint sprains (Fig. 19-25 and Box 19-8).

Treatment for grade I and grade II injuries is nonoperative, but treatment for grade III injuries is still controversial. Many physicians elect to treat grade III injuries nonoperatively and believe that outcomes are better with nonoperative management,[107,142] whereas others believe the joint needs to be stabilized surgically. Depending on the extent of damage a number of surgical measures are available including (1) stabilization of the clavicle to the coracoid process with a screw, (2) transarticular fixation of the acromioclavicular joint with pins after reduction, (3) resection of the outer end of the clavicle, and

(4) transposition of the coracoacromial ligament to the top of the acromioclavicular joint. Biomechanical studies[71] have indicated that the superior acromioclavicular ligament is the most important for stabilizing the acromioclavicular joint for normal daily activities. The conoid ligament is the most important for supporting the joint against significant injury.

Rehabilitation after first- and second-degree acromioclavicular separations consists of progressing motion as tolerated and beginning a PRE program when active range of motion is equal bilaterally. Modalities may be used in the early stages of healing to help decrease inflammation and pain. Third-degree separations treated nonoperatively usually require 2 to 4 weeks of immobilization, with a gradual progression of motion and strengthening exercises

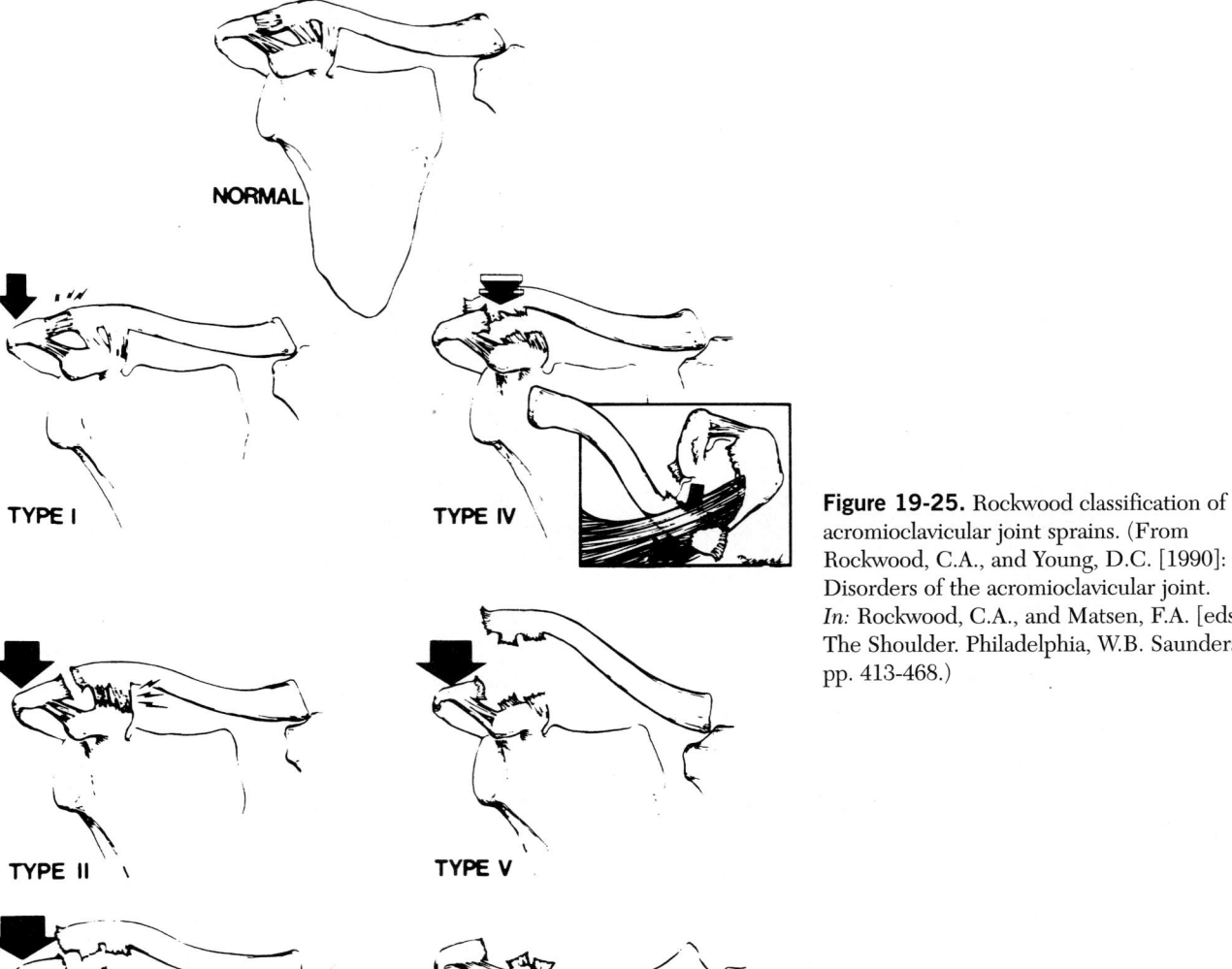

Figure 19-25. Rockwood classification of acromioclavicular joint sprains. (From Rockwood, C.A., and Young, D.C. [1990]: Disorders of the acromioclavicular joint. *In:* Rockwood, C.A., and Matsen, F.A. [eds.], The Shoulder. Philadelphia, W.B. Saunders, pp. 413-468.)

Box 19-8

Six Types of Acromioclavicular Joint Sprains

Type	Description
I	Injury to the acromioclavicular ligament
II	Involves injury to the acromioclavicular ligament and a sprain of the coracoclavicular ligament
III	Involves disruption of the acromioclavicular and coracoclavicular ligaments and some detachment of the deltoid and upper trapezius muscles from the distal clavicle
IV	Similar to type III injuries, except that in type IV acromioclavicular joint sprains, the clavicle displaces posteriorly through the trapezius muscle, and the deltoid and trapezius are detached
V	Significant displacement of the clavicle by 100% to 300%
VI	Involve the distal clavicle displacing inferiorly under the acromion

after immobilization. Pendulum exercises, elbow range-of-motion exercises, isometrics in all planes, and rope-and-pulley exercises for shoulder flexion and abduction can be initiated as tolerated after immobilization. Precautions in rehabilitation after a surgical repair of the acromioclavicular joint are similar to those after conservative care of grade III injuries, including limitation of

abduction and flexion to 90° for approximately 3 to 4 weeks. Pendulum and isometric exercises in all planes are encouraged in the initial stages of postsurgical rehabilitation. Range of motion is progressed to 90° in all planes as tolerated after 4 weeks. Rehabilitation should concentrate on strengthening the rotator cuff and scapula stabilizers and on restoring neuromuscular control and arthrokinematics, not unlike rehabilitation after other shoulder injuries.

GENERAL REHABILITATION GUIDELINES AFTER SURGERY

Injuries that do not respond to nonoperative care may require surgical intervention. Acromioplasty is commonly performed in conjunction with a rotator cuff repair. Rotator cuff tears seen and treated arthroscopically are most often incomplete tears that are noted on the undersurface of the muscle. Larger lesions may require repair with an open procedure. There are numerous surgical techniques to repair a full-thickness rotator cuff tear. The *deltoid-splitting procedure* is recommended to decrease morbidity and promote early range of motion. It typically involves arthroscopic débridement and open rotator cuff repair, using the deltoid-splitting or arthroscopy-assisted surgical procedure. The rehabilitation approach we take is based on the size of the tear and tissue quality; hence, in Tables 19-7 to 19-9, three different protocols, based on the size of the tear, are illustrated. These protocols can easily be adapted to other rotator cuff procedures, if necessary.

Table 19-7

Type I Rotator Cuff Repair Arthroscopic Assisted—Mini-Open Repair for Small to Medium Tears (1 cm or less)

I. Phase I: Immediate Postoperative Phase (Day 1 to 10)
Goals
 1. Maintain integrity of the repair
 2. Gradually increase passive range of motion
 3. Diminish pain and inflammation
 4. Prevent muscular inhibition
A. Day 1 to 6
 • Sling
 • Pendulum exercises 4 to 8 times daily (flexion, circles)
 • Active-assisted range of motion exercise (L-bar)
  • External/internal rotation in scapular plane
 • Passive range of motion
  • Flexion to tolerance
  • External/internal rotation in scapular plane
 • Elbow/hand gripping and range of motion exercises
 • Submaximal and pain-free isometrics
  • Flexion
  • Abduction
  • External rotation
  • Internal rotation
  • Elbow flexors
 • Cryotherapy for pain and inflammation

 • Ice 15 to 20 minutes every hour
 • Sleeping
  • Sleep in sling
B. Day 7 to 10
 • Discontinue use of sling at day 7 to 10
 • Continue pendulum exercises
 • Progress passive range of motion to tolerance
  • Flexion to at least 115°
  • External rotation in scapular plane to 45 to 55°
  • Internal rotation in scapular plane to 45 to 55°
 • Active-assisted range of motion Exercises (L-bar)
  • External/internal rotation in scapular plane
  • Flexion to tolerance (therapist provides assistance by supporting arm)
 • Continue elbow/hand range of motion and gripping exercises
 • Continue isometrics
  • Flexion with bent elbow
  • Extension with bent elbow
  • Abduction with bent elbow
  • External/internal rotation with arm in scapular plane
  • Elbow flexion

Continued

Table 19-7

Type I Rotator Cuff Repair Arthroscopic Assisted—Mini-Open Repair for Small to Medium Tears (1 cm or less)—cont'd

- May initiate external/internal rotation tubing at 0° abduction, if patient exhibits necessary active range of motion
- Continue use of ice for pain control
- Use ice at least 6 to 7 times daily
- Sleeping
- Continue sleeping in sling until physician instructs (usually day 7 to 10)
- Precautions:
  - No lifting of objects
  - No excessive shoulder motion behind back
  - No excessive stretching or sudden movements
  - No supporting of body weight by hands
  - Keep incision clean and dry

II. Phase II: Protection Phase (Day 11 to Week 5)

Goals
1. Allow healing of soft tissue
2. Do not overstress healing tissue
3. Gradually restore full passive range of motion (week 2 to 3)
4. Reestablish dynamic shoulder stability
5. Decrease pain and inflammation

A. Day 11 to 14
- Passive range of motion to tolerance
  - Flexion 0 to 145/160°
  - External rotation at 90° abduction to at least 75 to 80°
  - Internal rotation at 90° abduction to at least 55 to 60°
- Active-assisted range of motion to tolerance
  - Flexion
  - External/internal rotation in scapular plane
  - External/internal rotation at 90° abduction
- Dynamic stabilization drills
  - Rhythmic stabilization drills
    - External/internal rotation in scapular plane
    - Flexion/extension at 100° flexion
- Continue isotonic external/internal rotation with tubing
- Initiate active exercise prone rowing and elbow flexion
- Initiate active exercise flexion and abduction (day 15)
- Continue use of cryotherapy

B. Week 3 to 4
- Patient should exhibit full passive range of motion, nearing full active range of motion
- Continue all exercises listed above
- Initiate scapular muscular strengthening program
- Initiate side-lying external rotation strengthening (light dumbbell)
- Initiate isotonic elbow flexion
- Continue use of ice as needed
- May use pool for light range of motion exercises

C. Week 5
- Patient should exhibit full active range of motion
- Continue active-assisted range of motion and stretching exercises
- Progress isotonic strengthening exercise program
  - External rotation tubing
  - Side-lying external rotation
  - Prone rowing
  - Prone horizontal abduction

- Shoulder flexion (scapular plane)
- Shoulder abduction
- Biceps curls

Precautions
1. No heavy lifting of objects
2. No supporting of body weight by hands and arms
3. No sudden jerking motions

III. Phase III: Intermediate Phase (Week 6 to 12)

Goals
1. Gradual restoration of shoulder strength and power
2. Gradual return to functional activities

A. Week 6
- Continue stretching and passive range of motion (as needed to maintain full range of motion)
- Continue dynamic stabilization drills
- Progress isotonic strengthening program
- External/internal rotation tubing
- External rotation side-lying
- Lateral raises
- Full can in scapular plane
- Prone rowing
- Prone horizontal abduction
- Prone extension
- Elbow flexion
- Elbow extension
- If physician permits, may initiate *light* functional activities

B. Week 8 to 10
- Continue all exercise listed above
- Progress to independent home exercise program (fundamental shoulder exercises)
- Initiate interval golf program (slow rate of progression)

IV. Phase IV: Advanced Strengthening Phase (Week 12 to 20)

Goals
1. Maintain full non-painful active range of motion
2. Enhance functional use of upper extremity
3. Improve muscular strengthen and power
4. Gradual return to functional activities

A. Week 12
- Continue range of motion and stretching to maintain full range of motion
- Self-capsular stretches
- Progress shoulder strengthening exercises
- Fundamental shoulder exercises
- Initiate swimming or tennis program (if appropriate)

B. Week 15
- Continue all exercises listed above
- Progress Golf Program to playing golf (if appropriate)

V. Phase V: Return to Activity Phase (Week 20 to 26)

Goals
1. Gradual return to strenuous work activities
2. Gradual return to recreational sport activities

A. Week 20
- Continue fundamental shoulder exercise program (at least 4 times weekly)
- Continue stretching, if motion is tight
- Continue progression to sport participation

Table 19-8

Type II Rotator Cuff Repair Arthroscopic Assisted Mini-Open Repair for Medium to Large Tears (Greater than 1 cm, Less than 5 cm)

I. Phase I: Immediate Postoperative Phase (Day 1 to 10)

Goals
1. Maintain integrity of the repair
2. Gradually increase passive range of motion
3. Diminish pain and inflammation
4. Prevent muscular inhibition

A. Day 1 to 6
- Sling or slight abduction brace *(physician decision)*
- Pendulum exercises 4 to 8 times daily (flexion, circles)
- Active-assisted range of motion exercise (L-bar)
  - External/internal rotation in scapular plane
- Passive range of motion
  - Flexion to tolerance
  - External/internal rotation in scapular plane
- Elbow/hand gripping and range of motion exercises
- Submaximal painfree isometrics
  - Flexion
  - Abduction
  - External rotation
  - Internal rotation
  - Elbow flexors
- Cryotherapy for pain and inflammation
  - Ice 15 to 20 minutes every hour
- Sleeping
  - Sleep in sling or brace

B. Day 7 to 10
- Discontinue use of sling/brace at day 10 to 14
- Continue pendulum exercises
- Progress passive range of motion to tolerance
  - Flexion to at least 105°
  - External rotation in scapular plane to 35 to 45°
  - Internal rotation in scapular plane to 35 to 45°
- Active assisted range of motion exercises (L-bar)
  - External/internal rotation in scapular plane
  - Flexion to tolerance (therapist provides assistance by supporting arm)
- Continue elbow/hand range of motion and gripping exercises
- Continue isometrics
  - Flexion with bent elbow
  - Extension with bent elbow
  - Abduction with bent elbow
  - External/internal rotation with arm in scapular plane
  - Elbow flexion
- Continue use of ice for pain control
  - Use ice at least 6 to 7 times daily
- Sleeping
  - Continue sleeping in brace until physician instructs otherwise

Precautions
1. No lifting of objects
2. No excessive shoulder extension
3. No excessive stretching or sudden movements
4. No supporting of body weight by hands
5. Keep incision clean and dry

II. Phase II: Protection Phase (Day 11 to Week 6)

Goals
1. Allow healing of soft tissue
2. Do not overstress healing tissue
3. Gradually restore full passive range of motion (week 4 to 5)
4. Reestablish dynamic shoulder stability
5. Decrease pain and inflammation

A. Day 11 to 14
- Discontinue use of sling or brace
- Passive range of motion to tolerance
  - Flexion 0 *to* 125/145°
  - External rotation at 90° abduction to at least 45°
  - Internal rotation at 90° abduction to at least 45°
- Active-assisted range of motion to tolerance
  - Flexion
  - External/internal rotation in scapular plane
  - External/internal rotation at 90° abduction
- Dynamic stabilization drills
  - Rhythmic stabilization drills
    - External/internal rotation in scapular plane
    - Flexion/extension at 100° flexion
- Continue all isometric contractions
- Continue use of cryotherapy as needed
- Continue all precautions

B. Week 3 to 4
- Patient should exhibit full passive range of motion
- Continue all exercises listed above
- Initiate external/internal rotation strengthening using exercise tubing at 0° of abduction
- Initiate manual resistance external rotation supine in scapular plane
- Initiate prone rowing to neutral arm position
- Initiate isotonic elbow flexion
- Continue use of ice as needed
- May use heat before range of motion exercises
- May use pool for light range of motion exercises

C. Week 5 to 6
- May use heat before exercises
- Continue active-assisted range of motion and stretching exercises
- Initiate active range of motion exercises
  - Shoulder flexion scapular plane
  - Shoulder abduction
- Progress isotonic strengthening exercise program
  - External rotation tubing
  - Side-lying external rotation
  - Prone rowing
  - Prone horizontal abduction
  - Biceps curls

Precautions
1. No heavy lifting of objects
2. No excessive behind the back movements
3. No supporting of body weight by hands and arms
4. No sudden jerking motions

Continued

Table 19-8

Type II Rotator Cuff Repair Arthroscopic Assisted Mini-Open Repair for Medium to Large Tears (Greater than 1 cm, Less than 5 cm)—cont'd

III. Phase III: Intermediate Phase (Week 7 to 14)
Goals
1. Full active range of motion (week 8 to 10)
2. Full passive range of motion
3. Dynamic shoulder stability
4. Gradual restoration of shoulder strength and power
5. Gradual return to functional activities

A. Week 7
- Continue stretching and passive range of motion (as needed to maintain full range of motion)
- Continue dynamic stabilization drills
- Progress strengthening program
  - External/internal rotation tubing
  - External rotation side-lying
  - Lateral raises*
  - Full can in scapular plane*
  - Prone rowing
  - Prone horizontal abduction
  - Prone extension
  - Elbow flexion
  - Elbow extension

B. Week 8
- Continue all exercise listed above
- If physician permits, may initiate *light* functional activities

C. Week 14
- Continue all exercise listed above
- Progress to independent home exercise program (fundamental shoulder exercises)

IV. Phase IV: Advanced Strengthening Phase (Week 15 to 22)
Goals
1. Maintain full non-painful range of motion
2. Enhance functional use of upper extremity
3. Improve muscular strength and power
4. Gradual return to functional activities

A. Week 15
- Continue range of motion and stretching to maintain full range of motion
- Self-capsular stretches
- Progress shoulder strengthening exercises
  - Fundamental shoulder exercises
- Initiate interval golf program (if appropriate)

B. Week 20
- Continue all exercises listed above
- Progress golf program to playing golf (if appropriate)
- Initiate interval tennis program (if appropriate)
- May initiate swimming

V. Phase V: Return to Activity Phase (Week 23 to 30)
Goals
1. Gradual return to strenuous work activities
2. Gradual return to recreational sport activities

A. Week 23
- Continue fundamental shoulder exercise program (at least 4 times weekly)
- Continue stretching, if motion is tight
- Continue progression to sport participation

*Patient must be able to elevate the arm without shoulder or scapular hiking before initiating isotonics; if the patient is unable to do this, continue glenohumeral dynamic stabilization exercises.

Table 19-9

Type III Rotator Cuff Repair Arthroscopic Assisted Mini-Open Repair for Large to Massive Tears (Greater than 4 cm)

I. Phase I: Immediate Postoperative Phase (Day 1 to 10)
Goals
1. Maintain integrity of the repair
2. Gradually increase passive range of motion
3. Diminish pain and inflammation
4. Prevent muscular inhibition

A. Day 1 to 6
- Sling or slight abduction brace *(physician decision)*
- Pendulum exercises 4 to 8 times daily (flexion, circles)
- Active assisted range of motion exercise (L-bar)
  - External/internal rotation in scapular plane
- Passive range of motion
  - Flexion to tolerance
  - External/internal rotation in scapular plane (gentle range of motion)
- Elbow/hand gripping and range of motion exercises
- Submaximal gentle isometrics
  - Flexion
  - Abduction
  - External rotation
  - Internal rotation
  - Elbow flexors
- Cryotherapy for pain and inflammation
  - Ice 15 to 20 minutes every hour
- Sleeping
  - Sleep in sling or brace

B. Day 7 to 10
- Continue use of brace or sling
- Continue pendulum exercises
- Progress passive range of motion to tolerance
  - Flexion to at least 90°
  - External rotation in scapular plane to 35°
  - Internal rotation in scapular plane to 35°
- Continue elbow/hand range of motion and gripping exercises
- Continue submaximal isometrics

Table 19-9

Type III Rotator Cuff Repair Arthroscopic Assisted Mini-Open Repair for Large to Massive Tears (Greater than 4 cm)—cont'd

- Flexion with bent elbow
- Extension with bent elbow
- Abduction with bent elbow
- External/internal rotation with arm in scapular plane
- Elbow flexion
- Continue use of ice for pain control
  - Use ice at least 6 to 7 times daily
- Sleeping
  - Continue sleeping in brace until physician instructs otherwise

Precautions
1. Maintain arm in brace, remove only for exercise
2. No lifting of objects
3. No excessive shoulder extension
4. No excessive or aggressive stretching or sudden movements
5. No supporting of body weight by hands
6. Keep incision clean and dry

II. Phase II: Protection Phase (Day 11 to Week 6)

Goals
1. Allow healing of soft tissue
2. Do not overstress healing tissue
3. Gradually restore full passive range of motion (week 4 to 5)
4. Reestablish dynamic shoulder stability
5. Decrease pain and inflammation

A. Day 11 to 14
- Continue use of brace
- Passive range of motion to tolerance
  - Flexion 0 to approximately 125°
  - External rotation at 90° abduction to at least 45°
  - Internal rotation at 90° abduction to at least 45°
- Active assisted range of motion to tolerance
  - External/internal rotation in scapular plane
  - External/internal rotation at 90° abduction
- Dynamic stabilization drills
  - Rhythmic stabilization drills
    - External/internal rotation in scapular plane
    - Flexion/extension at 100° flexion
- Continue all isometric contractions
- Continue use of cryotherapy as needed
- Continue all precautions

B. Week 3 to 4
- Initiate active-assisted range of motion flexion in supine (therapist supports arm during motion)
- Continue all exercises listed above
- Initiate external/internal rotation strengthening using exercise tubing at 0° of abduction
- Progress passive range of motion till approximately full range of motion at week 4 to 5
- Initiate prone rowing to neutral arm position
- Initiate isotonic elbow flexion
- Continue use of ice as needed

- May use heat before range of motion exercises
- May use pool for light range of motion exercises
- Continue use of brace during sleeping until end of week 4
- Discontinue use of brace at end of week 4

C. Week 5 to 6
- May use heat before exercises
- Continue active-assisted range of motion and stretching exercises
- Initiate active range of motion exercises
  - Shoulder flexion scapular plane
  - Shoulder abduction
- Progress isotonic strengthening exercise program
  - External rotation tubing
  - Side-lying external rotation
  - Prone rowing
  - Prone horizontal abduction
  - Biceps curls

Precautions
1. No lifting
2. No excessive behind the back movements
3. No supporting of body weight by hands and arms
3. No sudden jerking motions

III. Phase III: Intermediate Phase (Week 7 to 14)

Goals
1. Full active range of motion (week 10 to 12)
2. Maintain full passive range of motion
3. Dynamic shoulder stability
4. Gradual restoration of shoulder strength and power
5. Gradual return to functional activities

A. Week 7
- Continue stretching and passive range of motion (as needed to maintain full range of motion)
- Continue dynamic stabilization drills
- Progress strengthening program
  - External/internal rotation tubing
  - External rotation side-lying
  - Lateral raises* (active range of motion only)
  - Full can in scapular plane* (active range of motion only)
  - Prone rowing
  - Prone horizontal abduction
  - Elbow flexion
  - Elbow extension

B. Week 8 to 10
- Continue all exercise listed above
- Progress to isotonic lateral raises and full can
- If physician permits, may initiate light functional activities

C. Week 14
- Continue all exercise listed above
- Progress to independent home exercise program (fundamental shoulder exercises)

Continued

Table 19-9

Type III Rotator Cuff Repair Arthroscopic Assisted Mini-Open Repair for Large to Massive Tears (Greater than 4 cm)—cont'd

IV. Phase IV: Advanced Strengthening Phase (Week 15 to 22)
Goals
1. Maintain full non-painful range of motion
2. Enhance functional use of upper extremity
3. Improve muscular strength and power
4. Gradual return to functional activities
A. Week 15
- Continue range of motion and stretching to maintain full range of motion
- Self-capsular stretches
- Progress shoulder strengthening exercises
- Fundamental shoulder exercises
B. Week 20
- Continue all exercises listed above

- Continue to perform range of motion stretching, if motion is not complete

V. Phase V: Return to Activity Phase (Week 23 to 30)
Goals
1. Gradual return to strenuous work activities
2. Gradual return to recreational sport activities
A. Week 23
- Continue fundamental shoulder exercise program (at least 4 times weekly)
- Continue stretching, if motion is tight
B. Week 26
- May initiate interval sport program (i.e., golf, etc.)

*Patient must be able to elevate the arm without shoulder or scapular hiking before initiating isotonics; if the patient is unable to do this, continue glenohumeral dynamic stabilization exercises.

An abduction pillow (Fig. 19-26) can be used after rotator cuff repair to alleviate stress on the cuff repair, because the adducted position may cause undue early stress on the repair, especially in large to massive tears. Lesion size and extent of repair determine whether an abduction pillow will be used and the duration of use. In most patients, an abduction pillow or splint is not used after rotator cuff repair (except in large tears). Use of the pillow can range from 2 to 5 weeks. Immediately after the repair, passive range-of-motion exercises should be performed to minimize the patient's chances of developing adhesive capsulitis or a stiff shoulder. AAROM may be initiated when the

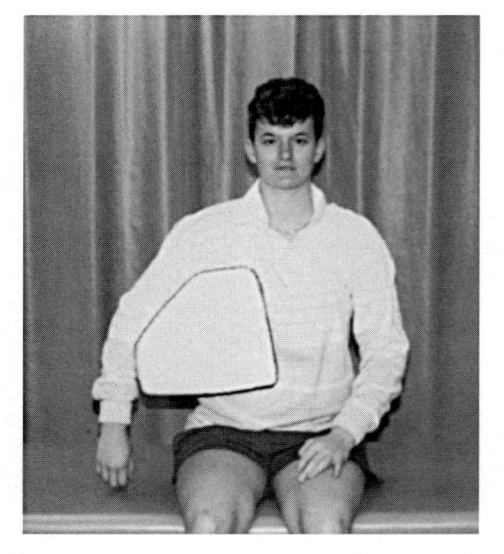

Figure 19-26. The use of an abduction pillow after rotator cuff repair can help alleviate stress placed on the repair.

physician feels that the repair has healed adequately. As active range of motion is restored, a PRE program should be initiated with a focus on posterior cuff and scapular stabilizer muscle strengthening. Postoperative rehabilitation depends on the extent of the cuff lesion, the tissue quality, and the procedure used for the repair. Recently, in the early 2000s arthroscopic rotator cuff repairs have become more popular. With arthroscopic repairs there is less scarring and loss of motion. However, we feel that the fixation which is currently available is not as secure as that for an open procedure; thus, rehabilitation is slower.

In all of our rehabilitation programs after shoulder stabilization surgery, we have a multiple-phase approach, with each phase consisting of specific goals and exercises (Table 19-10). We also use a criteria-based rehabilitation approach to help guide the rate of rehabilitation progression.

In the first phase, the immediate postoperative period, the rehabilitation goals are to (1) protect the healing soft tissues, (2) prevent the negative effects of immobilization, (3) reestablish dynamic joint stability, and (4) diminish postoperative pain and inflammation. Thus, during this maximal protection phase, we use early motion in a restricted and protected arc of motion. This early motion is intended to nourish the articular cartilage, assist in collagen tissue synthesis and collagen organization, and promote healing. Early motion will assist in decreasing the patient's pain through neuromuscular modulation.[59,80,168,178] Depending on the type of surgical procedure, method of fixation, and the patient's tissue status, a prescribed range of motion is outlined. The primary goal of this phase is to prevent excessive scarring but not allow too aggressive motion to compromise the surgical repair. Often after

Table 19-10

Rehabilitation Phases and Goals

I. Phase One: Acute Phase

A. Goals
- Diminish pain and inflammation
- Normalize motion
- Retard muscular atrophy
- Re-establish dynamic stability
- Control functional stress/strain

B. Exercises and Modalities
- Cryotherapy, ultrasound, electrical stimulation
- Flexibility and stretching for posterior shoulder muscles
- Rotator cuff strengthening (especially external rotators)
- Scapular muscles strengthening (especially retractors, protractors, depressors)
- Dynamic stabilization exercises (rhythmic stabilization)
- Closed kinetic chain exercises
- Proprioception training
- Abstain from throwing

II. Phase Two: Intermediate Phase

A. Goals
- Progress strengthening exercise
- Restore muscular balance (external/internal rotation)
- Enhance dynamic stability
- Control flexibility and stretches

B. Exercises and Modalities
- Continue stretching and flexibility
- Progress isotonic strengthening
  - Complete shoulder program
- Throwers' Ten Exercise Program
- Rhythmic stabilization drills
- Initiate core strengthening program
- Initiate leg program

III. Phase Three: Advanced Strengthening Phase

A. Goals
- Aggressive strengthening
- Progressive neuromuscular control
- Improve strength, power and endurance
- Initiate light throwing activities

B. Exercises and Modalities
- Flexibility and stretching
- Rhythmic stabilization drills
- Throwers' Ten Exercise Program
- Initiate plyometric program
- Initiate endurance drills
- Initiate short distance throwing program

IV. Phase Four: Return to Activity Phase

A. Goals
- Progress to throwing program
- Return to competitive throwing
- Continue strengthening and flexibility drills

B. Exercises
- Stretching and flexibility drills
- Throwers' Ten Exercise Program
- Plyometric program
- Progress interval throwing program to competitive throwing

anterior stabilization, motions such as extension and external rotation are limited or restricted because of the anterior capsule, whereas shoulder elevation in the scapular plane is encouraged instead of shoulder abduction. Dynamic stabilization exercises are performed to reestablish dynamic joint stability. These stability drills are performed with the patient maintaining a static position as the clinician facilitates a muscular co-contraction (Figs. 19-27 and 19-28). The static joint position should be carefully chosen by the clinician to prevent excessive stress on the stabilization procedure. Submaximal isometrics are performed for the rotator cuff to initiate voluntary muscular contractions of these muscles, which aids in preventing muscular atrophy and a loss of motor control. Wickiewicz and colleagues[190] reported that most human shoulder musculature is roughly a 50:50 mixture of slow-and fast-twitch muscle fibers. Immobilization has been shown to have a greater effect on slow-twitch fibers; thus, it is important for the patient to perform submaximal isometrics to prevent muscular atrophy. During this first week, we attempt to control the patient's pain and inflammation through guarded motion and isometric exercises and the judicious use of various therapeutic modalities (ice, electrical stimulation, etc.).

Phase II, the intermediate phase, emphasizes the advancement of shoulder mobility. Before the patient enters phase II, the following criteria must be met: (1) satisfactory static stability, (2) diminishing pain and inflammation, and (3) adequate muscular control and dynamic stability. During this phase, the patient's range of motion is gradually increased by using AAROM and PROM exercises, stretching, and joint-mobilization techniques. Guidelines for motion progression are based on the surgical procedure, method of fixation, and the patient's tissue status and are discussed throughout this chapter. Additionally, the rate of progression is based on the clinician's assessment of the quantity and endfeel of motion. For example, in a patient with less motion than desirable at that time and a firm or hard endfeel, stretch is more aggressive than in a patient who has a capsular or soft-endfeel. Joint-mobilization techniques are used to restore normal motion and to correct asymmetric capsular tightness; thus, the anterior capsule and posterior capsule should exhibit comparable flexibility. If one side of the capsule is excessively

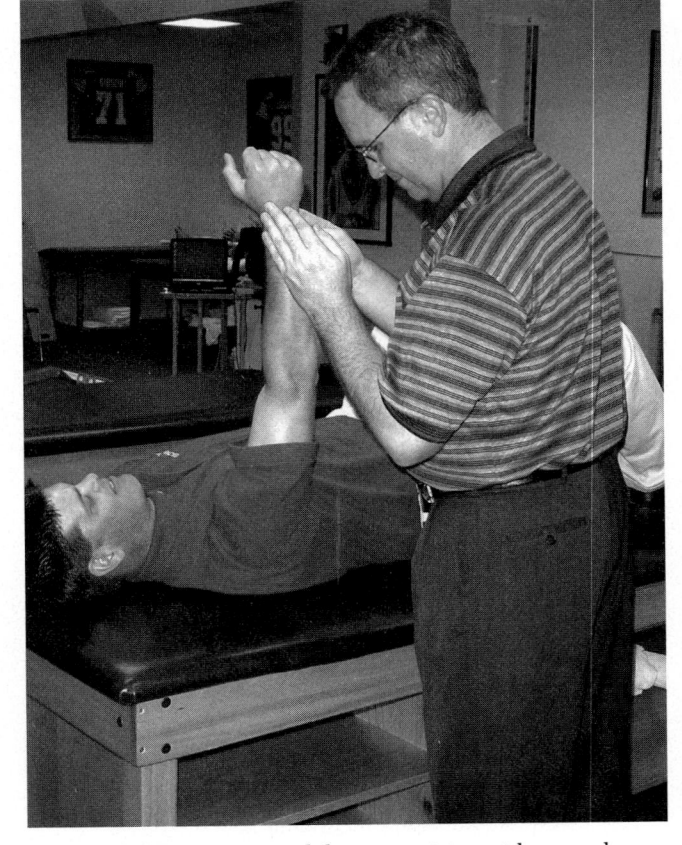

Figure 19-27. Dynamic stabilization training with manual resistance in the balanced shoulder position.

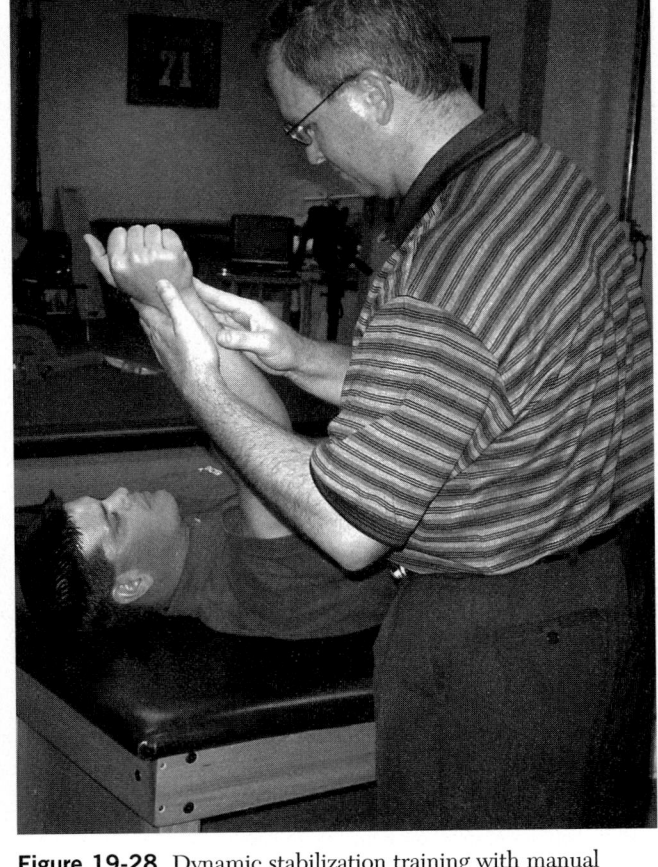

Figure 19-28. Dynamic stabilization training with manual resistance in 120° of glenohumeral elevation.

tight compared with the opposite side, this will result in the humeral head displacing excessively in the opposite direction, away from the tightness.[81,200] Thus, if the anterior capsule is excessively tight compared with the posterior capsule (after anterior stabilization surgery), the humeral head will tend to displace posteriorly during arm movements.[85] Correcting asymmetric capsular tightness should be a critical goal for the clinician. Other goals during this phase include improving muscular strength and enhancing neuromuscular control. To achieve these goals, we use PNF techniques with rhythmic stabilization,[199] neuromuscular control drills (Fig. 19-29)[199,200] and isolated muscular strengthening exercises for the rotator cuff and scapular muscles. In the overhead throwing athlete, toward the end of this phase, the clinician can begin aggressive stretching techniques to gradually increase motion past 90° of external rotation. External rotation of approximately 115 ± 5° is necessary for the these athletes to be able to begin throwing. Strengthening exercises are focused on reestablishing muscular balance, particularly the external rotation/internal rotation unilateral muscle ratio. During this phase we usually initiate the Throwers' Ten Exercise Program (Appendix A).

The third phase, the dynamic strengthening phase, is focused on improving the patient's strength, power, and endurance while maintaining a functional range of motion of the shoulder joint. The criteria that should be met before entering phase III are (1) full nonpainful functional motion, (2) muscular strength of at least 4 over 5 or of the good grade (manual muscle test), (3) satisfactory static stability on clinical examination, and (4) dynamic joint stability. Resistance exercises are progressed during this phase. The goal of this phase is to reestablish significant strength for the desired functional activities but also to reestablish muscular balance. Thus, a suitable ratio should exist between the posterior and anterior muscles, rotator cuff and deltoid muscles, and retractor and protractor scapular muscles. The muscular ratios we strive for are external rotation/internal rotation ratios of 62% to 70%, posterior rotator cuff (external rotation) to deltoid (abduction) ratio of 66% to 72%, and scapular retractor to protractor ratio of approximately 100%.[201] Muscular balance and dynamic joint stability should be achieved before aggressive strengthening exercises such as plyometrics or functional activities such as throwing and swimming are initiated to ensure that dynamic joint stability has been accomplished. During this phase, eccentric muscle training and proprioceptive training are emphasized. Muscular endurance training also is emphasized in this phase. This is a critical

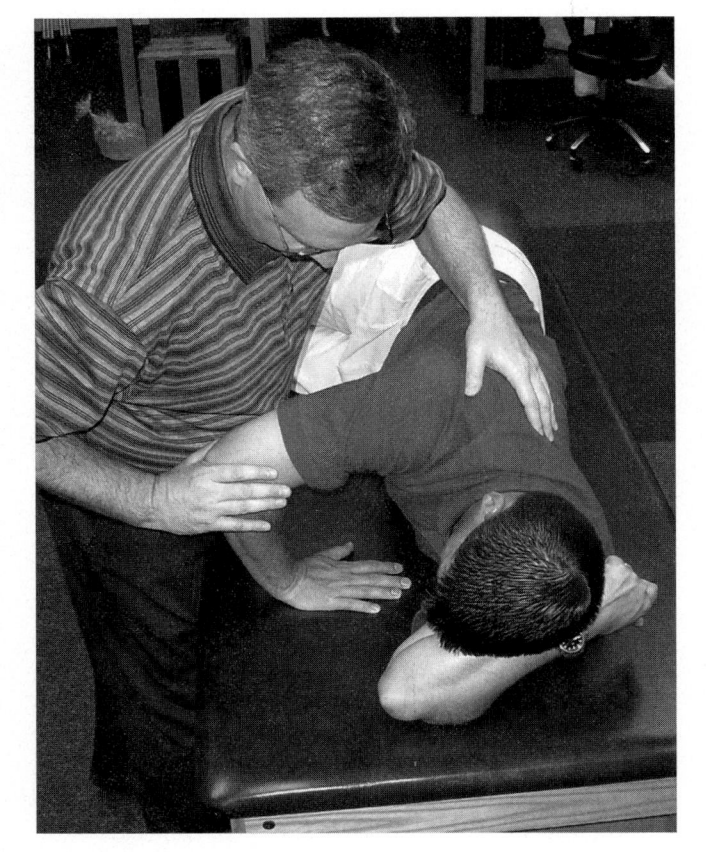

Figure 19-29. Side-lying manual neuromuscular control drills for scapulothoracic control.

element in the rehabilitation program. Wickiewicz and associates[189] showed that once the rotator cuff muscles have reached a significant level of fatigue, the humeral head displaces superiorly with simple arm movements such as shoulder abduction. The rehabilitation program should emphasize muscular endurance training to enhance dynamic functional joint stability and to prevent fatigue-induced subluxation.[192] Plyometric training drills are used in this phase to generally increase the athlete's shoulder motion and to gradually increase the functional stresses onto the shoulder joint.

Phase IV is referred to as the return-to-activity phase. The goal of this phase is to gradually and progressively increase the functional demands on the shoulder to return the patient to full, unrestricted sport or daily activities. The criteria established before a patient's return to sport activities are (1) full functional range of motion, (2) adequate static stability, (3) satisfactory muscular strength and endurance, (4) adequate dynamic stability, and (5) a satisfactory clinical examination. Once these criteria have been successfully met, the patient may initiate a gradual return to sport activity in a controlled manner. Healing constraints based on surgical technique and fixation, as well as the patient's tissue status, should be considered before a functional program is initiated. Other goals of this phase

are to maintain the patient's muscular strength, dynamic stability, and shoulder functional motion established in the previous phase. A stretching and strengthening program should be performed on an ongoing basis to maintain and continue to improve on these goals.

Rehabilitation after Thermal Capsular Shrinkage

Rehabilitation after thermal capsular shrinkage of the shoulder follows several key rehabilitation guidelines.[201] These rehabilitation guidelines include (1) the type of patient, (2) the patient's response to surgery, (3) the patient's tissue status, (4) the inflammatory reaction after surgery, (5) concomitant procedures, and (6) the patient's desired goals. The rehabilitation program must be adjusted to the type of patient and thus to the etiology of underlying instability.[20] Types of instability can include congenital atraumatic instability or acquired laxity, which is seen in athletes performing overhead movements. Another factor to consider is the patient's response to surgery, which includes not only the amount of motion, but also the feel at end range. Third, the program must be adjusted to the patient's tissue status. One technique to evaluate the patient's tissue status is to assess the contralateral shoulder. If a positive sulcus sign is seen on the uninvolved side or nonoperative shoulder, then we use a slower rate of progression through the rehabilitation program. Conversely, if a negative sulcus sign is present, then we follow our typical motion protocol. Another factor to consider is the patient's inflammatory response to the surgery. Hayashi and colleagues[88] demonstrated that an inflammatory reaction is present for at least 8 weeks and may be present as long as 3 to 6 months after a thermal procedure. This inflammatory reaction many times can lead to joint stiffness and soreness, which may limit the patient's progression in motion. Another factor to consider is concomitant procedures performed at the time of the thermal capsular shrinkage. Often, a SLAP repair or a rotator cuff débridement is performed concomitantly with the thermal capsular shrinkage. Also, the rehabilitation specialist must be cautious during the first 4 to 6 weeks to not include excessive stretching. Hecht and co-workers[89] demonstrated that during the first 8 weeks after a thermal procedure, the collagen tissue is extremely vulnerable to tissue stretch out; thus during the first 6 to 8 weeks the rehabilitation specialist must be cautious to not use overaggressive range-of-motion exercises. Schaefer and associates[170] demonstrated that use of overaggressive activities during the first 8 weeks after thermal application to patellar tendons in rabbits resulted in an overall increase in the resting length of the tendon. Lastly, the rehabilitation program must be adjusted to the patient's goals; thus, the professional athlete tends to follow a more aggressive type of rehabilitation program than the recreational athlete or the individual who has a congenitally laxed shoulder.

Ellenbecker and Mattalino[64] published a rehabilitation program for use after thermal capsular shrinkage and emphasized 2 to 4 weeks of immobilization. This was followed by range-of-motion exercises starting at week 4 and progressing to week 12. An aggressive strengthening program was then instituted at week 12 progressing to week 18. The authors emphasized no aggressive stretching for the first month to 6 weeks. Tyler and colleagues[183] published their rehabilitation program and emphasized the use of a sling for 4 weeks, allowing pendulum exercises but no stretching or active-assisted motion. At week 4, an AAROM program was used with range of motion being restored at week 12. A gradual return to sport was initiated at week 16.

Our rehabilitation program after thermal capsular shrinkage in athletes involved in overhead sports is presented in Table 19-11.[201] Immediately after surgery, we allow immediate motion but not stretching. We allow active-assisted flexion range of motion to be performed with a wand or L-bar to approximately 70°. We allow active-assisted internal and external rotation range of motion to be performed in the plane of the scapula at 30° of abduction, in a comfortable range. We do not allow excessive external rotation, elevation, or shoulder extension. This type of range-of-motion program is allowed during the first 2 weeks with a goal of immediate motion to stimulate proliferation of collagen tissue. It also assists in collagen synthesis, organization, alignment, and strength. Thus, we allow gradual progressive applied loads, but we caution against overaggressive stretching. At week 3, we allow internal/external rotation to be performed at 45° of abduction. We allow external rotation to approximately 30°. Internal rotation can be performed to touch the side. Active-assisted flexion is allowed to 90° and gradually progression past 90° during week 4. At week 5, we allow internal and external rotation to be performed at 90° of abduction. Our goal is by week 6 to have 75° of external rotation and by week 8 to have 90° external rotation at 90° of abduction. Usually by week 6 to 8, flexion is 170° to 180°. For the overhead throwing athlete, particularly a pitcher, we want to gain external rotation to approximately 115°. This goal is usually achieved no earlier than week 12. Wilk and co-workers[200] documented that professional pitchers exhibit 129° of external rotation. Thus, we allow stretching to 115° and functional activities to gain the rest of the motion necessary to throw. Therefore, by week 12, the overhead throwing athlete should have 115° of external rotation and approximately 60° to 65° of internal rotation.

Muscle training drills and exercises are performed immediately after surgery. These are done in the form of isometrics. Isometrics are performed in mid-range and are allowed to be performed submaximally for co-activation for the glenohumeral joint dynamic stabilizers. We allow isometrics for the first 7 to 10 days in a submaximal, sub-painful manner, usually allowing internal and external rotation, abduction, shoulder flexion, and biceps. At approximately 10 to 14 days postoperatively a light isotonic program will be allowed. We emphasize external rotation and scapular strengthening muscles. At week 5, the athlete is allowed to progress to the Throwers' Ten Exercise Program (Appendix A). Plyometrics are allowed at approximately 8 weeks postoperatively. Two-hand plyometric drills are permitted with restriction in the amount of external rotation. After 10 to 14 days, two-hand plyometric drills are progressed by incorporation of one-hand drills. An aggressive strengthening program is allowed starting at week 12, progressing to week 16. The program is adjusted according to the patient's response to the strengthening program and to surgery. A gradual return to throwing is instituted at week 16 in the form of a long toss throwing program (Appendix B). The interval throwing program is then progressed to mound throwing at week 22 to 24 (Appendix B).

Rehabilitation after thermal capsular shrinkage must be modified and adjusted to the patient's response to surgery. The program needs to be assessed and adjusted weekly, and not all patients appear to respond in the same manner after this surgical procedure. Some patients develop complications such as hyperelastic or looseness, whereas others may develop capsular stiffness. The program must be adjusted accordingly to prevent these complications from occurring. Dynamic stabilization, proprioception, and neuromuscular control should also be emphasized. This is to enhance dynamic stabilization of the glenohumeral joint during the throwing motion.

The results from this surgical procedure appear promising. Based on 2- to 3-year follow-up studies, it appears that 85% to 87% of all athletes return to their overhead sport after thermal capsular shrinkage.

Rehabilitation after Arthroscopic Stabilization Procedures

Another surgical procedure performed on overhead throwers is an arthroscopic stabilization technique to either repair a Bankart-type lesion or tighten the capsule. At our center, we use either a suture-anchor device or a cannulated absorbable fixation device* for the arthroscopic stabilization technique for repair of a Bankart lesion as described by Warner and Warren.[187] The overhead throwing athlete must exhibit specific criteria to be considered a candidate for arthroscopic stabilization.

The rehabilitation program after arthroscopic stabilization is significantly different from that after the open stabilization. The rate of progression immediately after surgery is much slower in the arthroscopically stabilized

---

*Available from Suretac, Acufex Microsurgical Inc., Mansfield, Massachusetts.

Table 19-11

Thermal Capsular Shrinkage: Athlete in Overhead Sports

I. Phase I: Protection Phase (Day 1 to Week 6)
Goals
1. Allow soft tissue healing
2. Diminish pain and inflammation
3. Initiate protected motion
4. Retard muscular atrophy

A. Week 0 to 2
- Sling use for 7 to 10 days
- Sleep in sling/brace for 7 days

Exercises
- Hand gripping exercises
- Elbow and wrist range of motion exercises
- Active range of motion cervical spine
- Passive and active-assisted range of motion exercises
  - Elevation to 75 to 90°
  - Internal rotation in scapular plane (45° by 2 weeks)
  - External rotation in scapular plane (25° by 2 weeks)
- Rope-and-pulley (flexion) active-assisted range of motion
- Cryotherapy to control pain
- Submaximal isometrics
- Rhythmic stabilization exercises at 7 days
- Proprioception and neuromuscular control drills

B. Week 3 to 4
- Range of motion exercises (active-assisted range of motion, passive range of motion, active range of motion)
  - Elevation to 125 to 135°
  - Internal rotation, in scapular plane, full motion
  - External rotation, in scapular plane 45 to 50° by week 4
  - At week 4, begin external/internal rotation at 90° abduction
- Strengthening exercises
  - Initiate *light* isotonic program
  - External/internal rotation exercise tubing (0° abduction)
  - Continue dynamic stabilization drills
  - Scapular strengthening exercises
  - Biceps/triceps strengthening
  - Proprioceptive neuromuscular facilitation D2 flexion/extension manual resistance
- Continue use of cryotherapy and modalities to control pain

C. Week 5 to 6
- Continue all exercises listed above
- Progress range of motion to the following:
  - Elevation to 145 to 160° by week 6
  - External rotation at 90° abduction (75 to 80°)
  - Internal rotation at 90° abduction (65 to 70°)
  - Initiate Throwers' Ten Exercise Program

II. Phase II: Intermediate Phase (Week 7 to 12)
Goals
1. Restore full range of motion (week 7)
2. Restore functional range of motion (week 10 to 11)
3. Normalize arthrokinematics
4. Improve dynamic stability, muscular strength

A. Week 7 to 8
- Progress range of motion to the following:
  - Elevation to 180°
  - External rotation at 90° abduction to 90 to 100° by week 8
  - internal rotation at 90° abduction to 70 to 75°
- Continue stretching program
- Strengthening exercises
- Continue Throwers' Ten Exercise Program
- Continue manual resistance, dynamic stabilization drills
- Initiate plyometrics (Two-handed drills)

B. Week 9 to 12
- Progress range of motion to the athlete's demands
  - Gradual progression from week 9 to 12
- Strengthening exercises
  - Progress isotonic program
  - May initiate more aggressive strengthening
    - Push-ups
    - Shoulder press
    - Bench press
    - Pull-downs
    - Single-arm plyometrics

III. Phase III: Advanced Activity and Strengthening Phase (Week 12 to 20)
Goals
1. Improve strength, power, and endurance
2. Enhance neuromuscular control
3. Functional activities

Criteria to Enter Phase III
1. Full range of motion
2. No pain or tenderness
3. Muscular strength 80% of contralateral side

A. Week 12 to 16
- Self-capsular stretches, active range of motion, passive stretching
- Continue all strengthening exercises
  - Isotonics
  - Plyometrics
  - Neuromuscular control/dynamic stabilization drills
- Initiate interval sport program (throwing, tennis, swimming, etc.)

B. Week 16 to 20
- Progress all exercises listed above
- May resume normal training program
- Continue specific strengthening exercises
- Progress interval program (throwing program to phase II)

IV. Phase IV: Return to Activity Phase (Week 22 to 26)
Goals
1. Gradual return to unrestricted activities
2. Maintain static and dynamic stability of shoulder joint

Criteria to Enter Phase IV
1. Full functional range of motion
2. No pain or tenderness
3. Satisfactory muscular strength (isokinetic test)
4. Satisfactory clinical exam

Exercises
1. Continue maintenance for range of motion
2. Continue strengthening exercises
3. Gradual return to competition

shoulder because of the method of fixation used. Shall and Crowley[172] reported the pull-out strength of various soft tissue fixation devices. The Suretac was found to fail ultimately at approximately 122 N (27 pounds), with the majority of failures (94%) occurring because of the tack pulling out from the bone. The investigators reported that the suture anchor (Mitek super-anchor)* was almost twice as strong (failing at 217 N). The Suretac is made of polyglyconate polymer that loses it strength over a 4- to 6-week period and gradually becomes reabsorbed during the next several months.[187] It is important for the clinician to realize that the strength of the arthroscopic tissue fixation method is somewhat tenuous for the first 4 to 6 weeks, and care should be taken not to disturb the soft tissue repair. For that reason, the initial postoperative rehabilitation is much slower for a shoulder undergoing arthroscopic stabilization than for a shoulder on which an open procedure was performed.

Several authors briefly outlined their postoperative rehabilitation programs after arthroscopic stabilization.[1,78,135,136] Some of them advocated postoperative immobilization for 4 to 6 weeks and a guarded motion program with a gradual restoration of motion. Wickiewicz and colleagues[190] suggested 4 weeks of immobilization followed by AAROM and PROM exercises from week 4 and full motion by approximately 2.5 months. Various authors suggested several time frames for immobilization. Some authors suggested 3 weeks of immobilization,[1,78,135] others 4 weeks,[78] and others 6 weeks after arthroscopic stabilization. Grana and associates[78] noted that some patients may not comply with long periods of strict immobilization because of minimal pain and less operative morbidity. These patients may return to some activities prematurely. Grana and associates[78] reported on 27 patients who underwent arthroscopic suture stabilization. The authors noted that 10 patients admitted removal of the immobilizer after the first week; for 8 of 10 of these patients results were rated as poor because of recurrent instability. Most investigators agree on restricting or limiting shoulder abduction and external rotation for several weeks (4 to 6 weeks), initiating a strengthening program at 4 to 8 weeks, and restricting contact sports or strenuous sports for 6 months.

The rehabilitation program of two of the authors (K.E.W. and C.A.) is divided into four specific phases (Table 19-12). The first phase is considered the maximal protection phase or restricted motion phase. Immediately after surgery, the patient's shoulder is placed in an immobilizer brace; this brace is used consistently for the first 2 to 3 weeks and is worn during sleep for 4 weeks after surgery. The patient will use a sling during daily activities from weeks 2 to 4. During the first 2 weeks, the patient is allowed to perform AAROM and PROM exercises. The

active-assisted motion is restricted to 60° of forward flexion, 45° of internal rotation, and 5 to 10° of external rotation with the arm placed in 20° of abduction. Additionally, PROM is performed for shoulder flexion and abduction to a maximum of 90° and internal rotation and external rotation, with the arm at 20° of abduction to tolerance. These ranges are strictly enforced to prevent potentially deleterious forces on the anteroinferior aspect of the glenohumeral capsule where the surgical procedure has been performed. During this phase, the patient also performs submaximal and subpainful isometrics for the shoulder musculature. Additionally, cryotherapy and other modalities may be used to reduce postoperative pain and inflammation.

At weeks 3 to 4, use of the sling is usually discontinued; this is based on the clinical assessment of the stability of the joint and the patient's response to surgery and pain level. Occasionally, the patient is encouraged to continue the use of the shoulder immobilizer while sleeping to restrict excessive uncontrolled shoulder motions and positioning. At this time, AAROM and PROM exercises are continued gradually to improve abduction and external rotation, as well as flexion and internal rotation. At 4 weeks, we increase but restrict active-assisted and passive abduction and flexion motion to 90° of shoulder abduction, which are limited to 15 to 20 and 60°, respectively. In addition, the patient will perform light strengthening exercises such as rhythmic stabilization exercises for the external rotation/internal rotation muscles and submaximal isometrics for all the shoulder musculature, both to restore dynamic joint stability.

At weeks 5 to 6, the goal is to gradually restore motion. The external rotation/internal rotation stretching and motion exercises are performed at 45° of abduction, which produces a mild stretch on the inferior capsule (during external rotation motion). The patient is encouraged to gradually improve shoulder flexion, progressing to 135 to 140° at 6 weeks. Also at this time, we will allow the patient to begin light resistance isotonic strengthening exercises. The external rotation/internal rotation muscles are exercised by using exercise tubing. Additionally, a lightweight (1 to 2 pounds) can be used to perform abduction to 90°, flexion to 90°, and scapular musculature strengthening.

During the first 6 weeks, we restrict motion to prevent overloading or overstressing the repaired capsule. Furthermore, we attempt to allow gradual restoration of motion, which helps prevent the negative effects of immobilization and assists in collagen formation and organization. During these first 6 weeks, care must be taken by the clinician not to overstress the healing tissue and the soft tissue fixation.

Phase II, the moderate protection phase, begins at week 6 and progresses to week 14. The goals of this phase are to (1) gradually restore full, nonpainful range of motion, (2) preserve the integrity of the surgical repair,

---

*Available from Mitek Surgical Products, Westwood, Massachusetts.

Table 19-12

Rehabilitation Protocol after Arthroscopic Anterior Bankart Repair

I. Phase I: Immediate Postoperative Phase "Restrictive Motion" (Week 0 to 6)

Goals
1. Protect the anatomic repair
2. Prevent negative effects of immobilization
3. Promote dynamic stability and proprioception
4. Diminish pain and inflammation

A. Week 0 to 2
- Sling for 2 to 3 weeks
- Sleep in immobilizer for 4 weeks
- Elbow/hand range of motion
- Hand gripping exercises
- Passive and gentle active assistive range of motion exercise
- Flexion to 70° week 1
- Flexion to 90° week 2
- External/internal rotation with arm 30° abduction
  - External rotation to 5 to 10°
  - Internal rotation to 45°
  NO active external rotation or extension or abduction
- Submaximal isometrics for shoulder musculature
- Rhythmic stabilization drills: external/internal rotation
- Proprioception drills
- Cryotherapy, other modalities as indicated

B. Week 3 to 4
- Discontinue use of sling
- Use immobilizer for sleep *(physician decision)*
- Continue gentle range of motion exercises (passive range of motion and active-assisted range of motion)
  - Flexion to 90°
  - Abduction to 90°
  - External/internal rotation at 45° abd in scapular plane
  - External rotation in scapular plane to 15 to 20°
  - Internal rotation in scapular plane to 55 to 60°
  NOTE: Rate of progression based on evaluation of the patient
- No excessive external rotation, extension, or elevation
- Continue isometrics and rhythmic stabilization (submaximal)
- Core stabilization program
- Initiate scapular strengthening program
- Continue use of cryotherapy

C. Week 5 to 6
- Gradually improve range of motion
  - Flexion to 145°
  - External rotation at 45° abduction: 55 to 50°
  - Internal rotation at 45° abduction: 55 to 60°
- May initiate stretching exercises
- Initiate exercise tubing external/internal rotation (arm at side)
- Scapular strengthening
- Proprioceptive neuromuscular facilitation manual resistance

II. Phase II: Intermediate Phase—Moderate Protection Phase (Week 7 to 14)

Goals
1. Gradually restore full range of motion (week 10)
2. Preserve the integrity of the surgical repair
3. Restore muscular strength and balance
4. Enhance neuromuscular control

A. Week 7 to 9
- Gradually progress range of motion
- Flexion to 160°
- Initiate external/internal rotation at 90° abduction
  - External rotation at 90° abduction: 70 to 80° at week 7
  - External rotation to 90° at weeks 8 to 9
  - Internal rotation at 90° abduction: 70 to 75°
- Continue to progress isotonic strengthening program
- Continue proprioceptive neuromuscular facilitation strengthening

B. Week 10 to 14
- May initiate slightly more aggressive strengthening
- Progress isotonic strengthening exercises
- Continue all stretching exercises
Progress Range of Motion to Functional Demands (i.e., Overhead Activity)
- Progress to isotonic strengthening (light and restricted range of motion)

III. Phase III: Minimal Protection Phase (Week 15 to 20)

Goals
1. Maintain full range of motion
2. Improve muscular strength, power, and endurance
3. Gradually initiate functional activities

Criteria to Enter Phase III
1. Full non-painful range of motion
2. Satisfactory stability
3. Muscular strength (good grade or better)
4. No pain or tenderness

A. Week 15 to 18
- Continue all stretching exercises (capsular stretches)
- Continue strengthening exercises:
  - Throwers' Ten Exercise Program or fundamental exercises
  - Proprioceptive neuromuscular facilitation manual resistance
  - Endurance training
  - Restricted sport activities (light swimming, half-golf swings)
- Initiate interval sport program (week 16 to 18)

B. Week 18 to 20
- Continue all exercises listed above
- Process interval sport program (throwing, etc.)

IV. Phase IV: Advanced Strengthening Phase (Week 21 to 24)

Goals
1. Enhance muscular strength, power and endurance
2. Progress functional activities
3. Maintain shoulder mobility

Continued

Table 19-12

Rehabilitation Protocol after Arthroscopic Anterior Bankart Repair—cont'd

Criteria to Enter Phase IV
1. Full non-painful range of motion
2. Satisfactory static stability
3. Muscular strength 75% to 80% of contralateral side
4. No pain or tenderness

A. Week 21 to 24
- Continue flexibility exercises
- Continue isotonic strengthening program
- Neuromuscular control drills
- Plyometric strengthening
- Progress interval sport programs

V. Phase V: Return to Activity Phase (Month 7 to 9)
Goals
1. Gradual return to sport activities
2. Maintain strength, mobility and stability

Criteria to Enter Phase V
1. Full functional range of motion
2. Satisfactory isokinetic test that fulfills criteria
3. Satisfactory shoulder stability
4. No pain or tenderness

Exercises
- Gradually progress sport activities to unrestricted participation
- Continue stretching and strengthening program

(3) restore muscular strength and endurance, and (4) allow some functional activities.

During this phase, all motions gradually progress. Shoulder flexion and abduction progress to 180°. Shoulder internal rotation and external rotation motion exercises are performed at 90° of abduction, and at 7 to 8 weeks, the patient should have 75 to 80° of external rotation and full internal rotation (70 to 75°). At weeks 9 to 10, we expect full range of motion; external rotation should be approximately 85° to 90°. At week 12, we begin aggressively to stretch the thrower's shoulder past 90° or external rotation with the goal of 115 to 125° of external rotation. During this phase, all strengthening exercises gradually progress with the goal of improving rotator cuff and scapular strength, restoring muscular balance, and enhancing dynamic stabilization of the glenohumeral joint complex. The patient is not allowed to perform isotonic exercises on weight-lifting equipment such as the bench press, pullovers, and so on.

Phase III is the minimal-protection phase, extending from weeks 14 through 20. The goals of this phase are to

(1) establish or maintain full range of motion, (2) improve strength and endurance, and (3) initiate functional activities gradually. At approximately 14 to 16 weeks, activities such as light swimming exercises at 90° of abduction, plyometrics, and golf swings are permitted. An interval throwing program or other interval sport programs may be initiated at week 18 if the criteria (Appendix B) have been met by the patient.

The advanced strengthening phase extends from weeks 22 through 26. This phase is characterized by aggressive strengthening exercises such as plyometrics, PNF drills, isotonic strengthening, and functional sports activities. In the overhead throwing athlete, throwing from the pitching mound may be initiated. Contact sports may also be permitted during this period. Competitive throwing is usually not permitted until 7 to 9 months after surgery.

In summary, the progression of the rehabilitation program after arthroscopic stabilization is much slower than that after open stabilization (Table 19-13), especially during the early phase, which allows soft tissue healing to

Table 19-13

Rehabilitation Protocol after Open Anterior Bankart Repair

I. Phase I: Immediate Postoperative Phase
Goals
1. Protect the surgical procedure
2. Minimize the effects of immobilization
3. Diminish pain and inflammation
4. Establish baseline proprioception and dynamic stabilization

A. Week 0 to 2
- Sling for comfort (1 week)
- May wear immobilizer for sleep (2 weeks) *(physician decision)*

- Elbow/hand range of motion
- Gripping exercises
- Passive range of motion and active-assistive range of motion (L-bar)
  - Flexion to tolerance 0 to 90° week 1, 0 to 100° week 2
  - External/internal rotation at 45° abduction in scapular plane
- Submaximal isometrics
- No internal rotation strengthening for 2 to 3 weeks
- Rhythmic stabilization

Table 19-13

Rehabilitation Protocol after Open Anterior Bankart Repair—cont'd

- External/internal rotation proprioception drills
- Cryotherapy modalities as needed

B. Week 3 to 4
- Gradually progress range of motion
  - Flexion to 120 to 140°
  - External rotation at 45° abduction in scapular plane to 35 to 45°
  - Internal rotation at 45° abduction in scapular plane to 45 to 60°
- Initiate light isotonics for shoulder musculature
  - Tubing for external/internal rotation
  - Abduction, full can, side-lying ER, prone rowing, biceps
  - Dynamic stabilization exercises, proprioceptive neuromuscular facilitation
- Initiate self-capsular stretching
- Core stabilization program

C. Week 5 to 6
- Progress range of motion as tolerated
  - Flexion to 160° (tolerance)
  - External/internal rotation at 90° abduction:
    - Internal rotation to 75°
    - External rotation to 70 to 75°
- Joint mobilization as necessary
- Continue self-capsular stretching
- Progress all strengthening exercises
- Continue proprioceptive neuromuscular facilitation diagonal patters
- Throwers' Ten Exercise Program
- Continue isotonic strengthening
- Dynamic stabilization exercises
- Initiate internal rotation strengthening
- Closed kinetic chain exercises
- Push-up on ball
- Wall stabilization
- Progress range of motion to:
  - External rotation at 90° abduction: 80 to 85°
  - Internal rotation at 90° abduction: 70 to 75°
  - Flexion: 165 to 175°

II. Phase II: Intermediate Phase

Goals
1. Reestablish full range of motion
2. Normalize arthrokinematics
3. Improve muscular strength
4. Enhance neuromuscular control

A. Week 8 to 10
- Progress to full range of motion (week 7 to 8)—flexion 180°, external rotation at 90 to 100°, internal rotation 75°
- Continue all stretching exercises
  - Joint mobilization, capsular stretching, passive and active stretching
  - In overhead athletes, maintain 90 to 100° ER
  - Continue strengthening exercises
- Throwers' Ten Exercise Program (for overhead athletes)
- Isotonic strengthening for entire shoulder complex

- Proprioceptive neuromuscular facilitation manual technique
- Neuromuscular control drills
- Isokinetic strengthening

B. Week 10 to 14
- Continue all flexibility exercises
- Continue all strengthening exercises
- Two-hand plyometrics (week 10)
- Chest pass
- Overhead
- Side to side
- One-hand plyometrics (week 12)
- 90/90 position
- Dribble
- May initiate light isotonic machine weight training (week 12 to 14)

III. Phase III: Advanced Strengthening Phase (Month 4 to 6)

Goals
1. Enhance muscular strength, power and endurance
2. Improve muscular endurance
3. Maintain mobility

Criteria to Enter Phase III
1. Full range of motion
2. No pain or tenderness
3. Satisfactory stability
4. Strength 70% to 80% of contralateral side

A. Week 14 to 20
- Continue all flexibility exercises
- Self-capsular stretches (anterior, posterior, and inferior)
- Maintain external rotation flexibility
- Continue isotonic strengthening program
- Emphasis muscular balance (external/internal rotation)
- Continue proprioceptive neuromuscular facilitation manual resistance
- May continue plyometrics
- Initiate interval sport program (physician approval necessary) (week 16)

B. Week 20 to 24
- Continue all exercise listed above
- Continue and progress all interval sport program (throwing off mound)

Goals
1. Gradual return to sport activities
2. Maintain strength and mobility of shoulder

Criteria to Enter Phase IV
1. Full non-painful range of motion
2. Satisfactory stability
3. Satisfactory strength (isokinetics)
4. No pain or tenderness

Exercises
- Continue capsular stretching to maintain mobility
- Continue strengthening program
- Either Throwers' Ten Exercise Program or a fundamental shoulder exercise program
- Return to sport participation (unrestricted)
- For contact sports, consider shoulder brace

bone. A period of immobilization is often advocated and has been shown to be a critical factor in preventing recurrent instability.[78] We have noted significantly less postoperative scarring after arthroscopic stabilization than after open stabilization procedures. Additionally, slower rehabilitation and progression are encouraged because of the somewhat weaker fixation methods currently used in arthroscopic stabilization procedures and the significantly weaker than normal appearance of the capsulolabral complex tissue. A period of strict immobilization of at least 3 to 4 weeks appears to be sufficient to allow adequate tissue healing after arthroscopic stabilization.[6,7,45,135] We advocate relative immobilization with early restricted and protected motion to expedite the functional return of the arm. We expect full motion at approximately 10 weeks after arthroscopic stabilization. The ultimate goals are similar to those of the open stabilization technique, with a return of full external rotation necessary to simulate the throwing motion at week 12 to 14. A return to strenuous and contact sports is usually permitted at 7 to 9 months after surgery, with a return to competitive throwing slightly later (9 to 12 months).

Rehabilitation after Anterior Capsular Shift Procedure

An open capsular shift procedure may be another type of surgical procedure performed in the overhead throwing athlete. This procedure requires a delicate balance between the surgical procedure and the postoperative rehabilitation program. In our experience with this type of surgical procedure postoperative management can be more aggressive. We use what we refer to as an accelerated rehabilitation approach, which is based on immediate restricted motion and a gradual return to the motion necessary for throwing activities (Table 19-14). Immediately after surgery, the patient's shoulder is passively moved, and the patient performs active-assisted motion. In the first phase, the protected motion phase, from weeks 1 through 6, the primary goals are to (1) restore motion gradually, (2) protect the repaired capsule, and (3) reestablish dynamic stability. During weeks 1 through 3, AAROM for external rotation/internal rotation is performed with the arm in 30° of abduction to patient tolerance. Shoulder flexion also is performed to tolerance, usually 100 to 125° by week 2. During the first 2 weeks, isometrics and rhythmic-stabilization exercises also are performed.

Table 19-14

Anterior Open Capsular Shift Rehabilitation Protocol (Accelerated)

The goal of this rehabilitation program is to return the patient/athlete to his or her activity/sport as quickly and safely as possible, while maintaining a stable shoulder. The program is based on muscle physiology, biomechanics, and anatomy and the healing process after surgery for a capsular shift.

In the capsular shift procedure, the orthopedic surgeon makes an incision into the ligamentous capsule of the shoulder, pulls the capsule tighter, and then sutures the capsule together.

The ultimate goal is a functional stable shoulder and a return to a preoperative functional level.

I. Phase I: Protection Phase (Week 0 to 6)

Goals
- Allow healing of sutured capsule
- Begin early protected range of motion
- Retard muscular atrophy
- Decrease pain/inflammation

A. Week 0 to 2

Precautions
1. Sleep in immobilizer for 2 weeks
2. No overhead activities for 4 weeks
3. Wean from immobilizer and into sling as soon as possible (orthopedist or therapist will tell the athlete when), usually 2 weeks

Exercises
- Wrist/hand range of motion and gripping
- Elbow flexion/extension and pronation/supination
- Pendulum exercises (nonweighted)
- Rope-and-pulley active-assisted exercises
  - Shoulder flexion to 90°
  - Shoulder abduction to 60°
- T-bar exercises
  - External rotation to 15 to 20° with arm in scapular plane
  - Internal rotation to 25° with arm abduction at 40°

- Shoulder flexion to 90°
- Active range of motion cervical spine
- Isometrics
  - Flexors, extensors, external rotation, internal rotation, abduction
- Rhythmic stabilization drills

B. Week 2 to 4

Goals
- Gradual increase in range of motion
- Normalize arthrokinematics
- Improve strength
- Decrease pain/inflammation
1. Range of motion exercises
   - L-bar active assisted exercises
   - External rotation at 45° abduction to 45°
   - Internal rotation at 45° abduction to 45°
   - Shoulder flexion to tolerance
   - Shoulder abduction to tolerance
   - Rope-and-pulley flexion
   - Pendulum exercises

All exercises performed to tolerance
   - Take to point of pain and/or resistance and hold
   - Gentle self-capsular stretches

Table 19-14

Anterior Open Capsular Shift Rehabilitation Protocol (Accelerated)—cont'd

2. Gentle joint mobilization to reestablish normal arthrokinematics to:
   - Scapulothoracic joint
   - Glenohumeral joint
   - Sternoclavicular joint
3. Strengthening exercises
   - Active range of motion week 3
   - May initiate tubing for external/internal rotation at 0° at week 3
   - Dynamic stabilization drills
4. Conditioning program for:
   - Trunk
   - Lower extremities
   - Cardiovascular system
5. Decrease pain/inflammation
   - Ice, nonsteroidal anti-inflammatory drugs, modalities

C. Week 4 to 5
   - Active-assisted range of motion flexion to tolerance (145°)
   - External/internal rotation at 90° abduction to tolerance
   - External rotation at 90° abduction to 60°
   - Internal rotation at 90° abduction to 45 to 50°
   - Initiate isotonic (light weight) strengthening
   - Gentle joint mobilization (grade III)

D. Week 6
   - Active-assisted range of motion; continue all stretching exercises
   - Progress external/internal rotation at 90° abduction
   - External rotation at 90°, abduction: 75°
   - Internal rotation at 90°, abduction: 65°
   - Progress shoulder flexion to 165 to 170°
   - Progress to Throwers' Ten Exercise Program

II. Phase II: Intermediate Phase (Week 7 to 12)

Goals
   - Full nonpainful range of motion at week 8
   - Normalize arthrokinematics
   - Increase strength
   - Improve neuromuscular control

A. Week 7 to 10
1. Range of motion exercise
   - Shoulder flexion to 180°
   - External rotation at 90°, abduction: 90°
   - Internal rotation at 90°, abduction: 65°
   - Horizontal adduction/abduction motion
   - L-bar active-assisted exercises
   - Continue all exercises listed above
   - Gradually increase range of motion to full range of motion week 8
     - External rotation at 90°, abduction 85 to 90°
     - Internal rotation at 90°, abduction: 70 to 75°
   - Continue self-capsular stretches
   - Continue joint mobilization
2. Strengthening exercises
   - Throwers' Ten Exercise Program
   - Continue dynamic stabilization
   - Closed kinetic chain exercises
   - Core stabilization drills

3. Initiate neuromuscular control exercises for scapulothoracic joint
   - Scapular muscular training

B. Week 10 to 12
1. Continue all exercises listed above
2. Continue all stretching exercises
   - Progress range of motion to thrower's motion
   - External rotation to 110 to 115°
   - Flexion to 180°
3. Continue strengthening exercises
   - Initiate progressive resistance exercise weight training
4. Initiate interval hitting program (week 12)
5. Initiate golf swing (week 10)

III. Phase III: Dynamic Strengthening Phase (Week 12 to 20)

Advanced strengthening phase

A. Week 12 to 16

Goals
   - Improve strength/power/endurance
   - Improve neuromuscular control
   - Maintain shoulder mobility
   - Prepare athlete to begin to throw

Criteria to Enter Phase III
   a. Full nonpainful range of motion
   b. No pain or tenderness
   c. Strength 70% or better compared with that of contralateral side
1. Continue all stretching and range of motion exercises
2. Continue all strengthening
   - Throwers' Ten Exercise Program
3. Initiate plyometrics
   - Two-hand drills (week 12)
   - One-hand drills (week 13 to 14)
4. Continue core stabilization drills

B. Week 16 to 20
   - Continue all exercises above
   - Continue stretching and range of motion exercises
   - Initiate interval sport program (week 16)

IV. Phase IV: Functional Activity Phase (Week 20 to 26)

Goals
   - Progressively increase activities to prepare patient for full functional return

Criteria to Progress to Phase IV
   1. Full range of motion
   2. No pain or tenderness
   3. Isokinetic test that fulfills criteria to throw
   4. Satisfactory clinical examination

Exercise
   - Continue interval sport program
   - Continue Throwers' Ten Exercise Program
   - Continue plyometric five exercises

Interval Throwing Program
   1. Long toss program (phase I) (week 16)
   2. Off the round program (phase II) (week 22)
   3. Simulated game (week 30)

During weeks 2 to 4, range of motion and stretching gradually progress. Active-assisted external rotation and internal rotation range-of-motion exercises are performed at 45° of abduction, with the goal of 45° of motion (external rotation and internal rotation) by week 4. During this time, tubing exercises may be initiated for the shoulder internal and external rotators; rhythmic-stabilization drills and co-contraction also are performed.

At weeks 4 to 5, external rotation/internal rotation stretching is performed at 90° of abduction. This progression is based on clinical assessment (degrees of motion and endfeel). At approximately 4.5 to 5 weeks, external rotation motion progresses more aggressively. By the end of week 6, our goal is 75° of external rotation in the overhead throwing athlete. The rate of progress (aggressiveness) of the stretching is determined by the clinical assessment and is based on the assessment of motion, stability, and endfeel. If the patient appears to be progressing slowly toward these goals, the program must be adjusted at week 6. In our opinion, all of these stretches are safe if performed with a gradual force, and force should not be applied rapidly. Stretches are usually initiated during week 7, and the clinician should consult the physician before their use. During this phase, isotonic strengthening exercises are performed for the entire shoulder complex. During weeks 3 to 4, rhythmic stabilization drills are emphasized with the goal of restoring dynamic stability. At week 5, external rotation/internal rotation strengthening may be performed at 90° of abduction.

The intermediate phase, weeks 7 through 12, is characterized by establishing full motion at week 8 and improving muscular strength and endurance. At week 8, the patient should exhibit full motion (90° of external rotation and 45 to 55° of horizontal abduction). From weeks 8 to 12, the overhead throwing athlete's stretching exercises progress to the amount of external rotation necessary to throw usually a minimum of 115 to 120° of external rotation. This is usually accomplished through physiologic stretching, capsular stretching, low-load, long-duration stretches, and controlled plyometric activities. During this phase all strengthening exercises, muscular balance, scapular strengthening, and endurance are emphasized.

The advanced strengthening phase begins at week 12 and progresses through week 20. The primary goals are to enhance muscular strength, power and endurance, while maintaining capsular mobility and glenohumeral joint stability. The patient is instructed to continue stretching to prevent capsular or muscular tightening or both caused by the aggressive strengthening exercises. The strengthening exercises consist of PNF, the Throwers' Ten Exercise Program (Appendix A), plyometrics, and neuromuscular-control drills.[55,196,192] At this time, the patient is carefully

evaluated and a determination is made as to when a throwing program can be initiated. A gradual throwing or sport program can usually be initiated between 14 and 16 weeks, depending on patient variables and progression in rehabilitation.

The return-to-activity phase is initiated at 21 weeks after surgery and represents a gradual return to sport activities. During this time, it is imperative that the athlete continues all strengthening and stretching exercises outlined in the previous phase. A return to unrestricted sports usually occurs between 6 and 9 months, depending on the patient's sport, position, skill level, and rate of progression.

Altchek and associates[6] reported on 40 patients (42 shoulders) in whom surgical stabilization was performed by using a T-plasty modification for multidirectional instability. Thirty-eight of 40 patients returned to sports at an average of 6.5 months (range, 5 to 10 months). Only 3 patients in the series were throwers; all 3 reported that they were unable to throw as fast as before the operation. Bigliani and co-workers[26] reported the results of an anteroinferior capsular shift performed on 63 athletic patients (68 shoulders). Of the 63 patients, 31 were overhead activity athletes, consisting of 16 baseball players. The results indicated that 50% returned to the same competition level. Kvitne and colleagues[120] reported on 105 patients who had undergone anterior capsulolabral reconstruction. In this series, 52 were baseball players, 35 of whom were pitchers, and 60% of the professional baseball pitchers were able to return to the same competition level.

The rehabilitation process after capsular tensioning in the overhead activity athlete is challenging to the clinician. Success rates vary greatly, depending on the sport and position. The reasons for failure are multifactorial. One commonly seen reason is a loss of external rotation. The rehabilitation program must be aggressive in restoring external rotation motion in the throwing athlete. Fleisig[68] determined the total arc of motion [late cocking (external rotation) to follow-through] as one of the critical factors in a pitcher's effectiveness. Thus, one of the primary and critical postoperative goals is a restoration of glenohumeral motion, particularly external rotation.

Rehabilitation after Glenoid Labrum Procedures

Labral lesions occur often in the overhead-throwing athlete due to the extremes in motion and tremendous muscular forces. The specific rehabilitation program after surgical intervention involving the glenoid labrum depends on the severity of the pathologic condition. For type I and type III SLAP lesions a simple arthroscopic débridement of the frayed labrum is used, and the rehabilitation program is similar. Because the biceps labral anchor is intact and no anatomic repair is necessary, the rehabilitation program is somewhat aggressive in restoring motion and function. Full range of motion is expected by 10 to 14 days postoperatively. Internal and external rotation tubing exercises are initiated at day 10 with gradual isotonic strengthening occurring between weeks 2 and 8. The athlete is allowed to begin an interval throwing program usually at week 8 to 12. This start date for throwing is often variable based on the time of season. The athlete who is undergoing rehabilitation during the sport season will begin throwing at an earlier date than the athlete who is undergoing rehabilitating during the off-season. The ultimate success depends on the athlete's dynamic stabilization of the glenohumeral joint.

Overhead throwing athletes commonly are seen with a type II SLAP lesion with the biceps tendon detached from the glenoid rim. Usually a peel-back lesion is present. Postoperative rehabilitation is delayed to allow healing of the anatomical repair to reattach the tendon. No isolated biceps strengthening is permitted for 6 to 8 weeks postoperatively to allow adequate healing. The athlete sleeps in a sling and swathe immobilizer and wears a sling in the daytime for the first 4 weeks. Protective range-of-motion activity is allowed for the first 4 weeks at less than 90° of elevation. During the first 2 weeks internal and external rotation is performed passively in the scapula plane to approximately 10 to 15° of external rotation and 45° of internal rotation. No excessive external rotation, extension, or abduction is allowed until week 5 to 6, when a light isotonic strengthening program is initiated. Internal and external rotation range of motion is progressed to 90° of abduction at week 5 to 6. Motion is gradually increased to restore full range by 8 to 10 weeks and progressed to thrower's motion through week 10 to 12. Restriction of motion is usually accomplished with little to minimal difficulty. Plyometric exercises are initiated at week 12 and an interval throwing program at week 16. Return to sport after surgical repair of a type II SLAP lesion occurs at approximately 9 to 11 months.

SUMMARY

Shoulder Injuries

- Mobility of the shoulder joint is acquired at the expense of stability.
- Shoulder injuries can be induced acutely through traumatic injuries, or they may arise with an insidious onset as a result of repetitive stresses over time.

- Overuse injuries to the shoulder are common in athletes whose endeavors require repetitive overhead activities, particularly throwers and swimmers.
- Most shoulder injuries occur during the late cocking, acceleration, and deceleration phases of throwing.
- The most common shoulder injuries include rotator cuff tendinitis or partial tears, compressive cuff disease, internal impingement syndrome, and shoulder instability (usually anterior).

Goals of Shoulder Rehabilitation

- The goals of shoulder rehabilitation are to prevent injuries through off-season and in-season conditioning programs that address flexibility, rotator cuff strength, scapular stability, and neuromuscular control of the shoulder girdle.
- The rehabilitation program should be progressive and systematic, using the principles of periodization.

General Shoulder Rehabilitation Principles

- Rehabilitation of these injuries should concentrate on developing dynamic joint stability.
- Those athletes who are susceptible to shoulder pathologic conditions should participate in an off-season shoulder flexibility and rotator cuff strengthening program to help prevent shoulder problems, and they should continue this stretching and strengthening program two or three times weekly during the season.
- Preventive and postinjury exercises should also be chosen to strengthen the rotator cuff muscles to dynamically stabilize the glenohumeral joint and the scapular stabilizers that help orient the glenoid fossa with the humeral head to maintain stability.
- Weakness in the scapula stabilizers can predispose the athlete to a variety of shoulder pathologic conditions.
- After shoulder surgery or injury, emphasis should be placed on addressing the inflammation process and restoring motion.
- After initiation of a rotator cuff strengthening program, PNF techniques may be implemented to help restore neuromuscular control.
- In the late phases of rehabilitation, eccentric, isokinetic, and plyometric exercises may be initiated.
- In the advanced strengthening phase, the goals of the program are to initiate sport-specific types of training for the shoulder joint complex.

THERAPEUTIC SHOULDER EXERCISE PROGRAM

Range-of-Motion Exercises

Circumduction Pendulum Swings. The athlete leans over the table, supporting the body with the uninvolved arm and allowing the involved arm to hang straight down in a relaxed position. The athlete gently swings the arm in circles clockwise and counterclockwise (Fig. 19-30*A*), in a pendulum motion forward and backward (Fig. 19-30*B*) and side to side, repeating one set of 10 repetitions each and progressing to 5 sets of 10 repetitions each, as tolerated.

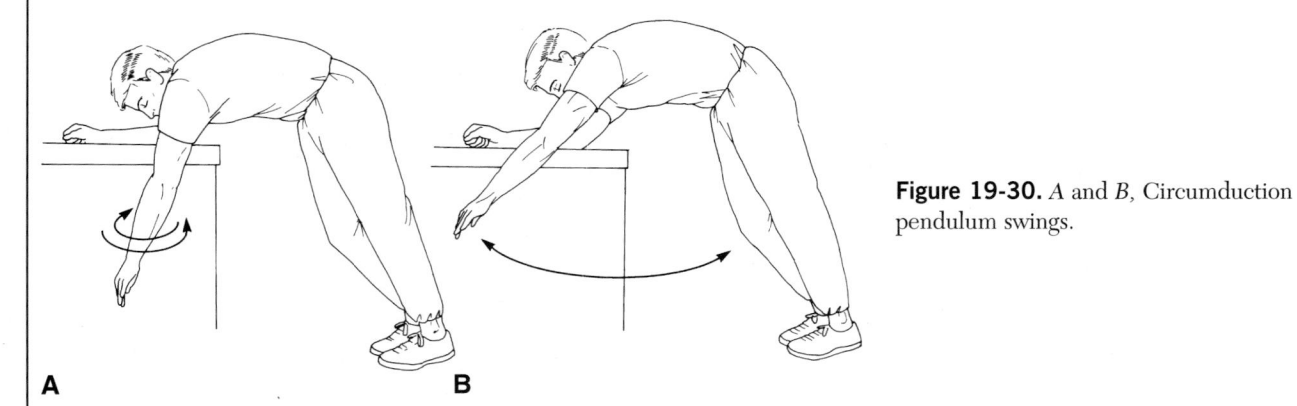

Figure 19-30. *A* and *B*, Circumduction pendulum swings.

A   **B**

Rope-and-Pulley Exercises. The overhead rope and pulley should be positioned in a doorway. The athlete sits in a chair with the back against the door, directly underneath the pulley.

Active-Assisted Flexion. With the elbow straight and the back of the hand facing upward, the athlete raises the involved arm to the front of the body as high as possible (Fig. 19-31*A*), assisting as needed by pulling with the uninvolved arm and holding for 5 seconds. The arm is lowered slowly, using the uninvolved arm to control lowering as needed. The athlete repeats one set of 10 repetitions, progressing to 5 sets of 10 repetitions as tolerated.

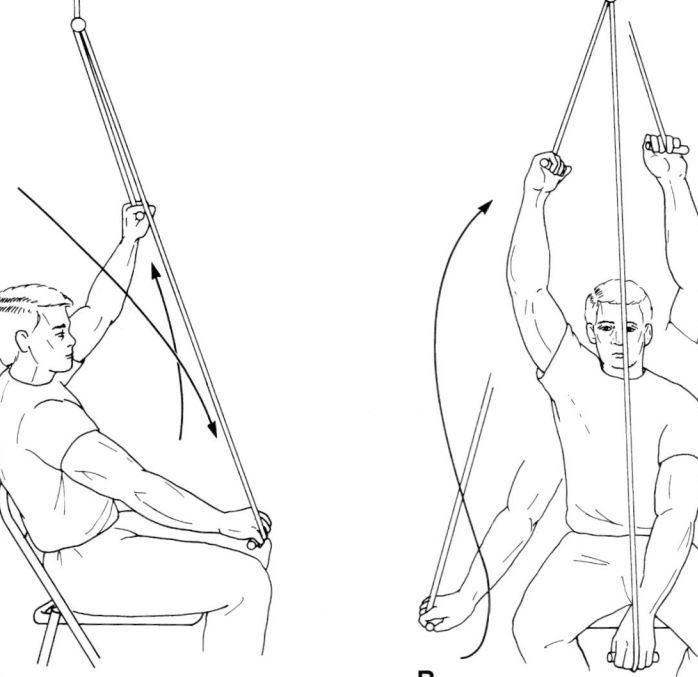
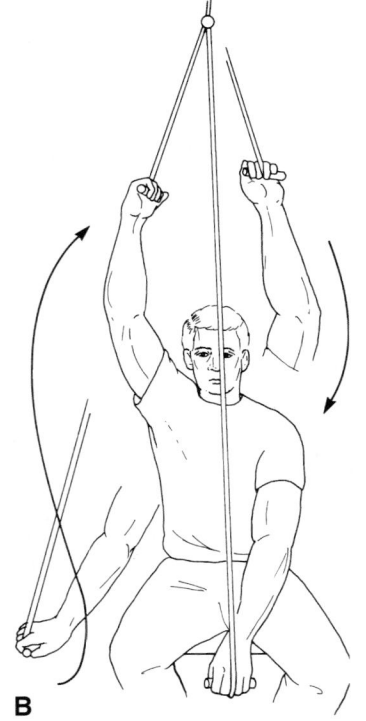

Figure 19-31. *A*, Active-assisted flexion. *B*, Active-assisted abduction.

A   **B**

Active-Assisted Abduction. With the elbow straight and the hand rotated outward as far as possible, the athlete raises the involved arm to the side of the body as high as possible (Fig. 19-31B), assisting as needed by pulling with the uninvolved arm and holding for 5 seconds. The arm is lowered slowly using the uninvolved arm to control lowering as needed. The athlete repeats one set of 10 repetitions, progressing to 5 sets of 10 repetitions as tolerated.

Supine Flexion. The athlete lies on the back, grips the bar in both hands with the palms up and arms straight (Fig. 19-32A), raises both arms overhead as far as possible (Fig. 19-32B), and holds for 5 seconds before returning to the starting position. This is repeated 10 to 15 times. This exercise may be performed with the thumb up as an alternate method, particularly if impingement syndrome is present.

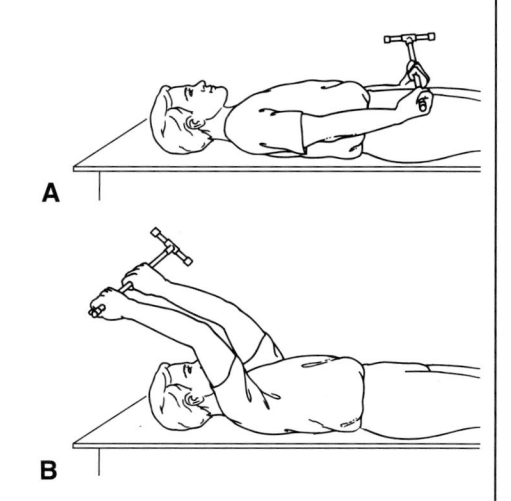

Figure 19-32. *A* and *B*, Supine flexion. (Redrawn from Wilk, K.E., Andrews, J.R., Arrigo, C.A. et al. [1997]: Preventive and Rehabilitative Exercises for the Shoulder and Elbow, 5th ed. Birmingham, AL, American Sports Medicine Institute.)

Supine Abduction. The athlete lies on the back with the involved arm at the side of the body, straightens the involved arm, and rotates the hand outward as far as possible. Then the athlete slides the arm along the table, bed, or floor, moving the arm away from the side as far as possible and using a T-bar to help push it up (Fig. 19-33A and B). This position is held for 5 seconds before the athlete returns to the starting position, and the exercise is repeated 10 to 15 times.

Figure 19-33. *A* and *B*, Supine abduction.

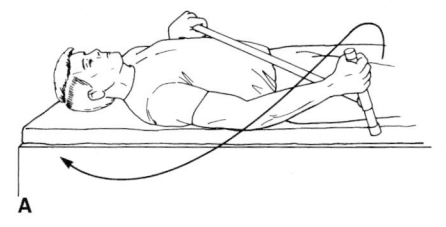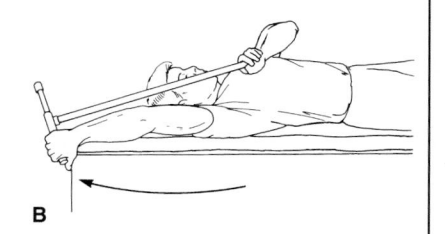

Supine External Rotation

External Rotation (0° Abduction). The athlete lies on the back with the involved arm against the body and the elbow bent at 90° (Fig. 19-34A). Gripping the T-bar handle with the uninvolved arm, the athlete pushes the involved shoulder into external rotation with the T-bar (Fig. 19-34B). This position is held for 5 seconds before the arm is returned to the starting position, and the exercise is repeated. A towel should be placed under the arm to stretch in the scapular plane.

Exercise Progression. Shoulder external rotation can be progressed by performing this exercise at 45° (Fig. 19-34C) and 90° (Fig. 19-34D) of shoulder abduction.

Standing External Rotation. With the involved arm overhead, the athlete holds a towel behind the neck and holds the other end of the towel with the uninvolved arm and pulls down (Fig. 19-35). As the left arm pulls in a downward direction, the right arm rotates externally. This position is held for 5 seconds before the arm is returned to the starting position, and the exercise is repeated 10 to 15 times.

Continued

THERAPEUTIC SHOULDER EXERCISE PROGRAM—cont'd

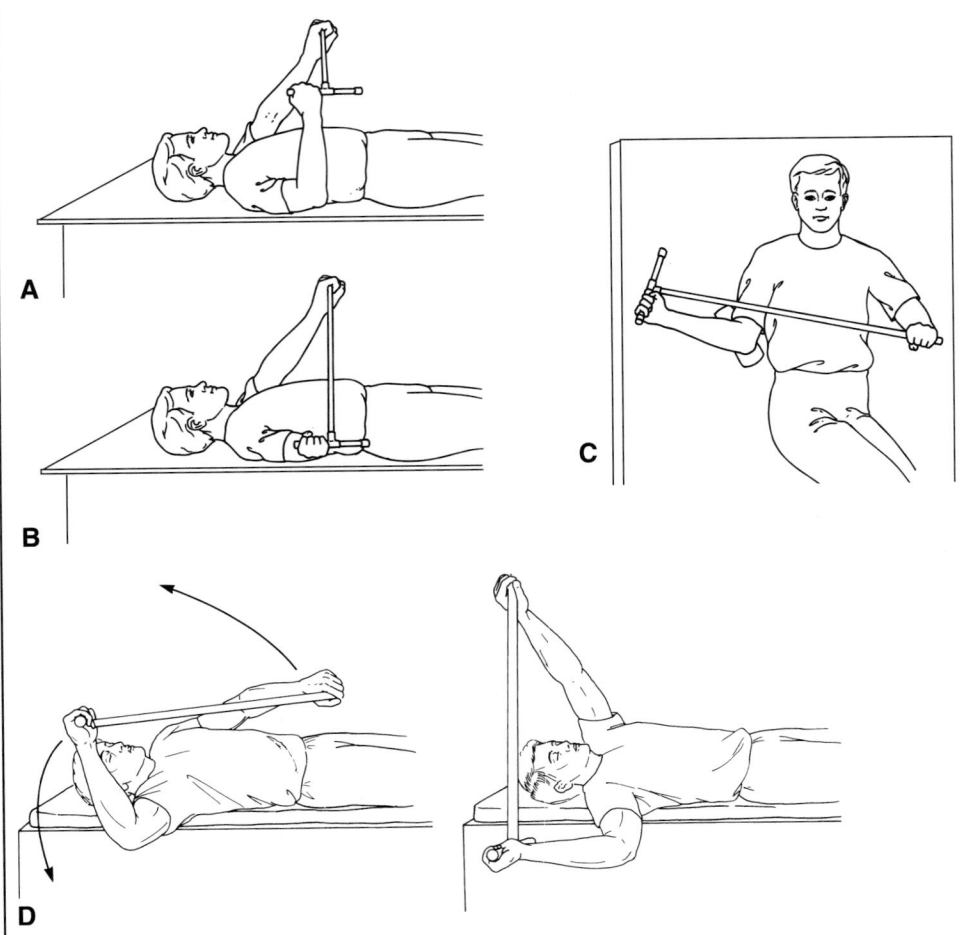

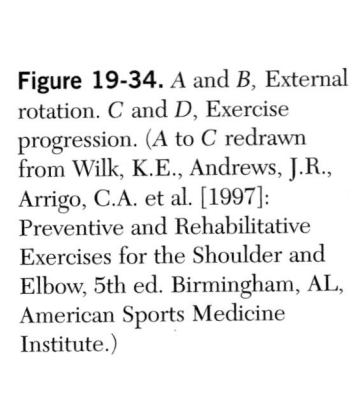

Figure 19-34. *A and B, External rotation. C and D, Exercise progression. (A to C redrawn from Wilk, K.E., Andrews, J.R., Arrigo, C.A. et al. [1997]: Preventive and Rehabilitative Exercises for the Shoulder and Elbow, 5th ed. Birmingham, AL, American Sports Medicine Institute.)*

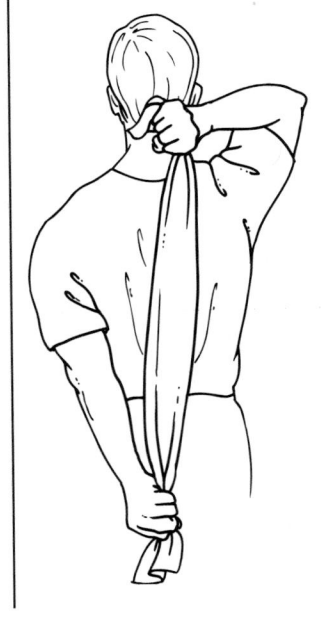

Figure 19-35. Standing external rotation. (Redrawn from Wilk, K.E., Andrews, J.R., Arrigo, C.A. et al. [1997]: Preventive and Rehabilitative Exercises for the Shoulder and Elbow, 5th ed. Birmingham, AL, American Sports Medicine Institute.)

Supine Internal Rotation. The athlete lies on the back with the involved arm out to the side of the body at 90° and the elbow bent at 90°. Gripping the T-bar in the hand of the involved arm and keeping the elbow in a fixed position, the athlete uses the uninvolved arm to push the involved arm into internal rotation with the T-bar (Fig. 19-36). This position is held for 5 seconds before the arm is returned to the starting position, and the exercise is repeated 10 to 15 times.

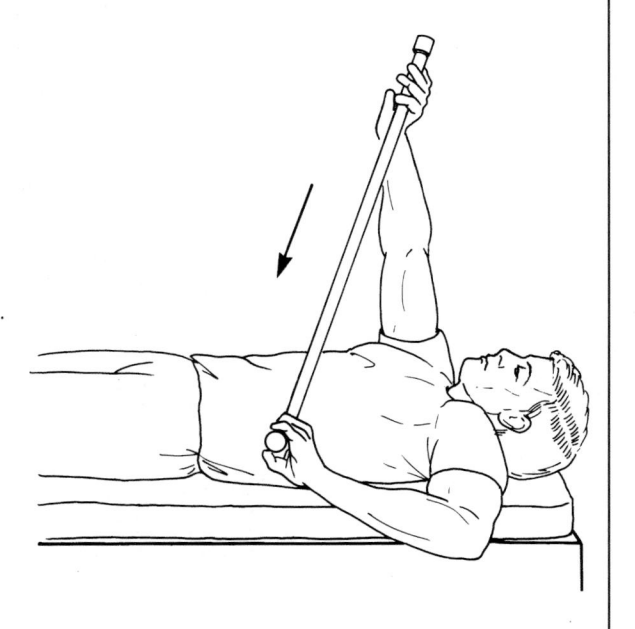

Figure 19-36. Supine internal rotation.

Standing Internal Rotation. The athlete's involved arm is behind the back holding a T-bar or a towel (Fig. 19-37). The uninvolved arm is overhead, pulling the bar or towel upward. This action will further rotate the shoulder inward, internally rotating the involved arm. This position is held for 5 seconds before the arm is returned to the starting position, and the exercise is repeated 10 to 15 times.

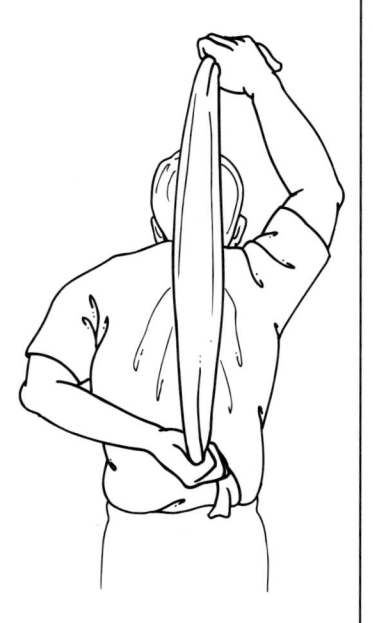

Figure 19-37. Standing internal rotation. (Redrawn from Wilk, K.E., Andrews, J.R., Arrigo, C.A. et al. [1997]: Preventive and Rehabilitative Exercises for the Shoulder and Elbow, 5th ed. Birmingham, AL, American Sports Medicine Institute.)

Horizontal Abduction-Adduction. The athlete lies on the back and holds the T-bar in front with the thumbs up (Fig. 19-38A). Keeping the arms straight, the athlete takes the arms as far as possible to one side of the body (Fig. 19-38B), holds for 5 seconds, and then take the arms as far as possible to the other side (Fig. 19-38C). Someone stabilizes the scapula on the affected side by holding the lateral border. This position is held for 5 seconds before the arm is returned to the starting position, and the exercise is repeated 10 to 15 times.

Continued

THERAPEUTIC SHOULDER EXERCISE PROGRAM — cont'd

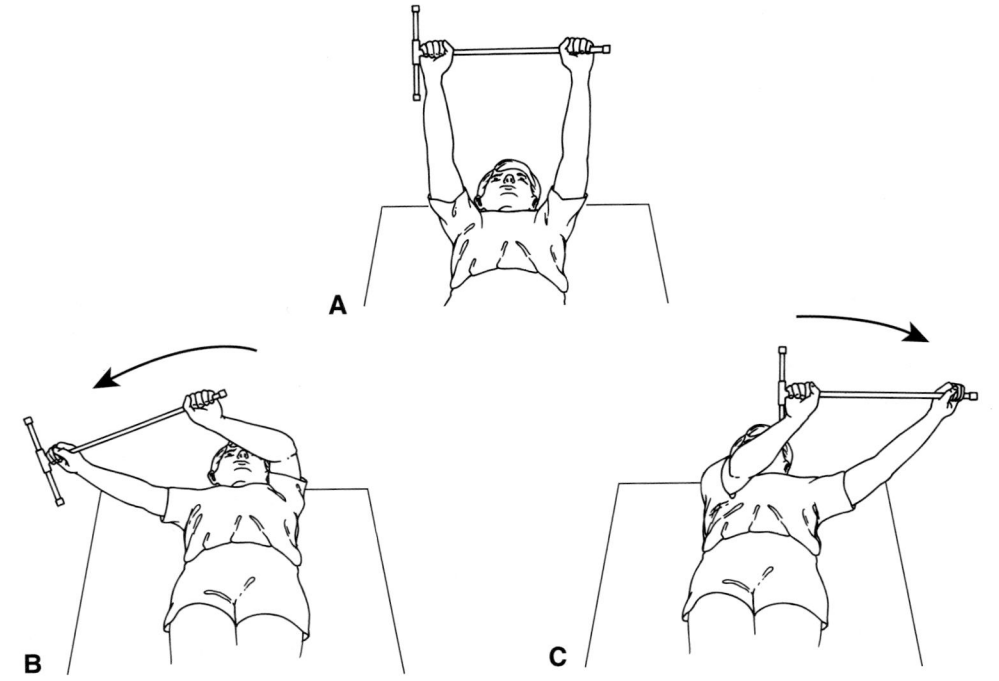

Figure 19-38. *A* to *C*, Horizontal abduction and adduction. (Redrawn from Wilk, K.E., Andrews, J.R., Arrigo, C.A. et al. [1997]: Preventive and Rehabilitative Exercises for the Shoulder and Elbow, 5th ed. Birmingham, AL, American Sports Medicine Institute.)

Posterior Capsular Stretch. The athlete grasps the elbow of the involved arm with the opposite hand and pulls the arm across the front of the chest (Fig. 19-39), holding for 5 seconds. The athlete then relaxes and repeats the exercise 10 to 15 times.

Inferior Capsular Stretch. The athlete holds the involved arm overhead with the elbow bent (Fig. 19-40*A*) and, using the uninvolved arm, stretches the arm farther overhead (Fig. 19-40*B*) until a stretching sensation is felt. This position is held for 5 seconds, and the exercise is repeated 10 to 15 times.

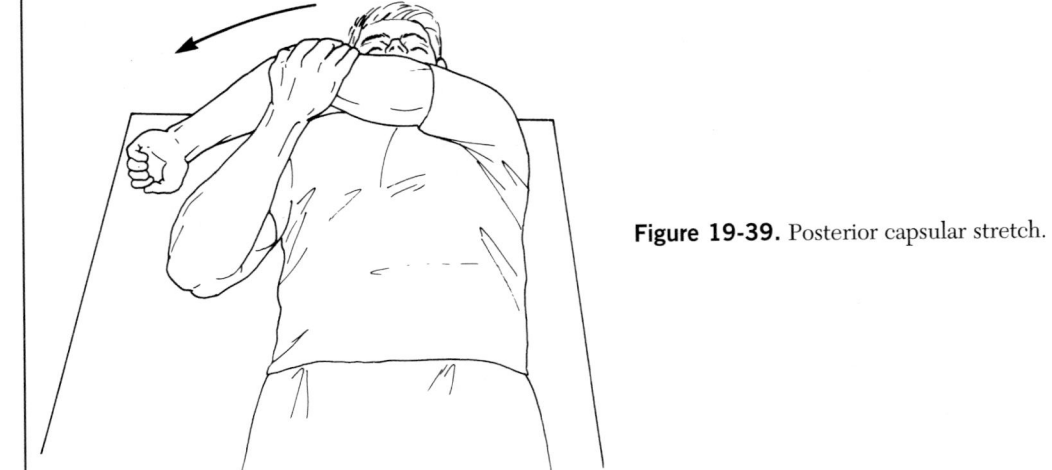

Figure 19-39. Posterior capsular stretch.

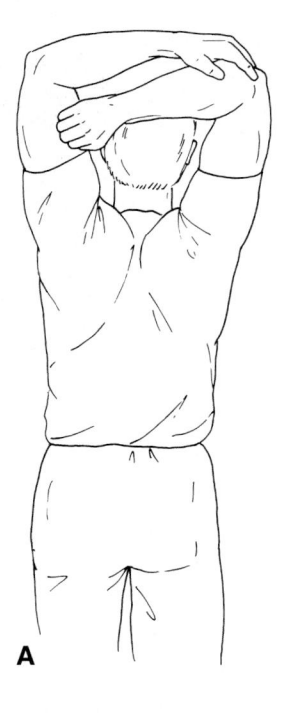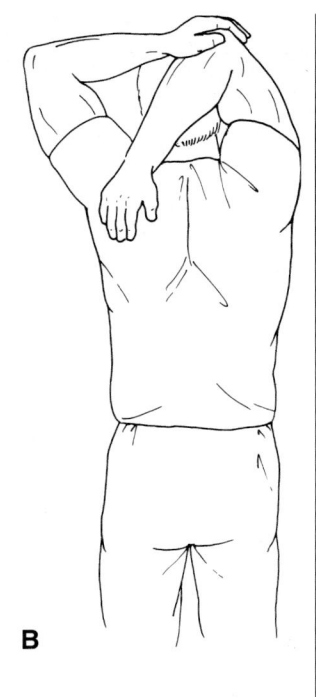

Figure 19-40. *A* and *B*, Inferior capsular stretch.

A   **B**

Anterior Capsular Stretch. The athlete stands in a doorway with the elbow straight and the shoulder abducted to 90° and externally rotated. With pressure on the arm, the arm is forced back to stretch the front of the shoulder (Fig. 19-41). This position is held for 5 seconds, and the exercise is repeated 10 to 15 times.

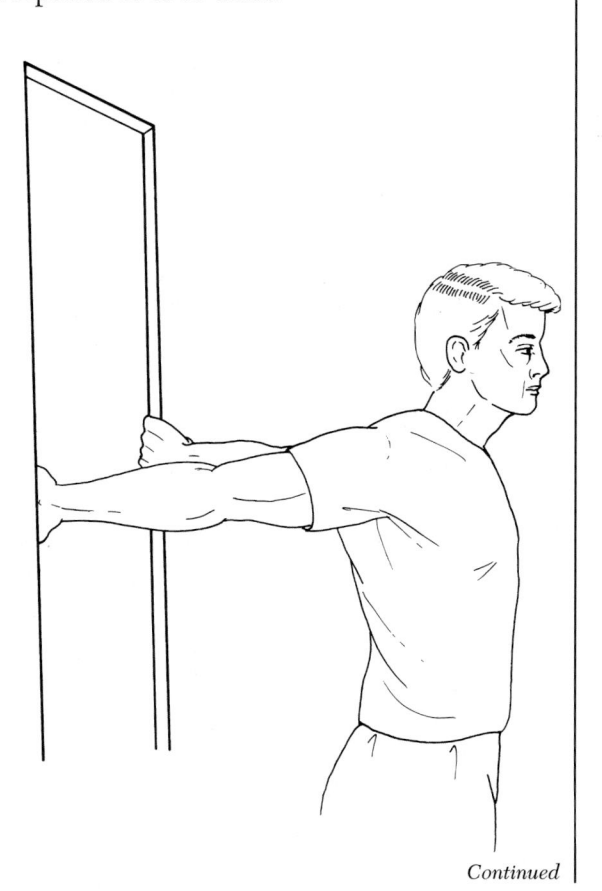

Figure 19-41. Anterior capsular stretch.

Continued

THERAPEUTIC SHOULDER EXERCISE PROGRAM—cont'd

Strengthening Exercises

ISOMETRICS

Flexion. The athlete stands facing out of a doorway, placing the involved arm in front (Fig. 19-42). The forearm and hand are placed on the door frame, and the athlete pushes as if to raise the arm overhead. The position is held at a submaximal force for 8 seconds, and the exercise is repeated.

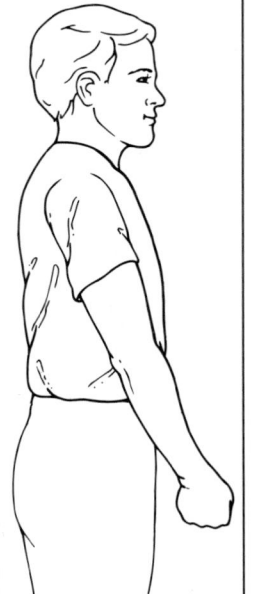

Figure 19-42. Flexion. (Redrawn from Wilk, K.E., Andrews, J.R., Arrigo, C.A. et al. [1997]: Preventive and Rehabilitative Exercises for the Shoulder and Elbow, 5th ed. Birmingham, AL, American Sports Medicine Institute.)

Abduction. The athlete stands against a wall or in a doorway with the involved arm at the side (Fig. 19-43) and presses back the forearm into the surface, keeping the arm at the side with the elbow straight. The position is held at a submaximal force for 8 seconds, and the exercise is repeated.

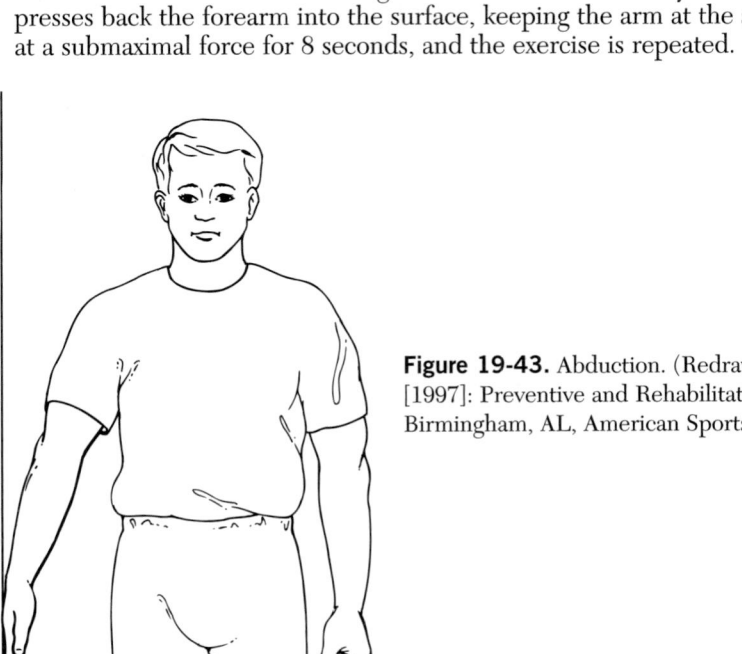

Figure 19-43. Abduction. (Redrawn from Wilk, K.E., Andrews, J.R., Arrigo, C.A. et al. [1997]: Preventive and Rehabilitative Exercises for the Shoulder and Elbow, 5th ed. Birmingham, AL, American Sports Medicine Institute.)

Extension. The athlete stands in a doorway in front of the door frame, places the involved arm slightly behind the body (Fig. 19-44), and pushes backward into the door frame. The position is held at a submaximal force for 8 seconds, and the exercise is repeated.

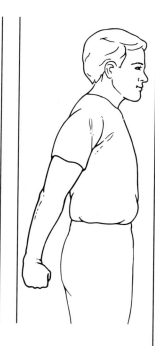

Figure 19-44. Extension. (Redrawn from Wilk, K.E., Andrews, J.R., Arrigo, C.A. et al. [1997]: Preventive and Rehabilitative Exercises for the Shoulder and Elbow, 5th ed. Birmingham, AL, American Sports Medicine Institute.)

External Rotation. The athlete stands against a wall or in a doorway with the arm at the side and the elbow bent to 90° (Fig. 19-45) and presses the back of the forearm into the surface. The position is held at a submaximal force for 8 seconds, and the exercise is repeated.

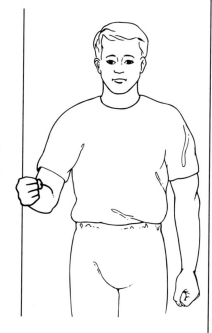

Figure 19-45. External rotation. (Redrawn from Wilk, K.E., Andrews, J.R., Arrigo, C.A. et al. [1997]: Preventive and Rehabilitative Exercises for the Shoulder and Elbow, 5th ed. Birmingham, AL, American Sports Medicine Institute.)

Internal Rotation. The athlete stands against a wall or in a doorway with the arm at the side and the elbow bent to 90° (Fig. 19-46) and presses the front of the forearm into the surface. The position is held at a submaximal force for 8 seconds, and the exercise is repeated.

Continued

THERAPEUTIC SHOULDER EXERCISE PROGRAM — cont'd

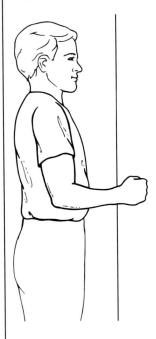

Figure 19-46. Internal rotation. (Redrawn from Wilk, K.E., Andrews, J.R., Arrigo, C.A. et al. [1997]: Preventive and Rehabilitative Exercises for the Shoulder and Elbow, 5th ed. Birmingham, AL, American Sports Medicine Institute.)

Elbow Flexion. The athlete uses the uninvolved arm to hold the involved elbow at angles of 45°, 90°, and 135° (Fig. 19-47) and flexes the elbow into the uninvolved hand, keeping the elbow still. The position is held at a submaximal force for 8 seconds, and the exercise is repeated.

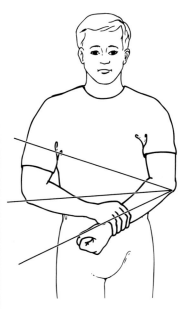

Figure 19-47. Elbow flexion. (Redrawn from Wilk, K.E., Andrews, J.R., Arrigo, C.A. et al. [1997]: Preventive and Rehabilitative Exercises for the Shoulder and Elbow, 5th ed. Birmingham, AL, American Sports Medicine Institute.)

ISOTONICS

Shoulder Flexion. The athlete stands with the elbow straight and the palm of the hand against the side, raises the involved arm out to the front of the body with the thumb up, and continues overhead as high as possible (Fig. 19-48). This position is held for 2 seconds, and the arm is slowly lowered.

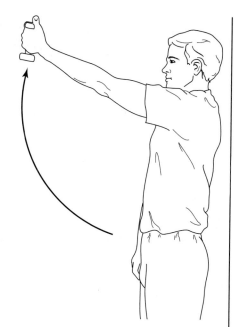

Figure 19-48. Shoulder flexion.

Shoulder Abduction. The athlete stands with the elbow straight and the hand rotated outward as far as possible and raises the involved arm to the side of body as high as possible (Fig. 19-49). This position is held for 2 seconds, and the arm is slowly lowered.

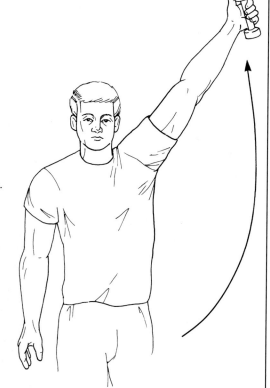

Figure 19-49. Shoulder abduction.

Supraspinatus Strengthening ("Empty Can" Position). The athlete stands with the elbow straight and the hand rotated inward as far as possible and raises the arm to be parallel to the floor at a 30° angle to the body (Fig. 19-50). This position is held for 2 seconds, and the arm is slowly lowered.

Continued

THERAPEUTIC SHOULDER EXERCISE PROGRAM—cont'd

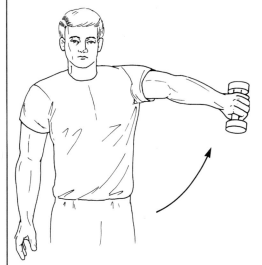

Figure 19-50. Supraspinatus strengthening ("empty can" position).

Supraspinatus, Rotator Cuff, and Deltoid Strengthening ("Full Can" Position). The athlete stands with the elbow extended and the thumb up and raises the arm to shoulder level at a 30° angle in front of the body (Fig. 19-51). The arm should not go above shoulder level. This position is held for 2 seconds, and the arm is slowly lowered.

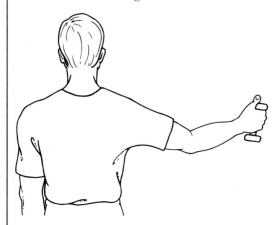

Figure 19-51. Strengthening, rotator cuff, and deltoid strengthening ("full can" position). (Redrawn from Wilk, K.E., Andrews, J.R., Arrigo, C.A. et al. [1997]: Preventive and Rehabilitative Exercises for the Shoulder and Elbow, 5th ed. Birmingham, AL, American Sports Medicine Institute.)

Prone Horizontal Abduction. The athlete lies on the table on the stomach, with the involved arm hanging straight to the floor. With the hand rotated outward as far as possible, the arm is raised out to the side, parallel to the floor (Fig. 19-52). This position is held for 2 seconds, and the arm is slowly lowered.

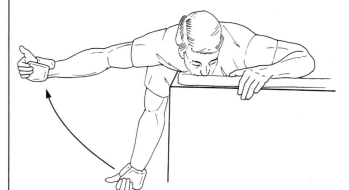

Figure 19-52. Prone horizontal abduction.

Prone Horizontal Abduction (100°). The athlete lies on the table on the stomach, with the involved arm hanging straight to the floor. With the hand rotated outward as far as possible and the shoulder at approximately 100° of abduction, the arm is raised out to the side, parallel to the floor (Fig. 19-53). This position is held for 2 seconds, and the arm is slowly lowered.

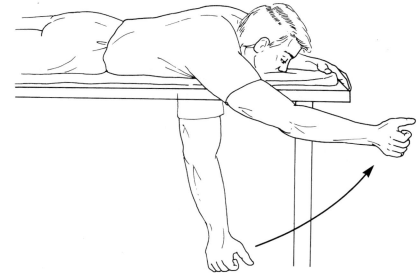

Figure 19-53. Prone horizontal abduction (100°).

Shoulder Extension. The athlete lies on the table on the stomach, with the involved arm hanging straight to the floor. With the hand rotated outward as far as possible, the arm is raised straight back into extension as far as possible (Fig. 19-54). When lifting the arm straight back, the athlete continues to rotate the extremity externally as far as possible through the entire range of motion. This position is held for 2 seconds, and the arm is slowly lowered.

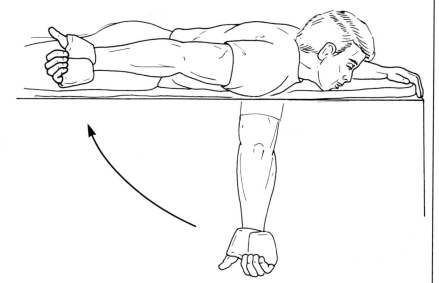

Figure 19-54. Shoulder extension.

Side-Lying External Rotation. The athlete lies on the uninvolved side, with the involved arm at the side of the body and the elbow bent at 90°. Keeping the elbow of the involved arm fixed to the side, the arm is rotated into external rotation (Fig. 19-55). This position is held for 2 seconds, and the arm is slowly lowered.

Continued

THERAPEUTIC SHOULDER EXERCISE PROGRAM — cont'd

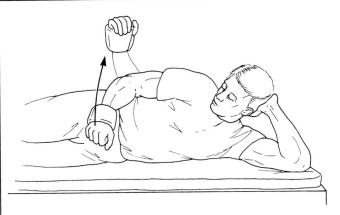

Figure 19-55. Side-lying external rotation.

Side-Lying Internal Rotation. The athlete lies on the involved side with the involved arm at the side of the body and the elbow bent at 90°. Keeping the elbow of the involved arm fixed to the side, the arm is rotated into internal rotation (Fig. 19-56). This position is held for 2 seconds, and the arm is slowly lowered.

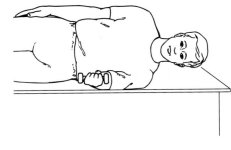

Figure 19-56. Side-lying internal rotation. (Redrawn from Wilk, K.E., Andrews, J.R., Arrigo, C.A. et al. [1997]: Preventive and Rehabilitative Exercises for the Shoulder and Elbow, 5th ed. Birmingham, AL, American Sports Medicine Institute.)

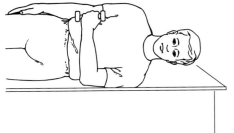

Shoulder Shrug. The athlete stands with the arms by the side, lifts the shoulders up to the ears, holds for 2 seconds (Fig. 19-57A), pulls the shoulders back, and pinches the shoulder blades together (Fig. 19-57B). This position is held for 2 seconds, the shoulders are relaxed, and the exercise is repeated.

Biceps Curl. The athlete supports the involved arm with the opposite hand and bends the elbow to full flexion. This position is held for 2 seconds, and the arm is then extended completely (Fig. 19-58).

French Curl (Triceps). The athlete raises the involved arm overhead, providing support at the elbow with the opposite hand, and straightens the arm overhead (Fig. 19-59). This position is held for 2 seconds, and the arm is then slowly lowered.

Progressive Push-up. The athlete starts with a push-up into the wall, gradually progressing to the tabletop (Fig. 19-60) and then to the floor, as tolerated.

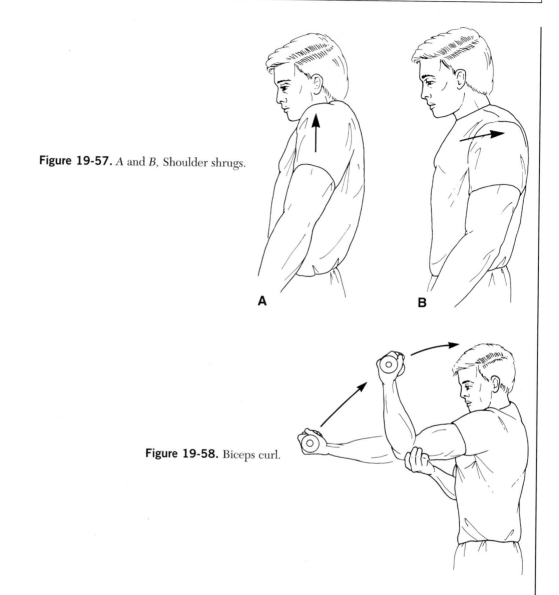

Figure 19-57. *A* and *B*, Shoulder shrugs.

Figure 19-58. Biceps curl.

Punch. The athlete lies on the back, holding a medicine ball or dumbbell, and punches the arm up toward the ceiling, allowing the shoulder blade to lift off the table (Fig. 19-61). The position is held for 2 seconds, the arm is slowly returned to the starting position, and the exercise is repeated.

Seated Rowing. The athlete sits in a chair facing a wall to which tubing has been affixed at shoulder level (Fig. 19-62A). The athlete brings the arm out to 90°, holds the tubing with palms down, pulls the elbows back, and squeezes the shoulder blades together (Fig. 19-62B). The position is held for 2 seconds, the arm is returned to starting position, and the exercise is repeated.

Advanced Strengthening Exercises

External Rotation at 0° Abduction. Standing, with the elbow at the side fixed at 90° of flexion and the involved arm across the front of the body, the athlete grips the tubing handle (the other end of the tubing is fixed) (Fig. 19-63A) and pulls out with the arm while keeping the elbow at the side (Fig. 19-63B). The tubing is returned slowly in a controlled manner.

Internal Rotation at 0° Abduction. Standing, with the elbow at the side fixed at 90° and the shoulder rotated out, the athlete grips the tubing handle (the other end of the tubing is fixed) (Fig. 19-64A) and pulls the arm across the body, keeping the elbow at the *side* (Fig. 19-64B). The tubing is returned slowly and in a controlled manner.

Continued

T H E R A P E U T I C S H O U L D E R E X E R C I S E
P R O G R A M — c o n t ' d

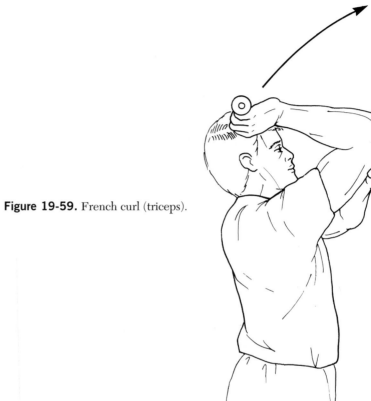

Figure 19-59. French curl (triceps).

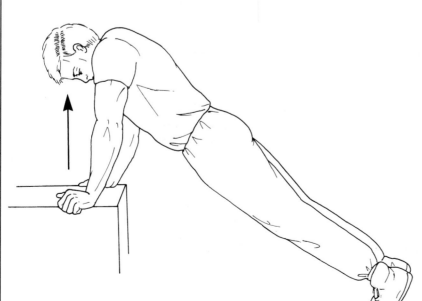

Figure 19-60. Progressive push-up.

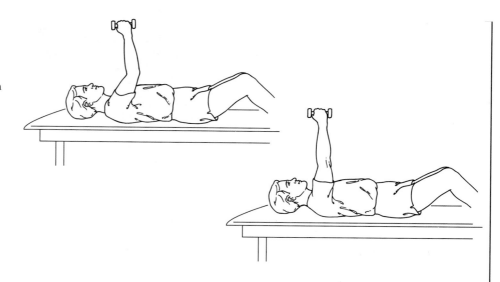

Figure 19-61. Punches. (Redrawn from Wilk, K.E., Andrews, J.R., Arrigo, C.A. et al. [1997]: Preventive and Rehabilitative Exercises for the Shoulder and Elbow, 5th ed. Birmingham, AL, American Sports Medicine Institute.)

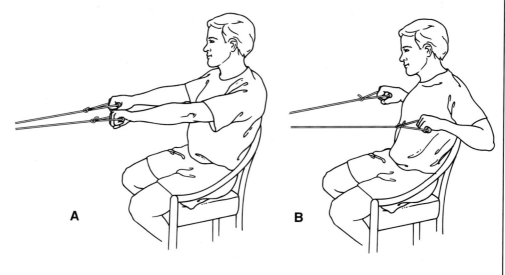

Figure 19-62. *A and B,* Seated rowing. (Redrawn from Wilk, K.E., Andrews, J.R., Arrigo, C.A. et al. [1997]: Preventive and Rehabilitative Exercises for the Shoulder and Elbow, 5th ed. Birmingham, AL, American Sports Medicine Institute.)

A   B

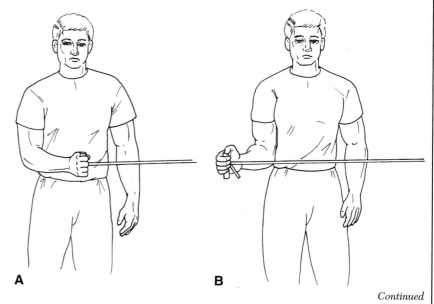

Figure 19-63. *A and B,* External rotation at 0° abduction.

A   B

Continued

T H E R A P E U T I C   S H O U L D E R   E X E R C I S E
P R O G R A M — c o n t ' d

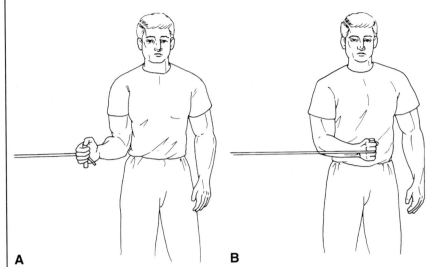

Figure 19-64. *A* and *B*, Internal rotation at 0° abduction.

A   B

External Rotation at 90° Abduction—Slow. The athlete stands with the shoulder abducted 90° and the elbow flexed 90° and grips the tubing handle (the other end of the tubing is fixed straight ahead) (Fig. 19-65*A* and *B*). Keeping the shoulder abducted, the athlete rotates the shoulder back (keeping the elbow at 90°), slowly returns to the starting position, pauses, and repeats the exercise.

External Rotation at 90° Abduction—Fast. This exercise is the same as the previous one except that the athlete externally rotates the shoulder quickly, keeping the elbow at 90°. The tubing and hand are returned to the starting position quickly and in a controlled manner.

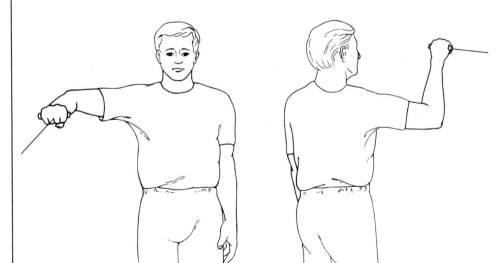

Figure 19-65. *A* and *B*, External rotation at 90° abduction.

A   B

Internal Rotation at 90° Abduction—Slow. The athlete stands with the shoulder abducted to 90° and externally rotated to 90° and the elbow flexed to 90° and grips the tubing handle (the other end of the tubing is fixed straight ahead) (Fig. 19-66*A* and *B*). Keeping the shoulder abducted, the athlete rotates the shoulder back (keeping the elbow at 90°), slowly returns to the starting position, pauses, and repeats.

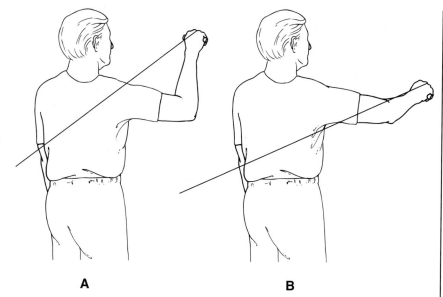

Figure 19-66. *A* and *B*, Internal rotation at 90° abduction.

Internal Rotation at 90° Abduction—Fast. This exercise is the same as the previous one except that the athlete internally rotates the shoulder quickly, keeping the elbow at 90°. The tubing and hand are returned to the starting position quickly and in a controlled manner.

Diagonal Pattern (D1) Flexion. The athlete grips the tubing handle in the hand of the involved arm. The athlete begins with the arm out 45° from the side and the palm facing backward (Fig. 19-67*A*). After turning the palm forward, the athlete proceeds to flex the elbow and brings the arm up and over the uninvolved shoulder (Fig. 19-67*B*), then turns the palm down, and reverses to take the arm to the starting position. The exercise should be performed in a controlled manner.

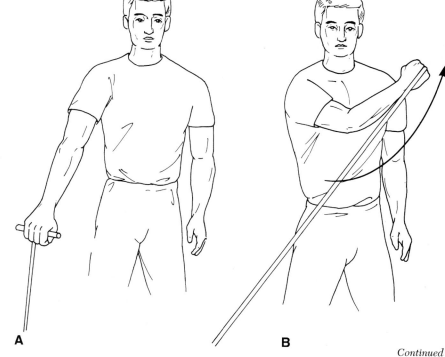

Figure 19-67. *A* and *B*, Diagonal pattern (D1) flexion.

Continued

THERAPEUTIC SHOULDER EXERCISE PROGRAM — cont'd

Diagonal Pattern (D2) Flexion. The athlete's involved hand grips the tubing handle across the body and against the opposite thigh (Fig. 19-68A). Starting with the palm down, the athlete rotates the palm up to begin, proceeds to flex the elbow, and brings the arm up and over the involved shoulder with the palm facing inward (Fig. 19-68B). The palm is turned down, and the movement is reversed to take the arm to the starting position. The exercise should be performed in a controlled manner.

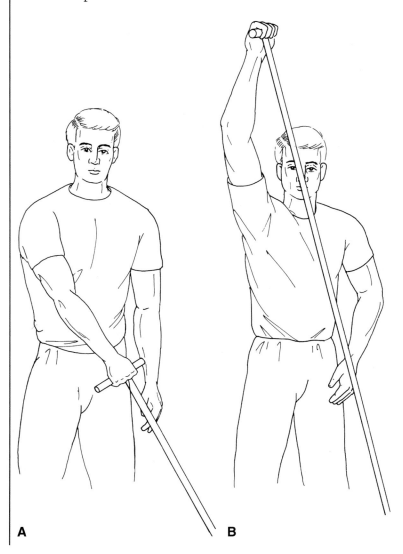

Figure 19-68. *A* and *B*, Diagonal pattern (D2) flexion.

A

B

Diagonal Pattern (D2) Extension. The athlete grips the tubing handle overhead and out to the side with the involved hand and pulls the tubing down and across the body to the opposite side of the leg (Fig. 19-69), leading with the thumb during the motion.

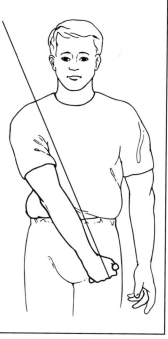

Figure 19-69. Diagonal pattern (D2) extension. (Redrawn from Wilk, K.E., Andrews, J.R., Arrigo, C.A. et al. [1997]: Preventive and Rehabilitative Exercises for the Shoulder and Elbow, 5th ed. Birmingham, AL, American Sports Medicine Institute.)

REFERENCES

1. Acerio, R.A., Wheeler, J.H., and Ryan, J.B. (1994): Arthroscopic Bankart repair vs. non-operative treatment for acute, initial anterior shoulder dislocations. Am. J. Sports Med., 22:589-594.

2. Ahmadain, A.M. (1987): The Magnuson-Stack operation for recurrent anterior dislocation of the shoulder. J. Bone Joint Surg. Br., 69:111-114.

3. Alderink, G.J., and Kuck, D.J. (1986): Isokinetic shoulder strength of high school and college aged pitchers. J. Orthop. Sports Phys., 7:163-172.

4. Altchek, D.W., Schwartz, E., and Warren, R.F. (1990): Radiologic measurement of superior migration of the humeral head in impingement syndrome. Presented at the annual meeting of the American Shoulder and Elbow Surgeons, New Orleans, LA, February 8-12.

5. Altchek, D.W., Skybar, M.J., and Warren, R.F. (1989): Shoulder arthroscopy for shoulder instability. Instr. Course Lect., 37:187-198.

6. Altchek, D.W., Warren, R.F., Skybar, M.J., and Ortiz, G. (1991): T-plasty modification of the Bankart procedure for multi-directional instability of the anterior and inferior types. J. Bone Joint Surg. Am., 73:105-112.

7. Allegrucci, M., Whitney, S.L., Lephart, S.M., et al. (1995): Shoulder kinesthesia in healthy unilateral athletes participating in upper extremity sports. J. Orthop. Sports Phys. Ther., 21:220-226.

8. Andrews, J.R. (1996): The pathomechanics of injury in the throwers' shoulder. Presented at the American Sports Medicine Institute Injuries in Baseball Course, Birmingham, AL, January 19.

9. Andrews, J.R., and Carson, W.G. (1984): The arthroscopic treatment of glenoid labrum tears in the throwing athlete. Orthop. Trans., 8:44-49.

10. Andrews, J.R., Carson, W.G., and McLeod, W.D. (1985): Glenoid labrum tears related to the long head of the biceps. Am. J. Sports Med., 13:337-341.

11. Andrews, J.R., Kupferman, S.P., and Dillman, C.J. (1985): Labral tears in throwing and racquet sports. Clin. Sports Med., 10:901-907, 1991.

12. Andrews, J.R., and Meister, K. (1993): Classification and treatment of rotator cuff injuries in the overhead athlete. J. Orthop. Sports Phys. Ther., 18:413-421.

13. Arnheim, D. (1985): Modern Principles of Athletic Training. St. Louis, C.V. Mosby.

14. Aronen, J.G. (1986): Anterior shoulder dislocation in sports. Sports Med., 3:224-234.

15. Aronen, J.G., and Regan, K. (1984): Decreasing the incidence of recurrence of first-time anterior shoulder dislocations with rehabilitation. Am. J. Sports Med., 12:283-291.

16. Baker, C.L., Uribe, J.W., and Whitman, C. (1990): Arthroscopic evaluation of acute initial anterior shoulder dislocations. Am. J. Sports Med., 18:25-28.

17. Bankart, A.S.B. (1923): The pathology and treatment of recurrent dislocation of the shoulder joint. Br. Med. J., 2:1132-1133.

18. Bankart, A.S.B. (1948): Discussion on recurrent dislocation of the shoulder. J. Bone Joint Surg., 30B:46-47.

19. Basmajian, J.V. (1963): The surgical anatomy and function of the arm-trunk mechanism. Surg. Clin. North Am., 43:1475-1479.

20. Basmajian, J.V., and Bazant, F.J. (1959): Factors preventing downward dislocation of the adducted shoulder joint. J. Bone Joint Surg., 41A:1182-1186.

21. Bartlett, L.R., Storey, M.D., and Simons, D.B. (1989): Measurement of upper extremity torque production and its relationship to throwing speed in the competitive athlete. Am. J. Sports Med., 17:89-91.

22. Bechtol, C. (1980): Biomechanics of the shoulder. Clin. Orthop., 146:37-41.

23. Berger, R.A. (1982): Applied Exercise Physiology. Philadelphia, Lea & Febiger, p. 267.

24. Bigliani, L.U. (1990): Multidirectional instability. Advances on the Knee and Shoulder. Cincinnati, Cincinnati Sports Medicine.

25. Bigliani, L.U., Codd, T.P., Connor, P.M., et al. (1997): Shoulder motion and laxity in the professional baseball player. Am. J. Sports Med., 25:609-612.

26. Bigliani, L.U., Kurzweil, P.R., Schwartzback, et al. (1994): Inferior capsular shift procedure for anterior-inferior shoulder instability in athletes. Am. J. Sports Med., 22:578-584.

27. Bigliani, L.U., Morrison, D., and April, E.W. (1986): The morphology of the acromion and its relationship to rotator cuff tears. Orthop. Trans., 10:228.

28. Blackburn, T.A. (1987): Throwing injuries to the shoulder. In: Donatelli R. (ed.), Physical Therapy of the Shoulder. New York, Churchill Livingstone.

29. Blackburn, T.A., McLeod, W.D., White, B.W., and Wofford, L. (1990): EMG analysis of posterior rotator cuff exercises. Athl. Train., 25:40-45.

30. Blasier, R.B., Carpenter, J.E., and Huston, L.J. (1994): Shoulder proprioception: effects of joint laxity, joint position, and direction of motion. Orthop. Rev. 23:45-50.

31. Bland, J. (1977): The painful shoulder. Semin. Arthritis Rheumatol., 7:21-47.

32. Boissonnault, W.G., and Janos, S.C. (1989): Dysfunction, evaluation, and treatment of the shoulder. In: Donatelli, R., and Wooden, M.J. (eds.), Orthopaedic Physical Therapy. New York, Churchill Livingstone.

33. Bost, F.C., and Inman, V.T. (1942): The pathological changes in recurrent dislocation of the shoulder; A report of Bankart's operative procedure. J. Bone Joint Surg., 24A:595-613.

34. Bowen, M.K., Deng, X.H., Hannafin, J.A., et al. (1992): An analysis of the patterns of glenohumeral joint contact and their relationship of the glenoid "bare area" (Abstract). Trans. Orthop. Res. Soc., 17:496, 1992.

35. Bowen, M.K., and Warren, R.F. (1991): Ligamentous control of shoulder stability based on selective cutting and static translation experiments. Clin. Sports Med., 10:757-782.

36. Braly, G., and Tullos, H.S. (1985): A modification of the Bristow procedure for recurrent anterior shoulder dislocation and subluxation. Am. J. Sports Med., 13:81-86.

37. Bratatz, J.H., and Gogia, P.P. (1987): The mechanics of pitching. J. Orthop. Sports Phys. Ther., 9:56-69.

38. Brewer, B.J. (1979): Aging of the rotator cuff. Am. J. Sports Med., 7:102-110.

39. Brewer, B.J., Wubben, R.G., and Carrera, G.F. (1986): Excessive retroversion of the glenoid cavity. J. Bone Joint Surg., 68A:724-726.

40. Brown, L.P., Niehues, S.L., Harrah, A., et al. (1988): Upper extremity range of motion and isokinetic strength of the internal and external shoulder rotators in major league baseball players. Am. J. Sports Med., 16:577-585.

41. Browne, A.O., Hoffmeyer, P., An, K.N., and Morrey, B.F. (1990): The influence of atmospheric pressure on shoulder stability. Orthop. Trans., 14:259-263.

42. Burkhardt, Morgan, C.D.

43. Caillet, R. (1966): Shoulder Pain. Philadelphia, F.A. Davis, 1966.

44. Cain, P.R., Mutschler, T.A., Fu, F.A., et al. (1987): Anterior stability of the glenohumeral joint: A dynamic model. Am. J. Sports Med., 15:144-148.

45. Caspari, R.B., and Savoie, F. (1991): Arthroscopic reconstruction of the shoulder: The Bankart repair. In: McGinty, J. (ed.), Operative Arthroscopy. New York, Raven Press, pp. 507-515.

46. Cave, E.F., Burke, J.F., and Boyd, R.J. (1974): Trauma Management. Chicago, Yearbook Medical, p. 437.

47. Chu, D. (1989): Plyometric exercises with a medicine ball. Livermore, CA, Bittersweet Publishing.

48. Clark, J.C., and Harryman, D.T. (1992): Tendons, ligaments, and capsule of the rotator cuff. J. Bone Joint Surg. Am., 74:713-719.

49. Clemente, C.A. (ed.) (1985): Gray's Anatomy of the Human Body, 30th ed. Philadelphia, (1993): Lea & Febiger, 1985.

50. Codman, E.A. (1934): The Shoulder, Boston: Thomas Todd.

51. Codman, E.A. (1934): Rupture of the supraspinatus tendon and other lesions in or about the subacromial bursa. *In:* Codman, E.A. (ed.), The Shoulder. Boston, Thomas Todd.

52. Colachis, S.C., and Strohm, B.R. (1971): The effect of suprascapular and axillary nerve blocks and muscle force in the upper extremity. Arch. Phys. Med. Rehabil., 52:22-29.

53. Colachis, S.C., Strohm, B.R., and Brechner, V.L. (1969): Effects of axillary nerve block on muscle force in the upper extremity. Arch. Phys. Med. Rehabil., 50:647-654.

54. Collins, K.A., Capito, C., and Cross, M. (1986): The use of the Putti-Platt procedure in the treatment of recurrent anterior dislocation. Am. J. Sports Med., 14:380-382.

55. Cook, E.E., Gray, U.L., Savinar-Nogue, E., et al. (1987): Shoulder antagonistic strength ratios: A comparison between college level baseball pitchers and non-pitchers. J. Orthop. Sports Phys. Ther., 8:451-461.

56. Davies, G.J., and Gould, J.A. (1985): Orthopaedic and Sports Physical Therapy. St. Louis, C.V. Mosby.

57. Davis, G.J., and Dickoff-Hoffman, S.D. (1993): Neuromuscular training and rehabilitation of the shoulder. J. Orthop. Sports Phys. Ther., 18:449-454.

58. DeDuca, C.J., and Forrest, W.J. (1973): Force analysis of individual muscles acting simultaneously on the shoulder joint during isometric abduction. J. Biomech., 6:385-393.

59. Dehre, E., and Tory, R. (1971): Treatment of joint injuries by immediate mobilization based upon the spinal adaption concept. Clin. Orthop., 77:218-232.

60. Dempster, W.T. (1965): Mechanisms of shoulder movement. Arch. Phys. Med. Rehabil., 46A:49.

61. DePalma, A.F. (1973): Surgery of the Shoulder, 2nd ed. Philadelphia, J.B. Lippincott.

62. DePalma, A.F., Callery, G., and Bennett, G.A. (1949): Variational anatomy and degenerative lesions of the shoulder joint. Instr. Course Lect., 6:255-281.

63. DiGiovine, N.M., Jobe, F.W., Pink, M., et al. (1992): An electromyographic analysis of the upper extremity in pitcher. J. Shoulder Elbow Surg., 1:15-25.

64. Ellenbecker, T.S., and Mattalino, A.J. (1999): Glenohumeral joint range of motion and rotator cuff strength following arthroscopic anterior stabilization with thermal capsulorraphy. J. Orthop. Sports Phys. Ther., 29:160-167.

65. Engle, R.P., and Canner, G.C. (1989): Posterior shoulder instability approach to rehabilitation. J. Orthop. Sports Phys. Ther., 10:488-494.

66. Ferrari, D.A. (1990): Capsular ligaments of the shoulder: Anatomical and functional study of the anterior superior capsule. Am. J. Sports Med., 18:20-24.

67. Flatow, E.L., Soslowsky, L.J., Ticker, J.B., et al. (1994): Excursion of the rotator cuff under the acromion: Patterns of subacromial contact. Am. J. Sports Med., 22: 779-788.

68. Fleisig, G.S. (1977): Ten years in twenty minutes: Conclusions from ASMI's research. Presented at 15th Annual Injuries in Baseball Course, American Sports Medicine Institute, Birmingham, AL, January 24.

69. Fleisig, G.S. (Exercise Abstract).

70. Fleisig, G.S., Dillman, C.J., and Andrews, J.R. (1997): Biomechanics of the shoulder during throwing. *In:* Andrews, J.R., and Wilk, K.E. (eds.), The Athlete's Shoulder. New York, Churchill Livingstone, pp. 355-368.

71. Fukuda, K., Craig, E.V., and An, K. (1986): Biomechanical study of the ligamentous system of the acromioclavicular joint. J. Bone Joint Surg. Am., 68:434-440.

72. Fukuda, H., Mikasa, M., Ogawa, K., et al. (1983): The partial-thickness tear of the rotator cuff. Orthop. Trans., 55:137.

73. Gambetta, V., and Odgers, S. (1991): The Complete Guide to Medicine Ball Training. Sarasota, FL, Optimum Sports Training.

74. Garth, W.P., Allman, F.L., and Armstrong, W.S. (1987): Occult anterior subluxations of the shoulder in non-contact sports. Am. J. Sports Med., 15:579-585.

75. Gibb, T.D., Sidles, J.A., Harryman, D.T., et al. (1991): The effect of capsular venting on glenohumeral laxity. Clin. Orthop., 268:120-127.

76. Glousman, R., Jobe, F., Tibone, J., et al. (1988): Dynamic electromyographic analysis of the throwing shoulder with glenohumeral instability. J. Bone Joint Surg. Am., 70: 220-226.

77. Gohlke, F., Essigkrug, B., and Schmitz, F. (1994): The pattern of the collagen fiber bundles of the capsule of the glenohumeral joint. J. Shoulder Elbow Surg., 3:111-128.

78. Grana, W., Buckley, P., and Yates, C. (1993): Arthroscopic Bankart suture repair. Am. J. Sports Med., 21: 348-353.

79. Habermeyer, P., Schuller, U., and Wiedemann, E. (1992): The intra-articular pressure of the shoulder: An experimental study on the role of the glenoid labrum in stabilizing the joint. Arthroscopy, 8:166-172.

80. Haggmark, T., Eriksson, E., and Jansson, E. (1986): Muscle fiber type changes in human muscles after injuries and immobilization. Orthopaedics, 9:181-189.

81. Harryman, D.T., II, Sidles, J.A., Clark, J.M., et al. (1990): Translation of the humeral head on the glenoid with passive glenohumeral motion. J. Bone Joint Surg. Am., 72:1334-1338.

82. Harryman, D.T., II, Sidles, J.A., Clark, J.A., et al. (1990): Translation of the humeral head on the glenoid with passive glenohumeral motion. J. Bone Joint Surg., 72A: 1334-1343.

83. Harryman, D.T., II, Sidles, J.A., Harris, S.L., and Matsen, F.A. (1992): Laxity of the normal glenohumeral joint: A qualitative in vivo assessment. J. Shoulder Elbow Surg., 1:66-76.

84. Harryman, D.T., II, Sidles, J.A., Harris, S.L., and Matsen, F.A. (1992): Role of the rotator interval capsule in passive motion and stability of the shoulder. J. Bone Joint Surg., 74A:53-66.

85. Hawkins, R.J., and Angelo, R.L. (1990): Glenohumeral osteoarthrosis: A late complication of the Putti-Platt procedure. J. Bone Joint Surg. Am., 72:1193-1197.

86. Hawkins, R., and Kennedy, J. (1980): Impingement syndrome in athletes. Am. J. Sports Med., 8:151-158.

87. Hawkins, R.J., Kippert, G., and Johnston, G. (1984): Recurrent posterior instability (subluxation) of the shoulder. J. Bone Joint Surg. Am., 66:169-174.

88. Hayashi, K., Massa, K.L., Thabit, G., et al. (1999): Histologic evaluation of the glenohumeral joint capsule after the

laser-assisted capsular shift procedure for glenohumeral instability. Am. J. Sports Med., 77:162-167.

89. Hecht, P., Hayashi, K., Lu, Y., et al. (1999): Monopolar
radiofrequency energy effect on joint capsular tissue: Potential
treatment for joint instability. An in vivo mechanical, morphological, and biomechanical study using an ovine model. Am. J.
Sports Med., 27:761-771.

90. Hill, H.A., and Sachs, M.D. (1940): The grooved defect of
the humeral head. A frequently unrecognized complication
of dislocations of the shoulder joint. Radiology, 35:
690-700.

91. Hinton, R.Y. (1988): Isokinetic evaluation of shoulder rotational
strength in high school baseball pitchers. Am. J. Sports Med.,
16:274-279.

92. Hollingshead, W.H. (1987): Anatomy for Surgeons, Vol. III.
The Back and Limbs. New York, Hoeber & Harper,
1958.

93. Hovelius L: Anterior dislocation of the shoulder in teenagers
and young adults. J. Bone Joint Surg. Am., 69:393-399.

94. Howell, S.M., and Galinet, S.J. (1989): The glenoid labral
socket: A constrained articular surface. Clin. Orthop.,
243:122-129.

95. Howell, S.M., Galinet, B.J., Renzi, A.J., and Marone, P.J.
(1988): Normal and abnormal mechanics of the glenohumeral
joint in the horizontal plane. J. Bone Joint Surg., 70A:
227-232.

96. Howell, S.M., Imobersteg, A.M., Segar, D.H., and Marone, P.J.
(1986): Clarification of the role of the supraspinatus
muscle in shoulder function. J. Bone Joint Surg. Am.,
68:398-404.

97. Hughston, J.C. (1989): Functional anatomy of the shoulder.
In: Zarins, B., Andrews, J.R., and Carson, W.G. (eds.), Injuries
to the Throwing Arm. Philadelphia, W.B. Saunders,
1985.

98. Iannotti, J.P., Swiontkowski, M., Esterhafi, J., and Boulas, H.F.
(1989): Intraoperative assessment of rotator cuff vascularity
using laser Doppler flowmetry (Abstract). Presented at the
Meeting of the American Academy of Orthopaedic Surgeons,
Las Vegas.

99. Inman, V., and Saunders, J.B. (1946): Observations of the
function of the clavicle. Calif. Med., 65:158-166.

100. Inman, V., Saunders, M., and Abbott, L. (1944): Observations
of the function of the shoulder joint. J. Bone Joint Surg. Am.,
26:1-30.

101. Jobe, C.M. (1995): Posterior superior glenoid impingement.
J. Shoulder Elbow Surg., 11:530-556.

102. Jobe, C.M. (1996): Superior glenoid impingement: current
concepts. Clin. Orthop., 330:98-107.

103. Jobe, C.M. (1997): Superior glenoid impingement. Orthop.
Clin. North Am., 28:137-143.

104. Jobe, F.W., and Jobe, C.M. (1983): Painful athletic injuries of
the shoulder. Clin. Orthop., 173:117-124.

105. Jobe, F.W., and Moynes, D.R. (1982): Delineation of diagnostic
criteria and a rehabilitation program for rotator cuff injuries.
Am. J. Sports Med., 10:336-339.

106. Jobe, F.W., Moynes, D.R., and Tibone, J.E. (1984): An EMG
analysis of the shoulder in pitching: A second report. Am. J.
Sports Med., 12:218-220.

107. Jobe, F.W., Tibone, J.E., Jobe, C.M., and Kvitne, R.S., Jr.
(1990): The shoulder in sports. In: Rockwood, C.A., and
Matsen, F.A., III (eds.), The Shoulder. Philadelphia, W.B.
Saunders.

108. Jobe, F.W., Tibone, J.E., Perry, J., et al. (1983): An EMG analysis of the shoulder in throwing and pitching: A preliminary
report. Am. J. Sports Med., 11:3-5.

109. Johnson, L. (1992): Patterns of shoulder flexibility among
college baseball players. J. Ath. Train., 27:44-49.

110. Kaltsas, D.S. (1983): Comparative study of the properties of
the shoulder joint capsule with those of other joint capsules.
Clin. Orthop., 173:20-26.

111. Kazar, B., and Relouszky, E. (1969): Prognosis of primary
dislocation of the shoulder. Acta. Orthop. Scand., 40:
216-219.

112. Kelly, B.T., Kadrmas, W.R., and Speer, K.P. (1996): The manual
muscle examination for rotator cuff strength. An electromyographic investigation. Am. J. Sports Med., 24B:
581-588.

113. Kennedy, J.C., and Willis, R.B. (1976): The effects of local
steroid injections on tendons: A biomechanical and microscopic
correlative study. Am. J. Sports Med., 4:11-21.

114. Kent, B. (1971): Functional anatomy of the shoulder complex:
A review. Phys. Ther., 51:867-887.

115. Kessel, L., and Watson, M. (1977): The painful arc syndrome.
J. Bone Joint Surg. Br., 59:166-172.

116. Kibler, W.B. (1991): Role of the scapular in the overhead
throwing motion. Contemp. Orthop., 22:525-532.

117. Kibler, W.B. (1998): The role of the athletic shoulder function.
Am. J. Sports Med., 26:325-337.

118. Kuland, D. (1982): The Injured Athlete. Philadelphia,
J.B. Lippincott.

119. Kumar, V.P., and Balasubramianium, P. (1985): The role of
atmospheric pressure in stabilizing the shoulder. An experimental study. J. Bone Joint Surg., 67B:719-721.

120. Kvitne, R.S., Jobe, F.W., and Jobe, C.M. (1995): Shoulder instability in the overhead or throwing athlete. Clin. Sports Med.,
14:917-935.

121. Lilleby, H. (1984): Shoulder arthroscopy. Acta. Orthop. Scand.,
55:561-566.

122. Lindblom, K. (1939): On pathogenesis of ruptures of the
tendon aponeurosis of the shoulder joint. Acta. Radiol.,
20:563-577.

123. Lippett, F.G. (1982): A modification of the gravity method
of reducing anterior shoulder dislocations. Clin. Orthop.,
165:259-260.

124. Lucas, D.B. (1973): Biomechanics of the shoulder joint. Arch
Surg. 107:425-432.

125. MacConnail, M., and Basmajian, J. (1969): Muscles and
Movement: A Basis for Human Kinesiology. Baltimore,
Williams & Wilkins.

126. Magnusson, S.P., Gleim, G.W., and Nicholas, J.A. (1994):
Shoulder weakness in professional baseball pitchers. Med. Sci.
Sports Exerc., 26:5-9.

127. Malanga, G.A., Jenp, Y.N., Growney, E.C., and An, K.N.
(1996): EMG analysis of shoulder positioning in testing and
strengthening the supraspinatus. Med. Sci. Sports Exerc.,
28:661-664.

128. Matsen, F.A., III (1980): Compartmental Syndromes. San Francisco, Grune & Stratton.

129. Matsen, F.A., III, and Arntz, C.T. (1990): Rotator cuff tendon failure. In: Rockwood, C.A., Jr., and Matsen, F.A., III (eds.), The Shoulder, Vol. II. Philadelphia, W.B. Saunders, pp. 647-677.

130. Matsen, F.A., III, and Arntz, C.T. (1990): Subacromial impingement. In: Rockwood, C.A., Jr., and Matsen, F.A., III (eds.), The Shoulder, Vol. II. Philadelphia, W.B. Saunders, pp. 623-646.

131. Matsen, F.A., Thomas, S.C., and Rockwood, C.A. (1985): Anterior glenohumeral instability. In: Rockwood, C.A., and Matsen, F.A. (eds.), The Shoulder, Philadelphia: W.B. Saunders.

132. McLeod, W.D.: The pitching mechanism. In: Zarins, B., Andrews, J.R., and Carson, W.G. (eds.), Injuries to the Throwing Arm. Philadelphia, W.B. Saunders, pp. 22-29.

133. McLeod, W.D., and Andrews, J.R. (1986): Mechanisms of shoulder injuries. Phys. Ther., 66:1901-1904.

134. Miller, L.S., Donahue, J.R., Good, R.P., and Staerk, A.J. (1984): The Magnuson-Stack procedure for treatment of recurrent glenohumeral dislocations. Am. J. Sports Med., 12:133-137.

135. Morgan, C.D. (1991): Arthroscopic transglenoid suture repair. Oper. Tech. Orthop. Surg., 1:171-179.

136. Morgan, C.D., and Bodenstab, A.B. (1987): Arthroscopic Bankart suture repair: Technique and early results. Arthroscopy, 3:111-122.

137. Morrison, D.S., and Bigliani, L.U. (1987): The clinical significance of variation in acromial morphology. Presented at the Third Open Meeting of the American Shoulder and Elbow Surgeons, San Francisco.

138. Moseley, H.F., and Goldie, I. (1963): The arterial pattern of rotator cuff of the shoulder. J. Bone Joint Surg. Br., 45: 780-789.

139. Moseley, H.F., and Overgaard, B. (1962): The anterior capsular mechanism in recurrent dislocation of the shoulder: Morphological and clinical studies with special reference to the glenoid labrum and glenohumeral ligaments. J. Bone Joint Surg., 44B:13-27.

140. Neer, C.S. (1972): Anterior acromioplasty for the chronic impingement syndrome in the shoulder: A preliminary report. J. Bone Joint Surg. Am., 54:41-50.

141. Neer, C.S. (1983): Impingement syndrome. Clin. Orthop., 173:70-77.

142. Neviaser, R.J. (1987): Injuries to the clavicle and acromioclavicular joint. Orthop. Clin. North Am., 18:433-438.

143. Norkin, C., and Levangie, P. (1983): Joint Structure and Function: A Comprehensive Analysis. Philadelphia, F.A. Davis.

144. Norwood, L.A. (1985): Posterior shoulder instability. In: Zarins, B., Andrews, J.R., and Carson, W.G. (eds.), Injuries to the Throwing Arm. Philadelphia, W.B. Saunders, pp. 153-159.

145. O'Brien, S.J. (1994): Glenoid labral lesions. Presented at Advances of the Knee and Shoulder, Hilton Head, SC, May.

146. O'Brien, S.J., Neves, M.C., and Arnoczky, S.J. (1990): The anatomy and histology of the inferior glenohumeral ligament complex of the shoulder. Am. J. Sports Med., 18: 449-456.

147. O'Brien, S.J., Neves, M.C., Arnoczky, S.P., et al.(1990): The anatomy and histology of the inferior glenohumeral ligament complex of the shoulder. Am. J. Sports Med., 18:449-456.

148. O'Brien, S.J., Schwartz, R.E., Warren, R.F., and Torzilli, P.A. (1988): Capsular restraints to anterior/posterior motion of the shoulder (Abstract). Orthop. Trans., 12:143.

149. Oveson, J., and Nielson, S. (1986): Anterior and posterior instability of the shoulder: A cadaver study. Acta Orthop. Scand., 57:324-327.

150. Pagnani, M.J., and Warren, R.F. (1994): Stabilizers of the glenohumeral joint. J. Shoulder Elbow Surg., 3:173-190.

151. Pappas, A.M., Zawacki, R.M., and Sullivan, T.J. (1985): Biomechanics of baseball pitching: A preliminary report. Am. J. Sports Med., 13:216-222.

152. Pavlov, H., Warren, R.F., Weiss, C.B., and Dines, D.M. (1985): The roentgenographic evaluation of anterior shoulder instability. Clin. Orthop., 194:153-158.

153. Perry, J. (1988): Muscle control of the shoulder. In: Rowe, C.R. (ed.), The Shoulder, pp. 17-34. New York: Churchill Livingstone.

154. Perry, J., and Glousman, R.E. (1990): Biomechanics of throwing. In: Nicholas, J.A., and Hershman, E.B. (eds.), The Upper Extremity in Sports Medicine. St. Louis, C.V. Mosby, pp. 727-751.

155. Podromos, C.C., Perry, J.A., and Schiller, J.A. (1990): Histological studies of the glenoid labrum from fetal life to old age. J. Bone Joint Surg. Am., 72:1344-1352.

156. Poppen, N.K., and Walker, P.S. (1976): Normal and abnormal motion of the shoulder. J. Bone Joint Surg. Am., 58: 195-201.

157. Poppen, N., and Walker, P. (1978): Forces at the glenohumeral joint in adduction. Clin. Orthop. 135:165-170.

158. Protzman, R.R. (1980): Anterior instability of the shoulder. J. Bone Joint Surg. Am., 62:909-918.

159. Rathbun, J.B., and Macnab, I. (1970): The microvascular pattern of the rotator cuff. J. Bone Joint Surg. Br., 52: 540-553.

160. Rockwood, C.A., and Young, D.C. (1990): Disorders of the acromioclavicular joint. In: Rockwood, C.A., and Matsen, F.A. (eds.), The Shoulder. Philadelphia, W.B. Saunders, pp. 413-468.

161. Rowe, C.R. (1956): Prognosis in dislocation of the shoulder. J. Bone Joint Surg., 38A:957-977.

162. Rowe, C.R. (1981): The Shoulder. New York, Churchill Livingstone, 1988.

163. Rowe, C.R. (1988): Tendinitis, bursitis, impingement, "snapping scapula" and calcific tendinitis. In: Rowe, C.R. (ed.), The Shoulder. New York, Churchill Livingstone, pp. 105-129.

164. Rowe, C.R., Patel, D., Southmayd, W.W. (1978): The Bankart procedure: A long term end-result study. J. Bone Joint Surg., 60A:1-16.

165. Rowe, C., and Zarins, B.: Recurrent transient subluxation of the shoulder. J. Bone Joint Surg. Am., 63:863-871.

166. Saha, A. (1961): Theory of Shoulder Mechanism: Descriptive and Applied. Springfield, IL, Charles C Thomas, 1961.

167. Saha, A.K. (1971): Dynamic stability of the glenohumeral joint. Acta Orthop. Scand., 42:491-505.

168. Salter, R.B., Hamilton, H.W., and Wedge, J.H. (1983): Clinical application of basic science research on continuous passive motion for disorders of injures and synovial joints. J. Orthop. Res., 1984;1:325-333.

169. Sarrafian, S. (1983): Gross and functional anatomy of the shoulder. Clin., Orthop., 173:11-19.

170. Schaefer, S.L., Ciarelli, M.J., Arnoczky, S.T., and Ross, H.E. (1997): Tissue shrinkage with the holmium:yttrium: aluminum:garnet laser: A postoperative assessment of tissue length, stiffness, and structure. Am. J. Sports Med., 25:841-848.

171. Schwartz, R.E., O'Brien, S.J., and Warren, R.F. (1988): Capsular restraints to anterior-posterior motion of the abducted shoulder: A biomechanical study (Abstract). Orthop. Trans., 12:727.

172. Shall, L.W., and Crowley, P.W. (1994): Soft tissue reconstruction in the shoulder: Comparison of suture anchors, absorbable staples and absorbable tacks. Am. J. Sports Med., 22:715-718.

173. Sigholm, G., Styf, J., Korner, L., and Herberts, P. (1988): Pressure recording in the subacromial bursa. J. Orthop. Res., 6:123-128.

174. Snyder, S.J., Karzel, R.P., DelPizzo, W., et al. (1990): SLAP lesions of the shoulder. Arthroscopy, 6:274-276.

175. Soslowsky, L.J., Flatow, E.L., Bigliani, L.U., et al. (1992): Quantitation of in situ contact areas and the glenohumeral joint: A biomechanical study. J. Orthop. Res., 10:524-535.

176. Steindler, A. (1955): Kinesiology of Human Body Under Normal and Pathological Conditions, Springfield, IL, Charles C Thomas, 1955.

177. Steindler, A. (1955): Kinesiology of the Human Body. Springfield, IL, Charles C Thomas.

178. Tipton, C.M., Mattes, R.D., and Maynard, J.A. (1975): The influence of physical activity on ligaments and tendons. Med. Sci. Sports Exerc., 7:165-175.

179. Townsend, H., Jobe, F.W., Pink, M., et al. (1992): EMG analysis of the glenohumeral muscles during a baseball rehabilitation program. Am. J. Sports Med., 19:264-269.

180. Travell, J.G., and Simons, D.G. (1983): Myofascial Pain and Dysfunction: The Trigger Point Manual. Baltimore, Williams & Wilkins.

181. Tullos, H.S., and King, J.W. (1973): Throwing mechanism in sports. Orthop. Clin. North Am., 4:709-721.

182. Turkel, S., Panio, M., Marshall, J., and Girgis, F. (1981): Stabilization mechanism preventing anterior dislocation of the glenohumeral joint. J. Bone Joint Surg. Am., 63: 1208-1217.

183. Tyler, T.F., Calabrese, G.J., Parker, R.D., and Nicholas, S.J. (2000): Electrothermally-assisted capsulorraphy (ETAC): A new surgical method for glenohumeral instability and its rehabilitation considerations. J. Orthop. Phys. Ther., 30: 390-400.

184. Walch, G., Boileau, P., Noel, E., and Donell, T. (1992): Impingement of the deep surface of the supraspinatus tendon on the glenoid rim. J. Shoulder Elbow Surg., 1:239-245.

185. Walsh, D.A. (1989): Shoulder evaluation of the throwing athlete. Sports Med. Update, 4:524-527.

186. Warner, J.J.P., Deng, X.P., Warren, R.F., and Torzilli, P.A. (1992): Static capsular ligamentous constraints to superior-inferior translation of the glenohumeral joint. Am. J. Sports Med., 20:675-685.

187. Warner, J.J.P., and Warren, R.F. (1991): Arthroscopic Bankart repair using a cannulated absorbable fixation device. Oper. Tech. Orthop. Surg., 1:192-198.

188. Wick, H.J., Dillman, C.J., Wisleder, D., et al. (1991): A kinematic comparison between baseball pitching and football passing. Sports Med. Update, 6:13-16.

189. Wickiewicz, T.L., Chen, S.K., Otis, J.C., and Warren, R.F. (1995): Glenohumeral kinematics in a muscle fatigue model: A radiographic study. Orthop. Trans., 18:126.

190. Wickiewicz, T.L., Pagnani, M.J., and Kennedy, K. (1993): Rehabilitation of the unstable shoulder. Sports Med. Arthrosc. Rev., 1:227-235.

191. Wilk, K.E. (1996): Conditioning and Training Techniques. In: Hawkins, R.J., and Misamore, G.W. (eds.), Shoulder Injuries in the Athlete. New York, Churchill Livingstone, pp. 339-364.

192. Wilk, K.E. (2000): Restoration of functional motor patterns and functional testing in the throwing athlete. In: Lephart, S.M., abd Fu, F.H. (eds.), Proprioception and Neuromuscular Control in Joint Stability. Champaign IL, Human Kinetics, pp. 415-438.

193. Wilk, K.E., and Andrews, J.R. (1993): Rehabilitation following arthroscopic shoulder subacromial decompression. Orthopedics, 16:349-355.

194. Wilk, K.E., and Andrews, J.R. (1993): Rehabilitation following arthroscopic subacromial decompression. Orthopaedics, 16:349-358.

195. Wilk, K.E., Andrews, J.R., Arrigo, C.A., et al. (1993): The strength characteristics of internal and external rotator muscles in professional baseball pitchers. Am. J. Sports Med., 21:61-69.

196. Wilk, K.E., Andrews, J.R., Arrigo, C.A. (1995): The abductor and adductor strength characteristics of professional baseball pitchers. Am. J. Sports Med., 23:307-311.

197. Wilk, K.E., Andrews, J.R., Arrigo, C.A., et al. (2001): Preventive and Rehabilitative Exercises for the Shoulder and Elbow, 6th ed. Birmingham, AL, American Sports Medicine Institute.

198. Wilk, K.E., and Arrigo, C.A. (1992): An integrated approach to upper extremity exercises. Orthop. Phys. Ther. Clin. North Am., 9:337-360.

199. Wilk, K.E., and Arrigo, C.A. (1993): Current concepts in the rehabilitation of the athletic shoulder. J. Orthop. Sports Phys. Ther., 18:365-378.

200. Wilk, K.E., Meister, K., and Andrews, J.R. (2003): Current concepts in the rehabilitation of the overhead athlete. Am. J. Sports Med., 30:136-151.

201. Wilk, K.E., Reinold, M.M., Dugas, J.R., and Andrews, J.R. (2002): Rehabilitation following thermal capsular shrinkage of the glenohumeral joint. J. Orthop. Sports Phys. Ther., 32:268-292.

202. Wilk, K.E., Voight, M., Keirns, M.A., et al. (1993): Stretch shortening drills for the upper extremity: Theory and clinical application. J. Orthop. Sports Phys. Ther., 17: 225-239.

203. Williams, P.L., and Warwick, R. (1986): Gray's Anatomy, 36th ed. (British). Philadelphia: W.B. Saunders.

204. Wilson, C.F., and Duff, G.L. (1943): Pathologic study of degeneration and rupture of the supraspinatus tendon. Arch. Surg., 47:121-135.

205. Wuelker, N., Wirth, C.J., Plitz, W., and Roetman, B. (1995): A dynamic shoulder model: Reliability testing and muscle force study. J. Biomech., 28:489-499.

206. Yamanaka, K., Fukuda, H., and Mikasa, M. (1987): Incomplete thickness tears of the rotator cuff. Clin. Orthop., 223: 51-58.

207. Zarins, B., and Rowe, C.R. (1984): Current concepts in the diagnosis and treatment of shoulder instability in athletes. Med. Sci. Sports Exerc., 16:444-448.

CHAPTER 20

REHABILITATION OF ELBOW INJURIES

Kevin E. Wilk, P.T.
Christopher A. Arrigo, M.S., P.T., ATC

CHAPTER OBJECTIVES

At the end of this chapter the reader will be able to:

■ Associate anatomical structures of the elbow to particular injuries based on the function of the structures during specific athletic endeavors.

■ Correlate the findings from a clinical examination to specific elbow injuries.

■ Incorporate biomechanical principles as they relate to the elbow in the prevention and postinjury rehabilitation of specific injuries.

■ Develop a rehabilitation program for specific elbow pathologic conditions that take into account the biomechanical function and healing parameters for the anatomical structures involved.

■ Progress an athlete through phases of rehabilitation based on specific criteria for advancement.

Elbow joint complex injuries are common occurrences in all types of athletic participation. Rehabilitation after these injuries is often challenging because of the unique anatomy of the elbow joint and the significant stress applied to this complex during sport-specific movements. The most common mechanisms of injuries are repetitive microtraumatic overuse and macrotraumatic overload forces.[91,92] Elbow complex injury patterns are typically sport specific because of the unique demands placed on the elbow during the sport or activity. Overhead throwing athletes such as pitchers and tennis players typically exhibit chronic stress overload or repetitive traumatic stress injuries.[23] Conversely, athletes participating in collision sports such as football, ice hockey, wrestling, and gymnastics are more susceptible to traumatic elbow injuries that include fractures and dislocations.

The ultimate goal of any rehabilitation program is to gradually restore function and return the athlete to symptom-free competition as quickly and safely as possible. Successful rehabilitation of the elbow joint is no different. It requires a thorough knowledge of the anatomy, biomechanics, and pathomechanics of athletic participation. In this chapter an overview of the anatomy and biomechanics of the elbow during sports, along with a detailed description of common clinical examination techniques for the injured athlete, will be provided. Several nonoperative and postoperative rehabilitation programs will be discussed for specific sport injuries, which use a multiphased, progressive rehabilitation approach based on current scientific research and clinical experience.

ANATOMY

Sport-specific applied anatomy of the elbow joint complex can be broken down and divided into the component osseous, capsuloligamentous, musculotendinous, and neurologic structures.

Osseous Structures

The elbow joint complex includes the humerus, radius, and ulna articulating together in concert to form four joints: the humeroulnar joint, the humeroradial joint, the proximal radioulnar joint and the distal radioulnar joints (Fig. 20-1).

The humeroulnar joint is generally considered a uniaxial, diarthrodial joint with 1° of freedom. It allows flexion and extension in the sagittal plane around a coronal axis. Morrey[51] described the humeroulnar joint as a modified hinge joint because of the small amounts of internal and external rotation that occur in the extreme end ranges of both flexion and extension. The anterior aspect of the distal humerus is composed of the convex trochlea. It is an hourglass-shaped surface covered with articular cartilage.

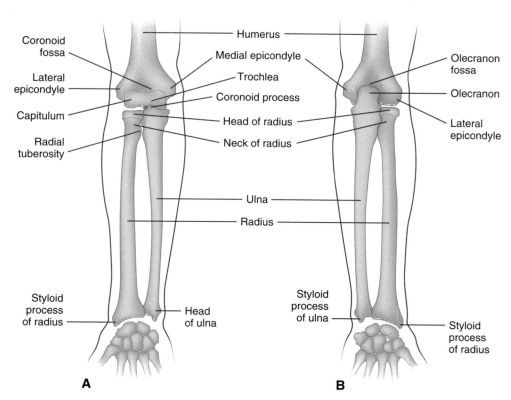

Figure 20-1. Osseous structures of the elbow.

The trochlear groove is located centrally within the trochlea and runs obliquely in an anterior-posterior direction. The distal end of the humerus is typically rotated anteriorly 30° with respect to the long axis of the humerus. Correspondingly, the proximal ulna is normally rotated 30° posteriorly in respect to the shaft of the ulna. This paired anatomical rotation of the humerus and ulna ensures the availability of end range elbow flexion to approximately 145 to 150°. It also serves to enhance the static stability of the elbow complex in full extension.[43]

The proximal ulna contains a central ridge that runs between two bony prominences, the coronoid process anteriorly and the olecranon posteriorly. Two fossas are located on each side of the corresponding articular surfaces of the humerus. Anteriorly, the coronoid fossa articulates with the coronoid process of the ulna during flexion. Posteriorly, the olecranon fossa receives the olecranon process of the ulna serving to limit extension. The congruency achieved via these articulations makes the humeroulnar joint one of the most stable joints in the human body.[54]

The medial epicondyle of the humerus also contributes significantly to the humeroulnar joint. Located proximal and medial to the trochlea, it serves as the site of origin for the flexor-pronator muscle group and the ulnar collateral ligament (UCL). Hoppenfeld[29] noted that both the size and prominence of the medial epicondyle provides an important mechanical advantage for the medial stabilizing structures of the elbow joint. The cubital tunnel is located posterior to the medial epicondyle and functions to protect the ulnar nerve as it transverses distally across the elbow joint complex.

Similarly, the humeroradial joint is a diarthrodial, uniaxial joint that allows elbow flexion and extension along with the humeroulnar joint. The humeroradial joint also pivots around a longitudinal axis to allow rotational movements in association with the proximal radioulnar joint, thus making the joint a combination hinge and pivot joint.[58]

The articular surfaces of the humeroradial joint include the concave radial head and the spherical convex capitellum at the distal aspect of the humerus.[36] The capitellum and trochlea are separated by a groove within the humerus, the capitulotrochlear groove. This groove guides the radial head as the elbow flexes and extends.

Immediately proximal to the capitellum on the anterior aspect of the humerus is the radial fossa. It receives the anterior aspect of the radial head when the elbow is in a maximally flexed position. The lateral epicondyle of the humerus lies just lateral to the radial fossa. It serves as the origin site for the wrist extensor muscle group. The radial tuberosity is located on the radius just distal to the radial head. It is the attachment site for the distal biceps brachii tendon.

The proximal and distal radioulnar joints are intimately related from a functional standpoint. Together they allow 1° of freedom in the transverse plane around a longitudinal axis, facilitating forearm supination and pronation. During these motions, the head of the radius rotates within a ring formed by the annular ligament and radial notch of the ulna. Little motion actually occurs in the ulna. The radius and ulna lie parallel to each other whereas the forearm is in a pronated position. As the forearm rotates into supination, the radius crosses over the ulna. The radius and ulna are connected midway between the two bony shafts by an interosseous membrane, which serves as an additional attachment site for the forearm musculature.

Functionally the bony articulation of the elbow joint forms the carrying angle of the elbow. This is defined as the angle formed by the long axis of the humerus and the ulna. It normally results in the abducted position of the forearm in relation to the humerus. The carrying angle is measured in the frontal plane with the elbow extended and averages 11 to 14° in males and 13 to 16° in females.[9,37] The carrying angle changes linearly as the elbow joint is flexed and extended, diminishing in flexion and increasing with extension.[51]

Capsuloligamentous Structures

The joint capsule is a relatively thin but strong structure, exhibiting significant strength from its transverse and obliquely oriented fibrous bands. The posterior portion of the capsule is a thin transparent structure that allows visualization of the bony prominences when the elbow is fully extended. The posterior capsule originates just above the olecranon fossa and inserts distally along the medial and lateral margins of the trochlea. The anterior capsule originates proximally above the coronoid and radial fossas, attaching distally at the anterior margin of the coronoid medially and into the annular ligament laterally. The anterior capsule is taut as the elbow is extended and lax in flexion. The greatest capsular laxity occurs at approximately 80° of elbow flexion.[35] A synovial membrane lines the joint capsule and is attached anteriorly above the radial and coronoid fossas to the medial and lateral margins of the

articular surface and posteriorly to the superior margin of the olecranon fossa.

The ligaments of the elbow consist of thickened parts of the medial and lateral capsules. The UCL is located on the medial aspect of the elbow. This ligamentous complex can be divided into three distinct portions, the anterior, posterior, and transverse bundles (Fig. 20-2). The anterior bundle originates from the inferior surface of the medial epicondyle and inserts at the medial aspect of the coronoid process. Because of the posterior orientation of this portion of the ligament in relation to the center of rotation of the elbow joint, the anterior bundle is taut throughout elbow range of motion (ROM). The anterior bundle can be further divided into two bands: the anterior band, which is taut in extension, and the posterior band, which tightens in flexion.[51,72] The anterior bundle of the UCL provides the main ligamentous support to valgus strain at the elbow.

The posterior bundle originates from the posteroinferior medial epicondyle and fans out to attach onto the posteromedial aspect of the olecranon. The transverse bundle of the UCL originates from the medial olecranon and inserts into the coronoid process. Several authors report that these two bundles provide minimal amounts of medial elbow stability.[53,54,72]

Laterally, the ligamentous complex helps stabilize the elbow against varus stress. It is made up of several components including the radial collateral ligament, the annular ligament, the accessory lateral collateral ligament, and the lateral ulnar collateral ligament.[51]

The characteristics of the radial collateral ligament are not as well defined as those for the UCL. Originating from the lateral epicondyle, the RCL fans out and inserts into the annular ligament (Fig. 20-2). The origin of the radial collateral ligament is in line with the axis of elbow joint rotation, allowing little change in length as the elbow moves through its full ROM.

Figure 20-2. The medial (A) and lateral (B) capsuloligamentous structures.

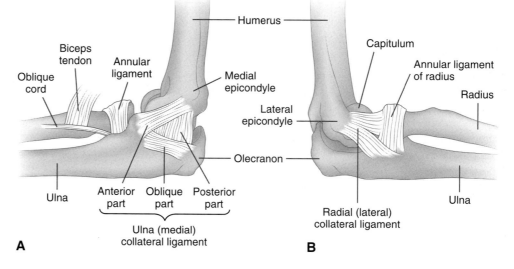

The annular ligament is a strong fibro-osseous ring that encircles and stabilizes the radial head within the radial notch of the ulna. Its origin and insertion occur along the anterior and posterior radial notch of the ulna. The anterior portion of this ligament becomes taut with supination whereas the posterior portion becomes taut with pronation.[75]

The accessory lateral collateral ligament originates from the inferior margin of the annular ligament and inserts discretely into the tubercle of the supinator crest of the ulna. The accessory lateral collateral ligament further assists the annular ligament in varus stabilization of the elbow joint complex.[47]

The lateral ulnar collateral ligament originates from the lateral epicondyle and inserts into the tubercle of the crest of the supinator. This ligament provides posterolateral stability for the humeroulnar joint.[61]

The elbow joint is one of the most congruent joints in the human body and therefore is also one of its most stable. Stability is provided by the interaction of the soft tissue and articular constraints. The static soft tissue stabilizers include the capsular and ligamentous structures. Table 20-1 summarizes the stabilizing influences of the ligamentous and articular components of the elbow joint.[54] When the elbow is in full extension, the anterior capsule provides approximately 70% of the restraint to joint distraction, whereas the UCL provides approximately 78% of the resistance to distractive forces at 90° of elbow flexion. The restraint to valgus displacement varies significantly, depending on the angle of elbow flexion. When the elbow is in full extension, the capsule provides 38% of the valgus restraint, the UCL provides 31%, and the osseous articulations provide the remaining 31%. Conversely, at 90° of elbow flexion, the primary restraint to valgus force is the UCL, which provides 54% of the restraint, followed by the osseous articulation (33%) and the capsule (13%). Varus stress is controlled in extension by the joint articulation (54%), lateral collateral ligament (14%), and joint capsule (32%). As the elbow flexes, the lateral collateral ligament and capsule contribute 9% and 13%, respectively, and the joint articulation provides 75% of the stabilizing force against varus stress.[54]

Musculotendinous Structures

The elbow joint musculature can be divided into six groups based on their functions. These groups include the elbow flexors, extensors, flexor-pronators, extensor-supinators, primary pronators, and primary supinators.

The three primary flexor muscles of the elbow are the biceps brachii, the brachioradialis, and the brachialis. The biceps brachii typically consists of a long and short head. The long head of the biceps brachii originates on the superior glenoid and glenoid labrum. It passes directly through the glenohumeral joint capsule and through the intertubercular groove of the humerus until it joins with the short head of the biceps brachii. The short head of the biceps originates from the coracoid process of the scapula. Together the two heads join to form a common attachment onto the posterior portion of the radial tuberosity and via the bicipital aponeurosis, which attaches to the anterior capsule of the elbow joint. The biceps is responsible for the vast majority of elbow flexion strength when the forearm is supinated and generates its highest torque values when the elbow is positioned between 80 and 100° of flexion.[58] The biceps also acts secondarily as a supinator of the forearm, principally when the elbow is in a flexed position.

The brachialis muscle originates from the lower half of the anterior surface of the humerus. It extends distally to cross the anterior aspect of the elbow joint and insert into both the ulnar tuberosity and coronoid process. The brachialis muscle is active in flexing the elbow in all positions of forearm rotation.[11]

The brachioradialis muscle originates from the proximal two thirds of the lateral supracondylar ridge of the humerus and along the lateral intermuscular septum just distal to the spiral groove. It inserts into the lateral aspect of the base of the styloid process of the radius. The muscular insertion of the brachioradialis is at a significant

Table 20-1

Forces Contributing to Displacement of the Elbow

Elbow Position	Stabilizing Structure	Distraction (%)	Varus (%)	Valgus (%)
Elbow extended (0°)	UCL	12		31
	LCL	10	14	
	Capsule	70	32	38
	Articulation		54	31
Elbow flexed (90°)	UCL	78		54
	LCL	10	9	
	Capsule	8	13	13
	Articulation		75	33

LCL, lateral collateral ligament; UCL, ulnar collateral ligament.

distance from the joint axis and, therefore, exhibits a substantial mechanical advantage as an elbow flexor.[58]

The triceps brachii and the anconeus muscles serve as the primary extensors of the elbow. The triceps brachii is a large three-headed (long, lateral, and medial) muscle that comprises almost the entire posterior brachium. The long head of the triceps originates from the infraglenoid tubercle whereas the other two heads, the lateral and medial heads, originate from the posterior and lateral aspects of the humerus. At the distal portion of the humerus, the three heads converge to form a common muscle that inserts into the posterior surface of the olecranon.

The small anconeus muscle originates from a broad area on the posterior aspect of the lateral epicondyle and inserts into the olecranon. The anconeus muscle covers the lateral portion of the annular ligament, the radial head, and the posterior surface of the proximal ulna. Electromyographic (EMG) activity of the anconeus muscle during the early phases of elbow extension has been noted, and this muscle appears to play a stabilizing role during both pronation and supination movements.[63]

The flexor-pronator muscles include the pronator teres, flexor carpi radialis, palmaris longus, flexor carpi ulnaris, and flexor digitorum superficialis. All these muscles originate completely or in part from the medial epicondyle and serve secondary roles as elbow flexors. Their primary roles are associated with movements at the wrist and hand. This muscle group may provide a limited amount of dynamic stability to the medial aspect of the elbow, resisting valgus stress.[34]

The extensor-supinator muscles include the brachioradialis, extensor carpi radialis brevis and longus, supinator, extensor digitorum, extensor carpi ulnaris, and extensor digiti minimi muscles. Each muscle originates near or directly from the lateral epicondyle of the humerus. Like the flexor-pronators, the primary functions of the extensor-supinator muscles involve the wrist and hand. They also provide dynamic support over the lateral aspect of the elbow. Both this muscle group and the flexor-pronator musculature are susceptible to various overuse conditions and muscular strains.

The pronator quadratus and pronator teres muscles act on the radioulnar joints to produce pronation. The pronator quadratus originates from the anterior surface of the lower ulna and inserts at the distal and lateral border of the radius. The pronator quadratus acts as a significant pronator in all elbow and forearm positions. The pronator teres, which possesses both humeral and ulnar heads, originates from the medial epicondyle and coronoid process of the ulna. The two heads join together and insert along the middle of the lateral surface of the radius. The pronator teres is a strong forearm pronator. It generates its highest contractile force during rapid or resisted pronation.[74] However, the contribution of the pronator teres to pronation strength diminishes when the elbow is positioned in

full extension.[58] The flexor carpi radialis and brachioradialis also act as secondary pronators.

The biceps brachii and the supinator muscles are the primary supinators of the forearm, whereas the brachioradialis acts as an accessory supinator. The supinator muscle originates from three separate locations: the lateral epicondyle, the proximal anterior crest and depression of the ulna distal to the radial notch, and the radial collateral and annular ligaments. The supinator muscle then winds around the radius to insert into the dorsal and lateral surfaces of the proximal radius. The supinator, although a significant supinator of the forearm, generally appears to be weaker than the biceps.[51] The supinator acts alone with unresisted slow supination in all elbow and forearm positions and with unresisted fast supination with the elbow extended.[36] The effectiveness of the supinator is not altered by elbow position; however, elbow position does significantly affect the biceps. Because the supinator does originate at the radial collateral and annular ligaments, it may also act as a supportive or stabilizing muscle to the lateral aspect of the elbow.

Neurologic Structures

The four nerves that play significant roles in normal elbow function are the median, ulnar, radial, and musculocutaneous nerves. Table 20-2 shows the effect of injury to each of these peripheral nerves.

The median nerve arises from branches of the lateral and medial cords of the brachial plexus. Nerve root levels include C5 to C8 and T1. This nerve proceeds distally over the anterior brachium, continuing to the medial aspect of the antecubital fossa. From the fossa, the nerve continues its course under the bicipital aponeurosis and passes most often between the two heads of the pronator teres. The median nerve can be compressed between these two heads or by the bicipital aponeurosis, resulting in either a pronator or anterior interosseous syndrome. Although relatively uncommon, highly repetitive and strenuous pronation movements of the forearm can also lead to entrapment of the median nerve.[45]

The ulnar nerve emanates from the C8 and T1 nerve root levels and descends into the proximal aspect of the upper extremity from the medial cord of the brachial plexus. The ulnar nerve passes from the anterior to posterior compartments of the brachium through the arcade of Struthers. This arcade represents a fascial bridging between the medial head of the triceps and medial intermuscular septum. The nerve continues distally, passing behind the medial epicondyle and through the cubital tunnel. At the cubital tunnel, the bony anatomy provides little protection for the nerve (Fig. 20-3). Ulnar nerve injury, which can occur by compression or stretching, takes place most often in the cubital tunnel. The cubital tunnel retinaculum flattens with elbow flexion, thus decreasing

Table 20-2

Effects of Injury to Specific Peripheral Nerves

Musculocutaneous nerve (C5)

Sensory supply	Lateral half of the anterior surface of the forearm from the elbow to the thenar eminence
Effect of injury	Severe weakness of elbow flexion
	Weakness of supination
	Loss of biceps deep tendon reflex
	Loss of sensation, cutaneous distribution

Radial nerve (C5, C6, C7, C8, and T1)

Sensory supply	Back of arm, forearm, wrist, radial half of the dorsum of the hand, back of thumb, index finger, and part of the middle finger
Effect of injury	Loss of triceps deep tendon reflex
	Weakness of elbow flexion
	Loss of supination (when elbow is extended)
	Loss of wrist extension
	Weakness of ulnar and radial deviation
	Loss of extension at the MCP joints
	Loss of extension and abduction of the thumb

Median nerve (C5, C6, C7, C8, and T1)

Sensory supply	Radial half of the palm, palmar surface of the thumb, index, middle, and radial half of the ring finger, and dorsal surface of the same fingers
Effect of injury	Loss of complete pronation (brachioradialis can bring the forearm to midpronation but not beyond)
	Weakness with flexion and radial deviation (ulnar deviation with wrist flexion)
	Loss of flexion at MCP joints
	Loss of thumb opposition or abduction, loss of flexion at IP and MCP joints

Ulnar nerve (C7, C8, and T1)

Sensory supply	Dorsal and palmar surfaces of the ulnar side of the hand, including the little finger, and ulnar half of the ring finger
Effect of injury	Weakness of wrist flexion and ulnar deviation (radial deviation with wrist flexion)
	Loss of flexion of DIP joints or ring and little fingers
	Inability to abduction or adduct fingers
	Inability to adduct thumb
	Loss of flexion of fingers, especially ring and little fingers at the MCP joints
	Loss of extension of fingers, especially ring and little fingers at the IP joint

DIP, distal interphalangeal; IP, interphalangeal; MCP, metacarpophalangeal.

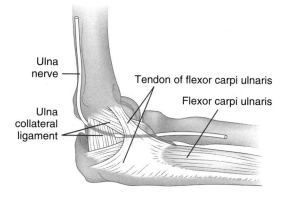

Figure 20-3. Ulnar nerve.

Ulna nerve

Tendon of flexor carpi ulnaris

Flexor carpi ulnaris

Ulna collateral ligament

the overall capacity within the cubital tunnel. This can be noted clinically when nerve symptoms are reproduced in elbow flexion, which typically occurs when osteophytes are present on the ulna or medial epicondyle.[77] Injury to the medial capsular ligaments can result in increased traction forces against the medial elbow, resulting in a change in length of the ulnar nerve. This change in length may result in neuropathy or ulnar nerve subluxation. The nerve enters the forearm by passing between the two heads of the flexor carpi ulnaris and continues distally between the flexor digitorum profundus and the flexor carpi ulnaris.

The radial nerve originates from the posterior cord of the brachial plexus and derives its nerve supply from the

C6, C7, and C8 nerve root levels with variable contributions from the C5 and T11 nerve root levels. At the midpoint of the brachium, the radial nerve descends laterally through the radial groove of the humerus and continues its course in a lateral and distal direction. The nerve descends anteriorly behind the brachioradialis and brachialis muscles to the level of the elbow where it divides into its posterior interosseous and superficial radial branches.

The musculocutaneous nerve originates from the lateral cord of the brachial plexus at nerve root levels C5 to C7. The nerve passes between the biceps and brachialis muscles to pierce the brachial fascia lateral to the biceps tendon. The nerve continues distally to terminate as the lateral antebrachial cutaneous nerve, which provides sensation over the anterolateral aspect of the forearm. Compression between the biceps tendon and the brachialis fascia can cause entrapment of the musculocutaneous nerve.

Sensory nerves innervate the elbow cutaneously and are derived from specific nerve root levels. The lateral arm is innervated by branches of the axillary nerve of the C5 nerve root level whereas the lateral forearm is innervated by the musculocutaneous nerve of the C6 nerve root level.[7] The medial arm is innervated by the brachial cutaneous nerve from the T1 nerve root level. The medial forearm is innervated by branches of the antebrachial cutaneous nerve from the C8 nerve root level.[7] The T2 dermatome extends from the axilla to the posteromedial elbow.[45] Variability does exist in the extent of innervation provided by each nerve root and overlap between dermatome distributions does occur.

BIOMECHANICS OF SPORT
Biomechanics of Baseball Pitching

The biomechanics of the elbow during overhead baseball pitching can be broken down into six phases: windup, stride, arm cocking, arm acceleration, arm deceleration, and follow-through. During the windup and stride, minimal elbow kinetics and muscle activity are present. As the foot contacts the ground, the elbow is flexed to approximately 85°.[86]

The arm-cocking phase begins as the foot comes into contact with the ground and continues until the point of maximum shoulder external rotation. As the arm moves into external rotation, a varus torque is produced at the elbow to prevent valgus stress.[86] Shortly before maximum external rotation, the elbow is flexed to 95° and a varus torque of approximately 64 Nm is produced.[23] At this critical instant, excessive valgus strain may cause injury to the medial stabilizing structures of the elbow, particularly the UCL. As previously discussed, Morrey and An[53] reported that at this moment the UCL is contributing approximately 54% of the resistance to this valgus strain moment. Assuming that the UCL absorbs 54% of the 64 Nm of valgus strain observed during the arm-cocking phase, 35 Nm of strain would be applied to the UCL in this position, approaching the maximum capacity of load before failure in the UCL.[22,23]

Also, as the elbow joint sustains this valgus strain, lateral compression is applied. This may lead to compressive injuries of the lateral compartment of the elbow as the radial head and humeral capitellum are approximated. This compression may lead to avascular necrosis, osteochondritis dissecans, and/or osteochondral chip fractures.

As the arm accelerates from maximal external rotation to ball release, the elbow extends at approximately 2500°/sec.[23] As the elbow extends and resists valgus strain simultaneously, the olecranon can impinge against the medial aspect of the trochlear groove and olecranon fossa,[22,23] which may lead to the formation of a posteromedial osteophyte and loose bodies. This type of compression under valgus stress was described by Wilson and associates[94] as valgus extension overload.

As the arm decelerates and continues into the follow-through phase, eccentric contraction of the elbow flexors must control the distractive forces at the elbow joint. Moderate activity of the biceps brachii and brachioradialis has been reported at this time.[86] Muscular activity of the elbow flexors may assist in the prevention of olecranon impingement as the elbow is rapidly extended. The elbow remains in a flexed position of approximately 20° as the arm continues into follow-through. Minimal kinetic and muscular activity at the elbow occurs during this final phase of throwing.

Biomechanics of the Elbow during Tennis

The kinematic and kinetic data during tennis vary depending on the type of stroke; therefore, the biomechanics of the serve and groundstrokes will be discussed separately. The overhead serve has been compared with the mechanics of overhead throwing.[23] The elbow has been reported to extend at 982°/sec and pronate at 347°/sec during the acceleration and deceleration phases of the tennis serve.[41] Morris and colleagues[55] reported high activity of the triceps and pronator teres during the tennis serve to produce significant racket velocity. Because of this excessive angular velocity, the eccentric contraction of the elbow flexors and supinators is critical for the prevention of injuries to the elbow during an overhead tennis serve.

During groundstrokes, both the forehand and the backhand, the wrist extensors are predominantly active as the athlete prepares the racquet for impact.[55] The extensor carpi radialis longus, brevis, and extensor communis musculatures are active during both strokes, with the forehand showing additional muscular activity of the biceps brachii and brachioradialis.[38,55,66] As the racquet comes into contact with the ball and begins the follow-through, there is continued activity of the extensor carpi radialis brevis. The backhand produces additional activity of the biceps brachii as the elbow decelerates into extension.[38,55,66]

Kelley and co-workers[38] compared the muscular activity of the elbow during the backhand stroke in subjects with and without lateral epicondylitis. Results indicated that the group of subjects exhibiting lateral epicondylitis showed a significant increase in EMG activity of the extensor carpi radialis longus and brevis, pronator teres, and flexor carpi radialis. These retrospective findings may have an impact on the explanation of the etiology of lateral epicondylitis.

Biomechanics of the Golf Swing

The biomechanics of the golf swing that pertain to elbow and wrist injuries can be broken down into five phases: the backswing, transition, downswing, impact, and follow-through. As the athlete swings the club, both the lead arm and back arm are susceptible to injuries at various moments during the swing.

The backswing phase produces few injuries to the elbow. As the backswing progresses, the lead wrist pronates, flexes, and radially deviates. The back arm flexes at the elbow and the wrist supinates, extends, and radially deviates. The wrist flexors exhibit minimal EMG activity, whereas the wrist extensors exhibit 33% of a maximum voluntary isometric contraction (MVIC).[25] As the clubhead approaches the top of the backswing, the musculature of the elbow must eccentrically contract to control the clubhead and transition from the backswing to the downswing. This motion places a great deal of stress of the stretched flexor-pronator mass of the back arm.[76]

As the downswing progresses, the wrists must uncoil to produce clubhead speed. The wrists and elbows uncoil to return to the neutral position initially observed at set-up to prepare for impact. The downswing is characterized by increased muscular activity of both the wrist extensors and flexors. The wrist extensors exhibit 45% MVIC and the wrist flexors 35% MVIC during the downswing. During impact the wrist and hands decelerate owing to the force of impact.[25] McCarroll and Gioe[50] reported that more than twice as many injuries occurred during the downswing than during the backswing because the elbows and wrists move approximately three times faster during the downswing. This deceleration of force places a great deal of strain on the forearm musculature as they attempt to maintain control of the club.[76] The majority of elbow injuries take place during impact as the lateral epicondyle of the lead arm and the medial epicondyle of the backarm are placed under significant strain. The lead elbow extensor mass has been reported to be under even greater stress at impact because of the compressive force of ball impact and divots.[49] At ball contact, the wrist flexor activity increases significantly to 91% MVIC. Additionally, the wrist extensors exhibit EMG activity of approximately 58% MVIC.[25]

After impact, the arm continues into the follow-through. Minimal injuries occur during this phase. The wrists and hands follow a reverse pattern as that seen during the backswing. The lead arm flexes at the elbow, supinates, extends and radially deviates at the wrist while the back arm pronates, flexes, and radially deviates at the wrist. During the follow-through, the EMG activity of the wrist extensors is approximately 60% to 70% MVIC The repetitive nature of elbow and wrist motion observed may be responsible for the golfing overuse injuries commonly seen in the forearm musculature.

When the muscular activity patterns of golfers with medial epicondylitis and golfers without injuries are compared, the golfers with medial epicondylitis exhibit significantly greater wrist flexor muscle activity during the backswing, transition, and downswing.[25]

CLINICAL EXAMINATION

The clinical examination of the elbow of an athlete requires a thorough history, extensive knowledge of the anatomy and biomechanics of the joint, and a well-organized physical examination. The goal of the examination is to identify the areas of dysfunction and determine an appropriate course of intervention.

History

Before the examination begins, a complete history is imperative.[8] The location, intensity, and duration of pain should be clearly identified. The date and mechanism of injury should be explained thoroughly, because this will assist in determining the structures involved. Other subjective information such as aggravating factors, previous injuries, and primary complaints should also be recorded to assist in the assessment and development of patient-specific treatment and goals.[8]

Observation

The patient should completely expose the trunk and arms for a comprehensive inspection to provide a full view of the neck, shoulder, and elbow. The skin should be evaluated for areas of contusion, ecchymosis, swelling, burns, surgical scars, redness, blanching, petechiae, and venous congestion. The carrying angle of the elbow should also be assessed during this portion of the examination.

Palpation

Palpation of the elbow begins with the identification of specific bony landmarks. The clinician should palpate each to determine whether tenderness or deformity exists.

The medial epicondyle may exhibit tenderness for various reasons including epicondylitis, muscle strains, and UCL injury. The medial supracondylar ridge should be examined for osteophytes, which may be entrapping the median nerve. The olecranon is easily palpated and is covered by the insertion of the triceps and the olecranon bursa, both of which may be tender if a pathologic condition exists. Osseous changes on the posteromedial olecranon may be associated valgus extension overload in overhead athletes. The ulnar border should also be palpated for stress fractures, which are sometimes present in the throwing population. The lateral epicondyle is often irritable when palpated in the presence of epicondylitis. Lastly, the radial head lies approximately 2 cm distally from the lateral epicondyle and should be palpated during passive supination and pronation.

When one palpates the soft tissues of the elbow, it is helpful to divide the elbow into four distinct regions: the medial, posterior, lateral, and anterior aspects.

The major structures of the medial aspect of the elbow include the ulnar nerve, flexor-pronator muscle group, the UCL, and the supracondylar lymph nodes. The clinician should manually determine whether the ulnar nerve is capable of being dislocated from within its bony sulcus. This is done by abducting and externally rotating the shoulder with the athlete in a supine position and the elbow flexed between 20 and 70°.[8] The medial epicondyle should also be palpated to determine tenderness to the flexor-pronator muscle mass or the UCL.

The posterior elbow contains the olecranon, which should be palpated for inflammation of a swollen bursa. The triceps insertion points should also be palpated for tenderness.

Laterally, the wrist extensor group is palpated. The brachioradialis is made prominent by having the patient close his or her fist, place the forearm in a neutral position, and resist elbow flexion. Resisted wrist flexion allows for easy palpation of the extensor carpi radialis longus and brevis.

The anterior structures of the elbow pass through the cubital fossa. These structures from medial to lateral are the median nerve, brachial artery, and the biceps tendon. The biceps can be made prominent by resisted elbow flexion.

Range of Motion

The normal ROM of the elbow is 0° of extension, 140 to 150° of flexion, 80° of pronation, and 80° of supination.[59] Passive ROM is assessed in each direction and is always compared with that of the contralateral side.

In addition, the endfeel of movement should be assessed. Normal endfeels of the elbow are different for each movement; elbow extension exhibits a bony endfeel, flexion has a soft tissue approximation, and forearm pronation and supination both have a capsular endfeel.[19]

Muscle Testing

Muscle testing of the elbow musculature begins with the patient seated.[40] The brachialis is tested with the elbow flexed and forearm pronated. The biceps is tested with the

forearm supinated and shoulder flexed to 45 to 50°. The brachioradialis is tested with the elbow flexed with neutral wrist rotation. Triceps extension is performed with the shoulder flexed to 90° and the elbow flexed 45 to 90°. Pronation and supination of the elbow are performed with the arm by the side and the elbow flexed to 90° and neutral wrist rotation. Resistance is applied at the distal forearm as the patient attempts to rotate in either direction. Wrist extension and flexion are performed with the elbow flexed to 30° and with the elbow fully extended. Isokinetic testing may also be applied to determine specific objective data of muscular strength, power, and endurance.

Special Tests

Special tests for the elbow joint are used in an attempt to elicit specific pathologic signs or symptoms. Laxity assessment is used to evaluate the integrity of the medial and lateral stabilizing structures. Varus and valgus testing may be performed by stabilizing the arm with one hand and applying a fulcrum at the elbow joint with the other. The clinician imparts a varus or valgus stress and notes the amount of gapping and the endfeel of motion. The tests are compared bilaterally and may be performed at 0° of extension and at 30° of flexion. Pain, excessive gapping, or a soft endfeel may all indicate a pathologic condition of the stabilizing structures.

There are several clinical tests that are used to test the integrity of the UCL. The two most common techniques are the supine and prone valgus stress tests. In the first, the athlete is positioned supine while the clinician holds the elbow and externally rotates the shoulder, blocking the upper extremity from further rotation (Fig. 20-4). The UCL is easily palpated in this position. The elbow is tested

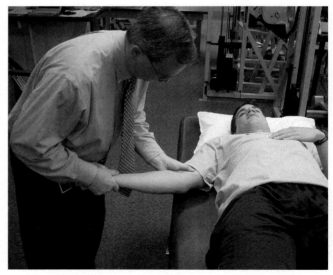

Figure 20-4. Clinical test for UCL instability in the supine position.

at 5° and 25 to 30° of flexion by applying a valgus stress to determine the integrity of the ligament. The amount of opening, or gapping, is assessed as well as the endfeel of motion. Excessive gapping, a soft endfeel, or localized medial pain may all indicate a UCL injury.[8]

Next, the athlete is placed in the prone position with the involved arm hanging over the edge of the table. The clinician internally rotates the shoulder and stabilizes the elbow and forearm in pronation before placing a valgus stress on the elbow at 5° and 25 to 30° of flexion (Fig. 20-5). Again the amount of opening and endfeel are assessed during the examination. The prone test is preferred by the authors because of its greater capacity for isolating the UCL and minimizing humeral rotation.

The clinical test for valgus extension overload is performed by the clinician grasping the elbow in a flexed position. As the clinician forces the elbow into extension, a valgus stress is simultaneously applied to the elbow. The clinician palpates the posteromedial joint for tenderness and/or crepitation. Pain over the posteromedial olecranon process signifies a positive test result.[94]

A lateral pivot shift test is used to assess posterolateral rotatory instability of the elbow.[61] Patients who have sustained an elbow dislocation often report a posterolateral rotatory mechanism of injury that is replicated during this test. The patient is supine, and the clinician holds the arm over the head with 90° of shoulder flexion and maximal external rotation.

The clinician applies a valgus and supination moment while flexing the elbow, resulting in the semilunar notch of the ulna displacing from the trochlea of the humerus. During this maneuver maximal displacement occurs at approximately 40°.[61] This test is often not tolerated by the patient without general anesthesia; however, signs of apprehension during testing indicate a positive clinical test result in the awake athlete.[39]

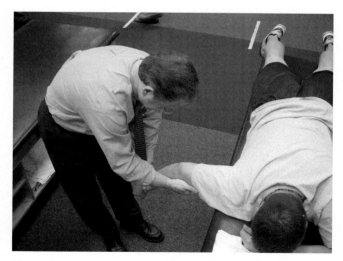

Figure 20-5. Clinical test for UCL instability in the prone position.

Neurologic Testing

The deep tendon reflexes that are significant to the examination of the elbow are the biceps reflex, brachioradialis reflex, and the triceps reflex, which are controlled by spinal levels C5, C6, and C7, respectively. A slight response is normal whereas an increased response could signify an upper motor neuron lesion and a decreased response may indicate the presence of a lower motor neuron lesion.

The biceps tendon reflex can be elicited with the elbow relaxed and in a flexed position; the clinician places the thumb over the biceps tendon in the cubital fossa and gently taps the thumb with a reflex hammer. The brachioradialis reflex is elicited by tapping the tendon at the lateral distal end of the radius with the flat edge of a reflex hammer. The triceps tendon reflex is elicited by tapping over the triceps tendon with a reflex hammer.

Sensory perception is assessed by using pinprick and light touch to the skin. The contralateral extremity is always used for comparison. The lateral arm is innervated by the axillary nerve (C5) and the lateral forearm is innervated by branches of the musculocutaneous (C6). The medial arm is innervated by the brachial cutaneous (C8) nerve and the medial forearm is innervated by the antebrachial cutaneous (T1) nerve.

Plain View Radiographs

Plain view radiographs may be a useful adjunct to the clinical examination. The views routinely taken of an elbow include both an anteroposterior and a lateral view. These views will allow the clinician to identify the presence of fractures or loose bodies. The internal and external oblique views may also provide further diagnostic information and are the best views to detect the presence of posterior olecranon osteophytes.

Computed Tomography Arthrogram

A diagnostic arthrogram is extremely useful when a UCL tear is suspected. Contrast dye is injected into the elbow, and radiographs are obtained to determine whether the dye has escaped the capsule through a tear. Complete tears of the UCL will provide a positive arthrogram. A computed tomographic scan, performed immediately after the arthrogram, can enhance visualization of a capsuloligamentous injury.

Magnetic Resonance Imaging

Magnetic resonance imaging (MRI) may prove to be beneficial in the differential diagnosis of various elbow pathologic conditions. An MRI scan of the elbow is helpful in diagnosing complete UCL tears, particularly when the elbow is injected with saline before testing. A UCL tear is indicated by a leakage of dye along the medial side of the elbow both proximally and distally along the medial olecranon. Timmerman and Andrews[78] referred to this occurrence as a "T-sign."

OVERVIEW OF ELBOW REHABILITATION

Rehabilitation after elbow injury or elbow surgery follows a sequential and progressive multiphased approach. The ultimate goal of elbow rehabilitation is to return the athlete to his or her previous functional level as quickly and safely as possible. Several key principles must be addressed when the athlete's elbow is rehabilitated: (1) the effects of immobilization must be minimized, (2) healing tissue must not be overstressed, (3) the patient must fulfill certain criteria to advance through each phase of the rehabilitation, (4) the program must be based on current scientific and clinical research, (5) the process must be adaptable to each patient and his or her specific goals, and (6) the rehabilitation program must be a team effort between the physician, physical therapist, athletic trainer,

and patient. Communication between each team member is essential for a successful outcome. The following section will provide an overview of the rehabilitation process after elbow injury (Table 20-3) and surgery (Table 20-4). Discussion of rehabilitation protocols for specific pathologies will follow this general overview. In Table 20-5 the rehabilitation goals and criteria for entering each phase of rehabilitation are summarized.

Phase I: Immediate Motion Phase

The first phase of elbow rehabilitation is the immediate motion phase. The goals of this phase are to minimize the effects of immobilization, reestablish nonpainful ROM, decrease pain and inflammation, and retard muscular atrophy. The rehabilitation specialist must not overstress healing tissues during this phase.

Early ROM activities are performed to nourish the articular cartilage and assist in the synthesis, alignment, and organization of collagen tissue.[18,21,28,60,64,69,70,79] ROM activities are performed for all planes of elbow and wrist

---

Table 20-3

General Elbow Rehabilitation Guidelines

Phase I: Immediate Motion Phase (Week 1)

Goals
- Improve pain-free range of motion
- Retard muscular atrophy
- Minimize pain and inflammation

Exercises
- Active and passive range of motion for wrist, elbow, and shoulder motions
- Grade I and II joint mobilization techniques
- Submaximal isometrics for the wrist, elbow and shoulder complexes
- Local modalities as appropriate

Phase II: Intermediate Phase (Week 2 to 4)

Goals
- Normalize motion (particularly elbow extension)
- Improve muscular strength, power, and endurance

Exercises

A. Week 2
- Isotonic strengthening program wrist and elbow musculature
- Elastic tubing exercises for shoulder musculature
- Local modalities as necessary

B. Week 3
- Advance isotonic strengthening program for the upper extremity
- Initiate upper extremity rhythmic stabilization drills
- Initiate isokinetic strengthening exercises for elbow flexion/extension, forearm pronation/supination and shoulder internal/external rotation

C. Week 4
- Emphasize eccentric biceps, flexor-pronation, and concentric triceps activities
- Initiate Thrower's Ten Exercise Program
- Advance endurance training activities
- Initiate light plyometric drills
- Begin swinging and/or hitting drills

Phase III: Advanced Strengthening (Week 4 to 8)

Goals
- Return to functional/athletic participation

Criteria to Enter Advanced Phase
- Full nonpainful range of motion
- No pain or tenderness on clinical examination
- Satisfactory clinical examination
- Satisfactory isokinetic test

A. Weeks 4 to 5
- Continue strengthening exercises, endurance drills, and flexibility activities
- Thrower's Ten Exercise Program
- Progress plyometric drills
- Progress swinging (hitting) drills

B. Weeks 6 to 8
- Initiate phase one of interval sport program
- Emphasize pathologic condition–specific maintenance program

Phase IV: Return to Activity (Week 6 to 9)
- Continue Thrower's Ten Exercise Strengthening Program
- Continue flexibility program
- Progress functional drills to unrestricted activity

Table 20-4

Postoperative Elbow Rehabilitation

PHASE I: Immediate Motion Phase (Week 1)

Goals

- Improve pain-free range of motion
- Decrease pain and swelling
- Retard muscular atrophy

A. Day of surgery: Initiate elbow range of motion gently in bulky dressing

B. Postoperative day 1 and 2:
- Remove bulky dressing and replace with elastic bandage
- Begin hand, wrist and elbow exercises:
  - Putty/grip strengthening
  - Wrist flexor stretching
  - Wrist extensor stretching
  - Wrist curls
  - Reverse wrist curls
  - Neutral wrist curls
  - Pronation/supination
  - Active/active-assisted elbow flexion/extension range of motion

C. Postoperative day 3 to 7:
- Passive range of motion elbow extension/flexion (to tolerance)
- Grade I/II joint mobilizations
- Begin 1-pound progressive resistance exercises:
  - Wrist curls
  - Reverse wrist curls
  - Neutral curls
  - Pronation/supination

PHASE II: Intermediate Phase (Week 2 to 4)

Goals

- Improve muscular strength and endurance
- Normalize elbow joint arthrokinematics (particularly elbow extension)

A. Week 2
- Range of motion exercises (overpressure in to extension)
- Add biceps curl and triceps extension
- Continue advancing progressive resistance exercises weight and repetitions as tolerated

B. Week 3
- Initiate biceps and triceps eccentric exercise program
- Initiate shoulder exercise program:
  - External rotators
  - Internal rotators
  - Deltoid
  - Supraspinatus
  - Scapulothoracic strengthening

PHASE III: Advanced Strengthening Phase (Week 4 to 8)

Goals

- Preparation for return to functional activities

Criteria to progress to advanced phase

- Full nonpainful range of motion
- No pain or tenderness on clinical examination
- Satisfactory clinical examination
- Satisfactory isokinetic test

Thrower's Ten Exercise Program

Initiate plyometric exercise drills

Advance drills to emphasize eccentric control, muscular strength and endurance

Initiate phase I interval throwing program

---

motions to prevent the formation of scar tissue and adhesions.[89,90] Reestablishing full elbow extension is the primary goal of early ROM activities. These interventions are designed to minimize the occurrence of elbow flexion contractures.[1,27,57] The elbow is predisposed to flexion contractures because of the intimate congruency of the joint articulations, the tightness of the joint capsule, and the tendency of the anterior capsule to develop adhesions after injury. The brachialis muscle also attaches to the capsule and crosses the elbow joint before becoming a tendinous structure. Injury to the elbow may cause excessive scar tissue formation of the brachialis muscle as well as functional splinting of the elbow.

Grade I and II joint mobilizations may be performed during this early phase of rehabilitation as tolerated. These grade I and II mobilization techniques are used to neuromodulate pain by stimulating type I and Type II articular receptors.[46,97] Posterior glides with oscillations are performed in the midrange of elbow motion to assist in regaining full extension. Aggressive mobilization techniques are not used until the later stages of rehabilitation when pain has subsided.

If the patient continues to have difficulty achieving full extension using ROM and mobilization techniques, a low-load, long-duration stretch may be performed to produce a creep of the collagen tissue, which will result in tissue elongation.[42,71,84,85] The authors find this intervention to be extremely beneficial in regaining full elbow extension.[88,89,93] The athlete lies supine with a towel roll placed under the brachium to act as a cushion and fulcrum. Light resistance exercise tubing is applied to the wrist of the patient and secured to the table or a dumbbell on the ground (Fig. 20-6). The patient is instructed to relax as much as possible for 10 to 12 minutes. The amount of resistance applied should be of low magnitude to enable the athlete to tolerate the stretch for the entire duration without pain or muscle spasm.

The aggressiveness of stretching and mobilization techniques is dictated by the healing constraints of the involved tissues as well as the amount of motion and endfeel of the joint complex. If the patient exhibits a

Table 20-5

Rehabilitation Goals for Each Phase of Elbow Rehabilitation

Phase I: Immediate Motion	Phase II: Intermediate Phase	Phase III: Advanced Strengthening	Phase IV: Return to Activity
	Criteria for entering this phase • Patient exhibits full range of motion • Minimal pain and tenderness • Good (4/5) manual muscle test of the elbow flexor and extensor musculature	*Criteria for entering this phase* • Full non-painful range of motion • No pain or tenderness • Strength that is 70% of the contralateral extremity	*Criteria for entering this phase* • Full range of motion • No pain or tenderness on clinical examination • Satisfactory isokinetic test • Satisfactory clinical examination
Goals	*Goals*	*Goals*	*Goals*
• Minimize the effects of immobilization • Reestablish nonpainful range of motion • Decrease pain and inflammation • Retard muscular atrophy The rehabilitation specialist must not overstress healing tissues during this phase	• Enhancing elbow and upper extremity mobility • Improving muscular strength and endurance • Reestablishing neuromuscular control of the elbow complex	• Involves a progression of activities to prepare the athlete for sport participation • Gradually increase strength, power, endurance, and neuromuscular control to prepare for a gradual return to sport	• Allows the athlete to progressively return to full competition using an interval return to sport program • Sport-specific functional drills performed to prepare the athlete for the stresses involved with each particular sport

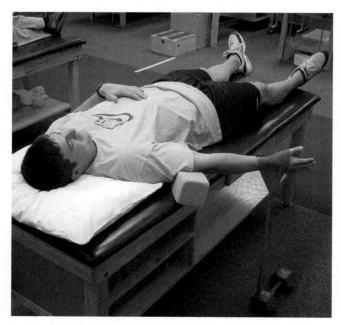

Figure 20-6. Low-load, long duration stretch into elbow extension.

decrease in motion and hard end-feel without pain, aggressive stretching and mobilization techniques may be used. Conversely, a patient exhibiting pain before resistance or an empty endfeel progression should be slow with gentle stretching.

Cryotherapy and high-voltage pulsed galvanic stimulation may be performed as required to assist in reducing pain and inflammation. Once the acute inflammatory phase has passed, moist heat, warm whirlpool, and/or ultrasound may be used at the onset of treatment to prepare the tissue for stretching and improve the extensibility of the capsule and musculotendinous structures.

The early phases of rehabilitation must also focus on retarding muscular atrophy. Subpainful and submaximal isometrics are performed initially for the elbow flexors and extensors, and for the wrist flexor, extensor, pronator, and supinator muscle groups. Isometrics should be performed at multiple angles for 2 to 3 sets of 10 repetitions, holding each contraction for 6 to 8 seconds. Shoulder isometrics may also be performed during this phase with caution against internal and external rotation exercises if painful.

Alternating rhythmic stabilization drills for shoulder flexion/extension/horizontal abduction/adduction and shoulder internal/external rotation are performed to begin reestablishing proprioception and neuromuscular control of the upper extremity.

Phase II: Intermediate Phase

Phase II, the intermediate phase, is initiated when the patient exhibits full ROM, minimal pain and tenderness, and a good (4 over 5) manual muscle test of the elbow flexor and extensor musculature. The emphasis in this phase includes enhancing elbow and upper extremity mobility, improving muscular strength and endurance, and reestablishing neuromuscular control of the elbow complex.

Stretching exercises are continued to maintain full elbow flexion and extension. Mobilization techniques may be progressed to more aggressive grade III techniques as needed to apply a stretch to the capsular tissue in end range. Flexibility activities are progressed during this phase to focus on wrist flexion, extension, pronation, and supination excursion. Shoulder flexibility is also maintained in athletes with emphasis on flexion, external and internal rotation, and horizontal adduction.

Strengthening exercises are advanced during this phase to include isotonic movements. Emphasis is placed on elbow flexion and extension, wrist flexion and extension, and forearm pronation and supination. The weight of the arm is initially used before progressing to a 1-pound dumbbell. Resistance is then advanced in a controlled progressive resistance fashion by 1 pound per week to gradually stress the involved tissues. The shoulder and scapular muscles are also included in a progressive resistance program during the later stages of this phase. Emphasis is placed on strengthening the shoulder external rotators and scapular muscles and training eccentric control of the elbow flexors. Shoulder internal and external rotation are performed with exercise tubing at 0° of abduction; standing scaption with external rotation (full can), standing abduction, prone horizontal abduction, and prone rowing are all included in this phase.

Muscular endurance activities are also incorporated during this phase of the rehabilitation program. High repetition, low resistance dumbbell exercises, and the upper body ergometer may be used to accomplish these goals.

Neuromuscular control exercises are initiated in this phase to enhance the ability of the muscle to control the elbow joint during athletic activities. These exercises include proprioceptive neuromuscular facilitation exercises with rhythmic stabilizations (Fig. 20-7) and slow reversal manual resistance elbow/wrist flexion drills (Fig. 20-8).

Phase III: Advanced Strengthening Phase

The third phase involves a progression of activities to prepare the athlete for sport participation. The goals of this

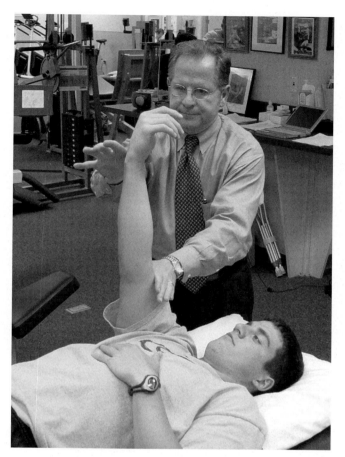

Figure 20-7. Manual proprioceptive neuromuscular facilitation D2 pattern with rhythmic stabilizations.

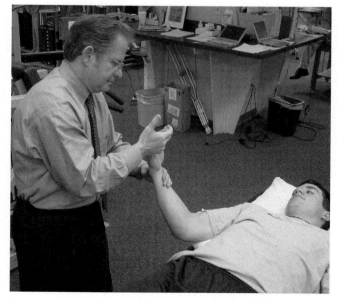

Figure 20-8. Manual resisted elbow and wrist flexion using both concentric and eccentric contractions of the elbow flexors.

phase are to gradually increase strength, power, endurance, and neuromuscular control to prepare the athlete for a gradual return to sport. Specific criteria that must be met before the athlete enters this phase include full nonpainful ROM, no pain or tenderness, and strength that is 70% of the contralateral extremity.

Advanced strengthening activities during this phase include aggressive strengthening exercises emphasizing high-speed and eccentric contractions as well as plyometric activities. Strengthening exercises are progressed to include the Thrower's Ten Exercise Program (Appendix A). These exercises were designed based on numerous electromyographic studies to strengthen all of the shoulder, scapular, elbow, and wrist muscles that are used during upper extremity athletic activities.[14,24,56,81] Internal and external rotation exercises with exercise tubing are progressed to a functional position of 90° of shoulder abduction with 90° of elbow flexion. Exercises should be performed at both slow and fast speeds. Scapulothoracic exercises are progressed to include prone horizontal abduction at 100° and full external rotation as well as prone rows into external rotation.

Elbow flexion exercises are advanced to emphasize eccentric control of elbow extension. The biceps muscle is an important stabilizer during the follow-through phase of overhead throwing to eccentrically control the deceleration of the elbow, preventing pathologic abutting of the olecranon within the fossa.[4,24] Elbow flexion can be performed with elastic tubing to emphasize slow and fast speed concentric and eccentric contractions.

Aggressive strengthening exercises with weight machines are also incorporated during this phase. These most commonly begin with bench press, seated rowing, and front latissimus dorsi pull-downs.

Neuromuscular control exercises are progressed to include side-lying external rotation with manual resistance. Concentric and eccentric external rotation is performed against the clinician's resistance with the addition of rhythmic stabilizations (Fig. 20-9). This manual resistance exercise may be progressed to standing external rotation with exercise tubing at 0° and finally at 90° of shoulder abduction (Fig. 20-10).

Plyometric drills are an extremely beneficial form of exercise for training the upper extremity musculature.[88,92] The physiologic principles of plyometric exercise use an eccentric prestretch of the muscle tissue, thereby stimulating the muscle spindle to produce a more forceful concentric contraction. Plyometric exercises are performed using a weighted medicine ball during the later stages of this phase to train the upper extremity musculature to develop and withstand high levels of stress. Plyometric exercises are initially performed with two hands performing a chest pass, side-to-side throw, and overhead soccer throw. These may be progressed to include one-hand activities such as 90/90 throws (Fig. 20-11), external and internal rotation throws at 0° of abduction (Fig. 20-12), and

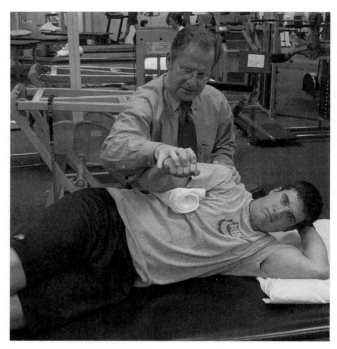

Figure 20-9. Manual resisted side-lying external resistance using both concentric and eccentric contractions of the external rotators.

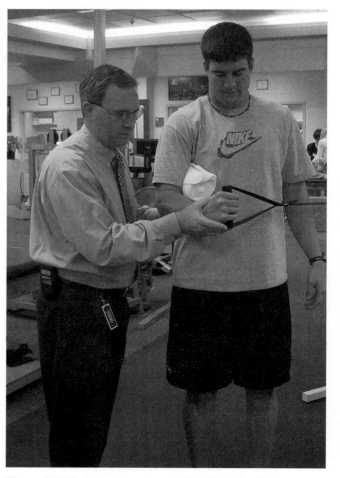

Figure 20-10. External rotation at 0° of shoulder abduction with tubing and manual resistance.

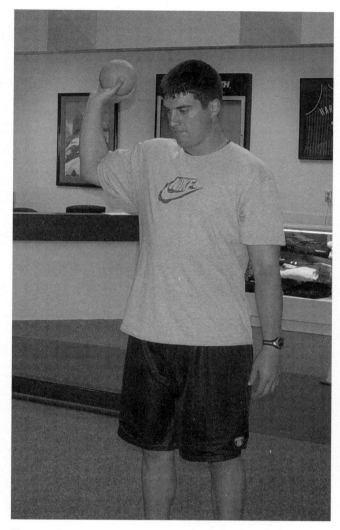

Figure 20-11. One-handed plyometric throws at 90° of shoulder abduction and 90° of elbow flexion using a 2-pound weighted ball.

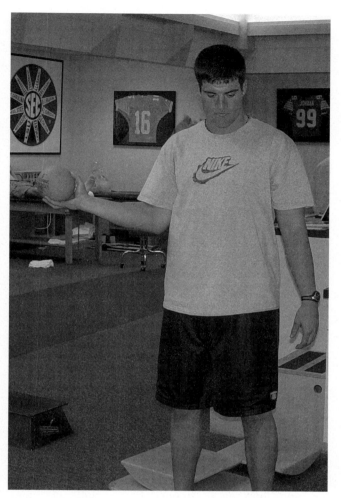

Figure 20-12. One-handed plyometric throws at 0° of abduction using a 2-pound weighted ball.

wall dribbles. Specific plyometric drills for the forearm musculature include wrist flexion flips (Fig. 20-13) and extension grips.

Phase IV: Return to Activity Phase

The final phase of elbow rehabilitation, the return to activity phase, allows the athlete to progressively return to full competition using an interval sport program. Sport-specific functional drills are performed to prepare the athlete for the stresses involved with each particular sport.

Before an athlete is allowed to begin the return to activity phase of rehabilitation, he or she must exhibit full ROM, no pain or tenderness on clinical examination, a satisfactory isokinetic test, and a satisfactory clinical examination. Isokinetic testing is commonly used to determine the readiness of the athlete to begin an interval sport program.

Athletes are routinely tested in elbow flexion/extension, shoulder internal/external rotation, and shoulder abduction/adduction at 180 and 300°/sec. Satisfactory isokinetic testing parameters are outlined in Table 20-6.

Upon achieving the criteria that have been outlined, a formal interval sport program should be initiated. The overhead thrower begins with a long-toss interval throwing program (Appendix B). The athlete throws three times per week with a day off from throwing in between. Each step is performed at least two times on separate days without symptoms before the athlete is allowed to advance to the next step. Throwing should be performed without pain or any significant increase in symptoms. If the athlete experiences symptoms at a particular step within the program, he or she is instructed to regress to the prior step until symptoms subside. It is important for the overhead athlete to perform stretching and an abbreviated strengthening program before and after performing the interval sport program. Typically, overhead throwers should warm-up, stretch, and perform one set of their exercise program before throwing, followed by two additional sets of

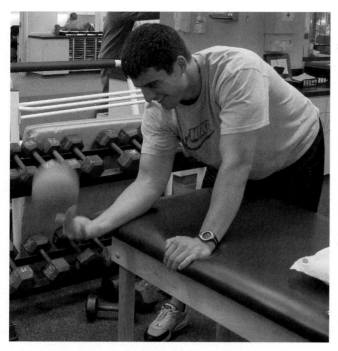

Figure 20-13. Plyometric wrist flips.

exercises after throwing. This provides an adequate warm-up but also ensures maintenance of necessary ROM and flexibility of the shoulder joint.

After completion of a long toss program, pitchers will progress to phase II of the throwing program, throwing off a mound (Appendix B). In phase II the number of throws, intensity, and type of pitches are progressed to gradually increase functional stress on the upper extremity.

Interval sport programs for tennis and golf follow the same guidelines as those for the baseball program. A specific interval program for tennis is outlined in Appendix B. As the athlete progresses through the program, the numbers of forehand and backhand shots are gradually increased. Overhead serving is typically initiated during the third week of the program, and games are allowed during the fourth week if symptoms have not exacerbated.

Appendix B outlines an interval golf program. The program begins with simple putting and chipping and progresses to include short iron swings by the end of week 1, medium iron swings by week 2, and long iron swings by week 3. Medium and long iron shots are hit using a tee to minimize the forces at the elbow observed in taking a divot. Use of woods are initiated at the end of week three and progressed to include drives by the fourth week. The athlete can play nine holes during the end of the fourth week if asymptomatic.

COMMON SPORT-RELATED INJURIES
Medial and Lateral Epicondylitis

Medial and lateral epicondylitis may result from numerous factors, many of which have been discussed earlier. The majority of causes are related to repetitive sports-specific microtrauma and poor biomechanics. Medially, overhead throwers most often exhibit pronator tendonitis and golfers have wrist flexor tendonitis, whereas lateral epicondylitis is most often seen in tennis players. Athletes most often are seen with tenderness near the epicondyle and along the flexor-pronator or extensor-supinator muscle masses, which may be exacerbated by contraction or stretching of the musculature.

Table 20-6

Satisfactory Isokinetic Test Results

Bilateral Comparisons

Velocity (°/deg)	Elbow (Flex)	Elbow (Ext)		
180	110-120%	105-115%		
300	105-115%	100-110%		
Velocity (°/deg)	Shoulder (ER)	Shoulder (IR)	Shoulder (Abd)	Shoulder (Add)
180	98-105%	110-120%	98-105%	110-128%
300	85-95%	105-115%	96-102%	111-129%

Unilateral Muscle Ratios

Velocity (°/deg)	Elbow (Flex/Ext)	Shoulder (ER/IR)	Shoulder (Abd/Add)	Shoulder (ER/Abd)
180	70-80%	66-76%	78-84%	67-75%
300	63-69%	61-71%	88-94%	67-75%

Peak Torque-to-Body Weight Ratios

Velocity (°/deg)	Shoulder(ER)	Shoulder (IR)	Shoulder (Abd)	Shoulder (Add)
180	18-23%	28-33%	26-33%	32-38%
300	12-20%	25-30%	20-25%	28-34%

Abd, abduction; Add, adduction; ER, external rotation; Ext, extension; Flex, flexion; IR, internal rotation.

During the clinical examination an attempt should be made to distinguish the involved structures. For medial epicondylitis, manual resistance of wrist flexion should be performed as well as pronation to determine whether a pronation strain has occurred. For lateral epicondylitis, testing of the extensor carpi radialis longus is performed with the elbow flexed to 30° and resistance given to the second metacarpal bone.[40] The extensor carpi radialis brevis is tested with the elbow fully flexed and resistance given to the third metacarpal bone.[40] In addition, the extensor carpi ulnaris can be differentiated by resisting ulnar deviation.[40]

The nonoperative approach for treatment of epicondylitis is outlined in Table 20-7. The program focuses on diminishing pain and gradually improving muscular strength. The primary goals of rehabilitation are to control the applied loads and create an environment for healing. The initial treatment consists of warm whirlpool, phonophoresis, transverse friction massage, stretching exercises, and light strengthening exercises to stimulate a healing response. High-voltage pulsed galvanic stimulation and cryotherapy are used after treatment to decrease pain and postexercise inflammation. The athlete should be cautioned against excessive gripping activities. When the athlete's symptoms have subsided, an aggressive stretching and strengthening program with emphasis on eccentric contractions can be initiated. Wrist flexion and extension activities should be performed initially with the elbow flexed 30 to 45° to decrease tissue stress. When the athlete

can perform these isotonic exercises with a 3-pound weight, they can be performed with the elbow fully extended. A gradual progression through plyometric activities precedes the initiation of an interval sport program. Because poor mechanics are often a cause of this condition, an analysis of sport mechanics and proper supervision through the interval sport program are critical for successful return to symptom-free athletic participation.

Ulnar Neuropathy

There are numerous theories about the cause of ulnar neuropathy of the elbow in athletes.[26] Ulnar nerve changes can result from tensile forces, compressive forces, or nerve instability. Any one or a combination of these mechanisms may be responsible for producing ulnar nerve symptoms.

A leading mechanism for tensile force on the ulnar nerve is valgus stress. This may also be coupled with an external rotation-supination stress overload mechanism. The traction forces are further magnified when underlying valgus instability from a UCL injury is present. Ulnar neuropathy is often a secondary pathologic consequence of UCL insufficiency.

Compression of the ulnar nerve is often due to hypertrophy of the surrounding soft tissues or the presence of scar tissue. The nerve may also be trapped between the two heads of the flexor carpi ulnaris.

Table 20-7

Epicondylitis Rehabilitation Program

Phase I (acute)
- Active rest
- Splint when necessary
- Modalities to reduce pain, inflammation, and edema and to promote healing
- Begin flexibility exercises when tolerated

Phase II
- Continue flexibility exercises
- Begin strengthening wrist flexors/forearm pronator
- Begin light multi-joint shoulder, scapula, and elbow strengthening (avoiding positions of elbow extension)
- Continue modalities as needed

Phase III
- Begin isolated wrist extension, radial deviation and supination strengthening if tolerated (elbow flexed)
- Continue strengthening for full upper extremity
- Continue flexibility exercises

Phase IV
- Begin wrist and forearm strengthening with elbow in extension if asymptomatic
- Continue aggressive upper extremity strengthening exercises
- Begin activity-specific function exercises and neuromuscular drills and endurance training
- Continue flexibility exercises

Phase V (return to activity)
- Begin sports-specific interval program
- Biomechanical or ergonomic assessment and alteration
- Maintenance program for strength and flexibility

Repetitive flexion and extension of the elbow with an unstable nerve can irritate or inflame the nerve. The nerve may subluxate or rest on the medial epicondyle, rendering it vulnerable to direct trauma. Complete dislocation of the nerve may occur anteriorly, leading to friction neuritis.

There are three stages of ulnar neuropathy.[2] The first stage includes an acute onset of radicular symptoms. The second stage is manifested by a recurrence of symptoms as the athlete attempts to return to competition. The third stage is associated with persistent motor weakness and sensory changes. When the athlete is seen in the third stage of injury, conservative management may not be effective.

Clinical examination often reveals tenderness along the cubital tunnel. Additionally, the clinician may perform a Tinel test by tapping on the cubital tunnel. A positive Tinel test result is paresthesia or tingling over the ulnar nerve distribution.

The nonoperative treatment of ulnar neuropathy focuses on diminishing ulnar nerve irritation, enhancing dynamic medial joint stability, and gradually returning the athlete to competition.

After the diagnosis of ulnar neuropathy, throwing athletes are instructed to discontinue throwing activities for at least 4 weeks. The athlete progresses through the immediate motion and intermediate phases of rehabilitation over the course of 4 to 6 weeks with emphasis placed on eccentric control and dynamic stabilization drills. Plyometric exercises are used to facilitate dynamic stabilization of the medial elbow. The athlete is allowed to begin an interval throwing program when the following criteria have been fulfilled: (1) full pain-free ROM, (2) a satisfactory clinical examination, (3) no neurologic symptoms, (4) adequate medial stability, and (5) satisfactory muscular performance. The athlete may gradually return to play if progression through an interval sport program does not reproduce further neurologic symptoms.

Ulnar Nerve Transposition

Surgical transpositioning of the ulnar nerve involves stabilizing the nerve with fascial slings. Caution is taken not to overstress the soft tissue structures involved with relocating the nerve. The rehabilitation process after an ulnar nerve transposition is outlined in Table 20-8. A posterior splint at 90° of elbow flexion is used for the first 2 weeks postoperatively to prevent excessive ROM and tension on the nerve while the facial slings heal. Use of the splint is discontinued at week 2, and light ROM activities are initiated. Full ROM is usually restored by weeks 3 to 4. Gentle isotonic strengthening is begun during week 4 and progressed to the full Thrower's Ten Exercise Program by 6 weeks after surgery. Aggressive strengthening including eccentric and plyometric training can typically be incorporated by week 7 to 8 and an interval sport program at week 8 to 9, if all previously outlined criteria have been met.

A return to competition can usually take place between postoperative week 12 and 16.

Valgus Extension Overload

Valgus extension overload occurs in repetitive sport activities such as throwing, tennis serving, and swimming. Injury usually occurs during the acceleration or deceleration phase as the olecranon wedges up against the medial olecranon fossa during elbow extension.[94] This mechanism may result in osteophyte formation and potentially can produce loose bodies. Repetitive extension stress from the triceps may further contribute to this injury. There is often a certain degree of underlying valgus elbow instability in these athletes, further facilitating osteophyte formation through compression of radiocapitellar joint and the posteromedial elbow.[3]

Athletes typically present with pain along the posteromedial aspect of the elbow that is exacerbated with forced extension and valgus stress. The clinical test for valgus extension overload involves the clinician grasping the elbow in a flexed position. As the clinician forces the elbow into extension, a valgus stress is simultaneously applied to the elbow (Fig. 20-14). The clinician palpates the posteromedial joint for tenderness and/or crepitation. Pain over the posteromedial olecranon process signifies a positive test result.[94]

A conservative treatment approach is often attempted before surgical intervention is considered. Initial treatment involves relieving the posterior elbow of pain and inflammation. As symptoms subside and ROM normalizes, strengthening exercises are initiated. Emphasis is placed on improving eccentric strength of the elbow flexors in an attempt to control the rapid extension that occurs at the elbow during athletic activities. Manual resistance exercises of concentric and eccentric elbow flexion as well as elbow flexion are performed with exercise tubing to accentuate the functional control required.

Posterior Olecranon Osteophyte Excision

Surgical excision of posterior olecranon osteophytes is performed using an osteotome or motorized burr. Approximately 5 to 10 mm of the olecranon tip is typically removed concomitantly and a motorized burr is used to contour the coronoid, olecranon tip, and fossa to prevent further impingement with extreme flexion and extension.[48]

The rehabilitation program after arthroscopic posterior olecranon osteophyte excision is slightly more conservative in restoring full elbow extension due to postsurgical pain. ROM is progressed within the athlete's tolerance. Normally by the tenth postoperative day the athlete should exhibit at least 15 to 100° of ROM and 10 to 110° by day 14. Full ROM is typically restored by day 20 to 25 after surgery. The

TABLE 20-8

Rehabilitation after Ulnar Nerve Transpositioning

Phase I: Immediate Postoperative Phase (Week 0 to 1)

Goals

- Allow soft tissue healing of relocated nerve
- Decrease pain and inflammation
- Retard muscular atrophy

A. Week 1

   1. Posterior splint at 90° elbow flexion with wrist free for motion (sling for comfort)
   2. Compression dressing
   3. Exercises such as gripping exercises, wrist range of motion, shoulder isometrics

B. Week 2

   1. Remove posterior splint for exercise and bathing
   2. Progress elbow range of motion (passive range of motion 15 to 120°)
   3. Initiate elbow and wrist isometrics
   4. Continue shoulder isometrics

Phase II. Intermediate Phase (Week 3 to 7)

Goals

- Restore full-pain free range of motion
- Improve strength, power, and endurance of upper extremity musculature
- Gradually increase functional demands

A. Week 3

   1. Discontinue posterior splint
   2. Progress elbow range of motion, emphasize full extension
   3. Initiate flexibility exercise for wrist extension/flexion, forearm supination/pronation, and elbow extension/flexion
   4. Initiate strengthening exercises for wrist extension/flexion, forearm supination/pronation, elbow extensors/flexors, and a shoulder program

B. Week 6

   1. Continue all exercises listed above
   2. Initiate light sport activities

Phase III: Advanced Strengthening Phase (Week 8 to 12)

Goals

- Increase strength, power, and endurance
- Gradually initiate sporting activities

A. Week 8

   1. Initiate eccentric exercise program
   2. Initiate plyometric exercise drills
   3. Continue shoulder and elbow strengthening and flexibility exercises
   4. Initiate interval throwing program

Phase IV: Return to Activity Phase (Week 12 to 16)

Goals

- Gradually return to sporting activities

A. Week 12

   1. Return to competitive throwing
   2. Continue Throwers' Ten Exercise Program

rate of ROM progression is most often limited by osseous structure pain and synovial joint inflammation.

The strengthening program is progressed in a similar fashion to that previously discussed. Isometrics are performed for the first 10 to 14 days. Isotonic strengthening is incorporated from week 2 to 6. The full Thrower's Ten Exercise Program is initiated by week 6. An interval sport program can typically be initiated by week 10 to 12. The rehabilitation focus is similar to that for nonoperative treatment of valgus extension overload, emphasizing eccentric control of the elbow flexors and dynamic stabilization of the medial elbow.

Andrews and Timmerman[6] reported on the outcome of elbow surgery in 72 professional baseball players. Sixty-five percent of these athletes exhibited a posterior olecranon osteophyte and 25% of the athletes who underwent an isolated olecranon excision later required an UCL reconstruction.[6] These results may suggest that subtle medial instability may accelerate osteophyte formation.

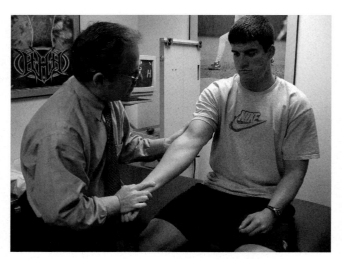

Figure 20-14. Clinical test for valgus extension overload. The clinician forcefully extends the elbow while applying a valgus stress.

Conversely, there is a certain amount of concern related to the effects of excising the posterior olecranon on medial elbow stability. Because this excision alters the static stability of the humeroulnar articulation, medial elbow stability may be compromised. Andrews and Heggland (unpublished work, 2001) examined the amount of stress applied to the anterior bundle of the UCL with varying amounts of posterior olecranon excisions. UCL strain was measured with intact olecranon and with 2-mm incremental resections of the medial olecranon up to 8 mm. A further resection of 13 mm was also performed. The UCL was then strained to failure during an applied valgus stress at varying degrees of elbow flexion from 50 to 100°. Results indicate no significant differences in strain on the UCL with changes in the extent of the osteotomy performed for a given applied load and angle of elbow flexion. Thus, it appears that UCL strain is not significantly increased with posterior olecranon resection.

Ulnar Collateral Ligament Injury

Injuries to the UCL are becoming increasingly more common in overhead throwing athletes, although the higher incidence of injury may be due to an improved ability to accurately diagnose these injuries. As described briefly in the biomechanics section, the elbow experiences a tremendous amount of valgus stress during overhead throwing. These stresses approach the ultimate failure load of the ligament with each throw. The repetitive nature of overhead sport activities such as baseball pitching, football passing, tennis serving, and javelin throwing further increase the susceptibility for UCL injury by exposing the ligament to repetitive microtraumatic forces.

The athlete with an injury to the UCL usually presents with pain and tenderness to the medial elbow. Generalized joint effusion may also be present. The athlete's subjective history typically reveals either recurring medial elbow symptoms or a single traumatic incident of medial elbow pain while throwing. The athlete recalls a sudden, sharp, medial elbow pain, often with a popping sensation. As described earlier, the physical examination and isolated analysis of UCL laxity via prone and supine valgus stress testing are critical for accurate assessment. Additionally, MRI scanning enhanced by an injection of intra-articular dye may be useful in the athlete with a suspected UCL injury. A UCL tear is indicated by a T-sign as previously discussed.[78]

Various opinions exist about the efficacy of nonoperative treatment for UCL strains or partial tears for the throwing athlete. If an injury to the UCL is suspected, the rehabilitation program outlined in Table 20-9 is initiated. ROM is initially permitted in a nonpainful arc of motion, usually 10 to 100°, to allow for a decrease in inflammation and the alignment of collagen tissue. A brace may be used to restrict motion and to prevent valgus strain. Isometric exercises are performed for the shoulder, elbow, and wrist to prevent muscular atrophy. Ice and anti-inflammatory medications are prescribed to control pain and inflammation.

ROM of both flexion and extension are gradually increased during the second phase of treatment as tolerated. Full ROM should be achieved by at least 3 to 4 weeks after surgery. Rhythmic stabilization exercises are initiated to develop dynamic stabilization and neuromuscular control of the upper extremity. As dynamic stability is advanced, isotonic exercises are incorporated for the entire upper extremity.

The advanced strengthening phase is usually initiated at 6 to 7 weeks postinjury. During this phase the athlete is progressed to the Thrower's Ten Exercise Program isotonic strengthening program and plyometric exercises. An interval sport program is initiated when the athlete regains full motion, adequate strength, and dynamic stability of the elbow. The athlete is allowed to return to competition after the asymptomatic completion of an appropriate interval sport program. If symptoms continue to persist, the athlete's condition is reassessed, and surgical intervention is considered.

Ulnar Collateral Ligament Reconstruction

The goal of surgical reconstruction of the UCL is to restore the stabilizing functions of the anterior bundle of the UCL.[95] The palmaris longus or an alternate graft source is harvested and passed in a figure-eight pattern through drill holes in the sublime tubercle of the ulna and the medial epicondyle.[5] An ulnar nerve transposition is often performed at the time of a UCL reconstruction.[5]

The rehabilitation program after UCL reconstruction varies based on the surgical technique, the method of transposition of the ulnar nerve, and the overall extent of

Table 20-9

Nonoperative UCL Rehabilitation

Acute Phase

Goals
- Diminish ulnar nerve inflammation
- Restore normal motion
- Maintain/improve muscular strength

1. Brace: (optional)
2. Range of motion: restore full nonpainful range of motion as soon as possible. Initiate stretching exercises for wrist, forearm and elbow musculature
3. Strengthening exercises: If elbow is extremely painful and/or inflamed use isometrics for approximately 1 week. Initiate isotonic strengthening.
   - Wrist flexion/extension
   - Forearm supination/pronation
   - Elbow flexion/extension
   - Shoulder program
4. Pain control/inflammation control
   - Warm whirlpool
   - Cryotherapy
   - High-voltage galvanic stimulation

Advanced Strengthening Phase (Week 3 to 6)

Goals
- Improve strength, power, and endurance
- Enhance Dyonic joint stability
- Initiate high-speed training

1. Exercise—Thrower's Ten Exercise Program
   - Eccentrics wrist/forearm muscles
   - Rhythmic stabilization drills for elbow joint
   - Isokinetics for elbow flex/extensor
   - Plyometric exercise drills
2. Continue stretching exercises

Return to Activity Phase (Week 4 to 6)

Goals
- Gradual return to functional activities
- Enhanced muscular performance

Criteria to begin throwing
- Full nonpainful range of motion
- Satisfactory clinical examination
- Satisfactory muscular performance

1. Initiate interval sport program
2. Continue Thrower's Ten Exercise Program
3. Continue all stretching exercise

---

injury to the elbow. The rehabilitation program currently used by the authors after UCL reconstruction is outlined in Table 20-10.[90,93] The athlete is placed in a posterior splint with the elbow immobilized at 90° of flexion for the first 7 days postoperatively. This allows adequate healing of the UCL graft and soft tissue slings involved in the nerve transposition. The athlete is allowed to perform wrist ROM, gripping, and submaximal isometrics for the wrist and elbow. The athlete is progressed from the posterior splint to an elbow ROM brace, which is adjusted to allow ROM from 30 to 100° of flexion. Motion is increased by 5° of extension and 10° of flexion thereafter to restore full ROM by the end of week 6 (0 to 145°). Use of the brace is discontinued by week 5 to 6 after surgery.

Isometric exercises are progressed to include light resistance isotonic exercises at week 4 and the full Thrower's Ten Exercise Program by week 6. Sport-specific exercises are incorporated at week 8 to 9. Focus is again placed on developing dynamic stabilization of the medial elbow. Due to the anatomical orientation of the flexor carpi ulnaris and flexor digitorum superficialis overlaying the UCL, isotonic and stabilization activities for these muscles may assist the UCL in stabilizing valgus stress at the medial elbow.

Aggressive exercises involving eccentric and plyometric contractions are included in the advanced phase, usually during weeks 9 through 14. An interval sport program is typically allowed 16 weeks postoperatively. In most cases, throwing from a mound is progressed within 4 to 6 weeks after the initiation of an interval throwing program and a return to competitive throwing at approximately 6 to 7 months after surgery.[10] Azar and associates[10] and later Cain and co-workers[17] reported 85% to 88% success rates (return to sports after UCL reconstruction in athletes).

ADOLESCENT ELBOW INJURIES

Skeletal immaturity in adolescents alters typical pathomechanics, resulting in a very different set of lesions at the elbow than those seen in the adult athlete. The elbow is the most common area of symptoms in the young baseball player and a vast majority of the osseous changes seen as a result of pitching occur at the radiohumeral joint.[83] The two most common injuries occurring at the adolescent elbow are osteochondritis dissecans and Little Leaguer's elbow.

Osteochondritis Dissecans

Osteochondritis dissecans of the elbow is a compression lesion of the radiocapitellar joint that results in bony and articular cartilage damage on the anterolateral surface of the capitellum.[33] Although it is most often seen in throwers, osteochondritis dissecans of the elbow has been reported as a result of participation in various athletic activities.[32,65,73] It is considered the leading cause of permanent elbow disability in the young pitching athlete.[31,80] Unlike lesions occurring to the medial side of the elbow, lateral lesions can result in permanent elbow

Table 20-10

Postoperative Rehabilitation After Ulnar Collateral Ligament Injury

Phase I. Immediate Postoperative Phase (0-3 weeks)

Goals
- Protect healing tissue
- Decrease pain/inflammation
- Retard muscular atrophy

A. Postoperative week 1
  1. Posterior splint at 90° elbow flexion
  2. Wrist active range of motion extension/flexion
  3. Elbow compression dressing (2 to 3 days)
  4. Exercises such as gripping exercises, wrist range of motion, shoulder isometrics (except shoulder external rotation), biceps isometrics
  5. Cryotherapy

B. Postoperative week 2
  1. Application of functional brace 30° to 100°
  2. Initiate wrist isometrics
  3. Initiate elbow flexion/extension isometrics
  4. Continue all exercises listed above

C. Postoperative week 3
  1. Advance brace 15° to 110° (gradually increase range of motion; 5° extension/10° flexion per week)

Phase II: Intermediate Phase (Week 4 to 8)

Goals
- Gradual increase in range of motion
- Promote healing of repaired tissue
- Regain and improve muscular strength

A. Week 4
  1. Functional brace set (10° to 120°)
  2. Begin light resistance exercises for arm (1 lb), wrist curls, extensions: pronation/supination elbow extension/flexion
  3. Progress shoulder program and emphasize rotator cuff strengthening (avoid external rotation until 6th week)

B. Week 6
  1. Functional brace set (0 to 130°); active range of motion 0 to 145° (without brace)
  2. Progress elbow strengthening exercises
  3. Initiate shoulder external rotation strengthening
  4. Progress shoulder program

Phase III: Advanced Strengthening Phase (Week 9 to 13)

Goals
- Increase strength, power, and endurance
- Maintain full elbow range of motion
- Gradually initiate sporting activities

A. Week 9
  1. Initiate eccentric elbow flexion/extension
  2. Continue isotonic program; forearm and wrist
  3. Continue shoulder program—Thrower's Ten Exercise Program
  4. Manual resistance diagonal patterns
  5. Initiate plyometric exercise program

B. Week 11
  1. Continue all exercises listed above
  2. May begin light sport activities (i.e., golf or swimming)

Phase IV: Return to Activity Phase (Week 14 through 26)

Goals
- Continue to increase strength, power, and endurance of upper extremity musculature
- Gradual return to sport activities

A. Week 14
  1. Initiate interval throwing program (phase I)
  2. Continue strengthening program
  3. Emphasis on elbow and wrist strengthening and flexibility exercises

B. Week 22 through 26
  1. Return to competitive throwing

damage and often shorten or terminate a throwing athlete's career.[83]

Although the exact cause of osteochondritis dissecans is unknown, it is believed that repeated traumatic impact of the radial head against the capitellum during the cocking and acceleration phases of throwing can result in a circulatory disturbance to the radiocapitellar joint. This disturbance produces primary changes to the bone and secondary changes to the articular cartilage.[61] Osteochondritis dissecans of the adolescent elbow is seen as aseptic necrosis of the radial head. This can result in the progressive formation of loose bodies, overgrowth of the radial head, and early arthritic changes.

Osteochondritis dissecans represents a major threat to the elbow joint, and it is important that it be diagnosed early. The athlete typically complains of anterolateral elbow tenderness along with decreased pronation and supination, suggesting radiocapitellar incongruity or radial head fracture.[82] The most common finding is a loss of full elbow extension that can be as much as a 20° loss of full extension.[16,80,96]

Conservative treatment consists of a period of active rest during which the athlete avoids all throwing and other exacerbating activities along with the use of local modalities to decrease pain and inflammation. When the athlete can tolerate it, an elbow rehabilitation program may be started; however, an overly aggressive approach can result in a progressive loss of motion. If avascular changes are noted on the lateral side of the elbow in the young thrower, abstinence from throwing should be maintained until revascularization of the affected area has occurred.

Most authors recommend surgical removal of symptomatic loose bodies and avoidance of other surgical procedures, unless there are changes that could compromise the architectural support of the capitellum.[62,96] Prognosis of osteochondritis dissecans after simple loose body removal is good if diagnosis is made early and there are no associated degenerative changes present. Recovery to normal function is slow, however, and some limitation of full extension is likely to remain. Tivnon and colleagues[80] reported an average preoperative elbow range of motion of 30 to 134° that improved to 11 to 136° after surgery. If ROM is to be reestablished or increased after loose body extraction in this condition, appropriate early mobilization is paramount.

Degenerative changes of the radiocapitellar joint have a poor prognosis for the athlete returning to pitching.[31] Although the osteophytes and loose bodies can be removed surgically, ankylosis of the elbow complex may result, leaving the young athlete unable to throw effectively.[30]

Little Leaguer's Elbow

Brogdon and Crow[15] first used the term *Little Leaguer's elbow* to describe an avulsion of the ossification center of the medial epicondyle caused by pitching in the adolescent athlete. Little Leaguer's elbow is now a catch-all term used to describe several pathologic conditions that occur at the elbow, including strain of the flexor-pronator muscle group, ulnar neuropathy, and osteochondritis dissecans.

Forces associated with this condition injure the epiphyseal plate because it is the weakest link in the adolescent kinetic chain. The injury is associated with repetitive throwing, which produces medial traction forces during the acceleration phase of the activity. Hypertrophy of the medial epicondyle develops as a physiologic response to throwing. A widened growth line or displacement of the epicondyle is evidence of a fracture.

Little Leaguer's elbow commonly presents with a history of medial elbow pain progressing over the course of a few weeks. These symptoms typically worsen with pitching and are relieved by rest. Additional signs and symptoms include limitation of complete extension, tenderness over the medial epicondyle, and pain with passive extension of the wrist and fingers. Radiographic changes include accelerated growth, separation, and fragmentation of the medial epicondylar epiphysis. Less commonly, the athlete may have dramatic symptoms, including the report of a popping sensation followed by medial elbow pain, the inability to throw because of pain, and swelling accompanied by medial elbow ecchymosis.

Prevention remains the best treatment for Little Leaguer's elbow. It is important that coaches and parents be educated about proper warm-up, conditioning, and off-season training of the adolescent pitcher. Also, the throwing of curve balls and other breaking pitches by pitchers in the 9- to 14-year-old age group should be prohibited, because stress associated with these pitches considerably increases the forces placed on wrist flexion and pronation.[20,62] Pitchers should be taught proper pitching mechanics and appropriate pitching limits or maximum should be established. Currently, Little League International pitching rules advise six innings per week, with 3 days of rest between pitching outings.[44] However, there are no rules or recommendations that govern the intensity and frequency of practice pitching that an athlete can engage in.

Treatment in the early stages of Little Leaguer's elbow includes rest from noxious stimuli, local modalities to decrease pain and inflammation and possibly immobilization. If radiographic findings reveal capitellum osteochondritis dissecans, it is recommended that the player stop pitching for the remainder of the baseball season. After initial conservative treatment, if the athlete returns to throwing and there is any recurrence of symptoms, he or she should completely abstain from throwing until the next season.

A medial epicondylar fracture that is displaced by more than 1 cm may occur in a small percentage of athletes. These injuries should be opened and fixed internally with a screw. With open and internal fixation, the elbow is immobilized for approximately 3 to 4 weeks, and the athlete should not engage in any throwing activity until the following season. Criteria for return to competition include no pain, normal elbow range of motion, and no weakness in muscle strength or endurance in all planes of wrist and elbow ROM. The return to throwing should be gradual and should follow the Little League interval throwing program (Appendix B). Fortunately, most elbow injuries in the adolescent thrower are adequately treated by rest and cause no permanent disability.

LESS-COMMON SPORT RELATED INJURIES
Osteochondritis Dissecans

Osteochondritis dissecans of the elbow may develop because of valgus strain on the elbow joint, which produces not only medial tension but also lateral compressive forces. This is observed as the capitellum of the humerus compresses with the radial head. Patients often complain of lateral elbow pain upon palpation and valgus stress. Morrey[52] described a three-stage classification of pathologic progression. Stage one included patients without evidence of subchondral displacement or fracture, whereas stage two referred to lesions showing evidence of subchondral detachment or articular cartilage fracture. Stage three lesions involved detached osteochondral fragments, resulting in intra-articular loose bodies. Nonsurgical treatment is attempted for patients with stage one lesions only and consists of relative rest and immobilization until elbow symptoms have resolved.

Nonoperative treatment includes 3 to 6 weeks of immobilization at 90° of elbow flexion. ROM activities for the shoulder, elbow, and wrist are performed 3 to 4 times a day. As symptoms resolve, a strengthening program is initiated with isometric exercises. Isotonic exercises are included after approximately 1 week of isometric exercise. Aggressive high speed, eccentric, and plyometric exercises are progressively included to prepare the athlete for the start of an interval sport program.

If nonoperative treatment fails or evidence of loose bodies exist, surgical intervention including arthroscopic abrading and drilling of the lesion with fixation or removal of the loose body is indicated.[68] Long-term follow-up studies regarding the outcome of patients undergoing surgery to drill or reattach the lesions have not produced favorable results, suggesting that prevention and early detection of symptoms may be the best form of treatment.[12,95]

Degenerative Joint Disease

Degenerative joint disease of the elbow may occur prematurely in certain athletes who participate in sport activities that repetitively load the articular surfaces of the elbow joint. Acceleration of joint degeneration and osteophyte formation may occur. Pain and joint effusion may be observed during examination as well as tenderness to palpation over the joint lines. Although this particular pathologic condition may not restrict normal function and activities of daily living, the pain and loss of motion associated with degenerative joint disease may restrict further participation in sports.

Conservative treatment is thus focused on first diminishing pain and inflammation and secondly improving ROM and soft tissue flexibility. Warm whirlpool treatment before stretching and gentle joint mobilization techniques may be beneficial to enhance soft tissue extensibility. As pain and ROM normalize, an overall enhancement of upper extremity strength and endurance is emphasized. If conservative treatment does not produce favorable results, an open or arthroscopic debridement may be indicated to alleviate symptoms.

Synovitis

Generalized joint synovitis may occur from the repetitive nature of throwing or other overhead sports. Athletes often complain of a diffuse joint pain not specific to one area and a flexion contracture is apparent upon examination. Initial treatment includes anti-inflammatory medications and activity modification to allow for a period of rest and recovery.

A rehabilitation program focused on restoring elbow extension is initiated. ROM, stretching, and mobilization exercises are performed as necessary to restore and maintain full ROM. The clinician must be cautioned against overaggressive stretching and mobilization during the acute phases of recovery to avoid contributing to the inflammatory synovial reaction. Tepid to warm whirlpool treatment may be used before ROM exercises. Contrast treatment (cold to warm) may also be beneficial. Submaximal isometric exercises are performed until the inflammatory response has diminished, followed by the initiation of an isotonic strengthening program. A return to sport-specific drills and an interval sport program are instituted once the athlete has achieved proper strength and has a satisfactory clinical examination.

Dislocations

Dislocations of the elbow joint most commonly occur in collision sports such as football and wrestling or in non-contact sports as the athlete lands onto an outstretched hand. A hyperextension injury occurs as the olecranon is forced into the olecranon fossa and the trochlea translates posteriorly or posterolaterally over the coronoid process.[7] Disruption of the UCL and possibly the lateral collateral ligament may occur during this type of severe injury. Concomitant fractures of the radial head or capitellum may also be produced.[7]

A lateral pivot shift test may be used to assess postero-lateral stability of the elbow.[61] Initial reduction of the injury may be performed by application of traction to the forearm and humerus with the elbow in 30° of flexion.[7] Neurovascular integrity should be assessed immediately, and surgical intervention may be necessary to repair concomitant ligament instability and osseous fractures.

Treatment depends greatly on the severity of injury and the associated injuries that are present. An initial period of rest and immobilization may be warranted to allow for soft tissue healing and a decrease in pain and inflammation. Early motion should be initiated within the first week after injury to minimize the chances of motion loss, which is one of the primary complications after elbow dislocation.[67] Rehabilitation follows a progressive sequence similar to that described earlier to regain motion and strength of the entire elbow and forearm complex.

Fractures

Various fractures of the elbow may occur in the athletic population, including extra- and intra-articular distal humerus fractures, radial head fractures, and olecranon fractures.[67] Stress fractures of the olecranon have been reported in overhead throwers and can occur in any part of the olecranon, especially in the mid-articular area.[13] The most likely cause of injury involves repetitive stresses applied to the olecranon as the elbow extends from triceps contraction during the acceleration, deceleration, and follow-through phases of throwing. Patients often subjectively report an insidious onset of pain in the posterolateral elbow while throwing. Symptoms appear similar to those of triceps tendinitis; however, tenderness over the involved site of the olecranon is often detected upon palpation. Plain radiographs are typically taken and diagnosis may be further enhanced with the aid of a bone and/or MRI scan.

Aggressive stretching and strengthening exercises are restricted for the first 6 to 8 weeks to allow adequate healing of the fracture site. The athlete should maintain motion with light ROM exercises. Heavy lifting, plyometrics, and sport-specific drills are not allowed until bony healing is seen on radiographic evaluation, typically by 8 to 12 weeks. When adequate healing has been documented, an interval sport program may be allowed. Complete recovery occurs in approximately 3 to 6 months after injury. An open reduction internal fixation may be indicated if conservative management fails.

Arthrolysis

Many of the pathologic conditions that have been discussed earlier involved motion loss as a primary complication. The elbow joint is one of the joints that most commonly develops a functional loss of motion due to injury or after surgery.[27,78] After injury, the elbow flexes in response to pain and hemarthrosis. The periarticular soft tissue and joint capsule become shortened and fibrotic and loss of motion develops. An arthroscopic arthrolysis may be necessary for patients whose injury does not respond to conservative treatment.

During the first postoperative week, the athlete is instructed to perform elbow and wrist ROM exercises hourly. Treatment to regain ROM at this time is cautiously aggressive.[87] Full motion should be obtained quickly; however, a pace that does not cause additional inflammation of the joint capsule is necessary to avoid further pain and reflexive splinting. Low-load long-duration stretching has been an extremely beneficial clinical treatment technique in these instances. Full passive ROM is usually restored by 10 to 14 days after surgery.

Isometric strengthening is begun during week 2 and progressed to isotonic dumbbell exercises during the third to forth week. Strengthening exercises are progressed as tolerated by the athlete. During the later phases of rehabilitation the emphasis on maintaining full motion is continued. Athletes are educated to continue a motion maintenance program several times per day and before and after sport activities for at least 2 to 3 months after surgery.

SUMMARY

- The elbow joint is a common site of injury in the athletic population.
- Injuries vary widely from repetitive microtraumatic injuries to gross macrotraumatic dislocations.
- A thorough understanding of the sport-specific anatomy and biomechanics of the joint is necessary for a successful clinical examination, assessment, and rehabilitation prescription.
- Rehabilitation of the elbow, whether postinjury or postsurgical, must follow a progressive and sequential order to ensure that healing tissues are not overstressed.
- A rehabilitation program that limits immobilization, achieves full range of motion early, progressively restores strength and neuromuscular control, and gradually incorporates sport-specific activities is essential to successfully return the athletes to their previous level of competition as quickly and safely as possible.

REFERENCES

1. Akeson, W.H., Amiel, D., and Woo, S.L.Y. (1980): Immobilization effects on synovial joints. The pathomechanics of joint contracture., Biorheology, 17:95-107.
2. Alley, R.M., and Pappas, A.M. (1995): Acute and performance-related injuries of the elbow. In: Pappas, A.M. (ed.), Upper Extremity Injuries in the Athlete. New York, Churchill Livingstone, pp. 339-364.
3. Anderson, K. (2001): Elbow arthritis and removal of loose bodies and spurs, and techniques for restoration of motion. In: Altchek

D.W., and Andrews, J.R. (eds.), The Athlete's Elbow. Philadelphia, Lippincott Williams & Wilkins, pp. 219-230.

4. Andrews, J.R., and Frank, W. (1985): Valgus extension overload in the pitching elbow. In: Andrews, J.R., Zarins, B., and Carson W.B. (eds.), Injuries to the Throwing Arm. Philadelphia, W.B. Saunders, pp. 250-257.

5. Andrews, J.R., Jelsma, R.D., Joyse, M.E., and Timmerman, L.A. (1996): Open surgical procedures for injuries to the elbow in throwers. Oper. Tech. Sports Med., 4:109-113.

6. Andrews, J.R., and Timmerman, L. (1995): Outcome of elbow surgery in professional baseball players. Am. J. Sports Med., 23:245-250.

7. Andrews, J.R., and Whiteside, J.A. (1993): Common elbow problems in the athlete. J. Orthop. Sports Phys. Ther., 17:289-295.

8. Andrews, J.R., Wilk, K.E., Satterwhite, Y.E., and Tedder, J.L. (1993): Physical examination of the thrower's elbow. J. Orthop. Sports Phys. Ther., 17:296-304.

9. Atkinson, W.B., and Elftman, H. (1945): The carrying angle of the human arm as a secondary sex character. Anat. Rec., 91:49-54.

10. Azar, F.M., Andrews, J.R., Wilk, K.E., and Groh, D. (2000): Operative treatment of ulnar collateral ligament injuries of the elbow. Am. J. Sports Med., 28:16-23.

11. Basmajian, J.V., and DeLuca, C.J. (1985): Muscles Alive: Their Function Revealed by Electromyography. Baltimore, Williams & Wilkins, pp. 279-280.

12. Baur, M., Jonsson, K., Josefson, P.O., et al. (1992): Osteochondritis dissecans of the elbow: A long-term follow-up study. Clin. Orthop., 284:156-160.

13. Bennett, G.E. (1941): Shoulder and elbow lesions of the professional baseball player. JAMA, 117:510-514.

14. Blackburn, T.A., McCleod, W.D., and White, B.: EMG analysis of posterior rotator cuff exercises. J. Athl. Train., 25:40-45, 1990.

15. Brogdon, B.S., and Crow, M.D. (1960): Little Leaguer's elbow. Am. J. Roentgenol., 85:671-677.

16. Brown, R., Blazina, M.E., Kerlan, R.K., et al. (1974): Osteochondritis of the capitellum. J. Sports Med., 2:27-46.

17. Cain, L., Andrews, J.R., and Wilk, K.E. (2002): Clinical follow-up of UCL reconstructions in the overhead athlete. Presented at the American Orthopaedic Society for Sports Medicine meeting, Orlando, FL, July 3.

18. Coutts, R., Rothe, C., and Kaita, J. (1981): The role of continuous passive motion in the rehabilitation of the total knee patient. Clin. Orthop., 159:126-132.

19. Cyriax, J. (1982): Textbook of Orthopedic Medicine, Vol. 1, Diagnosis of Soft Tissue Lesions, 8th ed. London, Bailliere Tindall, pp. 52-54.

20. DeHaven, K.E., and Evarts, C.M. (1973): Throwing injuries of the elbow in athletes. Orthop. Clin. North Am., 4:801-808.

21. Dehne, E., and Tory., R. (1971): Treatment of joint injuries by immediate mobilization based upon the spiral adaptation concept. Clin. Orthop., 77:218-232.

22. Fleisig, G.S., Andrews, J.R., Dillman, C.J., and Escamilla, R.F. (1995): Kinetics of baseball pitching with implications about injury mechanisms. Am. J. Sports Med., 23:233-239.

23. Fleisig, G.S., and Barrentine, S.W. (1995): Biomechanical aspects of the elbow in sports. Sports Med. Arthrosc. Rev., 3:149-159.

24. Fleisig, G.S., and Escamilla, R.F. (1996): Biomechanics of the elbow in the throwing athlete. Oper. Tech. Sports Med., 4(2):62-68.

25. Glazebrook, M.A., Curwin, S., Islam, M.N., et al. (1994): Medial epicondylitis. An electromyographic analysis and an investigation of intervention strategies. Am. J. Sports Med., 22:674-679.

26. Glousman, R.E. (1990): Ulnar nerve problems in the athlete's elbow. Clin. Sports Med., 9:365-377.

27. Green, D.P., and McCoy, H. (1979): Turnbuckle orthotic correction of elbow flexion contractures. J. Bone Joint Surg., 61A:1092.

28. Haggmark, T., and Eriksson, E. (1979): Cylinder or mobile cast brace after knee ligament surgery: A clinical analysis and morphologic and enzymatic studies of changes of the quadriceps muscle. Am. J. Sports Med., 7:48-56.

29. Hoppenfeld, S. (1976): Physical Examination of the Spine and Extremities. New York, Appleton-Century-Crofts, pp. 35-55.

30. Hunter, S.C. (1985): Little Leaguer's elbow. In: Zarins, B., Andrews, J.R., and Carson, W.G. (eds.), Injuries to the Throwing Arm. Philadelphia, W.B. Saunders, pp. 228-234.

31. Indelicato, P.A., Jobe, F.W., Kerlan, R.K., et al. (1979): Correctable elbow lesions in professional baseball players: A review of 25 cases. Am. J. Sports Med., 7:72-75.

32. Inoue, G. (1991): Bilateral osteochondritis dissecans of the elbow treated with Herbert screw fixation. Br. J. Sports Med., 25:142-144.

33. Jobe, F.W., and Nuber, G. (1986): Throwing injuries of the elbow. Clin. Sports Med., 5:621-636.

34. Jobe, F.W., Moynes, D.R., Tibone, J.E., and Perry, J. (1984): An EMG analysis of the shoulder in pitching. Am. J. Sports Med., 12:218-220.

35. Johansson, O. (1962): Capsular and ligament injuries of the elbow joint. Acta. Chir. Scand. Suppl., 287.

36. Kapandji, I.A. (1970): The Physiology of the Joints, Vol. 1. London, E & S Livingston, pp. 82-83, 112-117.

37. Keats, T.E., Teeslink, R., Diamond, A.E., and Williams, J.H. (1966): Normal axial relationships of the major joints. Radiology, 87:904.

38. Kelley, B.T., and Weiland, A.J. (2001): Posterolateral rotatory instability of the elbow. In: Altchek, D.W., and Andrews J.R. (eds.), The Athlete's Elbow. Philadelphia, Lippincott Williams & Wilkins, pp. 175-189.

39. Kelley, J.D., Lombardo, S.J., Pink, M., et al. (1994): EMG and cinematographic analysis of elbow function in tennis players with lateral epicondylitis. Am. J. Sports Med., 22:359-363.

40. Kendall, F.P., and McCreary, E.K. (1983): Muscles, Testing, and Function, 3rd ed. Baltimore, Williams & Wilkins, pp. 86-87.

41. Kibler, W.B. (1994): Clinical biomechanics of the elbow in tennis: implications for evaluation and diagnosis. Med. Sci. Sports Exerc., 26:1203-1206.

42. Kottke, F.J., Pauley, D.L., and Ptak, R.A. (1966): The rationale for prolonged stretching for connective tissue. Arch. Phys. Med. Rehab., 47:345-352.

43. Lehmkuhl, D.L., and Smith, L.R. (1983): Brunnstrom's Clinical Kinesiology. Philadelphia, F.A. Davis, pp. 149-170.

44. Little League International. (1996): Youth Baseball Handbook. Williamsport, PA, Little League International.

45. Magee, D.J. (1987): Orthopaedic Physical Assessment. Philadelphia, W.B. Saunders.

46. Maitland, G.D. (1977): Vertebral Manipulation. London, Butterworths, pp. 84-105.

47. Martin, B.F. (1958): The annular ligament of the superior radioulnar joint. J. Anat., 52:473.

48. Martin, S.D., and Baumgarten, T.E. (1996): Elbow injuries in the throwing athlete: Diagnosis and arthroscopic treatment. Oper. Tech. Sports Med., 4:100-108.

49. McCarroll, J.R. (1985): Golf. In: Schneider, R.C., et al. (eds.), Sports Injuries: Mechanisms, Prevention, and Treatment. Baltimore, Williams & Wilkins, pp. 290-294.

50. McCarroll, J.R., and Gioe, T.J. (1982): Professional golfers and the price they pay. Physician Sportsmed., 10:64-70.

51. Morrey, B.F. (1985): Anatomy of the elbow. In: Morrey, B.F. (ed.): The Elbow and Its Disorders. Philadelphia, W.B. Saunders, pp. 7-40.

52. Morrey, B.F. (1994): Osteochondritis dessicans. In: DeLee J.C., and Drez, D. (eds.), Orthopedic Sports Medicine. Philadelphia, W.B. Saunders, pp. 908-912.

53. Morrey, B.F., and An, K.N. (1983): Articular and ligamentous contributions to the static stability of the elbow joint. Am. J. Sports Med., 11:315-319.

54. Morrey, B.F., An, K.N., and Dobyns, J. (1985): Functional anatomy of the elbow ligaments. Clin. Orthop., 201:84.

55. Morris, M., Jobe, F.W., Perry, J., et al. (1989): EMG analysis of elbow function in tennis players. Am. J. Sports Med., 17:241-247.

56. Moseley, V.B., Jobe, F.W., and Pink, M. (1992): EMG analysis of the scapular muscles during a shoulder rehabilitation program. Am. J. Sports Med., 20:128-134.

57. Nirschl, R.P., and Morrey, B.F. (1985): Rehabilitation. In: Morrey, B.F. (ed.), The Elbow and Its Disorders. Philadelphia, W.B. Saunders, pp. 147-152.

58. Norkin, C., and Levangie, P. (1985): Joint Structure and Function: A Comprehensive Analysis. Philadelphia, F.A. Davis, pp. 191-210.

59. Norkin, C.C., and White, D.J. (1995): Measurement of Joint Motion: A Guide to Goniometry, 2nd ed. Philadelphia, F.A. Davis.

60. Noyes, F.R., Mangine, R.E., and Barber, S.E. (1987): Early knee motion after open and arthroscopic anterior cruciate ligament reconstruction. Am. J. Sports Med., 15:149-160.

61. O'Driscoll, S.W., Bell, D.F., and Morrey, B.F. (1991): Posterolateral rotatory instability of the elbow. J. Bone Joint Surg., 73A:440-446.

62. Pappas, A.M. (1982): Elbow problems associated with baseball during childhood and adolescence. Clin. Orthop., 164:30-41.

63. Pavly, J.E., Rushing, J.L., and Scheving, L.E. (1967): Electromyographic study of some muscles crossing the elbow joint. J. Anat., 159:47-53.

64. Perkins, G. (1954): Rest and motion. J. Bone Joint Surg., 35B:521-539.

65. Pintore, E., and Maffulli, N. (1991): Osteochondritis dissecans of the lateral humeral epicondyle in a table tennis player. Med. Sci. Sports Exerc., 23:889-891.

66. Rhu, K.N., McCormick, J., Jobe, F.W., et al. (1988): An electromyographic analysis of shoulder function in tennis players. Am. J. Sports Med., 16:481.

67. Richardson, J.K., and Iglarsh, Z.A. (1994): Clinical Orthopaedic Physical Therapy. Philadelphia, W.B. Saunders, pp. 227-230.

68. Roberts, W., and Hughes, R. (1950): Osteochondritis dissecans of the elbow joint: A clinical study. J. Bone Joint Surg., 32B:348-360.

69. Salter, R.B., Hamilton, H.W., and Wedge, J.H. (1984): Clinical application of basic research on continuous passive motion for disorders and injuries of synovial joints. A preliminary report of a feasibility study. J. Orthop. Res., 1:325-342.

70. Salter, R.B., Simmonds, D.F., Malcolm, B.W., et al. (1980): The effects of continuous passive motion on healing of full thickness defects in articular cartilage. J. Bone Joint Surg., 62A:1232-1251.

71. Sapega, A.A., Quedenfeld, T.C., Moyer, R.A., and Butler, R.A. (1976): Biophysical factors in range of motion exercise. Arch. Phys. Med. Rehab., 57:122-126.

72. Schwab, G.H., Bennett, J.B., Woods, G.W. (as quoted by Lanz), and Tullos, H.S. (1980): The biomechanics of elbow stability: the role of the medial collateral ligament. Clin. Orthop., 146:42.

73. Singer, K.M., and Roy, S.P. (1984): Osteochondrosis of the humeral capitellum. Am. J. Sports Med., 12:351-360.

74. Soderberg, G.L. (1981): Kinesiology Application to Pathological Motion. Baltimore, Williams & Wilkins, pp. 131-136.

75. Spinner, M., and Kaplan, E.B. (1970): The quadrate ligament of the elbow—Its relationship to the stability of the proximal radioulnar joint. Acta Orthop. Scand., 41:632.

76. Stanish, W.D., Loebenberg, M.I., and Kozey, J.W. (1994): The Elbow. In: Stover C. N., McCarroll, J.R., and Mallon, W. J. (eds.), Feeling up to Par: Medicine from Tee to Green. Philadelphia, F.A. Davis, pp. 143-149.

77. St. John, J.N., and Palmaz, J.C. (1986): The cubital tunnel in ulnar entrapment neuropathy. Musculoskelet. Radiol., 158:119.

78. Timmerman, L.A., and Andrews, J.R. (1994): Undersurface tears of the ulnar collateral ligament in baseball players. A newly recognized lesion. Am. J. Sports Med., 22:33-36.

79. Tipton, C.M., Mathies, R.D., and Martin, R.F. (1978): Influence of age and sex on strength of bone-ligament junctions in knee joints in rats. J. Bone Joint Surg., 60A:230-236.

80. Tivnon, M.C., Anzel, S.H., and Waugh, T.R. (1976): Surgical management of osteochondritis dissecans of the capitellum. Am. J. Sports Med., 4:121-128.

81. Townsend, H., Jobe, F.W., Pink, M., and Perry, J. (1991): Electromyographic analysis of the glenohumeral muscles during a baseball rehabilitation program. Am. J. Sports Med., 19:264-272.

82. Tullos, H.S., and Bryan, W.J. (1985): Examination of the throwing elbow. In: Zarins, B., Andrews, J.R., and Carson, W.G. (eds.), Injuries to the Throwing Athlete. Philadelphia, W.B. Saunders, pp. 201-210.

83. Tullos, H.S., and King, J.W. (1972): Lesion of the pitching arm in adolescents. JAMA, 220:264-271.

84. Warren, C.G., Lehmann, J.F., and Koblanski, J.N. (1971): Elongation of rat tail tendon: Effect of load and temperature. Arch. Phys. Med. Rehab., 52:465-474.

85. Warren, C.G., Lehmann, J.F., and Koblanski, J.N. (1976): Heat and stretch procedures: An evaluation using rat tail tendon. Arch. Phys. Med. Rehab., 57:122-126.

86. Werner, S., Fleisig, G.S., Dillman, C.J., et al. (1993): Biomechanics of the elbow during baseball pitching. J. Orthop. Sports Phys. Ther., 17:274-278.

87. Wilk, K.E. (1994): Rehabilitation of the elbow following arthroscopic surgery. In: Andrews J. R., and Soffer, S.R. (eds.), Elbow Arthroscopy. St. Louis, C.V. Mosby, pp. 109-116.

88. Wilk, K.E. (2000): Elbow injuries. In: Schenck, R.C. (ed): Athletic Training and Sports Medicine. Rosemont, IL, American Academy of Orthopaedic Surgeons, pp. 293-334.

89. Wilk, K.E., Arrigo, C.A., Andrews, J.R., and Azar, F.M. (1996): Rehabilitation following elbow surgery in the throwing athlete. Oper. Tech. Sports Med., 4:114-132.

90. Wilk, K.E., Azar, F.M., Andrews, J.R. (1995): Conservative and operative rehabilitation of the elbow in sports. Sports Med. Arthrosc. Rev., 3:237-258.

91. Wilk, K.E., Arrigo, C., and Andrews, J.R. (1993): Rehabilitation of the elbow in the throwing athlete. J. Orthop. Sports Phys. Ther., 17:305-317.

92. Wilk, K.E., and Levinson, M. (2001): Rehabilitation of the Athlete's Elbow. *In:* Altchek D. W., and Andrews, J.R. (eds.), The Athlete's Elbow. Philadelphia, Lippincott Williams & Wilkins, pp. 249-273.

93. Wilk, K.E., Voight, M., Keirns, M.D., et al. (1993): Plyometrics for the upper extremities: Theory and clinical application. J. Orthop. Sports Phys. Ther., 17:225-239.

94. Wilson, F.D., Andrews, J.R., Blackburn, T.A., and McClusky, G. (1983): Valgus extension overload in the pitching elbow. Am. J. Sports Med., 11:83-88.

95. Woodward, A.H., and Bianco, A.J., Jr. (1975): Osteochondritis dissecans of the elbow. Clin. Orthop., 110:35-41.

96. Woodward, A.H., and Bianco, A.J. (1975): Osteochondritis dissecans of the elbow. Clin. Orthop., 110:35-41.

97. Wyke, B.D. (1966): The neurology of joints. Ann. R. Coll. Surg. (Lond.), 41:25-29.

CHAPTER 21

REHABILITATION OF WRIST AND HAND INJURIES

Greg Pitts, M.S., O.T.R./L, C.H.T.
Jason Willoughby, O.T.R./L.
Tim L. Uhl, PhD, P.T. ATC

CHAPTER OBJECTIVES

At the end of this chapter the reader will be able to:

- Apply rehabilitation guidelines to sports-related wrist and hand injuries.
- Describe the mechanism of injury and clinical picture of common hand injuries.
- Identify treatment pitfalls to help avoid poor functional outcomes.
- Apply rehabilitation principles to progress an athlete from an acute phase of healing to return to sports for selected wrist and hand injuries.
- Choose appropriate splint types for specific wrist and hand injuries.

The purpose of this chapter is to provide a practical approach to treating athletes with injuries to their wrists, hands, and fingers. These injuries are often minimized or not given the full attention they deserve because athletes are often able to resume participation after minimal care. However, these injuries, if left untreated, can result in permanent disability.[11] The recovery of full function should always be a primary goal in the treatment of hand and wrist injuries. Fortunately, the progression of surgical techniques, rehabilitation techniques, and custom splinting allows earlier return of motion and functional tasks.

As with any other sport injury, the primary goal is to return the athlete to full participation as soon as possible without risking further injury or permanent disability.[19] However, formal informed discussion about the potential long-term outcome of an undertreated hand or wrist injury should be a primary goal of the initial evaluation. The primary emphasis of this chapter is the management of common wrist, hand, and finger injuries to minimize return to participation time and prevent permanent disability or deformity.

In this chapter, common mechanisms of injury, pathologic characteristics of the involved structures, and clinical assessment of the injury are briefly addressed. Practical management of the injury is presented with regard to protective splinting, taping, and initiation of rehabilitation. A summary of rehabilitation recommendations for each injury can be found in Table 22-10. Exercises are described to help the clinician return the athlete to participation and maximize full functional performance of the injured structure.

MALLET FINGER (DISTAL INTERPHALANGEAL TENDON INJURY)

Mallet injury occurs often in ball-catching sports such as football, basketball, baseball, and softball. Typically a ball or some object strikes the distal phalanx, forcing its hyperflexion while the extensor mechanism is active.[17,31,39] The mallet finger deformity is readily observed, because the athlete is unable to actively extend the distal phalanx. Additional clinical signs of this injury are listed in Box 21-1. McCue[26] classified this injury into five types (Table 21-1). Indications for physician referral include the following:

- Extensor lag of the distal interphalangeal (DIP) joint
- Passive range of motion greater than active range of motion extension of the DIP joint
- Pain and swelling focal to the DIP joint
- Ligamentous instability
- Painful passive compression of the finger; radiographs must be obtained to rule out fracture
- Need for surgical treatment for type IV and V injuries

Open injuries require surgical debridement to prevent infection of the bone and joint and need surgical repair of the damaged soft tissues.[53] Table 21-2 lists considerations for splint use and pitfalls in treatment of a mallet finger.

Mallet finger treatment depends on the type of injury the DIP and extensor mechanism have sustained. If the

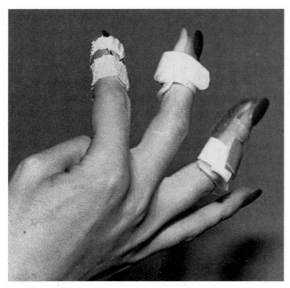

Figure 21-1. Three types of mallet finger splints: a dorsal splint on the index finger, a thermoplastic splint on the middle finger, and a stax splint on the ring finger. A variety of splints are often necessary to avoid skin maceration.

Data from McCue, F.C. (1982): The elbow, wrist, and hand. *In* Kulund, D.N. (ed.), The Injured Athlete. Philadelphia, J.B. Lippincott, pp. 295–329.

Table 21-1

Classification of Mallet Finger Type	Injury
I	Tendon stretch
II	Tendon rupture
III	Tendon rupture with avulsion of distal phalanx
IV	Distal phalanx fracture involving the articular surface
V	Epiphyseal fracture

Box 21-1

Signs of a Mallet Finger Injury

- The athlete is unable to actively extend the distal phalanx.
- Radiographs must be obtained to rule out presence of a fracture, but it is not generally necessary to acquire radiographs immediately.
- Crepitus and point tenderness in the distal phalanx are classic signs of a fracture.
- Along with the fracture, the digit may have a subungual hematoma.

dislocation is open, care is taken to prevent wound infection.[41] Initial swelling can be managed with the use of Coban wrap,* ice, elevation, and motion of the unaffected joints and digits. The athlete must be supervised and instructed to keep the DIP joint in full extension.

CLINICAL PEARL #1

Regular splint removal after a mallet finger injury is necessary to keep the area under the splint clean and dry to ensure skin integrity. It is imperative that the athlete maintains joint extension during this cleaning process.

---

*Available from 3M, St. Paul, Minnesota.

After the initial 8 weeks of continuous splinting, the athlete is advised to continue wearing the splint during athletic activities for 6 to 8 more weeks with assurance that return to play has been authorized by his or her physician.[20,29] Even with an aggressive rehabilitation program, complete reestablishment of full range of motion of the DIP joint is rare when there is a fracture through the joint. Consult Tables 21-9 and 21-10 for an expected timeline for return to sport.

JERSEY FINGER (FLEXOR DIGITORUM PROFUNDUS RUPTURE)

An athlete may sustain this injury when attempting to grasp an opponent or the opponent's jersey while he or she is breaking away. Forceful eccentric loading at the distal phalanx forces extension while the flexor digitorum profundus is active during grasp. This can cause an avulsion of the flexor digitorum profundus at the insertion of the distal phalanx.[5,21,47] The injury can occur at any finger, but most commonly involves the ring finger.[21,22]

Examination of this injury requires isolating the function of the flexor tendons.[45] The flexor digitorum profundus is isolated by blocking proximal interphalangeal (PIP) joint motion while actively flexing the DIP joint. Inability to isolate and actively flex the DIP joint should raise suspicion of flexor digitorum profundus injury.[46,53] Palpating for the retracted tendon along its path is important in identifying the level of retraction. Jersey finger is classified by Leddy and Packer[21] into three types of level of retraction (Table 21-3) with a type I injury being most severe.

Management of a jersey finger injury depends on the level of tendon retraction (available blood supply and vinculum status), time delay of the repair, athlete's participation level, point in the season, athlete's team position, future sports career plans, and philosophy of the treating physician. Common pitfalls that can occur in the management of this injury are described in Table 21-4.

Table 21-2

Splint Considerations and Treatment Pitfalls for Mallet Finger

Joint position	Conservative treatment by splinting the DIP joint in full extension[32]
Duration of splint wear	6 to 8 weeks of constant splinting, acute injury
Splinting for competition	3 additional weeks monitored by physician
Splint type	DIP dysfunction tendon injury: a variety of splints including commercially available dorsal or volar aluminum and custom-made thermoplastic stack splints (Fig. 21-1)[52]
Pitfalls of treatment	Poor compliance with treatment protocol
	Flexion occurring at any time during the immobilization phase: the 8-week immobilization period starts again from that day and may need to be longer
	Fracture malunion from poor compliance
	DIP joint splinted into hyperextension, which may cause an impairment of blood supply to the skin, resulting in a skin slough over the DIP joint[29]
	Heavy scar tissue formation
	The splint and skin must be kept dry to prevent maceration
	Infection or skin irritation due to poor splint fit.
Goals of treatment	Protect distal extensor mechanism, fracture, or joint dislocation
	Avoid deformity
	Preserve dexterity and strength
	Maintain independence with ADL tasks

Data from McCue, F.C., and Garroway, R.Y. (1985): Sport injuries to the hand and wrist. *In:* Schneider, R.C. (ed.), Sport Injuries: Mechanism, Prevention, and Treatment. Baltimore, Williams & Wilkins, pp. 743-764.
DIP, distal interphalangeal; ADL, activities of daily living.

Flexor tendon injuries should be monitored by a physician and a trained hand therapist to maximize the functional outcome. The Kleinert method of dynamic flexion should be used to assist all the digits (Fig. 21-2). Flexion assists attach to the tips of the DIP joints with hooks and adhesive. The fingertips are pulled into flexion to protect the tendon repair. For joints with excessive edema full passive flexion may not be obtained initially. These athletes should be seen more often to assure that full motion is achieved. A modified Klienert and Duran postoperative rehabilitation protocol is described in Table 21-5 for the repair of a torn flexor digitorum profundus (Fig. 21-3).[8,16] The pre- and postsurgical rehabilitation programs should include a focus on edema control with compression, elevation, and movement based upon the selected protocol (Fig. 21-4) as well as education of the athlete about long-term disabilities, precautions, and appropriate compliance with the rehabilitation protocol.

BOUTONNIÈRE INJURIES (EXTENSOR TENDON INJURY OF THE PROXIMAL INTERPHALANGEAL JOINT)

Common mechanisms of injury include a direct blow on the dorsum of the PIP joint or forced flexion of the PIP joint while the extensor mechanism is actively extending the joint (e.g., opening the hand to catch a pass and being struck on the dorsum of the hand at the same time). This deformity can occur as a result of swelling, which laterally displaces and shortens the ruptured extensor mechanism.

Anatomically, the central slip of the extensor mechanism is ruptured at the base of the middle phalanx. The extensor mechanism may glide volar to the axis of the PIP joint. The extensor mechanism will change the mechanical relationship and become flexors. This change coupled with the unopposed action of the flexor digitorum superficialis results in the boutonnière deformity.

In acute injuries, it is difficult to differentiate a PIP joint sprain from a boutonnière injury. With either injury, the athlete can have swelling, pain, and an inability to actively extend the PIP joint. A digital block performed by a physician can limit the inhibiting effect of the pain and assist in detection of a ruptured extensor mechanism.[3] The boutonnière deformity presents as a flexion deformity of the PIP joint with a hyperextension deformity of the DIP

Table 21-3

Classification of Jersey Finger Type	Amount of Retraction	Time to Repair
I	Retracted to palm	7 days
II	Retracted to PIP joint	10 days
III	Avulsion of distal phalanx	2 weeks

Data from Leddy, J.P., and Packer, J.W. (1977): Avulsion of the profundus tendon insertion in athletes. J. Hand Surg., 2:66–69.
PIP, proximal interphalangeal.

Table 21-4

Common Pitfalls in the Treatment of Jersey Finger

Human and anatomical factors	Compliance is poor.
	Adhesions of tendon in scar for finger may occur.
	Quadredgia (diminished ability to create movement due to adverse affect of the pathologic condition on common muscle belly performance) may occur.
	Intrinsic tightness will result in loss of fine motor dexterity.
	Extrinsic tightness will result in loss of gross motor dexterity.
Splinting	Awareness of flexion contractures of the PIP joint is inadequate.
Treatment	Injury is often missed due to soft tissue trauma.
	Postsurgically the athlete must have the capacity to passively flex all fingers to the palm and actively extend fingers to the dorsal block splint before leaving the first treatment session.[17]
	The athlete must be cautioned not to allow fingers or wrists to actively flex or extend outside the protected dorsal block splint.

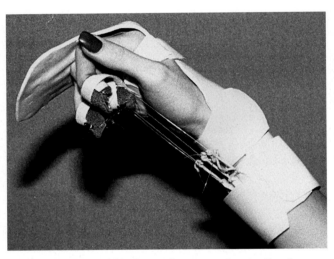

Figure 21-2. Dorsal blocking splint via a palmar pulley for flexor tendon repairs. This technique diminishes stress on flexor tendon repair.

joint. An extension lag at the PIP greater than 15° after injury due to joint or contractile tissue problems is an indication for referral to a specialist. Only those injuries that do not respond to splinting are considered for surgery. This option is rarely used because results are less predictable than with conservative management.[35] If this injury goes untreated or is treated as a PIP joint sprain by splinting the finger in slight flexion, a boutonnière deformity can occur. Other complications that may develop if this injury is not treated appropriately include volar plate tightness, oblique retinacular tightness, and adhesions of the lateral bands.

A variety of splinting techniques are used to treat this contracture. If there is a soft endfeel contracture of the PIP joint less than 35°, a prefabricated neoprene tube splint may be used. If a firm endfeel contracture is present and the athlete has active PIP joint flexion, a Joint Jack

splint or serial casting is recommended until the desired goal is obtained. If contracture is greater than 35°, a custom-made dorsal outrigger PIP joint extension splint is recommended (Fig. 21-5). All of these splints provide low-load progressive extension stretch to PIP joint volar soft tissue.[49] Splints should be provided by a qualified clinician. When full extension is achieved, the PIP joint is splinted continuously in full extension for 3 more weeks, and active range-of-motion exercises for the DIP and metacarpophalangeal (MCP) joints are then started.[46]

During the period of immobilization, the athlete is encouraged to perform active and passive range-of-motion exercises for the DIP and MCP joints to prevent joint contracture and assist in healing of the extensor mechanism.[47] Short-arc active range-of-motion exercises for the PIP joint are begun after the initial immobilization period. Splinting should continue until full pain-free motion is restored.[33]

If a loss of active extension develops, passive exercises should be discontinued and intermittent splinting restarted.[54] Strengthening exercises may commence once active extension is ensured. Consult Tables 21-9 and 21-10 for an approximate timeline for return to sport.

PROXIMAL INTERPHALANGEAL JOINT SPRAINS AND DISLOCATIONS

PIP joint sprains and dislocations are very common, so much so that they are often overlooked and undertreated. The mechanism of injury varies and is generally poorly reported by the athlete other than "I jammed my finger." Like DIP joint dislocations, many times PIP joint dislocations are reduced on the field and the player is then allowed to return to the game with buddy taping.[35] The problem with this approach is that the athlete may not have a simple dislocation but rather have a fracture or other soft tissue trauma such as a volar plate injury. If

Table 21-5

Modified Kleinert-Duran Protocol

Splint	3 Days-3 Weeks	4½ to 6 Weeks	6 Weeks	8-10 Weeks	10-12 Weeks
	Wrist placed in the dorsal block splint. Wrist placed in 20° of flexion. Metacarpal phalangeal joints placed in 60° flexion. Interphalangeal joints are placed in maximum extension. Dynamic traction via daytime palmar pulley with night resting strap	Dorsal block splint can be worn at night. A postoperative flexor tendon splint can be worn during the day. This splint provides finger pulley flex to palm all digits and allows wrist flexion and extension.	Dorsal block splint and postoperative flexor tendon splint discontinued	Protective distal interphalangeal joint splint at 30° flexion to be used with gross motor strengthening activities and athletic activities	Buddy tape for functional activities that exceed a medium physical demand level (25 lb) with one hand. Use protective distal interphalangeal joint splint when conducting competitive activities. *At 12 weeks all splints can be discontinued

Levels of Care	0	I	I and II	II	III
	3 Days-3 Weeks	4½ to 6 Weeks	6 Weeks	8-10 Weeks	10-12 Weeks
Exercise	Active extension of interphalangeal joints to the hood of the splint, 8 repetitions every hour without traction through the palmar pulley. Passive flexion of the digits, working toward full fist and isolated MCP, PIP, and DIP flexion, 10 repetitions 4-6 times a day in splint	Emphasize tendon gliding with basic four hand postures: dorsal compartment range of motion (elbow extended, pronated, full fist, actively flexed wrist)	Continue intrinsic and extrinsic compartment stretching. Passive overpressure exercise can be used in a protected posture (flexed wrist to stretch the lumbricals)	Start isometric and isotonic strengthening: Thera-Putty. Functional passive range of motion to restore intrinsic and extrinsic motion without protective posture	Continue progressive strengthening exercises. Continue stretching exercises to regain full motion

Continued

Table 21-5

Modified Kleinert-Duran Protocol—cont'd

	3 Days-3 Weeks	4½ to 6 Weeks	6 Weeks	7-10 Weeks	10-12 Weeks
		Volar compartment range of motion (elbow extended, supinated, fingers extended, actively extended wrist)		Start pushing activities (push-ups and bench press) and general conditioning tasks but avoid pulling exercises	Start sport-specific training activities including pulling exercises prep for to return to full sport participation
Precautions	No lift, carry, push, or pull done with the repaired hand	No lift, carry, push, or pull done with the repaired hand	Self-care activities at a sedentary physical level (not to exceed 5 lb)	Activity progressed to a light physical demand level (not to exceed 10 lb)	Ballistic pull tasks with force greater than 20 lb
Special considerations	Use Cobanwrap to control edema At 2 weeks postoperatively the fingers can be placed into a fist-like posture and AROM of wrist flexion and extension initiated (with therapist) Avoid the pain reflex with aggressive rehabilitation	Biofeedback training for fine motor and gross motor self-care tasks; need physician's clearance before starting AROM	Neuromotor reeducation Light resisted activities for increasing motor output of the flexor tendons	Explore correction of joint flexion deformity if present with physician's consent Scapular stabilization is key to focal movement of flexor tendons	Push tasks for conditioning can exceed pull tasks

AROM, active range of motion.

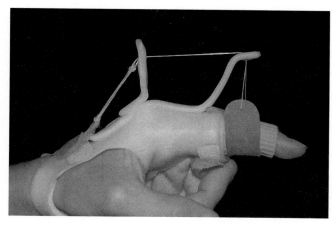

Figure 21-3. Dynamic hand-based splint option to provide low load for a long duration for proximal interphalangeal tendon and joint injuries.

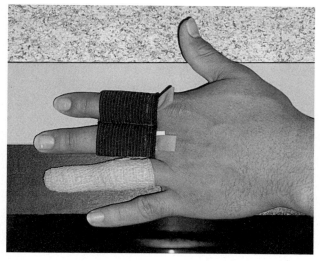

Figure 21-4. Cobanwrap for swelling on the ring finger and a double digi sleeve on the index and middle fingers. Buddy straps help initiate normal grasp and tendon gliding.

reduction of the dislocation occurs on the field, follow-up radiographs are required. Sotereanos and associates[49] advise that reduction should be delayed until a radiographic evaluation can be performed.

Examination of joint stability must be performed with the PIP joint in extension and flexion.[15] Anatomically, the collateral ligaments of the PIP joint are under the greatest tension when the joint is in full extension and maximum flexion.

There are three types of dislocations; the most common type is the dorsal dislocation. Dorsal dislocations involve dislocation of the middle phalanx dorsally, which often causes the volar plate to be torn from the insertion of the middle phalanx. A lateral dislocation damages the collateral ligaments and volar plate and a volar dislocation may cause an avulsion of the central slip of the extensor mechanism.[30] The dislocated PIP joint is typically treated with closed reduction. However, surgical intervention may be necessary, depending on the joint's stability after reduction or an inability to reduce the dislocation.

Treatment of collateral ligament sprains is successful with simple PIP joint splinting with 30° of flexion or buddy taping while the athlete continues sports participation. Continued use of the splint or taping during off-field activities for 3 weeks is critical to prevent small aggravations to the injured joint that can prolong recovery. Active exercises are begun as soon as possible and continued splinting or taping is recommended for 3 to 6 weeks during sports participation. As a result of this injury, flexor tendon adhesions commonly develop. It is important for the athlete to receive follow-up splinting so that a painful, stiff, or deformed finger does not develop 2 to 3 months later. This condition, which can develop without appropriate follow-up, has been termed "coach's finger."[32] Without this simple but appropriate care, these sprains can manifest themselves through the entire season. Splinting guidelines are listed in Box 21-2 and Tables 21-9 and 21-10 address an approximate timeline for return to sport.

Figure 21-5. Splints for boutonnière deformities. *From left to right:* custom-made proximal interphalangeal extension splint on index finger, safety pin splint, Joint Jack splint, and wire foam splint for severe flexion contractures. Care must be taken with proper fit to avoid additional injury.

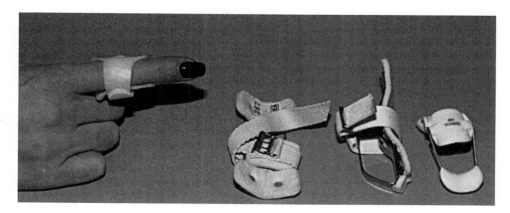

dynamic or static extension splinting may be used as in a boutonnière deformity (see Fig. 21-5). Additionally, referral to a hand therapist may be necessary.

Box 21-2

Splint Considerations for Proximal Interphalangeal Joint Sprains and Dislocations

Once reduction is performed:

- The finger is blocked with a dorsal extension gutter with the proximal interphalangeal (PIP) joint in 25° to 30° of flexion.[49]
- Edema should be controlled with 1-inch Coban wrap (Fig. 21-4).
- The athlete is instructed not to extend the PIP joint beyond the limits of the splint for 2 weeks to protect the volar plate and prevent hyperextension.
- After the protected phase, the athlete is instructed to progress to full active range-of-motion exercises.
- Strengthening exercises are initiated at 6 to 8 weeks postinjury.
- Protective splinting is continued during athletic events until complete, pain-free motion is achieved.

PSEUDOBOUTONNIÈRE DEFORMITY (VOLAR PLATE INJURY OF THE PROXIMAL INTERPHALANGEAL JOINT)

Pseudoboutonnière deformity occurs after a forceful hyperextension injury to the PIP joint involving the volar plate.[34] Its presentation is very similar to that of a boutonnière deformity, with flexion deformity of the PIP joint. The slight difference occurs in the DIP joint: a boutonnière deformity presents with the DIP joint in hyperextension, whereas a pseudoboutonnière deformity allows normal DIP joint motion.[34] If there is a flexion contracture greater than 45°, surgical intervention is usually necessary. If the athlete has flexion contractures less than 45°,

Rehabilitation includes initiation of active range-of-motion exercises during splinting to facilitate active flexion and extension. Splints should be removed to perform exercises four times per day.[30] Care must be taken to avoid injury with exercise. At 6 to 8 weeks, strengthening exercises are commenced for the PIP joint.[30] Consult Tables 21-9 and 21-10 for an approximate timeline for return to sport. Additionally, Table 21-6 provides a summary of splinting for boutonnière injuries, PIP joint sprains and dislocations, and pseudoboutonnière deformities.

METACARPAL FRACTURES

Metacarpal fractures may be the result of direct trauma, indirect compression, or rotational trauma.[13,39] Metacarpal fractures generally present with point tenderness and swelling within the hand. Careful inspection of rotation is done by having the athlete attempt to make a flat fist (a fist with MCP and PIP flexion and DIP extension) and observing whether all fingers have proper convergence. Radiographs are always necessary to confirm type, location, and angulation of the fracture.

Stabilization of a metacarpal fracture is dependent on the location, angulation, and rotation of the fracture. Stabilizing the fracture without bulky immobilization is critical to allowing the return of normal range of motion of the uninvolved joints, promoting healing, and maximizing function.[56] Thermoplastic splints have the advantage of being remolded as needed for changes. An ulnar or radial gutter cast or a custom-made thermoplastic splint can be used. Table 21-7 gives an outline of splinting guidelines for metacarpal fractures.

Table 21-6

Splinting Summary

	Boutonnière Injuries	PIP Sprains and Dislocations	Pseudoboutonnière Deformity
Splint type	Static custom finger-based splint	Custom dorsal block splint	Static progressive or dynamic splint to defeat flexor contracture
Joint position	PIP joint in extension while allowing MCP and DIP flexion	PIP joint in 15-30° of flexion	Maintain PIP joint at end range of extension
Duration of splint wear	Continuous splinting for 6 to 8 weeks, and participation in sports allowed[34]*	Dorsal block splint 3-8 weeks*	6 to 8 weeks*
Splinting for competition	Static finger- or hand-based splint at 10-12 weeks*	Static finger- or hand-based splint at 10-12 weeks*	Static finger- or hand-based splint at 10-12 weeks*

*Clearance from physician.
PIP, proximal interphalangeal.

Table 21-7	
Guidelines for Splinting Metacarpal Fractures	
Joint position	• Wrist 20 to 30° of extension • MCP joint 60 to 70° of flexion • PIP and DIP joints in full extension This position allows the MCP collateral ligaments to help stabilize the fracture and assists in preventing shortening of the fracture.[18]
Duration of splint wear	4 to 8 weeks, depending upon the severity of the fracture and the healing rate of the bone
Splinting for competition	Forearm-based custom splint in same position as described earlier
Goals of splint	Protect healing fracture by placing hand in a safe position and maintain length of supporting structures

DIP, distal interphalangeal; MCP, metacarpophalangeal; PIP, proximal interphalangeal.

CLINICAL PEARL #2

When a metacarpal fracture is splinted, caution must be taken to avoid malalignment or abnormal rotation, which can result in long-term dysfunction.

Poor stabilization and insufficient edema control and adhesion prevention may lead to complications during recovery. Edema should be managed using ice, elevation, and a compressive dressing during and after the splinting phase to facilitate motion and minimize the potential for adhesions. Rehabilitation of metacarpal fractures that are managed by closed reduction involves active range of motion of the unaffected joints during the initial immobilization of 3 to 6 weeks.[46] Passive motion may be initiated after clinical healing, at approximately 6 weeks.[46,57] Consult Tables 21-9 and 21-10 for an approximate timeline for return to sport.

BENNETT'S FRACTURE

Bennett's fracture is a small intra-articular fracture of the carpometacarpal joint of the thumb resulting from axial compression. Focal swelling at the carpometacarpal joint

of the thumb and pain with movement or palpation of the first metacarpal are clinical indications of this injury. Every athlete in whom this injury is suspected should be referred to a specialist. The small fragment fracture is generally treated with closed reduction and percutaneous pin fixation.[35] Splint considerations are presented in Table 21-8.

If the fracture is treated with rigid internal fixation, the player may return to sport earlier, with a protective forearm-based thumb spica splint.[43] Protective splinting is continued during competition until full strength and pain-free range of motion are reestablished.[35] Consult Tables 21-9 and 21-10 for an expected timeline for return to sport.

ULNAR COLLATERAL LIGAMENT INJURY OF THE THUMB

Commonly referred as "gamekeeper's thumb" or "skiers thumb," this injury is caused by forceful hyperabduction or hyperextension of the thumb or a combination of the two. The ulnar collateral ligament (UCL) injury is common in skiers who fall on a ski pole and football players and wrestlers who are attempting to grab their opponents.[17,18] Injury to the UCL proper, accessory UCL, adductor pollicis,

Table 21-8	
Splint Considerations for Bennett's Fracture	
Joint position	Thumb spica cast or splint applied and worn for 3 to 4 weeks continuously Thumb placed in mid position of abduction and extension
Duration of splint wear	4-8 weeks, depending on severity index and clinical healing
Splinting for competition	Additional 4 weeks with competition
Goals of splint	Protect healing structures at the base of the first metacarpal
Rehabilitation	At approximately 4 weeks, intra-articular pin removed and active motion of the thumb and wrist begun After 6 to 8 weeks, remaining pins removed and rehabilitation progressed to passive and resistance exercises[30] Protective splint for ADLs 4 wks; sports 8 weeks

Table 21-9

Hierarchical Plan for Functional Return: The Levels of Care[*26,41]

	Activity	Load	Pace	Goal
Level I: Restoration and balance phase (inflammatory and proliferation phase of healing)	• Rest with custom splint • ADL fine motor dexterity training (lacing, buttoning, pegboard) • Tendon glides (see Fig. 21-10) • Nerve glides (avoid increase of pain or symptoms) • Scapular and posture awareness (to increase proximal stability) • Resume cardiovascular training if no open wounds	• No load to avoid increasing the inflammatory phase of healing • Sedentary functional tasks conducted below shoulder level	• Therapist directed • Self-paced	• Athlete education on potential loss of function and need for compliance • Establish a balance of hand function to minimize potential for deformity • Maximize tendon excursion • Treat edema • Desensitize scar tissue • Maintain neuromotor control • Independence with self-care activities • Postural control
Level II: Load and correction phase (maturation phase of healing)	• Focus on strengthening in linear motion patterns of the wrist and arm below shoulder level • Thera-Putty • Isometric grip and hold • Isotonic wrist flexion and extension • Core stability of proximal stabilizers critical to establish during this rehabilitation phase • Closed kinetic chain exercises • Continue level I tasks	• Increase in physical demand level load from sedentary to light, light medium • Increase in duration of rehabilitation activity from 1 to 2 hours total	• Self-paced	• Increase motor control • Increase work capacity of injured structures in preparation for strength and conditioning program • Start measures to correct joint deformities • Eliminate compensatory movement patterns • Master postural control
Level III (return to sport phase); level considered to be the highest level of function	• Dynamic functional sport simulation tool use • Exposure to dynamic open kinetic chain strengthening tasks • Overhead weight lifting • Ulnar and radial deviation • Pronation and supination	• Increase in physical demand level load from medium to heavy	• Sport pace	• Maximize motor control • Safe return to sport

Data from Lindsay, M., and Lindsay, L., and Pitts, D.G. (1992): Levels of functional return. Personal communication, and Pitts, D.G., Hall, L.D., and Murray, P.M. (1999): Rehabilitation aspects of external fixation for distal radius fractures. Tech. Hand Upper Extremity Surg. 3:210-220.
[*]Based upon healing rates of involved tissues. The levels of care can provide clear communication on the hierarchical plan for functional return between clinicians and physicians during the rehabilitation process. This communication will help minimize the chance of overloading the recovering tissue, thereby producing a set-back, which occurs easily in hand rehabilitation. Consultation with the team physician should be considered before a change in level.
ADL, activities of daily living.

and volar plate or avulsion of the first proximal phalanx (Stener's lesion) is possible with this mechanism of injury.

A patient with a UCL injury to the thumb has pain and swelling in the web space or on the ulnar side of the MCP joint of the thumb.[36] Clinical examination of the UCL requires stressing the ligament in full extension to evaluate accessory UCL function and stressing it in flexion to evaluate proper UCL status.[2,36] Hyperextension laxity of the MCP joint would indicate volar plate involvement. Stress films are indicated for documenting abduction instability and identifying bony involvement.[38]

Surgical treatment and specialty care for these injuries are indicated for acute trauma with gross clinical instability, injuries that cannot be reduced because of bone or soft tissue obstruction, and injuries with significant articular surface fragment, bony displacement, or a rotation fracture fragment. Surgical management for chronic instability of the UCL is determined by the athlete's pain, instability of the MP joint, loss of pinch strength, and loss of ability to use a large grasp pattern.[35]

UCL sprains are generally treated with a hand-based thumb spica splint or cast with the thumb in slight adduction, approximately 40° from the palm, continuously for 3 weeks (Figs. 21-6 and 21-7). As healing progresses, active range-of-motion exercises are initiated after the immobilization period. Protective splinting is recommended for at least another 10 weeks to ensure complete healing.[28,38] Excessive stress to the UCL with early rehabilitation and every day tasks, noncompliance with splinting, and a poorly fit splint that does not control lateral motion of proximal phalanx can result in a poor outcome. Consult Tables 21-9 and 21-10 for an approximate timeline for return to sport.

SCAPHOID FRACTURE

Of all the carpal bones, the scaphoid is the most commonly fractured. Fracture usually results from falling on an outstretched hand with the wrist in extension.[7,54] Scaphoid fractures should be suspected in any athlete who has tenderness over the anatomic snuffbox, palmar side of the scaphoid, or radial side of the wrist. Pain with weight bearing, such as an inability to do push-ups with an open hand may indicate a previously missed fracture. The diagnostic radiographic series should include anteroposterior, lateral, right and left oblique, and clenched-fist views in maximal radial and ulnar deviation.[48,61] If the radiographs are normal but the athlete remains symptomatic, a bone scan should be ordered to evaluate the status of the scaphoid.[48] Nonunion of a scaphoid fracture after 6 months of conservative treatment requires surgical intervention.[48]

In a large number of scaphoid fractures, nonunion occurs or avascular necrosis develops.[15,39] Thirty percent of mid-third fractures and approximately 100% of proximal fractures develop avascular necrosis because the distal to proximal blood supply of the scaphoid is carried by a single artery arising from the dorsal branch of the radial artery. Scaphoid fractures can be broken down by anatomic distribution as follows[45]:

- 20% proximal pole
- 70% middle pole
- 10% distal pole

Continuous casting for 3 to 4 months, with radiographs and refitting of a cast every 3 to 4 weeks, is a standard treatment for scaphoid fractures as advocated by McCue.[35] The decision to use a bivalve cast for hygiene reasons depends on the compliance of the athlete and the preference of the sports medicine staff. Removing the cast for showering and wearing one cast for practice and another for activities of daily living can have a negative impact during the early healing period. Some physicians will choose a thumb spica cast or splint (Figs. 21-6 and 21-7). Compliance with treatment of all scaphoid fractures is critical because of poor healing rates. Consult Tables 21-9 and 21-10 for an approximate timeline for return to sport.

GANGLION CYSTS

Ganglion cysts generally arise from overuse of the musculotendinous and ligamentous structures around the wrist. They are most common on the radial side of the wrist, on either the volar or the dorsal surface. The ganglion cyst arises from the synovial lining of the tendon sheath or from the joint.[4] Ligamentous injuries to the wrist should be ruled out before return to sport. The athlete will complain of wrist pain with motion and wrist tenderness on palpation. Referral to a physician is needed to differentiate between a cyst and a tumor.

The conservative treatment of choice is rest with a wrist cock-up splint and activity modification along with nonsteroidal anti-inflammatory medications. Aspiration and surgical intervention are alternative treatments if conservative methods fail. Consult Tables 21-9 and 21-10 for an approximate timeline for return to sport.

TRIANGULAR FIBROCARTILAGE COMPLEX INJURY

The main function of the triangular fibrocartilage complex (TFCC) is to act as a strut, stabilizing the distal radioulnar joint during functional pronation and supination activities, and it is critical in the support of the ulnar carpus.[37,53] The TFCC supports approximately 20% of axial loading through the wrist, depending on position. The injury commonly occurs with a fall on the outstretched hand with the carpus in ulnar deviation. Therefore, this structure is commonly injured with distal radius fractures and wrist sprains. The TFCC can sustain injuries in both the medial meniscus disc area and the outer lateral disc areas.

Table 21-10

Treatment Guidelines Summary

Injury Name and Location	Key Anatomical structures	Splint Description	Splint Wear Schedule	Start Level I: AROM	Start Level I: PROM	Start Level II: Strength Program	Level III: Return to Sport
Mallet finger; fingertip	Terminal extensor mechanism	Custom stax splint with DIP joint in full extension	24 hours/day, 7 days/week for 8 weeks	8 weeks	10 weeks	10 weeks	S/P injury with physician consent
Jersey finger with FDP repair, fingertip	Rupture of FDP tendon	Dorsal block splint with wrist at 20-30° of flexion and dynamic finger flexion	24 hours/day, 7 days/week for 4.5-6 weeks	6 weeks	8-10 weeks with physician consent	8 weeks	8-10 weeks with protective splinting and physician consent
Boutonnière, deformity of PIP joint	Rupture of central slip	Finger-based splint PIP joint only in full extension disallowing movement	24 hours/day, 7 days/week for 2-4 weeks*	4 weeks	6-8 weeks only with physician consent	8-10 weeks with physician consent	S/P injury with physician consent
Pseudoboutonnière, PIP joint sprains and dislocations	Volar plate, collateral ligaments	Dorsal block splint with PIP joint in 30° of flexion	24 hours/day, 7 days/week for 4-6 weeks*	1-4 weeks	6-10 weeks	10-12 weeks	S/P injury with physician consent and protective splinting
Metacarpal fracture	Most common fourth or fifth metacarpal	Forearm based ulnar gutter splint with MCP joints in maximum flex and IPs in maximum extension	24 hours/day, 7 days/week for 4-6 weeks*	4-6 weeks	8-10 weeks	8-10 weeks	10-12 weeks
UCL sprain of the thumb	Sprain or rupture of the ulnar collateral ligament of the MCP joint of the thumb	Hand-based thumb spica splint with thumb in midabduction and extension	24 hours/day, 7 days/week for 4-6 weeks*	6-8 weeks	10-12 weeks	10-12 weeks	12 weeks

Injury	Description	Splint	Immobilization schedule	Phase A	Phase B	Phase C	Return to sport
Bennett's fracture	Fracture at the base of thumb	Hand-based thumb spica splint with thumb in mid-abduction and extension to protect web space	24 hours/day, 7 days/week for 6-8 weeks* Start rehab if cleared by physician	8-10 weeks Arom AOL therapy splint with sports	10-12 weeks Strengthen connective splinting		12 weeks Full sport if no pain and 80% strength
Scaphoid fracture	Fracture of scaphoid located just distal to the radius	Forearm-based thumb spica splint with thumb in midabduction and extension to protect web space	24 hours/day, 7 days/week for 12-16 weeks*	8-12 weeks Splint protect tender glide digits	12-16 weeks Arom wrist if healed Cleared by physician	14-16 weeks Progress strength tasks	
Ganglion cyst	Fluid-filled cyst normally appearing on the dorsal radius of wrist	Forearm-based wrist cock up splint with wrist in neutral to 10° of extension	24 hours/day, 7 days/week for 2 weeks*	0-2 weeks Arom	3-6 weeks Strength	7-10 weeks Full sports and splint	Return to sport with splint in 1 week with physician consent
Wrist sprain TFCC injury	Located at the distal ulna	Wrist gauntlet with wrist in neutral to 10° of extension	24 hours/day, 7 days/week for 8-12 weeks*	4-6 weeks Arom digits 3	8-12 weeks Arom digits	12 weeks Slow progress strength if cleared by physician	
de Quervain's tenosynovitis	Tendonitis of the first extensor compartment	Forearm-based thumb spica splint with thumb in midabduction and extension to rest the first extensor compartment	24 hours/day, 7 days/week for 4-6 weeks*	2-3 weeks Nest with splint	4-6 weeks Tendon glides Grip strength	6-8 weeks Work simulation	6-8 weeks

*Physician's approval should be obtained prior to progression by all.
DIP, distal interphalangeal; FDP, flexor digitorum profundus; IP, proximal interphalangeal; MCP, metacarpophalangeal; PIP, proximal interphalangeal; S/P, status-post; TFCC, triangular fibrocartilage complex; UCL, ulnar collateral ligament.

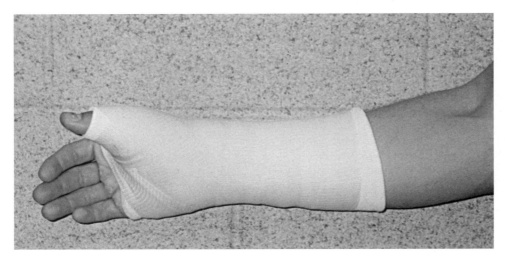

Figure 21-6. Thumb spica cast.

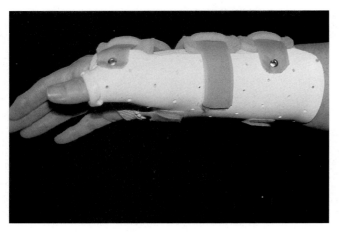

Figure 21-7. Thumb spica thermoplastic splint.

Palmer's[40] classification divides TFCC injuries into two types: type 1 traumatic injury, which results from an acute injury, and type 2 degenerative injury, which is attributed to degenerative processes such as arthritis. TFCC perforations increase with age with an estimated 7% incidence rate by age 30 and a 53% incidence rate by age 60.

These athletes will have pain and discomfort with palpation directly over the ulnar side of the wrist. They will also complain of painful catching and snapping of the wrist with tasks that require the wrist to be loaded and extended, forearm pronation and supination, wrist radial and ulnar deviation, and strengthening activities such as dips, bench press, overhead press, and dumbbell exercises because these activities have the elements of weight bearing and ulnar deviation.

Nonoperative treatment with rest to avoid painful activities should be the first treatment option.[30] The athlete should limit pronation, supination, and joint loading activities and avoid heavy lift/carry and push/pull activities. Overhead

and torquing tasks that incorporate radial/ulnar deviation and pronation/supination activities are also contraindicated.

Immobilization with a custom-fitted long-arm splint with the elbow at 90° of flexion, the forearm in a neutral position, and the wrist in 10° to 20° of extension is the treatment of choice.[31] A wrist gauntlet splint (10°-20° of wrist extension) is a second choice to support the wrist against ulnar and radial deviation for 4 to 6 weeks.

Having athletes start on pronation/supination and radial/ulnar deviation exercises too early without adequate control and wrist flexion/extension can result in a poor recovery from this injury. Improper wearing of splints is the main reason for poor functional outcomes. Consult Tables 21-9 and 21-10 for an approximate timeline for return to sport.

DE QUERVAIN'S TENOSYNOVITIS

de Quervain's tenosynovitis involves irritation of the tendons and sheath of the first dorsal extensor compartment encompassing the extensor pollicis brevis and abductor pollicis longus. It is usually caused by overuse, although it may occur from a direct blow to the first dorsal compartment. It is seen most often in players of racquet sports, gymnasts, and golfers.[24,52,55] The athlete presents with pain on the radial side of the wrist localized over the radial styloid area. A positive Finkelstein test result indicates a strong possibility of de Quervain's tenosynovitis. The test is performed by the athlete flexing the thumb into the palm and making a full fist; the wrist is then forcefully and passively deviated in an ulnar direction. The test is positive if the athlete feels excruciating pain over the radial styloid area.[10] Additionally, muscular tightness of the flexor pollicis longus and tenderness to palpation of the carpalmetacarpial joint should be assessed.

Conservative treatment consists of therapeutic modalities to decrease pain and inflammation and splinting with a forearm-based thumb spica to rest the area. The wrist is placed in approximately 15° of extension and the thumb in 40° of abduction and 10° flexion with the interphalangeal (IP) joint free, for up to 6 weeks[46] (see Fig. 21-7). Nonsteroidal anti-inflammatory medications may be prescribed, and steroid injections may also be considered.[48] If symptoms persist, surgery may be necessary to release the tendon sheath.[39] Flexor pollicis longus tightness, inappropriate work/rest cycles, and initiation of level II strengthening and level III torquing program before full active range of motion is mastered can have a detrimental impact on recovery. Consult Tables 21-9 and 21-10 for an approximate timeline for return to sport.

REHABILITATIVE EXERCISES

Level I (Inflammatory and Proliferation Phase of Healing)

ACTIVE MOTION EXERCISES FOR THE DIGITS AND UPPER EXTREMITY

Individual active range-of-motion exercises for the fingers are described below and can be used for all injuries when they are cleared for active range-of-motion exercises. These exercises establish a balance by maximizing excursion of tendons and eliminating muscle imbalance of the intrinsic and extrinsic muscle systems. If these exercises are performed while compensatory movements are eliminated, adhesion formation will be minimized. Each exercise is performed within the pain tolerance of the injured athlete. Sets and repetitions depend on the clinician's preference; generally 1 to 2 sets of 10 to 15 repetitions 4 to 6 times per day are used with these active exercises. Additionally, the injured athlete is educated in all appropriate exercises and has demonstrated proper exercise technique. The athlete is encouraged to take responsibility for performing the exercises several times a day independently.

Compensatory movement patterns are common with hand and wrist injuries. These learned abnormal movement patterns occur because of joint stiffness, tendon adhesions, pain, edema, or focal weakness. These patterns include scapular destabilization with protraction, elevation, and internal rotation. Compensatory hand patterns include thumb adduction and wrist flexion with grasp. These abnormal movement patterns are best addressed with rote functional tasks. These tasks defeat the pain reflex and restore natural motor patterns of the hand and upper extremities.

INTRINSIC HAND EXERCISES
Dorsal and Palmar Interossei Muscle Exercises

Interossei stretch. To stretch the interossei muscles the MCP joint is placed in slight hyperextension and the athlete's PIP joint only is slowly and passively moved into flexion. This stretch will improve flexibility around the MCP and PIP joints and help restore the natural grasp. Care should be taken not to overstretch the extensor hood with aggressive passive flexion exercises (Fig. 21-8).

Finger Abduction and Adduction. The athlete spreads the fingers apart and then places them together. This will facilitate a decrease in edema and working the interossei musculature of the hand.

Continued

REHABILITATIVE EXERCISES — cont'd

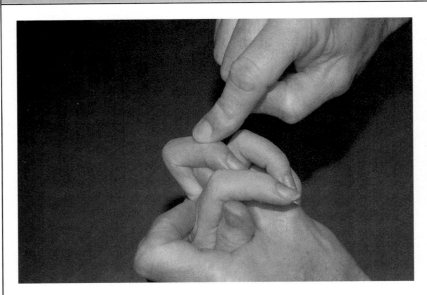

Figure 21-8. To stretch the interosseous muscles the metacarpophalangeal (MCP) joint is put into slight hyperextension and the athlete's proximal interphalangeal (PIP) joint only receives slow passive range of motion into flexion. This stretch will improve flexibility around the MCP and PIP joints and help restore the natural grasp.

Lumbrical Exercises

The athlete flexes the MCP joint to 90°, then alternately flexes and extends the IP joints into full flexion and full extension to facilitate the interossei and lumbricals (Fig. 21-9).[9] To stretch the lumbrical the MCP is positioned in slight hyperextension, and the athlete is asked to flex the DIP and PIP joints. This stretch will improve flexor digitorum profundus (FDP) function and help restore the natural grasp reflex. This exercise is recommended for all PIP joint injuries and any injuries that result in lack of PIP joint flexion.

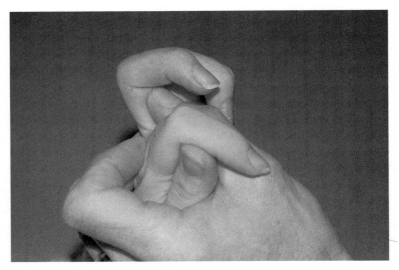

Figure 21-9. To stretch the lumbrical the metacarpophalangeal joint is put into slight hyperextension, and the athlete is asked to flex the distal interphalangeal and proximal interphalangeal joints. This stretch will improve flexor digitorum profundus function and help restore the natural grasp pattern. Level I.

Opposition

The athlete touches every fingertip with the thumb starting with the index finger and progressing by sliding the thumb down to the small finger into the palm of the hand to facilitate full flexion of the thumb.

EXTRINSIC HAND EXERCISES
Tendon Gliding Exercises or Staged Fisting

This exercise involves making various types of fists with the digits in a progression starting with full extension, followed by a tabletop (intrinsic-plus) position, a flat fist, a full fist without thumb, and finally a hook (intrinsic-minus) position (Fig. 21-10). These exercises are designed to facilitate the gliding of the flexor digitorum superficialis (FDS) and FDP tendons through zone II and to restore a balance between the intrinsic and extrinsic muscles.

Isolated Tendon Excursions or Joint-Blocking Exercises

These exercises are designed to isolate the FDS, FDP, and flexor pollicis longus (FPL) tendons to increase active range of motion of a specific joint (Fig. 21-11). The athlete holds the MCP joints of all fingers in extension. To

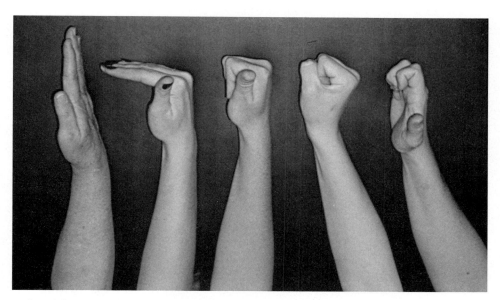

Figure 21-10. Tendon gliding exercises. *From left to right:* beginning position in full extension; a tabletop position (intrinsic-plus position); flat fist (flexor digitorum superficialis); full fist (flexor digitorum profundus); and a hook position (intrinsic-minus position to detect tightness of lumbricals). Level I.

Figure 21-11. Joint blocking for distal interphalangeal joint flexion of the index finger. This is focal tendon glide for flexor digitorum profundus. Level I.

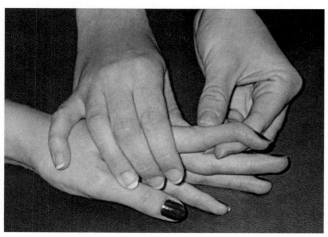

Continued

REHABILITATIVE EXERCISES — cont'd

isolate FDP tendon excursion, the athlete holds the finger below the DIP joint crease, then flexes and extends the DIP joint (see Fig. 21-11). To isolate the FDS, the athlete places the fingers beside the tested finger and then flexes and extends the PIP joint (Fig. 21-12). To isolate the FPL, the athlete holds the finger below the crease of the thumb IP joint, then flexes and extends the IP joint. It is critical that joints are properly stabilized during these exercises to prevent substitution.

EXTRINSIC FOREARM MUSCLE STRETCH

Extrinsic extensor stretch is conducted with the elbow extended, forearm pronated, a full fist, and wrist flexion stretching in conjunction with passive overpressure from the opposite hand This exercise stretches the extrinsic extensor muscles and improves grip strength and endurance (Fig. 21-13). Extrinsic flexor stretch is conducted with elbow in extension, forearm supinated, wrist in extension, and digits fully extended. This exercise will stretch the extrinsic flexor muscles and improve grip strength and endurance (Fig. 21-14).

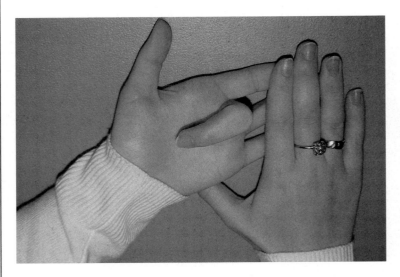

Figure 21-12. Isolation muscle test for flexor digitorum superficialis of the ring finger. This exercise helps avoid tendon adhesions and improves dexterity.

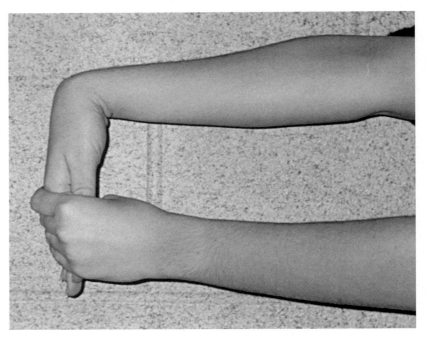

Figure 21-13. Passive wrist flexion to stretch the wrist extensors. This will improve motor control and endurance and minimize pain. Level I. (Stay below the pain reflex.)

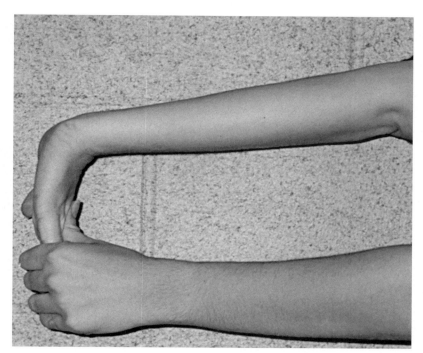

Figure 21-14. Passive wrist extension to stretch the wrist flexors. This will improve motor control and endurance and minimize pain. Level I.

PASSIVE MOTION EXERCISES FOR THE DIGITS

The goal of rehabilitation for digits is to obtain full flexion without losing extension. Pushing the joint beyond the pain threshold should be avoided, because this can cause an inflammatory reaction and slow progression. *Do not feed a pain reflex!* Passive range-of-motion exercises should be gentle and not be performed if extension of the digit is being compromised. Passive exercises are often combined with the active exercises described earlier and are performed with gentle overpressure by either the athlete or treating clinician. Hold a stretch for 5 to 10 seconds and repeat this 5 to 10 times as needed. Passive range-of-motion exercises are generally initiated after 2 weeks of active range-of-motion activities.

Treatment for Edema and Scar

Edema is a scar in evolution. Treat all hand injuries for edema and scar formation. There are several techniques that can be used to accomplish this. Overhead fisting should be performed at 5 to 10 repetitions per hour, which opens the lymphatic chain and allows edema to be pumped out of the hand. Overhead fisting also incorporates elevation and mobility to diminish the edema. The injured hand should be elevated above the heart level at all times, which allows gravity to have a positive impact on edema. Compression is obtained with a Coban wrap and edema glove to decrease edema in the digits and hand (see Fig. 21-4).

The use of thin silicone sheets or elastomere over a nonopen incision site for several hours a day will assist in scar management. Soft tissue massage is commonly prescribed to loosen a stiff joint or facilitate scar mobility. Mini-vibrators are also often used in the maturation phase to enhance this technique.

Level II (Maturation Phase of Healing)

STRENGTHENING EXERCISES

Rehabilitation should focus on a gradual ramping of load while maintaining focal excursion of affected structures. Care must be taken not to regress to the inflammatory stage. The athlete must be made aware of compensatory movement patterns and avoid them to have a complete and speedy recovery. Rehabilitation exercises should be conducted below shoulder level. Wrist and forearm strengthening should be conducted with linear motion planes. Core stability exercises are initiated to establish proximal strength and avoid compensation.

Continued

R E H A B I L I T A T I V E   E X E R C I S E S — c o n t ' d

All active range-of-motion exercises described earlier can be used for strengthening exercises with the use of manual resistance or light resistive elastic bands. Gripping exercises for strengthening the flexor tendons are common. Various devices can be used, including putty, soft rubber balls, wet washcloths, and resistive gripping devices.

CLINICAL PEARL #3

During the early stage of strengthening exercises the key is to ensure full excursion with no pain.

Soft Thera-Putty is ideal for early rehabilitation because it provides light biofeedback and allows full tendon excursion. Start with light resistance 3 to 5 minutes per day. Isometric grip and hold tasks help restore a natural grasp reflex with a controlled exposure to work without exposure to repetition. Start with a 30-second hold and 1-minute rest for 10 repetitions per day (Fig. 21-15). Wrist flexion and extension with resistance is a great way to restore a natural grasp. Start with 2 sets of 10 repetitions 3 times per day. (Figs. 21-16 and 21-17). Postural stability exercises are an effective way to enhance upper extremity function, which includes closed kinetic chain scapular stabilization exercises (Fig. 21-18). Progression should be guided by pain, maintenance of active excursion, and healing restraints of the particular injury.

Level III (Return to Sport Phase)

DYNAMIC STRENGTHENING EXERCISES FOR THE WRIST AND FOREARM

These exercises are considered the highest level of functional return. This group of exercises facilitates synergetic muscle recruitment to maximize motor control and coordination for return to sport. Exposure to forearm and wrist torquing exercises, overhead weight bearing tasks and kinetic chain exercises both open and closed are corner stones to this phase of rehabilitation. These types of exercises should only be attempted after the athlete masters level I and II tasks.

- Fast grips exercise is started with a 10-pound gripper with a set of 100 repetitions or fatigue (which ever occurs first) 1 per second followed by a 1-minute rest. This exercise will improve grip strength and endurance.
- Resistive radial deviation, ulnar deviation, supination, and pronation are considered to be high-level movement patterns and strengthening techniques (Figs. 21-19, 21-20, 21-21, and 21-22).

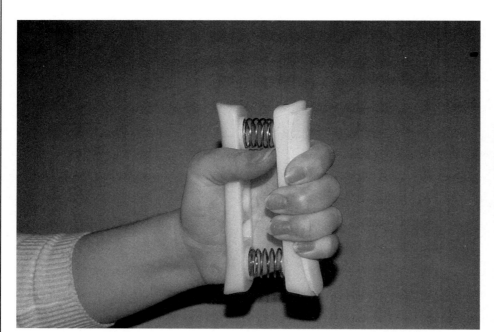

Figure 21-15. Grip and hold exercise. This exercise is used to improve grasp endurance and strength. Start slow at 10 pounds of resistance, holding 1 minute on and 1 minute off. Level II.

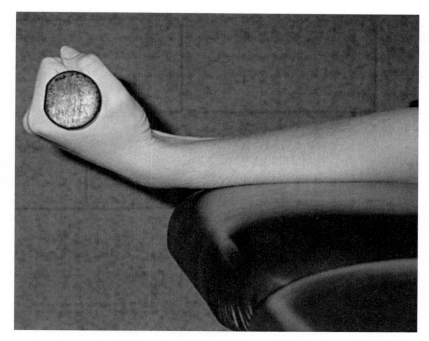

Figure 21-16. Resistive wrist flexion to strengthen the wrist flexors. This exercise will help improve grip strength and endurance. Level II.

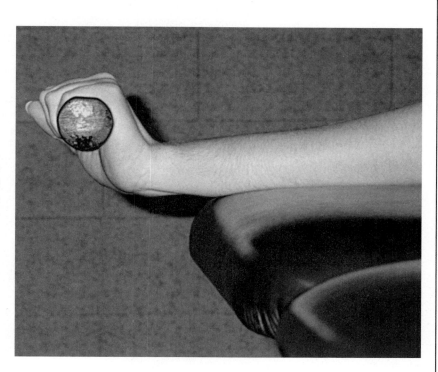

Figure 21-17. Resistive wrist extension to strengthen the wrist extensors. This exercise will help improve grip strength and endurance. Level II.

- Open kinetic chain tasks include but are not limited to weight lifting and Thera-Band° tasks.
- Closed kinetic chain tasks include but are not limited to stress loading and push-ups.

NOTE: All of these exercises are recommended for all wrist and hand injuries with physician consent.

°Available from The Hygenic Corporation, Akron, Ohio.

Continued

REHABILITATIVE EXERCISES — cont'd

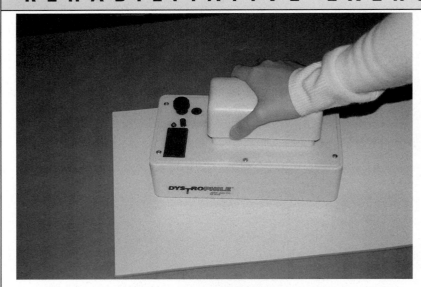

Figure 21-18. Stress loading exercise with the Dystrophile to enhance scapular stabilization with closed kinetic chain strengthening. Level II.

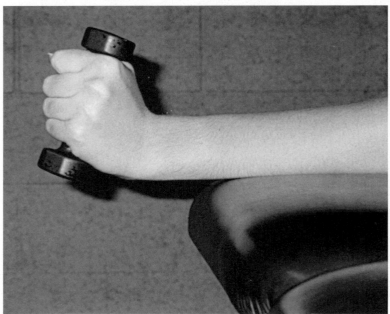

Figure 21-19. Resistive radial deviation. This movement is considered to be a high-level movement pattern and strengthening technique. Incorporate this exercise after successful completion of level II tasks. Level III.

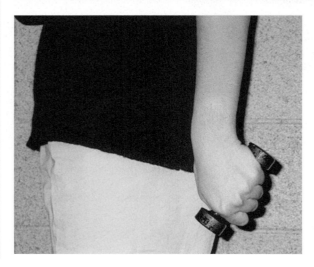

Figure 21-20. Resistive ulnar deviation. This movement is considered to be a high-level movement pattern and strengthening technique. Incorporate this exercise after successful completion of level II tasks. Level III.

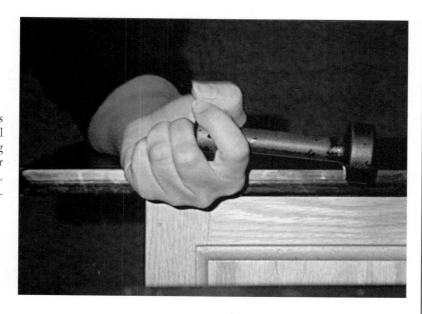

Figure 21-21. Resistive supination. This movement is considered to be a high-level movement pattern and strengthening technique. Incorporate this exercise after successful completion of level II tasks. Level III.

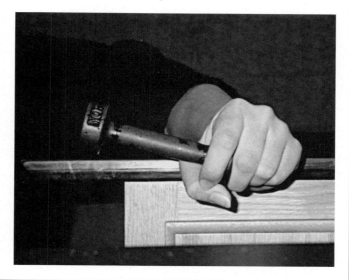

Figure 21-22. Resistive pronation. This movement is considered to be a high-level movement pattern and strengthening technique. Incorporate this exercise after successful completion of level II tasks. Level III.

SUMMARY

Hand injuries in the athlete pose many challenges to the health care profession. Pressure for early return to play and a good long term functional outcome can be difficult to accomplish. Advancement in surgical techniques of the hand increases the responsibility for early recognition of injuries and a clear understanding of rehabilitation goals. The following points of summary have proven to provide safe, reliable, and excellent functional outcomes.

- ■ "Do No Harm"— The hand is a complex system designed to produce power and dexterity. If mismanaged, dysfunction and poor outcome will occur.
- ■ Advanced upper extremity evaluation skills will enhance quality of care. These skills include; surface anatomy, postural analysis, joint function, nerve function, and the ability to determine between contractile and non-contractile tissue dysfunction.

- ■ "Don't feed a pain reflex"— Excessive passive range of motion can increase muscle guarding and decrease function.
- ■ Progress treatment based upon the stages of wound healing.
- ■ Seek to restore a balance of function.
  - ■ Treat the pitfalls prior to the development of these problems:
    - ■ Adhesions
    - ■ Intrinsic and extrinsic tightness
    - ■ Joint stiffness
    - ■ Pain reflex
- ■ "Edema is scar in evolution"— Use assertive edema management to prevent tendon adhesions, joint stiffness and painful scars. These techniques include:
  - ■ Elevation
  - ■ Compression

- ▦ Rest
- ▦ Movement
- ▦ Pressure on scar
- ▦ Use the hierarchy of hand rehabilitation to guide your treatment. This approach will help prevent pitfalls and restore function.
- ▦ Progress post surgical cases only with prior communication and consent of the physician.

Hand rehabilitation of the athlete can be rewarding and exciting. It requires hard work to meet the challenge of a growing area of practice.

REFERENCES

1. Abouna, J.M., and Brown, H. (1968): The treatment of mallet finger. The results in a series of 148 consecutive cases and a review of the literature. Br. J. Surg., 55:653-667.
2. Adams, B.D., and Muller, D.L. (1996): Assessment of thumb positioning in the treatment of ulnar collateral ligament injuries. A laboratory study. Am. J. Sports Med., 24:672-675.
3. Burton, R.I., and Eaton, R.G. (1973): Common hand injuries in the athlete. Orthop. Clin. North Am., 4:809-838.
4. Bush, D.C. (1995): Soft-tissue tumors of the hand. In: Hunter, J.M., Macken, E.J., and Callhan, A.B. (eds.), Rehabilitation of the Hand: Surgery and Therapy. St. Louis, Mosby-Year Book, pp. 1017-1033.
5. Carroll, R.E., and Match, R.M. (1970): Avulsion of the profundus tendon insertion. J. Trauma, 10:1109.
6. Colditz, J.C. (1995): Functional fracture bracing. In: Hunter, J.M., Macken, E.J., and Callhan, A.B. (eds.), Rehabilitation of the Hand: Surgery and Therapy. St. Louis, Mosby-Year Book, pp. 395-406.
7. Cooney, W.P., Linscheid, R.L., and Dobyns, J.H. (1996): Fracture and dislocation of the wrist. In: Rockwood, C.A., Green, D.P., and Bucholz, R.W. (eds.), Fracture in Adults. Philadelphia, Lippincott-Raven, pp. 745-867.
8. Duran, R., and Houser, R. (1975): Controlled passive motion following flexor tendon repair in zone 2 and 3. In: AAOS Symposium on Tendon Surgery in the Hand. St. Louis, C.V. Mosby.
9. Evans, R.B. (1995): An update on extensor tendon management. In: Hunter, J.M., Macken, E.J., and Callhan, A.B. (eds.), Rehabilitation of the Hand: Surgery and Therapy. St. Louis, Mosby-Year Book, pp. 565-606.
10. Finkelstein, H. (1930): Stenosing tendovaginitis at the radial styloid process. J. Bone Joint Surg., 12:509-540.
11. Foreman, S, and Gieck, J.H. (1992): Rehabilitative management of injuries to the hand. Clin. Sports Med., 11:239-252.
12. Gelberman, R.H., Panagis, J.S., Taleisnk, J., and Baumgaertner, M. (1983): The arterial anatomy of the human carpus. Part I. The extraosseous vascularity. J. Hand Surg., 8:367-375.
13. Hastings, H. (1992): Management of extraarticular fractures of the phalanges and metacarpals. In: Strickland, J.W., and Rettig, A.C. (eds.), Hand Injuries in Athletes. Philadelphia, W.B. Saunders, pp. 129-153.
14. Jahss, S.A. (1938): Fractures of the metacarpals: A new method of reduction and immobilization. J. Bone Joint Surg., 20:178-186.

15. Kapandji, I.A. (1982): The Physiology of Joints, Vol. I, Upper Limb. New York, Churchill Livingstone, pp. 1860-1891.
16. Kleinert, H.E., Kutz, J.E., and Cohen, M.J. (1975): Primary repair of zone 2 flexor tendon lacerations. In: AAOS Symposium on Tendon Surgery in the Hand. St. Louis, C.V. Mosby.
17. Kulund, D.N. (1982): The Injured Athlete. Philadelphia, J.B. Lippincott, pp. 295-329.
18. Lane, L.B. (1995): Acute ulnar collateral ligament rupture of the metacarpophalangeal joint of the thumb. In: Torg, J.S., and Shepard, R.J. (eds.), Current Therapy in Sports Medicine. St. Louis, C.V. Mosby, pp. 151-161.
19. Leadbeter, W.B., Buckwalter, J.A., and Gordon, S.L. (1990): Sport-Induced Inflammation: Clinical and Basic Science Concepts. Park Ridge, IL, American Academy of Orthopaedic Surgeons.
20. Leddy, J.F., and Dennis, T.R. (1992): Tendon injuries. In: Stricklan, J.W., and Rettig, A.C. (eds.), Hand Injuries in Athletes. Philadelphia, W.B. Saunders, pp. 175-207.
21. Leddy, J.P., and Packer, J.W. (1977): Avulsion of the profundus tendon insertion in athletes. J. Hand Surg., 2:66-69.
22. Lester, B. (1999): Sport Injuries. The Acute Hand. Stamford, CT, Appleton & Lange, pp. 361-390.
23. Lindsay, M., Lindsay, L., and Pitts, D.G. (1992): Levels of functional return. Personal communication.
24. Manske, P.R., and Lesker, P.A. (1978): Avulsion of the ring finger digitorum profundus tendon: An experimental study. Hand, 10:52-55.
25. Mayer, V.A., and McCue, F.C. (1995): Rehabilitation and protection of the hand and wrist. In: Nicholas, J.A., and Hershman, E.B. (eds.), The Upper Extremity in Sports Medicine, 2nd ed. St. Louis, Mosby-Year Book, pp. 591-634.
26. McCue, F.C. (1982): The elbow, wrist, and hand. In: Kulund, D.N. (ed.), The Injured Athlete. Philadelphia, J.B. Lippincott, pp. 295-329.
27. McCue, F.C., Andrew, J.R., and Hakala, M. (1974): The coach's finger. Am. J. Sports Med., 2:270-275.
28. McCue, F.C., and Bruce, J.F. (1994): Hand and wrist. In: DeLee, J.C., and Drez, D., Jr. (eds.), Orthopaedic Sports Medicine Principles and Practice, Vol. I. Philadelphia, W.B. Saunders, pp. 913-944.
29. McCue, F.C., and Cabrera, J.N. (1992): Common athletic digital joint injuries of the hand. In: Strickland, J.W., and Rettig, A.C. (eds.), Hand Injuries in Athletes. Philadelphia, W.B. Saunders, pp. 49-94.
30. McCue, F.C., and Garroway, R.Y. (1985): Sport injuries to the hand and wrist. In: Schneider, R.C. (ed.), Sport Injuries: Mechanism, Prevention, and Treatment. Baltimore, Williams & Wilkins, pp. 743-764.
31. McCue, F.C., Hakala, M.H., Andrews, J.R., and Gieck, J.H. (1974): Ulnar collateral ligament injuries of the thumb in athletes. J. Sports Med., 2:70-80.
32. McCue, F.C., Honner, R., and Gieck, J.H., et al. (1975): A pseudo-boutonniere deformity. Hand, 7:166-170.
33. McCue, F.C., Hussamy, O.D., and Gieck, J.H. (1996): Hand and wrist injuries. In: Zachazewski, J.E., Magee, D.J., and Quillen, W.S. (eds.), Athletic Injuries and Rehabilitation, Philadelphia, W.B. Saunders, pp. 585-597.
34. McCue, F.C., and Redler, M.R. (1990): Coach's finger. In: Torg, J.S., Welsh, P.R., and Shepard, R.J. (eds.), Current Therapy in Sports Medicine. Toronto, B.C. Decker, pp. 438-443.

35. McCue, F.C., and Wooten, S.L. (1986): Closed tendon injuries of the hand in athletics. Clin. Sports Med., 5:741-755.

36. Melone, C.P. (1990): Fracture of the wrist. *In:* Nicholas, J.A., and Hershman, E.B. (eds.), The Upper Extremity in Sports Medicine. St. Louis, C.V. Mosby, pp. 419-456.

37. Palmer, A.K. (1987): The distal radial ulnar joint. Anatomy, biomechanics, and triangular fibrocartilage complex abnormalities. Hand Clin., 3:31-40.

38. Pitts, D.G., Hall, L.D., and Murray, P.M. (1999): Rehabilitation aspects of external fixation for distal radius fractures. Tech. Hand Upper Extremity Surg. 3:210-220.

39. Posner, M.A. (1990): Hand injuries. *In:* Nicholas, J.A., and Hershman, E.B. (eds.), The Upper Extremity in Sports Medicine. St. Louis, C.V. Mosby, pp. 495-594.

40. Redler, M. (1989): Phalangeal and metacarpal fractures. Sport Injury Manage., 2:53-58, 1989.

41. Redler, M. (1989): Dislocation of the interphalangeal joints and metacarpophalangeal joints. Sport Injury Manage., 2: 59-66.

42. Rettig, AC. (1992): Closed tendon injuries of the hand and wrist in the athlete. Clin. Sports Med., 11:77-99.

43. Rettig, A.C., and Rowdon, G.A. (1995): Metacarpal fractures. *In:* Torg, J.S., and Shepard, R.J. (eds.), Current Therapy in Sports Medicine. St. Louis, C.V. Mosby, pp. 152-156.

44. Rosenthal, E.A. (1995): The extensor tendons: Anatomy and management. *In:* Hunter, J.M., Macken, E.J., and Callhan, A.B. (eds.), Rehabilitation of the Hand: Surgery and Therapy. St. Louis, Mosby-Year Book, pp. 519-564.

45. Russe, O. (1960): Fracture of the carpal navicular: Diagnosis, non-operative and operative treatment. J. Bone Joint Surg. Am., 42:759-768.

46. Sadler, J.A., and Koepfer, J.M. (1992): Rehabilitation and the splinting of the injured hand. *In:* Strickland, J.W., and Rettig, A.C. (eds.), Hand Injuries in Athletes. Philadelphia, W.B. Saunders, pp. 235-276.

47. Schneider, L.H. (1990): Tendon injuries of the hand. *In:* Nicholas, J.A., and Hershman, E.B. (eds.), The Upper Extremity in Sports Medicine. St. Louis, C.V. Mosby, pp. 595-618.

48. Shaw Wilgis, E.F., and Yates, A.Y. (1990): Wrist pain. *In:* Nicholas, J.A., and Hershman, E.B. (eds.), The Upper Extremity in Sports Medicine. St. Louis, C.V. Mosby, pp. 483-494.

49. Sotereanos, D.G., Levy, J.A., and Herndon, J.H. (1994): Hand and wrist injuries. *In:* Fu, F.H., and Stone, D.A. (eds.), Sport Injuries: Mechanisms, Prevention, Treatment. Baltimore, Williams & Wilkins, pp. 937-947.

50. Tubiana, R., Thomine, J.M., and Mackin, E. (1996): Functional anatomy. *In:* Examination of the Hand and Wrist. St. Louis, Mosby-Year Book, p. 12.

51. Weber, E.R., and Chao, E.Y. (1978): An experimental approach to the mechanism of scaphoid wrist fractures. J. Hand Surg., 3:142-148.

52. Weiker, G.G. (1992): Hand and wrist problems in the gymnast. *In:* Culzer, J.E. (ed.), Clinical Sports Medicine: Injuries of the Hand and Wrist. Philadelphia, W.B. Saunders, pp. 189-202.

53. Werner, F.M., Glisson, R.R., Murphy, D.J., and Palmer, A.K. (1986): Force transmission through the distal radioulnar carpal joint: Effect of ulnar lengthening and shortening. Handchir. Mikrochir. Plast. Chir. 18:304-308.

54. Wilson, R.L., and Hazen, J. (1995): Management of joint injuries and intraarticular fractures of the hand. *In:* Hunter, J.M., Macken, E.J., and Callhan, A.B. (eds.), Rehabilitation of the Hand: Surgery and Therapy. St. Louis, Mosby-Year Book, pp. 377-394.

55. Wright, H.H., and Rettig, A.C. (1995): Management of common sports injuries. *In:* Hunter, J.M., Macken, E.J., and Callhan, A.B. (eds.), Rehabilitation of the Hand: Surgery and Therapy. St. Louis, Mosby-Year Book, pp. 1809-1838.

56. Wright, S.C. (1990): Fracture and dislocation in the hand and wrist. *In:* Torg, J.S., Welsh, P.R., and Shepard, R.J. (eds.), Current Therapy in Sports Medicine. Toronto, B.C. Decker, pp. 443-446.

57. Wright, T.A. (1968): Early mobilization in fractures of the metacarpals and phalanges. Can. J. Surg., 11:491-498.

58. Zemmel, N.P., and Stark, H.H. (1986): Fractures and dislocations of the carpal bones. Clin. Sports Med., 5:709-724.

THROWERS' TEN EXERCISE PROGRAM

Kevin E. Wilk, P.T.

The Throwers' Ten Exercise Program* is designed to exercise the major muscles necessary for throwing. The goal of the program is to be an organized and concise exercise program. In addition, all exercises included are specific to the thrower and are designed to improve strength, power, and endurance of the musculature of the shoulder complex.

Diagonal Pattern (D2) Extension. The athlete grips the tubing handle overhead and out to the side with the involved hand. The athlete pulls the tubing down and across the body to the opposite side of the leg (Fig. A-1A). During the motion, the athlete leads with the thumb.

Diagonal Pattern (D2) Flexion. The athlete grips the tubing handle in the hand of the involved arm and brings the arm out 45° from the side, palm facing backward. After turning the palm forward, the athlete proceeds to flex the elbow and bring the arm up and over the uninvolved shoulder (Fig. A-1B). The palm is turned down and reversed to take the arm to the starting position. The exercise should be performed in a controlled manner.

External Rotation at 0° of Abduction. The athlete stands with the involved elbow fixed at the side, elbow at 90°, and the involved arm across the front of the body. The athlete grips the tubing handle (the other end of the tubing is fixed) and pulls out with the arm, keeping the elbow at the side (Fig. A-2A), and returns the tubing slowly and in a controlled manner.

Internal Rotation at 0° of Abduction. The athlete stands with the elbow at the side, fixed at 90°, with the shoulder rotated out. The athlete grips the tubing handle (the other end of the tubing is fixed) and pulls the arm across the body, keeping the elbow at the side (Fig. A-2B), and returns the tubing slowly and in a controlled manner.

External Rotation at 90° of Abduction. The athlete stands with the shoulder abducted to 90° and elbow flexed

to 90°. The athlete grips the tubing handle (the other end is fixed straight ahead, slightly lower than the shoulder). Keeping the shoulder abducted, the athlete rotates the shoulder back, keeping the elbow at 90° (Fig. A-2C). Slow- and fast-speed sets should be performed with the tubing. The clinician will need to change the tubing resistance as appropriate.

Internal Rotation at 90° of Abduction. The athlete stands with the shoulder abducted to 90°, externally rotated to 90°, and the elbow bent to 90°. Keeping the shoulder abducted, the athlete rotates the shoulder forward, keeping the elbow bent at 90° (Fig. A-2D), and then returns the tubing and hand to the starting position. Slow- and fast-speed sets should be performed with the tubing.

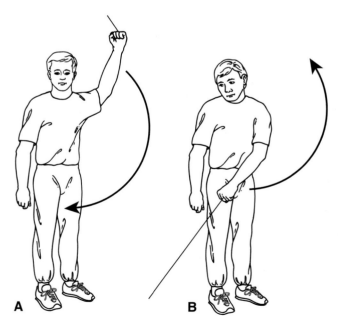

Figure A-1. Diagonal patterns. *A,* Extension. *B,* Flexion. (Redrawn from Wilk, K.E., Andrews, J.R., Arrigo, C.A., et al. [2001]: *Preventive and Rehabilitative Exercises for the Shoulder and Elbow,* 6th ed. Birmingham, AL, American Sports Medicine Institute.)

---

*Modified from Wilk, K.E., Andrews, J.R., Arrigo, C.A., et al. (2001): *Preventive and Rehabilitative Exercises for the Shoulder and Elbow,* 5th ed. Birmingham, AL, American Sports Medicine Institute.

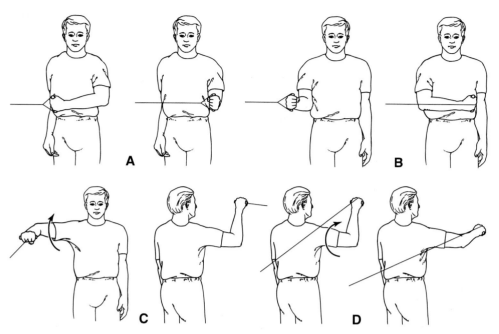

Figure A-2. *A,* External rotation at 0° abduction. *B,* Internal rotation at 0° abduction. *C,* External rotation at 90° abduction. *D,* Internal rotation at 90° abduction. (Redrawn from Wilk, K.E., Andrews, J.R., Arrigo, C.A., et al. [2001]: Preventive and Rehabilitative Exercises for the Shoulder and Elbow, 6th ed. Birmingham, AL, American Sports Medicine Institute.)

The clinician will need to change the tubing resistance as appropriate.

Shoulder Abduction to 90°. The athlete stands with the arm at the side, the elbow straight, and the palm against the side and raises the arm to the side, palm down, until the arm reaches 90° (shoulder level) (Fig. A-3). The athlete holds the position for 2 seconds and lowers the arm slowly.

Scaption, Internal Rotation. The athlete stands with the elbow straight and thumb down and raises the arm to shoulder level at a 30° angle in front of body (Fig. A-4), not going above shoulder height. The athlete holds the position for 2 seconds and lowers the arm slowly.

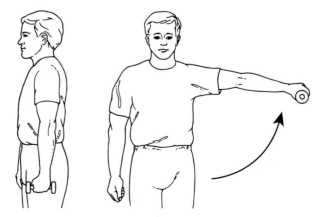

Figure A-3. Shoulder abduction to 90°. (Redrawn from Wilk, K.E., Andrews, J.R., Arrigo, C.A., et al. [2001]: Preventive and Rehabilitative Exercises for the Shoulder and Elbow, 6th ed. Birmingham, AL, American Sports Medicine Institute.)

Prone Horizontal Abduction (Neutral). The athlete lies on the table, face down, with the involved arm hanging straight to the floor and the palm facing down. The arm is raised out to the side, parallel to the floor (Fig. A-5*A*). The athlete holds the position for 2 seconds and lowers the arm slowly.

Prone Horizontal Abduction (Full External Rotation, 100° of Abduction). The athlete lies on the table, face down, with the involved arm hanging straight to the floor and the thumb rotated up (hitchhiker position). The arm is raised out to the side with the arm slightly in front of the shoulder, parallel to the floor (Fig. A-5*B*). The athlete holds the position for 2 seconds and lowers the arm slowly.

Press-ups. The athlete, seated on a chair or on a table, places both hands firmly on the sides of the chair or table, palm down and fingers pointed outward. The hands should be on a straight line with the shoulders. The athlete slowly pushes downward through the hands to elevate the body (Fig. A-6). The athlete holds the elevated position for 2 seconds and lowers the body.

Prone Rowing. The athlete lies on the stomach with the involved arm hanging over the side of the table, a dumbbell in the hand, and the elbow straight. The athlete slowly raises the arm, bending the elbow and bringing the dumbbell as high as possible (Fig. A-7). The athlete holds the position for 2 seconds and lowers the arm slowly.

Push-ups. The athlete starts in the down position with the arms in a comfortable position. The hands should be placed no more than shoulder-width apart. The athlete pushes up as high as possible, rolling the shoulders forward after the elbows are straight (Fig. A-8). The athlete can start with a push-up into the wall and can gradually progress to a table and eventually to the floor, as tolerated.

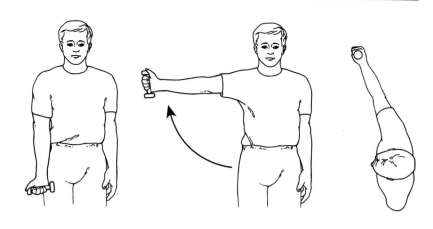

Figure A-4. Scaption external rotation. (Redrawn from Wilk, K.E., Andrews, J.R., Arrigo, C.A., et al. [2001]: Preventive and Rehabilitative Exercises for the Shoulder and Elbow, 6th ed. Birmingham, AL, American Sports Medicine Institute.)

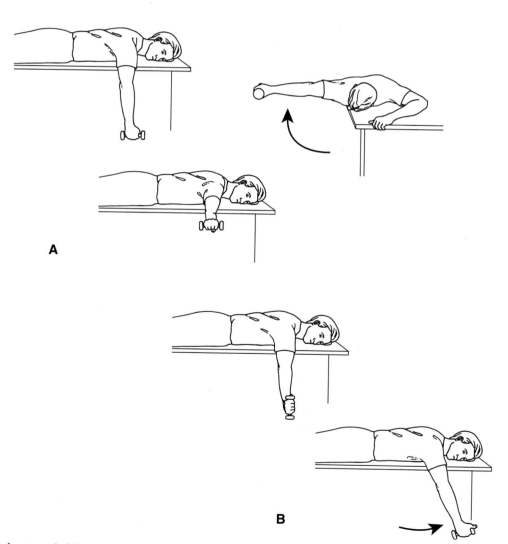

A

B

Figure A-5. Prone horizontal abduction. *A,* Neutral. *B,* Full external rotation, 100° abduction. (Redrawn from Wilk, K.E., Andrews, J.R., Arrigo, C.A., et al. [2001]: Preventive and Rehabilitative Exercises for the Shoulder and Elbow, 6th ed. Birmingham, AL, American Sports Medicine Institute.)

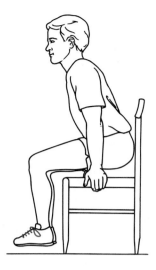

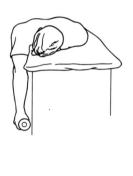

Figure A-6. Press-ups. (Redrawn from Wilk, K.E., Andrews, J.R., Arrigo, C.A., et al. [2001]: Preventive and Rehabilitative Exercises for the Shoulder and Elbow, 6th ed. Birmingham, AL, American Sports Medicine Institute.)

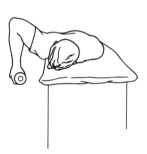

Figure A-7. Prone rowing. (Redrawn from Wilk, K.E., Andrews, J.R., Arrigo, C.A., et al. [2001]: Preventive and Rehabilitative Exercises for the Shoulder and Elbow, 6th ed. Birmingham, AL, American Sports Medicine Institute.)

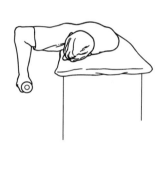

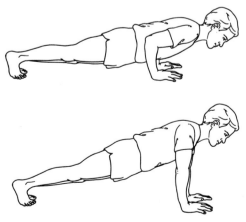

Figure A-8. Push-ups. (Redrawn from Wilk, K.E., Andrews, J.R., Arrigo, C.A., et al. [2001]: Preventive and Rehabilitative Exercises for the Shoulder and Elbow, 6th ed. Birmingham, AL, American Sports Medicine Institute.)

Elbow Flexion. With the arm against the side and the palm facing inward the athlete bends the elbow upward, turning the palm up as he or she progresses (Fig. A-9A). The athlete holds the position for 2 seconds and lowers the elbow slowly.

Elbow Extension. The athlete raises the involved arm overhead, with the uninvolved hand providing support at the elbow. The arm is straightened overhead (Fig. A-9B). The athlete holds the position for 2 seconds and lowers the arm slowly.

Wrist Extension. Supporting the forearm and with the palm facing downward, the athlete raises a weight in the hand as far as possible (Fig. A-10A). The athlete holds the position for 2 seconds and lowers the arm slowly.

Wrist Flexion. Supporting the forearm and with the palm facing upward, the athlete lowers a weight in the hand as far as possible and then curls it up as high as pos-

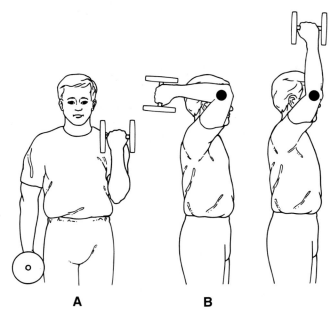

A   **B**

Figure A-9. *A,* Elbow flexion. *B,* Elbow extension. (Redrawn from Wilk, K.E., Andrews, J.R., Arrigo, C.A., et al. [2001]: Preventive and Rehabilitative Exercises for the Shoulder and Elbow, 6th ed. Birmingham, AL, American Sports Medicine Institute.)

sible (Fig. A-10*B*). The athlete holds the position for 2 seconds and lowers the arm slowly.

Supination. The athlete supports the forearm on a table, with the wrist in a neutral position. Using a weight or a hammer, the athlete rolls the wrist, taking the palm up. (Fig. A-10*C*). The athlete holds the position for 2 seconds, and the arm is returned to the starting position.

Pronation. The athlete supports the forearm on a table, with the wrist in a neutral position. Using a weight or hammer, the athlete rolls the wrist, taking the palm down (Fig. A-10*D*). The athlete holds the position for 2 seconds, and the arm is returned to the starting position.

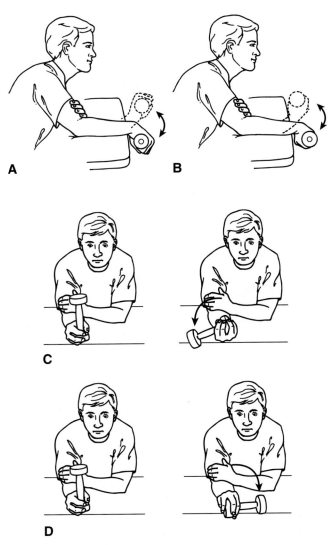

Figure A-10. *A,* Wrist extension. *B,* Wrist flexion. *C,* Wrist supination. *D,* Wrist pronation. (Redrawn from Wilk, K.E., Andrews, J.R., Arrigo, C.A., et al. [2001]: Preventive and Rehabilitative Exercises for the Shoulder and Elbow, 6th ed. Birmingham, AL, American Sports Medicine Institute.)

INTERVAL REHABILITATION PROGRAMS

Kevin Wilk, P.T.

INTERVAL THROWING PROGRAM FOR BASEBALL PLAYERS—PHASE I

The Interval Throwing Program (ITP) is designed to gradually return motion, strength, and confidence in the throwing arm after injury or surgery by slowly progressing through graduated throwing distances. The ITP is initiated upon clearance by the athlete's physician to resume throwing and performed under the supervision of the rehabilitation team (physician, physical therapist, and athletic trainer).

The program is set up to minimize the chance of reinjury and emphasize prethrowing warm-up and stretching. In development of the ITP, the following factors are considered most important.

1. The act of throwing the baseball involves the transfer of energy from the feet through the legs, pelvis, and trunk and out the shoulder through the elbow and hand. Therefore, any return to throwing after injury must include attention to the entire body.
2. The chance for reinjury is lessened by a graduated progression of interval throwing.
3. Proper warm-up is essential.
4. Most injuries occur as the result of fatigue.
5. Proper throwing mechanics lessen the incidence of reinjury.
6. Baseline requirements for throwing include:
   - Pain-free range of motion
   - Adequate muscle power
   - Adequate muscle resistance to fatigue

Because there is an individual variability in all throwing athletes, there is no set timetable for completion of the program. Most athletes, by nature, are highly competitive individuals and wish to return to competition at the earliest possible moment. Although this is a necessary quality of all athletes, the proper channeling of the athlete's energies into a rigidly controlled throwing program is essential to lessen the chance of reinjury during the rehabilitation period. The athlete may have the tendency to want to increase the intensity of the throwing program. This will increase the incidence of reinjury and may greatly retard the rehabilitation process. It is recommended that the athlete follow the program rigidly because this will be the safest route to return to competition.

During the recovery process the athlete will probably experience soreness and a dull, diffuse aching sensation in the muscles and tendons. If the athlete experiences sharp pain, particularly in the joint, he or she should stop all throwing activity until this pain ceases. If continued pain is present, the physician should be contacted.

Weight Training

The athlete should supplement the ITP with a high-repetition, low-weight exercise program. The strengthening regimen should be focused on a good balance between anterior and posterior musculature so that the shoulder will not be predisposed to injury. Special emphasis must be given to posterior rotator cuff musculature for any strengthening program. Weight training will not increase throwing velocity, but it will increase the resistance of the arm to fatigue and injury. Weight training should be done the same day as throwing; however, it should be after throwing is completed. The day in between throwing practice should be used for flexibility exercises and a recovery period. A weight training pattern or routine should be stressed at this point as a "maintenance program." This pattern can and should accompany the athlete into and throughout the season as a deterrent to further injury. It must be stressed that weight training is of no benefit unless accompanied by a sound flexibility program.

Individual Variability

The ITP is designed so that each level is achieved without pain or complications before the next level is started. This sets up a progression: a goal is achieved before advancement rather than advancement according to a specific time frame. Because of this design, the ITP may be used for individuals with different levels of skills and abilities from those in high school to professional levels. The reasons for performing the ITP will vary from person to person. For example, one athlete may wish to use alternate-day throwing with or without using weights in between; another athlete may have to throw every third or fourth day due to pain or swelling. A good rule to follow is, "Listen to your body—it will tell you when to slow down." Again, completion of the steps of the ITP will vary from person to person. There is no set timetable for days to completion.

Warm-up

Jogging increases blood flow to the muscles and joints, thus increasing their flexibility and decreasing the chance of re-injury. Because the length of the warm-up will vary from person to person, the athlete should jog until a light sweat develops and then progress to the stretching phase.

Stretching

Because throwing involves all muscles in the body, all muscle groups should be stretched before throwing. This should be done in a systematic fashion beginning with the legs and including the trunk, back, neck, and arms and continuing with capsular stretches and L-bar range-of-motion exercises.

Throwing Mechanics

A critical aspect of the ITP is maintenance of proper throwing mechanics throughout the advancement. The use of the crow-hop method simulates the throwing act, allowing emphasis on proper body mechanics. This throwing method should be adopted from the onset of the ITP. Throwing flat-footed encourages improper body mechanics, placing increased stress on the throwing arm and,

therefore, predisposing the arm to reinjury. The pitching coach and sports biomechanist (if available) may be valuable allies to the rehabilitation team with their knowledge of throwing mechanics.

Components of the crow-hop method are first a hop, then a skip, followed by the throw. The velocity of the throw is determined by the distance, whereas the ball should have only enough momentum to travel each designed distance. Again, emphasis should be placed upon proper throwing mechanics when the athlete beings phase II: "Throwing Off the Mound" or from the athlete's respective position, to decrease the chance of re-injury.

Throwing

Using the crow-hop method, the athlete should begin warm-up throws at a comfortable distance (approximately 30 to 45 feet) and then progress to the distance indicated for that phase (refer to the outline). The program consists of throwing at each step two to three times without pain or symptoms before progressing to the next step. The object of each phase is for the athlete to be able to throw the ball without pain the specified number of feet (45, 60, 90, 120, 150, and 180 feet), 75 times at each distance. After the athlete can throw at the prescribed distance without pain he or she will be ready for throwing from flat ground 60 feet, 6 inches in the normal pitching mechanics or return to their respective position (step 14). At this point, full strength and confidence should be restored in the athlete's arm. It is important to stress the crow-hop method and proper mechanics with each throw. Just as the advancement to this point has been gradual and progressive, the return to unrestricted throwing must follow the same principles. A pitcher should first throw only fast balls at 50%, progressing to 75%, and finally to 100%. At this time, the athlete may start more stressful pitches such as breaking balls. The position player should simulate a game situation, again progressing at 50% to 75% to 100%. Once again, if an athlete has increased pain, particularly at the joint, the throwing program should be backed off and readvanced as tolerated, under the direction of the rehabilitation team.

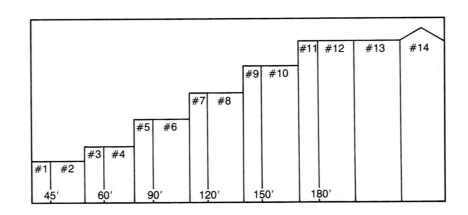

Batting

Depending on the type of injury that the athlete has, the time of return to batting should be determined by the physician. It should be noted that stress placed upon the arm and shoulder in the batting motion are very different from those for the throwing motion. A return to unrestricted use of the bat should also follow the same progression guidelines as seen in the training program. The athlete should begin with dry swings, progressing to hitting off the tee, then hitting a soft toss, and finally hitting live pitching.

Summary

In using the ITP in conjunction with a structured rehabilitation program, the athlete should be able to return to full competition status, minimizing any chance of reinjury. The program and its progression should be modified to meet the specific needs of each individual athlete. A comprehensive program consisting of a maintenance strength and flexibility program, appropriate warm-up and cool-down procedures, proper pitching mechanics, and progressive throwing and batting will assist the baseball player in returning safely to competition.

INTERVAL THROWING PROGRAM: THROWING OFF THE MOUND—PHASE II

After the athlete completes phase I of the ITP and can throw to the prescribed distance without pain, he or she will be ready for throwing off the mound or returning to competition. At this point, full strength and confidence in the athlete's arm should be restored. Just as the advancement to this point has been gradual and progressive, the return to unrestricted throwing must follow the same principles. A pitcher should first throw fast balls only at 50%, progressing to 75% and 100%. At this time, the athlete

A. 45-foot phase	B. 60-foot phase	C. 90-foot phase	D. 120-foot phase
1. Step 1 (a) Warm-up throwing (b) 45 feet (25 throws) (c) Rest 5 to 10 minutes (d) Warm-up throwing (e) 45 feet (25 throws) 2. Step 2 (a) Warm-up throwing (b) 45 feet (25 throws) (c) Rest 5 to 10 minutes (d) Warm-up throwing (e) 45 feet (25 throws) (f) Rest 5 to 10 minutes (g) Warm-up throwing (h) 45 feet (25 throws)	3. Step 3 (a) Warm-up throwing (b) 60 feet (25 throws) (c) Rest 5 to 10 minutes (d) Warm-up throwing (e) 60 feet (25 throws) 4. Step 4 (a) Warm-up throwing (b) 60 feet (25 throws) (c) Rest 5 to 10 minutes (d) Warm-up throwing (e) 60 feet (25 throws) (f) Rest 5 to 10 minutes (g) Warm-up throwing (h) 60 feet (25 throws)	5. Step 5 (a) Warm-up throwing (b) 90 feet (25 throws) (c) Rest 5 to 10 minutes (d) Warm-up throwing (e) 90 feet (25 throws) 6. Step 6 (a) Warm-up throwing (b) 90 feet (25 throws) (c) Rest 5 to 10 minutes (d) Warm-up throwing (e) 90 feet (25 throws) (f) Rest 5 to 10 minutes (g) Warm-up throwing (h) 90 feet (25 throws)	7. Step 7 (a) Warm-up throwing (b) 120 feet (25 throws) (c) Rest 5 to 10 minutes (d) Warm-up throwing (e) 120 feet (25 throws) 8. Step 8 (a) Warm-up throwing (b) 120 feet (25 throws) (c) Rest 5 to 10 minutes (d) Warm-up throwing (e) 120 feet (25 throws) (f) Rest 5 to 10 minutes (g) Warm-up throwing (h) 120 feet (25 throws)

E. 180-foot phase			Notes
11. Step 11 (a) Warm-up throwing (b) 180 feet (25 throws) (c) Rest 5 to 10 minutes (d) Warm-up throwing (e) 180 feet (25 throws)	12. Step 12 (a) Warm-up throwing (b) 180 feet (25 throws) (c) Rest 5 to 10 minutes (d) Warm-up throwing (e) 180 feet (25 throws) (f) Rest 5 to 10 minutes (g) Warm-up throwing (h) 180 feet (25 throws)	13. Step 13 (a) Warm-up throwing (b) 180 feet (25 throws) (c) Rest 5 to 10 minutes (d) Warm-up throwing (e) 180 feet (25 throws) Step 14: Begin throwing off the mound or return to respective position	(a) The throwing program should be performed every other day, unless otherwise specified by the physician or rehabilitation specialist. (b) Perform each step 2–3 times before progressing to next step.

F. Flat ground throwing	G. Flat throwing
(a) Warm-up throwing (b) Throw 60 feet (10 to 15 throws) (c) Throw 90 feet (10 throws) (d) Throw 120 feet (10 throws) (e) Throw 60 feet (flat ground) using pitching mechanics (20 to 30 throws)	(a) Warm-up throwing (b) Throw 60 feet (10 to 15 throws) (c) Throw 90 feet (10 throws) (d) Throw 120 feet (10 throws) (e) Throw 60 feet (flat ground) using pitching mechanics (20 to 30 throws) (f) Throw 60 feet (10 to 15 throws) (g) Throw 60 feet (flat ground) using pitching mechanics (20 throws)

A. Stage One: Fastballs Only

1. Step 1
   (a) Interval throwing
   (b) 15 throws off mound, 50%

2. Step 2
   (a) Interval throwing
   (b) 30 throws off mound, 50%

3. Step 3
   (a) Interval throwing
   (b) 45 throws off mound, 50%

4. Step 4
   (a) Interval throwing
   (b) 60 throws off mound, 50%

5. Step 5
   (a) Interval throwing
   (b) 70 throws off mound, 50%

6. Step 6
   (a) 45 throws off mound, 50%
   (b) 30 throws off mound, 75%

7. Step 7
   (a) 30 throws off mound, 50%
   (b) 45 throws off mound, 75%

8. Step 8
   (a) 65 throws off mound, 75%
   (b) 10 throws off mound, 50%

Notes

(a) Use interval throwing to 120-foot phase as warm-up.
(b) All throwing off the mound should be done in the presence of the pitching coach to stress proper throwing mechanics.
(c) Use a speed gun to aid in effort control.

B. Stage Two: Fastballs Only

9. Step 9
   (a) 60 throws off mound, 75%
   (b) 5 throws in batting practice

10. Step 10
    (a) 50 to 60 throws off mound, 75%
    (b) 30 throws in batting practice

11. Step 11
    (a) 45 to 50 throws off mound, 75%
    (b) 45 throws in batting practice

C. Stage Three

12. Step 12
    (a) 30 throws off mound, 75% warm-up
    (b) 15 throws off mound, 50% breaking balls
    (c) 45 to 60 throws in batting practice (fastball only)

13. Step 13
    (a) 30 throws off mound, 75%
    (b) 30 breaking balls, 75%
    (c) 30 throws in batting practice

14. Step 14
    (a) 30 throws off mound, 75%
    (b) 60 to 90 throws in batting practice (gradually increase the number of breaking balls)

15. Step 15
    (a) Simulated game—progressing by 15 throws per workout (pitch count)

may start more stressful pitches such as breaking balls. The position player should simulate a game situation, again progressing at 50% to 75% to 100%. Once again, if an athlete has increased pain, particularly at the joint, the throwing program should be backed off and readvanced as tolerated, under the direction of the rehabilitation team.

A. 30-foot phase
1. Step 1
    (a) Warm-up throwing
    (b) 30 feet (25 throws)
    (c) Rest 15 minutes
    (d) Warm-up throwing
    (e) 30 feet (25 throws)
2. Step 2
    (a) Warm-up throwing
    (b) 30 feet (25 throws)
    (c) Rest 10 minutes
    (d) Warm-up throwing
    (e) 30 feet (25 throws)
    (f) Rest 10 minutes
    (g) Warm-up throwing
    (h) 30 feet (25 throws)
B. 45-foot phase
1. Step 3
    (a) Warm-up throwing
    (b) 45 feet (25 throws)
    (c) Rest 15 minutes
    (d) Warm-up throwing
    (e) 45 feet (25 throws)
2. Step 4
    (a) Warm-up throwing
    (b) 45 feet (25 throws)
    (c) Rest 10 minutes
    (d) Warm-up throwing
    (e) 45 feet (25 throws)
    (f) Rest 10 minutes
    (g) Warm-up throwing
    (h) 45 feet (25 throws)

C. 60-foot phase
1. Step 5
    (a) Warm-up throwing
    (b) 60 feet (25 throws)
    (c) Rest 15 minutes
    (d) Warm-up throwing
    (e) 60 feet (25 throws)
2. Step 6
    (a) Warm-up throwing
    (b) 60 feet (25 throws)
    (c) Rest 10 minutes
    (d) Warm-up throwing
    (e) 60 feet (25 throws)
    (f) Rest 10 minutes
    (g) Warm-up throwing
    (h) 60 feet (25 throws)
D. 90-foot phase
1. Step 7
    (a) Warm-up throwing
    (b) 90 feet (25 throws)
    (c) Rest 15 minutes
    (d) Warm-up throwing
    (e) 90 feet (25 throws)
2. Step 8
    (a) Warm-up throwing
    (b) 90 feet (25 throws)
    (c) Rest 10 minutes
    (d) Warm-up throwing
    (e) 90 feet (25 throws)
    (f) Rest 10 minutes
    (g) Warm-up throwing
    (h) 90 feet (25 throws)

SUMMARY

In using the ITP in conjunction with a structured rehabilitation program, the athlete should be able to return to full competition status, minimizing any chance of reinjury. The program and its progression should be modified to meet the specific needs of each individual athlete. A comprehensive program consisting of a maintenance strength and flexibility program, appropriate warm-up and cool-down procedures, proper pitching mechanics, and progressive throwing and batting will assist the baseball player in returning safely to competition.

LITTLE LEAGUER INTERVAL TRAINING PROGRAM

The Little Leaguer Interval Throwing Program parallels the ITP in returning the Little Leaguer to a graduated progression of throwing distances. Warm-up and stretching should be performed before throwing.

INTERVAL TENNIS PROGRAM

The same principles should be followed with the Interval Tennis Program as for the Interval Throwing Program for baseball players. Proper warm-ups, stretching, and strengthening should still be implemented throughout the entire interval tennis rehabilitation program. As athletes begin the program, they should be reminded that mechanics play an important role in recovery and that questions should be directed to the physician or rehabilitation specialist.

INTERVAL GOLF PROGRAM

The same principles should be followed with the Interval Golf Program as for the Interval Throwing Program for baseball players. Proper warm-up, stretching, and strengthening should still be implemented throughout the entire Interval Golf Program. As athletes begin the program, they should be reminded that mechanics play an important role in recovery and that questions should be directed to the physician or rehabilitation specialist.

Week	Monday	Wednesday	Friday
1	12 FH	15 FH	15 FH
	8 BH	8 BH	10 BH
	10-minute rest	10-minute rest	10-minute rest
	13 FH	15 FH	15 FH
	7 BH	7 BH	10 BH
2	25 FH	30 FH	30 FH
	15 BH	20 BH	25 BH
	10-minute rest	10-minute rest	10-minute rest
	25 FH	30 FH	30 FH
	15 BH	20 BH	15 BH
3	30 FH	30 FH	30 FH
	25 BH	25 BH	30 BH
	10 OH	15 OH	15 OH
	10-minute rest	10-minute rest	10-minute rest
	30 FH	30 FH	30 FH
	25 BH	25 BH	15 OH
	10 OH	15 OH	10-minute rest
4	30 FH	30 FH	30 FH
	30 BH	30 BH	30 BH
	10 OH	10 OH	10 OH
	10-minute rest	10-minute rest	10-minute rest
	Play 3 games	Play set	Play 1½ sets
	10 FH	10 FH	10 FH
	10 BH	10 BH	10 BH
	5 BH	5 OH	3 OH

BH, backhand shots; FH, forehand shots; OH, overhead shots.

Week	Monday	Wednesday	Friday
1	10 putts	15 putts	20 putts
	10 chips	15 chips	20 chips
	5-minute rest	5-minute rest	5-minute rest
	15 chips	25 chipping	20 putts
			20 chips
			5-minute rest
			10 chips
			10 short irons
2	20 chips	20 chips	15 short irons
	10 short irons	15 short irons	20 medium irons (5 iron/tee)
	5-minute rest	10-minute rest	10-minute rest
	10 short irons	15 short irons	20 short irons
	15 medium irons (5 iron off tee)	15 chips	15 chips
		Putting	
		15 medium irons (5 iron/tee)	
3	15 short irons	15 short irons	15 short irons
	20 medium irons	15 medium irons	15 medium irons
	10-minute rest	10 long irons	10 long irons
	5 long irons	10-minute rest	10-minute rest
	15 short irons	10 short irons	10 short irons
	15 medium irons	10 medium irons	10 medium irons
	10-minute rest	5 long irons	10 long irons
	20 chips	5 wood	10 wood
4	15 short irons		
	15 medium irons		
	10 long irons	Play 9 holes	Play 9 holes
	10 drives		
	15-minute rest		
	Repeat		
5	9 holes	9 holes	18 holes

Chips
- Pitching wedge
- Short irons – W 9, 8
- Long irons – 4, 3, 2
- Woods – 3, 5
- Drives — driver

UPPER EXTREMITY PLYOMETRICS*

Kevin E. Wilk, P.T.

Chest Pass (Fig. C-1). The athlete stands facing a plyoback. Using both hands to hold a 3-pound medicine ball against the chest, the athlete pushes the ball away from the chest into the plyoback. The athlete's arm should return to the starting position as he or she catches the ball rebounding off the plyoback.

Two-Hand Overhead Soccer Throw (Fig. C-2). The athlete stands or kneels facing a plyoback. Holding a 3- to 5-pound medicine ball in both hands, the athlete raises the ball overhead, then throws it into the plyoback. The athlete should catch the ball overhead as it rebounds from the plyoback.

Two-Hand Side-to-Side Throw (Fig. C-3). The athlete stands facing a plyoback holding a 3- to 5-pound medicine ball with both hands, positioned over one shoulder. The athlete throws the ball into the plyoback, then catches it with both hands over the opposite shoulder. The athlete continues alternating sides. This exercise can also be used to train the rotators of the hips and trunk by allowing the body to rotate slightly as the ball is caught.

Baseball Toss at 90/90 (Fig. C-4). The athlete stands facing a plyoback with the arm at a 90°-angle away from the body and the elbow bent to 90° (cocking position). Holding a 1-pound medicine ball, the athlete forcefully throws the ball into the plyoback, then catches it as it rebounds, maintaining the same position of the arm and elbow. The exercise can also be used to train the legs and trunk to accelerate the arm by stepping out as the ball is thrown.

Backhand External Rotation at 0° (Fig. C-5). The athlete stands sideways with the involved side toward the plyoback and a 1- to 3-pound medicine ball in the involved hand. Keeping the upper arm against the body and the elbow bent to 90°, the athlete internally rotates the arm toward the chest, then forcefully externally rotates the arm, throwing the ball into the plyoback. The athlete should try catching the ball as it rebounds with the palm toward the body and upper arm close to the side.

Backhand Internal Rotation at 0° (Fig. C-6). The athlete stands sideways with the uninvolved side nearest the plyoback and a 1- to 3-pound medicine ball in the involved hand, keeping the upper arm of the involved side close to the body and the elbow bent to 90°. After the athlete externally rotates the arm, he or she forcefully throws the ball into the plyoback by internally rotating the arm. The athlete should catch the ball while maintaining the upper arm against the body.

Wall Dribbling (Fig. C-7). The athlete stands facing a wall, holding a 1- to 3-pound medicine ball slightly above shoulder level. The athlete should dribble the ball against the wall. This exercise can be progressed by dribbling the ball in an arch along the wall.

---

*From Wilk, K.E., Andrews, J.R., Arrigo, C.A., et al. (2001). Preventive and Rehabilitative Exercises for the Shoulder and Elbow. Birmingham, Alabama, American Sports Medicine Institute, pp. 32–33.

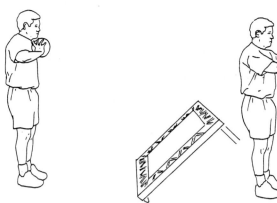
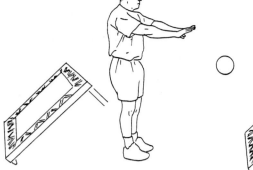
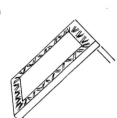

Figure C-1. Chest pass.

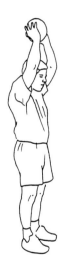
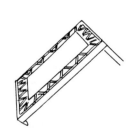

Figure C-2. Two-hand overhead soccer throw.

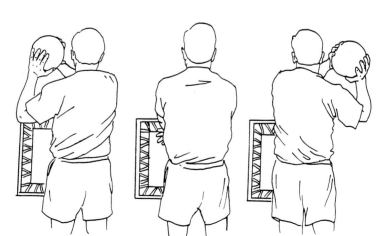

Figure C-3. Two-hand side-to-side throw.

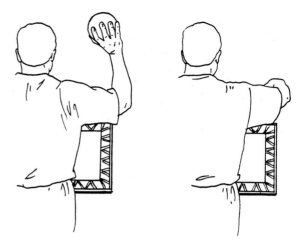

Figure C-4. Baseball toss at 90/90.

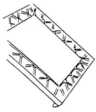
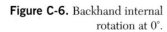
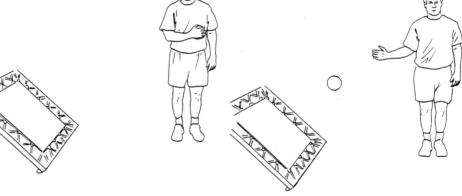

Figure C-5. Backhand external rotation at 0°.

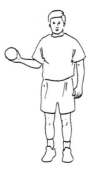
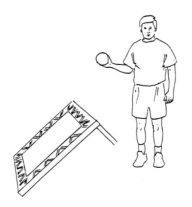
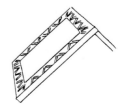

Figure C-6. Backhand internal rotation at 0°.

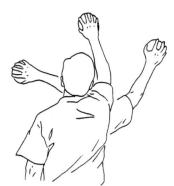

Figure C-7. Wall dribble.

INDEX

Joint mobilization-application techniques (*Continued*)
 glenohumeral joint inferior glide, 144f
 glenohumeral joint posterior glide, 145f
 hip joint posterior glide, 149f
 humeroulnar joint distraction, 146, 147f
 interphalangeal joint distraction, 148, 149f
 metatarsophalangeal joint distraction, 152f
 patellofemoral joint glides, 149, 150f
 proximal radioulnar joint glide, 146, 147f
 radiocarpal joint distraction, 147, 148f
 radiocarpal joint glide, 147–148, 148f
 scapulothoracic joint lateral glide, 145–146f
 talocrural joint anterior glide, 152f
 talocrural joint distraction, 151f
 talocrural joint posterior glide, 151f
 tibiofemoral joint glides, 150f
Joint oscillation exercises, 206–209
Joint position, 142, 143t
Joint position sense, 190t, 193–194, 196
Joint proprioception, 192–194
Joint range of motion, 101b, 103t, 104b
Joint range of motion-application techniques, 104b, 106–128
 ankle dorsiflexion, 120, 120f
 ankle eversion, 120, 121f
 ankle inversion, 120, 121f
 ankle plantar flexion, 119, 120f
 cervical extension, 122, 123f
 cervical flexion, 121, 122f
 cervical lateral flexion, 122, 123f
 cervical rotation, 122, 124, 124f
 elbow extension, 109, 110f
 elbow flexion, 109, 110f
 finger extension, 114f
 finger flexion, 114f
 forearm pronation, 109–110, 111f
 forearm supination, 110, 111f
 hip abduction, 116, 116f
 hip extension, 115, 115f
 hip external rotation, 118, 118f
 hip flexion, 114, 115f
 hip internal rotation, 116, 117f
 knee extension, 118–119, 119f
 knee flexion, 118, 119f
 lumbar extension, 124–126
 lumbar lateral extension, 126, 126f
 radial deviation, 112, 113f
 shoulder abduction, 107f
 shoulder adduction, 108f
 shoulder extension, 106f
 shoulder external rotation, 108f
 shoulder flexion, 106f
 shoulder internal rotation, 109f
 step-by-step procedure, 104b
 thoracicolumbar flexion, 124, 125f
 ulnar deviation, 113, 113f
 wrist extension, 112, 112f
 wrist flexion, 111, 112f
Joint range of motion exercise, 169
Joint receptors, 163
Joint-specific manual traction, 506f

Joint stiffness, 19
Joints of von Luschka, 480, 480f
Jump, 276
Jump from box, 282f
Jump or drop downs, 276
Jump training. *See* Plyometric training.

K
Kaltenborn's stages of traction, 140–141, 141t
Kinematic chain, 177
Kinesthesia, 176, 190t
Knee
 biomechanical considerations, 44–48
 injuries. *See* Knee injuries
 joint mobilization, 149–150
 plyometrics, 271b
 proprioception, 197–198
 range of motion, 103t, 118–119
Knee arthrometer, 132f
Knee braces, 408
Knee Dynasplint, 134f
Knee extension
 PCL, 46
 tibiofemoral joint, 47f
Knee flexion
 patellofemoral joint, 48
 PCL, 46
 tibiofemoral joint, 47f
Knee injuries, 377–428
 ACL. *See* ACL.
 arthrometry, 419–421
 articular cartilage injuries, 418–419
 basic principles, 385–392
 capsular restraints, 379–380
 combined injuries to knee, 415–418
 exercises, 386–392
 functional anatomy, 377–380
 functional tests, 422–423
 isokinetic testing, 421–422
 LCL, 379
 MCL, 379, 409, 412
 meniscus, 380, 412–415
 muscle function, 383–385
 patellofemoral biomechanics, 380–383
 patellofemoral dysfunction, 392–395
 PCL. *See* PCL.
Knee joint immobilization, 24
Kneeling hip flexor stretch, 472, 473f
Knowledge of performance (KP), 167t, 168
Knowledge of results (KR), 167t, 168
Konin, Jeff G., 129
KP, 167t, 168
KR, 167t, 168
KT-1000, 419, 419f

L
Labral lesions, 563
Laminar flow, 296
Landing, 270, 317
Lateral ankle instability, 362t